Gerontologic Nursing

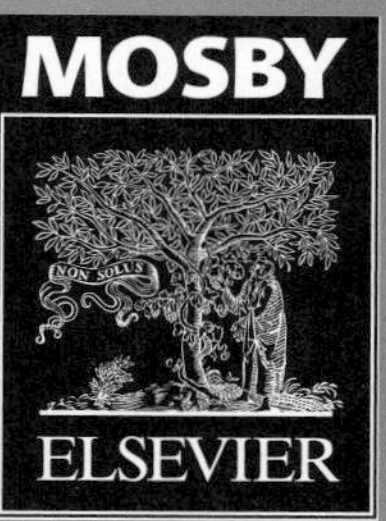

Gerontologic Nursing

Third Edition

Sue E. Meiner, EdD, APRN, BC, GNP
Nurse Practitioner in Private Practice
Las Vegas, Nevada;
President
Consultant on Health Issues, Inc.
Las Vegas, Nevada;

Formerly:
Assistant Professor
University of Nevada, Las Vegas
Las Vegas, Nevada

Annette G. Lueckenotte, MS, RN, BC, GNP, GCNS
Gerontologic Clinical Nurse Specialist
Barnes-Jewish West County Hospital
St. Louis, Missouri

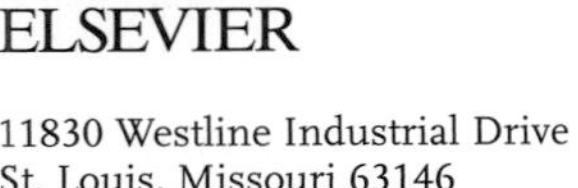

MOSBY
ELSEVIER

11830 Westline Industrial Drive
St. Louis, Missouri 63146

GERONTOLOGIC NURSING, THIRD EDITION
ISBN-13 978-0-323-03146-2
ISBN-10 0-323-03146-3

Notice

Knowledge and best practice in this field are constantly changing. As new research and experience broaden our knowledge, changes in practice, treatment and drug therapy may become necessary or appropriate. Readers are advised to check the most current information provided (i) on procedures featured or (ii) by the manufacturer of each product to be administered, to verify the recommended dose or formula, the method and duration of administration, and contraindications. It is the responsibility of the practitioner, relying on their own experience and knowledge of the patient, to make diagnoses, to determine dosages and the best treatment for each individual patient, and to take all appropriate safety precautions. To the fullest extent of the law, neither the Publisher nor the Authors assume any liability for any injury and/or damage to persons or property arising out or related to any use of the material contained in this book.

The Publisher

ISBN-13 978-0-323-03146-2
ISBN-10 0-323-03146-3

Executive Editor: Michael S. Ledbetter/Catherine Jackson
Senior Developmental Editor: Lisa P. Newton
Developmental Editor: Amanda Sunderman Politte
Editorial Assistant: Heather Bays
Publishing Services Manager: Deborah Vogel
Project Manager: Mary Drone
Designer: Amy Buxton
Cover Designer: Designers Collective

Printed in the United States of America

Last digit is the print number: 9 8 7 6 5 4 3 2 1

I have been very blessed to be able to do all of the things that bring joy to my life. Practicing nursing full-time, consulting in legal nursing part-time, and teaching both students and patients/families has been truly rewarding. Writing is an outlet for all of the wonderful findings that have been presented to me over a lifetime of nursing as my chosen career. This book is dedicated to my family (Robert, Diane, Suzanne, Tristyn, Braedyn, and Tony), my friends, colleagues, and all of the wonderful people that I have had the pleasure of meeting in this limited lifespan.

Sue E. Meiner

Contributors

Phyllis J. Atkinson, MS, RN, APRN, BC
General Nurse Practitioner
Evercare
Cincinnati, Ohio

Christopher Benjamin, MSN, RN, FNP
Lead Nurse Practitioner
Family Centered Care/Geriatrics
University of Virginia Health System
Charlottesville, Virginia

Lynn Ferebee, MSN, RN, FNP
Family Nurse Practitioner
Student Health Center
University of Nevada, Las Vegas
Las Vegas, Nevada

Kathleen Fletcher, MSN, RN, APRN-BC, GNP, FAAN
Gerontological Nurse Practitioner
Director Senior Services
Assistant Professor of Nursing
University of Virginia Health System
Charlottesville, Virginia

Sabrina Friedman, MSN, PhD, EdD, FNP
Associate Professor
Nevada State College
Henderson, Nevada

Catherine Hill, MSN, RN, GNP
Medicine Associates of North Texas
Virginia Henderson Fellow
Sigma Theta Tau
Dallas, Texas

Kristal Imperio PhD(c), RN, CS, ANP, GNP
Chairperson
Department of Nursing
Atlantic Union College
South Lancaster, Massachusetts

Kathleen F. Jett, PhD, APRN, GNP, BC
Assistant Professor
Gerontology Certificate Program, Coordinator
Christine E. Lynn College of Nursing
Florida Atlantic University
Boca Raton, Florida

Pamala D. Larsen, PhD, RN, CRRN
Director, School of Nursing
Associate Dean, College of Health and Human Services
University of North Carolina at Charlotte
Charlotte, North Carolina

Robyn A. Levy, MSN, RN, BC, ANP
Assistant Professor of Nursing
Barnes Jewish Hospital College of Nursing & Allied Health
St. Louis, Missouri

Margaret Louis, PhD, RN, BC
Associate Professor
School of Nursing
University of Nevada, Las Vegas
Las Vegas, Nevada

Sharon Roth Maguire, MS, APRN-BC, GNP, APNP
Senior Director, Healthcare and Resident Services
Alterra Healthcare Corporation
Milwaukee, Wisconsin
Clinical Assistant Professor
Marquette University College of Nursing
Milwaukee, Wisconsin

Susan A. Moore, PhD, RN
Professor of Nursing
New Hampshire Community Technical College
Manchester, New Hampshire

Elizabeth C. Mueth, MLS, AHIP
Resource Center and Archives Coordinator
Clinical Nursing Institute
Missouri Baptist Medical Center
St. Louis, Missouri

Eleanor Pusey-Reid, MS, MEd, RN, CCRN
Assistant Professor
Atlantic Union College
South Lancaster, Massachusetts

Mary J. Reed, PhD, APN, CS, BC
Advanced Practice Nurse
Southern Nevada Adult Mental Health Services
Las Vegas, Nevada

Barbara Resnick, PhD, CRNP, FAAN, FAANP
Associate Professor
University of Maryland School of Nursing
Baltimore, Maryland

Kathleen M. Rourke, PhD, RN, RD, CHES
Assistant Dean
Graduate College
Cincinnati, Ohio

Linda A. Stamm, APRN, BC, CON
Adult Nurse Practitioner
Wound/Ostomy Center
Barnes Jewish Hospital
St. Louis, Missouri

James R. Steele, MSN, RN, ANP-C
Lecturer in Adult Health Nursing
University of North Carolina at Charlotte
Planned Parenthood of Western North Carolina

Linda L. Steele, PhD, APRN, ANP-BC
Associate Professor of Nursing and Coordinator of Nurse Practitioner Programs
University of North Carolina at Charlotte
Charlotte, North Carolina
Nurse Practitioner
Planned Parenthood of Western North Carolina

Dianne Thames, DNS, RN
Dean, Academic Services
Charity School of Nursing
Delgado Community College
New Orleans, Louisiana

Reviewers

Patricia M. Burbank, DNSc, RN
Professor
College of Nursing
University of Rhode Island
Kingston, Rhode Island

Betty A. Maxwell, MSN, RN
Nursing Instructor
Associate Degree Nursing Program
St. Clair County Community College
Port Huron, MI

Linda Ritchie, PhD, RN
Associate Professor,
Chair Nursing Department
Brock University
St. Catharines Ontario
Canada

Debra L. Sietsema, PhD, RN
Chairperson
Department of Nursing
Hope College
Holland, MI

Meredith Wallace, PhD, APRN-BC
Associate Professor
School of Nursing
Fairfield University
Fairfield, CT

L. Diane Weed, PhD, FNP
Associate Professor
Nursing Department
Troy University
Troy, AL

Contributors to First and Second Editions

Gayle Andresen, MS, RN, A/GNP
Consultant & Educator
Former Senior Instructor
Department of Family Medicine
University of Colorado Health Sciences Center in Denver
Golden, Colorado

Myra A. Aud, PhD(c), RN
St. Louis, MO

Karen Baker, MSN, RN, C
Clinical Nurse Specialist
Clinical Center
National Institutes of Health
Bethesda, Maryland

Diana Ballard, MBA, JD, RN
Attorney at Law
Ballard Management Group
Cheshire, Connecticut

Martha Hains Bramlett, PhD, RN
Research Scientist
Gerontology Center
University of Georgia
Athens, Georgia

Sally Brozenec, PhD, RN
Assistant Professor
Rush University College of Nursing
Chicago, Illinois

Gina Marie Bufe, BSN, MSN(R), PhD, RNCS, ANCC, CS
Psychiatric Mental Health Clinical Nurse Specialist
Centerville, Massachusetts

Patricia M. Burbank, BS, MS, RN, DNSc
Associate Professor
University of Rhode Island College of Nursing
Kingston, Rhode Island

Pam Zurkowski Cacchione, PhD, RN, CSGNP
Gerontological Nurse Practitioner
St. Louis University
Division of Internal Medicine
Geriatric Medicine & School of Nursing
St. Louis, Missouri

Kathryn E. Christiansen, MA, BSN, DNSc
Assistant Professor
Department of Community Health
Rush University College of Nursing
Administrator
Rush Home Care Network
Chicago, Illinois

Marilyn Cummings, MS, RN
Clinical Nurse Specialist
Rush North Shore Medical Center
Skokie, Illinois

Brenda S. Gregory Dawes, MSN, RN, C[illegible]
Director
Surgical Services
St. Anthony's Hospital
St. Petersburg, Florida

Donna Deane, PhD, RN
Professor Emeritus of Nursing
Wright State University
Dayton, Ohio

Mary Ellen Dellefield, MS, RN
Instructor
University of Phoenix
San Diego, California

Sharon Dudley-Brown, MS, PhD, RN, C, FNP
Assistant Professor
Department of Nursing
The Chinese University of Hong Kong
Hong Kong

Janet Dugan, MS, RN
Coordinator
Continuing Education
Good Samaritan Hospital
Dayton, Ohio

Leann Eaton, MSN, RN, ANP
Assistant Professor
Jewish Hospital College of Nursing and Allied Health
Washington University Medical Center
St. Louis, Missouri

Sandra J. Hayes Engberg, MSN, PhD
University of Pittsburgh School of Nursing
Pittsburgh, Pennsylvania

Betty R. Ferrell, PhD, RN, FAAN
Associate Research Scientist
City of Hope National Medical Center
Duarte, California

Kathleen Fletcher, MSN, RN, CS, GNP
Director of Geriatric Services
University of Virginia Health System
Charlottesville, Virginia

Deborah K. Fultner, MS, RN, CS
Nursing Instructor
Texas Christian University
Fort Worth, Texas

Janet S. Fulton, BSN, MSN, PhD
Assistant Professor
Wright State University
College of Nursing & Health
Dayton, Ohio

Teresa M. Garrison, RN, BSN, MSN
Infection Control Supervisor
Barnes-Jewish Hospital
St. Louis, Missouri

Bernie Gorek, MA, RNC, GNP
Senior Learning Associate
The Evangelical Lutheran Good Samaritan Society
Sioux Falls, South Dakota

Carol Green-Nigro, MN, PhD, RN
Professor of Nursing
Johnson County Community College
Overland Park, Kansas

Sara H. Gueldner, DNSc, FAAN
Professor and Director of Doctoral Studies
College of Nursing
Medical University of South Carolina
Charleston, South Carolina

Joyce A. Guillory, PhD, RN
Assistant Professor and Director
Cancer Prevention Awareness Program
Deparment of Community Health/Preventive Medicine
Morehouse School of Medicine
Atlanta, Georgia

Sandra Lynne Hensel, MSN(R), RN, C
Clinical Nurse Specialist in Gerontological Nursing
Missouri Baptist Medical Center
St. Louis, Missouri

Mildred O. Hogstel, PhD, RN, C
Emeritus Professor of Nursing
Harris College of Nursing
Texas Christian University
Fort Worth, Texas

June Felice Johnson, BS, PharmD, BCPS
Associate Professor, Pharmacy Practice
Drake University
College of Pharmacy & Health Sciences
Des Moines, Iowa

Rhonda Kirk-Gardner, BSN, MSN, RN, BAd
Associate Professor
School of Nursing
Lakehead University
Thunder Bay, Ontario
Canada

Karen Van Dyke Lamb, BS, MS, ND, CS
Practitioner-Teacher, Associate Professor
Rush University, College of Nursing
Chicago, Illinois

Kem Louie, PhD, RN, CS, FAAN
Professor and Chairperson
Graduate Nursing Department
College of Mount Saint Vincent
Bronx, New York

Anita Lovell, BSN, RN, CCRN
RN Case Manager
University of Pittsburgh Medical Center
Pittsburgh, Pennsylvania

Ann Schmidt Luggen, PhD, RN, CNAA
Associate Professor, Nursing
Northern Kentucky University
College of Professional Studies
Highland Heights, Kentucky

Marjorie A. Maddox, EdD, MSN, ARNP, ANP-C
Associate Professor and Coordinator
Adult Nurse Practitioner Option
School of Nursing
University of Louisville
Louisville, Kentucky

Holly Evans Madison, MS, RN
Nursing Faculty
Southern Vermont College
Bennington, Vermont

Judith J. McCann, RN, DNSc
Assistant Professor in Gerontological Nursing
Rush University College of Nursing
Research Faculty
Rush Institute on Aging
Rush-Presbyterian—St. Luke's Medical Center
Chicago, Illinois

Beatrice Joan McDowell, BS, MPH, PhD
University of Pittsburgh School of Nursing
Pittsburgh, Pennsylvania

Sue E. Meiner, EdD, RN, CS, GNP
Gerontologist/Educator, Nurse Practitioner
Jewish Hospital College of Nursing and Allied Health
Washington University Medical Center
St. Louis, Missouri

Deanna Gray Miceli, MSN, RN, CS
Gerontological Nurse Practitioner
University of Medicine and Dentistry of New Jersey
School of Osteopathic Medicine
Stratford, New Jersey

Jean R. Miller, BS, MN, MA, PhD
Professor
University of Rhode Island, College of Nursing
Kingston, Rhode Island

Linda K. Mosel, MSN, RN, CS
Gerontology Clinical Nurse Specialist
Good Samaritan Hospital
Dayton, Ohio

Catherine E. O'Connor, DNSc, RN, CS
Former Associate Chief
Nursing Service for Long-Term Care
Veterans Administration
Miami, Florida

Marsha Evans Orr, MS, RN
CreativEnergy LLC
Healthcare Consulting Firm
Phoenix, Arizona

Ann Peterson, MSN, RN, CDE
Clinical Nurse Specialist
Clinical Center
National Institutes of Health
Bethesda, Maryland

Barbara M. Raudonis, PhD
Assistant Professor
The University of Texas at Arlington
School of Nursing
Arlington, Texas

Lynne M. Rivera, MSN, RN
Research Specialist
City of Hope National Medical Center
Duarte, California

Debbie Sanazaro, MSN, NP
Adjunct Instructor
St. Louis University School of Nursing
St. Louis, Missouri

Susan L. Sanders, MSN, RN, C, GNP
Nurse Practitioner
Midland Community Clinics
Midland, Texas

Vicki L. Schmall, PhD
Professor Emeritus
Oregon State University
Corvallis, Oregon

Darlene Stevens, BSN, BA, PhD, MHSA, RN
Associate Professor
School of Nursing
Lakehead University
Thunder Bay, Ontario
Canada

Tamara R. Tripp, AD, BSN, MSN
Gerontological/Adult Nurse Practitioner
Nalle Clinic University Family Practice
Charlotte, North Carolina

Meredith Wallace, MSN, RN
Assistant Professor
Southern Connecticut State University
New Haven, Connecticut
Heath Promotion Clinical Nurse Specialist
Hospital of St. Raphael
New Haven, Connecticut

Susan Mace Weeks, MS, RN, LMFT, LCDC
Instructor
Texas Christian University
Harris College of Nursing
Fort Worth, Texas

Ruth B. Weg, BA, MS, PhD
Professor Emeritus in Gerontology and Biology
Andrus Gerontology Center
University of Southern California
Los Angeles, California

Pamela Becker Weilitz, MSN(R), CS, ANP
Adult Nurse Practitioner
Washington University School of Medicine,
University Care
St. Louis, Missouri

Alice Welch, PhD, RN, CTN
Nursing Consultant
Associate Professor
School of Nursing
Indiana State University
Terre Haute, Indiana

Laurel Wiersema-Bryant, MSN, RN, CS
Clinical Nurse Specialist/Adult Nurse Practitioner
Barnes-Jewish Hospital
St. Louis, Missouri

Gail Wilkerson, MSN, RN, CS
Quality Practice Manager
Gerontological Clinical Specialist
Deaconess Home Health Services
St. Louis, Missouri

Carol Will, MA, RN
Will's Consulting
Keokuk, Iowa

Preface

The field of gerontologic nursing has blossomed over the past decades as the population of baby boomers nears or enters retirement age. The demand of health care for older adults is an ever-growing challenge. Age-appropriate and age-specific care is an expectation of current and future nurses across the globe. The many and varied issues related to health and wellness must be provided within a cost-effective and resource-sparse environment. The largest group of patients in hospitals (outside of obstetric and pediatric units) is older adults. Long-term and rehabilitation specialty facilities have predominantly older adults as residents. The specialty of gerontologic nursing is in greater demand now more than ever before.

Gerontologic Nursing, third edition, has been developed to provide today's students with a solid foundation to meet the future challenges of gerontologic nursing practice. This textbook provides comprehensive, theoretic, and practical information about basic and complex concepts and issues relevant to the care of older people across the care continuum. The extensive coverage of material provides the student with the information necessary to make sound clinical judgments while emphasizing the concepts, skills, and techniques of gerontologic nursing practice. Psychologic and sociocultural issues and aspects of older adult care are given special emphasis, but they are also integrated throughout the textbook, reflecting the reality of practice with this unique population. Care of both well and sick older people and their families and caregivers is included.

Intended for use by undergraduate nursing students in all levels of professional nursing programs, *Gerontologic Nursing* was developed for use in either gerontologic nursing or medical-surgical courses, or within programs that integrate gerontologic content throughout the educational program.

ORGANIZATION

The 31 chapters in *Gerontologic Nursing* are divided into six parts. Part One, Introduction to Gerontologic Nursing, includes four chapters that serve as the foundation for the remainder of the textbook. Chapter 1 introduces the student to the specialty by addressing historical developments, educational preparation and practice roles, future trends, and demographic factors relevant to the health and well being of older people. Basic tenets of selected biologic, sociologic, and psychologic theories of aging and their relevance to nursing practice are presented in Chapter 2. Chapter 3 presents an overview of practice standards, legal issues, and relevant laws applicable to the care of older adults across the care continuum and describes the principles of values and ethics associated with the care of older people. Chapter 4 discusses the importance of a nursing-focused assessment, special considerations affecting assessment of older people, and strategies and techniques for collecting a comprehensive health assessment. Functional, mental status, affective, and social assessment tools and techniques are included. Part Two, Influences on Health and Illness, includes chapters on cultural, family, and socioeconomic and environmental influences. Health promotion and illness/disability prevention are also included. The final chapter in this part presents an in-depth look at various health care delivery settings. Chapter 5 presents cultural concepts within the contexts of aging and the health and illness experiences of older people. Roles and functions of families, common family issues and decisions in later life, and family caregiving are described in Chapter 6. Specific tools and techniques for working with aging families, including crisis intervention, are also explained. Chapter 7 presents an overview of socioeconomic and environmental factors that affect health and illness, including issues associated with resource availability. Advocacy by and for older adults is included. Chapter 8 introduces the concepts of health promotion, protection, and disease prevention as it applies to older adults and includes strategies for health promotion activities with this population. Chapter 9 presents issues and trends associated with the care of older people in acute, home, hospice, and long-term care settings.

Part Three, Wellness Issues, details the needs and nursing care of older adults in the areas of nutrition, sleep and activity, safety, intimacy and sexuality, and mental health. Chapter 10 explores the role of nutrition in health and illness, including nutritional requirements, screenings and assessments, therapeutic diets, and other nutritional support and therapies. Age-related factors in maintaining a balance between sleep and activity and their effect on the older person's lifestyle are discussed in Chapter 11. Chapter 12 stresses the importance of a safe environment within the context of maintaining the older person's autonomy. Chapter 13 sensitively addresses the intimacy and sexuality needs of older adults, offering practical management strategies. In Chapter 14 the commonly occurring mental, emotional, and behavioral problems experienced by older people are discussed, including the availability of resources and trends in treatment and care. Each chapter in this section presents the age-related changes in structure and function and nursing interventions to promote healthy adaptation to the identified changes.

Part Four, Common Psychophysiologic Stressors, focuses on the special needs of older adults with pain, infection, cancer, chronic illness, and substance abuse, as well as nursing care related to loss and end-of-life issues. Chapter 15 provides an overview of pain and the special issues surrounding pain management in older people. The importance and significance of immunity and factors affecting immunocompetence in aging, as well as associated common problems and conditions, are explored in Chapter 16. Chapter 17 examines the concepts of chronic illness and rehabilitation in aging, as well as the related concepts of compliance, self-care, functional ability, psychosocial and physiologic needs, and the impact on family and caregiver. Chapter 18 includes risk factors, assessment tools and techniques, and nursing interventions for the most commonly abused substances. The nursing management of older adults with the most commonly occurring cancers is addressed in Chapter 19. Chapter 20 discusses the topics of loss and end-of-life issues. Differences between the loss and death experiences of older people and younger adults are reviewed. All of these chapters emphasize the nurse's role in effectively managing the nursing care of older clients with these problems.

Part Five, Diagnostic Studies and Pharmacologic Management, includes chapters on laboratory and diagnostic tests and pharmacologic management. Principles of laboratory testing in older adults, including age-related factors that influence laboratory values and age-specific values for hematologic, blood, and urine chemistry, are presented in Chapter 21. Chapter 22 contains current and comprehensive information on the critical issue of medications and the myriad of issues pertinent to drug use in this population.

Part Six, Nursing Care of Physiologic and Psychologic Disorders, contains nine chapters that detail nursing management of older adults with diseases or conditions of cardiovascular, respiratory, endocrine, gastrointestinal, musculoskeletal, urinary, cognitive and neurologic, integumentary, and sensory function.

In organizing the textbook every attempt was made to ensure a logical sequence by grouping related topics. However, it is not necessary to read the text in sequence. Material is cross-referenced throughout the text, and an extensive index is included. It is hoped that this approach provides the student with easy access to information of particular interest.

FORMAT

The third edition has been revised and reflects the growth and change of gerontologic nursing practice and the learning needs of today's student. The presentation of content has been designed for ease of use and reference. Consistent chapter pedagogy has been retained in this edition, and the textbook's visual appeal has been carefully planned to make it easy to read and follow. Content that is traditionally covered in fundamental or medical-surgical nursing courses has been deleted. The clinical examples still depict nurses practicing in many different roles at a wide variety of practice settings, reflecting current practice patterns.

Recognizing that there are differences of opinion regarding the use of the terms *client* and *patient*, *client* has been used throughout most of the textbook because it implies active participation by the person in encounters with the members of the health care team. *Patient* has been used in some chapters where it is reflective of the role of the older adult in that specific setting.

All body system chapters include an overview of age-related changes in structure and function. Common problems and conditions within each of the chapters are presented in a format that includes the definition, etiology, pathophysiology, and typical clinical presentation for each. The *Nursing Management* of the problems and conditions is central to each of these chapters and follows the five-step nursing process format of assessment, diagnosis, planning/expected outcomes, intervention, and evaluation. *Nursing Care Plans* for selected problems and conditions begin with a realistic clinical situation and emphasize nursing diagnoses pertinent to the situation, expected outcomes, and nursing interventions, all within an easy-to-reference, three-column format.

FEATURES

Each chapter begins with Learning Objectives to help the student focus on the important subject matter. Client/Family Teaching boxes are included where appropriate, providing key information on what to teach clients and families to enhance their knowledge and promote active participation in their care. Throughout the text, coupled with more content emphasizing health promotion and the needs of well older adults are Health Promotion boxes, which identify activities and interventions that promote a healthy lifestyle and prevent disease and illness. Nutrition boxes are found throughout the text to stress the importance of nutrition in the care of older adults. Research boxes are presented to emphasize the application of relevant study findings to current nursing practice and allow students to reflect on how to integrate research into everyday nursing practice. Cultural Awareness boxes are included where applicable to develop the student's cultural sensitivity and promote the delivery of culture-specific care. At the conclusion of the body system and clinical chapters, Home Care boxes provide pragmatic suggestions for care of the home-bound client and family. Finally, each chapter concludes with a brief Summary, followed by Key Points that highlight important principles discussed in the chapter. Critical Thinking Exercises at the end of every chapter stimulate the student to carefully consider the material learned and apply their knowledge to the situation presented.

As the scope of gerontologic nursing practice continues to expand, so must the knowledge guiding that practice reflect the most current standards and guidelines. Every effort has been made to incorporate the most current standards and guidelines from the AHCRQ, ANA, CDC, JCAHO, NANDA, OBRA, and CMS.

Acknowledgments

The development of this third edition would not have been possible without the combined efforts of many talented professionals who supported us throughout the entire process. The contributors were especially dedicated to reviewing the second edition, researching all of the information for current status of information as well as investigating any new and updated information on each of the topics selected. A special thank you to the contributors is in order in the face of tight deadlines and demands from all editors, including us.

A very special recognition goes to the editorial and production team at Mosby. This team of professionals worked extremely hard to assist us in meeting the deadlines. So many people were involved that we fear leaving someone out, so we will just say "Thank you so much" to the team.

Finally, we acknowledge our families, friends, and colleagues for the continual support they provided throughout this process.

Sue E. Meiner and Annette G. Lueckenotte

Detailed Contents

1 Overview of Gerontologic Nursing

SUE E. MEINER, EdD, APRN, BC, GNP, and ANNETTE G. LUECKENOTTE, MS, RN, BC, GNP, GCNP

Learning Objectives

On completion of this chapter, the reader will be able to:

1. Trace the historic development of gerontologic nursing as a specialty.
2. Distinguish the educational preparation, practice roles, and certification requirements of the gerontologic nurse generalist, nurse practitioner, and clinical nurse specialist.
3. Discuss the major demographic trends in the United States in relation to the older adult population. (Current information has not been updated since the 1998 profile compiled by the American Association of Retired Persons.)
4. Identify the factors responsible for the rapid growth of the older adult population.
5. Describe the effects of each of the following demographic factors on the health, well-being, and life expectancy of older adults:
   - Gender and marital status
   - Race/ethnicity
   - Housing/living situation
   - Educational status
   - Economic status
6. Explain why old age is considered a woman's problem.
7. Describe the effect of functional ability on the overall health status of older adults.
8. Discuss how the "aging of the aged" will affect health care delivery.
9. Explore future trends in gerontologic nursing care along the continuum of care.
10. Explore the concept of ageism as related to the care of older adults in various settings.
11. Identify the issues influencing gerontologic nursing education.
12. Analyze the issues affecting the development and future of gerontologic nursing research.

FOUNDATIONS OF THE SPECIALTY OF GERONTOLOGIC NURSING

The rich, diverse history of nursing has always been shaped by the population it serves. From the early beginnings of Florence Nightingale's experiences during the Crimean War to the present, as nurses care for the growing immigrant and prison populations, those with mental illnesses, those with substance abuse problems, teenage mothers, homeless individuals, and those infected with the human immunodeficiency virus (HIV), nurses are reminded that these clients and their problems define the knowledge and skills required for practice.

More than 34 million persons in the United States today who are 65 and older represent yet another group that has gradually shaped the practice of nursing, but only in recent decades has the impact been realized. The number of older adults has grown steadily since 1900, and they are now the fastest growing segment of the population. With a "gerontology boom" less than 15 years away, gerontologic nursing is finally being recognized as a specialty. The struggle for recognition can be traced back to the beginning of the twentieth century.

History and Evolution

Burnside (1988) conducted an extensive review of the *American Journal of Nursing (AJN)* for historic materials related to gerontologic nursing. Between 1900 and 1940, she found 23 writings, including works by Lavinia Dock, with a focus on older adults and covering such topics as rural nursing, almshouses, and private duty nursing, as well as early case studies and clinical issues addressing home care for fractured femur, dementia, and delirium. Burnside discovered an anonymous column in *AJN* entitled "Care of the Aged" that was written in 1925, and it is now thought be one of the earliest references to the need for a specialty in older adult care.

The modern health movement is constantly increasing life expectancy by its steady onslaught against preventable disease. Therefore nursing professionals must expect to care for relatively larger and larger numbers of patients with degenerative conditions. Perhaps it is time for nurses to consider creating yet another specialty.

During World War II and the postwar years (1940 to 1960), the population of older persons steadily increased, but articles about the care of older adults were general and not particularly comprehensive (Burnside, 1988). It was not until 1962, when the geriatric nursing conference group was established during the American Nurses Association (ANA) convention, that the question posed by the anonymous *AJN* columnist was finally addressed.

Professional Origins

In 1966 the ANA established the Division of Geriatric Nursing Practice and defined geriatric nursing as "concerned with the assessment of nursing needs of older people; planning and implementing nursing care to meet those needs; and evaluating the effectiveness of such care." In 1976 the Division of Geriatric Nursing Practice was changed to the Division of Gerontologic Nursing Practice to reflect the nursing roles of providing care to healthy, ill, and frail older persons. The division became the Council of Gerontologic Nursing in 1984 to encompass issues beyond clinical practice.

Standards of Practice

The years 1960 to 1970 were characterized by many "firsts," as the specialty devoted to the care of older adults began its exciting development (Table 1-1). Journals, textbooks, workshops and seminars, formal education programs, professional certification, and research with a focus on gerontologic nursing have since evolved. However, the singular event that truly legitimized the specialty occurred in 1969, when a committee appointed by the ANA Division of Geriatric Nursing Practice completed the first *Standards of Practice for Geriatric Nursing* (ANA, 1991). These standards were widely circulated during the next several years; in 1976 they were revised, and the title was changed to *Standards of Gerontological Nursing Practice.* In 1981 *A Statement on the Scope of Gerontological Nursing Practice* was published. The revised *Standards and Scope of Gerontological Nursing Practice* was published in 1987, reflecting the comprehensive concepts and dimensions of practice for the nurse working with older adults. On the 1993 recommendation of the ANA Board of Directors, the revision of the *Scope of Practice and Standards of Gerontological Nursing* was reassigned to the Council for Community, Primary, and Long Term Care Nursing Practice. In 1995 the newly revised *Scope and Standards of Gerontological Nursing Practice* was published. This document reflected the nature and scope of current gerontologic nursing practice but also incorporated the concepts of health promotion, health maintenance, disease prevention, and self-care. In 2004, all scope and standards of practice were combined into a set of three books known as the *Nursing Scope & Standards of Practice, Nursing's Social Policy Statement* (ANA, 2003) and the *Code of Ethics for Nurses with Interpretive Statements* (ANA, 2001). This merging of the standards of practice of all the specialties was an effort to outline the expectations of the professional role within which all registered nurses must practice nursing. According to the ANA (2004, p. vi), "These three resources provide a complete and definitive description for better understanding by specialty nursing organizations, policy makers, and the public of nursing practice and nursing's accountability to the public in the United States." These documents can be obtained from the ANA website: http://www. nursingworld.org/.

TABLE 1-1 Development of Gerontologic Nursing: 1960-1970

YEAR	EVENT
1961	Formation of a specialty group for geriatric nurses is recommended by the American Nurses Association (ANA).
1962	First national meeting of the ANA Conference on Geriatric Nursing Practice is held in Detroit, Mich.
	American Nurses' Foundation receives a grant for a workshop on the aged.
	First research in geriatric nursing is published in England (Norton D et al: *An investigation of geriatric nursing problems in hospital,* London 1962, National Corporation for the Care of Old People).
1966	First gerontologic clinical specialist nursing program is developed at Duke University by Virginia Stone.
	Geriatric Nursing Division of the ANA is formed; a monograph is published, entitled *Exploring Progress in Geriatric Nursing Practice.*
1968	Laurie Gunter is the first nurse to present a paper at the International Congress of Gerontology in Washington, DC.
	First gerontologic nursing interest group, Geriatric Nursing, is formed.
	Barbara Davis is the first nurse to speak before the American Geriatric Society.
	First article on nursing curriculum regarding gerontologic nursing is published (Delora JR, Moses DV: Specialty preferences and characteristics of nursing students in baccalaureate programs, *Nurs Res* March/April, 1969).
	The nine standards for geriatric nursing practice are developed.
1970	*Standards of Geriatric Nursing Practice* is first published.
	First gerontologic clinical nurse specialists graduate from Duke University.

Modified from Burnside IM: *Nursing and the aged: a self care approach,* ed 3, New York, 1988, McGraw-Hill.

Another hallmark in the continued growth of the gerontologic nursing specialty occurred in 1973, when the first gerontologic nurses were certified through the ANA. Certification is an additional credential granted by the ANA, providing a means for recognizing excellence in a clinical or functional area (ANA, 1995). Certification is usually voluntary, enabling the nurse to demonstrate to peers and others that a distinct degree of knowledge and expertise has been achieved. In some cases, certification can mean eligibility for third-party reimbursement for nursing services rendered. From the initial certification offering as a generalist in gerontologic nursing, to the first gerontologic nurse practitioner (GNP) examination offering in 1979, to the most recent gerontologic clinical nurse specialist (CNS) examination (first administered in 1989), this specialty has continued to grow and attract a high level of interest (Box 1-1).

Roles

The growth of the nursing profession as a whole, increasing educational opportunities, demographic changes, and changes in health care delivery systems have all influenced the development of the generalist role in gerontologic nursing, as well as the advanced practice roles of gerontologic CNS and GNP. The generalist in gerontologic nursing has completed a basic entry-level educational program. Since 1998 the baccalaureate degree has been required for the generalist certification examination (ANA, 2004). A generalist nurse may practice in a wide variety of environments, including the home and community. The challenge of the gerontologic nurse generalist is to identify older clients' strengths and assist them with maximizing their independence. Clients participate as much as possible in making decisions about their care. The generalist consults with the advanced practice nurse and other interdisciplinary health professionals for assistance in meeting the complex care needs of older adults.

The gerontologic CNS has a master's degree. The first program was launched in 1966 at Duke University. The gerontologic master's program typically focuses on the advanced knowledge and skills required to care for older adults in a wide variety of settings, and the graduate is prepared to assume a leadership role in the delivery of that care. The CNS functions as a clinician, educator, consultant, administrator, or researcher to plan care or improve the quality of nursing

BOX 1-1 American Nurses Credentialing Center Eligibility Requirements for Certification in Gerontologic Nursing

GERONTOLOGIC NURSE

The nurse must meet all of the following requirements:

1. Currently hold an active registered nurse (RN) license in the United States or its territories
2. Hold a baccalaureate or higher degree in nursing
3. Have practiced 2000 hours within the past 3 years (a requirement that may be met if engaged in direct client care or direct clinical management, supervision, education, or direction of other persons to achieve or help achieve client goals for the stated number of hours)
4. Have had 30 contact hours of continuing education applicable to gerontology/gerontologic nursing within the past 3 years

GERONTOLOGIC NURSE PRACTITIONER (GNP)

The nurse must meet all of the following requirements:

1. Currently hold an active RN license in the United States or its territories
2. Hold a master's or higher degree in nursing
3. Have been prepared as a nurse practitioner in either of the following:
   a. A GNP master's degree in nursing program
   b. A formal postgraduate GNP track or program within a school of nursing granting graduate-level academic credit (graduate, nonmatriculating program), with evidence of successful completion in the form of a certificate or letter from the program director; the educational program must have included didactic and clinical components, and verification by the program director is required.

CLINICAL SPECIALIST IN GERONTOLOGIC NURSING

The nurse must meet all the following requirements:

1. Currently hold an active RN license in the United States or its territories
   a. Hold a master's or higher degree in gerontologic nursing
   b. Hold a master's or higher degree in nursing with a specialization in gerontologic nursing
2. Have practiced a *minimum* of 12 months after completion of the master's degree
3. Meet the following requirements in current practice:
   a. If a clinical specialist, must have provided a *minimum* of 800 hours (post-master's) of direct client care or clinical management in gerontologic nursing within the past 24 months
   b. If a consultant, researcher, educator, or administrator, must have provided a minimum of 400 hours (post-master's) of direct client care or clinical management in gerontologic nursing within the past 24 months*

Modified from *American Nurses Credentialing Center Certification Catalog: 2004*, Washington DC, 2004, The Center. Accessed November 27, 2004 from website: at http://www.nursingworld.org/ancc/certify.htm. To keep current with the changing scope, standards, and education requirement, the eligibility criteria are reviewed yearly and subject to change. Therefore if applying to take a certification examination, a current catalog must be requested from the center, and compliance with the current eligibility criteria is required. Applications can be downloaded from the Internet.

*Supervision of student's client care fulfills the requirement for direct client care or clinical management only when the supervisor intervenes with the client and is personally responsible and accountable for the outcome of that intervention.

care for older adults and their families. Specialists provide comprehensive care based on theory and research. Today, CNSs can be found practicing in acute hospitals, long-term care or home care settings, or independent practices.

The GNP may be educationally prepared in numerous different ways. In the early 1970s the first GNPs were prepared primarily through continuing education programs. Another early group of GNPs received their training and clinical supervision from physicians. Only since the late 1980s has master's-level education with a focus on primary care been available. As a provider of primary care and a case manager, the GNP conducts health assessments, identifies nursing diagnoses, and plans, implements, and evaluates nursing care for older clients. A GNP has the knowledge and skills to detect and manage limited acute and chronic stable conditions; coordination and collaboration with other health care providers is a related essential function. The GNP's activities include interventions for health promotion, maintenance, and restoration. GNPs provide primary ambulatory care in an independent practice or a collaborative practice with a physician; they also practice in settings across the continuum of care, including the acute care hospital, subacute care center, and long-term care setting. Most recently, health maintenance organizations (HMOs) have begun including GNPs on their provider panels. Since 1992, nurses have been required to complete at least a master's degree in nursing to be eligible to take the GNP certification examination (ANA, 1990). Certification can elevate the status of the nurse practicing with older adults in any setting. More importantly, it enables the nurse to ensure the delivery of quality care to older adult clients.

Terminology

Any discussion of older adult nursing is complicated by the wide variety of terms used interchangeably to describe the specialty. Some terms are used because of personal preference or because they suggest a certain perspective. Still others are avoided because of the negative inferences they evoke. As described in the preceding overview of the evolution of the specialty, the terminology has changed over the years. The following are the most commonly used terms and definitions:

- **Geriatrics**—from the Greek *geras,* meaning "old age," geriatrics is the branch of medicine that deals with the diseases and problems of old age. Viewed by many nurses as having limited application to nursing because of its medical and disease orientation, the term *geriatrics* is generally not used when describing the nursing of older adults.
- **Gerontology**—from the Greek *geron,* meaning "old man," gerontology is the scientific study of the process of aging and the problems of aged persons; it includes biologic, sociologic, psychologic, and economic aspects.
- **Gerontologic nursing**—this specialty of nursing involves assessing the health and functional status of older adults, planning and implementing health care and services to meet the identified needs, and evaluating the effectiveness of such care. *Gerontologic nursing* is the term most often used by nurses specializing in this field.
- **Gerontic nursing**—this term was developed by Gunter and Estes in 1979 and is meant to be more inclusive than geriatric or gerontologic nursing because it is not limited to diseases or scientific principles. Gerontic nursing connotes the nursing of older persons—the art and practice of nurturing, caring, and comforting. This term has not gained wide acceptance, but it is viewed by some as a more appropriate description of the specialty.

These terms and their usage spark a great deal of interest and controversy among nurses practicing with older adults. As the specialty continues to grow and develop, it is likely the terminology will do so as well.

DEMOGRAPHIC PROFILE OF THE OLDER POPULATION

Far from the beginnings of gerontologic nursing practice in almshouses and nursing homes, nurses today find themselves caring for older adults in a wider variety of settings. Emergency rooms, medical-surgical and critical care units in hospitals, outpatient surgical centers, home care agencies, clinics, and rehabilitation centers are just some of the sites where nurses are caring for a older population that is rapidly growing. Nurses in any of these settings need only count the number of clients 65 and older to understand firsthand what demographers have termed the *graying of America.* Although this trend has already attracted the attention of the health care marketplace, it promises to become an even greater influence on health care organizations. It is clearly a trend that promises to shape the future practice of nursing in profound and dramatic ways.

Demography is the statistical science dealing with the distribution, density, and vital statistics of human populations. In the following review of basic demographic facts about older persons, the reader is cautioned against believing that age 65 automatically defines a person as being *old.* The rate and intensity of aging is highly variable and individual. It occurs gradually and in no predictable sequence.

Butler (1975), in his classic book, *Why Survive? Being Old in America,* cautions against using chronologic age as a measure of being old. He offers the following on why age 65 is the discretionary cutoff for defining old age:

> Society has arbitrarily chosen ages 60 to 65 as the beginning of late life (borrowing the idea from Bismarck's social legislation in Germany in the 1880s) primarily for the purpose of determining a point for retirement and eligibility for services and financial entitlements for the elderly.

When the social security program was established in 1935, it was believed that age 65 would be a reasonable age for the purpose of allocating benefits and services. Today, with so many older persons living productive, highly functional lives well beyond age 65, this age is obviously an inappropriate one for determining whether a person is old. However, demographic information and other forms of data are still reported using age 65 as the defining standard for "old." For example, older adults are categorized by cohort for some research and public policy purposes. Consequently, it is not uncommon to see older persons classified as *young-old, middle-old,* or *old-old.*

Although grouping older persons is useful in some circumstances, the nurse is cautioned against thinking of all persons over age 65 as similar. In fact, older persons are far from being a homogenous group. Landmarks for human growth and development are well established for infancy through middle age, whereas few norms have been as discretely defined for older adulthood. In fact, most developmental norms that have been described for later life categorize all older persons in the over-65 group. One could argue from a developmental perspective that as great a difference exists among 65-, 75-, 85-, and 95-year-olds as it does among 2-, 3-, 4-, and 5-year-olds. Yet no definitive standards for older adult development have been established. Consequently, the nurse is urged to view each older client as one would any client—a being with a richly diverse and unique array of internal and external variables that ultimately influence how the person thinks and acts. Understanding how the variables interact and affect older adults enables the nurse to provide individualized care. Additionally, the nurse is encouraged to use the individual client as the standard, comparing a client's previous level and pattern of health and function with the current status.

The Older Population

For several decades, the American Association of Retired Persons (AARP) maintained a yearly update of the profile of older adults in America. This organization is a nonprofit, nonpartisan membership organization for people age 50 and over. The AARP is dedicated to enhancing quality of life for all Americans as they age. The association acknowledges that its members receive a wide range of unique benefits, special products, and services. Additional information can be found at their website: www.aarp.org.

In 1997 the organization stopped compiling profile demographics and began to collect specific data, such as "Images of Aging in America, 2004: A Summary of Selected Findings." This AARP study included 1202 interviews. To increase minority participation, 314 interviews were with blacks and 318 were with Hispanic origin participants. The remaining 570 interviewees were white, Native and Alaskan Americans. and Pacific Islanders and Asian Americans. The final comprehensive report on the findings from this survey is now available. The following data is from the latest profile information.

Since 1900 the percentage of Americans ages 65 and older has more than quadrupled—from 3.1% in 1900 to 12.7% in 1997—and they now represent about one in every eight Americans (AARP, 1998). Not only has the *number* of persons over age 65 increased, but the *proportion* of this group in the total population has also increased. By 1996 the total number of older Americans had increased by 9.1% since 1990, compared with an increase of 7% for the under-65 population during that same period. The relatively high birth rate during the late nineteenth and early twentieth centuries accounts in part for the large number of older persons today (Burnside, 1988). Reduced infant and child mortality as a result of improved sanitation, advances in vaccination, and the development of antibiotics have also contributed. The large influx of immigrants before World War I is an additional important factor. The net effect, associated with a reduction in mortality for all ages and fertility rates at a replacement level, has been an increase in the older adult population.

Not only are large numbers of persons living to age 65, they are living to older ages. A child born in 1997 could expect to live 76.5 years, or about 29 years longer than a child born in 1900. This increase is largely a result of lower death rates for children and young adults. Life expectancy at age 65 increased by only 2.4 years between 1900 and 1960, but it has increased by 3.3 years since. In 1997 the *young-old,* or 65-to-74 age-group, was 8 times larger (18.5 million) than in 1900, but the *middle-old,* or 75-to-84 age-group, was 16 times larger (11.7 million), and the *old-old,* or 85-and-older group was 31 times larger (3.9 million) (AARP, 1998). The 3.9 million persons ages 85 and older represent the fastest growing subset, with a growth rate of nearly 3 times that of the overall older population. Occasionally termed the *aging of the aged,* this phenomenon is one of the greatest concerns and challenges for society and the health care system.

Persons in advanced age are more vulnerable to the multiple losses typically associated with aging, thus making them frailer. These frail older adults need more intensive care in all the health care settings in which they are found. Coupled with the growth of life-extending therapies and the continuous development of highly sophisticated treatment measures, the structure, services, and financing of the current health care delivery system are still not equipped to effectively manage the needs of this population segment.

As is discussed throughout the remaining chapters of this text, older adults have unique and varied responses to the interacting array of forces that affect their health status. It is well-documented that advancing age is associated with more physical frailty as a result of the increased incidence of chronic disease, greater vulnerability to illness and injury, diminished physical functioning, and the increased likelihood of developing cognitive impairment. Additionally, psychologic, social, environmental, and financial factors play a significant role in the level of frailty. Regardless, not *all* older adults are frail. The expectation of wellness, even in the presence of chronic illness and significant impairment, must be incorporated into the consciousness *and* practice of nurses who interact this population.

Projected Growth

It is expected that the older population will continue to grow, with those over age 65 expected to number nearly 39 million, or about 13% of the total population, by the year 2010. The most dramatic and rapid growth will occur between 2010 and 2030, when the "baby boom" generation reaches 65 years of age. Estimates for the year 2030 are that 79 million persons will be older than age 65, which is more than twice the number in 1997 (AARP, 1998) (Fig. 1-1). In 1997, minority populations represented 15% of the total older adult population; by 2030, this percentage is expected to climb to 25% (AARP, 1998). The greatest increases will be in the Hispanic and Asian/Pacific Islander races. Between 1997 and 2030 the White American, non-Hispanic population of older persons is projected to increase by 79%, whereas the Hispanic population will increase by 368% and the Asian/Pacific Islanders population by 354%. The black population is expected to increase by 134% during this same period (AARP, 1998).

Marital Status

In 1997, 74% of men over age 65 were married, compared with 42% of women (AARP, 1998). Widowhood for women also increases with advancing age—nearly half of all women over age 65 were widows in 1997, and 4 times more widows (8.5 million) than widowers (2.1 million) were living in the United States. Only 7% of all persons over age 65 were divorced. Blacks have higher divorce rates than whites and other minorities. Marital status is an important determinant of health and well-being, because it influences income, mobility, housing, intimacy, and social interaction.

Gender

Since 1930, women have been living longer than men as a result of reduced maternal mortality, a decreased death rate from infectious disease, and an increased death rate in men from chronic disease. Before that time, the number of older men and women was nearly equal. In 1997, 20.1 million older women and 14 million older men lived in the United States , which translates into a gender ratio of 143 women for every 100 men (AARP, 1998).

The discrepancy between proportions of older women and men is expected to continue to increase as the size of the over-85 age-group increases, a group in which women represent the clear majority. This demographic fact has important health care and policy implications, because the majority of older women are likely to be poor, live alone, and have a greater degree of functional impairment and chronic disease. The resulting increased reliance on social, financial, and health-related resources, coupled with emerging health care reforms, points to an uncertain future for older women. Because of these considerations, many gerontologists view aging as primarily a woman's problem. The nursing profession and gerontologic nurses in particular must assume a significant role in the political arena by advocating an agenda that addresses this important issue.

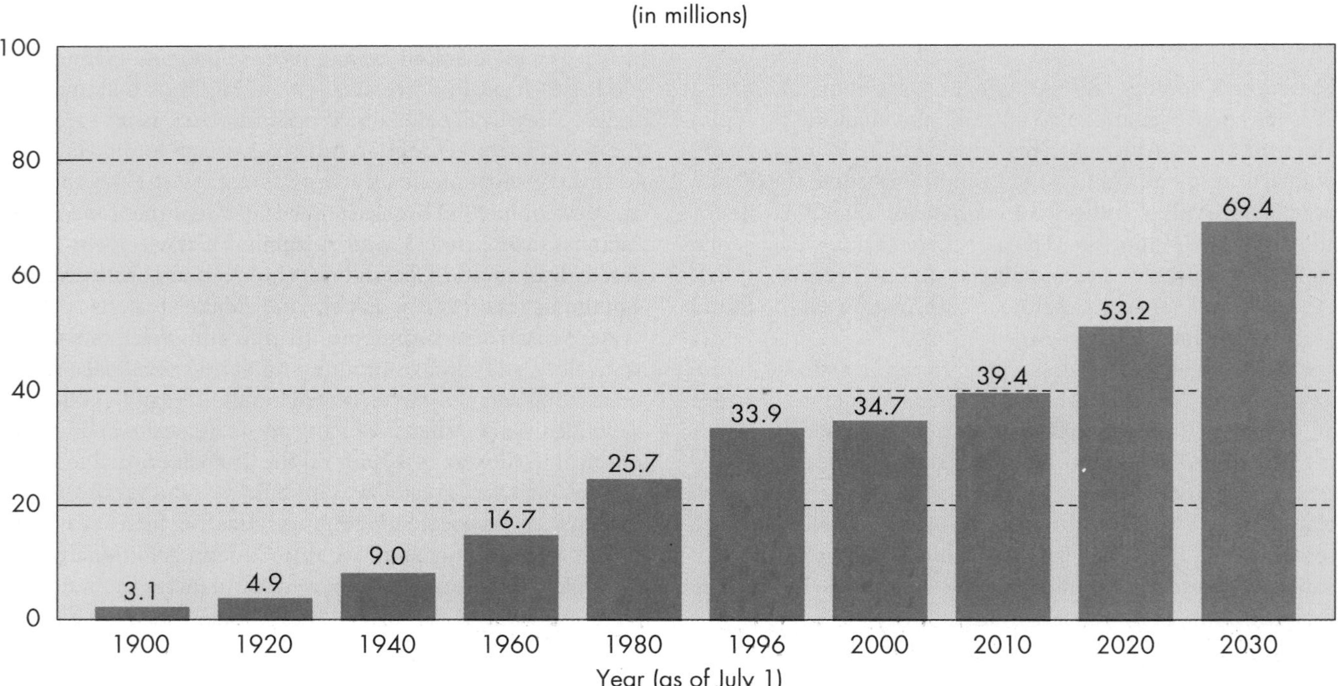

Fig. 1-1 Population trends of persons 65 and older: 1900-2030. (From American Association of Retired Persons: *A profile of older Americans: 1998,* Washington, DC, 1998, The Association.)

Living Arrangements and Housing

In 1997 the majority (66%) of older, noninstitutionalized persons over age 65 lived in a family setting (AARP, 1998)—approximately 80% (10.7 million) of older men and 57% (10.5 million) of older women. It is important to note that the proportion living in a family setting decreases with age. Approximately 8% of men and 17% of women were living with relatives other than a spouse; another 3% of men and 2% of women lived with nonrelatives. About 31% of all noninstitutionalized older persons in 1997 lived alone, representing approximately 41% of all older women and 17% of all older men. The number of older, noninstitutionalized persons living alone increased by 33% between 1980 and 1991, compared with 22% for the balance of the older population. This trend was reversed between 1990 and 1995, when the number of older persons living alone increased less rapidly (7%) than the balance of the older population (9%) (AARP, 1997) (Fig. 1-2).

About 1.4 million (4%) of persons over age 65 lived in nursing facilities in 1995 (AARP, 1998). The percentage increased dramatically with age: 1% for persons ages 65 to 74, 5% for persons ages 75 to 84, and 15% for persons ages 85 and older.

Of the 20.8 million households headed by older persons in 1995, 78% owned their homes and 22% rented (AARP, 1998). Roughly 53% of homes owned by older adults in 1995 were built before 1960, compared with 35% for younger owners. Overall the homes of older persons are typically older and less adequate than those of the rest of the population. The percentage of income spent on home maintenance and repair in 1995 was higher for older persons (34%) than for the younger population (27%). In 1995 the median value of homes owned by older persons was $81,956. Eighty percent of homeowners had completely paid for their homes; however, older persons were more likely to lose a home as a result of property taxes and maintenance costs that were difficult to pay on a fixed income.

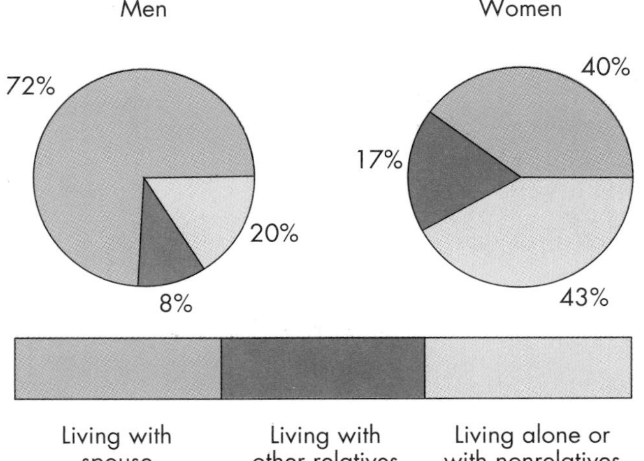

Fig. 1-2 Living arrangements of persons 65 and older: 1995. (From American Association of Retired Persons: *A profile of older Americans: 1998*, Washington, DC, 1998, The Association.)

A person's overall degree of health and well-being greatly influences the selection of housing in old age. Ideally housing should be selected to promote functional independence while emphasizing safety and social interaction needs.

Race and Ethnicity

Of the approximately 34 million Americans older than age 65 in 1997, approximately 90% were white, 8% were black, 4.9% were of Hispanic origin, 2% were Asian/Pacific Islander, and less than 1% were Native American or Native Alaskan (AARP, 1998). People of Hispanic origin may be of any race, but their origin is in the Spanish-speaking countries of Central or South America. They are counted in the census by racial groups, usually as white, black, or other. The higher proportion of older whites is expected to remain stable and continue into the 21st century, at which time the nonwhite segment of the population is expected to increase at a higher rate. Hispanics will continue to be one of the fastest growing segments, and the numbers of blacks, Native Americans, Native Alaskans, Asians, and Pacific Islanders will increase as well. The nursing profession must consider the impact of such changing demographic characteristics. Because people become more diverse as they age, it must be recognized that the increasing longevity of the nonwhite segment of the population will present unique nursing care challenges.

Geographic Distribution

In 1997, more than half (52%) of the population of persons 65 years of age and older lived in nine states: California (3.5 million); Florida (2.7 million); New York (2.4 million); and Pennsylvania, Texas, Illinois, Ohio, Michigan, and New Jersey (more than 1 million each) (AARP, 1998). Persons ages 65 and older constituted 14% or more of the total population in 10 states in 1997: Florida (18.5%), Pennsylvania and Rhode Island (15.9% each), West Virginia (15.1%), Iowa (15%), North Dakota and Connecticut (14.4% each), Arkansas and South Dakota (14.3% each), and Massachusetts (14.1%) (AARP, 1998). In 12 states the 65 and older population increased by 14% or more between 1990 and 1997. These states include Nevada (49%); Alaska (43%); Hawaii and Arizona (25% each); Utah and Colorado (19% each); Delaware (17%); North Carolina and Wyoming (15% each); and South Carolina, Florida, and Texas (14% each) (AARP, 1998). Persons 65 years of age and older were 4% less likely to live in metropolitan areas in 1997 than younger persons. About 29% of older persons lived in central cities, and 48% lived in the suburbs (AARP, 1998).

Older adults as a group are less likely to change residence than other age-groups. For many years, this phenomenon of *aging-in-place* has been an important factor in the growth of the 65 and older population in metropolitan and nonmetropolitan areas. Older adults tend to grow older wherever they reside, without moving. In 1997, only 5% of persons 65 years of age and older had moved since 1996 (compared with 18% of persons under 65). The majority of those (81%) had moved to another home in the same state.

Various factors can influence the decision to move. Dependency and health status may require older persons to move to be near caregivers. *Countermigration* describes the move some older adults make back to their home states after a previous migration to the Sunbelt states for retirement. Dwindling financial resources may necessitate a move to a more economical location; conversely, economic stability or affluence may afford the opportunity to move to a retirement community or a location with a temperate climate and recreational offerings.

Education

Although as a group, older adults are less educated than younger persons, the educational level of the older adult population has been steadily increasing. Between 1970 and 1997, the percentage who had completed high school increased from 28% to 66%. About 15% in 1995 had gone to college for 4 or more years (AARP, 1998). Educational levels are significantly different between whites and nonwhites. In 1997, 68% of whites had completed high school, whereas only 44% of blacks and 30% of Hispanics had completed the same level of education.

Low levels of education can impair older persons' abilities to live a healthy lifestyle, access service and benefit programs, recognize health problems and seek appropriate care, and follow recommendations for care. The educational level of older adult clients also affects the nurse-client health teaching process and so is an important consideration in health promotion and disease prevention (see Chapter 8).

Income and Poverty

The median income of older adults in 1996 was $17,768 for older men and $10,062 for older women. After adjusting for inflation, these figures actually represented an increase in real income from 1996 of 4.2% for men and 2.2% for women. For all older persons reporting income in 1997, which was 31.4 million persons, 37% reported less than $10,000 and only 21% reported $25,000 or more. The median income reported was $13,049. The major source of income for older individuals and couples in 1996 was Social Security (reported by 91% of older persons), a plan that was originally developed to be a supplemental source of income in old age. Other income sources in order of rank were income from assets (reported by 63%), public and private pensions (reported by 41%), earnings (reported by 21%), and public assistance (reported by 6%) (AARP, 1998).

Family households headed by persons 65 years of age and older had a median income in 1997 of $30,660. Nonwhites continue to have substantially lower incomes than their white counterparts. Blacks had a median income of $23,420 and Hispanics $22,677, whereas whites had a median income of $31,167. Fourteen percent of all family households headed by an older adult had annual median incomes of less than $15,000; 42% had incomes of $35,000 or more (Fig. 1-3).

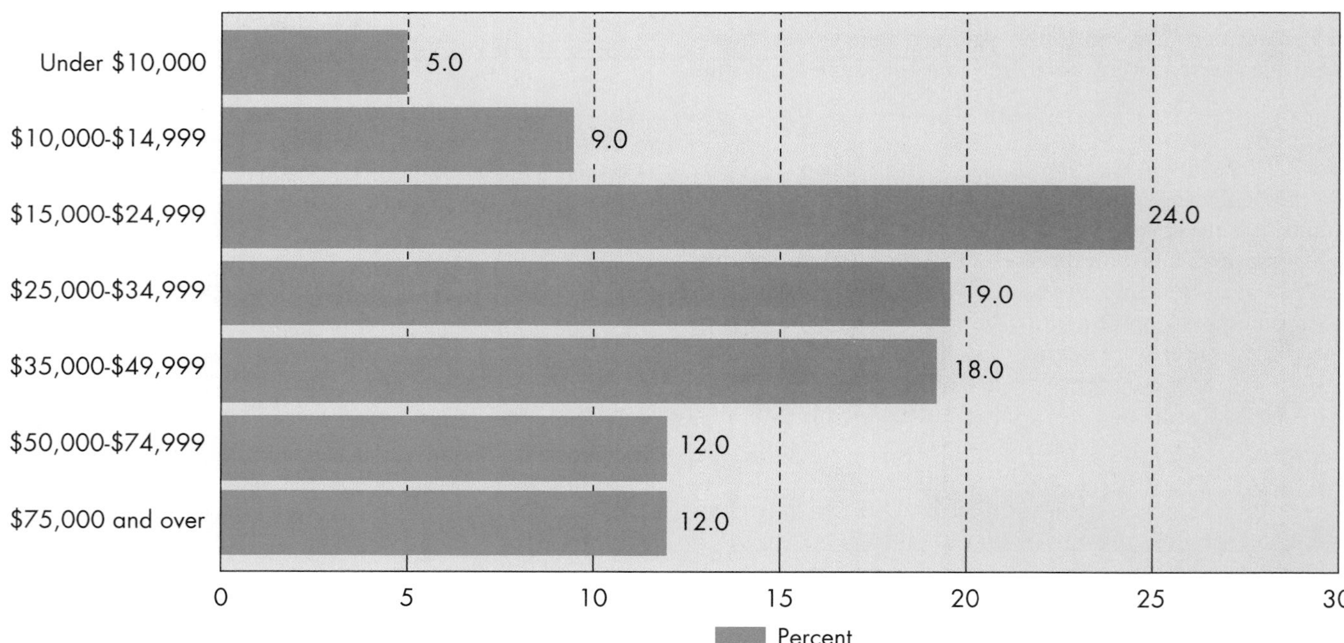

Fig. 1-3 Percentage distribution by income in households headed by persons 65 and older: 1997. (From American Association of Retired Persons: *A profile of older Americans: 1998*, Washington, DC, 1998, The Association.)

Approximately 3.4 million older adults were below the poverty level in 1997. Of note in this report is that the poverty rate for persons 65 years of age and older (10.5%) was *less* than the rate for persons 18 to 64 years of age (10.9%). Another 2.1 million older persons were classified as *near poor,* with incomes between the poverty level and 125% of the level. However, in 1997, 17% of the total older, noninstitutionalized population was poor or near poor (AARP, 1998).

Gender and race are significant indicators of poverty. Older women had a poverty rate nearly twice as high as older men in 1997. Only 9% of older whites were poor in 1997, compared with 26% of older blacks and 23.8% of older Hispanics.

The most important factors in the relationship between income and health are the lifestyle changes imposed by reduced or dwindling financial resources. Persons unable to meet their basic needs typically reduce the amount of or avoid spending any health-related dollars.

Employment

About 3.9 million older adults (12%) were classified as labor force participants (employed or actively seeking employment) in 1997, of which 17% were men and 9% women. In 1997 a little more than half of the workers 65 years of age and older worked part-time. In this same year, approximately 18% of older workers were self-employed, a rate 3 times as great as their younger counterparts. Nearly two thirds of older, self-employed workers were men. The labor force participation of older men has remained fairly constant since 1900, with only minor increases and decreases. The rate in 1996 was approximately 17%. The number of older women in the labor force was steady from 1900 to the 1950s, at which time the rate was 10.8% of the total labor force. A slight decrease occurred in 1985 to 7.3%, but it has been approximately 8% to 9% since 1988 (AARP, 1998).

HEALTH STATUS OF OLDER ADULTS

Before beginning a discussion of the health status of older adults, it is necessary to offer some words of caution: old age is *not* synonymous with disease. Although selected portions of this text address disease and disability in old age by emphasizing the provision of age-appropriate nursing care of persons with various conditions, the implication is not that disease is a normal, expected outcome of aging. Clearly, the risk of health problems and disability increases with age, but older adults are not necessarily incapacitated by these problems. They may have multiple, complex health problems resulting in sickness and institutionalization, but the nurse should not consider this the norm for this population.

Because of this high concentration of morbidity and frequent use of health services by certain high-risk groups of older adults, delivery systems are now being forced to more effectively manage resources. Strategies to maximize health and prevent disease in older persons are being incorporated into the emerging health care insurance plans. Incentives are prompting the development of innovative programs and services of care that improve outcomes and lower costs for healthy and chronically ill older adults. Such proactive developments hold much promise for the future care of older populations and provide opportunities to redefine gerontologic nursing practice. The notion of incorporating an expectation of wellness, even when treating those who have chronic disease and functional impairment, is one that can truly reshape the care of older adults. Accordingly, nurses are advised to remember that even older persons with disease, disability, or both may be considered healthy and well to some degree on the health-illness continuum. In fact, most older adults tend to already view their personal health positively, despite the presence of chronic illness, disease, and impairment.

Self-Assessed Health and Chronic Disease

In 1995, 28.3% of older persons assessed their own health as fair or poor, whereas nearly 72% rated it as excellent or good (AARP, 1998). More older blacks than older whites rated their health as fair or poor. Little difference between the genders was found. The proportion of adults reporting fair to poor health generally tends to increase with advancing age (Cohen and Van Nostrand, 1995).

More than 80% of persons older than 65 years of age are estimated to have at least one chronic condition, and many have multiple conditions. The most common conditions per 100 noninstitutionalized older adults in 1994 were arthritis (50), hypertension (36), heart disease (32), hearing impairments (29), cataracts (17), orthopedic impairments (16), sinusitis (15), and diabetes (10). The three leading causes of death for older persons in 1990 (in order) were heart conditions, malignant neoplasms, and cerebrovascular diseases (US Bureau of the Census, 1995b). Although death rates from heart disease have decreased for older adults since 1960, it remains the leading cause of death for this group. In contrast, death rates from cancer have increased since 1960.

Functional Status

The degree of functional ability is of greater concern to older adults and nurses than the incidence and prevalence of chronic disease. *Functional ability* is defined as the capacity to carry out the basic self-care activities that ensure overall health and well-being. Functional ability is classified in many measurement tools by activities of daily living (ADLs), such as bathing, dressing, eating, transferring, and toileting (Katz, 1963), and instrumental activities of daily living (IADLs), which include home-management activities such as shopping, cooking, housekeeping, laundry, and handling money (Lawton and Brody, 1969). The use of such measurement tools or scales to determine the effect of chronic disease and normal aging on physical, psychologic, and social function provides objective information about a person's overall degree of health. Assessment of the impact of chronic disease and age-related decreases in functional status enables the nurse to determine needs, plan interventions, and evaluate outcomes. Chronic disease and disability can impair physical and emotional health, self-care ability, and independence. Improving the health and functional status of older adults and preventing complications of chronic disease and disability may avert the onset of physical frailty and cognitive impairment, two conditions that increase the likelihood of institutionalization.

In 1994 to 1995, more than half of the older adult population (52.5%) reported having at least one disability that limited them in carrying out ADLs and IADLs; one third had a severe disability. The same year, it was estimated that more than 5 million older adults needed assistance of some type with ADLs (AARP, 1998). The number needing help increased sharply with advancing age, with those in the 85 and older group needing the most assistance (US Bureau of the Census, 1995a). For this same reporting period, more than 4.4 million (14%) had difficulty in carrying out ADLs, and 6.5 million (21%) reported difficulties with IADLs. In addition, the number of days in which usual activities were restricted because of illness or injury increased with age. Given the growth projections for older persons in the coming decades, the clear mandate is to transform the current care institutions into models of care delivery that are based on consumer characteristics, care needs, and environmental requirements (Kane, 1995-1996).

Health Care Expenditure and Use

The federal government funds the majority of health care in the United States for persons ages 65 and over. In 1995 33.1 million persons ages 65 and over were enrolled in Medicare; slightly more than 80% received health and medical services, with an average annual payment of $15,074 (excluding HMO enrollees). In the same year, more than 11 million older persons received services under the Medicaid program, with an average vendor payment for those 65 and over of $8868 (AARP, 1998).

In 1995 older persons accounted for 40% of all hospital stays and 49% of all days of care in hospitals. The average length of stay was 7.1 days for persons 65 and over, compared to 5.4 days for those under age 65. Contacts with doctors in 1995 for older persons averaged 11.1, versus 5 contacts for those under age 65 (AARP, 1998).

Managed care as another system of care for older adults is becoming more commonplace. By 1998, 346 Medicare risk contracts has been established nationwide, with 33 pending approval. In addition, slightly more than 6 million people were enrolled in Medicare health plans operated under these risk contracts through the Health Care Financing Administration (HCFA), at a cost of slightly more than $747 million per month (HCFA, 1999). The rapid escalation in enrollments in these plans is expected to continue for the next several years, promising to place Medicare managed care at the heart of continuing health care reform. In addition, several states are currently developing managed care structures for their Medicaid population.

Per capita public sector health-spending growth is expected to decelerate until 2002, primarily as a result of the Balanced Budget Act (BBA) of 1997 and its effect on Medicare (*Highlights of the National Health Care Expenditure Projections, 1997-2002,* 1999). The introduction of prospective payment systems, such as those just discussed, coupled with cutbacks in payment formulas, is expected to slow the rate of increase in Medicare expenditures. However, the growth in Medicare managed care enrollment is not expected to decrease the growth in overall Medicare spending.

The projected increases in the older adult population coupled with the current national concern about rising costs of government programs and health care will continue to force American leaders and policy makers to make tough decisions. The question of whether health care reform will meet the needs of older adults remains largely unanswered. For example, a major concern is whether Medicare managed care organizations, with their established incentives, are adequately serving their older enrollees. As the debate over these and other issues continues, nurses can expect to face numerous different dilemmas surrounding the delivery of health care to older persons.

Implications for Health Care Delivery

Although the future direction of health care is uncertain, it can confidently be surmised from the demographic profile that nurses in a wide variety of settings and roles will be challenged to provide care to an increasingly divergent, complex group of older persons. An urgent need exists for gerontologic nurses to (1) create roles that meet the needs of the older population across the continuum of care; (2) develop models of care delivery directed at all levels of prevention, with special emphasis on primary prevention and health promotion services in community-based settings; and (3) assume positions of leadership and influence not only in institutions and settings where care is currently provided to older persons but also in the political arena. The overriding fact to remember is that the majority of problems experienced by older adults fall within the scope of *nursing* practice.

The following descriptions of select settings of care are not intended to be inclusive. Rather, they represent the settings where the majority of older adult care is provided today (see Chapter 9).

Acute Care Setting

The time when the hospital was the hub of the health care delivery system has clearly passed. Political climate, market forces, technologic advances, and economics are a few of the major external forces that have brought about the significant changes seen in recent years in this traditional care setting. Although the shift is away from the acute care setting toward a wide array of community-based alternatives, a segment of the older adult population will continue to need care in a hospital setting. Acute conditions such as strokes, hip fractures, congestive heart failure, and infections are common in older adults and still treated in the hospital, as are critical medical and surgical health problems. However, few acute care hospitals adequately manage the care of their older adult clients by preventing functional decline and promoting independence, which is why the hospital setting continues to be one of the most dangerous for older persons.

In recent years, innovative hospital-based programs aimed at preventing functional decline and improving outcomes for older hospitalized clients have been developed and implemented. Progressive hospital organizations realize that their older clients are at higher risk for functional decline and adverse outcomes, and those economically viable mechanisms can be put into play to prevent such decline. Boult, Boult, and Pacala (1998) described various systems of care implemented by futuristic health care organizations that have shown promise in improving outcomes and reducing the costs of care of high-risk older adults. One such development is an acute care for elders (ACE) unit, which is a dedicated, physical unit within the hospital designed with special attention to the physical environment. An interdisciplinary team of gerontologic experts coordinates the care and uses client-centered protocols that focus on rehabilitation and prevention of prevalent problems such as delirium, immobility and falls, and urinary incontinence. Studies have documented the potential for such units to reduce functional decline with no additional costs to the hospital (Covinski et al, 1997; Landefeld et al, 1995; Palmer et al, 1994).

Subacute care units are another innovation aimed at the high-risk hospitalized older population. Such units typically provide interventions to eliminate or shorten the expensive hospital stays that are known to be so potentially hazardous for older adults. These units can be in freestanding facilities, be hospital-based, or located in a traditional nursing or rehabilitation facility that has upgraded the physical unit as well as the staff providing the care. The units provide such treatments as chemotherapy, wound care, intravenous therapy, and ventilator care. Studies reporting on the outcomes of subacute care are few and have limited generalizability, so additional studies of the processes and outcomes of care in subacute units are needed (Boult, Boult, and Pacala, 1998).

Case management is another intervention method that can reduce functional decline for high-risk hospitalized older adults. It, too, needs additional study to determine its effect on cost outcomes. Case management is typically provided for managed care enrollees and can include various different services. Data related to this form of intervention are largely anecdotal, but studies are underway to determine the effects of various case management strategies (Boult, Boult, and Pacala, 1998).

These interventions show promise, but additional data on cost effectiveness and outcomes are needed to make decisions about large-scale implementation. Regardless, the growing capitated Medicare market is forcing hospital organizations that are bearing the financial risk of caring for their enrollees to do something now. Incentives are in place for promoting good health and preventing illness and disease. Therefore exploring the *long-term* viability of these and other equally innovative initiatives is crucial.

Nurses in the acute care work force of today need to recognize immediately that because they are caring for a frail, high-risk older adult population, they should quickly acquire the necessary knowledge and skills for delivering timely, age-appropriate care—knowledge that includes (1) an understanding of normal aging and abnormal aging; (2) strong assessment skills to detect subtle changes that indicate impending, serious problems; (3) excellent communication skills for interacting with not only well older persons but also those with delirium, dementia, and depression; (4) a keen understanding of rehabilitation principles as they apply to the maintenance and promotion of functional ability in older adults; and (5) sensitivity and patience so that older adults are treated with dignity and respect. It is imperative for acute care nurses to incorporate this knowledge and these skills into their daily practice with older adult clients, because future hospitalized older adults will likely be even more frail than they are today.

Nursing Facilities

As discussed, the emphasis on reducing costs in the hospital setting through more rapid discharge has led to the shift of more acutely ill residents to nursing facilities, which are traditionally referred to as *nursing homes* or *long-term care facilities.* Unfortunately some of these facilities do not have an adequate number of qualified, professional nursing staff members to provide the complex care these residents require, or the staff does not have up-to-date knowledge and skills. In addition, the nursing staff mix may not be sufficient to meet the needs of this more acutely ill population. Finally, the physical environment and systems for delivering care in the traditional nursing facility may not be the most appropriate for meeting the needs of this more ill, more unstable population.

The increasing size of the over-85 segment of the population, members of which have decreased functional abilities, represents the group typically found in nursing facilities. Their care needs, coupled with those of the more acutely ill residents who are increasingly being placed in nursing facilities, have already placed greater demands on many of these institutions. In the immediate future, these forces promise to continue putting pressure on nursing facilities. Economics, particularly as driven by health care reform, will determine the future of these institutions.

In 1982 the Teaching Nursing Home Project (TNHP) was initiated with funding provided by the Robert Wood Johnson

Foundation and the American Academy of Nursing. This demonstration project consisted of affiliations between 11 university schools of nursing and 12 nursing facilities from across the country and was established to develop models of gerontologic nursing care delivery in nursing facilities that combined practice, education, and research. This landmark endeavor exemplifies the kind of creative activity needed to improve the long-term care of older adults and the education and training of nursing staff members in such facilities. Future efforts building on the findings of this initiative must continue to ensure the presence of nursing or long-term facilities that provide quality nursing care that meets the needs of the population being served. See the textbook *Teaching Nursing Homes: The Nursing Perspective* (1988), edited by Small and Walsh, for a complete report of this historic project.

In a 1998 article, Burggraf and Barry explored the future of gerontologic nursing and presented the visionary thinking of noted gerontologic nurses. The authors identified a decrease in the nursing facility or nursing home as it exists today. They noted that subacute care facilities were becoming more the norm than the traditional nursing home. In addition, numbers of special care units and centers are growing in response to the increase in *old-old* individuals, who are more likely to have dementia and other cognitive impairments. Specially designed environments that are tailored to maximize function and orientation, minimize environmental demand, and keep the individuals safe are generally much more appropriate than the traditional nursing home. Kane (1995-1996) noted that it is "urgent that typical long-term-care institutions be transformed into livable habitats for persons who relocate to them." The authors argue for a change from the "one-size-fits-all" environment, which currently places together older adults who are terminally ill, convalescing, comatose, rehabilitating, chronically physically impaired, and chronically cognitively impaired, to one that is more homelike and residential. The challenge, the authors note, is in devising a configuration that would allow older adults with the conditions identified to be treated—but in a residential setting.

Until such changes occur, nurses practicing in nursing facilities need to gain new knowledge and skills to care for the more acutely ill resident who, at least for the near future, will continue to be placed in these facilities. In some cases, the overall caliber of nurses needs to be better. Directors of nursing must alter environmental design elements and systems to accommodate this type of resident and support the safe delivery of nursing care. Innovative models of care delivery that go beyond the task approach are needed to improve the quality of care. An even stronger focus is needed on promoting the functional status of the resident, as is an emphasis on prevention and health promotion, to ensure that dependency is minimized and functional ability maximized.

As the role of the advanced practice nurse continues to take shape, opportunities for implementing various models of service delivery to nursing facility residents are growing. For example, GNPs are serving as case managers and coordinators of care in this setting. GNPs are also providing primary care services to residents, demonstrating the delivery of high-quality health care in nursing facilities (Burl et al, 1998; Fama and Fox, 1997). CNSs are providing staff education and training and serving as consultants to the nursing staff in assessing and planning nursing care for complex residents. Significant gains have been made in the quality of nursing facility resident care as a result of economic and legislative reforms that have allowed nurses to practice in these innovative ways. Although momentum is gaining, these advanced practice nurses are challenged to continue to serve as leaders in promoting continued reform and advocating higher standards of care.

Home Care

In 1995, about 4% of the population ages 65 and over resided in nursing facilities (AARP, 1998). The need for such institutional care will always exist for a small segment of the population, but most older persons need services that restore their health while allowing them to maintain their independence in their community. The desire and preference of most older persons to stay in their own homes for as long as possible is a major driving force influencing the need for increasing home care services. Additional factors are the recent economic, governmental, and technologic developments that have led to sicker clients going home from the hospital sooner, with needs for high-tech care and complex equipment (Potter, Perry, 2004).

Older home care clients have multiple, complex problems. In addition to possessing the knowledge and skills previously noted, home care nurses must be self-directed and capable of functioning with a multidisciplinary team that is widely dispersed throughout the community. Keen clinical judgment skills are essential, because the home care nurse is often called on to make decisions about whether clients should be referred to a physician. In addition to physical and psychosocial assessments, the home care nurse is responsible for determining older clients' functional status. Assessment of home safety considerations and family dynamics, knowledge and use of community resources, environmental factors, and knowledge of the treated conditions and lifestyle implications are also included. Excellent coordination and collaboration skills are necessary, because it is the home care nurse who is the primary resource of older clients and calls in other resources as warranted. Finally, a genuine respect for older clients' desires and rights to live at home is key.

Nurses caring for homebound older adults need to become increasingly more involved in conducting community assessments that focus specifically on the aged population. The data obtained from this type of assessment can be used to plan age-specific programs and services aimed at all levels of prevention but specifically at refinement of health screening, health promotion, and health maintenance activities. Linking these activities to community-based programs and organizations already used by older persons is a logical place to begin.

Community-based clinics that are operated and served by nurses are becoming more prevalent as the movement toward keeping frail and impaired older persons at home gains momentum. The four pilot community nursing organizations (CNOs) were established in 1994 as part of a demonstration project funded by HCFA to test nurse-managed models of care for Medicare recipients in community-based, ambulatory settings, and they are an example of how nurse-managed care can benefit older clients (Burtt, 1998). The models are all capitated plans that provide Medicare benefits such as home heath care, durable medical equipment, ambulance services, and outpatient therapies. They focus on health promotion and disease prevention while minimizing the need for hospitalization. The early successes demonstrated by the four models have resulted in Congress reauthorizing the project for an additional 2 years. With such success, coupled with continuing health care reform, even greater emphasis can be expected to be placed on the development of these types of models.

Continuum of Care

President Bill Clinton introduced the American Health Security Act in 1993. This proposed blueprint for health care reform was as sweeping a social change as the introduction of Social Security in 1935. The recommendations for change were massive and complex, and it ultimately failed to gain bipartisan support, but this proposed threat of change ultimately resulted in forcing the health care industry to begin making massive changes on its own. One of those changes, the organized health care of older persons, is one of the fastest growing aspects of health care reform. The increasing penetration into the Medicare market by managed care organizations presents many opportunities while simultaneously fueling debate over whether older adults will receive high-quality, comprehensive, coordinated, cost-effective, outcome-oriented care.

The shift from acute care, hospital-based organizations to fully integrated health systems has resulted in a highly competitive and intricate system of care. HMOs, preferred provider organizations (PPOs), provider service organizations (PSOs), and independent practice associations (IPAs) are just a few of the managed care systems that have arrived on the scene, and all indications are that they will continue to proliferate. More health care is being delivered on an ambulatory basis, a trend that is well established and likely to continue. With this shift to community-based care, greater emphasis is being placed on health promotion and disease prevention, with the goals of achieving maximum health and independence. Gerontologic nurses must advocate for *all* older persons along the continuum of care, promoting interventions that result in their highest level of wellness, functionality, and independence.

Continuing efforts to restructure the health care system for the older adult population must take into account the widely ranging levels of care needed by this group. The health care network that evolves for this population must integrate programs into coordinated systems of care that allow for ease of movement along the continuum. As eloquently stated by Ebersole and Hess in 1990, "Fragmented or superficial care is particularly dangerous to the elderly. Their functions become more and more interdependent as they age. A small disturbance is like a pebble in a still lake. The ripples extend outward in all directions." The future is uncertain, but older adults and their caregivers are anxiously awaiting the new choices that will be presented in hopes of more effectively meeting the needs of a growing and demographically changing population.

IMPACT OF AN AGING ADULT POPULATION ON GERONTOLOGIC NURSING

In view of the demographic projections presented previously in this chapter and the development of gerontologic nursing as a legitimate specialty, the current challenges are to (1) solidify the specialty as a major force within the health care arena, and (2) participate in the development of an appropriate health care delivery framework for older adults that considers their unique needs. Now is the time for all gerontologic nurses to create a new vision for practice, education, and research.

Ageism

Ageism is a term that was coined by Butler in 1969 to describe the deep and profound prejudice in American society against older adults. "Ageism reflects a deep-seated uneasiness on the part of young and middle-aged—a personal revulsion and distaste for growing old, disease, disability; and fear of powerlessness, 'uselessness,' and death." In a society that highly values youth and vitality, it is no surprise that ageism exists. Butler also likens ageism to bigotry: "Ageism can be seen as a process of systematic stereotyping of and discrimination against people because they are old, just as racism and sexism accomplishes this with skin color and gender. Ageism allows the younger generation to see older persons as different from themselves; thus they subtly cease to identify with their elders as human beings" (Butler, 1977).

Butler (1993) also discusses the development of a "new ageism" in recent years because of forces such as the economic gains of older adults, their increasing vigor and productivity, and their growing political influence. He added that for these and even more subtle reasons, the older population is considered a threat by many who fear their ever-increasing numbers will only further drain financial resources, slow economic growth, and create intergenerational conflict. Some of the suggestions Butler proposes to fight this "new ageism" (1993) include building coalitions among advocates of all agegroups; recognizing that older persons themselves are an economic market and developing ways to capitalize on it;

investing in biomedical, behavioral, and social research as a way to eliminate many of the costly chronic conditions of old age and strengthen social networks; and fostering the development of a healthy philosophy on aging. A sense of hope, pride, confidence, security, and integrity can greatly enhance the quality of life for older adults. Persons of *all* ages are stakeholders in developing strategies and solutions to this end. Only then will we be able to eliminate the negative attitudes and discriminatory practices that harm us all.

Unfortunately, the nursing profession is not immune to ageism. Because generally negative attitudes about older people are held by society at large—and nurses are members of society—it follows that nurses may have ageist views. Studies have found such attitudes among nursing recruits, a finding that has significant implications for practice, education, and research.

Nursing Practice

Gerontologic nursing practice is evolving as new issues concerning the health care delivery system in general and the health of older adults in particular demand attention. The continuing movement of health care away from acute care hospitals, economics as a driving force in health care delivery, the growth of managed care, the changing role of the registered nurse, and the use of unlicensed assistive personnel (UAPs) are some of the prominent health care industry trends that have implications for the future of nursing, especially for gerontologic nursing (Burggraf and Barry, 1998; Huston and Fox, 1998). In addition, today's older adult health care consumers are more knowledgeable and discerning and thus are better informed as they become more active decision-makers about their health and well-being. Because they have greater financial resources than they have had in the past, older adult consumers are able to exercise more options in all aspects of their daily lives.

As more care shifts from hospitals to ambulatory or community-based sites, older adults are demanding more programs and services aimed at (1) health maintenance and promotion and (2) disease and disability prevention. Gerontologic nurses will play an integral role in effecting these changes in the various emerging practice arenas. They will practice in clinics, the home care environment, and older adult living communities that range from independent homes to rehabilitation centers. Already, parish nurses are providing a wide range of services to older adults living in their service areas; this type of nursing practice is likely to continue to expand. Gerontologic nurses are also working as case managers in various practice sites, including hospitals and community-based ambulatory settings. As managed care grows, so will the opportunities associated with gerontologic nursing practice.

Some advanced practice gerontologic nurses are currently practicing independently in some areas, others work with a collaborating physician in a primary care office setting, and still others work in urgent care centers. Nurse-managed care is already found in many areas (Burtt, 1998; Lardner, 1998). Although practices such as these may soon become more common, gerontologic nurses must continue to educate older persons about their care options and lobby for legislation at the state and federal levels for expansion of reimbursement opportunities for advanced practice nurses who care for older adults.

In light of the increasing number of older adults requiring functional assistance to remain at home, in semiindependent living sites, or in other alternative settings, gerontologic nurses need to be vigilant as more care functions normally performed by RNs are transferred to UAPs. It is unclear whether the use of UAPs is a viable solution for providing safe, high-quality, cost-conscious care to the older population in *any* setting. However, with appropriate education and training, it may be possible to use UAPs in select situations. For this to be successful, nurses need to take a greater role in the education of such personnel within an appropriate practice framework and ensure that they meet established competency criteria. This would be an ideal role for a gerontologic nurse consultant, because it would encompass advocacy, education, and a standard setting.

Additional skills required by nurses to support home care of older adults and care through community-based services include the ability to teach families and other caregivers about safe and effective caregiving techniques, as well as about services and resources available. Because many of these older clients have varying degrees of functional impairment, nurses must have a comprehensive knowledge of functional assessment as well as intervention and management strategies from a rehabilitative perspective. Lifestyle counseling skills will also be needed by gerontologic nurses as the emphasis on health promotion and disease prevention grows and older persons assume more responsibility for their health. Most gerontologic nurses have had little experience with education and counseling related to preretirement planning, but they would be extremely helpful skills for assisting older adults. Gerontologic nurses could provide anticipatory guidance for the multiple possible psychologic reactions to such a relevant life experience as retirement.

Despite the aforementioned trends, the traditional medical model of care in the acute care setting and the nursing facility that focuses on the treatment of illness and disease continues to endure. However, older adults seldom seek care for a single symptom or disorder. Furthermore, even if older adults do have individual problems, they are likely to be intertwined with other variables. Consequently, future models of care must give greater consideration to the impact of many intervening variables on the health status of older adults. The psychologic, social, and financial needs must be considered commensurate with the presenting physical needs. The ability to comprehensively assess all of these areas will require the nurse to possess refined and highly discriminating assessment skills. This will become increasingly more important as nurses take on more responsibility for the care and treatment of older adults in all settings. Equally important will be the development of coordination and collaboration skills, communication and human relations skills, and the ability to influence others, because future practice models and sites will likely reflect a true team approach to older adult care.

Nursing Education

The need for adequately prepared nurses to care for the growing population of older adults continues to intensify. According to Alford (1987), between 1980 and 2030 the estimated number of RNs needed to care for older adults will increase by 466%. These figures, coupled with demographic forecasts, should prompt nursing faculty members to stop viewing gerontologic nursing content as a luxury and start considering it a necessary component of the curriculum.

The pioneering work of Gunter and Estes (1979) defined an educational program specific to five levels of nursing: nursing assistant/technician, licensed practical/vocational nurse, RN, graduate education at the master's degree level, and graduate education at the doctoral level. Although no reports in the nursing literature describe the use of this framework for curriculum development, this work has been an invaluable reference for nurse educators and in-service education staff members in various settings, because it is the first attempt to provide a conceptual framework, delineation, and definition for the specialty. Since the publication of this work, the published literature has cited some agreement among nurse educators as to what constitutes essential gerontologic content in the baccalaureate program. Through the Community College–Nursing Home Partnership Project, ideas about essential gerontologic nursing content in the associate degree program have been offered (Waters, 1991). However, despite the many recommendations that have been made, unanimous agreement as to what constituted *core* gerontologic nursing content at any level of nursing education did not exist until 1996, when the first edition of the *NGNA Core Curriculum for Gerontological Nursing* (Luggen, 1996) was published; the second edition was published in 2002 by Luggen and Meiner. These texts were developed in conjunction with the National Gerontological Nursing Association and were originally conceived as a tool to prepare candidates for the American Nurses Credentialing Center (ANCC) Certification Examination for the Gerontologic Nurse. Gerontologic nursing educational programs in colleges, universities, and nursing schools would do well to use the current text as a content outline for development of their programs.

One issue related to gerontologic nursing curriculum development is the preparation and expertise of the nurse faculty members who are leading the programs. A study conducted by Edel (1986) to determine the gerontologic nursing educational preparation of faculty members in baccalaureate nursing programs accredited by the National League for Nursing revealed a paucity of adequately prepared faculty members; only 4.41% of 4762 faculty members had completed course work in gerontology or gerontologic nursing. Findings of a recent study conducted by Yurchuck and Brower (1994) indicated that only 12% of faculty members have gerontologic nursing preparation; only 5% have master's preparation in gerontology/gerontologic nursing. The survey sample consisted of 211 undergraduate associate and baccalaureate nursing programs in the 15-state Southern Regional Education Board (SREB). Of the programs, 128 (61%) were associate degree programs, and 83 (39%) represented baccalaureate programs. If the number of gerontologic nursing–prepared faculty members continues to be limited, curriculum development, appropriate clinical site selection with faculty role models, student interest in the specialty, and research will continue to be hindered (Yurchuck and Brower, 1994). Related issues often cited in the literature that adversely influence the inclusion of gerontologic nursing content in the curriculum are found in Box 1-2.

The American Association of Colleges of Nursing (AACN) developed a position statement in 1993, *Nursing Education's Agenda for the 21st Century,* that "delineates a suggested role for nursing education in the context of *Nursing's Agenda for Health Care Reform,* the goals of *Healthy People 2000 & 2010,* and evolutions in health care delivery." The statement challenges nurse educators to anticipate and prepare for the changes indicated in the described documents (both of which address issues related to the care of older persons) and educate their students at the baccalaureate, master's, and doctoral levels for this new environment. In addition, the position statement identifies the need for curricular content that prepares nurses for roles in future health care systems, which includes acute care *and* health promotion and maintenance in relation to chronic conditions and older adult health. In terms of program evaluation and outcomes, the statement maintains that to meet the challenges set forth by

BOX 1-2 Issues Contributing to the Lack of Inclusion of Gerontologic Nursing Content in Nursing Curricula

- Reluctance to recognize gerontologic nursing as a legitimate academic and practice specialty
- Perceived low status compared with other areas of nursing practice
- Lack of adequate academic preparation of nurse faculty members in gerontologic nursing
- Questionable clinical competence of nongerontologic-prepared nurse faculty members
- Ageist attitudes of nongerontologic-prepared nurse faculty members
- Little consensus regarding gerontologic nursing content on NCLEX-RN
- Lack of requirement of a gerontologic nursing textbook

these documents and the evolutions in health care, "nursing curricula, instructional strategies, and clinical practice models should respond to major trends in health care." Nurse educators must develop clinical practice sites for students, outside the comfort of the institutional setting, that reflect the emerging trends of community-based care with a focus on health promotion, disease prevention, and the preservation of functional abilities. Nurse faculty members with formal preparation in the field of gerontologic nursing are imperative if students are to be adequately prepared to meet the needs of the projected older adult population. According to Morrissey (1995), nurse faculty members "need to get their heads out of the sand and accept the demographic reality of an aging population."

Assuring nursing students that they will be sufficiently prepared to practice in the future—a future that will undeniably include the care of older adults in a wide variety of settings—necessitates answering many questions concerning nursing education. The primary issue is not whether to include gerontologic nursing content but the extent of its inclusion. Until a sufficient number of nurse faculty members are prepared in the specialty, this question will remain unanswered, and students will continue to be inadequately prepared for the future of nursing.

Nursing Research

From 1967 to 1989 a total of nine reviews of gerontologic nursing research were found in the literature: Basson (1967), Gunter and Miller (1977), Brimmer (1979), Kayser-Jones (1981), Robinson (1981), Wolanin (1983), Burnside (1985), Cora and Lapierre (1986), and Haight (1989). Refer to each original source for a detailed discussion of the contents of the review and its findings. Although the methods of review were different, some similarities in the findings have implications for a future agenda for gerontologic nursing research.

Common conclusions of the reviews were that the studies had (1) an inconsistent or a lack of a theoretic or conceptual framework, (2) a lack of longitudinal and descriptive studies, (3) few replication studies, (4) imprecise descriptions of the age of subjects, (5) a primary focus on institutionalized older persons, (6) a high degree of interest in psychosocial-related issues, (7) a fair number of attitude studies, and (8) a lack of focus on clinical problems or outcomes of care. In recent years, more scientific studies have reported on clinical problems such as acute confusion, incontinence, restraint use, pressure ulcers, and falls. More studies such as these are needed to provide a broader database of information and generate new knowledge so that solutions can be found to the ongoing clinical problems of older persons. The specialty of gerontologic nursing still needs additional scientific knowledge for practice, and doctorally prepared nurses are needed to conduct this research. Both are urgently needed for the rapidly growing population of older adults to receive adequate nursing care.

The leading gerontologic nursing research questions for the future should be framed within larger issues such as client-centered outcomes, health promotion and maintenance, prevention of disease and disability, and early detection of disease and illness—all within traditional and alternative health care delivery systems. Knowledge built through research is imperative for the development of a safe and sound knowledge base that guides clinical practice, as well as for the promotion of the specialty.

SUMMARY

Despite the slow progress that has been made, nursing care of older adults is now recognized as a legitimate specialty. The important groundwork that has been laid now serves as the basis from which the specialty will forge into the future. Gerontologic nurses at all levels of educational preparation and in all settings of care must now venture into that future with creativity, pride, and determination as they meet their professional responsibility of providing quality care to older persons everywhere. Now is the time to seize the opportunity to advance gerontologic nursing practice, education, and research for the benefit of the older adult population—a population that continues to grow.

Key Points

- The growth of the nursing profession as a whole, increasing educational opportunities, demographic changes, and changes in health care delivery systems have all influenced the development of various gerontologic nursing roles.
- "Ages 65 and older" is widely accepted and used for reporting demographic statistics about older persons; however, turning 65 does not automatically mean a person is "old."
- The nurse is cautioned against thinking of all older persons as similar, despite the fact that most demographic data place all persons over age 65 into a single reporting group.
- Persons 65 years of age and older currently represent about 13% of the total population.
- The most rapid and dramatic growth for the older adult segment of the total U.S. population will occur between the years 2010 and 2030, when the "baby boom" generation reaches 65 years of age.
- Based on 1997 data, four times as many widows as widowers live in the United States.
- About 5% of persons over age 65 reside in nursing facilities, but the percentage increases dramatically with advancing age.
- More than half of all persons over age 65 live in only nine states: California, Florida, New York, Pennsylvania, Texas, Illinois, Ohio, Michigan, and New Jersey.
- Gender and race are significant indicators of poverty; older women have a poverty rate twice as high as older men, and a significantly higher percentage of blacks and Hispanics are poor than are whites.

- Estimates indicate that more than 80% of persons over 65 years of age have one or more chronic health conditions.
- The three leading causes of death for older persons, in order, are heart conditions, malignant neoplasms, and cerebrovascular diseases.
- Nurses in a wide variety of settings and roles are challenged to provide age-appropriate and age-specific care based on a comprehensive and scientific knowledge base.
- Ageism is prejudice against the old just because they are old.
- Gerontologic nursing content should be included in all basic nursing education programs.

Critical Thinking Exercises

1. Care of the older person today is considerably different than it was 50 years ago. Cite examples of how and why the care of older persons is different today than it was in the past.
2. When reporting for work, you note that you have been assigned to two 72-year-old women for the evening. Is it safe to assume that the care of these two women will be similar because they are the same age? Why or why not? How would their care be enhanced or be compromised if they were treated similarly?
3. As a student, you are often assigned to care for older persons. At what point in your education do you feel care of the older person should be included? Early in, later in, or throughout your nursing program? Support your position.

References

Alford D: Gerontological nursing: trends and transitions. In Pettengill MM, ed: *Society in transition: impact on nursing.* Proceedings of the eighth annual meeting and program, Midwest Alliance in Nursing, St Louis, Mo, Indianapolis, 1987, Midwest Alliance in Nursing.

American Association of Colleges of Nursing: *Position statement: nursing education's agenda for the 21st century,* Washington, DC, 1993, The Association.

American Association of Retired Persons: *Images of aging in America 2004: summary information,* Washington, DC, 2004, The Association.

American Association of Retired Persons: *A profile of older Americans: 1998,* Washington, DC, 1998, The Association.

American Association of Retired Persons: *A profile of older Americans: 1997,* Washington, DC, 1997, The Association.

American Nurses Association: *Nursing: scope & standards of practice,* Washington, DC, 2004, The Association.

American Nurses Association: *Nursing's social policy statement,* ed 2, Washington, DC, 2003, The Association.

American Nurses Association: *Code of ethics for nurses with interpretive statements,* Washington, DC, 2001, The Association.

American Nurses Association: *Scope and standards of gerontological nursing practice,* Washington, DC, 1995, The Association.

American Nurses Association: Nursing practice standards and guidelines, *Oasis: Council on Gerontological Nursing Practice* 8(4):2, 1991.

American Nurses Credentialing Center: *ANCC certification catalogue: 2004,* Washington, DC, 2004, The Center.

Basson P: The gerontological nursing literature search: study and results, *Nurs Res* 16:267-272, 1967.

Boult C, Boult L, Pacala JT: Systems of care for older populations of the future, *J Am Geriatr Soc* 46(4):499-505, 1998.

Brimmer P: The past, present and future in gerontological nursing research, *J Gerontol Nurs* 5(1):27-34, 1979.

Burggraf V, Barry R: Tomorrow: gerontological nursing in the 21st century, *J Gerontol Nurs* 24(4):29-35, 1998.

Burl JB et al: Geriatric nurse practitioners in long-term care: demonstration of effectiveness in managed care, *J Am Geriatr Soc* 46(4):506-510, 1998.

Burnside IM: *Nursing and the aged: a self care approach,* ed 3, New York, 1988, McGraw-Hill.

Burnside IM: Gerontological nursing research: 1975-1984. In National League for Nursing, ed: *Overcoming the bias of ageism in long-term care,* New York, 1985, The League.

Burtt K: Nurses step to forefront of elder care, *Am J Nurs* 98(7):52-54, 1998.

Butler RN: Dispelling ageism: the cross-cutting intervention, *Generations* 17(2):75-78, Spring/Summer 1993.

Butler RN: *Why survive? Being old in America,* New York, 1975, Harper & Row.

Butler RN: Age-ism: another form of bigotry, *Gerontologist* 9:243, 1969.

Butler RN, Lewis MI: *Aging and mental health,* ed 2, St Louis, 1977, Mosby.

Cohen RA, Van Nostrand JF: *Trends in the health of older Americans: United States, 1994,* National Center for Health Statistics, Vital and Health Statistics 3(30), 1995, US Department of Health and Human Services, Public Health Service, Centers for Disease Control and Prevention.

Cora V, Lapierre E: ANA speaks out (current research and ANA's statement on the Scope of Gerontological Nursing Practice), *J Gerontol Nurs* 12(6):21-26, 1986.

Covinski KE et al: Do acute care for elders units increase hospital costs? A cost analysis using the hospital perspective, *J Am Geriatr Soc* 45(6):729-734, 1997.

Ebersole P, Hess P: *Toward healthy aging: human needs and nursing response,* ed 3, St Louis, 1990, Mosby.

Edel MK: Recognizing gerontological content, *J Gerontol Nurs* 12(10):28-32, 1986.

Fama T, Fox PD: Efforts to improve primary care delivery to nursing home residents, *J Am Geriatr Soc* 45(5):627-632, 1997.

Gunter L, Estes C: *Education for gerontic nursing,* New York, 1979, Springer.

Gunter L, Miller J: Toward a nursing gerontology, *Nurs Res* 26:208-221, 1977.

Haight BK: Update on research in long-term care: 1984-1988. In National League for Nursing, ed: *Indices for quality in long-term care: research and practice,* New York, 1989, The League.

Health Care Finance Administration: HCFA benefit payments by major programs. Accessed via the Internet, Jan 2, 1999, at http://www.fedstats.gov.

Highlights of the National Health Care Expenditure Projections, 1997-2002. Accessed Jan 2, 1999, from website: http://www.hcfa.gov/stats/NHE-Proj/hilites.htm.

Huston CJ, Fox S: The changing health care market: implications for nursing education in the coming decade, *Nurs Outlook* 46(3):109-114, 1998.

Kane RA: Transforming care institutions for the frail elderly: out of one shall be many, *Generations* 19(4):62-68, Winter 1995-1996.

Katz L et al: Studies of illness in the aged. The index of ADL: a standardized measure of biological and psychosocial function, *JAMA* 185:94-98, 1963.

Kayser-Jones J: Gerontological nursing research revisited, *J Gerontol Nurs* 7:217-233, 1981.

Landefeld CS et al: A randomized trial of care in a hospital medical unit especially designed to improve the functional outcomes of acutely ill older adults, *N Engl J Med* 332:1338-1344, 1995.

Lardner J: For nurses, a barrier broken, *US News World Rep* pp 58-61, July 27, 1998.

Lawton MP, Brody EM: Assessment of older people: self maintaining and instrumental activities of daily living, *Gerontologist* 9:179, 1969.

Luggen AS: *NGNA core curriculum for gerontological nursing,* St Louis, 1996, Mosby.

Luggen AS, Meiner SE: *NGNA core curriculum for gerontological nursing,* ed 2, St Louis, 2002, Mosby.

Morrissey S: The best education and training: in nursing, a study in contradictions, *Generations* 19(2):18-20, Summer 1995.

Palmer RM et al: A medical unit for the acute care of the elderly, *J Am Geriatr Soc* 42:545-552, 1994.

Potter PA, Perry AG: *Fundamentals of nursing: concepts, process, and practice,* ed 5, St Louis, 2004, Mosby.

Robinson L: Gerontological nursing research. In Burnside IM, ed: *Nursing and the aged,* ed 2, New York, 1981, McGraw-Hill.

Small NR, Walsh MB, eds: *Teaching nursing homes: the nursing perspective,* Owings Mills, Md, 1988, National Health Publishing.

US Bureau of the Census: *Sixty-five plus in the United States: 1995, statistical brief,* Washington, DC, 1995a, Economics and Statistics Administration, US Department of Commerce.

US Bureau of the Census: *Statistical abstract of the United States: 1995,* Washington, DC, 1995b, US Government Printing Office.

Waters V, ed: *Teaching gerontology: the curriculum imperative,* New York, 1991, National League for Nursing Press.

Wolanin MO: Clinical geriatric research. In Werley H, Fitzpatrick J, eds: *Annual review of nursing research,* New York, 1983, Springer.

Yurchuck ER, Brower HT: Faculty preparation for gerontological nursing, *J Gerontol Nurs* 20(1):17-24, 1994.

2 Theories of Aging

SUE E. MEINER, EdD, APRN, BC, GNP

Learning Objectives

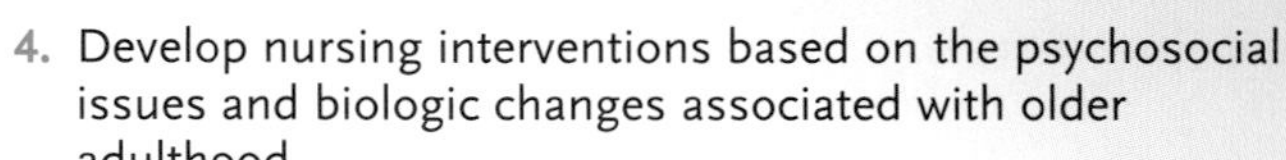

On completion of this chapter, the reader will be able to:

1. Define aging from a biologic, sociologic, and psychologic framework.
2. Analyze the prominent biologic, sociologic, and psychologic theories of aging.
3. Discuss the rationale for using an eclectic approach in the development of aging theories.
4. Develop nursing interventions based on the psychosocial issues and biologic changes associated with older adulthood.
5. Discuss several nursing implications for each of the major biologic, sociologic, and psychologic theories of aging.

Theories of aging have been debated since the time of the ancient Greeks. We have sought to embrace a theory that can explain the entire phenomenon. However, many scholars have concluded this quest is in vain and that no one definition or theory exists that explains all aspects of aging. Rather, scientists have found that several theories may be combined to explain various aspects of the complex phenomena we call aging (Gerhard and Cristofalo, 1992; Hayflick, 1996).

Theories function to help make sense of a particular phenomenon; they provide a sense of order and give a perspective from which to view the facts. Theories provide a springboard for discussion and research. Some theories are presented in this chapter because of their historical value; for the most part, they have been abandoned due to lack of empiric evidence. Other theories are the result of ongoing advances made in biotechnology and, as such, provide glimpses into our future.

Human aging is influenced by a composite of biologic, psychologic, social, functional, and spiritual factors. Aging may be viewed as a continuum of events that occur from conception to death (Ignatavicius and Workman, 2005). Biologic, social, and psychologic theories of aging attempt to explain and explore the various dimensions of aging. This chapter explores the *prominent theories* of aging as a guide for developing a holistic gerontologic nursing theory for practice application. No single gerontologic nursing theory has been accepted by this specialty, which requires nurses to use an eclectic approach from other disciplines as the basis of clinical decision making (Comfort, 1970) (Box 2-1).

By incorporating a holistic approach to the care of older adults, nurses can view this ever-increasing portion of the population more comprehensively. Interactions between gerontologic nurses and older adults are not limited to a specific disease or physiologic process, absolute developmental tasks, or psychosocial changes. Nurses have the ability to synthesize various aspects of the different aging theories, and they visualize older adults interfacing with their total environment, including physical, mental/emotional, social, and spiritual aspects. Therefore an eclectic approach provides an excellent foundation when planning high-quality care for older adults.

Theories of aging attempt to explain this phenomenon of aging as it occurs over the life span, which is thought to be a maximum of approximately 120 years (Cetron and Davies, 1998). Several basic assumptions and concepts have been accepted over the years as guiding research and clinical practice related to aging. Human aging is viewed as a total process that begins at conception. Because individuals have unique genetic, social, psychologic, and economic factors intertwined in their lives, the course of aging varies from individual to individual. *Senescence,* defined as a change in the behavior of an organism with age, leading to a decreased power of survival and adjustment, occurs as well. The recognition of the universal truths is what we attempt to discover through the theories of aging.

BIOLOGIC THEORIES OF AGING

Biologic theories are concerned with answering basic questions regarding the physiologic processes that occur in all living organisms as they chronologically age. These age-related changes occur independent of any external or pathologic influence. The primary question being addressed relates to the factors that trigger the actual aging process in organisms. These theories generally view aging as occurring from a molecular, cellular, or even a systems point of view. In addition, biologic

BOX 2-1 Theories of Aging

BIOLOGIC

Concerned with answering basic questions regarding physiologic processes that occur in all living organisms over time (Hayflick, 1996).

SOCIOLOGIC

Focused on the roles and relationships within which individuals engage in later life (Hogstel, 1995).

PSYCHOLOGIC

Influenced by both biology and sociology; address how a person responds to the tasks of his or her age.

MORAL/SPIRITUAL

Examine how an individual seeks to explain and validate his or her existence (Edelman and Mandle, 2003).

BOX 2-2 Biologic Theories of Aging

STOCHASTIC THEORIES

Error Theory

The error theory is based on the idea that errors can occur in the transcription of the synthesis of DNA. These errors are perpetuated and eventually lead to systems that do not function at the optimum level. The organism's aging and death are attributable to these events (Sonneborn, 1979).

Free Radical Theory

Free radicals are byproducts of metabolism. When these byproducts accumulate, they damage the cell membrane, which decreases its efficiency. The body produces antioxidants that scavenge the free radicals (Hayflick, 1996).

Cross-Linkage Theory

With age, according to this theory, some proteins in the body become cross-linked. This does not allow for normal metabolic activities, and waste products accumulate in the cells. The end result is that tissues do not function at optimum efficiency (Hayflick, 1996).

Wear and Tear Theory

The wear and tear theory equates humans with machines. It hypothesizes that aging is the result of use.

NONSTOCHASTIC THEORIES

Programmed Theory

Hayflick and Moorehead demonstrated that normal cells divide a limited number of times; therefore they hypothesized that life expectancy was preprogrammed (Hayflick, 1996).

Immunity Theory

Changes occur in the immune system, specifically in the T lymphocytes, as a result of aging. These changes leave the individual more vulnerable to disease (Phipps et al, 2003).

theories are not meant to be exclusionary. Theories may be combined to explain phenomena (Hayflick, 1996).

The foci of biologic theories include explanations of the following: (1) deleterious effects leading to decreasing function of the organism, (2) gradually occurring age-related changes that are progressive over time, and (3) intrinsic changes that can affect all members of a species because of chronologic age. The decreasing function of an organism may lead to a complete failure of either an organ or an entire system (Hayflick, 1996). In addition, according to these theories, all organs in any one organism do not age at the same rate, and any single organ does not necessarily age at the same rate in different individuals of the same species.

The biologic theories can be subdivided into two main divisions: stochastic and nonstochastic. Stochastic theories explain aging as events that occur randomly and accumulate over time, whereas nonstochastic theories view aging as certain predetermined, timed phenomena (Box 2-2).

Stochastic Theories

Error Theory. As a cell ages, various changes occur naturally in its deoxyribonucleic acid (DNA) and ribonucleic acid (RNA), the building blocks of the cell. DNA, found in the nucleus of the cell, contains the fundamental genetic code and forms the genes on all 46 human chromosomes (Black and Hawks, 2005).

In 1963 Orgel proposed the Error Theory, sometimes called the Error Catastrophe Theory. This theory's hypothesis is based on the idea that errors can occur in the transcription in any step of protein synthesis of DNA, and this eventually leads to either the aging or the actual death of a cell. The error would cause the reproduction of an enzyme or protein that was not an exact copy of the original. The next transcription would again contain an error. As the effect continued through several generations of proteins, the end product would not even resemble the original cell and its functional ability would be diminished (Sonneborn, 1979).

In recent years the theory has not been supported by research. Although changes do occur in the activity of various enzymes with aging, studies have not found that all aged cells contain altered or misspecified proteins, nor is aging automatically or necessarily accelerated if misspecified proteins or enzymes are introduced to a cell (Goldstein, 1993; Hayflick, 1996; Schneider, 1992).

Free Radical Theory. Free radicals are byproducts of fundamental metabolic activities within the body. Free radical production can increase as a result of environmental pollutants such as ozone, pesticides, and radiation. Normally, they are neutralized by enzymatic activity or natural antioxidants. However, if they are not neutralized, they may attach to other molecules. These highly reactive free radicals react with molecules in cell membranes, in particular cell membranes of unsaturated lipids such as mitochondria, lysosomes, and nuclear membranes. This action monopolizes the receptor sites on the membrane, thereby inhibiting the interaction with other substances that normally use this site; this chemical reaction is called lipid peroxidation. Therefore the mitochondria, for example, can no longer function as efficiently, and their cell membranes may become damaged, resulting in increased permeability. If excessive fluid is either lost or gained, the internal homeostasis is disrupted and cell death may result.

Other deleterious results are related to free radical molecules in the body. Although these molecules do not contain DNA themselves, they can cause mutations in the DNA-RNA transcription, thereby producing mutations of the original protein. In nervous and muscle tissue, to which free radicals have a high affinity, a substance called lipofuscin has been found and is thought to be indicative of chronologic age.

Lipofuscin, a lipid- and protein-enriched pigmented material, has been found to accumulate in older adults' tissues, and is commonly referred to as "age spots." As the lipofuscin's presence increases, healthy tissue is slowly deprived of oxygen and nutrient supply. Further degeneration of surrounding tissue eventually leads to actual death of the tissue. The body does have naturally occurring antioxidants or protective mechanisms. Vitamins C and E are two of these substances, which can inhibit the functioning of the free radicals or possibly decrease their production in the body.

Harman (1956) was the first to suggest that the administration of chemicals terminating the propagation of free radicals would extend the life span or delay the aging process. Animal research has demonstrated that administration of antioxidants did increase the average length of life, possibly because of the delayed appearance of diseases that may have eventually killed the animals studied. It appears that administration of antioxidants postpones the appearance of diseases such as cardiovascular disease and cancer, two of the most common causes of death. Antioxidants also appear to have an effect on the decline of the immune system and on degenerative neurologic diseases, both of which affect morbidity and mortality (Hayflick, 1996; Yu, 1998, 1993).

Cross-Linkage Theory. The cross-linkage theory of aging hypothesizes that with age some proteins become increasingly cross-linked or enmeshed and may impede metabolic processes by obstructing the passage of nutrients and wastes between the intracellular and extracellular compartments. According to this theory, normally separated molecular structures are bound together through chemical reactions. Primarily this involves collagen, which is a relatively inert long-chain macromolecule produced by fibroblasts. As new fibers are created, they become enmeshed with old fibers and form an actual chemical cross-link. The end result of this cross-linkage process is an increase in density of the collagen molecule but a decrease in the capacity to transport nutrients to, and to remove waste products from, the cells. Eventually, this results in a decrease in the structure's function. An example of this would be the changes associated with aging skin. The skin of a baby is soft and pliable, whereas aging skin loses much of its suppleness and elasticity. This aging process is similar to the process of tanning leather, which purposefully creates cross-links (Bjorkstein, 1976; Hayflick, 1996).

Cross-linkage agents have been found in unsaturated fats; in polyvalent metal ions like aluminum, zinc, and magnesium; and in association with excessive radiation exposure. Many of the medications ingested by the older population (such as antacids and coagulants) contain aluminum, as does the common cooking ingredient baking powder. Some research supports a combination of exercise and dietary restrictions in helping to inhibit the cross-linkage process, as well as the use of vitamin C prophylactically as an antioxidant agent (Bjorkstein, 1976).

Cerani has shown that blood glucose reacts with bodily proteins to form cross-links. He has found that the crystallin of the lens of the eye, membranes of the kidney, and blood vessels are especially susceptible to cross-linking under the conditions of increased glucose. Cerani suggests increased levels of blood glucose cause increased amounts of cross-linking, which accelerate lens, kidney, and blood vessel diseases (Schneider, 1992).

Cross-linkage theory proposes that as a person ages and the immune system becomes less efficient, the body's defense mechanism cannot remove the cross-linking agent before it becomes securely established. Cross-linkage has been proposed as a primary cause of arteriosclerosis, a decrease in efficiency of the immune system with age, and the loss of elasticity often seen in older adult skin. The cross-linkage theory has emerged from deductive reasoning, and aside from the previous examples there is little empiric evidence to support its claims (Hayflick, 1996).

Wear and Tear Theory. This theory proposed that cells wear out over time because of continued use. When this theory was first proposed in 1882 by Weisman, death was seen as a result of tissues being worn out because they could not rejuvenate themselves in an endless manner (Hayflick, 1988). Essentially, the theory reflects a belief that organs and tissues have a preprogrammed amount of available energy and wear out when the allotted energy is expended. Eventually this leads to the death of the entire organism.

Under this theory, aging is viewed as almost a preprogrammed process—a process thought to be vulnerable to stress, or an accumulation of injuries or trauma, which may actually accelerate it. "Death," said Weisman, "occurs because a worn out tissue cannot forever renew itself" (Hayflick, 1996).

Proponents of this theory cite microscopic signs of wear and tear that have been found in striated and smooth muscle tissue and in nerve cells. Researchers question this theory in light of research demonstrating increased functional abilities in individuals who exercise daily. This effect occurs even in persons with chronic limiting states such as rheumatoid arthritis. If exercise has been found to increase a person's level of functioning rather than decrease it, critics challenge, how can the wear and tear hypothesis be correct? This theory was developed during the Industrial Revolution, when people were attempting to explain and make sense of events in their world. These people were trying to equate humans with the marvelous machines they were producing. It eventually became clear just how different humans were from these machines.

Nonstochastic Theories

Programmed Theory or Hayflick Limit Theory. One of the first proposed biologic theories is based on a study completed in 1961 by Hayflick and Moorehead. This study included an experiment on fetal fibroblastic cells and their reproductive capabilities. The results of this landmark study changed the way scientists viewed the biologic aging process.

Hayflick and Moorehead's study showed that functional changes do occur within cells and are responsible for the aging of the cells and the organism. The study further supported the hypothesis that a cumulative effect of improper functioning of cells and eventual loss of cells in organs and tissues are therefore responsible for the aging phenomenon. This study contradicted earlier studies by Carrel and Ebeling in which chick embryo cells were kept alive indefinitely in a laboratory; the conclusion from this 1912 experiment was that cells do not wear out, but continue to function normally forever. An interesting aspect of the 1961 study was that freezing was found to halt the biologic cellular clock (Hayflick and Moorehead, 1961).

Based on this 1961 study, unlimited cell division was not found to occur; the immortality of individual cells was found to be more an abnormal than a normal occurrence. Therefore this study seemed to support the Hayflick Limit Theory. Life expectancy was generally seen as preprogrammed, within a species-specific range; this biologic clock for humans was estimated at 110 to 120 years (Gerhard and Cristofalo, 1992; Hayflick, 1996). Based on the conclusions of this experiment, the Hayflick Limit Theory is sometimes called the "Biologic Clock," "Cellular Aging," or "Genetic Theory."

Immunity Theory. The immune system is a network of specialized cells, tissues, and organs that provide the body with protection against invading organisms. Its primary role is to differentiate self from non-self, thereby protecting the organism from attack by pathogens. It has been found that as a person ages, the immune system functions less effectively. The term *immunosenescence* has been given to this age-related decrease in function.

Essential components of the immune system are T lymphocytes, which are responsible for cell-mediated immunity, and B lymphocytes, the antibodies responsible for humoral immunity. Both T and B lymphocytes may respond to an invasion of the organism, though one may provide more protection in certain situations. The changes that occur with aging are most apparent in the T lymphocytes, although changes also occur in the functioning capabilities of B lymphocytes. Accompanying these changes is a decrease in the body's defense against foreign pathogens, which manifests itself as an increased incidence of infectious diseases and an increase in the production of autoantibodies, which lead to a propensity to develop autoimmune-related diseases (Hayflick, 1996) (Box 2-3).

The changes in the immune system cannot be precisely explained by an exact cause-and-effect relationship, but they do seem to increase with advancing age. These changes include a decrease in humoral immune response, often predisposing older adults to (1) decreased resistance to a tumor cell challenge and the development of cancer, (2) decreased ability to initiate the immune process and mobilize the body's defenses against aggressively attacking pathogens, and (3) heightened production of autoantigens, often leading to an increase in autoimmune-related diseases.

Immunodeficient conditions, such as the human immunodeficiency virus (HIV) and the immune suppression of organ transplant recipients, have demonstrated a relationship between immunocompetence and cancer development. HIV has been associated with several forms of cancer, such as Kaposi's sarcoma. Recipients of organ transplants are 80 times more likely to contract cancer than the rest of the population (Black and Hawks, 2005).

BOX 2-3 Changes in Cell-Mediated Immune Function As a Result of Aging

- Increased autoantibodies as a result of altered immune system regulation. This predisposes an individual to autoimmune diseases such as lupus and rheumatoid arthritis.
- Low rate of T lymphocyte proliferation in response to a stimulus. This causes older adults to respond more slowly to allergic stimulants.
- Reduced response to foreign material, resulting in an increased number of infections. This is a result of a decrease in cytotoxic or killer T cells.
- Generalized T lymphocyte dysfunctions, which reduce the response to certain viral antigens, allografts, and tumor cells. This results in an increased incidence of cancer in older adults.

Emerging Theories

Neuroendocrine Control or Pacemaker Theory. The neuroendocrine theory examines the interrelated role of the neurologic and endocrine systems over the life span of an individual (Box 2-4). The neuroendocrine system regulates and controls many important metabolic activities. It has been observed that there is a decline, or even a cessation, in many of the components of the neuroendocrine system over the life span. The reproductive system, and its changes over the life of an individual, provides an interesting model for the functional capability of the neuroendocrine system.

Research has shown there are complex interactions between the endocrine and the nervous systems. It appears that the female reproductive system is governed not by the ovaries or the pituitary gland but by the hypothalamus. Men do not experience a reproductive event such as a menopause, though they do demonstrate a decline in fertility. The mechanisms that trigger this decline may offer a template for understanding the phenomena of aging (Hayflick, 1996).

Another hormone that has been receiving attention is dehydroepiandrosterone (DHEA). This hormone, secreted by the adrenal glands, diminishes over the lifetime of an individual. Administration of this hormone to laboratory mice showed it increased longevity, bolstered immunity, and made the animals appear younger. These mice also ate less, so there is some question whether DHEA-fed mice exhibit the effect of calorie restriction (Cupp, 1997; Guardiola-Lemaitre, 1997; Hayflick, 1996; Kendler, 1997)

Melatonin is a hormone being investigated for its role as a biologic clock. Melatonin is produced by the pineal gland, the function of which was a mystery until recently. Melatonin has been found to be a regulator of biologic rhythms and a powerful antioxidant that may enhance immune function. The level of melatonin production in the body declines dramatically from just after puberty until old age.

The belief that melatonin has a role in aging comes not only from its effect on the immune system and its antioxidant capability, but also from studies on rodents that demonstrated an increased life span when melatonin was administered. These studies also found that rodents fed supplementary melatonin restricted their calorie intake. More research needs to be performed regarding the safety and efficacy of melatonin. However, in the United States melatonin can already be sold as a dietary supplement, so there is little financial incentive for conducting research. In Europe melatonin is considered a neurohormone, so there would be more financial gain to determining its role in the aging process. At this time, no individual should take melatonin without his or her primary health care provider's knowledge (Guardiola-Lemaitre, 1997; Hayflick, 1996).

BOX 2-4 Emerging Theories of Aging

NEUROENDOCRINE CONTROL OR PACEMAKER THEORY

The neuroendocrine system controls many essential activities with regard to growth and development. Scientists are studying the roles that the hypothalamus and the hormones DHEA (dehydroepiandrosterone) and melatonin play in the aging process (Guardiola-Lemaitre, 1997; Hayflick, 1996).

METABOLIC THEORY OF AGING/CALORIC RESTRICTION

The role of metabolism in the aging process is being investigated (Hayflick, 1996).

DNA-RELATED RESEARCH

Two developments are occurring at this time in relationship to DNA and the aging process. First, as scientists continue to map the human genome, they are identifying certain genes that play a role in the aging process (Schneider, 1992). Second is the discovery of telomeres, located at the ends of chromosomes, which may function as the cells' biologic clocks (Hayflick, 1996).

Metabolic Theory of Aging/Caloric Restriction. This theory proposes that all organisms have a finite metabolic lifetime and that organisms with a higher metabolic rate have a shorter life span. Evidence for this theory comes from research showing that certain fish, when the water temperature is lowered, live longer than their warm water counterparts. Extensive experimentation on the effects of caloric restriction on rodents has demonstrated that caloric restriction increases the life span and delays the onset of age-dependent diseases (Hayflick, 1996; Schneider, 1992).

DNA-Related Research. Two major developments are occurring at the time of this writing in relation to our understanding of the role DNA plays in the aging process. The first involves the process of mapping, or identification, of the human genome, with the hope that this task will be accomplished early in the twenty-first century. It is believed that there may be as many as 200 genes responsible for controlling aging in humans (Schneider, 1992). Investigation into the "aging" genes in select body systems, such as the immune system, may lead to greater understanding of the process of aging.

The second development that has occurred is in relation to the discovery of telomeres, which are the regions at the ends of chromosomes that may function as biologic clocks (Fig. 2-1). It has been found that with each cell division that takes place in cultured, normal human cells, part of the telomere is lost. This discovery explains why normal cells have a limited capacity to divide. Abnormal cells, such as cancer cells, seem to have found a way to keep from shortening at each division, which confers a type of "immortality" on them. These "abnormal" cells produce an enzyme called telomerase. The enzyme telomerase actually adds telomere sequences to the ends of each chromosome at each cell division. The immediate benefit of this discovery was the development of tests to detect the

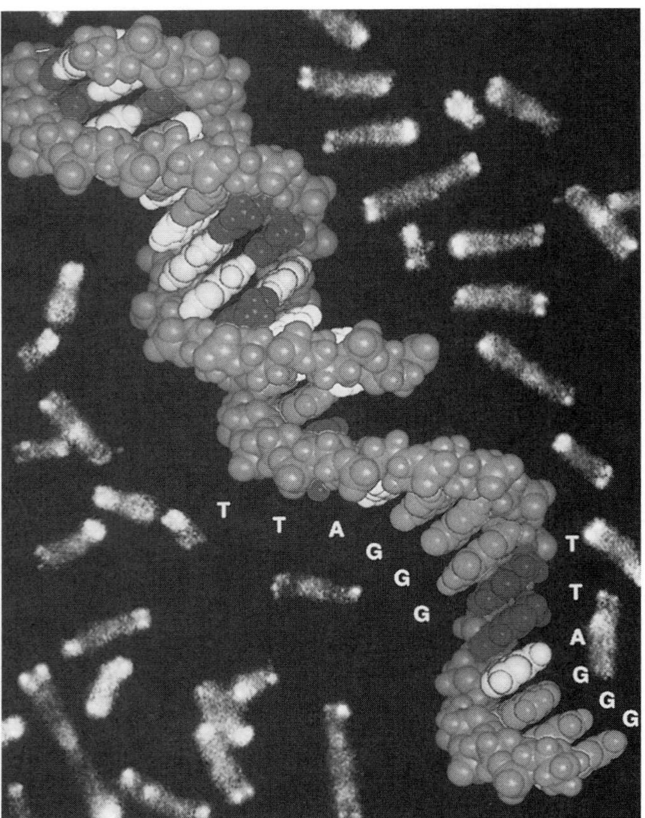

Fig. 2-1 A DNA model against a background of chromosomes. The light ends on the chromosomes are telomeres. (Used with permission from The University of Texas Southwestern Medical Center at Dallas; Office of News and Publications; 5323 Harry Hines Boulevard; Dallas, TX 75235.)

enzyme telomerase, thereby identifying abnormal cells. Research is proceeding to develop substances that would inhibit the production of telomerase in an effort to prevent cancer cells from multiplying (Gupta and Han, 1996; Hayflick, 1996; Keys and Marble, 1998).

Implications for Nursing

When interacting with the older population, caregivers must relate the key concepts of the biologic theories to the care being provided. Although these theories do not provide *the answer,* they certainly can explain some of the changes seen in the aging individual. Aging and disease do not necessarily go hand in hand, and the nurse caring for older adults needs to have a clear understanding of the difference between age-related changes and those that may actually be pathologic. Nurses must remember that scientists are still in the process of discovering what is "normal" aging.

Among biologic theories of aging, two concepts have gained wide acceptance: (1) there may be a limited replicative capacity for certain cells that causes overexpression of damaged genes and oxidative damage to cells, and (2) free radicals may cause damage to cells over time. Based on these concepts, gerontologic nurses can promote the health of older adult clients in a number of ways. Providing assistance with smoking cessation would be one example of health promotion. Cigarette smoking causes increased cell turnover in the oral cavity, bronchial tree, and alveoli. Smoking also introduces carcinogens in the body that may result in an increased rate of cell damage that can lead to cancer. Using the same principles, nurses could develop a health promotional activity for education regarding sun exposure. Excessive exposure to ultraviolet light is another example of a substance causing rapid turnover of cells, which may lead to mutations and finally malignancies. In an effort to reduce free radical damage, nurses can also advise clients to ingest a varied, nutritious diet using the food pyramid as a guide, and suggest supplementation with antioxidants such as vitamins C and E (Goldstein, 1993). Activity continues to play an important role in the lives of older adults. Daily routines need to incorporate opportunities that capitalize on existing abilities, strengthen muscles, and prevent further atrophy of muscles because of disuse. Encouraging older adults to participate in activities may prove a challenge to nurses interacting with these clients (see Research box, p. 25).

Performing activities of daily living (ADLs) requires functional use of extremities. Daily exercises that enhance upper arm strength and hand dexterity contribute to older adults' ability to successfully perform dressing and grooming activities. Even chair-based activities, like deep breathing, increase the oxygen flow to the brain, thereby promoting clear mental cognition, minimizing dizziness, and increasing stamina with activity.

Encouraging older adults to participate in daily walking, even on a limited basis, facilitates peripheral circulation and promotes the development of collateral circulation. Walking can also help with weight control, which often becomes a problem in older adults. Additional benefits of walking include (1) replacement of fat with muscle tissue, (2) prevention of muscle atrophy, and (3) a generalized increase in the person's sense of well-being.

The health care delivery system is beginning to focus on disease prevention and health promotion. Older adults must be included in this focus. Stereotypic views that older adults are "too old to learn new things" must be replaced by factual knowledge about the cognitive abilities of older adults. It is necessary for client teaching to stress the concept that certain conditions or diseases are not inevitable just because of advancing years. A high level of wellness is needed to help minimize the potential damage caused by disease in later years. Although aging brings with it a decrease in the normal functioning of the immune system, older adults should not suffer needlessly from infections or disease. Encouraging preventive measures like an annual influenza vaccine or a one-time inoculation with the pneumococcal vaccine is

Research

SAMPLE/SETTING

A nonrandomized study of 184 male veterans, older than 65, and not living in an institution.

METHODS

The Interaction Model of Client Health Behavior (Cox, 1982) was administered. The independent variables were age, education, race, marital status, children, siblings, income, spiritual well-being, functional status, motivation, health conceptions, and loneliness. The dependent variable was Schwirian's (1992) active composure, conceptualized as activities producing rest, relaxation, and anxiety and stress reduction. A multiple regression model explained 49% of the variance in active composure. Race, income, religious aspect of spiritual well-being, instrumental activities of daily living (IADLs), and loneliness were significant predictors.

FINDINGS

The findings of this study demonstrated that higher levels of active composure occurred to nonwhite individuals who perceived that they had adequate incomes, and had higher religious aspects of spiritual well-being, greater independence in IADLs, and lower levels of loneliness. The ability to perform IADLs in older adulthood appears to be a better predictor of active composure than age alone. It is possible that health behaviors are more socially defined and less influenced by education than other forms of health behavior. Areas that did not correlate with the findings were age, education, marital status, number of children and siblings, spiritual well-being, motivation, and health conception.

IMPLICATIONS

Nurses are challenged to promote the health of an older, community-living population with chronic illnesses. As the cohort of older adults increases, a proactive approach to health through appropriate health promotion strategies can be an effective means of reducing health care costs and supporting community-living status.

Carter KF: Behaviors of Older Men Living in the community: correlates producing active composure, *J Gerontol Nurs* 29(10):37, 2003.

essential to providing a high-quality life experience for the older population.

Other applications of biologic theories to practice include the recognition that life stress, both physical and psychologic, has an impact on the aging process. In planning interventions, nurses should pay attention to the various stress factors in an older person's life. Activities to minimize stress and to promote healthy coping mechanisms must be included in the client teaching plan for older adults.

BOX 2-5 Sociologic Theories of Aging

DISENGAGEMENT THEORY

As individuals age, they withdraw from society and society supports this withdrawal (Cumming and Henry, 1961).

ACTIVITY/DEVELOPMENTAL TASK THEORY

Individuals need to remain active to age successfully. Activity is necessary to maintain life satisfaction and a positive self-concept (Havighurst, Neugarten, and Tobin, 1963).

CONTINUITY THEORY

Individuals will respond to aging in the same way they have responded to previous life events. The same habits, commitments, preferences, and other personality characteristics developed during adulthood are maintained in older adulthood (Havighurst, Neugarten, and Tobin, 1963).

AGE STRATIFICATION THEORY

Society consists of groups of cohorts that age collectively. The people and roles in these cohorts change and influence each other, as does society at large. Therefore a high degree of interdependence exists between older adults and society (Riley, 1985).

PERSON-ENVIRONMENT FIT THEORY

Each individual has personal competencies that assist the person in dealing with the environment. These competencies may change with aging, thus affecting the older person's ability to interrelate with the environment (Lawton, 1982).

Teaching the basic techniques of relaxation, guided imagery, visualization, distraction, and music therapy can facilitate a sense of control over potential stress-producing situations. Additional options involving the application of hot or cold, therapeutic touch, and massage therapy might be explored. Being aware of individual cultural preferences and sharing these with other health care professionals will further promote positive interactions with older adults in all settings.

SOCIOLOGIC THEORIES OF AGING

Sociologic theories focus on changing roles and relationships (Box 2-5). In some respects, sociologic theories relate to various social adaptations in the lives of older adults. One of the easiest ways to view the sociologic theories is within the context of the societal values at the time in which they were developed. The early research was carried out largely on institutionalized and ill older persons, skewing the information obtained. Contemporary research is being conducted in a variety of more naturalistic environments, reflecting more accurately the diversity of the aging population.

During the 1960s sociologists focused on the losses of old age and the manner in which individuals adjusted to these losses in the context of their roles and reference groups. A decade later, society began to have a broader view of aging as reflected in the aging theories proposed during this period. These theories focused on more global, societal, and structural factors that influenced the lives of aging persons. The 1980s and 1990s again brought another change in focus, as sociologists began to explore interrelationships, especially those between older adults and the physical, political, environmental, and even socioeconomic milieu in which they lived.

Disengagement Theory

When the disengagement theory was introduced by Cumming and Henry in 1961, the theory sparked immediate controversy. These two theorists viewed aging as a developmental task in and of itself, with its own norms and appropriate patterns of behavior. The identified appropriate patterns of behavior were conceptualized as a mutual agreement between older adults and society on a reciprocal withdrawal. Individuals would change from being centered on society and interacting in the community to being self-centered persons withdrawing from society, by virtue of becoming "old." Social equilibrium would be the end result (Cumming and Henry, 1961).

The idea that older adults preferred to withdraw from society and to voluntarily decrease their interactions with others was not readily accepted by the general public, much less the older population. Although the theory oversimplified the aging process, its lasting benefit relates to the controversy it created. The theory itself is no longer supported, but the discussion and the research stemming from its premise continue today.

Activity Theory or Developmental Task Theory

Whereas one group of theorists proposed that older adults need to disengage from society, other sociologists proposed that people need to stay active if they are to age successfully. In 1953 Havighurst and Albrecht first proposed the idea that aging successfully means staying active. It was not until 10 years later that the phrase "activity theory" was coined by Havighurst and his associates (Havighurst, Neugarten, and Tobin, 1963).

This theory sees activity as necessary to maintain a person's life satisfaction and positive self-concept. By remaining active, the older person stays young and alive and does not withdraw from society because of an age parameter. Essentially the person actively participates in a continuous struggle to remain "middle-aged." This theory is based on three assumptions: (1) it is better to be active than inactive, (2) it is better to be happy than unhappy, and (3) an older individual is the best judge of his or her own success in achieving the first two assumptions (Havighurst, 1972). Within the context of this theory, activity can be viewed broadly as physical or intellectual. Therefore, even with illness or advancing age, the older person can remain "active" and achieve a sense of life satisfaction (Havighurst, Neugarten, and Tobin, 1963).

Continuity Theory

The continuity theory dispels the premises of both the disengagement and activity theories. According to this theory, being active, trying to maintain a sense of being middle-aged, or willingly withdrawing from society does not necessarily bring happiness. Instead, the continuity theory proposes that how a person has been throughout life is how that person will *continue* to be through the remainder of life (Havighurst, Neugarten, and Tobin, 1963).

Old age is not viewed as a terminal or final part of life separated from the rest of life. According to this theory, the latter part of life is a continuation of the earlier part and therefore an integral component of the entire life cycle. When viewed from this perspective, the theory can be seen as a developmental theory. Simply stated, the theory proposes that as people age, they try to maintain or continue previous habits, preferences, commitments, values, beliefs, and all the factors that have contributed to their personalities (Havighurst, Neugarten, and Tobin, 1963).

Age Stratification Theory

Beginning in the 1970s, theorists on aging began to focus more broadly on societal and structural factors that influenced how the older population was being viewed. The age stratification theory is only one example of a theory addressing societal values. The key societal issue being addressed in this theory is the concept of interdependence between the aging person and society at large (Riley, Johnson, and Foner, 1972).

This theory views the aging person as an individual element of society and also as a member, with peers, interacting in a social process. The theory attempts to explain the interdependence between older adults and society and how they constantly influence each other in a variety of ways.

Riley (1985) identifies the five major concepts of this theory: (1) each individual progresses through society in groups of cohorts that are collectively aging socially, biologically, and psychologically; (2) new cohorts are continually being born, and each of them experiences their own unique sense of history; (3) society itself can be divided into various strata according to the parameters of age and roles; (4) not only are people and roles within every stratum continuously changing, but so is society at large; and (5) the interaction between individual aging people and the entire society is not stagnant but remains dynamic.

Person-Environment Fit Theory

Another aging theory relates to the individual's personal competence within the environment in which he or she interacts. This theory, proposed by Lawton (1982), examines the concept of interrelationships among the competencies of a group of persons, older adults, and their society or environment.

All people, including older persons, have certain personal competencies that help mold and shape them throughout life. Lawton (1982) identified these personal competencies as including ego strength, motor skills, individual biologic health, and cognitive and sensory-perceptual capacities. All these help people deal with the environment in which they live.

As a person ages, there may be changes or even decreases in some of these personal competencies. These changes influence the individual's abilities to interrelate with the environment. If a person develops one or more chronic diseases, such as rheumatoid arthritis or cardiovascular disease, then competencies may be impaired and the level of interrelatedness may be limited.

The theory further proposes that, as a person ages, the environment becomes more threatening and he or she may feel incompetent dealing with it. In a society constantly making rapid technologic advances, this theory helps explain why an older person might feel inhibited and may retreat from society.

Implications for Nursing

It is important to remember that all older adults cannot be grouped collectively as just *one* segment of the population. There are differences within the aged population. The young-old (ages 65 to 74), the middle-old (ages 75 to 84), the old-old (more than 85), and the elite-old (more than 100 years old) are four distinct cohort groups, and the individuals within each of these cohort groups have their own history. There is variation among even the same cohort group based on culture, life experiences, gender, and health and family status. Nurses need to be aware of the fact that whatever similarities exist among the individuals of a cohort group, they are still individuals. Older adults are not a homogeneous sociologic group, and care needs to be taken not to treat them as if they were.

Older adults respond to current experiences based on their past life encounters, beliefs, and expectations. If their "typical" reaction to stress, challenges, or fear is to disengage from interactions, then current situations often produce the same responses. Because older adults are individuals, their responses must be respected. However, it is within the nurse's scope of practice to identify maladaptive responses and intervene to protect the integrity of the person.

Withdrawal by older adults may be a manifestation of a deeper problem, such as depression. Using assessment skills and specific tools, nurses can further investigate and plan appropriate interventions to help resolve a potentially adverse situation. Older adults may refuse to engage in a particular activity because of fear of failure or frustration at not being able to perform the activity. Planning realistic activities for particular client groups is crucial to successful group interaction. The successful completion of a group activity provides an opportunity for increasing an older person's self-confidence, whereas frustration over an impossible task further promotes feelings of inadequacy and uselessness.

By examining the past and being aware of significant events or even beliefs about health and illness, the health care provider can develop a deeper understanding of *why* these particular older adults act or believe the way they do. The health care provider can also gain insight into how a particular group of older adults responds to illness and views healthy aging. This knowledge and insight can certainly assist in planning not only activities but also meaningful client teaching.

Another application of the sociologic theories relates to helping adults adapt to various limitations and securing appropriate living arrangements. Following the passage of the 1990 Americans With Disabilities Act, a majority of buildings are now easily accessible to individuals with special needs. These special needs may include doorways that are wide enough for wheelchairs, ramps instead of stairs, handrails in hallways, and working elevators. Although these changes assist younger members of society with limited physical capabilities, they also benefit older adults. In addition, older adults might consider the installation of medical alert devices, preprogrammed or large-numbered phones, and even special security systems.

Helping older adults adjust to limitations, while accentuating positive attributes, may enable them to remain independent and may perpetuate a high quality of life during later years. These adaptations may encourage older adults to remain in the community, perhaps even in the family home, instead of being prematurely institutionalized. Older adults continue to feel valued and viewed as active members of society when allowed to maintain a sense of control over the living environment.

In some cities, multigenerational communities are developing, fostering a sharing of different cultures as well as generations. Schools are promoting "adopt a grandparent" programs, day care centers are combining services for children and older adults, and older volunteers visit hospitalized children or phone "latchkey" children after school. These are examples of the application of sociologic aging theories in practice. Older adults are continuing to be active, engaging or disengaging as they wish, and remaining valued members of society.

PSYCHOLOGIC THEORIES OF AGING

The basic assumption of the psychologic theories of aging is that development does not end when a person reaches adulthood, but remains a dynamic process throughout the life span (Box 2-6). As a person passes from the middle to the later life roles, abilities, perspectives, and belief systems enter a stage of transition. The nurse, by providing holistic care, seeks to employ strategies to enhance clients' quality of life (Hogstel, 1995). The psychologic theories of aging are much broader in scope than the previous theories because they are influenced by both biology and sociology. Therefore psychologic aging cannot readily be separated from biologic and sociologic influences.

As a person ages, various adaptive changes help him or her cope with or accept some of the biologic changes. Some of the adaptive mechanisms include memory, learning capacity, feelings, intellectual functioning, and motivations to perform or not perform particular activities (Birren and Cunningham, 1985). Psychologic aging, therefore, includes not only behavioral changes but also developmental aspects related to the lives of older adults. How does behavior change in relation to advancing age? Are these behavioral changes consistent in pattern from one individual to another? Theorists are searching for answers to questions such as these.

Maslow's Hierarchy of Human Needs

According to this theory, each individual has an innate internal hierarchy of needs that motivates all human behaviors (Maslow, 1954). These human needs have different orders of priority. When people achieve fulfillment of their elemental needs, they strive to meet those needs on the next level, continuing on until the highest order of needs is reached. These human needs are often depicted as a pyramid, with the most elemental needs at the base (Fig. 2-2).

The initial human needs each person must meet relate to physiologic needs, needs for basic survival. Initially a starving person worries about obtaining food to survive. Once this need is met, the next concern is about safety and security. These needs must be met, at least to some extent, before the person becomes concerned with the needs for love, acceptance, and a feeling of belonging. According to Maslow (1968), as each succeeding layer of needs is addressed, the individual is motivated to look to the needs at the next higher step.

Maslow's fully developed, self-actualized person displays high levels of all the following characteristics: perception of reality; acceptance of self, others, and nature; spontaneity; problem-solving ability; self-direction; detachment and the desire for privacy; freshness of peak experiences; identification with other human beings; satisfying and changing relationships with other people; a democratic character structure; creativity; and a sense of values (Maslow, 1968). Maslow's ideal self-actualized person is probably only attained by about 1% of the population (Thomas and Chess, 1977). Nevertheless, the person developing in a healthy way is always moving toward more self-fulfilling levels.

BOX 2-6 Psychologic Theories of Aging

MASLOW'S HIERARCHY OF HUMAN NEEDS

Human motivation is viewed as a hierarchy of needs that are critical to the growth and development of all people. Individuals are viewed as active participants in life, striving for self-actualization (Carson and Arnold, 1996).

JUNG'S THEORY OF INDIVIDUALISM

Development is viewed as occurring throughout adulthood, with self-realization as the goal of personality development. As an individual ages, he or she is capable of transforming into a more spiritual being.

ERIKSON'S EIGHT STAGES OF LIFE

All people experience eight psychosocial stages during the course of a lifetime. Each stage represents a crisis, where the goal is to integrate physical maturation and psychosocial demands. At each stage the person has the opportunity to resolve the crisis. Successful mastery prepares an individual for continued development. Individuals always have within themselves an opportunity to rework a previous psychosocial stage into a more successful outcome (Carson and Arnold, 1996).

PECK'S EXPANSION OF ERIKSON'S THEORY

Seven developmental tasks are identified as occurring during Erikson's final two stages. The final three of these developmental tasks identified for old age are (1) ego differentiation versus work role preoccupation, (2) body transcendence versus body preoccupation, and (3) ego transcendence versus ego preoccupation (Ignatavicius and Workman, 2005).

SELECTIVE OPTIMIZATION WITH COMPENSATION

Physical capacity diminishes with age. An individual who ages successfully compensates for these deficits through selection, optimization, and compensation (Schroots, 1996).

Jung's Theory of Individualism

The Swiss psychologist Carl Jung (1960) proposed a theory of personality development throughout life: childhood, youth and young adulthood, middle age, and old age. An individual's personality is composed of the ego, the personal uncon-

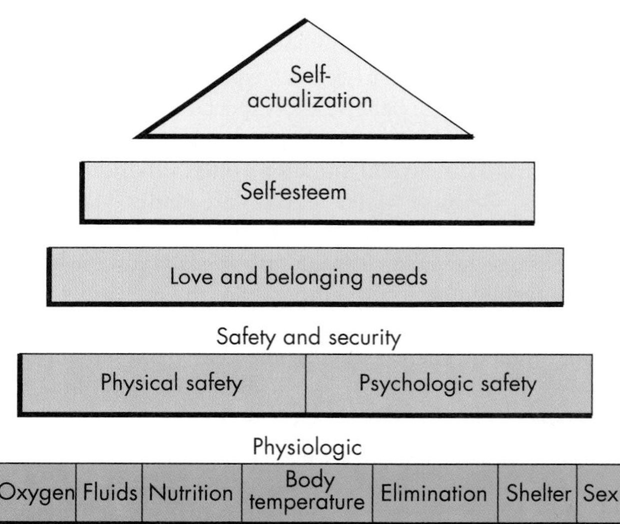

Fig. 2-2 Maslow's hierarchy of needs. (From Maslow AH et al: Motivation and personality, ed 3, Upper Saddle River, NJ, ©1987, Reprinted by permission of Pearson Education, Inc.)

sciousness, and the collective unconsciousness. According to this theory, a person's personality is visualized as oriented either toward the external world (extroversion) or toward subjective, inner experiences (introversion). A balance between these two forces, which are present in every individual, is essential for mental health.

Applying Jung's theory to individuals as they progress through life, Jung proposed that it is at the onset of middle age that the person begins to question values, beliefs, and possible dreams left undone. The phrase "midlife crisis," popularized by this theory, refers to a period of emotional, and sometimes behavioral, turmoil that heralds the onset of middle age. This period may last for several years, with the exact time and duration varying from person to person.

During this period, the individual often searches for answers about reaching goals, questioning whether a part of his or her personality or "true self" has been neglected and whether time is running out for the completion of these quests. This may be the first time the individual becomes aware of the effects of the aging process and the fact that the first part of the adult life is over. This realization does not necessarily signal a time of trauma. For many people, it is just another "rite of passage."

As the person ages chronologically, the personality often begins to change from being outwardly focused, concerned about establishing oneself in society, to becoming more inward, as the individual begins to search for answers from within. Successful aging, when viewed from Jung's theory, is when a person looks inward and values himself or herself for more than just current physical limitations or losses. The individual accepts past accomplishments and limitations (Jung, 1960).

Eight Stages Of Life

Erikson (1993) proposed a theory of psychologic development that reflects cultural and societal influences. The major focus of development in this theory is with an individual's ego structure, or sense of self, especially in response to the ways in which society shapes its development. In each of the eight stages identified by Erikson, a "crisis" occurs that affects the development of the person's ego. The manner in which a person masters any particular stage influences future success or lack of success in mastering the next stage of development.

When considering older adults, one must focus attention on the developmental tasks of both middle and older adulthood. The task of middle adulthood is resolving the conflict between generativity and stagnation. During older adulthood, the developmental task needing resolution is balancing the search for integrity and wholeness with a sense of despair (Table 2-1).

In 1968 Peck expanded Erikson's original theory regarding the eighth stage of older adulthood. Erikson grouped all individuals together into "old age" beginning at age 65, not anticipating that a person could live another 30 to 40 years beyond this milestone. Since people were living longer, there was an obvious need to identify additional stages for older adults. Peck (1968) expanded the eighth stage, ego integrity versus despair, into three stages: ego differentiation versus work role preoccupation, body transcendence versus body preoccupation, and ego transcendence versus ego preoccupation (Ignatavicius and Workman, 2005).

During the stage of ego differentiation versus work role preoccupation, the task for older adults is to achieve identity and feelings of worth from sources other than the work role. The onset of retirement and termination of the work role may reduce feelings of self-worth. In contrast, a person with a well-differentiated ego, who is defined by many dimensions, can replace the work role as the major defining source for self-esteem.

The second stage, body transcendence versus body preoccupation, refers to the older person's view of the physical changes that occur as a result of the aging process. The task is to adjust to or transcend the declines that may occur in order to maintain feelings of well-being. This task can be successfully

TABLE 2-1 Summary of Erikson's Theory: Middle and Older Adulthood

STAGES AND AGES	CHARACTERISTICS OF STAGES	THEORY ADDENDUM
GENERATIVITY VS. SELF-ABSORPTION OR STAGNATION		
40 to 65 years old; middle adulthood Mode: nurturing Virtue: care	Mature adults are concerned with establishing and guiding the next generation. Adults look beyond the self and express concern for the future of the world in general.	Self-absorbed adults will be preoccupied with their personal well-being and material gains. Preoccupation with self leads to stagnation of life.
EGO INTEGRITY VS. DESPAIR		
65 years to death; older adulthood Mode: acceptance Virtue: wisdom	Older adults can look back with a sense of satisfaction and acceptance of life and death.	Unsuccessful resolution of this crisis may result in a sense of despair in which individuals view life as a series of misfortunes, disappointments, and failures.

Modified from Potter PA, Perry AG: *Fundamentals of nursing,* ed 5, St Louis, 2004, Mosby.

resolved by focusing on the satisfaction obtained from interpersonal interactions and psychosocial activities.

The third and final task, ego transcendence versus ego preoccupation, involves acceptance of the individual's eventual death without dwelling on the prospect of it. Remaining actively involved with a future that extends beyond a person's mortality is the adjustment that must be made to achieve ego transcendence.

Selective Optimization With Compensation

Baltes (1987) has conducted a series of studies on the psychologic processes of development and aging from a life-span perspective and formulated a psychologic model of successful aging. This theory's central focus is that individuals develop certain strategies to manage the losses of function that occur over time. This general process of adaptation consists of three interacting elements. First, there is the element of selection, which refers to an increasing restriction of one's life to fewer domains of functioning because of an age-related loss. The second element, optimization, reflects the view that people engage in behaviors to enrich their lives. The third element, compensation, also results from restrictions caused by aging, requiring older adults to compensate for any losses by developing suitable, alternative adaptations (Schroots, 1996).

The lifelong process of selective optimization with compensation allows people to age successfully. Schroots (1996) used the famous pianist Rubinstein to illustrate an application of these elements. As he grew older, Rubinstein said he first reduced his repertoire and played a smaller number of pieces (selection); second, he practiced these more often (optimization); and third, he slowed down his playing right before fast movements, producing a contrast that enhanced the impression of speed in the fast movements (compensation). These concepts of selection, optimization, and compensation can be applied to any aspect of older adult life to demonstrate successful coping with declining functions.

Implications for Nursing

Integrating the psychologic aging theories into nursing practice becomes increasingly important as the population continues to age. Present and future generations can learn from the past. Older adults should be encouraged to engage in a "life review" process; this can be accomplished using a variety of techniques like reminiscence, oral histories, and story telling. Looking back over life's accomplishments or failures is crucial in assisting older adults to accomplish developmental tasks (as in ego integrity), to promote positive self-esteem, and to acknowledge that one "did not live in vain."

As nurses apply the psychologic theories to the care of older adults in any setting, they help dispel many of the myths about being old. If an older person is talking about retirement, worrying about physical living space, or even planning funeral arrangements, these are all part of the developmental tasks appropriate for this age group. Instead of trying to change the topic or encouraging the person not to be so "morbid," the nurse must understand that each stage of life has specific developmental tasks to achieve. Instead of hampering, the nurse should facilitate their achievement.

Nurses also need to keep in mind that intellectual functioning remains intact in the majority of older adults. A younger person can gain much by observing older persons, listening to how they have coped with life experiences, and discussing their plans for the future with them.

As did other humanistic psychologists, Maslow focused on the human potential, which sets an effective and positive foundation for nurse-client interactions. Maslow's theory also sets priorities for the nurse in relationship to client needs. Employing Maslow's theory, the nurse recognizes that the essential elements such as food, water, oxygen, elimination, and rest must be met prior to self-actualization needs. The nurse recognizes, for example, that client education will be more successful if clients are well rested (Carson and Arnold, 1996).

In planning activities for older adults, nurses need to remember that all individuals enjoy feeling needed and respected and being considered contributing members of society. Perhaps activities like collecting an oral history, creating a mural, or quilting a particular event or even an individual's lifetime could be included. Not only would such activities demonstrate that the individual is valued, but they would also serve to pass on information from one generation to the next; this is an important task that is often forgotten.

Programs promoting interaction between older adults and younger children might prove beneficial to all concerned. For some older adults, caring for small children represented a happy time in their lives. Rocking, cuddling, and playing with children might bring back feelings of being valued and needed. The touching aspects of this activity are also important in relieving stress; many older adults no longer experience any type of meaningful physical contact with others, yet all individuals need this type of contact.

As eyesight and manual dexterity diminish, many older adults enjoy the opportunity to cook or to work in a garden. Often the feel of dirt between the fingers is relaxing and brings back memories of beautiful flowers and prize vegetables. For the older woman in particular, preparing a meal may be an activity she has not been able to do for several years and, with assistance, she may find baking cookies a pleasant activity filled with memories of holidays and loved ones, or prizes at the county fair. Older men may also enjoy cooking and should not be left out of this activity. Preparing muffins for a morning snack would be an activity in which everyone could participate.

MORAL/SPIRITUAL DEVELOPMENT

Human beings seek to explain and validate their existence in the world. For many individuals this occurs through their development as moral and spiritual thinkers. Kolberg has postulated a theory of moral development that is based on interviews with young persons. He found there to be distinct sequential stages of moral thinking. Although he did not study older adults, parallels could be drawn between his highest stage of moral development, Universal Ethical Principles, and Maslow's highest level of Self-Transcendent Needs. In each instance only a small segment of the population reaches this highest level of development, where their personal needs are sublimated for the greater good of society (Edelman and Mandle, 2003; Levin and Chatters, 1998; Mehta, 1997).

It is important for the nurse to acknowledge the spiritual dimension of a person and support spiritual expression and growth (Hogstel, 1995). *Spirituality* no longer merely denotes religious affiliation; it synthesizes a person's contemplative experience. Illness, a life crisis, or even the recognition that our days on earth are limited may cause a person to contemplate spirituality. The nurse can assist clients in finding meaning in their life crises. Research has begun to explore the relationship between client-centered outcomes and spirituality. A correlation between successful outcomes and spirituality has been demonstrated in some of this research. Regardless of outcomes, nurses need to address spirituality as a component in holistic care (Phipps et al, 2003).

SUMMARY

When interacting with older adults, the nurse often plays a key role as the coordinator of the health care team. Nurses have the background to incorporate information from a variety of sources when planning care for older adults. By using an eclectic approach to aging theories, the nurse will have a broad background from which to draw specific details to provide clarity, explanations, or additional insight into a particular situation.

Biologic theories help the nurse understand how the physical body may change with advancing years and what factors may increase older adults' vulnerability to stress or disease. The nurse will also be able to develop health promotional strategies on behalf of older clients. Understanding sociologic theories broadens the nurse's view of older adults and their interactions with society. Psychologic theories provide an understanding of the values and beliefs an older person may possess. These theories enable a nurse to understand the phases of the life span and the developmental tasks faced by the aged population. By integrating the various components of these theories, nurses can plan high-quality care for older adults. As the population continues to age, nurses with the capability to understand and apply theories of aging from several disciplines will be the leaders of gerontologic nursing. These nurses will contribute to increasingly holistic care and an improved quality of life for older adults.

Key Points

- There is no one theory that explains the biologic, sociologic, or psychologic aging processes.
- An eclectic approach incorporating concepts from biology, sociology, and psychology was used in developing aging theories.
- Biologic theories must address what factors actually trigger the aging process in organisms.
- Humans are thought to have a maximum life span of 110 to 120 years.
- A change in the efficiency of immune processes may predispose individuals to disease with advancing age.
- Biologic theories alone *do not* provide a comprehensive explanation of the aging process.
- Reminiscence is supported by sociologic theories and assists older adults in appreciating past memories.
- Each individual, no matter what age, is unique. Older adults are not a homogeneous population.
- The activity theory remains popular because it reflects current societal beliefs about aging.
- As a person ages, various adaptive changes occur that may assist the person in coping with or accepting some of the biologic changes.
- Human development is a process that occurs over the life span.

Critical Thinking Exercises

1. Discuss how sociologic theories of aging may be influenced by changing societal values (e.g., advanced technology or a community health care focus) in the next decade.
2. A 62-year-old woman believes that heart disease and poor circulation are inevitable consequences of growing older and is resistant to altering her ADLs and dietary regimen. How would you respond?
3. Think of various programs and institutions in your community that care for older persons. Identify two and discuss the sociologic aging theories exemplified in each example.
4. A 74-year-old man repeatedly talks about how he wishes he were as strong and energetic as he was when he was younger. His family consistently changes the topic or criticizes him for being so grim. How would you intervene in this situation?
5. What health promotion strategies would you recommend to promote successful aging?
6. Imagine yourself at age 75. Describe your appearance, your health issues, and your lifestyle.

REFERENCES

Baltes PB: *Life-span development and behavior,* vol 7, 1987, Lawrence Erlbaum.

Birren JE, Cunningham WR: Research on the psychology of aging. In Birren JE, Scheie KW, editors: *Handbook of the psychology of aging,* New York, 1985, Van Nostrand Reinhold.

Bjorkstein J: The crosslinkage theory of aging: clinical implications, *Compr Ther* 11:65, 1976.
Black JM, Hawks JH: *Medical-surgical nursing: clinical management for positive outcomes,* Philadelphia, 2005, WB Saunders.
Carson VB, Arnold EN: *Mental health nursing, the nurse-patient journey,* Philadelphia, 1996, WB Saunders.
Carter KF: Behaviors of older men in the community: correlates producing active composure, *J Gerontal Nurs* 29(10): 37, 2003.
Cetron M, Davies O: Extended lifespans: are you ready to live to 120 or more? *Futurist* 32(3):17, 1998.
Comfort A: Biological theories of aging, *Human Development* 13:127, 1970.
Cumming E, Henry W: *Growing old: the process of disengagement,* New York, 1961, Basic Books.
Cupp MJ: Melatonin, *Amer Fam Phys* 56(5):1421, 1997.
Edelman CL, Mandle CL: *Health promotion throughout the lifespan,* ed 5, St Louis, 2003, Mosby.
Erikson E: *Childhood and society,* ed 35, New York, 1993, WW Norton.
Gerhard G, Cristofalo V: The limits of biogerontology, *Generations* 16(4):55, 1992.
Goldstein S: The biology of aging: looking to defuse the time bomb, *Geriatrics* 48(9):76, 1993.
Guardiola-Lemaitre B: Toxicology of melatonin, *J Biol Rhythms* 12(6):693, 1997.
Gupta J, Han LP: Development of retinoblastoma in the absence of telomerase activity, *J Amer Cancer Institute* 8(16):1152, 1996.
Harman D: Aging: a theory based on free radical and radiation chemistry, *J Gerontol* 11:298, 1956.
Havighurst RJ: *Developmental tasks and education,* ed 3, New York, 1972, David McKay.
Havighurst RJ, Albrecht R: *Older people,* New York, 1953, Longmans, Green.
Havighurst RJ, Neugarten BL, Tobin SS: Disengagement, personality and life satisfaction in the later years. In Hansen P, editor: *Age with a future,* Copenhagen, 1963, Munksgoasrd.
Hayflick L: *How and why we age,* New York, 1996, Ballantine Books.
Hayflick L: Why do we live so long? *Geriatrics* 43(10):77, 1988.
Hayflick L, Moorehead PS: The serial cultivation of human diploid all strains, *Exp Cell Res* 25:585, 1961.
Hogstel MO: *Geropsychiatric nursing,* ed 2, St Louis, 1995, Mosby.
Holstein M: Qualitative gerontology, *Res Aging* 17(1):114, 1995.
Ignatavicius DD, Workman ML: *Medical-surgical nursing: critical thinking for collaborative care,* ed 5, St Louis, 2005, Saunders.
Jung C: The stages of life. In *Collected works: the structure and dynamics of the psyche,* vol 8, New York, 1960, Pantheon Books.
Kendler BS: Melatonin: media hype or therapeutic breakthrough, *Nurs Pract: Amer J Primary Health Care* 22(2):66, 71, 77, 1997.
Keys SW, Marble M: In vivo data demonstrates critical role for telomeres, *Cancer Weekly Plus* May 4, 1998, p 11.
Lawton MP: Competence, environmental press, and the adaptation of older people. In Lawton MP, Windley PG, Byerts TO, editors: *Aging and the environment: theoretical approaches,* New York, 1982, Springer.
Levin JS, Chatters LM: Religion, health, and psychological well-being in older adults: findings from three national surveys, *J Aging Health* 10(4):504, 1998.
Maslow A: *Toward a psychology of being,* ed 2, Princeton, NJ, 1968, Van Nostrand Reinhold.
Maslow A: *Motivation and personality,* New York, 1954, Harper & Row.
Mehta KK: The impact of religious beliefs and practices on aging: a cross-cultural comparison, *J Aging Studies* 11(2):101, 1997.
Peck R: Psychological development in the second half of life. In Neugarten B, editor: *Middle age and aging,* Chicago, 1968, University of Chicago Press.
Phipps WJ et al: *Medical-surgical nursing: health and illness perspectives,* ed 7, St Louis, 2003, Mosby.
Riley MW: Age strata in social systems. In Binstock RH, Shanas E, editors: *Handbook of aging and social sciences,* New York, 1985, Van Nostrand Reinhold.
Riley MW, Johnson M, Foner A: *Aging and society: a sociology of age stratification,* vol 3, New York, 1972, Russel Stage Foundation.
Schneider E: Biological theories of aging, *Generations* 16(4):7, 1992.
Schroots E: Theoretical developments in the psychology of aging, *Gerontologist* 36(6):742, 1996.
Sonneborn T: The origin, evolution, nature and causes of aging. In Behnke J, Finch CE, Moment C, editors: *The biology of aging,* New York, 1979, Plenum Press.
Thomas A, Chess S: *Temperament and development,* New York, 1977, Brunner/Masel.
Yu BP: *Methods in aging research,* Boca Raton, Fla, 1998, CRC Press.
Yu BP: *Free radicals in aging,* Boca Raton, Fla, 1993, CRC Press.

3 Legal and Ethical Issues

SUE E. MEINER, EdD, APRN, BC, GNP

Learning Objectives

On completion of this chapter, the reader will be able to:

1. Discuss how professional standards are used to measure the degree to which the legal duties of nursing care of clients are met.
2. State the sources and definitions of laws, such as statutes, regulations, and case law, as well as the levels of laws, such as federal, state, and local.
3. Explore why older adults are considered a vulnerable population, why this is legally significant, and the legal implications of such a designation.
4. Discuss the reasons behind the sweeping nursing facility reform legislation known as the Omnibus Budget Reconciliation Act of 1987, and understand its continuing significance and impact for residents and caregivers in nursing facilities.
5. Identify the Omnibus Budget Reconciliation Act's three major parts, and describe the key areas addressed in each.
6. Discuss the legal history of the doctrine of autonomy and self-determination, and cite major laws that have influenced contemporary thought and practice.
7. Identify the three broad categories of elder abuse, define seven types of abuse, and discuss the responsibility of the nurse in responding to suspected abuse of older adults.
8. Name and state the purpose of the legal tools known as "advance directives," and list the major points that should be addressed in a Do Not Resuscitate policy.
9. Explain the requirements of the four major provisions of the Patient Self-Determination Act and the nurse's responsibility with respect to advance directives.
10. Describe the values history and how it can help clients and health care professionals in preparing for end-of-life decisions.
11. Identify at least three ethical issues nurses may face in caring for older adults, considering the areas of care of the terminally ill, organ donation, and self-determination.
12. State the function and role, as well as the recommended membership composition, of an institutional ethics committee.
13. Relate at least three major reasons why the skillful practice of professional nursing can improve the quality of life for older adults in health care settings.

The needs of older adults have come to the forefront as the nation's demographics change, with a significant increase in the U.S. population over the age of 65. According to the Social Security Administration, there will be between 64 million and 74 million older adults in the United States by the year 2030, when the baby boomer generation enters its 70s and 80s—more than twice the older adult population of 1980 (American Association of Retired Persons [AARP], 1998). According to the U.S. Bureau of the Census, this will amount to approximately 21% of the total U.S. population. For most situations discussed in this chapter, older adults are defined as those age 65 or older.

During the Social Security "crisis" of 1982, certain implications of this aging population in the United States became apparent (Manton, 1991). Realization that the projections of life span used to forecast the use of the Social Security Trust Fund had significantly underestimated the size of the older adult population in future years was finally apparent.

The conclusion that there would be many more older Americans in future years raised major concerns about the economic effects on Social Security and Medicare. Health changes occur more often as people age. Nearly a fourth of the older adult population has some form of disability for which they require assistance (Scanlon, 1998). The aging of the population will lead to a tremendous increase in the older adult population in the next 3 decades and an even larger increase in the 85-and-over population, who are more likely to require long-term care services (Scanlon, 1998).

Medicaid, a government payment program for the needy, is the largest single payer for nursing facility care. Although Medicare pays for only a limited duration of nursing facility care, it is still a substantial source of coverage for most other types of general health and rehabilitation care for older persons (Krauss et al, 1997). For example, the federal government paid nursing facilities nearly $28 billion in 1997 (GAO/HEHS Report 98-202, 1998). In 2002 payments to skilled nursing facilities increased by an additional $1.5 billion as the result of "Medicare Program; Prospective payment system and consolidated billing for skilled nursing facilities update" (RIN:

0938-AK47). The government's concerns over whether there will be enough money available to continue to provide service to older adults, who consume the largest percentage of these services, has led to measures designed to improve efficiency and to reduce the cost of specific services, while the overall costs increase.

An important example is the Prospective Payment System (PPS). PPS was initially designed to control Medicare hospitalization costs by establishing reimbursement through diagnosis-related groups (DRGs). Medicare payment under a prospective system began in 1983. DRGs group and classify diseases and establish in advance what the reimbursement level will be for a person receiving treatment for that specific condition. As a result of this program, a reported $18 billion was saved by the year 1990 (Manton, 1991). Similar systems will continue to be implemented and expanded into other areas of government-reimbursed services to older adults, such as home care and nursing facility care.

Simply stated, programs such as the PPS save money by changing reimbursement principals and reconfiguring the manner in which services are provided. Some of the results are already visible—shorter hospital stays, older persons discharged sooner to the home or long-term care facility, and the enactment of strict rules governing the use of resources in providing their care.

The implications for nurses are significant. Older, sicker clients leave hospitals more rapidly. They return home or to institutional settings sicker than before, and high-quality care must be provided even with restrictions in reimbursement that can limit resource availability.

More recently, Medicare Part C has been introduced. Established as a part of the Balanced Budget Act of 1997, Medicare Part C provides beneficiaries access to a wide array of health plans from which to receive their Medicare benefits (Grimaldi, 1997). In addition to the fee-for-service plans and health maintenance organizations (HMOs) that have served Medicare beneficiaries, these initiatives are cost-cutting measures; the Medicare program may benefit from a wider range of potential service providers, thus reaping some of the benefits of cost competition.

Thus there is good reason to be concerned about how the health needs of older adults will be met. Their unique characteristics and needs present meaningful questions of legal and ethical significance. As their functional independence is compromised and they become more reliant on health care that is paid for through public funds, the policies that accompany the flow of money can interfere in many ways with their personal autonomy (Kane and Kane, 1990).

Older adults depend more than younger persons on the health care system to deliver the care that optimizes their health status and functional capabilities. Thus their quality of life often depends on the type and quality of nursing care they receive (Northrop and Kelly, 1987). This chapter focuses on the issues and legal concerns of nurses who care for older adults.

PROFESSIONAL STANDARDS: THEIR ORIGIN AND LEGAL SIGNIFICANCE

Health care providers have a general obligation to live up to accepted or customary standards of care, which may be determined on either a regional or a national basis (*Health care facility management*, 1990). Nurses are responsible for providing care to the degree, skill, and diligence measured and recognized by applicable standards of care. The duty of care rises as clients' physical and mental conditions and ability for self-care decline (Strauss et al, 1990).

Nursing standards of practice are measured according to the expected level of professional practice of those in similar roles and clinical fields. For example, the standards of practice of a gerontologic nurse practicing at the generalist level would be measured against the practice of other nurse generalists practicing in the area of gerontology. The advanced practice gerontologic nurse, who has at least a master's degree in an applicable field, would be expected to conform to standards established for similarly situated advanced practice nurses.

A standard of care is a guideline for nursing practice and establishes an expectation for the nurse to provide safe and appropriate care (Potter and Perry, 2004). It is used to evaluate whether care administered to clients meets the appropriate level of skill and diligence that can reasonably be expected, given the nurse's level of skill, education, and experience.

Standards originate from many sources. Both state and federal statutes may help establish standards, although conformity with a state's minimum standards does not necessarily prove that due care was provided. Conformity with local standards or comparison with similar facilities in the region may be considered evidence of proper care (Strauss et al, 1990).

The published standards of professional organizations, representing the opinion of experts in the field, are important in establishing the proper standard of care. The *Scope and Standards of Gerontological Nursing Practice,* published by the American Nurses Association (ANA) in 1995, is one example. However, in 2004 the ANA combined the scope and standards of practice into one book for all practice areas (ANA, 2004). Nurses who care for older clients should be familiar with these standards and those from all relevant sources.

Most health care facilities, at some point, seek accreditation status. This means that they voluntarily undergo a detailed survey by an organization with the skill and expertise to evaluate their services. One of the best known accreditation organizations is the Joint Commission on Accreditation of Healthcare Organizations (JCAHO). Since it is a well-known and long-existing organization, the standards established and used by the JCAHO to review health care facilities are often referred to in court cases to ascertain the appropriate standard of care. Thus the JCAHO is often considered the "industry standard," even for facilities that are not accredited (Schreiber, 1990).

Federal and state statutes require nursing facilities to have written health care and safety policies, which have been used successfully to establish a standard of care in court cases. Bylaws and internal rules and policies also help establish the standard of care in an organization, although, depending on the circumstances, their importance may vary. In any event, it is important for nurses to be aware of their organization's policies; failure to follow "your own rules" clearly poses a liability risk—both to the nurse and the organization.

OVERVIEW OF RELEVANT LAWS

Sources of Law

Statutes are laws created by legislation and can be enacted at the federal and state level. Common laws are principles and rules of action, which derive authority from judgments and decrees of the court, and are also known as case law (Black, 1979). Regulations are rules of action and conduct developed to explain and interpret statutes and to prescribe methods for carrying out statutory mandates. Regulations are also promulgated at the federal and state levels.

Federal and State Laws

The federal government, under the Social Security Act, has the primary responsibility for providing medical services to certain aged and indigent Americans. The government fulfills this obligation through the Medicare and Medicaid programs (Schabes, 1991). These programs were enacted as part of the Social Security Amendments of 1965 (P.L. No. 89-97, July 30, 1965).[1]

The U.S. Department of Health and Human Services (DHHS) promulgated regulations for the Medicare and Medicaid programs until July 1, 2001. At that time the Health Care Financing Administration (HCFA) became the Centers for Medicare and Medicaid Services, with the acronym CMS. The restructured agency aims to increase emphasis on responsiveness to the beneficiaries and providers, with quality improvement as a goal. Then Health and Human Services Secretary Tommy G. Thompson made the announcement on June 14, 2001. "We're making quality service the number one priority in this agency," said Thompson.

Two levels of care are generally associated with nursing facilities: intermediate and skilled. Skilled nursing facilities (SNFs) provide technical and complex care and offer more skilled levels of professional staff. Medicare pays only for skilled care, which includes nursing, physical therapy, occupational therapy, and speech therapy, for Medicare-insured persons in long-term care facilities. Medicaid pays for both intermediate and skilled care for indigent persons. Intermediate care is custodial and is supervised by professional nurses.

The Omnibus Budget Reconciliation Act of 1987 (OBRA), refers to SNFs only in relation to Medicare facilities and has merged the distinctions *skilled* and *intermediate* into the single term *nursing facility* for Medicaid purposes (as of OBRA's effective date, October 1, 1990). For survey purposes a single set of survey requirements is used. However, these designations are used for reimbursement and survey purposes only and are presented here to assist in understanding what is meant by the terms in connection with reimbursement or survey activities.

Survey and certification procedures, and the process by which CMS evaluates and determines whether a provider is in compliance with the Medicare and Medicaid requirements, are the responsibilities of the Health Standards and Quality Bureau within CMS.

Continued public policy interest in the welfare and quality of life of older adults in the United States is expressed in other legislation such as the Older Americans Act (OAA), which requires states to maintain a minimum bureaucratic system to perform various services for older adults. The objectives of the OAA are to secure basic rights for all older adults in the United States. It defines older adults as those over the age of 60.

The *OAA Amendments* (1988) increase states' responsibilities for maintaining an effective long-term care ombudsman program. Ombudsmen are usually trained volunteers. Their role is to receive and resolve health and human services complaints affecting residents in nursing facilities. Nursing facilities must cooperate with and must provide access for the ombudsman to meet with residents. The OAA programs continue to operate even though the act, which was originally enacted in 1965, expired in 1995. As of the 105th Congress in 1998, Congress has not reauthorized the act. The result is that while programs for older adults continue, funding levels have suffered. At the direction of the President, CMS sought a long-term reauthorization from Congress in 1999 to ensure the availability of ombudsmen to assist in monitoring the care of older Americans in the nations' nursing facilities (HCFA, 1998).

Health Insurance Portability and Accountability Act of 1996 (HIPAA)

Recent changes in federal law now give additional, though limited, protections to individuals and their family members when they need to buy, change, or continue their health insurance. These important laws can affect the health benefits of millions of working Americans and their families. It is important that nurses understand these new protections, as well as laws in their state, to help them make more informed choices for themselves or to inform their patients of the options available. The Health Insurance Portability and Accountability Act of 1996 (HIPAA) may:

1. Increase a person's ability to get health care coverage when the person begins a new job
2. Lower the chance of losing existing health coverage, whether the coverage is through a job or through individual health insurance

[1]42 U.S.C. § 3001 (1965).

3. Help maintain continuous health coverage when a change of job occurs
4. Help purchase health insurance coverage individually if the coverage is lost under an employer's group health plan and no other health coverage is available (HIPPA, 2004)

Among the specific protections of HIPAA, it:

1. Limits the use of preexisting condition exclusions
2. Prohibits group health plans from discriminating by denying coverage or charging extra for coverage based on the person's or a family member's past or present poor health
3. Guarantees certain small employers, and certain individuals who lost job-related coverage, the right to purchase health insurance
4. Guarantees, in most cases, that employers or individuals who purchase health insurance can renew the coverage regardless of any health conditions of individuals covered under the insurance policy (HIPAA, 2004)

There are several misunderstandings about what HIPAA provides. Note that:

1. HIPAA does *not* require employers to offer or pay for health coverage for employees or family coverage for spouses and dependents.
2. HIPAA does *not* guarantee health coverage for all workers.
3. HIPAA does *not* control the amount an insurer may charge for coverage.
4. HIPAA does *not* require group health plans to offer specific benefits.
5. HIPAA does *not* permit people to keep the same health coverage they had in their old job when they move to a new job.
6. HIPAA does *not* eliminate all use of preexisting condition exclusions.
7. HIPAA does *not* replace the state as the primary regulator of health insurance (HIPAA, 2004).

OLDER ADULT ABUSE AND PROTECTIVE SERVICES

It has already been noted that the incidence of illness and disability increases with age. Old-old adults, those over age 85, make up the fastest growing group (Zedlewski et al., 1989), and their health status often leads to changes in living arrangements both in homes and in institutions. These changes affect not only older adults, but often their family and others who must see to their care and living needs (see Chapter 1). These conditions can lead to neglect, deliberate abuse, or exploitation of older adults.

As older adults' abilities to manage their affairs are compromised, the necessity of turning the management of certain activities over to others may open the door to mistreatment. The legal recognition of this vulnerability is reflected in laws enacted specifically to protect older adults.

This need to protect older adults from abuse is a subject of growing public policy interest. In 1981 researchers estimated that 10% of the U.S. older adult population, or 2.5 million people, were victims of various forms of elder abuse. In 1996 it was estimated that there were between 820,000 and 1,860,000 abused elders in the country (National Center for Elder Abuse [NCEA], 1998). However, given the potential for hiding incidents of elder abuse in domestic settings as a "family secret," the incidents of elder abuse are likely grossly underreported.

Elder abuse is defined by state laws, which vary from state to state. However, there are three basic categories of elder abuse: (1) domestic elder abuse, (2) institutional elder abuse, and (3) self-neglect or self-abuse (NCEA, 1998). Domestic elder abuse refers to forms of maltreatment by someone who has a special relationship with the elder, such as a family member or caregiver. Institutional abuse refers to abuse that occurs in residential institutions such as nursing facilities, usually by someone who is a paid caregiver, such as a nursing facility staff member. Within these three broad categories are a number of recognized types of elder abuse.

An analysis of existing state and federal definitions of elder abuse, neglect, and exploitation conducted by the NCEA (National Center for Elder Abuse, 1998) identified seven different kinds of elder abuse:

1. Physical abuse—use of physical force that may result in bodily injury, physical pain, or impairment
2. Sexual abuse—nonconsensual sexual contact of any kind with an older adult
3. Emotional abuse—infliction of anguish, pain, or distress through verbal or nonverbal acts
4. Financial and material exploitation—illegal or improper use of an elder's funds, property, or assets
5. Neglect—the refusal or failure of a person to fulfill any part of his or her obligations or duties to an older adult
6. Abandonment—the desertion of an older adult by an individual who has physical custody of the elder or by a person who has assumed responsibility for providing care to the elder
7. Self-neglect—behaviors of an older adult that threaten the elder's health or safety

Elder abuse generally occurs as the result of a number of complex factors. Abuse may be a result of caregiver stress. The physical and emotional demands of caring for a physically or mentally impaired person can be great, and the caregiver may not be prepared to undertake the responsibility. Supportive resources may also be lacking. It has been found that abuse tends to occur when the caregiver's stress level is heightened by the elder person's worsening condition (NCEA, 1998).

Nurses must be alert to signs and symptoms of abuse. Signs of physical abuse may be visible, such as bruises, wounds, or fractures. They may also be less apparent, such as an elder's report of being hit or mistreated or a sudden change in behavior. Sexual abuse may be detectable by signs such as bruises in the genital area or unexplained vaginal bleeding. But other forms of abuse such as the taking of pornographic photographs may be more difficult to detect. Signs of neglect may include living in unclean conditions or being malnourished or dehydrated. In addition, the nurse should be alert to signs of financial or material exploitation such as the unexplained disappearance of funds or valuable possessions.

Because signs and symptoms of elder abuse in its many forms can be difficult to detect, the nurse must be educated in this regard and must be alert to the actions of others involved in the care of older adults, such as nursing attendants. It has been shown that the primary abusers of nursing facility residents are nurse aides and orderlies who have never received training in stress management, and who are working in facilities that show evidence of administrative problems such as high staff turnover (Keller, 1996).

A training program designed specifically for nurse aides in long-term care facilities, providing information about abuse, including possible causes and conflict intervention strategies, was tested on 216 nurse aides in the Philadelphia area. In this study, training was shown to bring about significant improvement in attitudes toward residents, conflict with residents, resident aggression toward staff, and self-reported abuse actions by staff (Keller, 1996). This may suggest that training can serve as an effective abuse prevention strategy, and expansion to other care settings may be important in preventing abuse of older adults.

"Adult protective services" refers to the range of laws and regulations enacted to deal with abusive situations. The laws and regulations are typically administered by an agency within the state, such as the Department of Social Services, which receives and investigates complaints. Specific responses to safeguard abused or at-risk elders can include protective orders issued to shield older adults from abusive members of their households; elder abuse statutes, which outlaw harmful acts that victimize older adults; and laws to protect older residents of nursing facilities from abuse (Strauss et al, 1990).

Elder abuse laws levy criminal penalties against those who commit harmful acts against older adults. Many states' laws enhance the penalties for criminal offenses against older persons, such as violent or property-related offenses, and some outlaw any acts that victimize older adults (e.g., see Conn. Gen. Statutes Ann. § 46a-15). These laws typically apply to the abuse of older adults in the community.

States may also levy penalties for acts of elder abuse committed by those who are responsible for the care of older adults in nursing facilities or other institutions (Strauss et al, 1990). These laws are in addition to those already in effect to protect the rights of clients in facilities governed by federal regulation. Most states have mandatory reporting requirements for nurses, other health care workers, and facility employees who have a reasonable suspicion of elder abuse.

The definition of what constitutes elder abuse under these statutes varies. For example, emotional abuse can be acts such as "ridiculing or demeaning . . . or making derogatory remarks to a . . . resident"[2]; "any non-accidental infliction of physical injury, sexual abuse, or mental injury"[3]; and "unauthorized use of physical or chemical restraint, medication, or isolation."[4]

For the purposes of these types of statutes, some states define older adults as those ages 60 and older. It is important for a nurse to know the legal requirements relating to the abuse of older adults for the state in which he or she practices.

Most states designate certain professionals or other caregivers as "mandated reporters." This means that the mandated reporter is *required* by law to report suspected cases of abuse, neglect, or exploitation. Failure to report as required under this law can result in imposition of civil and/or criminal penalties.

In 1996, 22.5% of all domestic elder abuse reports came from physicians and other health care professionals, while another 15.1% came from service providers, such as the staff of agencies providing services to older adults (NCEA, 1998).

A report of suspected abuse may be required on a "reasonable suspicion." This implies that actual knowledge or certainty is not necessary. Most states provide immunity from civil liability for anyone reporting older adult abuse based on reasonable suspicion and in good faith, even if it is later shown that the reporter was mistaken. However, it is interesting to note that the majority of elder abuse reports are in fact substantiated after investigation. In 1996, 64.2% of all reports made were substantiated (NCEA, 1998).

In most care settings, the nurse is a mandated reporter. To be responsive to this legal obligation and because there is great variation among the states, the nurse should determine the specific reporting requirements of his or her jurisdiction, including where reports and complaints are received and in what form they must be made.

Nurses must be aware at all times of the responsibility to respect and to preserve the autonomy and individual rights of older adults. All people, including older adults, have the right to decide what is to be done to them, as well as the right to exercise maximum control of their personal environments and living conditions. The nurse's responsibility in this regard emanates from both legal and professional standards.

The fact of ongoing legislative responses to the identification and preservation of these rights underscores this point. The nurse is often the health professional closest to older clients and therefore may be in the best position to communicate and understand their wishes. This presents both an unequaled opportunity and a legally recognizable and indisputable responsibility to advocate on their behalf. Thus the need to be legally informed and professionally conscientious is greater than ever.

[2]Delaware Title 16 § § 1132 and 1135.

[3]Illinois Chapter $111^1/_2$¶ 4161-176.

[4]California Welfare and Institutions § § 15600-15637.

NURSING FACILITY REFORM

In 1985 5% of the older adult population resided in nursing facilities (1.5 million persons) (Collier, 1990). Over 1.6 million older adults and disabled persons receive care in approximately 16,800 nursing facilities across the United States (HCFA, 1998). CMS estimates that by the year 2010, 10.8% of the older adult population will reside in nursing facilities. Half of persons over the age of 85 require long-term care.

During the 1970s disturbing evidence emerged from studies, reports, and books suggesting widespread abuse of residents in the nation's nursing facilities, and suggesting that state and federal officials were lax in regulating the facilities (Hamme, 1991). In 1983 the DHHS contracted with the Institute of Medicine of the National Academy of Sciences to conduct a comprehensive study of federal and state regulations and policies for nursing facility certification and to formulate recommendations for legislative and agency action (Hamme, 1991). This study served as the impetus for nursing facility reform (*Suffering in silence,* 1993), and many of the recommendations of the study were adopted by the U.S. Congress when it enacted OBRA in 1987 (Hamme, 1991). Coupled with the increasing challenges of meeting the needs of the aging population, Congress passed OBRA, a sweeping new form of legislation that brought about dramatic changes in the way nursing facilities in this country are run.

OBRA applies to all Medicare- and Medicaid-certified nursing facilities, including (1) beds in acute care hospitals certified to be used as long-term nursing care beds at times when they are not needed for acute care purposes (so-called swing beds), and (2) beds in acute care hospitals certified as separate units for Medicare-approved services (so-called distinct part units) (Collier, 1990). It is the most sweeping reform affecting Medicare and Medicaid nursing facilities since the programs began.

Since OBRA was enacted, there have been amendments and new regulations. The discussion of OBRA in this chapter encompasses any changes made as of the printing of this text, including OBRA '90 and any subsequent modifications.

There is clear evidence that the health and safety of nursing facility residents has improved as a result of these tough regulations and sweeping reforms. Such improvements, among other things, include less overuse of antipsychotic drugs, a reduction in the inappropriate use of restraints, and a reduction in the inappropriate use of indwelling urinary catheters. Since 2001, CMS has increased the number of penalties levied on poor quality nursing facilities (CMS, 2004).

However, CMS has also identified areas requiring greater regulatory oversight. Nursing facility surveys are too predictable and are rarely conducted on weekends or during evening hours. Some states rarely cite nursing facilities for substandard care, an indication that their inspections may be inadequate. Nursing facility residents continue to suffer from pressure ulcers and skin breakdown, malnutrition and dehydration, and various forms of abuse (CMS, 2004). For these reasons, new enforcement tools are being added to the regulatory oversight of the nations' nursing facilities. Some of these additional measures are discussed in the following section.

OBRA'S Three Major Parts

OBRA provisions are divided into three parts: (1) provision of service requirements for nursing facilities, (2) survey and certification process, and (3) enforcement mechanisms and sanctions.

The provision of service requirements for nursing facilities includes resident assessments, preadmission and annual screening of residents, maintenance of minimal nurse staffing levels, required and approved nurse aide training programs and competency levels, professional social worker services in facilities with 120 or more beds, and the important focus on specifying and ensuring resident rights.

The survey and certification process was substantially revised with the enactment of OBRA. New types of surveys were established to evaluate facilities. In brief, each facility is subject to a standard annual survey. Any change in facility management or ownership is further evaluated by a "special" survey. If any survey suggests that care may be substandard, the facility may be subject to a more detailed "extended" survey. States are also evaluated for the effectiveness of their survey process through a "validation" survey. Furthermore, the federal authorities may make an independent and binding determination of a facility's compliance through a "special compliance" survey.

OBRA also brought a new range of enforcement mechanisms and sanctions. Thus a number of corrective measures can be applied to repair deficiencies, based on the severity of the risk to residents. These three OBRA provisions are discussed further in the following sections.

Overall the regulations focus on the quality of life of nursing facility residents and emphasize their individual rights. OBRA has created a new regulatory environment by empowering residents, giving them a greater say in these quality of life issues (Salkin, 1991).

Provision of Service Requirements

Quality of Care. Nursing facility residents must be assessed to identify medical problems, describe their capacity to perform daily life functions, and note any significant impairments in their functional capacity. In Medicare- and Medicaid-certified long-term care facilities, physicians evaluate residents at the time of admission, at 30 days and 90 days, when a change in condition occurs, and at 1 year. The government's final regulations permitted certified nurse practitioners to certify the necessity for skilled nursing services for residents of nursing facilities (Vaca and Daake, 1998). A state-specified instrument must be used to conduct the assessment, which is based on a uniform data set, referred to as the minimum data set (MDS), established by the DHHS.

The assessment is used to develop a written and comprehensive plan of care for each resident. The plan must quantify expected levels of functioning and must be reviewed quarterly. MDS assessment categories include resident background, daily pattern of activity, cognition, physical functioning, psychosocial status, health problems, and specific body systems. Certain responses on the MDS, called resident assessment protocols (RAPs), are designed to prompt more thorough assessment and evaluation of common clinical problems (Vaca and Daake, 1998).

A similar uniform approach to assessment of adult home care clients, known as the Outcome and Assessment Information Set (OASIS), is being tested in a number of locations across the country. The goal of this tool is to provide a set of essential data items necessary for measuring client outcomes that have utility for such purposes as outcome monitoring, clinical assessment, and care planning. CMS is likely to issue new rules relating to home health agencies that include the required collection of OASIS data.

The assessment and planning of care for nursing facility residents is a most important role for the professional nurse. As can be seen from this discussion of nursing facility reform, it is a central point for determining the care and services that particular residents will need. Careful assessment and planning are time consuming and also require the professional nurse to be skilled and knowledgeable in carrying out these functions.

Because of the complexity of the rules and regulations governing nursing facilities, the current trend is to employ better qualified administrators and nursing directors. However, since most nursing facilities rely to a great degree on reimbursement from Medicare and Medicaid, which may not pay for some of these services, the numbers of nursing facility staff have been reduced to keep expenses at an acceptable level (Conely and Campbell, 1991).

The advent of OBRA and nursing facility reform has ushered in a new phase of professional accountability. It has increased the demands on nursing time and performance, has forced nursing facilities to change the structure of their operation, and has resulted in a different image of what nursing facilities are and how they care for their residents.

Medicare SNFs and Medicaid nursing facilities must have licensed nursing services available 24 hours a day, 7 days a week. A registered professional nurse must be on duty at least 8 hours a day, 7 days a week.

Nursing assistants must be trained according to regulatory specifications and pass state-approved competency evaluations. They must receive classroom training before any contact with residents and must receive training in areas such as interpersonal skills, infection control, safety procedures, and resident rights (Hamme, 1991). They also must have 6 hours of in-service education each quarter to ensure ongoing competency (Vaca and Daake, 1998).

Nursing assistants often make up the largest number of employees in nursing facilities. In addition, they have the greatest turnover rate of any employee group. In 1993 the turnover rate of nursing assistants (or nurse aides) was 43.7% (Marion Merrell Dow Inc, 1994); the rate is much higher or lower in some locations. Since they provide most of the direct care for nursing facility residents, it is not surprising that stringent requirements for their training and evaluation have been enacted.

Resident Rights. A primary thrust of OBRA's nursing facility reform provisions is to protect and promote the rights of residents to enhance their quality of life. Thus the legislation contains numerous requirements to ensure the preservation of a resident's rights.[5]

OBRA imposed new disclosure obligations on nursing facilities to apprise residents of their rights; these require that residents be notified, both orally and in writing, of their rights and responsibilities and of all rules governing resident conduct. This notification and disclosure must take place before or up to the time of admission and must be updated and reviewed during the course of residents' stays. Box 3-1 shows a sample of OBRA's resident bill of rights statements, as adapted from the Code of Federal Regulations.

Most facilities have developed a contract for new residents (or a family member or other responsible person) to sign at the time of admission. This is usually called the admission

BOX 3-1 Resident Bill of Rights

A facility must protect and must promote the exercise of rights for all residents.

The following are some of those rights:

1. The right to select a personal attending physician and to receive complete information about one's care and treatment, including access to all records pertaining to the resident
2. Freedom from physical or mental abuse, corporal punishment, involuntary seclusion, and any unwarranted physical or chemical restraints
3. Privacy with regard to accommodations, medical treatment, mail and telephone communication, visits, and meetings of family and resident groups
4. Confidentiality regarding personal and clinical records
5. Residing in a facility and receiving services with reasonable accommodation of individual needs and preferences
6. Protesting one's treatment or care without discrimination or reprisal, including the refusal to participate in experimental research
7. Participation in resident and family groups
8. Participation in social, religious, and community activities
9. The right to examine the federal or state authorities' surveys of a nursing facility

Modified from 42 CFR § 483.10.

[5]OBRA '87 at § 4211(a), 42 U.S.C.A. § 139r(c) (West Supp 1989).

agreement. This agreement sets forth the rights, obligations, and expectations of each party. It is a good way to inform residents of a facility's rules, regulations, and philosophy of care. Thus it is a practical way to meet OBRA's notification and disclosure requirements.

As with any agreement, it can only be a valid contract if the parties entering into the agreement are capable of understanding its provisions. If a resident is not capable of doing this, then a family member or other responsible person may sign on the resident's behalf. The laws of the particular state should be explored to determine who has standing to contract on behalf of the resident.

OBRA limits the ability of a facility to transfer or discharge residents to the following situations: (1) if the facility cannot meet the residents' needs, (2) if their stay is no longer required for their medical condition, (3) if they fail to pay for their care as agreed to, or (4) if the facility ceases to operate. These provisions are designed to establish the basic right of a resident to remain in a facility and not be transferred involuntarily unless one of these conditions exists; they also ensure that a resident has been given proper notice with the opportunity to appeal the decision. This was, in part, a response to situations in which older residents of nursing facilities were "ousted" without notice and perhaps without regard to the detrimental effects (both physical and emotional) of being uprooted from familiar surroundings.

The requirement for a bill of rights for residents is not an entirely new item on the landscape. Many states have had such provisions in their facility licensure statutes for many years. Medicare and Medicaid regulations have included resident rights requirements for some time as well. OBRA strengthened and enhanced the importance of these requirements by enforcing them as part of the facility survey process. Although the specific contents of resident's rights laws vary considerably from state to state, both the state and federal contents have some similarities. In particular, both are concerned with participation in medical decision making, privacy, dignity, access to visitors and services, ability to pursue grievances, selection of a physician, and transfer and discharge rights (Johnson, 1991).

Unnecessary Drug Use and Chemical and Physical Restraints. OBRA requires that nursing facility residents be free from unnecessary drugs of all types; from chemical restraints, commonly thought of as psychotropic drugs; and from physical restraints. Chemical restraints are drugs that are used to limit or inhibit specific behaviors or movements. Physical restraints are appliances that inhibit free physical movement, such as limb restraints, vests, jackets, and waist belts. Wheelchairs, geriatric chairs, and side rails can, in some circumstances, also be forms of physical restraint (Conely and Campbell, 1991).

OBRA's guidelines for unnecessary drug use pertain to the use of antipsychotics, benzodiazepines, other anxiolytic and sedative drugs, and hypnotics. As of this writing, CMS has not developed guidelines concerning antidepressant use, since it is believed that depression is undertreated and underrecognized in nursing facilities.

The drug use guidelines are based on the principles that certain problems can be handled with nondrug interventions and that such forms of treatment must be ruled out before drug therapy is initiated. Furthermore, when used, drugs must maintain or improve a resident's functional status.

OBRA's guidelines detail doses but do not set maximum dosage limitations. The dosage detailing is a way to draw attention to the need for comprehensive assessment and review of drug use. Surveyors review the duration of drug therapy regimens and look for documentation of indications for use of the drug therapy. Nurses should also carefully document observed effects of drug therapy.

This is an area where the nurse should exercise skill and leadership by working with others on the resident's care team to ensure that the resident is not overmedicated or unnecessarily medicated. For example, the nurse can work with the interdisciplinary care team to plan nondrug interventions. The nurse is also in a position to inform a resident's physician about OBRA's unnecessary drug use guidelines. Not only may this be new information for the physician, but it may also provide a sound explanation for the physician to use with a resident's family members who may be requesting drug interventions. In fact, the nurse is in the best position to work with residents and family to provide information and reinforcement about this important approach to care.

Research has shown that many psychoactive drugs have been misused (Cooper, 1990). They have been administered based on clients' symptoms rather than their underlying conditions. Psychoactive drugs are rarely beneficial as chemical restraints and are often harmful to clients (Cooper, 1990).

Drug toxicities have been underestimated, and at times drugs have been used to meet the desires of nurses or other facility staff for "environmental control," such as to settle residents down for sleep. The need to manage the environment can pose a genuine dilemma for nurses, since certain resident behaviors such as yelling or wandering into other residents' rooms can be disruptive. Such behaviors may cause family members to pressure nurses to quiet such residents or take other steps to stop the bothersome behavior. Nursing facility residents can be challenging in spite of a nursing staff's intent to provide good care and to identify causes of residents' disturbing behavior (Cooper, 1990). However, drug therapy may not be used for environmental control.

Physical restraints may be used only when there are specific medical indications and when a physician has written a specific order for their use. The order must include the type of restraint, the condition or specific behavior for which it is to be applied, and a specified time or duration for its use. Orders for a restraint must be reevaluated and, if use is to be continued, periodically reassessed.

The nurse must carefully document the behavior or condition that led to the order for a restraint and monitor the resident's ongoing condition, noting responses to the application of a restraint and changes in condition. When physical restraints are used, the resident must be observed and the restraints released at regular intervals. Records documenting these activities must be kept.

OBRA guidelines require that antipsychotic drugs be used at the minimum dose necessary. This minimization must be ensured through careful monitoring and documentation by the staff to identify why a behavioral problem may exist and whether the antipsychotic treatment is actually effecting a change in the target symptom.

Residents receiving an antipsychotic drug must have an indication for use of the drug based on one of 12 conditions. The conditions include schizophrenia or schizoid-affective disorder; delusional disorder; acute psychosis or mania with psychotic mood; brief reactive psychosis; atypical psychosis; Tourette's syndrome; Huntington's chorea; short-term symptomatic treatment of nausea, vomiting, hiccups, or itching; or dementia associated with psychotic or violent features that represent a danger to the clients or others.

Reasons for the use of antipsychotic drugs must be documented in the physician's orders and in the resident care plan. They should not be used for behaviors such as restlessness, insomnia, yelling or screaming, inability to manage the resident, or wandering.

OBRA mandates a 25% reduction in dose trial, unless the drug has been tried previously and resulted in decompensation of the resident or the resident has 1 of the 12 conditions listed above. A "reduction in dose trial" consists of a reduction in the dose of the drug coupled with observations to note the return of symptoms or any adverse side effects. The dose is gradually increased until optimum effectiveness in treatment response and minimum necessary dose are achieved.

The physician's order must include specific information as to (1) the reasons for the use of antipsychotic drugs, including medical indications; (2) the target behaviors that the drug therapy is intended to treat; (3) the goals of therapy; and (4) common side effects. These notations must also be entered in the resident's care plan. The observations and charting made by the nurse must address these specific points as well.

A facility is not absolved from regulatory liability by the mere presence of a physician's written order for restraints of any kind. The nursing staff is professionally responsible for challenging questionable orders (Johnson, 1991). For example, statement three and its interpretation in the Code for Nurses identify the nurses' responsibility to "safeguard the client," and to act on any "questionable practice in the provision of health care." Nurses should participate in the development of problem-solving procedures, established to provide constructive and effective ways to resolve disputes involving client care issues. Such procedures generally provide an avenue of communication that can be used to resolve questions or disagreements that arise between health care professionals. When a question or issue does arise, the nurse must institute the dispute-resolution procedure promptly.

Reductions in the use of physical restraints and almost universal use of CMS's resident assessment system are indications that nursing facility reform is working (*Suffering in silence*, 1993). Recent studies indicate that antipsychotic drug use is down, resulting in economic benefits and improving the quality of life for nursing facility residents (CMS, 2004; Starr, 1992).

Nurses have been successful in employing practices directed toward avoiding the use of chemical or physical restraints. Some of these techniques are companionship; increased client supervision; meeting physical needs such as toileting, exercise, or hunger; modifying staff attitudes; and other psychosocial approaches. Again, it can be seen that nurses are in a unique position to positively affect the quality of life of institutionalized older adults. Nurses should continue to educate others about these behavior management techniques. According to Wayne Ray, a Vanderbilt University researcher, "When the nursing staff had the knowledge and techniques to deal with maladaptive behavior that comes from dementia, they didn't have to use physical or chemical restraints" (Starr, 1992).

Urinary Incontinence. Urinary incontinence is one of three key reasons older adults enter nursing facilities (*Suffering in silence*, 1993). In fact, more than half of nursing facility residents are incontinent. Left untreated, this condition can lead to other physical problems such as infections and skin breakdown.

Since this is a prevalent condition and one that has implications for the quality and enjoyment of life, it can be expected to remain a major area of regulatory scrutiny. Under OBRA, nursing facilities are required to include incontinence in the comprehensive assessment of a resident's functions and to provide the necessary treatment.

Furthermore, state Division of Aging surveyors are being instructed to focus on this problem by evaluating its occurrence in the nursing facilities they survey and assessing the extent to which residents are in bladder training programs.

Nurses should be familiar with guidelines and procedures for management of incontinence, such as the Agency for Health Care Policy and Research Guidelines. (Refer to Chapter 28 for more information.) Charting should be specific to reflect the presence and extent of the problem of incontinence, and it should note the treatment plan that has been established and the effects of the treatment. From the OBRA perspective, behavioral approaches are preferable to more intense mechanical or chemical therapies.

Facility Survey and Certification. CMS is determined to see that every nursing facility implement and comply with the letter and spirit of OBRA's requirements. This determination is enforced through a process of surveying facilities and based on the results of the survey, which certifies a facility's compliance with OBRA laws and regulations.

OBRA's enactment created a new survey process. In general, the standard survey is conducted to review the quality of care by evaluating criteria such as medical, nursing, and rehabilitative care; dietary services; infection control; and the physical environment.

Written care plans and resident assessments are evaluated for their adequacy and accuracy, and the surveyors look for compliance with residents' rights (Hamme, 1991). OBRA's long-term care survey processes have a renewed emphasis on the outcome of resident care, rather than mere paper compliance with regulatory requirements (Schabes, 1991).

By contractual arrangement with DHHS, state survey agencies are authorized to certify the compliance of facilities. States are also required to educate facility staff as to the survey process, and are further authorized to investigate complaints of all types. Based on reports of persistent problems in nursing facilities, CMS will strengthen federal oversight of nursing facility quality and safety standards. These steps will include more frequent inspections for repeat offenders or facilities with serious violations; more inspections carried out on weekends and evenings; targeting of states with weak inspections systems; and assurance that state surveyors enforce CMS's policies to sanction nursing facilities with serious violations (CMS, 2004).

Surveys are conducted by a multidisciplinary survey team of professionals, including at least one registered professional nurse. Survey participants include facility personnel, residents and their families, and the state's long-term care ombudsman. (For more on ombudsman, refer to the discussion of the OAA earlier in this chapter.) Surveyors interview residents and ask them about facility policies and procedures. They observe staff in the performance of their duties, and staff may be asked to complete forms required by the survey team.

Enforcement Mechanisms and Sanctions. DHHS and the states may apply sanctions or penalties against a facility for failure to meet requirements and standards. Such sanctions can include civil monetary penalties, appointment of a temporary manager to run a facility while deficiencies are remedied, or even closure of a facility or transfer of residents to another facility (or both). In addition, CMS plans to publish individual nursing facility survey results and violation records on the Internet to increase accountability and flag repeat offenders for families and the public (CMS, 2004).

The sanctions applied must be appropriate to the facility deficiency. This often depends on whether an immediate threat to the health and safety of residents exists. Sanctions may also be increased if there are repeat or uncorrected deficiencies. Deficiencies are analyzed based on the scope of the deficiency—that is, whether it constitutes a pattern of activity or whether it is an isolated or sporadic occurrence—and the severity of the deficiency—that is, the extent to which it presents a threat to the safety and welfare of residents. To assist in analysis, the scope and severity factors are laid out on a "grid" and sanctions are applied based on the result of this analysis.

It is important for the nurse to understand that officials authorized by the state or federal agencies that oversee the operation of nursing facilities (or any licensed health care institution or setting) may enter and review activities at any time. They are not required to announce the visit in advance (in fact, OBRA regulations specifically prohibit this for the annual standard survey), and the nurse must respond to their questions and requests for information and records.

The director of nursing has an important role in the survey process. If requested to do so by the surveyor, the director may participate in rounds or other activities of the surveyor; the director is also present at a closing conference where the overall results of the survey are discussed. Often, the surveyors follow up the visit by telephone, or they may return for additional visits to a facility if further information is needed.

A written report of the survey is ultimately sent to the facility, and if there are deficiencies or violations, the director of nursing and other members of the nursing staff may participate in formulating a plan of correction to submit to the regulatory officials.

In the course of an inspection a surveyor may find information suggesting that the practice of a licensed nurse may have been improper or may not have met the proper standard of care. For example, a particular nurse may have a high incidence of medication errors or may not have taken proper action when a client experienced a change in condition. In such cases the surveyor may forward the record showing the relevant findings to the appropriate state agency or board for review of the nurse's practice, requesting a determination as to whether the nurse may have violated the state's nurse practice act. The board may find no basis for further action and not proceed, or it may require a hearing or other measures that could lead to disciplinary action. Disciplinary action could range from reprimand, to required educational remediation, to suspension or revocation of the nurse's license. This again underscores the need for nurses to be diligent and conscientious in their professional practice and to remember that they will be held accountable for their individual performance.

Proposed Legislative Changes

The federal government, while recognizing certain improvements in the care of nursing facility residents, has also been alarmed by reports of persistent serious problems. In part, this concern is the result of a report by DHHS, which was the subject of congressional hearings in the summer of 1998. Changes made to achieve CMS goals are addressing these issues.

Congress has taken some steps to ensure a safe environment for nursing facility residents. For example, OBRA requires all states to establish and maintain a registry of nurse aides who are unfit to provide care because of abusive or criminal histories. In addition, 33 states currently require nursing facilities to do criminal background checks on new job applicants. However, most states require only checks of the states' own criminal database and not a national database. This permits unsuitable workers to gain employment by crossing state lines.

In July 1998, using existing authority, President Bill Clinton ordered a step-up in nursing facility survey and enforcement activities. Specifically, he announced steps to make facility inspections less predictable by ordering state officials to inspect the facilities at night and on weekends. He further instructed officials to focus these enforcement activities on facility operators with a history of poor performance. And, through emphasis on training of nursing assistants, he stepped up initiatives to enhance the ability to care for residents with pressure ulcers, dehydration, and nutrition problems (Pear, 1998). CMS will likely continue to develop action plans to improve these areas.

AUTONOMY AND SELF-DETERMINATION

The right to self-determination has its basis in the doctrine of informed consent. Informed consent is the process by which competent individuals are provided with information that enables them to make a reasonable decision about any treatment or intervention that is to be performed on them.

A great deal of legal analysis has been put to the question, "What is enough information for a person to make a reasonable decision?" It is generally accepted that for consent to be valid and legally sufficient, a standard of disclosure must be met that includes the diagnosis, the nature and purpose of the treatment, the risks of the treatment, the probability of success of the treatment, available treatment alternatives, and the consequences of not receiving the treatment.

Informed consent has developed out of strong judicial deference toward individual autonomy, reflecting a belief that individuals have a right to be free from nonconsensual interference with their persons, and a basic moral principle that it is wrong to force others to act against their will (Furrow et al, 1987). The judicial system's strong deference toward individual autonomy in the medical context was articulated long ago by Justice Benjamin Cardozo:

> Every human being of adult years and sound mind has a right to determine what shall be done with his own body.
>
> *Schloendorf v. Society of New York Hospital,* 211 N.Y. 125, 129 (1914)

The right to self-determination, then, has a longstanding basis in the common or case law and has roots under the right of liberty guaranteed by the U.S. Constitution. These common law rights, to a large extent, have been codified, acted on by legislatures, and enacted into statutory law. The codification of these legal rights should serve to make the legal tools of self-determination more readily available to the citizenry. Nurses should take care, though, since sometimes the opposite effect occurs. Rather than making mechanisms for the exercise of consent more available, the codification of these rights sometimes results in a view that the absence of a legal, written tool or directive, such as a living will or a signed consent form, means that a client's decision has not been made. But there may in fact be other sources of information that express a person's wishes, and caregivers should not presume that the absence of a written document is the same as a lack of consent. Rather, nurses must remember that the right to decide what shall be done for and to oneself is a fundamental right, and legal tools should be used to assist, not detract, from that basic human right. The nurse's role as advocate has a high degree of importance in this regard.

The right to self-determination covers all decisions about one's care and treatment, including the removal of life support or life-sustaining treatments and life-prolonging or life-saving measures. These issues are particularly relevant to older adults. Although individuals of all ages are concerned with these matters and young persons do die, incapacity and infirmity are more common in old age. Therefore more frequent discussion of the need to preserve the right to self-determination occurs among older adults.

The doctrine and standards of informed consent are intended to apply to the decision-making capability of one who is competent to make such a decision. In this context, *competent* means one who is able to understand the proposed treatment or procedure and thereby make an informed decision.

When a person is not competent, the decision may be made by a surrogate. This is known as "substituted" judgment. More discussion on this point appears later in the chapter.

Do Not Resuscitate Orders

A Do Not Resuscitate (DNR) order is a specific order from a physician, entered on the physician order sheet, which instructs health care providers not to use or order specific methods of therapy, which are referred to as cardiopulmonary resuscitation (CPR) (Lieberson, 1992).

CPR generally includes those measures and therapies used to restore cardiac function or to support ventilation in the event of a cardiac or respiratory arrest[6] and to handle emergencies caused by sudden loss of oxygen supply to the brain as a result of lung or heart failure.

DNR orders have been used for many years. In 1974 the American Medical Association (AMA) recommended that decisions not to resuscitate a client be formally entered into the medical record, a practice that had already become widespread (Lieberson, 1992). The concept of withholding resuscitation in appropriate circumstances is widely accepted (Schreiber, 1990).

---

[6]McKinney's consolidated laws of New York annotated, Public Health Law § § 2961(4).

New York is one of only a few states that have passed specific codified procedures covering DNR orders, and this statute is useful to look to for guidelines.[7] The law applies to clients in general hospitals and in nursing facilities.[8] In New York, consent to CPR is presumed unless a DNR order has been issued.[9] As is customary, there is also a presumption of competency to make such a decision.[10] Competent individuals may choose to forego any treatment or care, even if the choice will result in death.

To determine whether a person can choose to accept or reject medical care, a determination must be made of whether the person is competent. The reluctance of courts to articulate a standard for competence has resulted in very few reported opinions that state any formal opinion of competency. Rather, courts prefer to involve physicians, often psychiatrists, and other caregivers in testifying about the mental state of a person, and the courts base the determination of competency on that information (Furrow et al, 1987).

The capacity to make decisions is applicable only to the decision being made at the time. Even if a person has appointed an agent to manage his or her affairs, this does not necessarily mean that the person is incompetent in any total sense. "It is ethically inappropriate to assign blanket 'incapacity to decide' to the [older adult] client based on isolated areas of irrationality."[11]

In a court determination of competency, the nurse may be called on to testify and will be asked to offer information relative to the client's behavior or verbalizations that may offer evidence as to the person's state of mind. The medical record is extremely important in this type of proceeding, and the nurse will want to use it to back up any testimony given.

Older adults are more often faced with issues concerning the right to self-determination and that in such matters, the clients' statements and other indications of their wishes, as well as their state of mind, are critical. Nurses should keep these points in mind when they are responsible for the care of older adults, and they should make certain that records and notations, assessments, and other ongoing observations are carefully, objectively, and accurately documented. If a time comes when a nurse needs to refer to records to testify in a court proceeding, the information provided will be used to help determine how an individual's basic rights are being addressed. A nurse can be secure in knowing that everything has been done to see that the resident's rights are respected.

[7]McKinney's consolidated laws of New York annotated, Public Health Law § § 2960 to 2979, as amended by Ch. 370, L. 1991, effective July 15, 1991. See also Florida Statutes § 765.101(2) and Colorado Revised Statutes § 15-18.6-101(1).

[8]McKinney's consolidated laws of New York annotated, Public Health Law § § 2800(1) and (3) (McKinney, 1993).

[9]McKinney's consolidated laws of New York annotated, Public Health Law § 2962(1) (McKinney, 1993).

[10]McKinney's consolidated laws of New York annotated, Public Health Law § 2963(1) (McKinney, 1993).

[11]Lieberson AD, Advance Medical Directives, Vol 1 Pub. 9/97, Sec 30.3, p 453.

Guidelines for DNR Policies in Nursing Facilities. Nurses often raise questions and are faced with dilemmas about DNR policies because there is inconsistency or uncertainty either in the existing policy or in the application of procedures. Since the nurse may be the only health care professional present in the nursing facility at any given time, it is imperative for the nurse to request that the facility have a detailed and specific policy to provide the necessary guidance.

If a facility does develop a DNR policy, the following guidelines should be considered. Whatever policies are adopted should be well communicated to the staff and should be adhered to scrupulously. The policy should indicate:

- That a facility must have competently trained staff available 24 hours a day to provide CPR (Schreiber, 1990).
- Whether CPR will be performed unless there is a DNR order.
- The conditions under which the facility will issue DNR orders. These factors should be in compliance with applicable state law; thus it is necessary to examine the DNR provisions of the jurisdiction. Considerations include required physician consultations regarding medical condition and documented discussions with the client and family members.
- That competency is established, again with proper documentation or medical consultation, as may be indicated by applicable state law.
- The origin of consent for the order: via the client, while competent; by an advance medical directive (AMD); or by a substitute or surrogate decision maker.
- Provision for renewal of DNR orders at appropriate intervals with ongoing documentation of condition to note changes.
- As required by the JCAHO standards, the roles of various staff members. The policy should be approved through all appropriate channels (see Standard CP 1.5.18 and its subsections; *Long Term Care Standards Manual*, 1989).

Advance Medical Directives

AMDs are documents that permit people to set forth in writing their wishes and preferences regarding health care. AMDs are used to indicate their decisions if the time should come when they are unable to speak for themselves. Some advance directives also permit people to designate someone to convey their wishes in the event they are rendered unable to do so. AMDs are helpful to professionals, since they provide information and guidance when treatment decisions are made.

A number of issues pose problems to the professional in honoring advance directives. To begin, an advance directive is not operative until the client is no longer capable of decision making (Lieberson, 1997). Therefore the first decision must be whether a client is capable of making a decision, or whether the advance directive must be followed. At times the client may be awake and responsive but not clear in his or her ability to think or communicate (Lieberson, 1997). However, if a determination of incapacity is made, then an advance directive can be looked to and can speak when the person cannot.

Sometimes, the policy of the provider or the judgment of the treating physician may not be in accord with the client's wishes. In such cases it is necessary to advise the client of this. For example, if a nursing facility does not offer CPR and the client desires that option, then the facility must advise the client and offer the option of transfer. In the same way, a physician who does not agree with or cannot carry out the client's wishes must advise the client of this and must then transfer the care of the client to another physician as soon as practical.

Remember, the right to self-determination is well grounded in the common law and is interpreted in the U.S. Constitution under the right of liberty. The statutory developments and codification of these principles promote communication and make it easier for individuals to exercise their right to autonomy. For more information on the role of the nurse regarding advance directives, see Nurses' Responsibilities, p. 49.

Legal Tools

Living Wills or Designation of Health Care Agents. Living wills are intended to provide written expressions of a client's wishes regarding the use of medical treatments in the event of a terminal illness or condition (Doukas et al, 1991). Health care agent designations entail appointing a trusted person to express the client's wishes regarding the withholding or withdrawal of life support.

Allowing for variations among states, living wills are generally not effective until (1) the attending physician has the document and the client has been determined to be incompetent, (2) the physician has determined the client has a terminal condition or a condition such that any therapy provided would only prolong dying, and (3) the physician has written the appropriate orders in the medical record (Lieberson, 1992).

States vary in the type of written instruments used for these purposes. For example, New York does not have a living will statute as such, but does have a health care proxy provision, which combines the elements of the living will and the designation of a health care agent.

General Provisions in Living Wills. Living wills may be executed by any competent adult. Most statutes contain specific language excluding euthanasia and declaring that withholding care in compliance with the document does not constitute suicide.

Most statutes require that the client's signature be witnessed. The witness usually does not have to attest to the client's mental competence; however, many forms require that the witness indicate that the principal "appeared" to be of sound mind.

In general, it is also prohibited for an owner or employee of a facility in which a client resides to serve as a witness to a signature, unless the owner is a relative. In some states a person who has an interest in the client's estate may not serve as witness or be designated the health care agent.

Pain and comfort measures may not be withheld. A living will may be revoked at any time and by any means.

Durable or General Power of Attorney: Differences and Indications. The durable power of attorney is a legal instrument by which a person can designate someone else to make health care decisions at a time in the future when he or she may be rendered incompetent. This is called a springing power, one that comes into effect in the future on occurrence of a specific event—in this case, the incompetence of the client.

The person delegating the power of attorney is called the principal, whereas the person to whom the power is granted is known as the agent. A durable power of attorney is different from a general power of attorney in that a general power of attorney would become invalid on incompetence of the principal.

Thus the durable power of attorney allows the designation of a legally enforceable surrogate decision maker. The role of the designated surrogate in this situation is to make the decisions that most closely align with the client's wishes, desires, and values.

The durable power of attorney has an advantage over the living will, in that the designated agent can assess the current situation, ask questions, and gather information to assist in determining the probable wishes of the client (Peters, 1987). The living will, on the other hand, speaks for clients who cannot speak themselves; obviously, it cannot ask questions.

All states now have laws providing for types of living will documents, durable powers of attorney, or both. Since specifics of the laws vary from state to state, it is important for the nurse to be knowledgeable of the laws in the state in which he or she practices. Furthermore, since this is a developing area of the law, the nurse should keep abreast of changes. Depending on a nurse's work environment, resources for this information may be the facility administration, risk management staff, legal counsel, or another appropriate source.

Decision Diagram

The decision diagram assists in understanding the thought process that should be followed when trying to analyze end-of-life decision-making situations (Box 3-2).

If clients are competent, then they are capable of making their own decisions. While competent, a person can prepare for possible future incompetence by executing AMDs and by discussing personal wishes with health care professionals and family members so that they fully understand that person's specific preferences for future care and treatment.

When the time comes for AMDs to be used, a verification of incompetence will be made. This can normally be accomplished by medical judgment and family discussion. Laws of any jurisdiction should be evaluated to see what documentation and procedures are required.

Once a person is deemed incompetent, substituted decision-making alternatives must be chosen. If a person has not executed AMDs, other people are looked to for their knowledge about the client's wishes. If all agree about the client's medical condition, then the statutory order of priority for surrogates can be looked to for designation of the decision maker. In New York, for example, decision makers are selected in this order (their willingness is also considered): spouse, son or daughter over age 18, parent, brother or sister over age 18, or close friend.

If there are executed AMDs, and there is agreement among health care professionals and family, then the wishes may be carried out according to the directives. There is comprehensive immunity from civil liability for physicians who, in good faith, rely on AMDs in carrying out treatment directives.

Where there is lack of agreement or confusion, it may be necessary to seek a court-ordered conservator. (This person is sometimes referred to as a *guardian*; the word *conservator* is used here, but jurisdictions may assign varied meanings to these terms.) The conservator then acts as the surrogate and decides according to the client's wishes as can best be determined by available information. The conservator also makes such decisions in the best interest of the client. This refers to a conservator of the person, as opposed to a conservator of the property, who deals with matters related to an individual's property and belongings and thus is not a subject of this discussion.

The court-appointed conservator has priority over other decision makers. The conservator may be a spouse, parent, or other family member. It may also be any other person the court determines may best serve the interests of the client. For a paradigm of end-of-life decision making, see Box 3-2.

An example of a typical living will document is presented in Box 3-3, and an example of a document concerning appointment of a health care agent is presented in Box 3-4. States usually provide forms for these purposes, but may not require that the specific form be used. Rather, most simply require that the executed documents be in substantially the same form. In any event, the laws of the jurisdiction should be reviewed to see if a specific form or document is required.

BOX 3-2 End-of-Life Decision Diagram

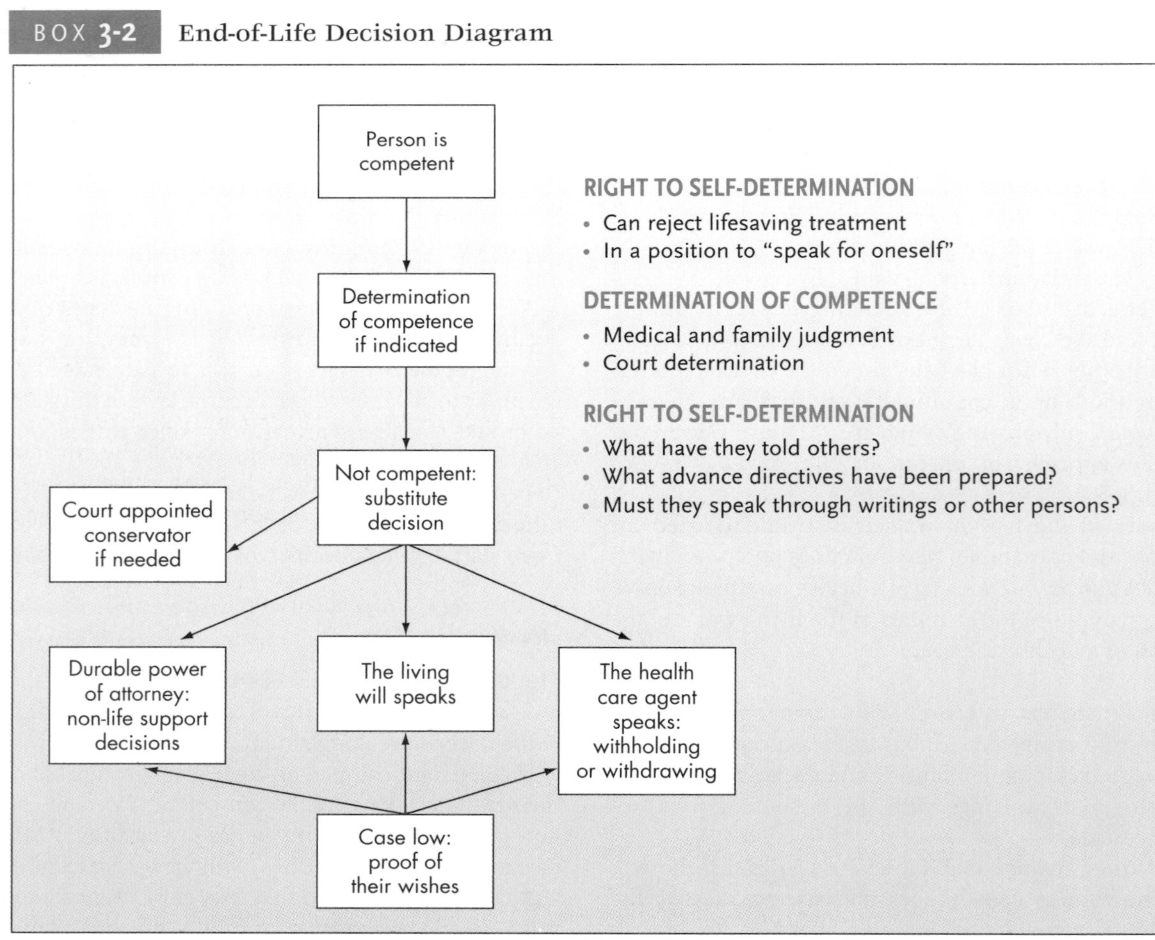

BOX 3-3 Living Will: Connecticut General Statutes § 19a-575. Form of Document

Any person 18 years of age or older may execute a document which shall contain directions as to specific life support systems which such person chooses to have administered. Such document shall be signed and dated by the maker with at least two witnesses and may be substantially in the following form:

DOCUMENT CONCERNING WITHHOLDING OR WITHDRAWAL OF LIFE SUPPORT SYSTEMS

If the time comes when I am incapacitated to the point where I can no longer actively take part in decisions for my own life, and am unable to direct my physician as to my own medical care, I wish this statement to stand as a testament of my wishes.

"I .... (NAME) request that, if my condition is deemed terminal or if it is determined that I will be permanently unconscious, I be allowed to die and not be kept alive through life support systems. By terminal condition, I mean that I have an incurable or irreversible medical condition which, without the administration of life support systems, will, in the opinion of my attending physician, result in death within a relatively short time. By permanently unconscious I mean that I am in a permanent coma or persistent vegetative state which is an irreversible condition in which I am at no time aware of myself or the environment and show no behavioral response to the environment. The life support systems that I do not want include, but are not limited to:

Artificial respiration
Cardiopulmonary resuscitation
Artificial means of providing nutrition and hydration
(Cross out any initial life support systems you want administered.)

I do not intend any direct taking of my life, but only that my dying not be unreasonably prolonged.

Other specific requests:

This request is made, after careful reflection, while I am of sound mind.

.... (Signature)
.... (Date)

This document was signed in our presence, by the above-named . . .(NAME) who appeared to be 18 years of age or older, of sound mind, and able to understand the nature and consequences of health care decisions at the time the document was signed.

.... (Witness)
.... (Address)
.... (Witness)
.... (Address)

BOX 3-4 Health Care Agent: Connecticut Health Care Agent (C.G.S. § 19a-577)

(a) Any person 18 years of age or older may execute a document that may, but need not be in substantially the following form:

DOCUMENT CONCERNING THE APPOINTMENT OF HEALTH CARE AGENT

I appoint .... (NAME) to be my health care agent. If my attending physician determines that I am unable to understand and appreciate the nature and consequences of health care decisions and to reach and communicate an informed decision regarding treatment, my health care agent is authorized to:

(1) convey to my physician my wishes concerning the withholding or removal of life support systems.
(2) take whatever actions are necessary to ensure that my wishes are given effect.

If this person is unwilling or unable to serve as my health care agent, I appoint .....(NAME) to be my alternative health care agent.

This request is made, after careful reflection, while I am of sound mind.

.... (Signature)
.... (Date)

This document was signed in our presence, by the above-named .....(NAME) who appeared to be 18 years of age or older, of sound mind, and able to understand the nature and consequences of health care decisions at the time the document was signed.

.... (Witness)
.... (Address)
.... (Witness)
.... (Address)

Conflicts Between Directives and Family Desires

Families may disagree with the directives of a family member. Often, family members express the desire to have more care than is requested by a client. The law upholds the expressed desires of a client over those of the family, but families can exert influence that sometimes is contrary to the client's expressed wishes (Lieberson, 1997). This puts physicians and nurses in confusing and conflicting situations.

Although the law consistently upholds the expressed desires of clients, families continue to exert influence over medical decisions, even when they support decisions known to be contrary to the client's wishes (Lieberson, 1997). Designated health care agents may also find themselves in conflict with family members who question the control of the agent and may not understand why the agent has been given this control.

Most AMD statutes specifically provide immunity for physicians who follow, in good faith, the wishes of a client as expressed therein. Nurses should note that in most cases this immunity applies only to the physician and not to the nurse, since the physician is given the legal duty to put into effect the client's wishes. Consequently, the nurse must rely on effective communication with the physician, client, and family, and on the quality of the facility's policies and procedures, to be sure that his or her actions are consistent with the legally required steps. In addition, an effective ethical process for discussion and problem solving, discussed elsewhere in this chapter, is critical in these situations.

THE PATIENT SELF-DETERMINATION ACT

The Patient Self-Determination Act[12] (PSDA) became effective December 1, 1991. The intent of this law is to ensure that clients are given information about the extent to which their rights are protected under state law. The PSDA itself does not create any new substantive legal right for individuals regarding their decision making. Rather, its focus is on education and communication.

The PSDA requires hospitals, nursing facilities, and other health care providers who receive federal funds such as Medicare or Medicaid to give clients written information explaining their legal options for refusing or accepting treatment should they become incapacitated.

Background: the Cruzan Case

On January 11, 1983, Nancy Cruzan, a healthy 25-year-old woman, was seriously injured in an automobile accident; she became comatose, in a persistent vegetative state. Seven years later, the U.S. Supreme Court considered whether her life support could be withdrawn. Her parents, who had also been designated her coguardians by a judgment of the court, sought a court order to withdraw the artificial feeding and hydration equipment after it became apparent that she had virtually no chance of regaining her cognitive facilities.[13]

In June 1990, in a 5-to-4 decision, the Court held that because there was no clear and convincing evidence of Nancy's desire to have life-sustaining treatment withdrawn under such circumstances, her parents lacked the authority to carry out such a request.[13] The Court affirmed that the Missouri Supreme Court was within its rights to request more evidence to indicate what Nancy's decision would be if she were in a position to make that decision herself. It was in this decision that the Court permitted the state of Missouri (and thus made it constitutionally permissible) to require "clear and convincing proof" as the standard needed to determine a person's wishes regarding the withdrawal of life support.

Most states have not adopted this rigorous standard of proof for such decisions. In fact, as of this writing, only two states—Missouri and New York—use the "clear and convincing" standard. In most jurisdictions, family members, those close to the individual, or other surrogate decision makers may make decisions for a client who has not left specific oral or written instructions (Coleman, 1994).

[12]42 U.S.C. §§ 1395 and 1396 (1990), as amended, 60 FR 33262, June 27, 1995.

[13]*Cruzan v Director, Missouri Dept. of Health* (1990, US), 111 L Ed 2d 224, 234, 110 S Ct 2841.

Clear and Convincing Proof

It is difficult, if not impossible, to come up with a precise meaning of "clear and convincing proof." Although this standard is not applied in most states, a discussion is presented here to provide insight into the Cruzan case, to help one understand the significance of the Court's decision to initiate AMD legislation nationwide and to enact the PSDA, and to provide some clarification for understanding a lesser standard of proof.

The clear and convincing standard is an intermediate standard of evidence, higher than a "preponderance of the evidence" but below "certainty beyond a reasonable doubt." A clear and convincing presentation should provide enough facts to produce in the mind of the adjudicator a "firm belief or conviction" regarding the events to be established (Black, 1979).

An AMD may help to meet this standard. However, in the absence of an AMD, the evidence required to meet this standard is somewhat cloudy. Writings such as a living will would be accorded more weight than oral statements.

In re Westchester County Medical Center on Behalf of O'Connor[14] described the clear and convincing standard as "a firm and settled commitment . . . under circumstances like those presented"; it must be "more than immediate reactions to the unsettling experience of seeing or hearing another's unnecessarily prolonged death."[15]

The Cruzan decision must be examined for the areas of clarification it provides. While it does not declare a "right to die" as such, it does provide much stimulus for the development of state legislation to clarify the existing rights to self-determination. In addition, it also served as the catalyst for the enactment of the PSDA:

> A competent person has a constitutionally protected right under the Fourteenth Amendment to refuse medical treatment, even life saving nutrition and hydration; an incompetent or incapacitated person may have that right exercised by a surrogate.
>
> *Cruzan v. Director, Missouri Department of Health*, 111 L Ed 2d 224, 110 S Ct 2841 (1990)

In her concurring opinion, U.S. Supreme Court Justice Sandra Day O'Connor made the following points (the interpretation is the author's analysis of points taken from the concurring opinion of O' Connor; modified from *Cruzan v. Director, Missouri Department of Health* [1990, US] 111 L Ed 2d 224, 247-251, 110 S Ct 2841):

> Artificial provision of nutrition and hydration involves intrusion and restraint and invokes the same due process concerns as any other medical treatment.
>
> One does not by incompetence lose one's due process liberty interests.
>
> The U.S. Constitution may require the states to implement the decision of a client's duly appointed surrogate.

[14]72 NY2d 517, 534 NYS2d 886, 531 NE2d 607 (1988).

[15]72 NY2d 517, 534 NYS2d 886, 531 NE2d 607 (1988) at 903.

The Four Significant Provisions of the PSDA

The PSDA has four significant provisions:

1. It requires hospitals, SNFs, home health agencies, hospice programs, and HMOs that participate in Medicare and Medicaid programs to maintain written policies and procedures guaranteeing that every adult receiving medical care is given written information regarding his or her involvement in treatment decisions. This information must include (1) individual rights under state law, either statutory or case law; and (2) written policies of the provider or organization regarding the protection of such rights. When state advance directive laws change, facilities must update their materials accordingly, but no later than 90 days after the changes in state laws.

   The information must be provided by hospitals at the time of admission, nursing facilities at the time of admission as a resident, hospice programs at the time of the initial receipt of hospice care, HMOs at the time of enrollment, and home health agencies in advance of the individual coming under the agencies' care.

   The PSDA further requires distrubtion of written information that describes each facility's policy for protecting the rights of clients. *Each client's medical record must document whether the client has executed an AMD.*

   The PSDA also provides protection against discrimination or refusal to provide care based on whether an individual has executed an AMD.

   A facility may engage a contractor to perform services required by the PSDA, but it retains the legal obligations for compliance with the law.

   If a patient or resident is incapacitated at the time of admission, the required information may be furnished to the family member or responsible party, but the client or resident must be provided with the material at such time as he or she is no longer incapacitated.
2. The provider must provide for education of staff and community on issues concerning AMDs but is not required to provide the public with the same material it provides clients.
3. States are required to develop a written description of the law concerning AMDs in their respective jurisdictions, and to distribute the material to providers who provide it to clients according to the requirements of the PSDA.
4. The secretary of DHHS was also required to develop and implement a national campaign to inform the public of the option to execute AMDs and of the client's right to participate in and direct his or her health care decisions.

Nurses' Responsibilities

The ANA (1997) published the following statement made by its board of trustees, articulating the nurse's important role in implementation of the PSDA: "Nurses should know the laws of the state in which [they] practice . . . and should be familiar with the strengths and limitations of the various forms of advance directive. The nurse has a responsibility to facilitate informed decision making, including but not limited to advance directives."

The ANA recommends that the following questions be part of the nursing admission assessment:

- Do you have basic information about advance care directives, including living wills and durable power of attorney?
- Do you wish to initiate an advance care directive?
- If you have already prepared an advance care directive, can you provide it now?
- Have you discussed your end-of-life choices with your family or designated surrogate and health care team workers (ANA, 1992)?

Problems and Ethical Dilemmas Associated With Implementation of the PSDA

Although public and medical professionals overwhelmingly support AMDs, clients have historically been reluctant to complete them. Even distribution of forms and information has failed to increase the participation rate.

During the first 2 years after the passage of the PSDA, only about 5% to 15% of clients completed an advance directive or were even familiar with their rights of self-determination (Parkman, 1997). By the end of 1994, 90% of Americans reportedly supported advance directives, yet only 10% to 20% had actually written one (Parkman, 1997). Overall, data suggest that despite passage of the PSDA, most clients still do not complete advance directives (Lieberson, 1997).

Other research indicates that care of dying clients may not be keeping pace with national guidelines or legal decisions upholding clients' rights to accept or refuse treatment. Physicians may be reluctant to discuss advance directives with their clients. The major barriers to this communication process are a lack of knowledge about advance directives and the belief that advance directives are not necessary for young healthy clients. Other studies have found that clients' personal desires do not always get attention, and physicians try to avoid discussion of grim subjects (Parkman, 1997).

Questions arise about the effectiveness of AMDs in situations where, for example, the person is away from home, a person changes his or her mind, or a situation arises that is not anticipated. Some approaches have been advised regarding these issues.

For example, some states have included in the language of living will provisions that a validly executed living will from another jurisdiction will be honored. However, if there is any uncertainty, it is probably wise to have people from another state execute a new document as soon as possible.

AMD provisions appropriately provide that people can change their minds at any time and by any means. Nurses need to be alert to any indications from a client. Based on the person's medical condition, subtle signs such as a gesture or a nod of the head may be easily overlooked.

The protocols established by facilities to comply with the PSDA may turn the "tangible indicators of extremely important and personal decisions into just another piece of paper." AMDs must be part of a clinical process, not an administrative one (LaPuma, Orrentlicher, and Moss, 1991). These very personal and difficult questions may be asked along with routine questions about finances and next of kin. The meaning and importance of these issues may be undermined if they become merely a familiar administrative procedure.

Many have questioned whether the time of admission to a hospital or a nursing facility is the best time to discuss advance directives. At such times, clients may be fearful, uncomfortable, in pain, and anxious. These emotional states may affect a client's understanding and level of competence. It is important for the nurse to facilitate this process using the professional skills and understanding necessary to comply with the PSDA in such circumstances.

Conflicts between medical judgment and client choices are bound to become more common. It will be necessary to take steps to ensure that the directives of clients are accorded appropriate compliance, and that the judgment of health care professionals is respected.

As discussed previously, both the PSDA and OBRA require a facility or a physician who is unable to comply with the client's wishes notify that client when it is appropriate to be transferred to another facility or to the care of another physician. This ensures that the client's wishes are respected and preserves the integrity of the medical practitioner and provider. The medical record should reflect only the facts of such a situation. It is neither necessary nor appropriate to "make a case" in the record as to which party was right or wrong. It is appropriate only to show that proper procedures were followed and that all relevant matters were fully explained.

There are still many unanswered questions in the PSDA that will have to be sorted out over time. For example, the exact time of admission may be unclear. How is the matter handled with those who are illiterate? What should the nurse do if clients refuse to produce their AMDs?

In the case of surrogate decision makers, what about the response of a designated agent who is then called on to decide about the removal of life support? If and when the time comes, will the person be able to carry out the principal's wishes? Will the instructions left be clear enough to ensure that those wishes are carried out (Ballard, 1993)?

The responsibility to make these truly awesome decisions may arise at times of great personal difficulty and may in fact be more demanding than the agent ever thought possible. A realistic approach to these points at the time such instruments are executed will help resolve such dilemmas. The nurse should be alert for opportunities to gain information from both clients and their families or health agents to gauge their level of understanding. The nurse's role in clarifying matters and in explaining information may help alleviate the emotional dilemma associated with carrying out end-of-life decisions.

VALUES HISTORY

AMDs such as living wills and durable powers of attorney are easing some of the difficult situations faced by health care professionals and families when making decisions about treatment to prolong life. However, one criticism of such documents is that they may not offer insight into the person's own values or underlying beliefs regarding such directives (Doukas et al, 1991).

A values history may help add this dimension to advance health care decision making. The values history is an instrument that asks questions related to quality versus length of life and tries to determine what values a person sees as important to maintain during terminal care. The instrument asks people to specify their wishes regarding several types of medical situations. It presents the types of treatment that may be available in each situation and describes with whom these matters have been discussed in the past and who should be involved in the actual decision making.

As a practical matter, its use may be limited by the time required for discussion with the physician, or the physician's discomfort or reluctance to directly address the issues. But this should not serve as a reason to abandon this potentially useful tool.

The values history has important implications for the nurse. The values history, although a document with questions and answers, is really more than that. It is a process of "reflection and communication that can take place over a lifetime" (Lieberson, 1992). Nurses' close interpersonal relationships with clients and families and high degree of communication skills speak to the critical role they can play in this process. As life-and-death situations become more complex, demanding real knowledge of the client's wishes, the values history may help preserve the autonomy of the individual.

The values history may encourage extended conversation between individuals and their physicians and other health care professionals. This type of instrument may increase autonomy by providing a better basis for representing the clients' desires when they can no longer express their wishes. A copy of the values history developed at the University of New Mexico is included in Appendix 3A, p. 57.

NURSES' ETHICAL CODE AND END-OF-LIFE CARE

Ethics relate to the moral actions, behavior, and character of an individual. Nurses occupy a most trusted place in society, and conforming to a code of ethics gives evidence of acceptance of that responsibility and trust. A code of ethical conduct offers general principles to guide and to evaluate nursing actions (ANA, 1995).

The role of the health care professional is to maintain patient autonomy, maintain or improve health status, and do no harm (Sabatini, 1998). The nurse-patient relationship is built on trust, and nurses should understand key ethical principles as the basis of a trusting relationship. The key ethical principles should serve as a framework and basis for nursing decision making and application of professional judgment. These key ethical principles are autonomy or self-determination, beneficence (doing good), nonmaleficence (avoiding evil), justice (allocation of resources), and veracity (truthfulness) (Sabatini, 1998). Issues of ageism, ethnicity, sexual orientation, gender, physical or mental disability, and race are critical areas of difference that may affect the provider-patient relationship (Sabatini, 1998). These factors must be acknowledged and addressed if the moral and ethical principles of the provider-patient relationship are to be respected.

Scope and Standards of Gerontological Nursing Practice, Professional Performance Standard V, states that a gerontologic nurse's practice is guided by the Code for Nurses (Box 3-5), established by the ANA as the guide for ethical decision making in the practice of nursing (ANA, 2001). The code explains the values and ideals that serve as a framework for the nurses' ethical decision making and conduct (Rushton and Scanlon, 1998). A violation of the ethical code may not by itself be a violation of law. The state's nursing association may take action against a nurse in violation of the ethical code. More important, the ethical code serves to regulate professional practice from within the profession and ensure ethical conduct in the professional setting. Maintaining mutual respect among practitioners in the field is arguably one of the best ways to bring respect to a profession and to oneself.

Ethical directives can guide and direct the nurse who is caring for dying patients. As in other aspects of nursing care, care of the terminally ill and dying should be done with professional and ethical deliberation. The code of ethical conduct for nurses prohibits nurses from participating in assisted suicide. ANA's position statement holds that "nurses, individually and collectively, have an obligation to provide comprehensive and compassionate end-of-life care which includes the promotion of comfort and the relief of pain, and at times, foregoing life sustaining treatments" (*American Nurses Association praises supreme court for suicide ruling*, 1997).

BOX 3-5 Code of Ethics for Nurses

1. The nurse, in all professional relationships, practices with compassion and respect for the inherent dignity, worth, and uniqueness of every individual, unrestricted by considerations of social or economic status, personal attributes, or the nature of health problems.
2. The nurse's primary commitment is to the patient, whether an individual, family, group, or community.
3. The nurse promotes, advocates for, and strives to protect the health, safety, and rights of the patient.
4. The nurse has responsibility and accountability for individual nursing practice and determines the appropriate delegation of tasks consistent with the nurse's obligation to provide optimum patient care.
5. The nurse owes the same duties to self as to others, including the responsibility to preserve integrity and safety, to maintain competence, and to continue personal and professional growth.
6. The nurse participates in establishing, maintaining, and improving health care environments and conditions of employment conducive to the provision of quality health care and consistent with the values of the profession through individual and collective action.
7. The nurse participates in the advancement of the profession through contributions to practice, education, administration, and knowledge development.
8. The nurse collaborates with other health professionals and the public in promoting community, national, and international efforts to meet health needs
9. The profession of nursing, as represented by associations and their members, is responsible for articulating nursing values, for maintaining the integrity of the profession and its practice, and for shaping social policy.

Reprinted with permission from ANA: *Code for nurses with interpretive statements*, Washington, DC, 2001, The Association.

Ethical Dilemmas and Considerations

Euthanasia, Suicide, and Assisted Suicide. Michigan's Dr. Jack Kevorkian notwithstanding, the issue of physician-assisted suicide has become a front burner national debate. (The debate on euthanasia was nationally renewed with the highly publicized case of Dr. Kevorkian, who invented a "suicide machine," first used by client Janet Adkins to take her own life in June 1990.) Opinions on this issue are varied and changing. There may be signs of increased public support for aid-in-dying. A report released in 1992 (Blendon et al, 1992) shows an increase in approval for physician aid-in-dying on request of the client and family; approval rose from 34% to 63% between 1950 and 1991. Other polls suggest over 60% of Americans now support some legalized form of physician-assisted dying (Lieberson, 1997). Associated views and issues are controversial. However, efforts to change and shape public policy on this issue will continue.

The AMA has maintained its opposition to physician-assisted suicide. The ANA applauded the U.S. Supreme Court decision that found no constitutionally protected rights to physician-assisted suicide (*American Nurses Association praises supreme court for suicide ruling*, 1997).

However, many citizens, some physicians, and some other health care professionals believe that doctors should be allowed to help severely ill persons take their own lives (Lieberson, 1992). In most states, assisted suicide is considered an illegal act. However, an act of affirmative euthanasia (actual administration of the instrumentality that causes death) constitutes an illegal criminal offense in all 50 states.

On November 8, 1994, Oregon voters approved ballot Measure 16, otherwise known as Oregon's Death with Dignity Act. Despite legal challenges, the measure was reaffirmed by Oregon voters in 1997. Under the Oregon law, physicians may prescribe life-ending medication to anyone who is mentally competent and diagnosed as having less than 6 months to live. The patient may take the lethal dose only after a 15-day waiting period. The law does not specify what medications may be used (Maier, 1997). In March 1998 an Oregon woman dying of breast cancer became the first person to use the law by ingesting physician-prescribed medication to end her own life (*American Nurses Association praises supreme court for suicide ruling*, 1997). Oregon proponents of the law cite improvements in end-of-life care since passage of the measure in 1994.

Precise information as to the incidence of "assisted dying" type activities is not available. If such acts occur, they may be handled with subtlety and thus may be unlikely to be recognized as affirmative euthanasia. Actions such as failure to take steps to prevent a suicide, deliberate administration of a medication in a dosage that will suppress respiration and cause death, or the heavy doses of pain medications needed to comfort a terminally ill client may be intentional or inadvertent acts of assisting suicide or euthanasia. The nurse in particular may be in the middle of the conflict between the therapeutic necessity of treatment and the likely outcomes. Unlike an act of affirmative euthanasia, where the nurse's actions are clear, in situations where there are competing interests (e.g., therapeutic necessity and likely outcomes), the nurse must rely on the clients' needs and his or her own professional judgment. The nurse should not hesitate to request assistance from the institutional ethics committee to help cope with such dilemmas.

What about the person who, although not terminally ill or in a persistent vegetative state, is in her 80s and wishes to stop eating or drinking with the intent of causing her own death? In a 1987 case, *In re Application of Brooks* (NY Sup CT, Albany County, June 10, 1987), the court denied the petition of a nursing facility administrator to authorize forced feeding. Although physicians disagreed regarding the resident's competence, the court decided she was competent and thus had a right to determine what was to be done with her body. It found that failing to force feed is not abetting suicide.

In these challenging times the nurse may be confronted with unanswered questions, ambiguity, and decisional conflicts in the clinical setting (Rushton and Scanlon, 1998). Nurses must sharpen their ethical and analytical skills to deal effectively with these situations, and look to the learning tools and information available to them.

Reference has already been made to the Code for Nurses, which establishes the ethical framework for nursing practice. In addition, nurses should look to their client's statements, either written or verbal. Nurses should be alert to their own visceral reaction—that is, does the situation "feel right"?—and try to clarify what issues about the matter are causing concern (Rushton and Scanlon, 1998). By answering such questions, and by proceeding in a cautious and deliberate manner, nurses can usually determine the proper action steps. A most disturbing interruption to this process can emerge when there is disagreement or conflict, and the nurse may have to stop and reassess all factors before proceeding on the planned course of action (Rushton and Scanlon, 1998).

Experimentation and Research

As previously discussed, nursing facility residents are accorded specific rights with respect to their treatment. The patient/resident bill of rights entitles them to choose a primary physician if desired. Furthermore, they have the right to be informed about their medical condition and proposed plan of treatment.

Nursing facility residents, or any clients, may refuse to participate in experimental research (e.g., see Annotated code of Maryland, 1957, § 19-344(f); and Vermont statutes annotated, Title 18 § 1852(a)(10) and Title 33 § 3781(3), as redesignated by Act 219, L. 1990, effective July 1, 1990), and they may refuse to be examined, observed, or treated by students or other staff without jeopardizing their access to care (e.g., see 1990 edition, General laws of Massachusetts, supplemented by the 1991 Supplement, Chapter 111: 70E9h).

The goals of research are different from the goals of care. Research seeks to acquire knowledge with no intended benefit to the subjects, because much of clinical research is conducted to determine effective treatments or potential benefits of new drugs and medical devices. The goal of client care, on the other hand, is to provide benefit only to a specific client (Brett et al, 1991). This is a complex and controversial subject. Key points to consider in such issues are the goals and value of the research, conflicts between institutional interests and researchers, and the medical interests of the individual.

DHHS regulations may permit waiving the right to informed consent under the following specific circumstances: the research poses only a minimum risk; there will be no adverse effects on the rights and welfare of the subjects; the research could not effectively be carried out without the waiver; and whenever possible, the participants are provided with pertinent information during or after participation.

Only a full review of the research that includes legal analysis determines whether a waiver of informed consent can be justified. It may be that the right to informed consent cannot be waived even when the research poses minimum risk.

Research involving humans should be examined by an appropriate review board (Brett et al, 1991). All aspects of the proposed study must be evaluated to ensure that the research is justified and is of benefit, and that the individual rights of all persons, including volunteer participants, are not sacrificed. Nurses, as a professional group closely involved with the clinical aspects of human research, should be represented on the review board.

There are both state and federal regulatory provisions governing human research investigations. The diligent efforts of the research review board consider not only these laws and regulations but also their application to the particular benefits of the proposed research. A nurse involved in any aspect of human research should ask to see the details of the proposed study and the deliberations and decision of the institutional review board. It is not improper for a nurse to ask to attend a meeting of the review board if the nurse is involved in carrying out any aspect of the research or has any information that is of importance to the board's deliberations. Furthermore, the nurse should report to the board any time issues arise with respect to the research, if it appears that individual rights are in question.

Organ Donation

Technologic and medical advances have facilitated the successful transplantation of vital organs, and such procedures have become routine at many medical centers. But this success has exacerbated the ethical questions involving the allocation of scarce donor organs (Giuliano, 1997).

Which individuals should have priority for receiving donated organs? Should relatives, for example, be permitted to donate kidneys? What about the risks of such procedures to the donors? The psychologic issues and family dynamics? Should donors be compensated or should recipients pay for their organs? What about animal organ transplants?

Recognizing there are many more recipients waiting than there are donors, the federal government has taken steps to promote organ donation. Hospitals in the United States are now required to report *all* deaths to the local organ procurement agency (OPO). This would permit the nation's 63 OPOs, which collect organs and coordinate donation daily, to determine whether a person is a suitable donor (Neus, 1998). DHHS believes that this measure, which is now a condition for participating in the Medicare program, will save lives by substantially increasing organ donations in the United States.

Clearly there are more questions than answers. Still, there are some legal guidelines. For example, the 1984 National Organ Transplant Act prohibits selling organs in the United States (Giuliano, 1997). Standards of informed consent must be adhered to with respect to both donors and recipients. Even when an individual has signed an organ donor card, the consent of survivors is still needed (US HHS, 1998).

In dealing with the ethical issues faced in these situations, the answers are not clear cut and may depend on individual values (Giuliani, 1997). However, when it is necessary to sort out conflicts or report anything believed to be illegal or unethical, the nurse should consider obtaining guidance from an institutional ethics committee or other ethical resource.

Ethics Committees

Institutional biomedical ethics committees can play a pivotal role in dealing with sensitive conflicts about treatment decisions. They can help resolve conflicts that might otherwise force treatment decisions "from the bedside to the courtroom" (McCormick, 1991). Their objective is to carefully evaluate differing positions to achieve a consensus that is ethically and legally acceptable to all parties (Houge, 1993).

Ethics committees do not have any legal authority. Their main purpose is to create a forum where clients, client representatives, and providers can express and consider different points of view.

Two thirds of general hospitals with more than 200 beds have such panels. Their presence in nursing facilities is not as widespread. Membership on ethics committees should be diverse to minimize a group's tendency to view the task as technical, to help maintain a balanced view among professionals and special interest groups, and to offer a variety of perspectives to those seeking guidance (Hollerman, 1991). The nurse's role is crucial. Representation should be diverse and include administrative and staff nurses, as well as nurses practicing in specialty areas. It is recommended that nurses make up approximately one third of committee members (Hollerman, 1991).

Ethics committees' primary purposes are to (1) provide education and help guide policy making regarding ethical issues, (2) facilitate the resolution of ethical dilemmas, and (3) take an activist role in involving all interested parties in promoting the best care for clients (Houge, 1993).

Issues and topics that might be discussed by an ethics committee include euthanasia; patient competency and decision-making capacities; guardianship issues; DNR orders and policies; patient refusal of treatment; starting, continuing, or stopping treatment; informed consent; use of feeding tubes; and use of restraints. In fact, the list could be almost endless.

An organization considering the establishment of an ethics committee should be prepared to make the necessary commitment of time and resources. A committee should be visible and available and should publish clear notice of means to obtain access. Ethics committees provide a process, not a decision.

Home Care

- Remember that home care agencies' standards are based on the *Scope and Standards of Gerontological Nursing Practice,* published by the ANA (1995).
- Assess for older adult abuse and notify the proper authorities (e.g., local elderly protective services or ombudsmen program).
- On initial assessment, inform homebound older adults and their caregivers of home care client rights. Have them sign a copy that documents they have been informed of their rights.
- Inform caregivers and homebound older adults of their right to self-determination. Document that homebound older adults and/or caregivers have been informed by obtaining signatures. Advance directives must be part of a clinical assessment.
- Obtain a copy of homebound older adults' advance directives and keep them on file in their charts. Send copies to the physicians to file.
- Remember that a DNR order must be signed by the physician within 48 hours as specified by Medicare regulations.
- To help caregivers and homebound older adults make decisions about treatment used to prolong life, consider using a values history. The values history is an instrument that asks questions related to quality versus length of life and the values that persons see as important to maintain during terminal care.

SUMMARY

This chapter presented the legal and ethical issues associated with the nursing care of older adults. Professional standards of practice were identified as the legal measure against which nursing practice is judged, and sources of such standards were identified. Laws applicable to older adults generally were presented, and since older adults who reside in nursing facilities are particularly vulnerable, comprehensive coverage of nursing facility regulations was covered, including issues involving quality of life and rights of residents.

Issues associated with autonomy and self-determination were described, including physician-assisted dying, DNR orders, advance directives, end-of-life decision making, and organ donation. Ethical considerations were discussed, including issues associated with euthanasia and human research investigation. Nurses have an important role in helping to meet the health care needs of older adults, whose unique characteristics, vulnerabilities, and needs present great and varied challenges. The older person's quality of life is affected to a great extent by the quality of nursing care he or she receives.

Key Points

- The nurse's duty to clients is to provide care according to a measurable standard. When clients' physical and mental conditions, and their ability to care for themselves, decline, the duty of care rises.
- Older adults, and in particular infirm older adults, are considered a vulnerable population; therefore their treatment in licensed health care institutions and other settings (including the home) is carefully regulated.
- Evidence provided to the U.S. Congress in 1983 suggested widespread abuse of residents in nursing facilities and resulted in the enactment of OBRA '87, the most sweeping reform affecting Medicare and Medicaid nursing facilities since those programs began. Results of the reforms are mixed, and reports of continuing problems affecting quality of care for older adults persist, causing Congress to consider closer regulation and more stringent enforcement.
- OBRA focuses on the quality of life of residents in nursing facilities and assurances of the preservation of their human rights and due process interests. The regulations address virtually every element of life in a nursing facility. OBRA's regulations are enforced through a survey process that focuses on the outcomes of residential care and includes sanctions designed to force compliance, analyzed according to the scope and severity of violations.
- There is a strong judicial deference toward individual autonomy. This ensures every human being the right to determine what shall be done with his or her own body. These rights are guaranteed in the U.S. Constitution and have been additionally interpreted in case law and state laws.
- Legal tools and instruments such as advance directives, DNR orders, designation of health care agents, and durable powers of attorney help people plan for future decision making so that their wishes can be carried out even when they are no longer able to speak for themselves. The presence or absence of these instruments may add to the information available about an individual's wishes, but care should be taken to avoid equating the instruments themselves with the existence of these fundamental human rights.
- The right to self-determination was given even more emphasis with the passage of the PSDA, which went into effect in December 1991. This law requires health care providers to inform and educate clients about their rights as they exist under the laws of each state.
- Physician-assisted suicide and issues surrounding the care of terminally ill older persons are subjects of national interest and debate, as well as judicial and legislative interest, and the role and obligation of the nurse in such matters must be carefully monitored.
- The technologic advancements that help people live longer also contribute to the complicated ethical dilemmas that exist in the care of older adults. Ethics committees can help in these matters by responding to the need for the education of and communication between caregivers and clients.

- It is preferable to resolve client care dilemmas at the bedside rather than in the courtroom. The courts prefer such matters to be handled by clients, their families, and health care professionals. With careful guidance and discussion, this can often be achieved.

Critical Thinking Exercises

1. An 80-year-old man has been able to care for himself with minimum assistance until recently. Should he and his family decide that it is time for him to move to a long-term care facility? How will his rights as an individual be protected, since he will be giving up his independence? Explain.
2. A 94-year-old man resides in a long-term care facility. He has signed an AMD in case he becomes seriously ill. A 72-year-old woman is being treated in the hospital for a recent cerebral vascular accident that has left her severely incapacitated. Her family has requested a DNR order. How do these two instruments differ? In what ways do they protect each person's rights?
3. You are the nurse in charge of a wing of a nursing facility. During rounds one evening an older, sometimes confused resident tells you that a nurse aide "pushed her around" during dinner that evening. What issues are presented and what actions should you take?

References

American Association of Retired Persons: *A profile of older Americans: 1998*, Washington, DC, 1998, The Association.

American Nurses Association: *Scope and Standards of Practice*, Washington, DC, 2004, The Association.

American Nurses Association: *Scope and standards of gerontological nursing practice*, Washington, DC, 1995, The Association.

American Nurses Association: *Position statement on nursing and the Patient Self-Determination Act*, Washington, DC, 1992, The Association.

American Nurses Association: *Code for nurses with interpretive statements*, Washington, DC, 2001, The Association.

American Nurses Association praises supreme court for suicide ruling, *US Newswire*, June 26, 1997.

Ballard D: Don't leave final decisions to doctors, *Hartford Courant*, May 17, 1993.

Black HC: *Black's law dictionary*, ed 5, St Paul, Minn, 1979, West Publishing.

Blendon RI et al: Should physicians aid their patients in dying? *JAMA* 267(19):2658, 1992.

Breaux JS: Background checks of nursing home staff, Congressional Testimony, Sept 14, 1998.

Brett A et al: Ethical aspects of human experimentation in health services research, *JAMA* 265(14):1854, 1991.

Centers for Medicare and Medicaid Services: *Protecting your health insurance coverage*, Washington, DC, 2004, The Agency.

Coleman CH: Surrogate decision-making in New York: the legislative proposal of the New York State Task Force on Life and the Law. In *American Bar Association: Newsletter of the Medicine and Law Committee*, Chicago, 1994, The Association.

Collier HG: Current issues in federal regulation of long-term care. In Gosfield AG, editor: *Health law handbook*, New York, 1990, Clark Boardman Callaghan.

Conely GC, Campbell LA: The use of restraints in caring for the elderly: realities, consequences and alternatives, *Nurs Pract* 16(12):51, 1991.

Cooper JW: OBRA regulations and chemical restraints, *Nurs Homes Sen Cit Care* 39:5, 1990.

Department of Health and Human Services, Centers for Medicare and Medicaid Services [DHHS and CMS]: Prospective payment system and consolidated billing for skilled nursing facilities—update, 2004, Washington DC, www.go.gov/decisions/majrule/d011047r.htm, downloaded on Nov 28, 2004, The Agency.

Doukas DJ et al: The values history: the evaluation of the patient's values and advance directives, *Fam Pract* 32(2):145, 1991.

Furrow BR et al: *Health law: cases, materials and problems*, St Paul, Minn, 1987, West Publishing.

GAO/HEHS Report 98-202: *California nursing homes report to the special committee on aging*, US Senate, 1998.

Giuliano KK: Organ transplants: tackling the tough ethical questions . . ., *Nursing* 27(7):34, 1997.

Grimaldi PL: Medicare Part C means more choices, *Nurs Manag*, Feb 1, 1997.

Hamme JM: An overview of OBRA '87 and '90. In National Health Lawyers Association: *Long term care handbook*, Washington, DC, 1991, The Association.

Health care facility management, Chicago, 1990, Commerce Clearing House, 1060.

Health Care Financing Administration (HCFA): *Fact Sheet*, July 21, 1998.

HIPAA: Health Insurance Portability and Accountability Act of 1996, Washington, DC, 2004, http://hipaa.hcfa.gov., and www.cms.hhs.gov/hipaa/hipaa1/contant/protect.pdf, downloaded on Nov 28, 2004, The Agency.

Hollerman CE: Membership of institutional ethics committees, *Phys Exec* 17(3):34, 1991.

Houge EE: Ethics committees help facilities to cope with the PSDA, *Brown Univ Long Term Care Newsletter* 5(3):5, 1993.

Johnson SH: Residents' rights under OBRA of 1987. In National Health Lawyers Association: *Long term care handbook*, Washington, DC, 1991, The Association.

Kane RL, Kane RA: The impact of long-term-care financing on personal autonomy, *Generations* 14(suppl):86, 1990.

Keller HB: Training course reduces abuse in nursing homes (preventing abuse in nursing homes), *Aging* 3:110, 1996.

Krauss NA et al: *Nursing home update, 1996, MEPS (Medical Expenditure Panel Survey) highlights*, No. 2, July 1997, Agency for Health Care Policy and Research.

LaPuma J, Orrentlicher D, Moss RJ: Advance directives on admission: clinical implications and analysis of the Patient Self-Determination Act, *JAMA* 266:402, 1991.

Lieberson AD: *Advance medical directives*, vol 1, Sept 1997.

Lieberson AD: *Advance medical directives*, New York, 1992, Clark Boardman Callaghan.

Long Term Care Standards Manual 1990, Chicago, 1989, Joint Commission on Accreditation of Healthcare Organizations.

Maier T: Election 97/death by choice/Oregon voters back MD-aided suicides, *Newsday*, 1997, p A05.

Manton KG: The dynamics of population aging: demography and policy analysis, *Milbank Q* 69(2):309, 1991.

Marion Merrell Dow, Inc: *Managed care digest, long term care edition*, Kansas City, Mo, 1994, SMG Marketing Group.

McCormick B: Right to die dilemma: are ethics committees equipped to fill their roles? *Am Med News* 34(42):3, 1991.

National Center for Elder Abuse: Statistics: elder abuse information series 1, 1998, The Center.

Neus E: Hospital must report all deaths to find more organ donors, *Gannett News Service*, June 17, 1998.

Northrop CE, Kelly ME: *Legal issues in nursing*, St Louis, 1987, Mosby.

Older Americans Act Amendments of 1988, Public Law 100-175.

Parkman CA: The Patient Self-Determination Act: measuring its outcomes, *Nurs Manag* 28(5):44 Oct 1, 1997.

Pear R: Clinton orders crackdown on substandard nursing homes, *New York Times,* July 22, 1998.

Peters: Advance medical directives: the case for the durable power of attorney for health care, *Legal Med* 8J:437, 451, 1987.

Potter PA, Perry AG: *Fundamentals of nursing: concepts and clinical practice,* ed 5, St Louis, 2004, Mosby.

Rushton HC, Scanlon C: A road map for navigating end-of-life care, *Med Surg Nurs* 7(3):57, 1998.

Sabatini MM: Health care ethics: models of the provider-patient relationship, *Dermatol Nurs* 10(5):201, June 1998.

Salkin S: Do you know about OBRA? It could affect your sales to nursing homes, *Institut Distrib* 27(7):78, 1991.

Scanlon WJ: Speech before the special committee on aging, US Senate, March 3, 1998.

Schabes AE: LTC surveys. In National Health Lawyers Association: *Long term care handbook,* Washington, DC, 1991, The Association.

Schreiber JC: Decision-making in treatment issues. In Gosfield AG, editor: *Health law handbook,* New York, 1990, Clark Boardman Callaghan.

Starr C: Consultants and OBRA regs: an Rx for better care, *Drug Top* 136(23), 1992.

Strauss PJ et al: *Aging and the law,* Chicago, 1990, Commerce Clearing House.

Suffering in silence, *Long Term Care Manag,* June 2, 1993.

Twenty-eight percent would aid suicide, *Hartford Courant,* April 15, 1993.

US HHS: HHS announces new hospital rules to increase organ donation, *M2 PressWIRE,* June 18, 1998.

Vaca BL, Daake CJ: Review of nursing home regulations, *Med Surg Nurs* 7(6):165, 1998.

Zedlewski SR et al: *Needs of the elderly in the 21st century,* Washington, DC, 1989, Urban Institute.

APPENDIX 3A

Values History Form

Name: ________________________________

Date: ________________________________

If someone assisted you in completing this form, please fill in his or her name, address, and relationship to you.

Name: ________________________________

Address: ________________________________

____

Relationship: ________________________________

The purpose of this form is to assist you in thinking about and writing down what is important to you about your health. If you should at some time become unable to make health care decisions for yourself, your thoughts as expressed on this form may help others make a decision for you in accordance with what you would have chosen.

The first section of this form asks whether you have already expressed your wishes concerning medical treatment through either written or oral communications and if not, whether you would like to do so now. The second section of this form provides an opportunity for you to discuss your values, wishes, and preferences in a number of different areas, such as your personal relationships, your overall attitude toward life, and your thoughts about illness.

From Center for Health and Law Ethics, Institute of Public Law, University of New Mexico, Albuquerque.

SECTION 1

A. Written Legal Documents

Have you written any of the following legal documents?

___

If so, please complete the requested information.

Living Will
Date written: ___

Document location: ___

Comments: (e.g., any limitations, special requests, etc.)

___

Durable Power of Attorney
Date written: ___

Document location: ___

Comments: (e.g., whom have you named to be your decision maker?) ___

Durable Power of Attorney for Health Care Decisions
Date written: ___

Document location: ___

Comments: (e.g., whom have you named to be your decision maker?) ___

Organ Donations
Date written: ___

Document location: ___

Comments: (e.g., any limitations on which organs you would like to donate) ___

B. Wishes Concerning Specific Medical Procedures

If you have ever expressed your wishes, either written or orally, concerning any of the following medical procedures, please complete the requested information. If you have not previously indicated your wishes on these procedures and would like to do so now, please complete this information.

Organ Donation
To whom expressed: ___

If oral, when? ___

If written, when? ___

Document location: ___

Comments: ___

Kidney Dialysis
To whom expressed: ___

If oral, when? ___

If written, when? ___

Document location: ___

Comments: ___

Cardiopulmonary Resuscitation (CPR)
To whom expressed: ___

If oral, when? ___

If written, when? ___

Document location: ___

Comments: ___

Respirators

To whom expressed: ______________________________

If oral, when? ______________________________

If written, when? ______________________________

Document location: ______________________________

Comments: ______________________________

Artificial Nutrition

To whom expressed: ______________________________

If oral, when? ______________________________

If written, when? ______________________________

Document location: ______________________________

Comments: ______________________________

Artificial Hydration

To whom expressed: ______________________________

If oral, when? ______________________________

If written, when? ______________________________

Document location: ______________________________

Comments: ______________________________

C. General Comments

Do you wish to make any general comments about the information you provided in this section?

____

SECTION 2

A. Your Overall Attitude toward Your Health

1. How would you describe your current health status? If you currently have any medical problems, how would you describe them? ______________________________
2. If you have current medical problems, in what ways, if any, do they affect your ability to function? ______________________________
3. How do you feel about your current health status? ______________________________
4. How well are you able to meet the basic necessities of life—eating, food preparation, sleeping, personal hygiene, etc.? ______________________________
5. Do you wish to make any general comments about your overall health? ______________________________

B. Your Perception of the Role of Your Doctor and Other Health Caregivers

1. Do you like your doctors? ______________________________
2. Do you trust your doctors? ______________________________
3. Do you think your doctors should make the final decision concerning any treatment you might need? ______________________________

4. How do you relate to your caregivers, including nurses, therapists, chaplains, social workers, etc.?

5. Do you wish to make any general comments about your doctor and other health caregivers?

C. Your Thoughts about Independence and Control

1. How important are independence and self-sufficiency in your life?

2. If you were to experience decreased physical and mental abilities, how would that affect your attitude toward independence and self-sufficiency?

3. Do you wish to make any general comments about the value of independence and control in your life?

D. Your Personal Relationships

1. Do you expect that your friends, family, and/or others will support your decisions regarding medical treatment you may need now or in the future?

2. Have you made any arrangements for your family or friends to make medical treatment decisions on your behalf? If so, who has agreed to make decisions for you and in what circumstances?

3. What, if any, unfinished business from the past are you concerned about (e.g., personal and family relationships, business and legal matters)?

4. What role do your friends and family play in your life?

5. Do you wish to make any general comments about the personal relationships in your life?

E. Your Overall Attitude toward Life

1. What activities do you enjoy (e.g., hobbies, watching TV)?

2. Are you happy to be alive?

3. Do you feel that life is worth living?

4. How satisfied are you with what you have achieved in your life? ____________________

5. What makes you laugh/cry? ____________________

6. What do you fear most? What frightens or upsets you?

7. What goals do you have for the future? ____________________

8. Do you wish to make any general comments about your attitude toward life? ____________________

F. Your Attitude toward Illness, Dying, and Death

1. What will be important to you when you are dying (e.g., physical comfort, no pain, family members present)? ____________________

2. Where would you prefer to die? ____________________

3. What is your attitude toward death? ____________________

4. How do you feel about the use of life-sustaining measures in the face of:
   Terminal illness? ____________________

   Permanent coma? ____________________

   Irreversible chronic illness (e.g., Alzheimer's disease)?

5. Do you wish to make any general comments about your attitude toward illness, dying, and death?

G. Your Religious Background and Beliefs

1. What is your religious background? ____________________

2. How do your religious beliefs affect your attitude toward serious or terminal illness? ____________________

3. Does your attitude toward death find support in your religion? ____________________

4. How does your faith community, church, or synagogue view the role of prayer or religious sacraments in an illness? ____________________

5. Do you wish to make any general comments about your religious background and beliefs?

H. Your Living Environment

1. What has been your living situation over the last 10 years (e.g., lived alone, lived with others)? ________

2. How difficult is it for you to maintain the kind of environment for yourself that you find comfortable? Does any illness or medical problem you have now mean that it will be harder in the future? ________

3. Do you wish to make any general comments about your living environment? ________

I. Your Attitude Concerning Finances

1. How much do you worry about having enough money to provide for your care? ________

2. Would you prefer to spend less money on your care so that more money can be saved for the benefit of your relatives and/or friends? ________

3. Do you wish to make any general comments concerning your finances and the cost of health care? ________

J. Your Wishes Concerning Your Funeral

1. What are your wishes concerning your funeral and burial or cremation? ________

2. Have you made your funeral arrangements? If so, with whom? ________

3. Do you wish to make any general comments about how you would like your funeral and burial or cremation to be arranged or conducted? ________

Optional Questions

1. How would you like your obituary (announcement of your death) to read? ________

2. Write yourself a brief eulogy (a statement about yourself to be read at your funeral). ________

Suggestions for Use

After you have completed this form, you may wish to provide copies to your doctors and other health caregivers, your family, your friends, and your attorney. If you have a Living Will or Durable Power of Attorney for Health Care Decisions, you may wish to attach a copy of this form to those documents.

4 Gerontologic Assessment

SHARON ROTH MAGUIRE, MS, APRN-BC, GNP, APNP

Learning Objectives

On completion of this chapter, the reader will be able to:

1. Explain the interrelationship between the physical and psychosocial aspects of aging as it affects the assessment process.
2. Describe how the nature of illness presentation, changes in homeostatic mechanisms, and the lack of normative standards for older adults affect the assessment process.
3. Compare and contrast the clinical presentation of delirium and dementia.
4. Describe the assessment modifications that may be necessary when assessing older adults.
5. Describe strategies and techniques to ensure collection of relevant and comprehensive health histories for older adults.
6. Identify the basic components of health histories for older adults.
7. List the principles to observe when conducting physical examinations of older adults.
8. Explain the rationale for assessing functional status in older adults.
9. Describe the elements of a functional assessment.
10. Describe the basic components of a mental status assessment.
11. Discuss the rationale for conducting affective assessments on older adults.
12. Explain the rationale for assessing social function in older adults.
13. Conduct a comprehensive health assessment on an older adult client.

The nursing process is a problem-solving process that provides the organizational framework for the provision of nursing care. Assessment, the crucial foundation on which the remaining steps of the process are built, includes the collection and analysis of data and results in a nursing diagnosis. A nursing-focused assessment is crucial in determining nursing diagnoses that are amenable to nursing intervention. Unless the approach to assessment maintains a *nursing* focus, the sequential steps of the nursing process—diagnosis, planning, implementation, and evaluation—cannot be carried out.

A nursing focus evolves from an awareness and understanding of the purpose of nursing. This purpose was defined in the 1980 American Nurses Association (ANA) publication, *Nursing: A Social Policy Statement*, as "the diagnosis and treatment of human responses to actual or potential health problems." In 1995 ANA developed *Nursing's Social Policy Statement*, which elaborated on the above purpose of nursing based on the growth of nursing science "and its integration with the traditional knowledge base for diagnosis and treatment of human responses to health and illness." Although providing no specific definition of nursing, this policy statement cited three "essential features of contemporary nursing practice" that are common to most definitions:

- Attention to the full range of human experiences and responses to health and illness without restriction to a problem-focused orientation.
- Integration of objective data with knowledge gained from an understanding of the client or group's subjective experience.
- Application of scientific knowledge to the processes of diagnosis and treatment. Provision of a caring relationship that facilitates health and healing (ANA, 1995).

It is clear from these elements that the nurse collects subjective and objective data about the client to assist in determining the client's response to health and illness. A comprehensive, *nursing-focused* assessment of these responses establishes a database about a client's ability to meet the full range of physical and psychosocial needs. Client responses that reveal an inability to satisfactorily meet these needs indicate a need for nursing care, or the "caring relationship that facilitates health and healing" (ANA, 1995).

Nursing-focused assessment of older people occurs in the traditional settings of the hospital, home, or long-term care facility, as well as in nontraditional settings such as senior centers, congregate living units, hospice facilities, and independent or group nursing practices. The setting dictates the way data collection and analysis should be managed to serve clients best. Although the setting may vary, the purpose of nursing-focused assessment of older clients remains that of determining the older person's ability to meet any health- and illness-related needs. Specifically, the purpose of older adult assessment is to identify client strengths and limitations so that effective and appropriate interventions can be delivered to support, promote, and/or restore optimum function and to prevent disability and dependence.

Gerontologic nurses recognize that assessing older adult clients involves the application of a broad range of skills and abilities, as well as consideration of many complex and varied issues. Nursing-focused assessment based on a sound, scientific gerontologic knowledge base, coupled with repeated practice to acquire the *art* of assessment, is essential for the nurse to recognize client responses that reflect unmet needs. Many frameworks and tools are available to guide the nurse in assessing older adults. Regardless of the framework or tool used, the nurse should collect the data while observing the following key principles: (1) use of an individual, person-centered approach; (2) a view of clients as participants in health monitoring and treatment; and (3) an emphasis on clients' functional ability.

SPECIAL CONSIDERATIONS AFFECTING ASSESSMENT

Nursing assessment of older adults is a complex and challenging process that must take into account the following points to ensure an age-specific approach.

INTERRELATIONSHIP BETWEEN PHYSICAL AND PSYCHOSOCIAL ASPECTS OF AGING

The health of people of all ages is subject to the influence of any number and kind of physical and psychosocial factors within the environment. The balance that is achieved within that environment of many factors greatly influences a person's health status. Factors such as reduced ability to respond to stress, increased frequency and multiplicity of loss, and physical changes associated with normal aging can combine to place older adults at high risk for loss of functional ability. Consider the following case, which illustrates how the interaction of select physical and psychosocial factors can seriously compromise function.

Ms. L, age 81, arrives in the emergency room after being found in her home by a neighbor. The neighbor had become concerned because he noticed Ms. L had not picked up her newspapers for the past 3 days. She was found in her bed, weak and lethargic. She stated that she had the flu for the past week, so she was unable to eat or drink much because of the associated nausea and vomiting. Except for her mild hypertension, which is medically managed with an antihypertensive agent, she had enjoyed relatively good health before this acute illness. She is admitted to the hospital with pneumonia.

Because of the emergent nature of the admission, Ms. L does not have any personal belongings with her, including her hearing aid, glasses, and dentures. She develops congestive heart failure after treatment of her dehydration with intravenous fluids. She then becomes confused and agitated, and begins receiving haloperidol (Haldol). Her impaired mobility, resulting from the chemical restraint, has caused her to become incontinent of urine and stool, and she has developed a stage 2 pressure ulcer on her coccyx. She needs to be fed because of her confusion and eats very little. She sleeps at intervals throughout the day and night, and when she is awake, she is usually crying.

Table 4-1 depicts the many serious consequences of the interacting physical and psychosocial factors in this case. A word of caution: undue emphasis should not be placed on individual decrements. In fact, it is imperative that the gerontologic nurse search for the client's strengths and abilities, and build the plan of care on these. However, in a situation such as that of Ms. L, the nurse should be aware of the potential for the consequences illustrated here. A single problem is not likely, since multiple conditions are often superimposed. In addition, the cause of one problem is often best understood in view of the accompanying problems. Careful consideration, then, of the interrelationships between physical and psychosocial aspects in every client situation is essential.

TABLE 4-1 Effect of Selected Variables on Functional Status

VARIABLE	EFFECT
Visual and auditory loss	Apathy Confusion, disorientation Dependency, loss of control
Multiple strange and unfamiliar environments	Confusion, agitation Dependency, loss of control Sleep disturbance Relocation stress
Acute medical illness	Mobility impairment Dependency, loss of control Sleep disturbance Pressure ulcer Inadequate food intake
Altered pharmacokinetics and pharmacodynamics	Persistent confusion Drug toxicity Potential for further mobility impairment, loss of function, and altered patterns of bowel and bladder elimination Loss of appetite, in turn affecting wound healing, bowel function, and energy level; dehydration Sleep disturbance (oversedation)

Adapted from Lueckenotte AG: *Pocket guide to gerontologic assessment*, ed 3, St Louis, 1998, Mosby.

NATURE OF DISEASE AND DISABILITY AND THEIR EFFECTS ON FUNCTIONAL STATUS

Aging does not necessarily result in disease and disability. Although the prevalence of chronic disease increases with age, most older people remain functionally independent. However, what cannot be ignored is that chronic disease increases older adults' vulnerability to functional decline. Comprehensive assessment of physical and psychosocial function is important because it can provide valuable clues to a disease's effect on functional status. Also, the self-report of vague signs and symptoms such as lethargy, incontinence, decreased appetite, and weight loss can be an indicator of functional impairment. Ignoring older adults' vague symptomatology exposes them to an increased risk of physical frailty. Physical frailty, or impairments in the physical abilities that are needed to live independently, is a major contributor to the need for long-term care. Therefore it is essential to comprehensively investigate the report of nonspecific signs and symptoms to determine whether there are underlying conditions that may contribute to the older person's frailty.

Declining organ and system function and diminishing physiologic reserve with advancing age are well documented in the literature. Such normal changes of aging may make the body more susceptible to disease and disability, the risk of which increases exponentially with advancing age. It can be difficult for the nurse to differentiate normal age-related findings from indicators of disease or disability. In fact, it is not uncommon for nurses and older adults alike to mistakenly attribute vague signs and symptoms to normal aging changes or just "growing old." However, it is essential for the nurse to determine what is "normal" versus what may be an indicator of disease or disability so that treatable conditions are not disregarded.

Decreased Efficiency of Homeostatic Mechanisms

Declining physiologic function and increased prevalence of disease, particularly in the old-old (ages 85 and older), are in part a result of a reduction in the body's ability to respond to stress through all of its homeostatic mechanisms, most importantly the immune system. Older persons' adaptive reserves are reduced and their homeostatic mechanisms weakened; these factors result in a decreased ability to respond to physical and emotional stress.

The immune system, as the body's major defense against illness and disease, has a decreased ability to provide protection with aging (see Chapter 16). Although scientists have attempted to identify which age-related immune system changes cause the decline in immunocompetence, it has been difficult to do so since immunocompetence is affected by multiple other factors.

Increasing consideration has also been given in recent years to the potential impact of psychosocial stress on the older adult immune system. This growing consideration, coupled with the knowledge about factors affecting physiologic immunocompetence, has potential clinical relevance that is a current source of controversy. The reader is referred to an immunology text for a more complete discussion of the effect of aging on the immune response.

The important point is that older adults often encounter profound and repeated losses; the time between the occurrences of these losses is often short, resulting in an inadequate period for resolution and return to a baseline state. Older adults have less ability than younger people to cope with assaults such as infection, blood loss, a high-technology environment, or loss of a significant person (see Chapter 20). The nurse should therefore assess older adults for the presence of physical and psychosocial stressors and their physical and emotional manifestations.

Lack of Standards for Health and Illness Norms

Determining older adults' physical and psychosocial health status is not easy, because norms for health and illness are always being redefined. Established standards for what is normal versus abnormal are changing as more scientific studies are conducted and the knowledge base is expanded.

One area where scientific study is changing how health care providers interpret normal versus abnormal status is with laboratory values. Relying on established norms for laboratory values when analyzing older adults' assessment data could lead to incorrect conclusions. Fasting blood glucose of 80 mg/100 ml may be within the normal range for a young adult, but an older person with that same level may experience symptoms of hypoglycemia. Polypharmacy and the multiplicity of illness and disease are only two variables that may affect laboratory data interpretation for older adults (see Chapters 21 and 22).

In addition, there are no definitive aging norms for many pathologic conditions. For example, controversy has existed over what constitutes isolated systolic hypertension in older people. Is a high systolic pressure simply a function of age, or does it require treatment? *The Seventh Report of the Joint National Committee on Detection, Evaluation, and Treatment of High Blood Pressure* (JNC VII) states that cardiovascular morbidity and mortality in older people have been reduced with antihypertensive drug therapy (National High Blood Pressure Education Program, 2003). As more studies are conducted in this and other areas, norms for older adults will continue to be redefined.

Landmarks for human growth and development are well established for infancy through middlescence, whereas few norms are defined for older adulthood. Developmental norms that have been described for later life categorize all older people in the "over-65" group. However, it could easily be argued from a developmental perspective that as great a difference exists among adults ages 65, 75, 85, and 95 as it does among children ages 2 through 5. In fact, given the demographic facts and predictions, there is a pressing need to know the developmental characteristics of older people for each decade of life. This is an important area for scientific inquiry.

To compensate for the lack of definitive standards, the nurse should first assume heterogeneity rather than homogeneity when caring for older people. It is crucial to respect the uniqueness of each person's life experiences and to preserve the individuality created by those experiences. The older person's experiences represent a rich and vast background that the nurse can use to develop an individualized plan of care. Second, the nurse can compare the older person's own previous patterns of physical and psychosocial health and function with the current status, using the individual as the standard. Finally, the nurse must have a complete, current, scientific knowledge base and skills in gerontologic nursing to apply to each individual older adult client.

Altered Presentation of and Response to Specific Diseases

With advanced age the body does not respond as vigorously to illness or disease because of diminished physiologic reserve. The diminished reserve poses no particular problems for older people as they carry out their daily routines. However, in times of physical and emotional stress, older people will not always exhibit the expected or "classic" signs and symptoms. The characteristic presentation of illness in older adults is more commonly one of blunted or atypical signs and symptoms.

The atypical presentation of illness can be displayed in various ways. For example, the signs and symptoms may be modified in some way, as in the case of pneumonia, when older adults may exhibit dry coughs instead of the classic productive coughs. Also, the presenting signs and symptoms may be totally unrelated to the actual problem, such as the confusion that may accompany a urinary tract infection. Finally, the expected signs and symptoms may not be present at all, as in the case of a myocardial infarction that includes no chest pain (Table 4-2). All these atypical presentations challenge the nurse to conduct careful and thorough assessments and analyses of symptoms to ensure appropriate treatment. Again, a simple and safe strategy is to compare the presenting signs and symptoms with the older adult's normal baselines.

Cognitive Impairment. As can be seen in Table 4-2, delirium is one of the most common, atypical presentations of illness in older adults, representing a wide variety of potential problems.

Confusion, mental status changes, cognitive changes, and *delirium* are some of the terms used to describe one of the most common manifestations of illness in old age. Foreman (1986) advocates use of the term *acute confusional state* (ACS) to describe "an organic brain syndrome characterized by transient, global cognitive impairment of abrupt onset and relatively brief duration, accompanied by diurnal fluctuation of simultaneous disturbances of the sleep-wake cycle, psychomotor behavior, attention, and affect." Unfortunately, the ageist views of many health care providers cause them to believe that an ACS is a normal, expected outcome of aging, thus robbing older adults of complete and thorough workups of this syndrome. The nurse as an advocate for older persons may need to remind other team members that a sudden change in cognitive function is often the result of illness, not aging. Knowing older adults' baseline mental status is key to avoid overlooking a serious illness manifesting itself as an ACS. Box 4-1 outlines the multivariate causes of an ACS that the nurse must consider during assessment.

One of the more challenging aspects of older adult assessment is distinguishing a reversible ACS from irreversible cognitive changes such as those seen in dementia and related disorders. In contrast to the characteristics of an ACS noted previously, dementia is a global, sustained deterioration of cognitive function in an alert client. Other diagnostic features of dementia include memory impairment and one or more of the following cognitive disturbances: aphasia, apraxia, agnosia, or disturbance in executive functioning (e.g., planning, organizing, sequencing, abstracting) (American Psychiatric Association, 1994). Primary dementias include senile dementia of the Alzheimer's type, Lewy body disease, Pick's disease, Creutzfeldt-Jakob disease, and multi-infarct dementia. Secondary dementias that have the same presenting symptoms but are often reversible with *early* diagnosis include normal pressure hydrocephalus, intracranial masses or lesions, pseudodementia, and Parkinson's dementia. Table 4-3 depicts the distinguishing features of an ACS and dementia. See Chapter 29 for a complete description of these primary and secondary dementing diseases.

Assessment can be complex because of the multiple associated characteristics of an ACS and dementia. In fact, it is not uncommon for an ACS to be superimposed on dementia. In this case the symptoms of a new illness may be accentuated or may be masked, thus confounding assessment. Therefore the nurse must have a clear understanding of the differences between an ACS and dementia, and must recognize that only subtle evidence may be present to indicate the existence of a problem. Also, it may not be possible or desirable to complete the total assessment during the first encounter with the client. In conducting the initial assessment of the course of the presenting symptoms, the nurse should remember that families and friends of the client can be valuable sources of data regarding the onset, duration, and associated symptoms.

TAILORING THE NURSING ASSESSMENT TO THE OLDER PERSON

The health assessment may be collected in a variety of physical settings, including hospital, home, office, day care

TABLE 4-2 How Illness Changes With Age

PROBLEM	CLASSIC PRESENTATION IN YOUNG PATIENT	PRESENTATION IN ELDERLY PATIENTS
Urinary tract infection	Dysuria, frequency, urgency, nocturia	Dysuria often *absent;* frequency, urgency, nocturia *sometimes* present. Incontinence, delirium, falls, and anorexia are other signs.
Myocardial infarction	Severe substernal chest pain, diaphoresis, nausea, dyspnea	Sometimes *no* chest pain, or atypical pain location such as in jaw, neck, shoulder, epigastric area. Dyspnea may or may not be present. Other signs are tachypnea, arrhythmia, hypotension, restlessness, syncope, and fatigue/weakness. A fall may be a prodrome.
Bacterial pneumonia	Cough productive of purulent sputum, chills and fever, pleuritic chest pain, elevated white blood cell (WBC) count	Cough may be productive, dry, or absent; chills and fever and/or elevated WBCs also may be absent. Tachypnea, slight cyanosis, delirium, anorexia, nausea and vomiting, and tachycardia may be present.
Congestive heart failure	Increased dyspnea (orthopnea, paroxysmal nocturnal dyspnea), fatigue, weight gain, pedal edema, nocturia, bibasilar crackles	All the manifestations of young adult *and/or* anorexia, restlessness, delirium, cyanosis, and falls. Cough.
Hyperthyroidism	Heat intolerance, fast pace, exophthalmos, increased pulse, hyperreflexia, tremor	Slowing down (apathetic hyperthyroidism), lethargy, weakness, depression, atrial fibrillation, and congestive heart failure.
Hypothyroidism	Weakness, fatigue, cold intolerance, lethargy, skin dryness and scaling, constipation	Often presents without overt symptoms; majority of cases are subclinical. Delirium, dementia, depression/lethargy, constipation, weight loss, and muscle weakness/unsteady gait are common.
Depression	Dysphoric mood and thoughts, withdrawal, crying, weight loss, constipation, insomnia	Any of classic symptoms *may or may not* be present. Memory and concentration problems, cognitive and behavioral changes, increased dependency, anxiety, and increased sleep. Muscle aches, abdominal pain or tightness, flatulence, nausea and vomiting, dry mouth, and headaches. Be alert for congestive heart failure, diabetes, cancer, infectious diseases, and anemia. Cardiovascular agents, anxiolytics, amphetamines, narcotics, and hormones can also play a role.

Modified from Henderson ML: Altered presentations, *Am J Nurs* 15:1104, 1986.

center, and long-term care facility. Any of these settings can be adapted to be conducive to the free exchange of information between the nurse and an older adult. The overall atmosphere established by the nurse should be one that conveys trust, caring, and confidentiality. The following general suggestions related to preparation of the environment and consideration of individual client need foster the collection of meaningful data (see Cultural Awareness box, p. 69).

Environmental modifications made during the assessment should take into account sensory and musculoskeletal changes. The following points should be considered in preparation of the environment:

- Provide adequate space, particularly if the client uses a mobility aid.
- Minimize noise and distraction such as those generated by television, radio, intercom, or other nearby activity.
- Set a comfortable, sufficiently warm temperature with no drafts.
- Use diffuse lighting with increased illumination; avoid directional or localized light.
- Avoid glossy or highly polished surfaces, including floors, walls, ceilings, and furnishings.
- Place the client in a comfortable seating position that facilitates information exchange.
- Maintain proximity to a bathroom.
- Keep water or other preferred fluids available.
- Provide a place to hang or store garments and belongings.
- Maintain absolute privacy.
- Plan the assessment, taking into account the older adult's energy level, pace, and adaptability. More than one session may be necessary to complete the assessment.
- Be patient, relaxed, and unhurried.

BOX 4-1 Physiologic, Psychologic, and Environmental Causes of Acute Confusional States in Hospitalized Older Adults

PHYSIOLOGIC

A. Primary Cerebral Disease

1. Nonstructural factors
   a. Vascular insufficiency—transient ischemic attacks, cerebrovascular accidents, thrombosis
   b. Central nervous system infection—acute and chronic meningitis, neurosyphillis, brain abscess
2. Structural factors
   a. Trauma—subdural hematoma, concussion, contusion, intracranial hemorrhage
   b. Tumors—primary and metastatic
   c. Normal pressure hydrocephalus

B. Extracranial Disease

1. Cardiovascular abnormalities
   a. Decreased cardiac output state—myocardial infarction, arrhythmias, congestive heart failure, cardiogenic shock
   b. Alterations in peripheral vascular resistance—increased and decreased states
   c. Vascular occlusion—disseminated intravascular coagulopathy, emboli
2. Pulmonary abnormalities
   a. Inadequate gas exchange states—pulmonary disease, alveolar hypoventilation
   b. Infection—pneumonias
3. Systemic infective processes—acute and chronic
   a. Viral
   b. Bacterial—endocarditis, pyelonephritis, cystitis, mycosis
4. Metabolic disturbances
   a. Electrolyte abnormalities—hypercalcemia, hyponatremia and hypernatremia, hypokalemia and hyperkalemia, hypochloremia and hyperchloremia, hyperphosphatemia
   b. Acidosis and alkalosis
   c. Hypoglycemia and hyperglycemia
   d. Acute and chronic renal failure
   e. Volume depletion—hemorrhage, inadequate fluid intake, diuretics
   f. Hepatic failure
   g. Porphyria
5. Drug intoxications—therapeutic and substance abuse
   a. Misuse of prescribed medications
   b. Side effects of therapeutic medications
   c. Drug-drug interactions
   d. Improper use of over-the-counter medications
   e. Ingestion of heavy metals and industrial poisons
6. Endocrine disturbance
   a. Hypothyroidism and hyperthyroidism
   b. Diabetes mellitus
   c. Hypopituitarism
   d. Hypoparathyroidism and hyperparathyroidism
7. Nutritional deficiencies
   a. B vitamins
   b. Vitamin C
   c. Protein
8. Physiologic stress—pain, surgery
9. Alterations in temperature regulation—hypothermia and hyperthermia
10. Unknown physiologic abnormality—sometimes defined as pseudodelirium

PSYCHOLOGIC

1. Severe emotional stress—postoperative states, relocation, hospitalization
2. Depression
3. Anxiety
4. Pain—acute and chronic
5. Fatigue
6. Grief
7. Sensory/perceptual deficits—noise, alteration in function of senses
8. Mania
9. Paranoia
10. Situational disturbances

ENVIRONMENTAL

1. Unfamiliar environment creating a lack of meaning in the environment
2. Sensory deprivation or environmental monotony creating a lack of meaning in the environment
3. Sensory overload
4. Immobilization—therapeutic, physical, pharmacologic
5. Sleep deprivation
6. Lack of temporospatial reference points

Modified from Foreman MD: Acute confusional states in hospitalized elderly: a research dilemma, *Nurs Res* 35(1):34, 1986.

- Allow the client plenty of time to respond to questions and directions.
- Maximize the use of silence to allow the client time to collect thoughts before responding.
- Be alert to signs of increasing fatigue such as sighing, grimacing, irritability, leaning against objects for support, dropping of head and shoulders, and progressive slowing.
- Conduct assessment during client's peak energy time.

Regardless of the degree of decrement and decline an older adult client may exhibit, there are assets and capabilities that allow the client to function within the limitations imposed by

TABLE 4-3 **Differentiating Dementia and ACS**

CLINICAL FEATURE	ACS	DEMENTIA
Onset	Acute/subacute; depends on cause; often occurs at twilight	Chronic, generally insidious; depends on cause
Course	Short; diurnal fluctuations in symptoms; worse at night, dark, and on awakening	Long; no diurnal effects; symptoms progressive, yet relatively stable over time
Duration	Hours to less than 1 month	Months to years
Awareness	Fluctuates, generally reduced	Generally clear
Alertness	Fluctuates—reduced or increased	Generally normal
Attention	Impaired, often fluctuates	Generally normal
Orientation	Fluctuates in severity, generally impaired	May be impaired
Memory	Recent and immediate memory impaired; unable to register new information or recall recent events	Recent and remote memory impaired; loss of recent memory is first sign; some loss of common knowledge
Thinking	Disorganized, distorted, fragmented, slow, or accelerated	Difficulty with abstraction and word finding
Perception	Distorted, illusions, delusions, or hallucinations	Misperceptions often absent
Sleep-wake cycle	Disturbed, cycle reversed	Fragmented

Modified from Foreman MD: Acute confusional states in hospitalized elderly: a research dilemma, *Nurs Res* 35(1):34, 1986.

that decline. During the assessment the nurse must provide an environment that gives the older adult the opportunity to demonstrate those abilities. Failure to do so could result in inaccurate conclusions about the client's functional ability, which may lead to inappropriate care and treatment:

- Assess more than once and at different times of day.
- Measure performance under the most favorable of conditions.
- Take advantage of natural opportunities that would elicit assets and capabilities; collect data during bathing, grooming, and mealtime.
- Ensure that assistive sensory devices (glasses, hearing aid) and mobility devices (walker, cane, prosthesis) are in place and functioning correctly.
- Interview family, friends, and significant others who are involved in the client's care to validate assessment data.
- Use body language, touch, eye contact, and speech to promote the client's maximum degree of participation.
- Be aware of the client's emotional state and concerns; fear, anxiety, and boredom can lead to inaccurate assessment conclusions regarding functional ability.

Cultural Awareness

CULTURAL ASSESSMENT

Cultural or culturologic nursing assessment refers to a systematic appraisal or examination of older adult individuals, groups, and communities in relation to their cultural beliefs, attitudes, values, behaviors, and practices to determine explicit nursing needs and interventions within the cultural context of the people being evaluated. Because they deal with cultural values, belief systems, and lifestyles, cultural assessments tend to be broad and comprehensive, though it is possible to focus on a smaller segment.

Cultural assessment consists of both process and content. The process aspect concerns the nurse's approach to clients, taking into account verbal and nonverbal communication, meaning and context of speech, spatial behavior and spatial needs, relevance of social versus clock time, environmental control issues, and biologic variations. The sequence or order in which data are gathered is often critical, and the order of the assessment may need to be varied depending on the cultural group and the clients' individual needs. The content of the cultural assessment consists of the actual data categories in which information about clients is gathered.

THE HEALTH HISTORY

The nursing health history and interview, as the first phase of a comprehensive, nursing-focused health assessment, provide a subjective account of the older adult's current and past health status. The interview forms the basis of a therapeutic nurse-client relationship, in which the client's well-being is the mutual concern. Establishing this relationship with the older adult is essential to gathering useful, significant data. The data obtained from the health history alert the nurse to focus on key areas of the physical examination that require further investigation. By talking with the nurse about health concerns, the older adult increases his or her awareness of health, and topics for health teaching can be identified. Finally, the process of recounting a client's history in a purposeful, systematic way can have the therapeutic effect of serving as a life review.

Although a number of formats exist for the nursing health history, all have similar basic components (Box 4-2). In addition, the nursing health history for the older adult should include assessment of functional, cognitive, affective, and

Text continues on p. 73

BOX 4-2 Sample Older Adult Health History Format

1. Client Profile/Biographic Data
Name ______ Address ______
Telephone ______ Date and place of birth/age ______
Sex ____ Race ______ Religion ______ Marital status ______
Education ______ Nearest contact person ______
Address/telephone ______
Advance directives: Living will: ______
Code status: ______
DPOA-Health care: ______ POA-Finance: ______

2. Family Profile
Spouse(s) ______
Living ______
Health status ______
Age ______
Occupation ______
Deceased ______
Year of death ______
Cause of death ______

Children ______
Living ______
Names and addresses ______
______
______
______
Deceased ______
Year of death ______
Cause of death ______

3. Occupational Profile
Current work status ______
______
Previous occupations ______
______
Source(s) of income and adequacy for needs ______
______

4. Living Environment Profile
Type of dwelling ______
Number of rooms ______ Number of levels ______
Number of people living in dwelling ______
Degree of privacy ______ Nearest neighbor ______
Address/telephone ______
______

5. Recreation/Leisure Profile
Hobbies/interests ______
Organizational memberships ______
Vacations/travel ______

6. Resources/Support Systems Used
Religious preference/affiliation ______
Confidants ______
Who helps when need arises ______
Physician(s) ______
______
Hospital ______
Clinic ______
Home health agency ______
Meals on Wheels ______
Adult day care ______
Other ______
______

7. Description of Typical Day (Include Usual Bedtime Ritual)
______

8. Present Health Status
General health status during past year ______
______
General health status during past 5 years
______
Chief complaint ______
______
Knowledge, understanding, and management of health problems (e.g., special diet, dressing changes) ______
______
Overall degree of function relative to health problems and medical diagnoses ______
______

MEDICATIONS

Name(s) ______
______
Dosage ______
______
How/when taken ______
______
Prescribing physician ______
Date of prescription ______
Problems with adherence (complicated regimen with large number and variety of drugs, visual deficits, unpleasant side effects, perception of effectiveness, difficulty obtaining, and affordability)

IMMUNIZATION STATUS (NOTE DATE OF MOST RECENT IMMUNIZATION)

Tetanus, diphtheria ______
PPD ______
Influenza ______
Pneumovax ______

ALLERGIES (NOTE SPECIFIC AGENT AND REACTION)

Drugs ______
Foods ______
Contact substances ______
Environmental factors ______

NUTRITION

24-hour diet recall (include fluid intake)
Special diet, food restrictions, or preferences ______
______

BOX 4-2 Sample Older Adult Health History Format—cont'd

History of weight gain/loss ______

Food consumption patterns (e.g., frequency, alone or with others) ______

Problems affecting food intake (e.g., inadequate income, lack of transportation, chewing/swallowing problems, emotional stress) ______

Habits ______

9. Past Health Status

Childhood illnesses ______

Serious or chronic illnesses ______

Trauma ______

Hospitalizations (note reason, date, place, duration, physician[s]) ______

Operations (note type, date, place, reason, physician[s]) ______

Obstetric history ______

10. Family History

Draw pedigree (identify grandparents, parents, aunts, uncles, siblings, spouse[s], children)

Survey the following: cancer, diabetes mellitus, heart disease, hypertension, seizure disorder, renal disease, arthritis, alcoholism, mental health problems, anemia

11. Review of Systems

Check yes or no for each symptom and include full symptom analysis on positive responses at end of each system.

GENERAL	YES	NO
Fatigue		
Weight change in past year		
Appetite change		
Fever		
Night sweats		
Sleeping difficulty		
Frequent colds, infections		

Self-rating of overall health status ______

Ability to carry out activities of daily living (ADLs) ______

INTEGUMENT	YES	NO
Lesions/wounds		
Pruritus		

INTEGUMENT, cont'd	YES	NO
Pigmentation changes		
Texture changes		
Nevi changes		
Frequent bruising		
Hair changes		
Nail changes		
Corns, bunions, calluses		
Chronic sun exposure		

Healing pattern of lesions, bruises ______

HEMATOPOIETIC	YES	NO
Abnormal bleeding/bruising		
Lymph node swelling		
Anemia		

Blood transfusion history ______

HEAD	YES	NO
Headache		
Past significant trauma		
Dizziness		
Scalp itching		

EYES	YES	NO
Vision changes		
Glasses/contact lenses		
Pain		
Excessive tearing		
Pruritus		
Swelling around eyes		
Floaters		
Diplopia		
Blurring		
Photophobia		
Scotomata		
History of infections		

Date of most recent vision examination ______

Date of most recent glaucoma check ______

Impact on ADL performance ______

EARS	YES	NO
Hearing changes		
Discharge		
Tinnitus		
Vertigo		
Hearing sensitivity		
Prosthetic device(s)		
History of infection		

Date of most recent auditory examination ______

Usual ear care habits ______

Impact on ADL performance ______

NOSE AND SINUSES	YES	NO
Rhinorrhea		
Discharge		
Epistaxis		
Obstruction		

Continued

BOX 4-2 Sample Older Adult Health History Format—cont'd

NOSE AND SINUSES, cont'd	YES	NO
Snoring		
Pain over sinuses		
Postnasal drip		
Allergies		
History of infections		

Self-rating of olfactory ability ______________________

____

MOUTH AND THROAT	YES	NO
Sore throat		
Lesions/ulcers		
Hoarseness		
Voice changes		
Difficulty swallowing		
Bleeding gums		
Caries		
Altered taste		
Difficulty chewing		
Prosthetic device(s)		
History of infections		

Date of most recent dental examination ______________________

Brushing pattern ______________________

____

Flossing pattern ______________________

____

Denture cleaning routine and problems ______________________

____

NECK	YES	NO
Stiffness		
Pain/tenderness		
Lumps/masses		
Limited movement		

BREASTS	YES	NO
Lumps/masses		
Pain/tenderness		
Swelling		
Nipple discharge		
Nipple changes		

Breast self-examination pattern ______________________

____

Date and results of most recent mammogram ______________________

RESPIRATORY	YES	NO
Cough		
Shortness of breath		
Hemoptysis		
Wheezing		
Asthma/respiratory allergy		

Date and results of most recent chest x-ray examination

____

CARDIOVASCULAR	YES	NO
Chest pain/discomfort		
Palpitations		
Shortness of breath		

CARDIOVASCULAR, Cont'd	YES	NO
Dyspnea on exertion		
Paroxysmal nocturnal dyspnea		
Orthopnea		
Murmur		
Edema		
Varicosities		
Claudication		
Paresthesias		
Leg color changes		

GASTROINTESTINAL	YES	NO
Dysphagia		
Indigestion		
Heartburn		
Nausea/vomiting		
Hematemesis		
Appetite changes		
Food intolerances		
Ulcers		
Pain		
Jaundice		
Lumps/masses		
Change in bowel habits		
Diarrhea		
Constipation		
Melena		
Hemorrhoids		
Rectal bleeding		

Usual bowel pattern ______________________

____

URINARY	YES	NO
Dysuria		
Frequency		
Dribbling		
Hesitancy		
Urgency		
Hematuria		
Polyuria		
Oliguria		
Nocturia		
Incontinence		
Painful urination		
Stones		
Infections		

GENITOREPRODUCTIVE—MALE	YES	NO
Lesions		
Discharge		
Testicular pain		
Testicular mass(es)		
Prostate problems		
Venereal disease(s)		
Change in sex drive		
Impotence		
Concerns re: sexual activity		

BOX 4-2 Sample Older Adult Health History Format—cont'd

GENITOREPRODUCTIVE—FEMALE	YES	NO
Lesions		
Discharge		
Dyspareunia		
Postcoital bleeding		
Pelvic pain		
Cystocele/rectocele/prolapse		
Venereal disease(s)		
Infections		
Concerns re: sexual activity		

Menstrual history (age of onset, date of last menstrual period) ______

Menopausal history (age, symptoms, postmenopausal problems) ______

Date and result of most recent Pap test ______

GR ______ P ______ A ______

MUSCULOSKELETAL	YES	NO
Joint pain		
Stiffness		
Joint swelling		
Deformity		
Spasm		
Cramping		
Muscle weakness		
Gait problems		
Back pain		
Prosthesis(es)		

Usual exercise pattern ______

Impact on ADL performance ______

CENTRAL NERVOUS SYSTEM	YES	NO
Headache		
Seizures		
Syncope/drop attacks		

CENTRAL NERVOUS SYSTEM, Cont'd	YES	NO
Paralysis		
Paresis		
Coordination problems		
Tic/tremor/spasm		
Paresthesias		
Head injury		
Memory problems		

ENDOCRINE SYSTEM	YES	NO
Heat intolerance		
Cold intolerance		
Goiter		
Skin pigmentation/texture changes		
Hair changes		
Polyphagia		
Polydipsia		
Polyuria		

PSYCHOSOCIAL	YES	NO
Anxious		
Depressed		
Insomnia		
Crying spells		
Nervous		
Fearful		
Trouble with decision making		
Difficulty concentrating		

Statement of general feelings of satisfaction/frustration ______

Usual coping mechanisms ______

Current stresses ______

Concerns about death ______

Impact on ADL performance ______

From Lueckenotte AG: *Pocket guide to gerontologic assessment,* ed 3, St Louis, 1998 Mosby.

social well-being. Specific tools for the collection of these data are addressed later in this chapter.

The physical, psychosocial, cultural, and functional aspects of the older adult client, coupled with a life history filled with people, places, and events, demand adaptations in interviewing styles and techniques. Making adaptations that reflect a genuine sensitivity toward the older adult and a sound, theoretic knowledge base of aging enhances the interview process.

The Interviewer

The interviewer's ability to elicit meaningful data from the client depends on the interviewer's attitudes and stereotypes about aging and older people. The nurse must be aware of these factors because they affect nurse-client communication during the assessment (see Cultural Awareness boxes, p. 74).

Attitude is a feeling, value, or belief about something that determines behavior. If the nurse has an attitude that characterizes older people as less healthy and alert and more dependent, then the interview structure will reflect this attitude. For example, if the nurse believes that dependence in self-care normally accompanies advanced age, the client will not be questioned about strengths and abilities. The resulting inaccurate functional assessment will do little to promote client independence. Myths and stereotypes about older

Cultural Awareness

CULTURAL CONSIDERATIONS DURING THE INTERVIEW: INTRODUCTIONS AND NAMES

Because initial impressions are important in all human relationships, if a mutually respectful relationship is to be established, nurses should introduce themselves and should indicate to clients how they prefer to be addressed (by first name, last name, or title). They should then elicit the same information from the clients, because this enables nurses to address persons in a manner that is culturally appropriate; this could actually spare considerable embarrassment. For example, it is the custom among some Asian and European cultures to write the last name first; the nurse must make sure to have a client's name correct. Avoid the use of nicknames (e.g., Grandma, Pop, Dear) that may be offensive to older adult clients. Regardless of the nurse's good intentions, older adults may construe the use of such terms as overly familiar, ill mannered, or inappropriate.

Cultural Awareness

CULTURAL CONSIDERATIONS AND THE INTERVIEWER

- Be respectful of, interested in, and understanding of other cultures without being judgmental.
- Avoid stereotyping by race, gender, age, ethnicity, religion, sexual orientation, socioeconomic status, and other social categories.
- Know the traditional health-related beliefs and practices prevalent among members of a client's cultural group, and encourage clients to discuss their cultural beliefs and practices.
- Learn about the traditional or folk illnesses and folk remedies common to clients' cultural groups.
- Try to understand client perceptions of appropriate wellness and illness role behaviors and expectations of health care providers in times of health and illness.
- Study the cultural expressions and manifestations of caring and noncaring behaviors expected by clients.
- Avoid stereotypic associations with violence, poverty, crime, low level of education, "noncompliant" behaviors, and nonadherence to time-regimented schedules, and avoid any other stereotypes that may adversely affect nurse-client relationships.
- Be aware that clients who have lived in the United States for a number of years may have become increasingly westernized and have fewer remaining practices of their birth culture.
- Learn to value the richness of cultural diversity as an asset rather than a hindrance to communication and effective intervention.

adults also can affect the nurse's questioning. For example, believing that older people do not participate in sexual relationships can result in the nurse's failure to interview the client about sexual health matters (see Chapter 13). The nurse's own anxiety and fear of personal aging, as well as a lack of knowledge regarding older people, contribute to commonly held negative attitudes, myths, and stereotypes about older people. Gerontologic nurses have a responsibility to themselves and to their older adult clients to improve their understanding of the aging process and aging people.

To ensure a successful interview, the nurse should explain the reason for the interview to the client and should give a brief overview of the format to be followed. This alleviates anxiety and uncertainty, and the client can then focus on telling the story. Another strategy that can be employed in some settings is to give the client selected portions of the interview form to complete *before* meeting with the nurse. This allows clients sufficient time to recall their long life histories, thus facilitating the collection of important health-related data.

Older people have lengthy and often complicated histories. A goal-directed interviewing process helps the client share the pertinent information, but the tendency to reminisce may make it difficult for the client to stay focused on the topic. *Guided reminiscence,* however, can elicit valuable data and can promote a supportive therapeutic relationship. Using such a technique helps the nurse balance the need to collect the required information with the client's need to relate what is personally important. For example, the client may relate a story about a social outing that seems irrelevant, but may reveal important information about available resources and support systems. The interplay of the previously noted factors may necessitate more than one encounter with the client to complete the data collection. Setting a time limit in advance helps the client focus on the interview and aids with the problem of diminished time perception. Keeping a clock that is easy to read within view of the client may be helpful.

Because of the need to structure the interview, there is a tendency for the nurse to exhibit controlling behavior with the client. To promote client comfort and sharing of data, the nurse and client should mutually establish the organization of the interview. In addition, the nurse should seek the client's permission to take notes during the interview. The client should feel that the nurse is a caring person who treats others with respect. Self-esteem is enhanced if the client feels included in the decision-making process.

At the beginning of the interview, the nurse and client need to determine the most effective and comfortable distance and position for the session. The ability to see and hear within a comfortable territory is critical to the communication process with an older adult, and adaptations to account for any deficits must include consideration of personal space requirements (see Cultural Awareness box, p. 75, left).

Also, the appropriate use of touch during the interview can reduce the anxiety associated with the initial encounter.

Cultural Awareness

SPACE AND DISTANCE

Both the older adult's and the nurse's sense of spatial distance is significant in cross-cultural communication, with the perception of appropriate distance zones varying widely among cultural groups. Although there are individual variations in spatial requirements, persons of the same culture may act similarly. For example, white nurses may find themselves backing away from clients of Hispanic, East Indian, or Middle Eastern origins, who often invade the nurse's personal space in an attempt to bring the nurse into the space that is comfortable to them. Although nurses may be uncomfortable with the physical proximity of these clients, the clients may be perplexed by the nurse's distancing behaviors and may perceive the nurse as aloof and unfriendly.

Because individuals are usually not consciously aware of their personal space requirements, they often have difficulty understanding a different cultural pattern. For example, sitting closely may be perceived by one client as an expression of warmth and friendliness but by another as a threatening invasion of personal space. Findings from some research suggest that American, Canadian, and British clients require the most personal space, whereas Latin American, Japanese, and Middle Eastern clients need the least.

The importance of and comfort with touch is highly individual, but older persons need and appreciate it. Burnside (1988) advises that the nurse does not have to be overly professional and cautious about the use of touch with the older adult client. However, a word of caution: do not use touch in a condescending manner (see Cultural Awareness box at right). Touch should always convey respect, caring, and sensitivity. Nurses should not be surprised if an older person reciprocates because of an unmet need for intimacy.

Finally, the nurse does not have to obtain the entire history in the traditional manner of a seated, face-to-face interview. In fact, this technique may be inappropriate with the older adult, depending on the situation. The nurse should not overlook the natural opportunities available in the setting for gathering information. Interviewing the client at mealtime, or even while participating in a game, hobby, or other social activity, often provides more meaningful data about a variety of areas.

The Client

Several factors influence the client's ability to participate meaningfully in the interview. The nurse must be aware of these factors because they affect the older adult's ability to communicate all the information necessary for determining appropriate, comprehensive interventions. Sensory-perceptual deficits, anxiety, reduced energy level, pain, multiple and interrelated health problems, and the tendency to reminisce are the major client factors requiring special consideration while the nurse elicits the health history (see Cultural Awareness boxes, p. 76). Table 4-4 contains recommendations for managing these factors.

Cultural Awareness

CULTURE AND TOUCH

Although recognizing the many reported benefits of establishing rapport with clients through touch (including the promotion of healing through therapeutic touch), nurses must understand that physical contact with clients conveys various meanings cross-culturally. In many cultures (e.g., Middle Eastern, Hispanic) male health care providers may be prohibited from touching or examining either all or certain parts of the female body. Older women (e.g., those having a gynecologic examination) may prefer female health care providers over male ones and may actually refuse to be examined by a man. Nurses should be aware that clients' significant others may also exert pressure on nurses by enforcing these culturally meaningful norms in the health care setting.

The following beliefs concerning touch are stereotypes that should be validated with clients to ascertain individual beliefs, practices, and preferences.

HISPANICS

Highly tactile
Very modest (men and women)
May request health care provider of same gender
Women may refuse to be examined by male health care providers.

ASIAN/PACIFIC ISLANDERS

Avoid touching (patting the head is strictly taboo).
Touching during an argument equals loss of control (shame).
Putting feet on furniture is both impolite and disrespectful.
Public displays of affection toward members of same gender are permissible, but not toward members of the opposite gender.

BLACKS

Do not touch without permission.

NATIVE AMERICANS

Usually shake hands lightly
Do not touch without permission.

The Health History Format

The components of the sample format for collecting a health history (see Box 4-2) are extensive, and they focus on the special needs and concerns of the older adult client. Although the entire format may seem overwhelming and repetitive in places, remember that this population may have many physical and psychosocial conditions, some of which may overlap.

Cultural Awareness

OVERCOMING LANGUAGE BARRIERS: USE OF AN INTERPRETER

- Before locating an interpreter, be sure that the language the client speaks at home is known, since it may be different from the language spoken publicly (e.g., French is sometimes spoken at home by well-educated and upper-class members of certain Asian or Middle Eastern cultures).
- Avoid interpreters who are not actually from the client's native state, region, or nation (e.g., a Palestinian who knows Hebrew may not be the best interpreter for a Jewish client).
- Be aware of gender differences between interpreter and client. In general, the same gender is preferred.
- Be aware of age differences between interpreter and client. In general, an older, more mature interpreter is preferred to a younger, less experienced one.
- Be aware of evident socioeconomic differences between interpreter and client.
- Ask the interpreter to translate as closely to verbatim as possible.
- An interpreter who is a nonrelative may seek compensation for services rendered.
- An interpreter who is a relative may change the meaning of what is said out of concern for the older family member's well-being.

RECOMMENDATIONS FOR INSTITUTIONS

- Maintain a computerized list of interpreters who may be contacted as needed.
- Network with area hospitals, colleges, universities, and other organizations that may serve as resources.
- Use the translation services provided by telephone companies (e.g., AT&T).

Cultural Awareness

OVERCOMING LANGUAGE BARRIERS: NO INTERPRETER

- Be polite and formal.
- Greet the person using the appropriate title (e.g., Mr., Mrs., Ms., Dr., Rev., Col.) and last or complete name. Gesture to yourself and say your name. Offer a handshake or nod. Smile.
- Proceed in an unhurried manner. Pay attention to any effort by the client or family to communicate.
- Speak in a low, moderate voice. Avoid talking loudly. Remember that there is a tendency to raise the volume and pitch of your voice when the listener either speaks another language or appears not to understand. The listener may perceive that the nurse is shouting or angry.
- Use any words known in the client's language. This indicates that the nurse is aware of and respects the client's culture.
- Use simple words such as "pain" instead of "discomfort." Avoid medical jargon, idioms, and slang. Avoid using contractions (e.g., don't, can't, won't). Use nouns repeatedly instead of pronouns.
- Avoid negative interrogatives. Example: Do not say, "He has not been taking his medicine, has he?" Say, "Does Juan take medicine?"
- Pantomime words and simple actions while verbalizing them.
- Give instructions in the proper sequence. Example: Do not say, "Before you rinse the bottle, sterilize it." Say, "First, wash the bottle. Second, rinse the bottle."
- Discuss one topic at a time. Avoid using conjunctions. Example: Do not say, "Are you cold and in pain?" Say, "Are you cold (while pantomiming)? Are you in pain?"
- Validate client understanding by having him or her repeat instructions, demonstrate the procedure, or act out the meaning.
- Write out several short sentences in English and determine the person's ability to read them.
- Try a third language. Many Southeast Asians speak French. Europeans often know three or four languages. Try Latin words or phrases if you are familiar with that language.
- Ask if anyone among the client's family and friends could serve as an interpreter.
- Obtain phrase books from a library or bookstore, or make or purchase flash cards with commonly used words.

Depending on the setting and purpose, not every client needs to be asked every question. The suggested format can be used as a reference from which to proceed in collecting data from each client. The order of the components enables the nurse to begin with the less threatening "get-acquainted" type of questioning, which eases the tension and anxiety and builds trust. The nurse then gradually moves to the more personal and sensitive questions. Box 4-3 is a discussion of each of the components. When possible, refer to old records to obtain information that will lessen the time required of both the client and the interviewer.

Client Profile/Biographic Data. This profile is basic, factual data about the older adult. In this section, it is often useful to comment on the reliability of the information source. For example, if the client's cognitive ability prevents giving accurate information, secondary sources such as family, friends, or other medical records should be consulted. Knowledge of the source of the data alerts the reader or user to the context within which he or she must consider the information. Take time to clarify advance directives such as the existence of a living will, powers of attorney for health care and finances, and code status.

TABLE 4-4 Client Factors Affecting History Taking and Recommendations

FACTOR	RECOMMENDATIONS
Visual deficit	Position self in full view of client. Provide diffused, bright light; avoid glare. Ensure client's glasses are worn, in good working order, and clean. Face client when speaking; do not cover mouth.
Hearing deficit	Speak directly to client in clear, low tones at a moderate rate; do not cover mouth. Articulate consonants with special care. Repeat if client does not understand question initially, then restate. Speak toward "good" ear. Reduce background noises. Ensure client's hearing aid is worn, on, and working properly.
Anxiety	Give sufficient time to respond to questions. Establish rapport and trust by acknowledging expressed concerns. Determine mutual expectations of interview. Use open-ended questions that indicate an interest in learning about the client. Explain why information is needed. Use a conversational style. Allow for some degree of life review. Offer a cup of coffee, tea, or soup. Call the client often by name.
Reduced energy level	Position comfortably to promote alertness. Allow for more than one assessment encounter; vary the meeting times. Be alert to subtle signs of fatigue, inability to concentrate, reduced attention span, restlessness, posture. Be patient; establish a slow pace for the interview.
Pain	Position comfortably to reduce pain. Ask client about degree of pain; intervene before interview or reschedule. Comfort and communicate through touch. Use distraction techniques. Provide a relaxed, "warm" environment.
Multiple and interrelated health problems	Be alert to subjective and objective cues about body systems and emotional and cognitive function. Give client opportunity to prioritize physical and psychosocial health concerns. Be supportive and reassuring about deficits created by multiple diseases. Complete full analysis on all reported symptoms. Be alert to reporting of new or changing symptoms. Allow for more than one interview time. Compare and validate data with old records, family, friends, or confidants.
Tendency to reminisce	Structure reminiscence to gather necessary data. Express interest and concern for issues raised by reminiscing Put memories into chronologic perspective to appreciate the significance and span of client's life.

From Lueckenotte AG: *Pocket guide to gerontologic assessment,* ed 3, St Louis, 1998, Mosby.

Family Profile. This information about immediate family members gives a quick overview of who may be living in the client's home or who may represent important support systems for the client. These data also establish a basis for a later description of family health history.

Occupational Profile. Information about work history and experiences can alert the nurse to possible health risks or exposures, lifestyle or social patterns, activity level, and intellectual performance. Retirement concerns may also be identified. Obtaining the client's perception of the adequacy of income for meeting daily living needs can have implications for designing nursing interventions. Financial resources and health have an interdependent relationship.

Living Environment Profile. Any nursing interventions for the client must be planned with consideration of the living environment. Degree of function, safety and security, and feelings of well-being are a few of the areas affected by a client's living environment.

BOX 4-3 Basic Components of a Nursing Health History

Client Profile/Biographic Data: Address and telephone number; date and place of birth, age; gender; race; religion; marital status; education; name, address, and telephone number of nearest contact person; advance directives
Family Profile: Family members' names and addresses, year and cause of death of deceased spouse and children
Occupational Profile: Current work or retirement status, previous jobs, source(s) of income and perceived adequacy for needs
Living Environment Profile: Type of dwelling; number of rooms, levels, and people residing; degree of privacy; name, address, and telephone number of nearest neighbor
Recreation/Leisure Profile: Hobbies or interests, organization memberships, vacations or travel
Resources/Support Systems Used: Names of physician(s), hospital, clinics, and other community services used
Description of Typical Day: Type and amount of time spent in each activity
Present Health Status: Description of perception of health in past 1 and 5 years, health screenings, chief complaint and full symptom analysis, prescribed and self-prescribed medications, immunizations, allergies, eating and nutritional patterns
Past Health Status: Previous illnesses throughout life, traumatic injuries, hospitalizations, operations, obstetric history
Family History: Health status of immediate and living relatives, causes of death of immediate relatives, survey for risk of specific diseases and disorders
Review of Systems: Head-to-toe review of all body systems and review of health promotion habits for same

Recreation/Leisure Profile. Identifying what the client does to relax and have fun, and how the client uses free time, can provide clues to some of the client's social and emotional dimensions.

Resources/Support Systems Used. Obtaining information about the various health care providers and agencies used by the client can alert the nurse to patterns of use of health care and related services, perceptions of such resources, and attitudes about the importance of health maintenance and promotion. The importance of religion in all its dimensions, including participation in church-related activities, is an important area to assess. Frequently, the church "family" is a significant source of support for the older adult.

Description of Typical Day. Identifying the activities of a client during a full 24-hour period provides data about practices that either support or hinder healthy living. Analysis of the usual activities carried out by the client can serve to explain symptoms that may be described later in the Review of Systems section (see Box 4-2). Clues about the client's relationships, lifestyle practices, and spiritual dimensions may also be uncovered.

Present Health Status. The client's perception of health in both the past year and past 5 years, coupled with information about health habits, reveals much about his or her physical integrity. Based on how the client responds, the nurse may be able to ascertain whether the client needs health maintenance, promotion, or restoration.

The chief complaint, stated in the client's own words, enables the nurse to identify specifically why the client is seeking health care. It is best to ask about this using terms other than *chief complaint,* however, since clients may take offense at that choice of words. If a symptom is the reason, usually its duration is included as well. A complete and careful symptom analysis can be carried out for the chief complaint by collecting information on the factors identified in Box 4-4. When the client does not display specific symptomatology, but instead has broader health concerns, the nurse should identify those concerns to begin establishing potential nursing interventions.

BOX 4-4 Symptom Analysis Factors

DIMENSIONS OF A SYMPTOM	QUESTIONS TO ASK
1. Location	"Where do you feel it? Does it move around? Does it radiate? Show me where it hurts."
2. Quality or character	"What does it feel like?"
3. Quantity or severity	"On a scale of 1 to 10, with 10 being the worst pain you could have, how would you rate the discomfort you have now?" "How does this interfere with your usual activities?" "How bad is it?"
4. Timing	"When did you first notice it? How long does it last? How often does it happen?"
5. Setting	"Does this occur in a particular place or under certain circumstances? Is it associated with any specific activity?"
6. Aggravating or alleviating factors	"What makes it better? What makes it worse?"
7. Associated symptoms	"Have you noticed other changes that occur with this symptom?"

From Barkauskas VH et al: *Health and physical assessment,* ed 2, St Louis, 1998, Mosby.

Information about the client's knowledge and understanding of current health state, including treatments and management strategies, helps the nurse to focus on possible areas of health teaching and reinforcement, to identify a client's access to and use of resources, to discover coping styles and strategies, and to determine health behavior patterns. Data about the client's perception of functional ability in light of perceived health problems and medical diagnoses provide valuable insight into the individual's overall sense of physical, social, emotional, and cognitive well-being.

Medications. Assessment of the older adult's current medications is usually accomplished by having the client bring in *all* prescription and over-the-counter drugs, as well as regularly and occasionally used home remedies. The nurse should also inquire about the client's use of herbal and other related products. Be sure to ask about all routes of medications, including oral, topical, inhaled, etc. Obtaining the medications in this manner allows the nurse to examine medication labels, which may show the use of multiple physicians and pharmacies. Also, the nurse can determine the client's pattern of drug taking (including compliance), his or her knowledge of medications, the expiration dates of medications, and the potential risk for drug interactions.

Immunization and Health Screening Status. The older adult's immunization status for specific diseases and illnesses is particularly important because of the degree of risk for this age group. More attention is increasingly being paid to the immunization status of the older adult population, primarily because of inappropriate use and underuse of vaccines in the past, especially the influenza and pneumococcal vaccines. (See Chapter 24 for a more complete discussion of influenza and pneumonia.) Tetanus and diphtheria toxoids (Td) are recommended as a booster at 10-year intervals for adults who have been previously immunized as adults or children. Older adults should still participate in health screenings for the most recent recommendations. Tuberculosis, a disease that was once fairly well controlled, is now exhibiting resurgence in this country. Older adults who may have had a tubercular lesion at a young age can experience a reactivation as a result of age-related immune system changes, chronic illness, and poor nutrition. Particularly vulnerable are frail and institutionalized older adults who should be screened for exposure or active disease through an annual purified protein derivative (PPD) test.

Allergies. Determining the older adult's drug, food, and other contact and environmental allergies is essential to planning nursing interventions. It is particularly important to note their reactions to the allergen and usual treatments.

Nutrition. A 24-hour diet recall is a useful screening tool that provides information about the intake of daily requirements, including the intake of "empty" calories, the adherence to prescribed dietary therapies, and the practice of unusual or "fad" diets. The nurse should also assess the time meals and snacks are eaten. If a 24-hour recall cannot be obtained or the information gleaned raises more questions, having the client keep a food diary for a select period may be indicated. The diets of older adults may be nutritionally inadequate because of advanced age, multiple chronic illnesses, lack of financial resources, mobility impairments, dental health problems, and loneliness (see Chapter 10). The diet recall and diary provide nutritional assessment data that reflect the client's overall health and well-being (see Cultural Awareness box below).

Past Health Status. Since a person's present health status can depend on past health conditions, it is essential to gather data about common childhood illnesses, serious or chronic illnesses, trauma, hospitalizations, operations, and obstetric history. The client's history of measles, mumps, rubella, chickenpox, diphtheria, pertussis, tetanus, rheumatic fever, and poliomyelitis should be obtained to identify potential risk factors for future health problems.

Cultural Awareness

CULTURAL ASSESSMENT OF NUTRITIONAL NEEDS

- What is the meaning of food and eating to the client?
- What does the client eat during:
  - — A typical day?
  - — Special events such as secular or religious holidays (e.g., Muslims fast during the month of Ramadan; some blacks may eat moderately during the week but consume large, heavy meals on weekends)?
- How does the client define food (e.g., unless rice is served, many from India do not consider the ingestion of food to be a meal; some Vietnamese clients consume large quantities of calcium-rich pork bones and shells, which offsets their lower intake of milk products)?
- What is the timing and sequencing of meals?
- With whom does the client usually eat (e.g., alone, with others of the same gender, with spouse)?
- What does the client believe constitutes a "healthy" versus "unhealthy" diet? Any hot/cold or yin/yang beliefs (see Chapter 5)?
- From what sources does the client obtain food items (e.g., ethnic grocery store, home garden, restaurant)? Who usually does the grocery shopping?
- How are foods prepared (e.g., type of preparation; cooking oil used; length of time foods are cooked; amount and type of seasoning added before, during, and after preparation)?
- Has the client chosen a particular nutritional practice such as vegetarianism or abstinence from alcoholic beverages?
- Do religious beliefs and practices influence the client's diet or eating habits (e.g., amount, type, preparations, or designation of acceptable food items or combinations)? Ask the client to explain the religious calendar and guidelines that govern these dietary practices, including exemptions for older adults and the sick.

An older adult client may not know what diseases are considered major, or may not fully appreciate why it is important to screen for the presence of certain diseases. In such cases the nurse should ask the client directly about the presence of specific diseases. It is also important to note the dates of onset or occurrence and the treatment measures prescribed for each disease.

For the older adult the history of traumatic injuries should be completely described, noting date, time, place, circumstances surrounding the incidents, and impact of the incidents on the client's overall function. Based on the information gathered about previous hospitalizations, operations, and obstetric history, additional data may be needed to gain a complete picture of the older client's health status. The client may need to be guided through this process because of forgetfulness or because of a lengthy, complicated personal history.

Family History. Collecting a family health history provides valuable information about inherited diseases and familial tendencies, whether environmental or genetic, for the purposes of identifying risk and determining need for preventive services. In surveying the health of blood relatives, the nurse should note the degree of overall health, the presence of disease or illness, and age; if deceased, note the cause of death. By collecting these data, the nurse may also be able to identify the existence and degree of family support systems. Data are usually recorded in a family tree format.

Review of Systems. The review is generally a head-to-toe screening to ascertain the presence or absence of key symptoms within each of the body systems. It is important to question the client in lay terminology, and if a positive response is elicited, conduct a complete symptom analysis to clarify the course of the symptomatology (see Box 4-4). To reduce confusion and to ensure the collection of accurate data, the nurse should ask the client for only one piece of information at a time. Information obtained here alerts the nurse about what to focus on during the physical examination.

The Physical Examination Examination Approach and Sequence

The objective information acquired in the physical examination adds to the subjective database already gathered. Together, these components serve as the basis for establishing nursing diagnoses and planning, developing interventions, and evaluating nursing care.

Physical examination is typically performed after the health history. The approach should be a systematic and deliberate one that allows the nurse to (1) determine client strengths and capabilities, as well as disabilities and limitations; (2) verify and gain objective support for subjective findings; and (3) gather objective data not previously known.

There is no single right way to put together the parts of the physical examination, but a head-to-toe approach is generally the most efficient. The sequence used to conduct the physical examination within this approach is a highly individual one, depending on the older adult client. In all cases, however, a side-to-side comparison of findings is made using the client as the control. To increase mastery in conducting an integrated and comprehensive physical examination, the nurse should develop a method of organization and should use it consistently.

Ultimately the practice setting and client condition together determine the type and method of examination to be performed. For example, an older adult admitted to an acute care hospital with a medical diagnosis of congestive heart failure initially requires respiratory and cardiovascular system assessments to plan appropriate interventions for improving activity tolerance. In the home care setting, assessment of the client's musculoskeletal system is a priority for determining potential for fall-related injury and the ability to perform basic self-care tasks. The frail, immobile client in a long-term care setting requires an initial skin assessment to determine risk for pressure ulcer development and preventive measures required. Regular examination of the skin thereafter is necessary to assess effectiveness of the prevention measures instituted.

In all the above situations, complete physical examinations are important and should eventually be carried out, but the client and setting dictate priorities. Consider the subjective client data already obtained in terms of the urgency of the situation, the acute or chronic nature of the problem, the extent of the problem in terms of body systems affected, and the interrelatedness of physical and psychosocial factors in determining where to begin.

General Guidelines. Regardless of the approach and sequence used, the following principles should be considered during the physical examination of an older adult:

- Recognize that the older adult may have no previous experience with a nurse conducting a physical examination; an explanation may be warranted. The examiner needs to project warmth, sincerity, and interest to allay any anxiety or fear.
- Be alert to the older client's energy level. If the situation warrants it, complete the most important parts of the examination first, and complete the other parts of the examination at another time. Generally it should take approximately 30 to 45 minutes to conduct the examination.
- Respect the client's modesty. Allow privacy for changing into a gown; if assistance is needed, assist in such a way as to not expose the client's body or cause embarrassment.
- Keep the client comfortably draped. Do not unnecessarily expose a body part; expose only the part to be examined.

- Sequence the examination to keep position changes to a minimum. Clients with limited range of motion and strength may require assistance. Be prepared to use alternative positions if the client is unable to assume the usual position for examination of a body part.
- Develop an efficient sequence for examination that minimizes both nurse and client movement. Variations that may be necessary will not be disruptive if the sequence is consistently followed. Working from one side of the client, generally the right side, promotes efficiency.
- Ensure comfort for the client. Offer a blanket for added warmth, or a pillow or alternative position for comfort.
- Explain each step in simple terms. Give clear, concise directions and instructions for performing required movements.
- Warn of any discomfort that might occur. Be gentle.
- Probe painful areas last.
- For reassurance, share findings with the client when possible. Encourage the client to ask questions.
- Take advantage of "teachable moments" that may occur while conducting the examination (e.g., breast self-examination).
- Develop a standard format on which to note selected findings. Not all data need to be recorded, but the goal is to reduce the potential for forgetting certain data, particularly measurements.

Equipment and Skills

Because the older adult client may become easily fatigued during the physical examination, the nurse should ensure proper function and readiness of all equipment before the examination begins to avoid unnecessary delays. Place the equipment within easy reach and in the order in which it will be used. The traditional techniques of inspection, palpation, percussion, and auscultation are used with older adults, with age-specific variations for some areas. See Chapters 23 through 31 for these variations.

ADDITIONAL ASSESSMENT MEASURES

Obtaining the health history as described previously does not always provide sufficient data for planning nursing care for the older adult. Assessment of all the dimensions of the older adult is essential to establishing baseline functional ability and providing individualized care.

The extremely delicate balance of homeostatic mechanisms the older adult is able to achieve is vulnerable to assault from a variety of sources, thus increasing the risk of impairment or disability. The primary reason for such a precarious situation is that the physical, mental, emotional, and social well-being of the older adult are all closely interrelated. Medical diagnoses alone do not provide a reliable measure of functional ability. In fact, a lengthy medical problem list may not correlate at all with any degree of functional loss. Therefore what is crucial for the nurse to know is how the older person has adapted to manage all dimensions of life with the diagnosed illnesses and medical problems. Standardized tools and measures of functional status that enable health care providers to objectively determine the older person's ability to function independently despite disease and mental, emotional, and social disability are important adjuncts to traditional assessment. These assessments include determination of the client's ability to perform activities of daily living (ADLs) and instrumental activities of daily living (IADLs), as well as the client's cognitive, affective, and social level of function. Obtaining these additional data provides a more comprehensive view of the impact of all the interrelated variables on the older adult's total functioning.

Functional Status Assessment

Functional status is considered a significant component of an older adult's quality of life. Assessing functional status has long been viewed as an essential piece of the overall clinical evaluation of an older person. Functional status assessment is a measurement of the older adult's ability to perform basic self-care tasks, or ADLs, and tasks that require more complex activities for independent living, referred to as IADLs (Kane and Kane, 1981). Determination of the degree of functional independence in these areas can identify a client's abilities and limitations, leading to appropriate interventions.

The client's situation determines the location and time when any of the scales or tools should be administered, as well as the number of times the client may need to be tested to ensure accurate results. Many tools are available, but the nurse should use only those which are valid, reliable, and relevant to the practice setting. The following is a description of tools appropriate for use with older adults in most settings.

The Katz Index of ADLs (Katz et al, 1963) is a tool widely used to determine the results of treatment and the prognosis in older and chronically ill people (Box 4-5). The index ranks adequacy of performance in the six functions of bathing, dressing, toileting, transferring, continence, and feeding. A dichotomous rating of independence or dependence is made for each of the functions. One point is given for each dependent item. Only people who can perform the function without any help at all are rated as independent; the actual evaluation form merely shows the rater how a dependent item is determined. The order of items reflects the natural progression in loss and restoration of function, based on studies conducted by Katz and his colleagues (Kane and Kane, 1981). The Katz Index is a useful tool for the nurse because it describes the client's functional level at a specific point in time and objectively measures the effects of treatment intended to restore function. The tool takes only about 5 minutes to administer and can be used in most settings.

The Barthel Index (Mahoney and Barthel, 1965), another tool used for measuring functional status, rates self-care

BOX 4-5 Katz Index of Activities of Daily Living

INDEX OF INDEPENDENCE IN ACTIVITIES OF DAILY LIVING

The Index of Independence in Activities of Daily Living is based on an evaluation of the functional independence or dependence of clients in bathing, dressing, going to toilet, transferring, continence, and feeding. Specific definitions of functional independence and dependence appear below the index.

A—Independent in feeding, continence, transferring, going to toilet, dressing, and bathing
B—Independent in all but one of these functions
C—Independent in all but bathing and one additional function
D—Independent in all but bathing, dressing, and one additional function
E—Independent in all but bathing, dressing, going to toilet, and one additional function
F—Independent in all but bathing, dressing, going to toilet, transferring, and one additional function
G—Dependent in all six functions
Other—Dependent in at least two functions, but not classifiable as C, D, E, or F

Independence means without supervision, direction, or active personal assistance, except as specifically noted below. This is based on actual status and not on ability. A client who refuses to perform a function is considered as not performing the function, even though he or she is deemed able.

BATHING (SPONGE, SHOWER, OR TUB)

Independent: assistance only in bathing a single part (such as back or disabled extremity) or bathes self completely
Dependent: assistance in bathing more than one part of body, assistance in getting in or out of tub, or does not bathe self

DRESSING

Independent: gets clothes from closets and drawers; puts on clothes, outer garments, braces; manages fasteners; act of tying shoes is excluded
Dependent: does not dress self or remains partly undressed

GOING TO TOILET

Independent: gets to toilet; gets on and off toilet; arranges clothes; cleans organs of excretion (may manage own bedpan used at night only and may or may not be using mechanical supports)
Dependent: uses bedpan or commode or receives assistance in getting to and using toilet

TRANSFER

Independent: moves in and out of bed independently and moves in and out of chair independently (may or may not be using mechanical supports)
Dependent: assistance in moving in or out of bed and/or chair; does not perform one or more transfers

CONTINENCE

Independent: urination and defecation entirely self-controlled
Dependent: partial or total incontinence in urination or defecation; partial or total control by enemas, catheters, or regulated use of urinals and/or bedpans

FEEDING

Independent: gets food from plate or its equivalent into mouth (precutting of meat and preparation of food, as buttering bread, are excluded from evaluation)
Dependent: assistance in act of feeding (see above); does not eat at all, or parenteral feeding

EVALUATION FORM

Name ____________________ Date of evaluation __________

For each area of function listed below, check the description that applies. (The word "assistance" means supervision, direction of personal assistance.)

BATHING

Either sponge bath, tub bath, or shower

- Receives no assistance (gets in and out of tub by self if tub is usual means of bathing)
- Receives assistance in bathing only one part of the body (such as back or a leg)
- Receives assistance in bathing more than one part of the body (or not bathed)

DRESSING

- Gets clothes from closets and drawers—including underclothes, outer garments, and using fasteners (including braces if worn)
- Gets clothes and gets completely dressed without assistance
- Gets clothes and gets dressed without assistance except for assistance in tying shoes
- Receives assistance in getting clothes or in getting dressed, or stays partly or completely undressed

TOILETING

- Goes to the "toilet room" for bowel and urine eliminations; cleans self after elimination and arranges clothes
- Goes to "toilet room," cleans self, and arranges clothes with assistance (may use object for support such as cane, walker, or wheelchair, and may manage night bedpan or commode, emptying same in morning)
- Receives assistance in going to "toilet room," in cleansing self, or in arranging clothes after elimination, or in use of night bedpan or commode
- Does not go to "toilet room" for the elimination process

TRANSFER

- Moves in and out of bed as well as in and out of chair without assistance (may be using object for support such as cane or walker)
- Moves in or out of bed or chair with assistance
- Does not get out of bed

From Katz S et al: Studies of illness in the aged: the index of ADL—a standardized measure of biological and psychological function, *JAMA* 185:914, 1963.

BOX 4-5 Katz Index of Activities of Daily Living—cont'd

CONTINENCE
- Controls urination and bowel movement completely by self
- Has occasional "accidents"
- Supervision helps keep urine or bowel control; catheter is used, or is incontinent

FEEDING
- Feeds self without assistance
- Feeds self except for cutting meat or buttering bread
- Receives assistance in feeding or is fed partly or completely by using tubes or intravenous fluids

abilities in the areas of feeding, moving, toileting, bathing, walking, propelling a wheelchair, using stairs, dressing, and controlling bowel and bladder (Box 4-6). For each item the individual is rated based on ability to perform the task independently or with help; more points are scored for independence, with a maximum score of 100 indicating independence on all items. However, the instrument developers note that a score of 100 does not necessarily mean one could live alone or without assistance. The Barthel Index is most appropriate for use in rehabilitation settings for documenting improvement in performance and ability.

IADLs represent a range of activities more complex than the self-care tasks described in the above tools (Kane and Kane, 1981). Lawton and Brody (1969) described the Philadelphia Geriatric Center Instrumental Activities of Daily Living Scale as one that measures complex activities such as using a telephone, shopping, preparing food, housekeeping, doing laundry, using transportation, taking medication, and handling finances (Box 4-7). The scale's limitations include an absence of instructions for summing up the items and an emphasis on tasks traditionally performed by women, especially given today's cohort of older people (Kane and Kane, 1981). Its usefulness is that it may identify people living in the community who need help, which enables the nurse to match services and other sources of support for clients.

Older adults in most health care settings can benefit from functional status assessment, but those in acute care settings are particularly in need of such an assessment because of their typically advanced age, level of acuity, comorbidity, and risk for iatrogenic conditions such as urinary incontinence, falls, delirium, and polypharmacy. The hospitalization experience for older adults can cause loss of function and self-care ability because of the many extrinsic risk factors associated with this setting, including aggressive treatment interventions, forced bed rest, restraint use, lack of exercise, insufficient nutritional intake, and iatrogenic infection. Box 4-8 provides a clinical practice protocol to guide acute care nurses in the functional assessment process for older adults (Kresevic et al, 1997). Nurses in this setting are in a key position to assess the older adult's function and implement interventions aimed at preventing decline. Specialized care units known as acute care for elders (ACE) units have been developed in hospitals around the country to better address these issues. Research is being conducted to determine the impact of this age-specific, comprehensive approach on reducing morbidity and mortality associated with hospitalizing older adults.

Nurses practicing in all settings should begin incorporating the tools noted above, as well as others described in the comprehensive text by Kane and Kane (1981), into routine assessments to determine a client's baseline functional ability. However, with all the previously mentioned tools, the nurse should remember the following points:

- Scores will be affected by the environment in which the tool is administered.
- The client's affective and cognitive state will affect performance.
- The result represents but one piece of the total assessment.

Cognitive/Affective Assessment

The purpose of mental status assessment in the older adult is to determine the client's level of cognitive function (which implies all those processes associated with mentation or intellectual function) and the effect of the assessed degree of impairment on functional ability. This assessment is usually integrated into the interview and physical examination, with testing conducted in a natural, nonthreatening manner with consideration of ethnicity. Table 4-5 identifies typical areas to assess in a mental status assessment. Note that this mental status assessment provides a baseline that identifies the need for the administration of one of the standardized mental status examinations.

The multiple physiologic, psychologic, and environmental causes of cognitive impairment in older adults, coupled with the view that mental impairment is a normal, age-related process, often lead to incomplete assessment of this problem. Standardized examinations test a variety of cognitive functions, aiding the identification of deficits that affect overall functional ability. Formal, systematic testing of mental status can help the nurse determine which behaviors are impaired and warrant intervention.

The Short Portable Mental Status Questionnaire (SPMSQ) (Box 4-9), used to detect the presence and degree of intellectual impairment, consists of 10 items to assess orientation, memory in relation to self-care ability, remote memory, and mathematic ability (Pfeiffer, 1975). The simple scoring method rates the level of intellectual function, which aids in making clinical decisions regarding self-care capacity.

BOX 4-6 Barthel Index

ACTION	WITH HELP	INDEPENDENT
1. Feeding (if food needs to be cut up = help)	5	10
2. Moving from wheelchair to bed and return (includes sitting up in bed)	5-10	15
3. Personal toilet (wash face, comb hair, shave, clean teeth)	0	5
4. Getting on and off toilet (handling clothes, wipe, flush)	5	10
5. Bathing self	0	5
6. Walking on level surface (or if unable to walk, propel wheelchair)	0*	5*
7. Ascend and descend stairs	5	10
8. Dressing (includes tying shoes, fastening fasteners)	5	10
9. Controlling bowels	5	10
10. Controlling bladder	5	10

A client scoring 100 BDI is continent, feeds himself, dresses himself, gets up out of bed and chairs, bathes himself, walks at least a block, and can ascend and descend stairs. This does not mean that the client is able to live alone: the client may not be able to cook, keep house, and meet the public but may be able to get along without attendant care.

DEFINITION AND DISCUSSION OF SCORING

1. Feeding
   - 10 = Independent. The client can feed himself a meal from a tray or table when someone puts the food within his reach. He must put on an assistive device if this is needed, cut up the food, use salt and pepper, spread butter, etc. He must accomplish this in a reasonable time.
   - 5 = Some help is necessary (with cutting up food, etc., as listed above).
2. Moving from wheelchair to bed and return
   - 15 = Independent in all phases of this activity. Client can safely approach the bed in her wheelchair, lock brakes, lift footrests, move safely from bed, lie down, come to a sitting position on the side of the bed, change the position of the wheelchair, if necessary, to transfer back into it safely and return to the wheelchair.
   - 10 = Either some minimal help is needed in some step of this activity or the client needs to be reminded or supervised for safety of one or more parts of this activity.
   - 5 = Client can come to a sitting position without the help of a second person but needs to be lifted out of bed, or if she transfers, with a great deal of help.
3. Doing personal toilet
   - 5 = Client can wash hands and face, comb hair, clean teeth, and shave. He may use any kind of razor but he must put in blade or plug in razor without help, as well as get it from the drawer or cabinet. Female clients must put on own makeup, if used, but need not braid or style hair.
4. Getting on and off toilet
   - 10 = Client is able to get on and off toilet, fasten and unfasten clothes, prevent soiling of clothes, and use toilet paper without help. She may use a wall bar or other stable object for support if needed. If it is necessary to use a bed pan instead of toilet, he must be able to place it on a chair, empty it, and clean it.
   - 5 = Client needs help because of imbalance, in handling clothes, or in using toilet paper.
5. Bathing self
   - 5 = Client may use a bathtub or a shower or take a complete sponge bath. He must be able to do all the steps involved in whichever method is employed without another person being present.
6. Walking on a level surface
   - 5 = Client can walk at least 50 yards without help or supervision. She may wear braces or prostheses and use crutches, canes, or a walkerette but not a rolling walker. She must be able to lock and unlock braces if used, assume the standing position and sit down, get the necessary mechanical aids into position for use, and dispose of them when she sits. (Putting on and taking off braces is scored under Dressing.)

6a. Propelling a wheelchair
   - 5 = If a client cannot ambulate but can propel a wheelchair independently, he must be able to go around corners, turn around, maneuver the chair to a table, bed, toilet, etc. He must be able to push a chair at least 50 yards. Do not score this item if the client gets a score for walking.

7. Ascending and descending stairs
   - 10 = Client is able to go up and down a flight of stairs safely without help or supervision. She may and should use handrails, canes, or crutches when needed. She must be able to carry canes or crutches as she ascends or descends stair.
   - 5 = Client needs help with or supervision of any one of the above items.
8. Dressing and undressing
   - 10 = Client is able to put on and remove and fasten all clothing, and tie shoe laces (unless it is necessary to use adaptations for this). This activity includes putting on and removing and fastening corset or braces when these are prescribed. Such special clothing as suspenders, loafer shoes, or dresses that open down the front may be used when necessary.
   - 5 = Client needs help in putting on and removing or fastening any clothing. He must do at least half the work himself. He must accomplish this in a reasonable time.

*Score only if unable to walk.

BOX 4-6 Barthel Index—cont'd

Women need not be scored on use of a brassiere or girdle unless these are prescribed garments.

9. Continence of bowels
   - 10 = Client is able to control her bowels and have no accidents. She can use a suppository or take an enema when necessary (as for spinal cord injury patients who have had bowel training).
   - 5 = Client needs help using a suppository or taking an enema or has occasional accidents.
10. Controlling bladder
   - 10 = Client is able to control his bladder day and night. Spinal cord injury clients, who wear an external device and leg bag, must put them on independently, clean and empty bag, and stay dry day and night.
   - 5 = Client has occasional accidents, cannot wait for the bed pan, cannot get to the toilet in time, or needs help with an external device.

The total score is not as significant or meaningful as the breakdown into individual items, since these indicate where the deficiencies are.

Any applicant to a chronic hospital who scores 100 BDI should be evaluated carefully before admission to see whether such hospitalization is indicated. Discharged clients with 100 BDI should not require further physical therapy but may benefit from a home visit to see whether any environmental adjustments are indicated.

Modified from Mahoney FI, Barthel DW: Functional evaluation: the Barthel Index, *Maryland State Med J* 14:61, 1965.

BOX 4-7 Instrumental Activities of Daily Living Scale

	Score
1. Ability to use telephone	
A. Operates telephone on own initiative—looks up and dials numbers, etc.	1
B. Dials a few well-known numbers	1
C. Answers telephone but does not dial	1
D. Does not use telephone at all	0
2. Shopping	
A. Takes care of all shopping needs independently	1
B. Shops independently for small purchases	0
C. Needs to be accompanied on any shopping trip	0
D. Completely unable to shop	0
3. Food preparation	
A. Plans, prepares, and serves adequate meals independently	1
B. Prepares adequate meals if supplied with ingredients	0
C. Heats and serves prepared meals, or prepares meals but does not maintain adequate diet	0
D. Needs to have meals prepared and served	0
4. Housekeeping	
A. Maintains house alone or with occasional assistance (e.g., "heavy work—domestic help")	1
B. Performs light daily tasks such as dishwashing and bedmaking	1
C. Performs light daily tasks but cannot maintain acceptable level of cleanliness	1
D. Needs help with all home maintenance tasks	1
E. Does not participate in any housekeeping tasks	0
5. Laundry	
A. Does personal laundry completely	1
B. Launders small items—rinses socks, stockings, etc.	1
C. All laundry must be done by others	0
6. Mode of transportation	
A. Travels independently on public transportation or drives own car	1
B. Arranges own travel via taxi but does not o therwise use public transportation	1
C. Travels on public transportation when assisted or accompanied by another	1
D. Travel limited to taxi or automobile with assistance of another	0
E. Does not travel at all	0
7. Responsibility for own medications	
A. Is responsible for taking medication in correct dosages at correct time	1
B. Takes responsibility if medication is prepared in advance in separate dosages	0
C. Is not capable of dispensing own medication	0
8. Ability to handle finances	
A. Manages financial matters independently (budgets, writes checks, pays rent, bills, goes to bank), collects and keeps track of income	1
B. Manages day-to-day purchases but needs help with banking, major purchases, etc.	1
C. Incapable of handling money	0

From Lawton HP, Brody EM: Assessment of older people: self maintaining and instrumental activities of daily living, *Gerontologist* 9:179, 1969.

BOX 4-8 Nursing Standard of Practice Protocol: Assessment of Function in Acute Care

The following nursing care protocol has been designed to assist bedside nurses to monitor function in older patients, prevent decline, and to maintain the function of older adults during acute hospitalization.
Objective: The goal of nursing care is to maximize the physical functioning and prevent or minimize decline in ADL function.

I. BACKGROUND

A. Functional status of individuals describes the capacity to safely perform ADL. Functional status is a sensitive indicator of health or illness in older adults and therefore a critical nursing assessment.
B. Some functional decline may be prevented or ameliorated with prompt and aggressive nursing intervention (e.g., ambulation, enhanced communication, adaptive equipment).
C. Some functional decline may occur progressively and is not reversible. This decline often accompanies chronic and terminal disease states such as Parkinson's disease and dementia.
D. Functional status is influenced by physiologic aging changes, acute and chronic illness, and adaptation. Functional decline is often the initial symptom of acute illness such as infections (pneumonia, urinary tract infection). These declines are usually reversible.
E. Functional status is contingent on cognition and sensory capacity, including vision and hearing.
F. Risk factors for functional decline include injuries, acute illness, medication side effects, depression, malnutrition, and decreased mobility (including the use of physical restraints).
G. Additional complications of functional decline include loss of independence, loss of socialization, and increased risk for long-term institutionalization and depression.
H. Recovery of function can also be a measure of return to health such as those individuals recovering from exacerbations of cardiovascular disease.

II. ASSESSMENT PARAMETERS

A. A comprehensive functional assessment of older adults includes independent performance of basic ADLs, social activities, or IADLs; the assistance needed to *accomplish* these tasks; and the sensory ability, cognition, and capacity to ambulate.
   1. Basic ADLs
      a. Bathing
      b. Dressing
      c. Grooming
      d. Eating
      e. Continence
      f. Transferring
   2. IADLs
      a. Meal preparation
      b. Shopping
      c. Medication administration
      d. Housework
      e. Transportation
      f. Accounting
B. Elderly patients view their health in terms of how well they can function rather than in terms of disease alone.
C. The clinician should document functional status and recent or progressive declines in function.
D. Function should be assessed over time to validate capacity, decline, or progress.
E. Standard instruments selected to assess function should be efficient to administer, be easy to interpret, and provide useful, practical information for clinicians.
F. Multidisciplinary team conferences should be scheduled.

III. CARE STRATEGIES

A. Strategies to maximize function
   1. Maintain individual's daily routine. Help to maintain physical, cognitive, and social function through physical activity and socialization: encourage ambulation; allow flexible visitation, including pets; and encourage reading the newspaper.
   2. Educate older adults and caregivers on the value of independent functioning and the consequences of functional decline.
      a. Physiologic and psychologic value of independent functioning
      b. Reversible functional decline associated with acute illness
      c. Strategies to prevent functional decline—exercise, nutrition, and socialization
      d. Sources of assistance to manage decline
   3. Encourage activity including routine exercise, range of motion, and ambulation to maintain activity, flexibility, and function.
   4. Minimize bed rest.
   5. Explore alternatives to physical restraint use.
   6. Judiciously use psychoactive medications in geriatric dosages.
   7. Design environments with handrails, wide doorways, raised toilet seats, shower seats, enhanced lighting, low beds, and chairs.
   8. Help individuals regain baseline function after acute illnesses by use of exercise, physical therapy consultation, and increasing nutrition.
   9. Obtain assessment for physical and occupational therapies needed to help regain function.
B. Strategies to help individuals cope with functional decline
   1. Help older adults and family determine realistic functional capacity with interdisciplinary consult.
   2. Provide caregiver education and support for families of individuals when decline cannot be ameliorated in spite of nursing and rehabilitative efforts.
   3. Carefully document all intervention strategies and patient responses.
   4. Provide information to caregivers on causes of functional decline related to the patient's disorder.

BOX 4-8 Nursing Standard of Practice Protocol: Assessment of Function in Acute Care—cont'd

5. Provide education to address safety care needs for falls, injuries, and common complication. Alternative care settings may be required to ensure safety.
6. Provide sufficient protein and caloric intake to ensure adequate intake and prevent further decline.
7. Provide caregiver support and community services, such as home care, nursing, and physical and occupational therapy services, to manage functional decline.

IV. EXPECTED OUTCOMES

A. Patients can:
  1. Maintain safe level of ADL and ambulation.
  2. Make necessary adaptations to maintain safety and independence, including assistive devices and environmental adaptations.

B. Provider can demonstrate:
  1. Increased assessment, identification, and management of patients susceptible to or experiencing functional decline.
  2. Ongoing documentation of capacity, interventions, goals, and outcomes.
  3. Competence in preventive and restorative strategies for function.

C. Institution can demonstrate:
  1. Decrease in incidence and prevalence of functional decline in all care settings.
  2. Decrease in morbidity and mortality rates associated with functional decline.
  3. Decreased use of physical restraints.
  4. Decreased incidence of delirium.
  5. Increase in prevalence of patients who leave hospital with baseline functional status.
  6. Decreased readmission rate.
  7. Increased use of rehabilitative services (occupational and physical therapy).
  8. Support of institutional policies/programs that promote function.
     a. Caregiver educational efforts
     b. Walking programs
     c. Continence programs
     d. Self-feeding initiatives
     e. Elder group activities

Modified from Kresevic DM et al: Assessment of function: critically important to acute care of elders, *Geriatr Nurs* 18(5):216, 1997.

TABLE 4-5 Mental Status Assessment

EXAM COMPONENT	AREA TO ASSESS
General appearance	Observe physical appearance, coordination of movements, grooming and hygiene, facial expression, and posture as measures of mental function.
Alertness	Note level of consciousness (alert, lethargic, obtunded, stuporous, or comatose).
Mood or affect	Note verbal and nonverbal behaviors for appropriateness, degree, and range of affect.
Speech	Evaluate comprehension of and ability to use the spoken language; note volume, pace, amount, and degree of spontaneity.
Orientation	Note awareness of person, place, and time.
Attention and concentration	Note ability to attend to or concentrate on stimuli.
Judgment	Note ability to evaluate a situation and determine appropriate reaction or response.
Memory	Note ability to accurately register, retain, and recall data or events (may need to verify with collateral sources).
Perception	Note presence or absence of delusions or visual and auditory hallucinations.
Thought content and processes	Observe for organized, coherent thoughts; note ability to relate history in a clear, sequential, and logical manner.

Since the SPMSQ is given orally, it is easy to memorize. It can be administered as a screening assessment for older people in acute, community-based, and long-term care settings. Based on the score, a more complete mental status assessment and neuropsychiatric evaluation may be warranted.

The MiniMental State Examination (MMSE) (Box 4-10) tests the cognitive aspects of mental functions: orientation, registration, attention and calculation, recall, and language (Folstein, Folstein, and McHugh, 1975). The highest possible score is 30, with a score of 21 or less generally indicative of cognitive impairment requiring further investigation. The examination takes only a few minutes to complete and is easily scored, but it cannot be used alone for diagnostic purposes. Because the MMSE quantifies the severity of cognitive impairment and demonstrates cognitive changes over time and with treatment, it is a useful tool for assessing client progress in relation to interventions. As with the SPMSQ, if the MMSE score demonstrates the client is impaired, addi-

BOX 4-9 Short Portable Mental Status Questionnaire (SPMSQ)

Instructions: Ask questions 1-10 in this list, and record all answers. Ask question 4a only if patient does not have a telephone. Record total number of errors based on 10 questions.

+	−	
___	___	1. What is the date today? ___________ Month Day Year
___	___	2. What day of the week is it?
___	___	3. What is the name of this place?
___	___	4. What is your telephone number?
___	___	4a. What is your street address? (Ask only if patient does not have a telephone.)
___	___	5. How old are you?
___	___	6. When were you born?
___	___	7. Who is the President of the United States now?
___	___	8. Who was the President just before him?
___	___	9. What was your mother's maiden name?
		10. Subtract 3 from 20 and keep subtracting 3 from each new number, all the way down.
	___	Total Number of Errors

TO BE COMPLETED BY INTERVIEWER

Patient's name: ______________________ Date__________

Sex: _____ Male Race: _____ White
_____ Female _____ Black
_____ Other

Years of education: _________ Grade School
High School
Beyond High School

Interviewer's name:

____

Instructions for Completion of the Short Portable Mental Status Questionnaire (SPMSQ)

All responses to be scored as correct must be given by subject without reference to calendar, newspaper, birth certificate, or other aid to memory.

Question 1 is to be scored as correct only when the exact month, exact date, and the exact year are given correctly.

Question 2 is self-explanatory.

Question 3 should be scored as correct if any correct description of the location is given. "My home," correct name of the town or city of residence, or the name of hospital or institution if subject is institutionalized are all acceptable.

Question 4 should be scored as correct when the correct telephone number can be verified, or when the subject can repeat the same number at another point in the questioning.

Question 5 is scored as correct when stated age corresponds to date of birth.

Question 6 is to be scored as correct only when the month, exact date, and year are all given.

Question 7 requires only the last name of the President.

Question 8 requires only the last name of the previous President.

Question 9 does not need to be verified. It is scored as correct if a female first name plus a last name other than subject's last name is given.

Question 10 requires that the entire series must be performed correctly in order to be scored as correct. Any error in the series or unwillingness to attempt the series is scored as incorrect.

Scoring of the Short Portable Mental Status Questionnaire (SPMSQ)

The data suggest that both education and race influence performance on the Mental Status Questionnaire and they must accordingly be taken into account in evaluating the score attained by an individual.

For the purposes of scoring, three educational levels have been established: (1) persons who have had only a grade school education; (2) persons who have had any high school education or who have completed high school; (3) persons who have had any education beyond the high school level, including college, graduate school, or business school.

For white subjects with at least some high school education, but not more than high school education, the following criteria have been established:

0-2 errors	Intact intellectual functioning
3-4 errors	Mild intellectual impairment
5-7 errors	Moderate intellectual impairment
8-10 errors	Severe intellectual impairment

Allow one more error if subject has had only a grade school education.

Allow one less error if subject has had education beyond high school.

Allow one more error for black subjects, using identical education criteria.

From Pfeiffer E: A short portable questionnaire for the assessment of organic brain deficit in elderly patients, *J Am Geriatr Soc* 23:433, 1975.

tional diagnostic testing and mental status examination are indicated.

The Mini-Cog (Fig. 4-1) is an instrument that combines a simple test of memory with a clock drawing test. It was created by researchers at the University of Washington led by Soo Borson. The Mini-Cog is both quick and easy to use and has been found to be as effective as longer, more time-consuming instruments in accurately identifying cognitive impairment (Borson et al, 2003). It is relatively uninfluenced by education level or language.

Affective status measurement tools are used to differentiate the type of serious depression that affects many domains of function from the low mood common to many people. Depression is common in older adults and is often associated

BOX 4-10 MiniMental State Examination

MiniMental LLC

NAME OF SUBJECT ______________________ Age ____________

NAME OF EXAMINER ______________________ Years of School Completed ____

Date of Examination ________

Approach the patient with respect and encouragement.
Ask: Do you have any trouble with your memory? ☐ Yes ☐ No
May I ask you some questions about your memory? ☐ Yes ☐ No

SCORE	ITEM
5 ( )	TIME ORIENTATION Ask: What is the year ________ (1), season ________ (1), month of the year ________ (1), date ________ (1), day of the week ________ (1)?
5 ( )	PLACE ORIENTATION Ask: Where are we now? What is the state ________ (1), city ________ (1), part of the city ________ (1), building ________ (1), floor of the building ________ (1)?
3 ( )	REGISTRATION OF THREE WORDS Say: Listen carefully. I am going to say three words. You say them back after I stop. Ready? Here they are– PONY (wait 1 second), QUARTER (wait 1 second), ORANGE (wait 1 second). What were those words? ________ (1) ________ (1) ________ (1) Give 1 point for each correct answer, then repeat them until the patient learns all three.
5 ( )	SERIAL 7s AS A TEST OF ATTENTION AND CALCULATION Ask: Subtract 7 from 100 and continue to subtract 7 from each subsequent remainder until I tell you to stop. What is 100 take away 7? ____ (1) Say: Keep Going. ________ (1), ________ (1), ________ (1), ________ (1).
3 ( )	RECALL OF THREE WORDS Ask: What were those three words I asked you to remember? Give one point for each correct answer ________ (1), ________ (1), ________ (1).
2 ( )	NAMING Ask: What is this? (show pencil) ________ (1), What is this? (show watch) ________ (1).

For more information or additional copies of this examination, call (617) 587-4215.

Continued

BOX 4-10 MiniMental State Examination—cont'd

1 ( ) REPETITION

Say:

Now I am going to ask you to repeat what I say. Ready? No ifs, ands, or buts.

Now you say that ______________________________ (1)

3 ( ) COMPREHENSION

Say:

Listen carefully because I am going to ask you to do something:

Take this paper in your left hand (1), fold it in half (1), and put it on the floor. (1)

1 ( ) READING

Say:

Please read the following and do what it says, but do not say it aloud. (1)

Close your eyes

1 ( ) WRITING

Say:

Please write a sentence. If patient does not respond, say: Write about the weather. (1)

____

____

1 ( ) DRAWING

Say: Please copy this design.

TOTAL SCORE __________ Assess level of consciousness along a continuum

____

Alert Drowsy Stupor Coma

	YES	NO
Cooperative:	☐	☐
Depressed:	☐	☐
Anxious:	☐	☐
Poor Vision:	☐	☐
Poor Hearing:	☐	☐
Native Language:		

____

	YES	NO
Deterioration from previous level of functioning:	☐	☐
Family History of Dementia:	☐	☐
Head Trauma:	☐	☐
Stroke:	☐	☐
Alcohol Abuse:	☐	☐
Thyroid Disease:	☐	☐

FUNCTION BY PROXY

Please record date when patient was last able to perform the following tasks. Ask caregiver if patient independently handles:

	YES	NO	DATE
Money/Bills:	☐	☐	______
Medication:	☐	☐	______
Transportation:	☐	☐	______
Telephone:	☐	☐	______

From Folstein MF, Folstein SE, McHugh PR: Mini-mental state: a practical method for grading the cognitive state of patients for the clinician, *J Psychiatr Res* 12(3):189, 1975.

DATE________ PT INITIALS________ #____________ AGE___ GENDER M F CLINIC NAME ______________ PROVIDER ____________ TESTED BY __________

MINI-COG™

1) **GET THE PATIENT'S ATTENTION, THEN SAY: "I am going to say three words that I want you to remember. The words are**
Banana Sunrise Chair.
Please say them for me now." (Give the patient 3 tries to repeat the words. If unable after 3 tries, go to next item.)
(Fold this page back at the TWO dotted lines BELOW to make a blank space and cover the memory words. Hand the patient a pencil/pen.)
2) **SAY ALL THE FOLLOWING PHRASES IN THE ORDER INDICATED: "Please draw a clock in the space below. Start by drawing a large circle."** (When this is done, say) **"Put all the numbers in the circle."** (When done, say) **"Now set the hands to show 11:10 (10 past 11)."**

3) **SAY: "What were the three words I asked you to remember?"**

________ ________ ________ (Score 1 point for each) 3-Item Recall Score ☐

Score the clock (see other side for instructions): Normal clock 2 points; Abnormal clock 0 points. Clock Score ☐

Total Score = 3-item recall plus clock score ☐ ***0, 1, or 2 possible impairment; 3, 4, or 5 suggests no impairment***

CLOCK SCORING

NORMAL CLOCK

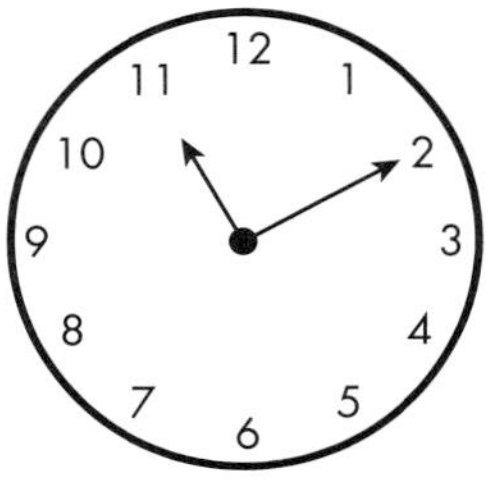

A NORMAL CLOCK HAS ALL OF THE FOLLOWING ELEMENTS:

All numbers 1-12, each only once, are present in the correct order and direction (clockwise).

Two hands are present, one pointing to 11 and one pointing to 2.

ANY CLOCK MISSING EITHER OF THESE ELEMENTS IS SCORED ABNORMAL. REFUSAL TO DRAW A CLOCK IS SCORED ABNORMAL.

SOME EXAMPLES OF ABNORMAL CLOCKS (THERE ARE MANY OTHER KINDS)

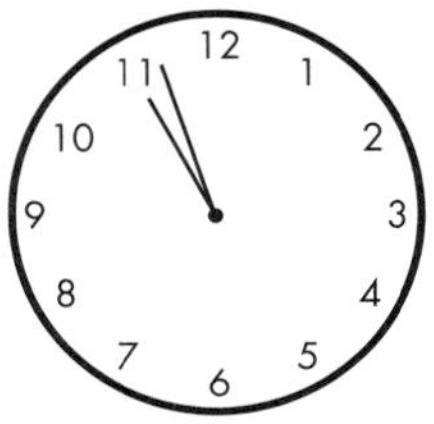

Abnormal Hands

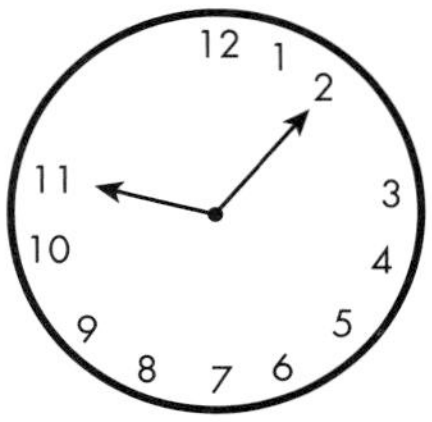

Abnormal Spacing

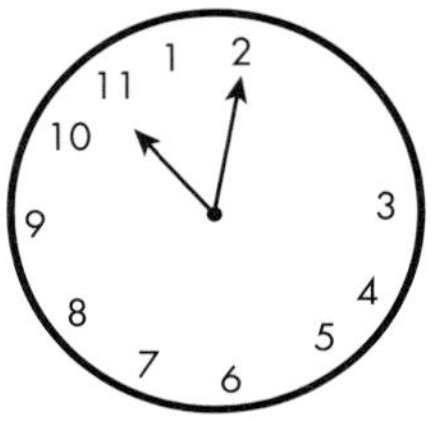

Abnormal Spacing/Numbers

Fig. 4-1 Mini-Cog test. (Mini-Cog™ [Versions 1.0 and 2.0], Copyright 2000 and 2003, Soo Borson and James Scanlan. All rights reserved. Reprinted under license from the University of Washington solely for use as a clinical or teaching aid. Any other use is strictly prohibited without permission from Dr. Borson, soob@u.washington.edu.)

with confusion and disorientation, so depressed older people are often mistakenly labeled demented. It is important to note here that people who are depressed usually respond to items on mental status examinations by saying, "I don't know," which leads to poor performance. Since mental status examinations are not able to distinguish between dementia and depression, a response of "I don't know" should be interpreted as a sign that further affective assessment is warranted.

The Beck Depression Inventory contains 13 items describing a variety of symptoms and attitudes associated with depression (Beck and Beck, 1972). Each item is rated using a 4-point scale to designate the intensity of the symptom. The tool is easily scored and can be self-administered or given by the nurse in about 5 minutes. Depending on the degree of impairment, the number of responses for each item could be confusing or could create difficulty for the older client. The nurse may need to assist clients experiencing this problem with the tool. The scoring cutoff points aid in estimating the severity of the depression.

The short form Geriatric Depression Scale (Box 4-11), derived from the original 30-question scale, is a convenient instrument designed specifically for use with older people to screen for depression (Yesavage and Brink, 1983). Questions answered as indicated score one point. A score of 5 or more may indicate depression.

The instruments described here for assessing cognitive and affective status are valuable screening tools the nurse can use to supplement other assessments. They may also be used to monitor a client's condition over time. The results of any screening mental or affective status examination should never be accepted as conclusive; they are subject to change based on further workup or after treatment interventions have been implemented.

BOX 4-11 Yesavage Geriatric Depression Scale, Short Form

1. Are you basically satisfied with your life? (no)
2. Have you dropped many of your activities and interests? (yes)
3. Do you feel that your life is empty? (yes)
4. Do you often get bored? (yes)
5. Are you in good spirits most of the time? (no)
6. Are you afraid that something bad is going to happen to you? (yes)
7. Do you feel happy most of the time? (no)
8. Do you often feel helpless? (yes)
9. Do you prefer to stay home at night, rather than go out and do new things? (yes)
10. Do you feel that you have more problems with memory than most? (yes)
11. Do you think it is wonderful to be alive now? (no)
12. Do you feel pretty worthless the way you are now? (yes)
13. Do you feel full of energy? (no)
14. Do you feel that your situation is hopeless? (yes)
15. Do you think that most persons are better off than you are? (yes)

Score 1 point for each response that matches the yes or no answer after the question. A score of 5 or more may indicate depression.

From Yesavage JA, Brink TL: Development and validation of a geriatric depression screening scale: a preliminary report, *J Psychiatr Res* 17:37, Elsevier Science Ltd, Pergamon Imprint, Oxford, England, 1983.

Social Assessment

There are several legitimate reasons why health care providers should screen for social function in older people, despite the diverse concepts of what constitutes social function (Kane and Kane, 1981). First, social function is correlated with physical and mental function. Alterations in activity patterns can negatively affect physical and mental health, and vice versa. Second, an individual's social well-being can positively affect his or her ability to cope with physical impairments and ability to remain independent. Third, a satisfactory level of social function is a significant outcome in and of itself. The quality of life an older person experiences is closely linked to social function dimensions such as self-esteem, life satisfaction, socioeconomic status, and physical health and functional status.

The relationship the older adult has with family plays a central role in the overall level of health and well-being. The assessment of this aspect of the client's social system can yield vital information about an important part of the total support network. Contrary to popular belief, families provide substantial help to their older members (see Chapter 6). Consequently, the level of family involvement and support cannot be disregarded when collecting data.

Support for people outside the family plays an increasingly significant role in the lives of many older persons today. Faith-based community support, especially in the form of the parish nurse program, is evolving as a meaningful source of help for older persons who have no family or who have family in distant geographic locations (see Chapter 13). The nurse must regard these "nontraditional" sources of social support as legitimate when assessing the older adult's social system.

A short screening tool that can be used to assess the older person's social function is the Family APGAR (Smilkstein, Ashworth, and Montano, 1982). Adaptation, partnership, growth, affection, and resolve (APGAR) are the aspects of family function that the tool assesses (Box 4-12). The tool can be easily adapted for use with clients who have more intimate social relationships with friends than family by simply substituting the term "friends" for "family" in the statements. A score of less than 3 suggests a highly dysfunctional family; a score of 4 to 6 suggests a moderately dysfunctional family. The use of this screening instrument with a new client, or following a serious, stressful life event, is appropriate.

One of the components of the Older Adults Resources and Services (OARS) Multidimensional Functional Assessment

BOX 4-12 Family APGAR

1. I am satisfied that I can turn to my family (friends) for help when something is troubling me. *(adaptation)*
2. I am satisfied with the way my family (friends) talks over things with me and shares problems with me. *(partnership)*
3. I am satisfied that my family (friends) accepts and supports my wishes to take on new activities or directions. *(growth)*
4. I am satisfied with the way my family (friends) expresses affection and responds to my emotions, such as anger, sorrow, or love. *(affection)*
5. I am satisfied with the way my family (friends) and I share time together. *(resolve)*

Scoring:
Statements are answered *always* (2 points), *some of the time* (1 point), *hardly ever* (0 points). A score of less than 3 suggests a highly dysfunctional family; a score of 4 to 6 suggests a moderately dysfunctional family.

From Smilkstein G, Ashworth C, Montano MA: Validity and reliability of the Family APGAR as a test of family function, *J Fam Prac* 15:303, 1982. Reprinted with permission from Appleton & Lange.

Questionnaire, developed at Duke University, is the Social Resource Scale (Duke University Center for the Study of Aging and Human Development, 1988) (Box 4-13). This scale is one of the better-known measures of general social function for older adults. The questions extract data about family structure, patterns of friendship and visiting, availability of a confidant, satisfaction with the degree of social interaction, and availability of a helper in the event of illness or disability. Different questions (noted in italics in Box 4-13) are used for clients residing in institutions. The interviewer rates the client using a 6-point scale ranging from "excellent social resources" to "totally socially impaired" based on the responses to the questions.

Many other measures of social function can be found in the literature, but a lack of consensus by experts as to which are most suitable for use with older adults makes it difficult to recommend any one with certainty. Therefore the nurse should use these tools with caution and care, remembering that it is crucial to attempt to screen for those older people at social risk.

For all the additional assessment measures discussed above, the nurse should bear in mind that these are meant to augment the traditional health assessment, not replace it. Care needs to be taken to ensure the tools are used appropriately with regard to purpose, setting, timing, and safety. Doing so can lead to a more accurate appraisal on which to base nursing diagnostic statements and to plan suitable and effective interventions.

Home Care

1. Include social support systems, as well as environmental and safety needs, in the assessment of the older adult.
2. Assessing and intervening when an older adult has vague signs and symptoms can reduce the risk of hospitalization.
3. Laboratory data are important indicators of the older adult's compliance with the medication regimen.
4. Obtain subjective assessment data from family members if the older adult has an acute confusional state (ACS) or dementia to ensure collection of reliable information.

LABORATORY DATA

The last component of a comprehensive assessment is evaluation of laboratory tests. The results of laboratory tests can validate history and physical examination findings, and can also identify potential health problems not pointed out by the client or the nurse. Data are considered with regard to established norms based on age and gender. See Chapter 21 for a comprehensive discussion of age-related changes in laboratory tests.

SUMMARY

This chapter presented the components of a comprehensive nursing-focused assessment for an older adult, including special considerations to ensure an age-specific approach, as well as pragmatic modifications for conducting the assessment with this unique age group. Components of the health history and physical examination were discussed, with consideration given to additional functional status assessment measures that can be used with older adults. Compiling an accurate and thorough assessment of an older adult client, which serves as the foundation for the remaining steps of the nursing process, involves the blending of many skills and is an art not easily mastered.

Key Points

- The less vigorous response to illness and disease in older adults as a result of diminished physiologic reserve, coupled with the diminished stress response, causes an atypical presentation of and response to illness and disease.
- Standards for what constitutes normal and abnormal in health and illness for older adults are constantly changing as the scientific knowledge base grows.
- Cognitive change is one of the most common manifestations of illness in old age.
- An abrupt onset ACS in the older adult requires a complete workup to identify the cause so that appropriate interventions can be developed to reverse it.

BOX 4-13 **OARS Social Resource Scale**

Now I'd like to ask you some questions about your family and friends.

Are you single, married, widowed, divorced, or separated?

1 Single 3 Widowed 5 Separated
2 Married 4 Divorced ___ Not answered

If "2" ask following:
Does your spouse live here also?
1 yes
0 no
___ Not answered

Who lives with you?
(Check "yes" or "no" for each of the following.)

Yes	No	
______	______	No one
______	______	Husband or wife
______	______	Children
______	______	Grandchildren
______	______	Parents
______	______	Grandparents
______	______	Brothers and sisters
______	______	Other relatives (does not include in-laws covered in the above categories)
______	______	Friends
______	______	Nonrelated paid help (includes free room)
______	______	Others (specify)

In the past year about how often did you leave here to visit your family and/or friends for weekends or holidays or to go on shopping trips or outings?
1 Once a week or more
2 1-3 times a month
3 Less than once a month or only on holidays
4 Never
___ Not answered

How many people do you know well enough to visit with in their homes?
3 Five or more
2 Three to four
1 One to two
0 None
___ Not answered

About how many times did you talk to someone—friends, relatives, or others—on the telephone in the past week (either you called them or they called you)? (If subject has no phone, question still applies.)
3 Once a day or more
2 Twice
1 Once
0 Not at all
___ Not answered

How many times during the past week did you spend some time with someone who does not live with you, that is, you went to see them, or they came to visit you, or you went out to do things together?

How many times in the past week did you visit with someone, either with people who live here or people who visited you here?
3 Once a day or more
2 Two to six
1 Once
0 Not at all
___ Not answered

Do you have someone you can trust and confide in?
1 Yes
0 No
___ Not answered

Do you find yourself feeling lonely quite often, sometimes, or almost never?
0 Quite often
1 Sometimes
2 Almost never
___ Not answered

Do you see your relatives and friends as often as you want to, or not?
1 As often as wants to
0 Not as often as wants to
___ Not answered

Is there someone *(outside this place)* who would give you any help at all if you were sick or disabled (e.g., your husband/wife, a member of your family, or a friend)?
1 Yes
0 No one willing and able to help
___ Not answered

If "yes," ask A and B.

A. Is there someone *(outside this place)* who would take care of you as long as needed, or only for a short time, or only someone who would help you now and then (e.g., taking you to the doctor, or fixing lunch occasionally)?
3 Someone who would take care of subject indefinitely (as long as needed)
2 Someone who would take care of subject for a short time (a few weeks to six months)
1 Someone who would help subject now and then (taking him to the doctor or fixing lunch, etc.)
___ Not answered

B. Who is this person?
Name ______________________
Relationship ______________________

RATING SCALE

Rate the current social resources of the person being evaluated along the 6-point scale presented below. Circle the *one* number that best describes the person's present circumstances.

1. *Excellent Social Resources:* Social relationships are very satisfying and extensive; at least one person would take care of him (her) indefinitely.
2. *Good Social Resources:* Social relationships are fairly satisfying and adequate and at least one person would take care of him (her) indefinitely, or

BOX 4-13 OARS Social Resource Scale—cont'd

Social relationships are very satisfying and extensive, and only short-term help is available.

3. *Mildly Socially Impaired:* Social relationships are unsatisfactory, of poor quality, few; but as least one person would take care of him (her) indefinitely, or
   Social relationships are fairly satisfactory and adequate, and only short-term help is available.
4. *Moderately Socially Impaired:* Social relationships are unsatisfactory, of poor quality, few; and only short-term care is available, or
   Social relationships are at least adequate or satisfactory, but help would only be available now and then.
5. *Severely Socially Impaired:* Social relationships are unsatisfactory, of poor quality, few; and help would be available only now and then, or
   Social relationships are at least satisfactory or adequate, but help is not available even now and then.
6. *Totally Socially Impaired:* Social relationships are unsatisfactory, of poor quality, few; and help is not available even now and then.

From Duke University Center for the Study of Aging and Human Development: *OARS multidimensional functional assessment: questionnaire,* Durham, NC, 1988, Duke University.

- Conducting a health assessment with an older adult requires modification of the environment, consideration of the client's energy level and adaptability, and opportunity for demonstrating assets and capabilities.
- Sensory-perceptual deficits, anxiety, reduced energy level, pain, multiple and interrelated health problems, and the tendency to reminisce are the major factors requiring special consideration by the nurse while conducting the health history with the older adult.
- An older adult's physical health alone does not provide a reliable measure of functional ability; assessment of physical, cognitive, affective, and social function provides a comprehensive view of the older adult's total degree of function.
- The purpose of a nursing-focused assessment of the older adult is to identify client strengths and limitations so that effective and appropriate interventions can be delivered to promote optimum function and to prevent disability and dependence.
- An older adult's reduced ability to respond to stress, the increased frequency and multiplicity of loss, and the physical changes associated with normal aging combine to place the older adult at high risk for loss of functional ability.
- A comprehensive assessment of an older adult's report of nonspecific signs and symptoms is essential to determine the presence of underlying conditions that may lead to functional decline.
- To compensate for the lack of definitive standards for what constitutes "normal" in older adults, the nurse can compare the older client's own previous patterns of physical and psychosocial health and function with the client's current status.

Critical Thinking Exercises

1. You are interviewing a 78-year-old man who was just admitted to the hospital. He states he is hard of hearing; you note that he is restless and apprehensive. How would you revise your history-taking interview based on these initial observations?
2. Three individuals, ages 65, 81, and 98, have blood pressure readings of 152/88, 168/90, and 170/92 mm Hg, respectively. The nurse infers that all older people are hypertensive. Analyze the nurse's conclusion. Is faulty logic being used in this situation? What assumption(s) did the nurse make with regard to older people in general?

References

American Nurses Association: *Nursing's social policy statement,* Washington, DC, 1995, The Association.

American Nurses Association: *Nursing: a social policy statement,* Kansas City, Mo, 1980, The Association.

American Psychiatric Association: *Diagnostic and statistical manual of mental disorders,* ed 4, Washington, DC, 1994, The Association.

Beck AT, Beck RW: Screening depressed patients in family practice: a rapid technique, *Postgrad Med* 52:81, 1972.

Borson S et al: The Mini-Cog as a screen for dementia: validation in a population-based sample, *J Am Geriatr Soc* 51(10):1451, 2003.

Burnside IM: *Nursing and the aged: a self-care approach,* ed 3, New York, 1988, McGraw-Hill.

Duke University Center for the Study of Aging and Human Development: *OARS multidimensional functional assessment: questionnaire,* Durham, NC, 1988, Duke University.

Folstein MF, Folstein SE, McHugh PR: Mini-mental state: practical method for grading the cognitive state of patients for the clinician, *J Psychiatr Res* 12:189, 1975.

Foreman MD: Acute confusional states in hospitalized elderly: a research dilemma, *Nurs Res* 35(1):34, 1986.

Kane RA, Kane RL: *Assessing the elderly: a practical guide to measurement,* Lexington, Mass, 1981, Lexington Books.

Katz S et al: Studies of illness in the aged: the index of ADL—a standardized measure of biological and psychosocial function, *JAMA* 185:914, 1963.

Kresevic DM et al: Assessment of function: critically important to acute care of elders, *Geriatr Nurs* 18(5):216, 1997.

Lawton HP, Brody EM: Assessment of older people: self maintaining and instrumental activities of daily living, *Gerontologist* 9:179, 1969.

Mahoney FI, Barthel DW: Functional evaluation: the Barthel Index, *Maryland State Med J* 14:61, 1965.

National High Blood Pressure Education Program, US Department of Health and Human Services, Public Health Service: *The seventh report of the Joint National Committee on Detection, Evaluation, and Treatment of High Blood Pressure,* Washington, DC, 2003, National Institutes of Health, National Heart, Lung, and Blood Institute.

Pfeiffer E: A short portable mental status questionnaire for the assessment of organic brain deficit in elderly patients, *J Am Geriatr Soc* 23:433, 1975.

Smilkstein G, Ashworth C, Montano MA: Validity and reliability of the Family APGAR as a test of family function, *J Fam Prac* 15:303, 1982.

Yesavage JA, Brink TL: Development and validation of a geriatric depression screening scale: a preliminary report, *J Psychiatr Res* 17:37, 1983.

5 Cultural Influences

KATHLEEN F. JETT, PhD, APRN, GNP, BC

Learning Objectives

On completion of this chapter, the reader will be able to:

1. Discuss the major demographic trends in the United States in relation to the various older adult ethnic populations.
2. Analyze the nursing implications of ethnic demographic changes.
3. Differentiate among culture, ethnicity, and race.
4. Identify potential barriers to care for the ethnic older person.
5. Discuss cultural variations in beliefs about health and illness and treatment.
6. Describe how one's orientation to time can affect health care practices.
7. Describe how differences in cultural patterns may result in a potential conflict between a gerontologic nurse and an older person or his or her family member.
8. Propose how to increase the quality of the interaction between the nurse and the older adult through the nurse's knowledge of the concept of context as it relates to relationships and behavior.
9. Apply linguistically appropriate techniques in communicating with an ethnic older person.
10. Discuss ways in which planning and implementation of nursing interventions can be adapted to older adults' ethnicity.

DIVERSITY OF THE OLDER ADULT POPULATION IN THE UNITED STATES

The United States has seen a significant shift in the percentage of persons who identify themselves with ethnic groups other than those classified as white, of European descent. It is projected that by 2050 those persons from groups that have long been counted as statistical minorities will assume membership in what can be called the emerging majority.

Although older adults of color will still be outnumbered by their white counterparts for years to come, tremendous growth is anticipated. The largest growth in the older adult population is occurring among persons who consider themselves Hispanic—from less than 5% of the total older adult population in 2000 to 16.4% by 2050. The number of older black persons will grow from 8% of the over 65 population to 12.2%. The percentage of older Asian or Pacific Islanders is projected to increase from 2.4% to 6.5%; Native Americans and Alaskans from 0.4% to 0.5% (Administration on Aging, 2004). It must be noted, however, that these and many of the figures we have today are drawn from the U.S. Census, in which persons of color are often underrepresented and those who are here illegally are not included at all. In reality the numbers of ethnic older adults in the United States may be or become substantially higher.

Furthermore, within the broad census racial and ethnic categories there is considerable diversity. The broad terms are useful statistically, but considerably less useful for the gerontologic nurse caring for the ethnic older person. One who identifies himself or herself as a "Native American" is a member of 1 of over 500 tribal groups, each with both common and unique cultural features. An elder identified as Asian/Pacific Islander may be from one of over a dozen countries that rim the Pacific Ocean and speak 1 (or more) of over 1000 languages or dialects.

Adding to the diversity in the United States is the number of persons immigrating from an increasing number of countries. The immigrant population is growing at a faster rate than that of the native born. In 2003 Gelfand reported that the median age of those born elsewhere was 52, persons who will soon need the care of gerontologic nurses. Although access to the United States varies with global politics, older adults are continually being reunited with their adult offspring, where they assist with homemaking and care for younger children in the family and are cared for themselves. It is becoming increasingly common for communities to support senior centers with activities and meals reflective of their diverse participants.

Certain communities and regions in the United States are decidedly more diverse than others. The states with the largest numbers of ethnic, immigrant, or refugee elders are California, Illinois, Florida, Nevada, New Jersey, Massachusetts, Arizona, Virginia, and Michigan (Gelfand, 2003). Figs. 5-1 to 5-4 provide information about the geographic distribution of older persons from each census group. Gerontologic nursing in these states is likely to be a cross-cultural experience. Today and in the

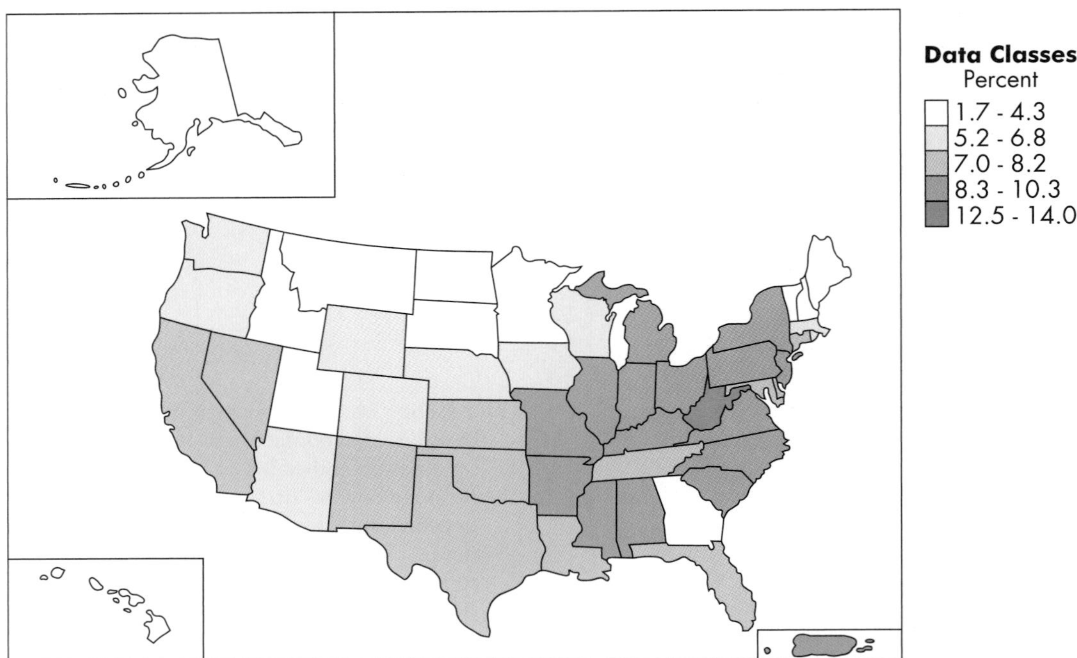

Fig. 5-1 Percent of persons 65 years and over (black or African-Americans alone). (From US Bureau of the Census, 2000.)

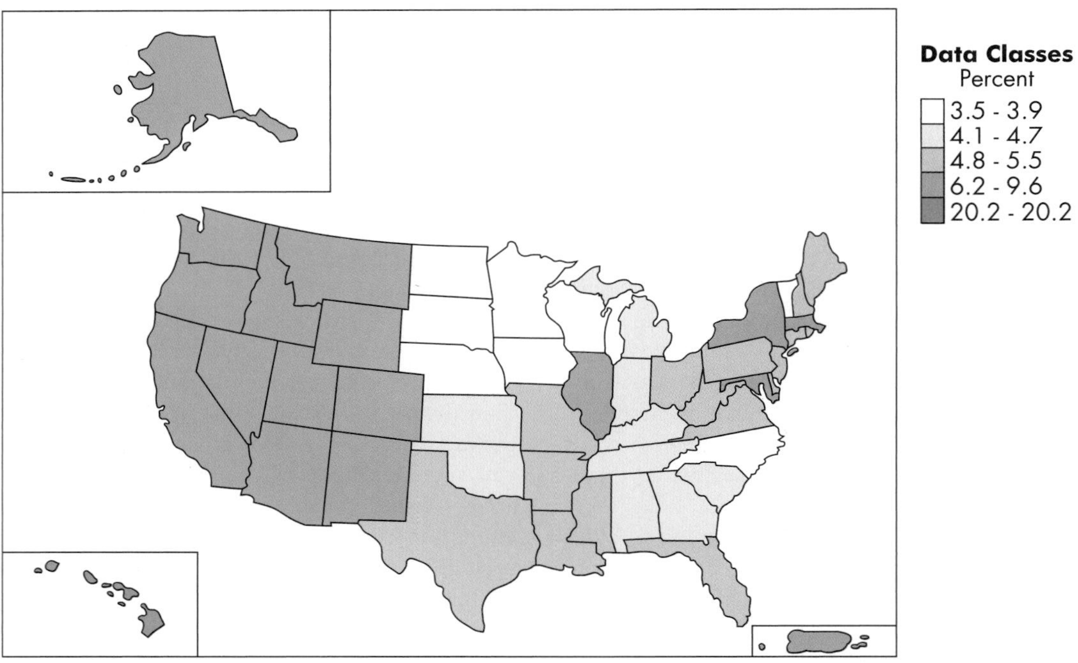

Fig. 5-2 Percent of persons 65 and over (Asian alone). (From US Bureau of the Census, 2000.)

future, nurses may provide care to older adults from several ethnic groups in the course of a single day.

IMPLICATIONS OF ETHNIC DEMOGRAPHIC CHANGES FOR GERONTOLOGIC NURSING

The diversity of values, beliefs, languages, and historical life experiences of older adults today challenges nurses to gain new awareness, knowledge, and skills to provide culturally and linguistically appropriate care.

Nurses must be aware of and understand the considerable problems that many persons from ethnic groups encounter in the pursuit and receipt of health care, and the considerable disparities in health outcomes. Through this awareness, nurses can provide more compassionate and relevant care.

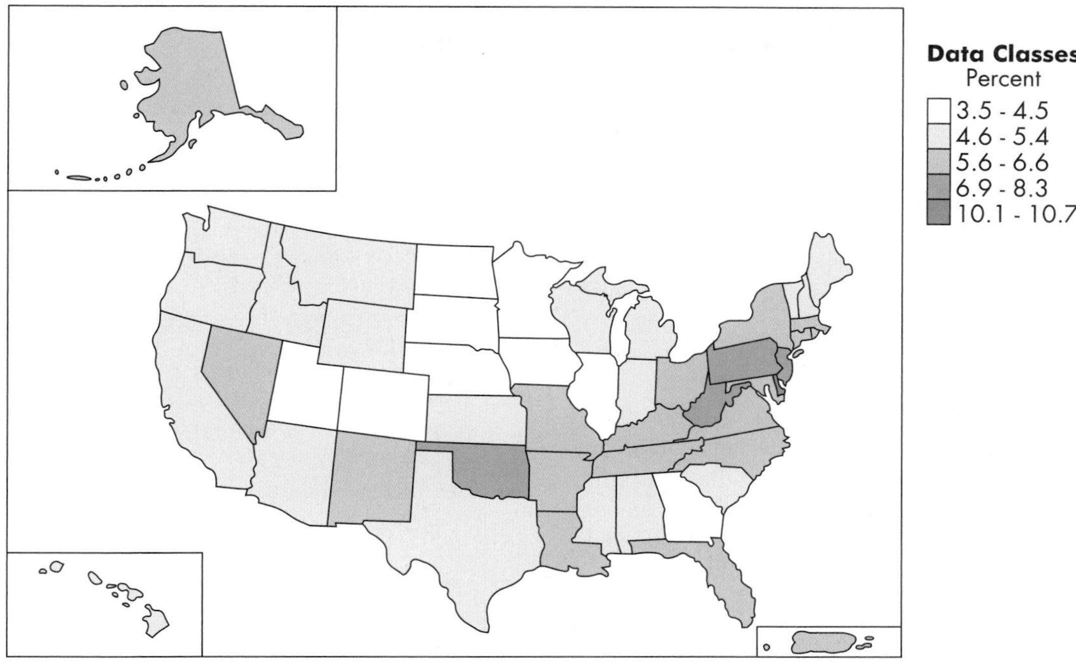

Fig. 5-3 Percent of persons 65 and over (American Indian or Alaskan native only). (From US Bureau of the Census, 2000.)

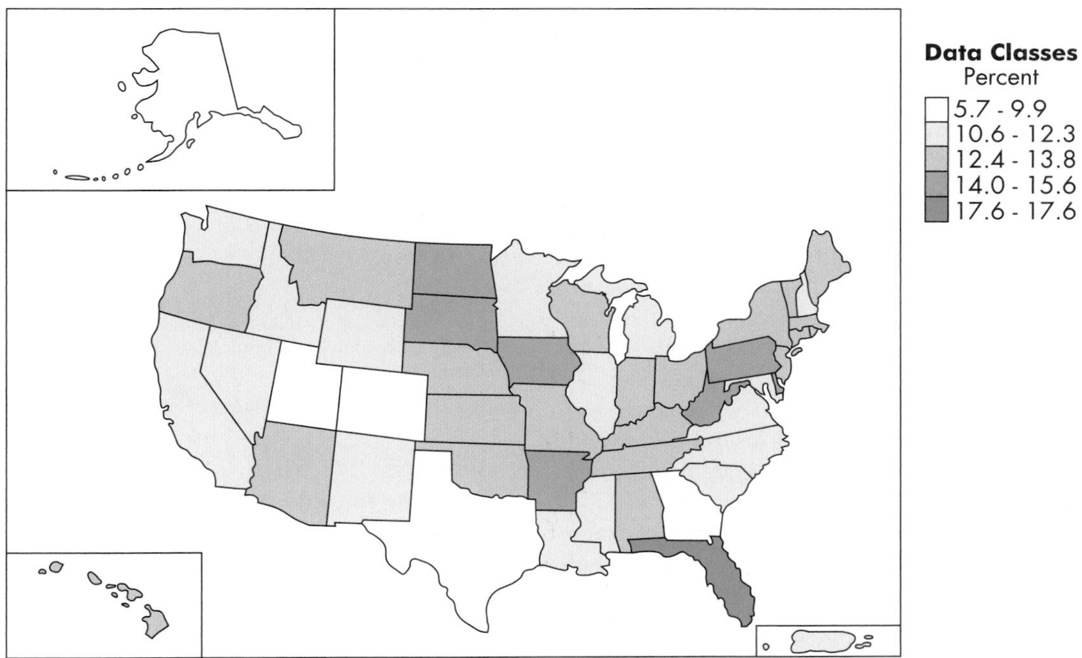

Fig. 5-4 Percent of persons 65 and over (Hispanic or Latino, any race). (From US Bureau of the Census, 2000.)

Cross-cultural knowledge can minimize frustration and cultural conflict between older adult clients, nurses, and other health care providers. Courses in anthropology (political, economic, and cultural), world religions, intercultural communication, scientific health and folk care systems, cross-cultural nutrition, and languages are relevant. Such information can help schools of nursing, students, practitioners, and health care institutions become more culturally sensitive to the diversity of their present and potential client population. It will allow the nurse to improve client health outcomes.

The nursing skills required to work across cultures include the application of the new knowledge. Leininger's theory and her Sunrise Model (Leininger, 1995; Leininger, 1991) provide different frameworks for comprehensive assessment of culture and the person. The Explanatory Model offered by

Kleinman, Eisenberg, and Good (1978) and the LEARN Model (Berlin and Folkes, 1992) are useful in the day-to-day interaction with persons from diverse backgrounds.

Finally, the gerontologic nurse caring for ethnic older adults would benefit from increased skills in the basics of cross-cultural communication, especially how to work with interpreters.

Increasing awareness, knowledge, and skills are the tools needed to begin to overcome the barriers to culturally competent care and, as a consequence, to reduce health disparities.

Awareness

The development of competence begins with increased awareness of our own beliefs and attitudes and those commonly seen in the community at large and in the community of health care. Awareness of one's thoughts and feelings about others who are culturally different from oneself is necessary. These thoughts and feelings can be hidden from you, but may be evident to clients. To be aware of these thoughts and feelings about others, one can begin to share or write down personal memories of those first experiences of cultural differences. Questions such as, "How did it happen? How did I feel? How did they react?" are a good starting point to begin the process of cultural self-discovery.

Cultural awareness has several levels. The first is the self-level, requiring self-understanding of one's experiences and values. The second level involves the ability to work with and build relationships with a member from another cultural group. The third level is the recognition of factors beyond culture such as health, safety, and poverty that affect members of a cultural group. On the fourth level, it is important to understand how one's own community history affects how others are viewed, and on the last level, one must be able to step outside of cultural bias and accept that other cultures have different ways of perceiving the world that are as valid as our own.

Conducting a cultural self-assessment before assessing clients of other cultural groups can be a useful exercise to identify one's beliefs about aging and immigrant populations coming to this country as older adults. The questions found in the Cultural Self-Assessment and Culture Care Questions (see Cultural Awareness boxes) may serve as a starting point.

Awareness is also enhanced through the acquisition of new knowledge about culture and the common barriers to high-quality health care too often faced by persons from ethnically distinct groups.

Please review information in Chapter 4 related to cultural considerations during the nursing assessment process.

Knowledge

Increased knowledge is a prerequisite for increased cultural competence in the care of ethnic older adults.

Cultural Awareness

CULTURAL SELF-ASSESSMENT

- What are my personal beliefs about older adults from different cultures?
- What experiences have influenced my values, biases, ideas, and attitudes toward older adults from different cultures?
- What are my values as they relate to health, illness, and health-related practices?
- How do my values and attitudes affect my clinical judgments?
- How do my values influence my thinking and behaving?
- What are my personal habits and typical communication patterns when interacting with others? How would these be perceived by older adults of different cultures?

Cultural Awareness

CULTURAL CARE QUESTIONS

- How has this problem or change affected your life?
- Do you know anyone else who has had this problem or change? What did he or she do about it? What kinds of treatments were used?
- Do you think there is any way to keep this from happening again?
- What treatments have you tried?
- What do you think I (or we) can do for you?
- Is there someone in your family whom you would like to be involved in conversations about this problem or the plan for what to do about the problem?
- Does anyone else need to be involved in your healing?

From the Explanatory Model for Gerontological Nurses, adapted from Kleinman A, Eisenberg L, Good B: Culture, illness and care: clinical lessons from anthropological and cross-cultural research, *Annals Intern Med* 88:251, 1978.

Beginning to Understand Culture. Several key terms and concepts are discussed here in an attempt to clarify those which are often used incorrectly or interchangeably in any discussion related to culture and ethnicity.

Culture is the shared and learned beliefs, expectations, and behaviors of a group of people. Style of dress, food preferences, language, and social systems are expressions of culture. Beliefs about aging may be relatively consistent within one culture group (Jett, 2003). Cultural knowledge is transmitted from one member to another through the process called *enculturation*. It provides individuals with a sense of security and a blueprint for interacting within the family, community, and country. Culture allows members of the culture to predict each other's behavior and respond appropriately (Boxes 5-1 to 5-4).

BOX 5-1 Anglo-American (European-American) Culture (Mainly U.S. Middle and Upper Class)

CULTURAL VALUES	CULTURE CARE MEANINGS AND ACTION MODES
Individualism—focus on a self-reliant person	Alleviating stress
Independence and freedom	• Physical means
Competition and achievement	• Emotional means
Materialism (items and money)	Personalized acts
Technologic dependence	• Doing special things
Instantaneous actions	• Giving individual attention
Youth and beauty	Self-reliance (individualism) by:
Equal sex rights	• Reliance on self
Leisure time	• Reliance on self (self-care)
Reliance on scientific facts and numbers	• Becoming as independent as possible
Less respect for authority and older adults	• Reliance on technology
Generosity in time of crisis	Health instruction
	• Explaining how "to do" this care for self
	• Giving the "medical" facts

From Leininger M, editor: *Culture care diversity and universality: a theory of nursing*, Sudbury, Mass, 1991, National League for Nursing, Jones and Bartlett.

BOX 5-2 Appalachian Culture

CULTURAL VALUES	CULTURE CARE MEANINGS AND ACTION MODES
Keeping ties with kin from the "hollows"	Knowing and trusting "true friends"
Personalized religion	Being kind to others
Folk practices as "the best lifeways"	Being watchful of strangers or outsiders
Guarding against "strangers"	Doing for others; less for self
Being frugal; always using home remedies	Keeping with kin and local folks
Staying near home for protection	Using home remedies "first and last"
Mother as decision maker	Taking help from kin as needed (primary care)
Community interdependency	Helping people stay away from the hospital—"the place where people die"

From Leininger M, editor: *Culture care diversity and universality: a theory of nursing*, Sudbury, Mass, 1991, National League for Nursing, Jones and Bartlett.

BOX 5-3 Black Culture

CULTURAL VALUES	CULTURE CARE MEANINGS AND ACTION MODES
Extended family networks	Concern for "my brothers and sisters"
Religion (many are Baptists)	Being involved
Interdependence with blacks	Providing a presence (physical)
Daily survival	Family support and "get-togethers"
Technology (e.g., radio, car)	Touching appropriately
Folk (soul) foods	Reliance on folk home remedies
Folk healing modes	Reliance on Jesus to "save us" with prayers and songs
Music and physical activities	

From Leininger M, editor: *Culture care diversity and universality: a theory of nursing*, Sudbury, Mass, 1991, National League for Nursing, Jones and Bartlett.

Culture is universal. It is a phenomenon found in all parts of the world. It is unique. No two cultures are exactly alike; there are similarities, but there are distinct differences as well.

Culture is adaptive. It is responsive to changes in the environment, availability of resources, contact with other cultures, and technologic development.

Culture exists at the micro level in terms of the individual or family and at the macro level in terms of a region, country, or religious group. A *subculture* is a distinguishable subgroup of people within a larger cultural group who share unique characteristics that may be different from those of the larger group; one example is gerontologic nurses.

Cultural beliefs about what is right and what is wrong behavior are known as *values*. Values provide a standard from which judgments are made, are learned early in childhood, and are expressed throughout the lifespan.

BOX 5-4 Arab-American Muslim Culture

CULTURE CARE MEANINGS AND ACTION MODES

Providing family care and support—a responsibility
Offering respect and private time for religious beliefs and prayers (five times each day)
Respecting and protecting cultural differences in gender roles
Knowing cultural taboos and norms (e.g., no pork, alcohol, or smoking)
Recognizing honor and obligation
Helping others to "save face" and preserve cultural values
Obligation and responsibility to visit the sick
Following the teachings of the Koran
Helping children and elderly when they are ill

From Leininger M, editor: *Culture care diversity and universality: a theory of nursing*, Sudbury, Mass, 1991, National League for Nursing, Jones and Bartlett.

Acculturation is a process that occurs when a member of one cultural group adopts the values, beliefs, expectations, and behaviors of another group, usually in an attempt to become recognized as a member of the new group. This is particularly relevant for ethnic older persons. Many emigrate to join their children's families who have established themselves in the United States. They may live in ethnically homogeneous neighborhoods of "Little Italy," "Little Havana," "Chinatown," etc. They may have little interest or need in acculturation to mainstream United States. Their children, on the other hand, may live in two cultures, that of their parents and that of the workplace. They would be described as bicultural.

Assimilation is the extreme case of acculturation, when a member of one culture becomes completely accepted by the host culture and is no longer seen as distinct. Full assimilation requires (1) the disappearance of outward behavior traits that distinguish an individual as different from a member of the host culture, and (2) the disappearance of exclusive and discriminatory behavior among members of the host culture toward the newcomer (Smedley, Stith, and Nelson, 2003). Unless the individual develops the outward physical appearance of the members of the host group, complete assimilation may not be possible.

Race is defined as "a division of the species which differs from other divisions by the frequency with which certain hereditary traits appear among its members" (Bruce, 1977). Hereditary traits, the product of one's genetic makeup, include skin and eye color, facial structures, hair texture, and body shape and proportions. There are four major racial groups worldwide: Caucasian, Mongoloid, Negro, and Australoid, often referred to in terms of underlying skin tones as white, red, black, and yellow, respectively. However, the relative importance of race is diminishing due to widespread mixing of the gene pool so that it is becoming increasingly uncommon for any one person to be genetically homogeneous (Gelfand, 2003). Acknowledgment of this heterogeneity was demonstrated when a new racial category of "mixed" was finally added to the 2000 census.

Ethnicity, in contrast to race, is not based on genetics or skin tones, but on socialization and identification. Ethnicity is defined as a social differentiation of people based on group membership, shared history, and some common characteristics. For example, the term *Hispanic* is often applied to persons who share the Spanish language and often the Catholic religion. However, one who self-identifies as Hispanic may have been born in one of several countries and be of any race. *Ethnic identity* refers to the individual's willingness to identify himself or herself as a member of the group. Ethnic identity cannot be assumed by appearance, language, or other outward features. I once asked an older black women, "May I assume you identify yourself as an African American?" To which she replied, "Well, no—I have always thought of myself as just an American and don't think in terms of 'African American.'"

Barriers to Providing Culturally Appropriate Care. Gerontologic nursing care is provided to persons in all situations, without regard to personal characteristics. However, there is evidence of racial and ethnic disparities in health care and health outcomes across the range of illness and services and all age groups. While socioeconomic factors account for some of these differences, in too many well-controlled studies only race explains the disparities. Significantly for older adults, alarming differences are seen in the rate of angioplasty, use of pain medication, timing of mammograms, and mortality associated with prostate cancer, to name only a few (Kim, Hofer, and Kerr, 2003; Mudano, Casebeer, and Patino, 2003; Smedley, Stith, and Nelson, 2003) (see Research box).

Gerontologic nurses who provide culturally competent care will contribute to the reduction of health disparities through awareness of, and sensitivity to, both overt and covert barriers to our caring. Among these barriers are ethnocentrism, racism, and discrimination. As a result of any of these, we may see cultural conflict in the nursing situation.

Ethnocentrism is a belief that one's own ethnic group is superior to that of another's. In nursing we have a unique culture and usually expect our clients to adapt to us. We expect them to be on time for appointments, follow our instructions, and listen to what we have to say. If we are caring for older adults in an institutional setting, we expect they will agree to the frequency of prescribed bathing, eating (and timing of this), sleep and rest cycles, etc. The better acculturated an older person is to the institution's culture, the more content he or she will appear. The resident will eat the meals provided even if the food does not look like or taste like what he or she has always eaten. A non–English speaking resident will cooperate with the staff, with or without an interpreter.

Research

Kressin NR, Petersen LA: Racial differences in the use of invasive cardiovascular procedures: review of the literature and prescription for future research, *Ann Intern Med* 135(5):352, 2001.

It has long been suspected that white men receive significantly more invasive cardiac procedures (catheterizations, percutaneous transluminal angioplasty [PCTA], and coronary artery bypass graft [CABG]) than men of color. This article reviewed the literature about these discrepancies that appeared between 1966 and 2000; the review included 61 studies. When patients with similar levels of disease were compared, a white patient had a 94% chance of receiving a cardiac catheterization compared with a 41% chance for a black patient; findings were similar for PTCAs and CABGs, and for Hispanic or Asian patients. The higher frequency of lower levels of education in patients of color explained only a part of the discrepancy. A full explanation of the difference has not been found, but health care provider bias appears to be a factor. Patients working with persons they can trust may make a difference.

IMPLICATIONS

The gerontologic nurse can be instrumental in reducing discrepancies such as these. The use of cultural knowledge and optimum intercultural communication and advocacy may help all persons seek the optimum care and intervention available.

Racism is the assumption of negative beliefs, attitudes, or behavior toward a person or groups of persons based solely on skin color. Racism results in hostile attitudes of prejudice and the differential treatment and behavior of discrimination that is directed at a specific ethnic or minority group.

A gerontologic nurse responded to a call from an older patient's room. For some unknown reason the patient, repeatedly and without comment, dropped his watch on the floor while talking to the nurse. She calmly picked it up, handed it back to him, and continued talking. During one of the droppings an aide walked in the room, picked up the watch, and attempted to hand it back to him. The patient immediately started yelling and cursing at the aide for attempting to steal his watch. When telling this story, the nurse thought the whole situation odd, but not too remarkable. It was not until she learned about subtle racism in health care settings that she recognized the patient's harmful, racist behavior: he was white and so was she, but the aide was black.

There are many "isms" that interfere with the pursuit and receipt of health care, including ageism; sexism; (social) classism; and the negative beliefs, attitudes, and behaviors toward a person or a group of persons based on one of these characteristics.

Discrimination is the differential treatment of individuals because they belong to a specific racial, ethnic, religious, or social group. The results of differential treatment are inequitable experiences and opportunities for the disadvantaged group and advantages for the perpetrator.

Cultural conflict is the anxiety experienced when people interact with individuals who have different beliefs, values, customs, languages, and lifeways than their own. For example:

An immigrant Korean nurse is instructed to walk with an 80-year-old black client. The client says that he is tired and wants to remain in bed this morning. The nurse does not insist. The European American nurse manager reprimands the immigrant Korean nurse for not walking with the client as ordered. The immigrant Korean nurse says to another Korean nurse: "Those Americans do not respect their elders; they talk to them as if they were children." The European American nurse tells the physician that "those Asian nurses allow men to run all over them."

In the Korean culture, men are the decision makers, and older adults are revered. Those from the culture known as mainstream American, or European American, do not usually consider age or gender in these circumstances. In the responses of both nurses, each denigrated the other's culturally prescribed behavior to underscore that their own cultural response was "correct."

Home Care. When home care nursing is ordered or requested for a client with unknown cultural barriers, the nurse needs to ascertain whether the older adult came to the United States as a child, young adult, or older adult, or was born in America, since this will affect his or her level of acculturation and eligibility for benefits and services. The nurse should refer to the appropriate agency or social worker for assistance if necessary. Knowledge of the differences and similarities of values of homebound clients can minimize tension and cultural conflict within the home care setting. The nurse should adapt communication styles and techniques so they are ethnically appropriate, reducing the potential for conflict. The nurse should assess the caregiver's and client's own concepts of health and illness. Finally, the nurse needs to assess the home environment for evidence of cultural values. These data are incorporated into the plan of care to meet the cultural needs of the client and family.

Cultural Knowledge. There are many ways to increase one's cultural knowledge. One of the most common is the encyclopedic approach. The nurse selects a culture of interest and learns as much as possible about the group. This may include language; dress; diet; religion; history; and beliefs about aging, health, and illness. There are multiple sources for this information, but the nurse must be cautious about the validity of the source, and take care not to use such knowledge in perpetuating negative stereotypes. The positive stereotypic information, such as common health beliefs or death practices, can be used as a starting point for communication. For example, the nurse might ask, "It is my understanding that remaining active in the church is important to many in the black community. Is this important to you? If so, how is your stroke affecting this aspect of your life?"

Another approach is to use particular clinical issues, and how they are usually dealt with in a particular culture, as a point of reference. Issues of special interest to the gerontologic nurse include beliefs about end of life (Baker, 2000; Braun, Pietsch, and Blanchette, 2000; Kobylarz, Hernandez, and Hurwitz, 2002; Mazanec and Tyler, 2003), death practices (Irish, Lundquist, and Nelsen, 1993), caregiving (Farran, Paun, and Elliott, 2003; Lee, 2004), help seeking (Jett, 2002), specific disease processes (Rhoades and Buchwald, 2003), and drug metabolism (Burroughs, Maxey, and Levy, 2002). This approach is particularly helpful for nurses working with older adults in specialty settings such as nursing homes, hospices, and oncology units, or in the community.

A third approach to knowledge is to consider perspectives that may cross and transcend cultures and significantly influence the older person's behavior and present potential sources of conflict in the health care setting. These include health and illness beliefs, time orientation, and cultural patterns and context.

Beliefs About Health and Illness

Although the standard World Health Organization (1947) definition of health states, "Health is the complete physical, mental, and social well-being and not merely the absence of disease," the definitions held by many people of the world differ. Beliefs about health and illness are also closely tied to beliefs about treatment (Spector, 2004).

Beliefs about health, illness, and treatments can be loosely divided into three theoretical categories: magico-religious, balance/harmony, and biomedical. The individual's perception of illness is influenced by others within the family and culture. Older adults have lifelong experiences with illness of self, family, and others within their ethnic groups. The significance they attach to illness symptoms and their reactions are related to the outcomes they have experienced or observed in the past.

In the *magico-religious theory,* both illness and disease are caused by the actions of a higher power (e.g., God, gods, or supernatural forces or agents). Health is viewed as a blessing or reward of God and illness as a punishment for breaching rules, breaking a taboo, or displeasing the source of power. Beliefs about illness and disease causation attributed to the wrath of God are prevalent among members of the Holiness, Pentecostal, and Fundamental Baptist churches. Examples of magical causes of illness are voodoo, especially among persons from the Caribbean; root work among southern black Americans; hexing among Mexican Americans and blacks; and Gaba among Filipino Americans (Box 5-5). Treatments may involve religious practices such as praying, meditating, fasting, wearing amulets, burning candles, and establishing family altars. Such practices may be used both curatively and preventively.

Significant conflict with nurses may result when a patient refuses biomedical treatments because doing so is viewed as a sign of disrespect for God, as challenging God's will. Although this belief is more common in certain groups, most of us are believers of this approach to some extent. How many nurses and their older patients have prayed to a higher power that health be restored or maintained?

Many people view health as a sign of *balance*—of the right amount of exercise, food, sleep, evacuation, interpersonal relationships, or geophysical and metaphysical forces in the universe, such as chi. Disturbances in this balance result in disharmony and subsequent illness. The appropriate interventions, therefore, are methods that restore balance, such as following a strict American Dietetic Association diet or one in which the sodium intake does not upset the fluid balance. A common manifestation of this theoretical approach is in the yin/yang of ancient China and in the hot/cold theory common throughout the world.

The yin/yang theory is an ancient Chinese theory that has been used continuously for the past 5000 years. It is common throughout Asia and is gaining acceptance in the United States. Chinese and other Asian groups apply it along with practices of Western medicine. The theory posits that all organisms and things in the universe consist of yin or yang energy forces. The seat of the energy forces is within the autonomic nervous system. Health is a state of perfect balance between the yin and the yang. When a person is in balance, he or she experiences a feeling of inner and outer peace. Illness represents an imbalance of yin and yang. Balance may be restored by herbs, acupuncture (insertion of the needles into points along the body's meridians), acupressure (application of pressure or massage to the same meridian points), or controlled deep-breathing exercises.

Hot/cold theory posits that illness can be classified as either hot or cold. The treatments (including food) provided must balance the illness to be effective. Hot foods and treatments are needed for cold illnesses and cold foods and treatments for hot illnesses. The culturally caring nurse can ask older adults if they have a belief about the hotness or coldness of a condition and what accommodations are needed. While caring for a newly emigrated Vietnamese couple in my practice as a gerontologic nurse practitioner, I asked if a hot or cold treatment was needed for the management of bronchitis and was told that hot medication was needed. My two choices were Biaxin, a white pill, and Ziythromax, a dark pink pill. I chose the Zithromax as my best guess.

The third theoretic perspective is called *biomedical* or *Western.* The body is viewed as a functioning machine. A part may fall into disrepair and need adjustment or become susceptible to object intrusion, that is, infection by germs. Health is a state of optimum function and the absence of microorganisms such as bacteria or viruses. The microorganisms enter the body and overpower the natural resistance, causing an inflammatory response. Treatment is directed at removal of the damaged part or use of drugs to kill or to retard the growth of the causative organism or intruder. Some non-Western cultures believe that inanimate or animate objects

BOX 5-5 Religious Beliefs of 23 Different Groups That Can Affect Nursing Care

ADVENTIST (SEVENTH DAY ADVENTIST; CHURCH OF GOD)

May believe in divine healing and practice anointing with oil and use of prayer
May desire communion or baptism when ill
Believe in human choice and God's sovereignty
May oppose hypnosis as therapy

BAPTIST (27 GROUPS)

Laying on of hands (some groups)
May resist some therapies, such as abortion
Believe God functions through physician
May believe in predestination; may respond passively to care

BLACK MUSLIM

Faith healing unacceptable
Always maintain personal habits of cleanliness

BUDDHIST CHURCHES OF AMERICA

Believe illness to be a trial to aid development of soul; illness due to karmic causes
May be reluctant to have surgery or certain treatments on holy days
Believe cleanliness to be of great importance
Family may request Buddhist priest for counseling

CHURCH OF CHRIST SCIENTIST (CHRISTIAN SCIENCE)

Deny the existence of health crisis; see sickness and sin as errors of mind that can be altered by prayer
Oppose human intervention with drugs or other therapies; however, accept legally required immunizations
Many believe that disease is a human mental concept that can be dispelled by "spiritual truth" to the extent that they refuse all medical treatment

CHURCH OF JESUS CHRIST OF LATTER DAY SAINTS (MORMON)

Devout adherents believe in divine healing through anointment with oil, laying on of hands by certain church members holding the priesthood, and prayers
Medical therapy not prohibited; members have free will to choose treatments

EASTERN ORTHODOX (IN TURKEY, EGYPT, SYRIA, ROMANIA, BULGARIA, CYPRUS, ALBANIA, AND OTHER COUNTRIES)

Believe in anointing of the sick
No conflict with medical science

EPISCOPAL (ANGLICAN)

May believe in spiritual healing
Rite for anointing sick available but not mandatory

FRIENDS (QUAKERS)

No special rites or restrictions

GREEK ORTHODOX

Each health crisis handled by ordained priest; deacon may also serve in some cases
Holy Communion administered in hospital
May desire Sacrament of the Holy Unction performed by priest

HINDU

Illness or injury believed to represent sins committed in previous life
Accept most modern medical practices

ISLAM (MUSLIM/MOSLEM)

Faith healing not acceptable unless patient's psychologic condition is deteriorating; performed for morale
Ritual washing after prayer; prayer takes place five times daily (on rising, midday, afternoon, early evening, and before bed); during prayer, face Mecca and kneel on prayer rug

JEHOVAH'S WITNESS

Generally absolutely opposed to transfusions of whole blood, packed red blood cells, platelets, and fresh or frozen plasma, including banking of own blood; individuals can sometimes be persuaded in emergencies
May be opposed to use of albumin, globulin, factor replacement (hemophilia), and vaccines
Not opposed to nonblood plasma expanders

JUDAISM (ORTHODOX AND CONSERVATIVE)

May resist surgical procedures on Sabbath, which extends from sundown Friday until sundown Saturday
Seriously ill and pregnant women exempt from fasting
Illness as grounds for violating dietary laws (e.g., patient with congestive heart failure does not have to use kosher meats, which are high in sodium)

LUTHERAN

Church or pastor notified of hospitalization
Communion may be given before or after surgery or similar crisis

MENNONITE (SIMILAR TO AMISH)

No illness rituals
Deep concern for dignity and self-determination of individual; would conflict with shock treatment or medical treatment affecting personality or will

METHODIST

Communion may be requested before surgery or similar crisis

NAZARENE

Church official administers communion and laying on of hands
Believe in divine healing, but without excluding medical treatment

Continued

BOX 5-5 Religious Beliefs of 23 Different Groups That Can Affect Nursing Care—cont'd

PENTECOSTAL (ASSEMBLY OF GOD, FOUR-SQUARE)

No restrictions regarding medical care

Deliverance from sickness provided for by atonement; may pray for divine intervention in health matters and seek God in prayer for themselves and others when ill

ORTHODOX PRESBYTERIAN

Communion administered when appropriate and convenient

Blood transfusion accepted when advisable

Pastor or elder should be called for ill person

Believe science should be used for relief of suffering

ROMAN CATHOLIC

Encourage anointing of sick, although older members of the church may see this as equivalent to "extreme unction," or "last rites"; may require careful explanation if reluctance is associated with fear of imminent death

Traditional church teaching does not approve of contraceptives or abortion

RUSSIAN ORTHODOX

Cross necklace is important and should be removed only when necessary and replaced as soon as possible

Believe in divine healing, but without excluding medical treatment

UNITARIAN UNIVERSALIST

Most believe in general goodness of fellow humans and appreciate expression of that goodness by visits from clergy and fellow parishioners during times of illness

Adapted from Wong DL et al: *Whaley and Wong's nursing care of infants and children*, ed 6, St Louis, 1998, Mosby; Beliefs that can affect therapy, *Pediatr Nurs* 5(3):40, 1979; and Spector RE: *Cultural diversity in health and illness*, ed 4, New York, 1996, Appleton and Lange.

enter the body and must be removed through direct or indirect methods, which may be a variation of the germ theory.

In most cultures older adults are likely to treat themselves informally for familiar or chronic conditions they have successfully treated in the past, based on one or several of the beliefs noted previously. When self-treatment fails, a person will consult with others he or she knows to be knowledgeable or experienced with the problem, such as a community healer. Only when this fails do most people seek professional help within the formal health care system.

Immigrant older adults and those living in ethnically homogeneous communities (e.g., Appalachia, Chinatown) often establish the same type of health care services found in their native land or communities or based on long-enduring traditions (Purnell and Paulanka, 2003). Preparation of medications for self-care is a part of life. Older immigrants may be accustomed to brewing certain herbs, grasses, plants, and leaves to make herbal teas, drinks, solutions, poultices, decoctions, and medicines to prevent and treat illness. Many of the same drugs prescribed by physicians are prepared by older adult immigrants at less expense than buying the drug at the pharmacy. When these people come to America, they can obtain many of the same plants, leaves, buds, and grasses in ethnic grocery stores and botanicas. Others grow their own treatments in potted plants and backyard herb and vegetable gardens (Spector, 2004).

Time Orientation. Another cultural perspective is that of time orientation. Time orientation has long been theoretically recognized but is often overlooked as a factor influencing the use of health care, especially preventive practices (Lukwago et al, 2001). Older adults are more likely to use the orientation of their culture of origin, which may contrast significantly with that of the health care system in the United States.

Time orientation refers to one's primary focus—toward the past, present, or future. An older person who is future oriented is in congruency with mainstream U.S. health care, or Western medicine. Holders of this belief accept that what we do now can affect our future health. This means that a problem noted today can "wait" until an office appointment with a health care provider tomorrow—that the problem will still be there and that the delay will not necessarily affect the outcome. This also means that health screenings will help detect a problem today for potentially better health at a later time, days, weeks, or years ahead. The strength and acceptance of this orientation is seen in the influence of the document *Health People 2010* (US DHHS, 2000) as the national agenda for health care.

Quite different from a future orientation are those of the past and present. Persons oriented to the present experience a problem now and expect treatment now. The outcome is seen as current and not future. Preventive actions are not consistent with this approach.

Persons oriented to the past see present health as dependent on past actions, either from a past life, earlier in this life, or events or circumstances of one's ancestors. Dishonoring ancestors by failing to perform certain rituals may result in illness. Illness may also be viewed as a punishment for past deeds. Thus present health is as a matter of fate, of reward or punishment.

Conflicts between the future-oriented Westernized world of the nurse and clients with past or present orientations are not hard to imagine. Such clients are likely to be labeled as noncompliant for failure to keep appointments or for failure to participate in preventive measures, such a turning schedule for a bedbound patient or immunizations.

The nurse can, however, listen closely to the ethnic older person, find out which orientation he or she values most, and find ways to work with it rather than try (often unsuccessfully) to continue to expect the person to conform. In this way we reach beyond our ethnocentrism to improve the quality of the care we provide.

Cultural Patterns. Another useful perspective is the consideration of cultural patterns. Among these is the individualist or collectivist pattern (Hofstede and Pedersen, 2002). White Americans of European descent tend to highly value autonomy and individuality, with identity bound to the self. In a large, classic study Rathbone-McCune (1982) found that European American older persons would go to great lengths and live with significant discomfort rather than ask for help. To seek or receive help was considered a sign of weakness and dependence, things to be avoided at all costs. The reliance on the individual is institutionalized in the passing of the Patient Self-Determination Act of 1990. It articulates the rights and responsibilities of the individual to participate in all decisions regarding his or her health.

This pattern is in sharp contrast to that of the collectivist, also known as familialism (Lukwago et al, 2001). Those from a collectivist perspective derive their identity from affiliation with and participation in a social group such as a family or ethnic group. The group is more important than the individual, decisions are made for the benefit of the group rather than the individual, and exchanges of help are common place. Jett (2002) found that help seeking among frail, elderly black women was a common experience. The receipt of help was considered a sign of the love of others, a reflection of the status of the older person. The greater the affection of others, the higher the level of help received, and that ". . . good things will come to you" (p. 384).

When a European American nurse who values individuality provides care for an elder who has a collectivist perspective, there is the potential for cultural conflict, illustrated by the following scenario:

An older Filipino woman is seen in her home by a public health nurse and found to have a blood pressure of 210/100 mmHg, and a blood glucose level of 380 mg/100 ml. The nurse insists on calling the client's physician and arranging immediate transportation to the health facility of the physician's choice. The older Filipino insists that she must wait until her son-in-law and daughter get off work to tell them of her condition. The daughter and her husband must decide where and when the client will go for treatment. She is concerned about the family's welfare and wants to ensure that income is not lost by their leaving work early. The family also jointly decides if they can afford a doctor's visit and a possible hospitalization, since the client does not have health insurance. The nurse's main concern is the health of the woman, and the woman's concern is her family. The nurse is operating from the value that says an individual is independent and responsible for personal health care decisions.

Context. A final perspective is that of context. High and low context refers to the characteristics of relationships and behaviors toward others (Hall 1990; Hall, 1977). When a person from a high-context culture interacts with the nurse, the person's family and community are involved. It is important for the nurse to ask about the family members and appear friendly and genuinely interested in the person first, and be concerned with what might be called nursing tasks second. Body language is more important than spoken words, because therein the true meaning is considered to reside. The quality of the relationship between the nurse and the person is more important, perhaps, than the needs of the person. The majority of cultures across the globe are high context in nature.

In stark contrast are those whose relationships and behaviors are low context, such as the culture of Western medicine and nursing, drawn from English and German roots. Low-context health care encounters are task oriented and only secondarily concerned about the relationship between the nurse and the older adult. Individual identity is not as important; Ms. Gomez is not the 82-year-old immigrant from Mexico, mother of seven and grandmother of 30, but is the "fractured hip in 203." For the person who is low context, small talk may be considered a waste of time; a direct approach is expected, with a literal message, "Just tell me what is wrong with me!" There is a low use of nonverbal communication, and verbal communication is kept to that which is necessary.

The culturally competent nurse is skilled enough to assess the patterns of those cared for and skillful enough to move between the contexts in the provision of the highest quality of caring.

SKILLS FOR CULTURALLY COMPETENT CARE

Increased awareness is the first tool in the development of the skills needed to provide culturally competent and appropriate care to ethnic elders. Increased awareness can lead to increased cultural sensitivity. Increased knowledge has the potential to further increase skills. However, the application of cultural knowledge may require new skills as well. The most important skills are those associated with intercultural communication. The linguistically competent gerontologic nurse will be able to appropriately use the conventions of the handshake, silence, and eye contact. She or he will also have fundamental skills related to working with interpreters.

Handshake

A handshake, the customary greeting in the business world in the United States, consists of smiling warmly, extending the hand, and grasping the other person's hand. The quality of the handshake is open to varied interpretation. A firm handshake in European American culture is a sign of good character and strength. Many Native American older adults interpret a vigorous handshake as a sign of aggression. They may offer their hand, but it is more of a passing of the hand with light touch, which could be misinterpreted as a sign of not being welcome or of weakness.

To Soviet older adult immigrants, a handshake may be interpreted as insolent and frivolous (Tripp-Reimer and Lauer, 1987). Handshakes also raise gender issues with older adults from the Middle East. Same-gender individuals may shake hands, but touch outside of marriage is forbidden by individuals of the opposite gender. If the nurse is of the same gender as the older adult, then a handshake will be received.

Silence

The value, use, and interpretation of silence also vary markedly from one culture to another. Generally, Eastern cultures value silence over the use of words; in Western cultures, the opposite is true. For older adults of many Eastern cultural groups, especially those which embrace the Confucian philosophy, silence is a sign of respect for the wisdom and expertise of the speaker. Silence is expected by young family members and by family members who have less authority. In traditional Japanese and Chinese families, silence during a conversation may indicate the speaker is giving the listener time to ponder what has been said, before moving on to another idea. In Native-American cultures it is believed that one learns self-control, courage, patience, and dignity from remaining silent. Silence during a conversation may signify that the listener is reflecting on what the speaker has just said. French, Spanish, and Soviet older adult immigrants may interpret silence as a sign of agreement (Purnell and Paulanka, 2003; Tripp-Reimer and Lauer, 1987).

Eye Contact

In the European American culture, direct eye contact is a sign of being honest, trustworthy, straightforward, and truthful. Nursing students are taught to establish and to maintain eye contact when interacting with clients, but this behavior may be misinterpreted by older adults of different ethnic groups. The less "Western" acculturated Native American older adults may not allow the nurse to make eye contact with them. They may move their eyes slowly from the floor to the ceiling and around the room. This behavior may lead the nurse to erroneous conclusions.

In many Asian cultures, looking one directly in the eyes implies equality. Older adults may avoid eye contact with physicians and nurses because they view health care professionals as authority figures. Direct eye contact is considered disrespectful in most Asian cultures.

There are gender issues in maintaining eye contact as well. In Middle Eastern cultures, direct eye contact between the sexes is forbidden, except between husband and wife. It is interpreted as a sexual invitation. Nurses may want to avoid direct eye contact with clients and physicians of the opposite gender from a Middle Eastern culture.

Use of Interpreters

The gerontologic nurse can increase the linguistic competence of care through the appropriate use of interpreters. *Interpretation* is the processing of oral language in a manner that preserves the meaning and tone of the original language without adding or deleting anything. The interpreter's job is to work with two different linguistic codes in a way that will produce equivalent messages (Haffner, 1992). The interpreter tells the older person what the nurse has said and the nurse what the older person has said without altering meaning or adding opinion.

An interpreter is needed any time the nurse and the client speak different languages, when the client has limited English proficiency, or when cultural tradition prevents the client from speaking directly to the nurse. The more complex the decision making, the more important the interpreter is, such as when determining the older person's wishes regarding life-prolonging measures.

It is ideal to engage persons who are trained in medical interpretation and are the same sex and social status of the older person. Ideally the interpreter would be a mature individual to avoid potential problems of age differentials. However, often children are called on to act as interpreters. In such cases the nurse must realize that the child or the older person may "edit" his or her comments because of cultural restrictions about the content (i.e., what is or is not appropriate to speak to parent or child about).

When working with an interpreter, the nurse first introduces herself or himself to the client and the interpreter and sets down guidelines for the interview. Sentences should be short, employ the active tense, and avoid metaphors, since they may be impossible to convert from one language to another. The nurse asks the interpreter to say exactly what is being said, and directs all conversation to the client.

For more information related to the Cultural Awareness box, refer to the detailed guidelines and protocols available from Enslein and colleagues at the University of Iowa (Enslein et al, 2002; Enslein et al, 2001).

PUTTING IT TOGETHER

Leininger's Theory

Leininger's theory of cultural care diversity and universality (1991) is unique and appropriate for use with the older adult population; it was designed primarily to assist nurses in discovering ways to provide culturally congruent care to people who have different lifeways from those of the professional nurse.

Leininger's theory uses worldview, social structure, language, ethnohistory, environmental context, folk systems,

Cultural Awareness

TRADITIONAL, FOLK, OR INDIGENOUS HEALERS

Older adults from culturally diverse backgrounds may seek the assistance of traditional, folk, or indigenous healers. The following is a partial listing of healers used by selected cultural groups.

GROUP	HEALER	SCOPE OF PRACTICE
Black Americans	Voodoo priest(ess)	Recommends herbal remedies for voodoo illnesses. Also treats Mexican Americans and Native Americans. May be called "root doctors."
	Spiritualist	Treats physical, mental, and spiritual problems. Most prevalent in urban communities.
	Grannies	Older adult women who gives advice on childrearing and common illnesses in children and adults. Practices in both urban and rural settings.
Chinese American	Herbalist	Diagnoses illnesses after interviewing, palpating pulses, auscultating, and inspecting. Prescribes herbal remedies; sometimes owns a small store in Chinatown area.
	Acupuncturist	Treats painful conditions and provides regional anesthesia by passing long thin needles through the skin to specific points; free end of needle is twirled and used to conduct a weak electric current or transmit heat (called moxibustion).
	Acupressurist	Same as acupuncturist, only uses pressure instead of needle.
	Bone setter	Specializes in setting fractures; sometimes skillful as an herbalist as well.
Hispanic	Curandero (male)	Treats traditional illnesses using herbs, diet, massage, and rituals.
	Curandera (female)	Trained in an apprenticeship; usually enjoys respect of community members.
	Espiritualista	Emphasizes prevention of illness or bewitchment with use of religious medals, amulets, and prayers; can analyze dreams and foretell future events; born with special gifts, which may be developed through apprenticeship with an older practitioner.
	Sabador	Treats musculoskeletal conditions using massage and manipulation of bones and muscles.
	Santero	Diagnoses and treats mental disorders, which are caused by spirits outside the body; client may be taken to a psychiatrist to be "calmed down" in preparation for treatment by a santero.
	Yerbo	Consulted for preventive and curative use of herbs for both traditional and Western illnesses; no formal training.
Native American	Medicine man Medicine woman Herbalist Shaman	With 510 federally recognized tribes, wide variation exists; three major categories are (1) preventive measures, (2) treatment regimens, and (3) health maintenance.

and professional systems as the framework for looking at the influences on cultural care and well-being. The components of cultural and social structure dimensions are technologic, religious, philosophic, kinship, social, political, legal, economic, and educational factors, as well as cultural values and lifeways.

The theory identifies three modes of action for the professional nurse to provide culturally congruent care: (1) cultural care preservation or maintenance, (2) cultural care accommodation or negotiation, and (3) cultural care repatterning or restructuring. Leininger defines the three modes of nurse decisions and actions as follows:

1. Cultural care preservation or maintenance refers to those assistive, supporting, facilitative, or enabling professional actions and decisions that help people of a particular culture to retain and to maintain their well-being, to recover from illness, or to face handicaps or death.
2. Cultural care accommodation or negotiation refers to those assistive, supporting, facilitative, or enabling creative professional actions and decisions that help people of a designated culture to adapt to or negotiate with others for a beneficial or satisfying health outcome.
3. Cultural care repatterning or restructuring refers to those assistive, supporting, facilitative, or enabling professional actions and decisions that help clients reorder, change, or greatly modify their lifeways for new, different, and beneficial health care patterns while respecting clients' cultural values and beliefs and still providing

beneficial or healthier lifeways than existed before the changes were established (Leininger, 1991).

This theory can be used with individuals, families, groups, communities, and institutions in diverse health care delivery systems. Leininger has developed the Sunrise Model to depict the components of the theory and the interrelationship of its components. This model can be used as a visual and cognitive map to guide the nurse in teasing out the essential data from all the dimensions of the influencers so as to gain clues for providing culturally congruent care (Fig. 5-5).

The Explanatory Model

Kleinman, Eisenberg, and Good presented a far-reaching proposition in 1978. They suggested that to provide culturally competent care, the health care professional (e.g., the gerontologic nurse) tries to find out the meaning of the health situation from the patient's perspective. This was a radical approach at the time and one that is becoming more relevant with the growing diversity in the United States.

See Boxes 5-1 to 5-4 for questions the gerontologic nurse might use in coming to know the older adult from a culture different from that of the nurse.

The Learn Model

The LEARN Model (Berlin and Folkes, 1992) uses the same perspective as the explanatory model and expands it to the person-nurse interaction. The LEARN Model is a useful tool in guiding the nurse in the clinical setting who is interacting with older adults of any ethnicity. Through it, the nurse increases his or her cultural sensitivity and becomes instrumental in providing more culturally competent care and consequently contribute to the reduction of health disparities. The model consists of these steps:

L Listen carefully to what the older person is saying. Attend not just to the words but to the nonverbal communication and the meaning behind the stories. Listen to the person's perception of the situation, desired goals, and ideas for treatment.

E Explain your perception of the situation and the problems.

A Acknowledge and discuss both the similarities and the differences between your perceptions and goals and those of the older person.

R Recommend a plan of action that takes both perspectives into account.

N Negotiate a plan that is mutually acceptable.

SUMMARY

Gerontologic nurses need to develop awareness, sensitivity, knowledge, and skills to deliver culturally and linguistically competent care to the diversifying older adult population. Conducting a cultural self-assessment can be a useful exercise to enable the nurse to provide culturally sensitive and relevant nursing care. In addition, the body of knowledge related to transcultural nursing is continuing to grow, making it possible for nurses to provide culturally competent nursing care.

Members of ethnic or racial cultures across the country are suffering from compromised outcomes in the receipt and pursuit of their health care. Gerontologic nurses can take the lead to provide culturally and linguistically appropriate care. In doing so, they can contribute to the national agenda to reduce health disparities.

Home Care

1. Ascertain whether the older adult came to the United States as a child, young adult, older adult, or was born in America, because this affects his or her level of acculturation and eligibility for benefits and services. Refer to the appropriate agency or social worker for assistance if necessary.
2. Knowledge of the differences and similarities of values of homebound clients can minimize tension and cultural conflict in the home care setting. Adapt communication styles as needed to reduce the potential for conflict.
3. Assess the caregiver's and client's own concepts of health and illness.
4. Communication between culturally different clients and nurses must be ethnically appropriate.
5. Assess the home environment for evidence of cultural values, and determine views on health and illness concepts. Incorporate these data into the care plan to meet the cultural needs of the client and family.

Key Points

- The current older adult population in the United States is more culturally diverse than ever in history.
- Culture is a universal phenomenon that is learned and transmitted from one generation to another, providing the blueprint for a person's beliefs, behaviors, attitudes, and values.
- Culture affects all dimensions of health and well-being, so the nurse must consider clients' cultures when planning, delivering, and evaluating nursing care.
- Ethnocentrism, discrimination, and racism contribute to health disparities.
- Cultural competence requires awareness, new knowledge, and new skills.
- The nurse should be knowledgeable about the predominant characteristics of the cultural groups for which care is provided, but he or she should still individualize the care rather than generalize about all clients in any given group.
- Cultural assessment tools and instruments need to be free from bias and previously tested on the ethnic group for whom they are intended.

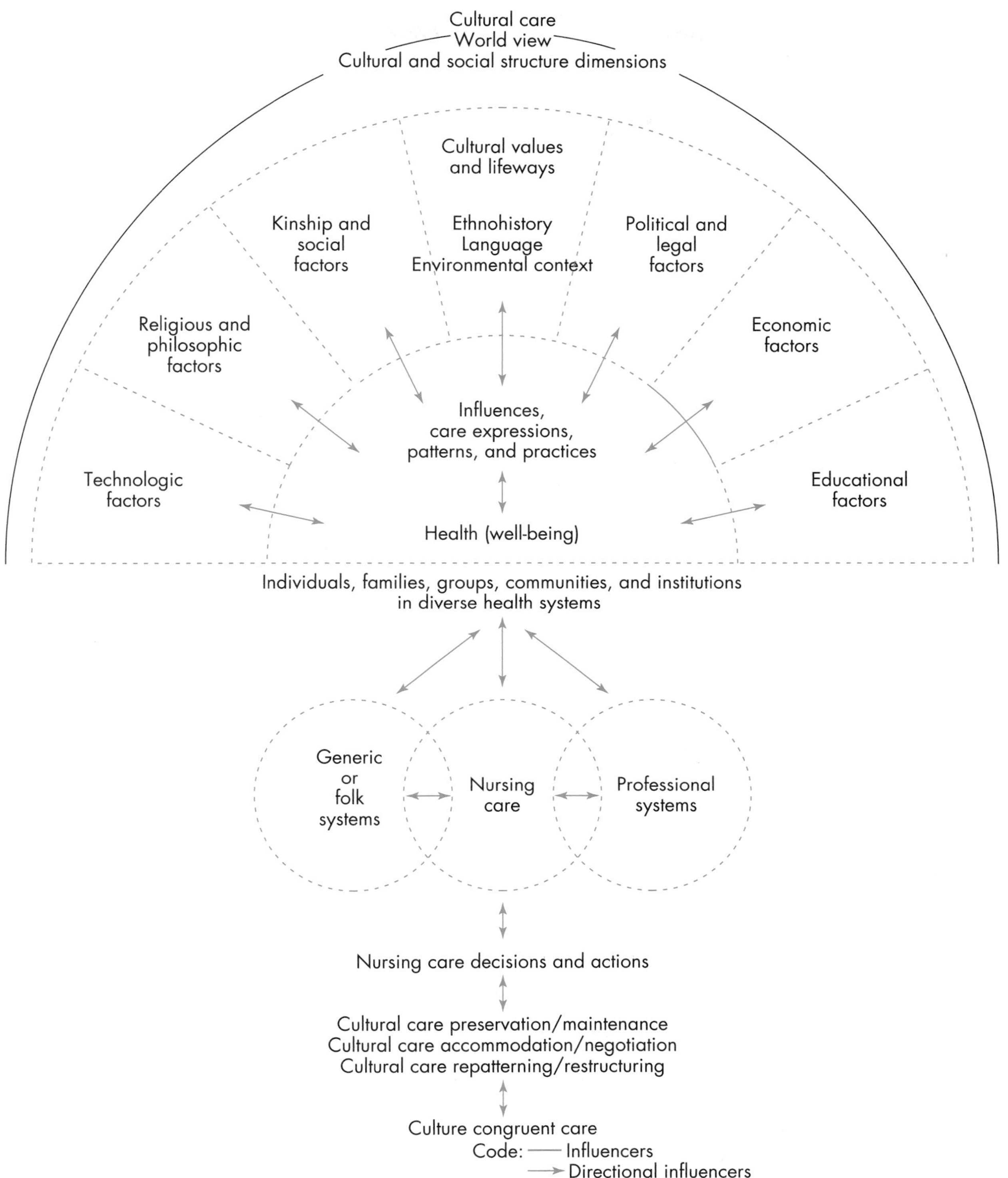

Fig. 5-5 Leininger's model for discovering transcultural nursing care and performing cultural assessments. (From Leininger M, editor: *Culture care diversity and universality: a theory of nursing*, Sudbury, Mass, 1991, National League for Nursing, Jones and Bartlett.)

- Nurses caring for older adults from diverse ethnic and cultural backgrounds should be aware that nurse-client relationships may be based on different orientations to communication than the typical Western mode.
- Nurses should conduct a cultural self-assessment to determine how they are influenced by their own cultures and how their cultures affect their interactions with people of different cultures.
- Nursing interventions should be adapted to meet the cultural needs of older adult clients.

Critical Thinking Exercises

1. In what ways do you value diversity in the world around you?
2. What are the limitations of using only race or ethnicity in identifying older clients?
3. Interview two or more older clients from the same ethnic group and discuss their cultural adaptation.
4. Identify your ethnocentric views toward certain groups and the basis on which you have formulated them.
5. What knowledge must the nurse possess to avoid stereotyping or generalizing about older clients?
6. How would you respond to a colleague who just made a racist remark or joke?
7. How would you recognize cultural conflict? How would you respond to it?
8. What are the nurse's responsibilities when discussing the use of alternative healing practices, medicines, and nutrition with older clients?
9. What responsibilities do you have with an older client who does not speak English?
10. Discuss the ethical conflicts that may arise among older clients whose values and beliefs are different from yours.
11. What specific cultural nursing skills are needed in caring for older clients from another ethnic group?

References

Administration on Aging: *A profile of older Americans: 2002,* accessed June 16, 2004, www.aoa.gov/prof/statistics/profile/5.asp.

Baker M: Cultural differences in the use of advance directives: a review of the literature, *African Amer Res Perspect* 6(3):35, 2000.

Berlin E, Folkes W: A teaching framework for cross-cultural health care: application in family practice, *Western J Med* 39:934, 1992.

Braun KL, Pietsch JH, Blanchette PL: *Cultural issues in end-of-life decision making,* Thousand Oaks, Calif, 2000, Sage.

Bruce AM: *People and races,* New York, 1977, Macmillan.

Burroughs V, Maxey R, Levy R: Racial and ethnic differences in response to medicines: towards individualized pharmaceutical treatment, *J National Med Assoc* 94(10, suppl):1, 2002.

Enslein J et al: Evidence-based protocol: interpreter facilitation for individuals with limited English proficiency, *J Gerontol Nurs* pp 5-13, 2002.

Enslein J et al: *Evidence-based protocol: interpreter facilitation for persons with limited English proficiency,* 2001, Research Dissemination Core Product, available for the University of Iowa Gerontological Nursing Interventions Research Center

Farran CJ, Paun O, Elliott MH: Religion, spirituality, and ethnicity: what it means for caregivers of persons with Alzheimer's disease, *Dementia* 2(3):353, 2003.

Gelfand D: *Aging and ethnicity: knowledge and service,* ed 2, New York, 2003, Springer.

Haffner L: Translation is not enough—interpreting in a medical setting, *West J Med* 157(3):255, 1992.

Hall ET: *Understanding cultural differences,* Yarmouth, Me, 1990, Intercultural Press.

Hall ET: *Beyond culture,* Garden City, NY, 1977, Anchor Press.

Hofstede G, Pedersen P: *Exploring culture: exercises, stories and synthetic culture,* Yarmouth, Me, 2002, Intercultural Press.

Irish DP, Lundquist KF, Nelsen VJ: *Ethnic variations in dying, death, and grief: diversity in universality,* Philadelphia, 1993, Taylor & Francis.

Jett KF: The meaning of aging and the celebration of years among rural African American women, *Geriatric Nurs* 24(5):290, 2003.

Jett KF: Making the connection: seeking and receiving help by elderly African Americans, *Qualitative Health Res* 12(3):373, 2002.

Kim C, Hofer T, Kerr E: Review of evidence and explanations for suboptimal screening and treatment of dyslipidemia in women, *J General Intern Med* 18:854, 2003.

Kleinman A, Eisenberg L, Good B: Culture, illness and care: clinical lessons from anthropological and cross-cultural research, *Annals Intern Med* 88:251, 1978.

Kobylarz F, Hernandez G, Hurwitz E: Culturally-sensitive decision making in end-of-life care, *Annals Long-Term Care* 10(8):40, 2002.

Lee RLT: Caring for family members with stroke: Chinese family caregivers' experiences, *Asian J Nurs Studies* 7(1):18, 2004.

Leininger M: *Transcultural nursing: concepts, theories and practice,* ed 2, New York, 1995, McGraw-Hill.

Leininger M: The theory of culture care diversity and universality. In Leininger M, editor: *Culture care diversity and universality: a theory of nursing,* Sudbury, Mass, 1991, National League for Nursing, Jones and Bartlett.

Lukwago S et al: Development and validation of brief scales to measure collectivism, religiosity, racial pride, and time orientation in urban African American women, *Fam Community Health 2001,* Oct 1, 2001.

Mazanec P, Tyler MK: Cultural considerations in end-of-life care, *AJN* 103(3):50, 2003.

McGrath B: Illness as a problem of meaning: moving culture from the classroom to the clinic, *Advan Nurs Sci* 21(2):7, 1998.

Mudano A, Casebeer L, Patino F: Racial disparities in osteoporosis prevention in managed care, *Southern Med J* 96(5):445, 2003.

Purnell LD, Paulanka, BJ: *Transcultural health care: a culturally competent approach,* ed 2, Philadelphia, 2003, FA Davis.

Rathbone-McCune E: *Isolated elders: health and social intervention,* Rockville, Md, 1982, Aspen.

Rhoades DA, Buchwald D: Hypertension in older urban Native-American primary care patients, *J Amer Geriatrics Soc* 51:774, 2003.

Smedley B, Stith A, Nelson A, editors: *Unequal treatment: confronting racial and ethnic disparities in health care,* 2003, Institute of Medicine, National Academy Press. Special report.

Spector R: *Cultural diversity in health and illness,* ed 6, Upper Saddle River, NJ, 2004, Prentice-Hall.

Tripp-Reimer T, Lauer GM: Ethnicity and families with chronic illness. In Wright LM, Leahy M, editors: *Families and chronic illness,* Springhouse, Pa, 1987, Springhouse.

US Department of Health and Human Services: *Healthy People 2010,* ed 2, vols 1 and 2, Washington, DC, November 2000, US Government Printing Office.

World Health Organization: *Chronicle of WHO,* 1:1-2, New York, 1947, The Organization.

6 Family Influences

ELIZABETH C. MUETH, MLS, AHIP

Learning Objectives

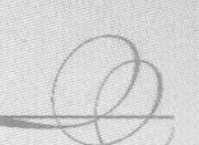

On completion of this chapter, the reader will be able to:

1. Gain an understanding of the role of families in the lives of older adults.
2. Identify demographic and social trends that affect families of older adults.
3. Understand common dilemmas and decisions older adults and their families face.
4. Develop approaches that can be suggested to families faced with specific aging-related concerns.
5. Identify common stresses that family caregivers experience.
6. Identify interventions to support families.
7. Plan strategies for working more effectively one-on-one with families of older adult clients.

What would you do if you were faced with the following situations?

- You have been married 45 years. Your husband recently had a severe stroke and cannot communicate. He managed the family finances and made the family decisions. You do not know anything about your financial affairs.
- Your mother, 86, is mentally competent, but her physical condition means she cannot manage alone in her home. She refuses all offers of help and rejects any other living situation.
- Your father is dying. You promised that no heroic measures would be taken to prolong his life; he did not want to die "with tubes hooked up to my body." Your brother demands the physician use all possible measures to keep your father alive.
- Your father's reactions and eyesight are poor. You don't want your children with him when he is driving. He always takes the grandchildren to get ice cream and will be hurt if you say the children cannot ride with him.

Although each situation involves medical considerations, these are tough issues and decisions that extend beyond medical aspects (Schmall, 1994):

- How independent and risk-taking do I allow my family member to be?
- Is my family member fully capable of making his or her own decisions?
- When, if ever, should I step in and take control of the situation?
- What should I do if my family member refuses help or to make a change?
- What should I do if my family member's actions are putting himself or others at risk?

The nurse needs to be aware of the various roles families play in the lives of older adults, to be sensitive to family needs as well as those of the older person, and to recognize and accept that some families are limited in the level of support and caregiving they can provide.

ROLE AND FUNCTION OF FAMILIES

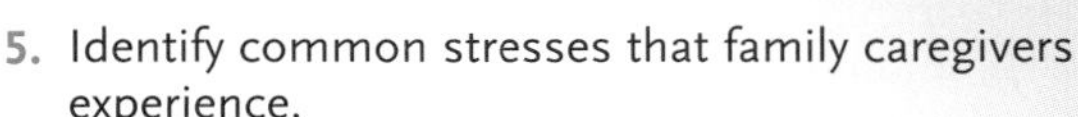

Families play a significant role in the lives of most older persons. When family is not involved, it generally is because the older person has no living relatives nearby or there have been longstanding relationship problems. In the early to mid-1990s only 5.7% of elderly in the United States were in residential care (Kinsella and Velkoff, 2001). This means that the majority of long-term care for the elderly is provided by the family. Community services generally are used only after a family's resources have been depleted. However, several demographic and social trends have affected families' ability to provide support. These trends include:

- **Increase in the old-old.** The over-85 age-group is the fastest growing segment of the older population. In the United States in 1900, only 13% of all 65-year-olds were expected to reach age 85. By 2000 the percentage had increased to 42% (Costa, 2003). The U.S. population will age rapidly when the "baby boomers" (born between 1946 and 1964) start to reach age 65 in the year 2010. By 2050 the percentage of the population who are over age 65 is projected to be 20% compared with about 13% today (Kinsella and Velkoff, 2001). Because of the increased life expectancy, many of the old-old will have children who are over age 65.
- **Decrease in fertility.** A declining birth rate means fewer adult children are available to share in the support of aging parents.

- **Increase in employment of women.** Traditionally women have been the primary caregivers. However, women are increasingly employed (Doty, Jackson, and Crown, 1998; National Alliance for Caregiving, 1997; Neal, Ingersoll-Dayton, and Starrels, 1997). Although employed women often provide as much support as their unemployed counterparts, they often sacrifice personal time. A fairly small percentage (10%) leave the work force or take an early retirement to provide care, but many rearrange work schedules, reduce work hours, or take a leave of absence without pay. Changes in employment status have implications for the financial security of these women in their own later years.
- **Increase in mobility of families.** Families today may live not only in a different city from their older relative but in a different state, region, or country. Geographic distance makes it more difficult to directly provide the ongoing assistance an older family member may need (Greenwell and Bengston, 1997).
- **Increase in divorce and remarriage.** Since the 1950s divorce rates have risen not only among the young, but also among older adults. In 1990 there were 20.9 divorces for every 1000 married women over 15 years of age (Hughes, 2004). Divorce and remarriage can increase the complexity of family relationships and decision making and affect helping patterns. Difficulties can arise from family conflicts, the different perspectives of birth children and stepchildren, and the logistics of caring for two persons who do not live together. However, in some situations, remarriage increases the pool of family members available to provide care.
- **Elderly providing as well as receiving support.** Many elderly receive financial help from adult children, but many older adults give support (money, child care, shelter) to their adult children and grandchildren. Studies suggest that elderly parents are more likely to provide financial help than to receive it (Kinsella and Velkoff, 2001).

For more on the family views of various cultures regarding older adults, see the Cultural Awareness boxes at left and p. 115.

COMMON LATE-LIFE FAMILY ISSUES AND DECISIONS

When changes occur in an older person's functioning, family members are generally involved in making decisions about the person's living situation, arranging for social services and health care, and caregiving (Noelker, 1994). They also can facilitate, obstruct, or prohibit the older family member's access to care and services.

Some of the most common issues and difficult decisions families face include changes in living arrangements, nursing facility placement, financial and legal concerns, end-of-life health care decisions, vehicle driving issues, and family caregiving.

Changes in Living Arrangements

Many families face the question, "What should we do?" when an older family member begins to have problems living alone. Common scenarios heard from families include the following (Schmall, 1994):

- "Dad is so unsteady on his feet. He's already fallen twice this month. I'm scared he'll fall again and really injure himself the next time. He refuses help, and he won't move. I don't know what to do."
- "Mom had a stroke and the doctor says she can't return home. It looks like she will have to live with us or go to a nursing facility. We have never gotten along, but she'll be very angry if we place her in a nursing facility."
- "Grandmother has become increasingly depressed and isolated in her home. She doesn't cook, and she hardly eats. She has outlived most of her friends. Wouldn't she be better off living in a group setting where meals, activities, and social contact are provided?"

Family members are often emotionally torn between allowing a person to be as independent as possible and creating a more secure environment. They may wonder whether they should force a change, particularly if they believe the person's choice is not in his or her best interest. The family may be focused on the advantages of a group living situation (e.g., good

Cultural Awareness

CULTURAL ATTITUDES TOWARD OLDER ADULTS

Blacks	Greater respect for older adults and their role in the family compared with whites Value placed on kinship and extended family bonds
Whites	Less respect for older adults and their role in the family Tendency for men and women to share more equally in family; democratic family structure Aging parents expected to be self-sufficient and not overly dependent on adult children
East Asians	High level of respect for older adults Hierarchic family roles and ascribed status (related to age and gender) Oldest son assuming responsibility for aging parents as part of filial duty
Hispanics	More overt respect for older adults than whites Tendency toward a more patriarchal family structure Aging parents invited to live in household that consists of extended family members
Native Americans (540 federally recognized tribes)	High level of respect for older adults and their years of accumulated wisdom and knowledge; sought after for advice

Cultural Awareness

MYTHS AND THE REALITY OF AGING

Myth In the past, three-generation households were the most common living arrangement.

Reality Coresidence of three generations has never been the dominant living arrangement in the United States. Most households consisted of nuclear, not extended, families.

Myth Most older persons want to live with their children.

Reality Most older persons, as long as they can manage independently, prefer to live in households separate from their children. "Intimacy at a distance" is preferred both by older persons and their adult children.

Myth Older persons are often abandoned by their families.

Reality The family is still the top provider of support and caregiving to older persons. Even when bedridden or homebound, older persons are twice as likely to be cared for by a relative at home than by professionals in an institution. Extended family members—for example, nieces, nephews, or grandchildren—often help when older persons do not have spouses or adult children. Also, brothers and sisters often play an important role in the lives of older persons who are widowed or have never married.

Myth Families use nursing facilities as a "dumping ground" for frail older family members.

Reality Most persons in care facilities are greatly impaired and need comprehensive care. Older persons who do not have children and live alone are the most vulnerable to nursing facility placement. Approximately half of all nursing facility residents are single women or widows without close family. Families do not suddenly "dump" and abandon their older family members in care facilities. The reality is that most families use nursing facilities as a last resort, only after they have exhausted other alternatives.

Myth If family-oriented services are made readily available, families will be less likely to provide caregiving.

Reality Policymakers sometimes fear that requests for services will be overwhelming if respite and adult day care programs are subsidized; yet studies show that caregivers, in general, are willing to pay for what they can afford and are modest in their use of services.

nutrition, socialization, and security). However, an older person may view a move as a loss of independence or as being "one step closer to the grave."

The nurse plays an important role in:

- Providing an objective assessment of an older person's functional ability
- Exploring with families ways to maintain an older relative in his or her home, and the advantages and disadvantages of other living arrangement options
- Helping families understand the older person's perspective of the meaning of home, and the significance of accepting help or moving to a new environment

It can be particularly frustrating when a family knows an older relative has difficulty functioning independently yet refuses to accept help in the home. Yet, as long as the older person has the mental capacity to make decisions, he or she cannot be forced to accept help. To deal successfully with resistance, a family first must understand the reasons underlying the resistance. Encourage the family to ask themselves the following questions (Schmall, Cleland, and Sturdevant, 1999):

- Is my family member concerned about the cost of the service and its impact on personal financial resources?
- Does my relative think he or she does not have a problem?
- Does my family member view agency assistance as "welfare," "charity," or "going on the dole?"
- Does my family member fear having a stranger in the house or having possessions stolen?
- Does my relative believe that the tasks I want to hire someone to do are ones that he or she can do, or that "family should do"?
- Does my family member view accepting outside help as a loss of control and independence?
- Are the requirements of community agencies—financial disclosure, application process, interviews—overwhelming to my family member?

Depending on the answers to these questions, it may be helpful to share one or more of the following suggestions with the family (Schmall, Cleland, and Sturdevant, 1999):

- **Deal with your relative's perceptions and feelings.** For example, if your older mother thinks she does not have any problems, be objective and specific in describing your observations. Indicate that you know it must be hard to experience change. If your father views government-supported services as "welfare," emphasize that he has paid for the service through taxes.
- **Approach your family member in a way that prevents him or her from feeling helpless.** Many people, regardless of age, find it difficult to ask for or accept help. Try to present the need for assistance in a positive way, emphasizing how it will enable the person to live more independently. Generally, emphasizing the ways in which a person is dependent only increases resistance.
- **Suggest only one change or service at a time.** If possible, begin with a small change. Most people need time to think about and accept changes. Introducing ideas slowly rather than pushing for immediate action increases the chances of acceptance.
- **Suggest a trial period.** Some people are more willing to try a service when they initially see it as a short-term arrange-

ment rather than a long-term commitment. Some families have found that giving a service as a gift works.

- **Focus on your needs.** If an older person persists in asserting, "I'm okay. I don't need help," it can be helpful to focus on the family's needs rather than the older person's needs. For example, saying, "I would feel better if . . ." or "I care about you and I worry about . . .; will you consider trying this for me so I will worry less?" sometimes makes it easier for a person to try a service.
- **Consider who has "listening leverage."** Sometimes an older person's willingness to listen to a concern, consider a service, or think about moving from his or her home is strongly influenced by who initiates the discussion. For example, an adult child may not be the best person to raise a particular issue with an older parent. An older person may "hear" the information better when it is shared by a certain family member, a close friend, or a doctor (Box 6-1; Fig. 6-1).

Making a Decision About a Care Facility

The decision to move an older family member into a care facility is difficult for most families. It is often a decision filled with guilt, sadness, anxiety, doubt, and anger—even

BOX 6-1 John A. Hartford Foundation Institute for Geriatric Nursing at New York University

MISSION

The John A. Hartford Foundation Institute for Geriatric Nursing (www.hartfordign.com) is the only nurse-led organization in the country seeking to shape the quality of the nation's health care for older Americans by promoting geriatric nursing excellence to the nursing profession and to the larger health care community. The Hartford Institute seeks to positively influence both the skills of individual nurses and the quality of the systems in which they learn and work.

BEST NURSING PRACTICES IN CARE FOR OLDER ADULTS: INCORPORATING ESSENTIAL GERONTOLOGIC CONTENT INTO STAFF DEVELOPMENT

Because of our increasingly aging patient population, all nurses can expect to care for older adults at some time in their careers. Thus, all nurses should be trained in the essentials of care for older adults whether or not they have chosen to specialize in gerontological nursing.

The Best Nursing Practices Partner Program includes a curriculum guide, implementation manual, teaching slides, hospital nursing competencies, and a feedback form. All are conveniently available on a CD.

The curriculum is designed using the "less is more" philosophy. Although it covers more than 20 topics, only those promoting concern for the issue of quality of life in older adults were included. The material is organized to allow use of all or part of any chapter. Chapters include instruments and scales, case studies, evaluation strategies, resources, and experiential exercises in addition to the content materials. It is encouraged that nurses share the materials with their colleagues.

In addition to the curriculum manual, there is a set of PowerPoint slides and overhead projection materials.

Topics covered in the curriculum guide include:

- Attitudes about Aging (includes Aging Sensitivity exercises)
- Cross-cultural Influences on Older Adults
- Sensory Changes and Communication with Older Adults
- Functional Assessment of Older Adults
- Cognitive/Mental Assessment of Older Adults
- Depression, Delirium, Dementia in Older Adults
- Pressure Ulcers in Older Adults
- Nutrition: Eating/Feeding of Older Adults
- Sleep/Rest for Older Adults
- Pain/Palliation of Older Adults
- Urinary Continence of Older Adults
- Falls of Older Adults
- Polypharmacy and Older Adults
- Physical Restraint Reduction for Older Adults
- Ethical Issues of Elder Care
- Caregiving/Elder Mistreatment
- Teaching Older Adults
- Financing Health Care for Older Adults
- Living Arrangements of Older Adults
- Interdisciplinary Collaboration for Elder Care
- Resources for Gerontology and Gerontological Nursing

From *Partners Program: best nursing practices in care for older adults*, New York, 2003, John A. Hartford Foundation Institute for Geriatric Nursing at New York University.

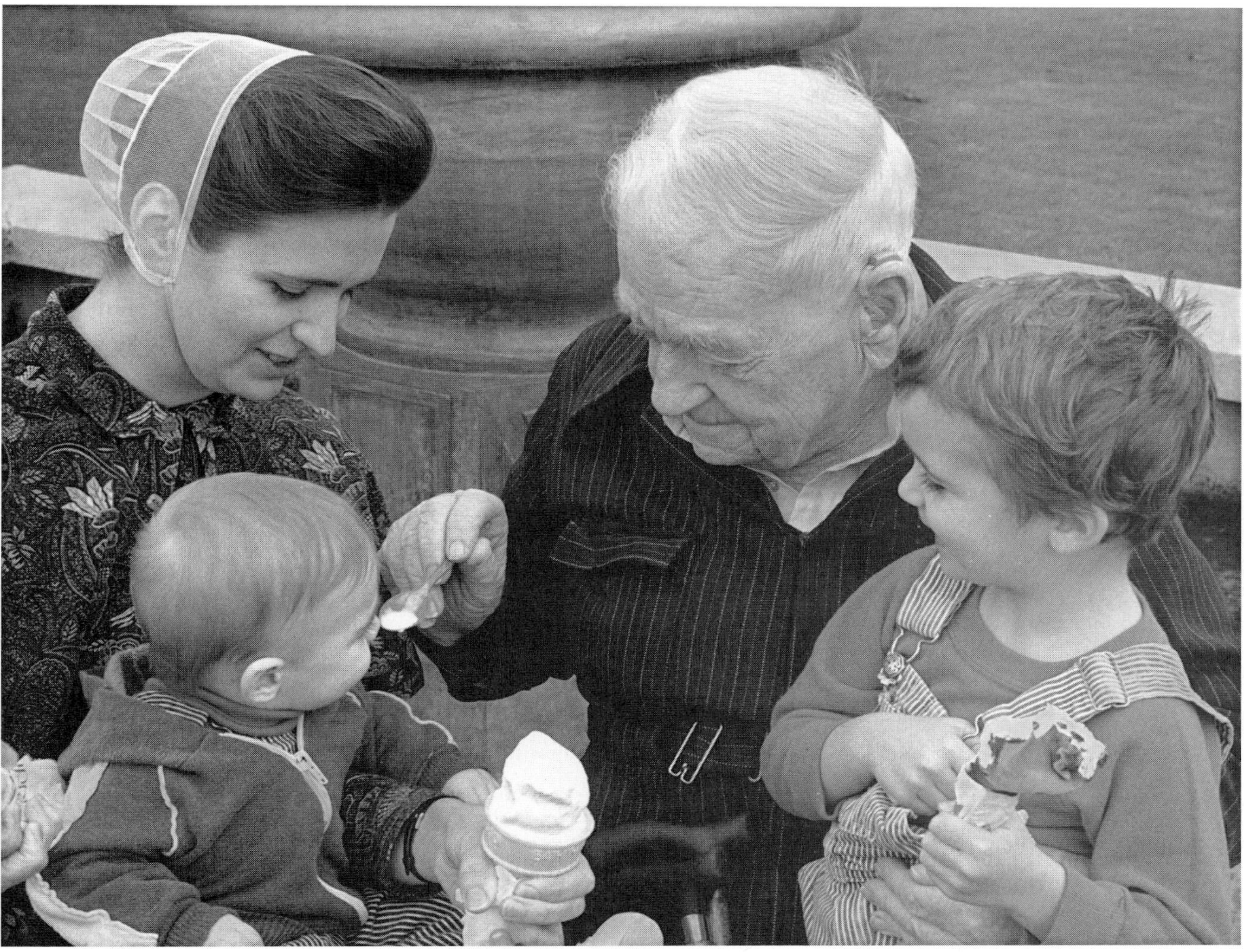

Fig. 6-1 Grandfather helping with responsibilities of feeding baby. (Courtesy Rod Schmall, West Linn, Oregon.)

when the older person makes the decision. The difficulty of the decision is reflected in these comments:

- "It was easier to bury my first husband than to place my second husband in a nursing home."
- "On a scale of 1 to 10, the difficulty of the decision was a 10+ for me, even though the doctor said my mother needed the care a nursing home provides."

As important as stressing the need for long-term care is dealing with the family's feelings about placement. Many families view facilities negatively because of what they have seen in the media concerning neglect, abuse, and abandonment.

A common feeling families express when faced with care facility placement is guilt. Guilt may come from several sources, including (1) pressures and comments from others ("I would never place my mother in a care facility," or "If you really loved me, you would take care of me"); (2) family tradition and values ("My family has always believed in taking care of its own—and that means you provide care to family members at home"); (3) the meaning of nursing facility placement ("I'm abandoning my husband," "I should be able to take care of my mother. She took care of me when I needed care," or "You do not put someone you love in a nursing facility"); and (4) promises ("I promised Mother I would always take care of Dad," or "When I married, I promised 'till death do us part'").

It can help to talk with family members about the potential benefits of a care facility. For many people it is not easy walking into a care facility for the first time. It is helpful to prepare families about what to expect and to give guidelines for evaluating facilities, moving an older family member into a care facility, and helping an older family member adjust to the changes (see Research box).

For more information, see Questions to Consider When Moving from Independent Living to a Supervised Living Facility (Box 6-2) and, Internet Resources (Table 6-1).

Research

SAMPLE/SETTING

The convenience sample consisted of five African-American and five European-American individuals who were primary caregivers before placing older adults in nursing facilities; placement occurred 6 to 12 months before the interview. The African Americans were associated with one predominantly African-American nursing facility and the European Americans with one predominantly European-American nursing facility. Both facilities had reputations for providing excellent care.

METHODS

Face-to-face interviews were conducted with caregivers in their homes. Each caregiver was asked to tell about his or her experience with placing a relative in the nursing facility. Then probing questions were asked about the decision-making process and how things had gone since placement. Responses were audiotaped and transcribed verbatim. Latent content analysis was used to identify major themes.

FINDINGS

Few differences were observed between the African-American and European-American caregivers. However, African-American caregivers were more likely to view caregiving as an extended family responsibility rather than a solely personal responsibility. When assistance was not forthcoming from extended family members or they had to assume sole responsibility, they were more likely to express anger and resentment.

The circumstances that led to nursing facility placement were similar for both groups. These included inadequate resources, conflicts with their own or the family's needs, deterioration in the health of the older adults, and changes in the caregiver health and capabilities. Caregivers also reported that even when they qualified for or could pay for community services, the services often did not meet their needs. Caregivers found that it was often more of an ordeal than a relief to arrange for others to provide care. Lack of consistency in service providers was problematic.

All caregivers reported that they were the primary decision makers about placement and that the care recipient was generally included in decisions. Caregivers did not seek or value the advice of family members who were not involved in caregiving. The caregivers sometimes used professional advice to validate their decisions.

The post-placement experience of the caregivers revolved around three themes: (1) relief and reinvolvement, (2) regrets and losses, and (3) continuing a caregiver role in the care facility. The caregivers' personal experiences with the nursing facilities generally had been more positive than their expectations.

IMPLICATIONS

It is important for nurses to understand a caregiver's experiences, the meaning he or she attaches to these experiences, and the influence of cultural values. To work most effectively with families in either home care or institutional settings, nurses should use individualized approaches, based on careful assessment, and take a family-centered perspective, not just focus on the older adult's needs.

The study also suggested that nurses need to recognize that nursing facility placement can have positive outcomes for both older adults and their families. Some caregivers reported that the message received from health care professionals about nursing facility placement was that they "could expect to feel guilty after placement" or that the older adults would "inevitably go downhill" after entering a facility. The experience of these caregivers was far more positive than what they had been led to expect.

It is also important for a nurse to determine the role caregivers want to have in a care facility and to acknowledge and support the caregivers' continuing roles. As the researchers point out, caregivers' "expert knowledge of the resident over a lifetime can be invaluable to staff members in seeking approaches to the resident's care."

Fink SV, Picot SF: Nursing home placement decisions and post-placement experiences of African-American and European-American caregivers, *J Gerontol Nurs* 21(12):35, Dec 1995.

Financial and Legal Concerns

Major financial issues some families face include paying for long-term care, helping an older person who has problems managing money, knowing about and accessing resources for the older family member whose income is not sufficient, responding when an older family member is depleting financial resources on "prize contests" and scams, and planning for and talking about potential incapacity (Schmall, Cleland, and Sturdevant, 1999).

One of the most important things a nurse can do is to become knowledgeable about the community resources that can help families who are faced with financial and legal concerns, eligibility requirements for programs, program access issues, and options for older persons who need assistance in managing their finances. If a family and their older relative have not already discussed potential financial concerns, encourage them to do so.

Many families do not discuss finances before a crisis—and then it is often too late. However, talking about finances is not easy for many families (Goetting and Schmall, 1993). Sometimes adult children hesitate to discuss financial concerns for fear of appearing overly interested in inheritance. After all, talking about inheriting Mom and Dad's money usually means talking about the circumstances under which it will be transferred. Few people feel comfortable starting a conversation with "Dad, when you die . . .," or "Mom, if you become unable to make decisions . . . ."

When a person has been diagnosed with Alzheimer's disease or a related disorder, it is critical that the family make financial and legal plans while the older person is able to participate. Once the person becomes incapacitated, if plans have not been made, the options are fewer, more complex, and more intrusive. A family may need to seek a conservatorship, which requires court action.

Seeking a conservatorship (or a guardian of the estate) is usually emotionally painful for both the family and the older person (Schmall, 1993). The older person, if present, must listen to the evidence concerning his or her own mental decline. The family must publicly declare the loss of capacity experienced by their older relative. The older person's situation and intimate family matters are exposed, particularly if a court trial is held. The conservatorship process is also expensive, involving attorney and court filing fees.

Older persons with limited mobility, diminished vision, or loss of hand dexterity may need only minimum assistance with finances—for example, help with reading fine print, balancing a checkbook, preparing checks for signature, or dealing with Medicare or other benefit programs. Others who are homebound because of poor health but who still are able to direct their finances may need someone to implement their directives. In such situations a family's objective should be to assist, not to take away control. The goal is to choose the least intrusive intervention that will enable the older person to remain as independent as possible.

BOX 6-2 Questions To Consider When Moving From Independent Living to a Supervised Living Facility

1. Is the move permanent or temporary?
2. Does the patient view the facility as a safety net or dumping ground?
3. Who is in control of the patient's finances?
4. What are the personal space needs of the patient?
5. Will these needs be met in the facility?
6. Does the patient understand the diagnosis and prognosis of the illness that is precipitating the placement?
7. What has the patient's living situation been (did the patient live alone or with others)?
8. Does the patient have long-term friends and associates in reasonable proximity to the facility to allow visiting?
9. Does the patient have a pet or pets whose care must be arranged, or does the facility allow pets?

From Baldwin K, Shaul M: When your patient can no longer live independently: a guide to supporting the patient and family, *J Gerontol Nurs* 27(11):10, 2001.

TABLE 6-1 Internet Resources for Caregivers

ORGANIZATION	URL	RESOURCES
Administration on Aging	http://www.aoa.gov	Information about insurance, lifestyle management, finances, nursing homes, assisted living, and living independently.
AARP	http://www.aarp.org	An excellent site with many topics and links of interest to older persons and their families.
American Health Care Association	http://www.ahca.org/info/pubthink.htm	Association for long-term care includes guide to choosing a nursing facility. The guide is similar to the one from Medicare but has an extensive assessment guide to help in the decision.
Centers for Medicare and Medicaid Services	http://www.medicare.gov	"Guide to Choosing a Nursing Home," which includes long-term care options, definitions, payment for services and care, how to assess a nursing home, and issues of nursing home living.
National Association of Professional Geriatric Care Managers	http://www.caremanager.org	Describes role, qualifications, and education of care managers; guidance on selection of a qualified person; and search for care manager by zip code function.
National Family Caregivers Association	http://www.nfcacares.org	Information about caregiving and chat rooms for caregivers.

Modified from Baldwin K, Shaul M: When your patient can no longer live independently, *J Gerontol Nurs* 27(11):10, 2001.

End-of-Life Health Care Decisions

The use of life-sustaining procedures is another difficult decision, especially when family members are uncertain about the older person's wishes or they disagree about "what Mom (or Dad) would want." Yet, when an older person is ill and unable to make health care decisions, the family generally is asked about what the client would want (Oregon Health Care Decisions, 1995).

It is important for the nurse to realize that life's final developmental stage ultimately ends in death. Thus, end-of-life decisions are common for most patients and their families. Often this process does not begin until after the patient has lost the ability to participate in the decision. Advance directives are one method for the patient to be assured his or her wishes are understood. However, the nurse should encourage ongoing discussions with the family about end-of-life care to avoid negative feelings (Norton and Talerico, 2000).

Adult children approaching a parent about end-of-life decisions need to remember that mental incapacity is not related just to aging and illness. A debilitating accident can happen to anyone, regardless of age. Parents may be more likely to listen to adult children who have also done advance planning themselves (Goetting and Schmall, 1993).

The Issue of Driving

Driving is a critical issue for seniors—and for this country. Older drivers are more likely to get in multiple-vehicle accidents than younger drivers, including teenagers. The elderly are also more likely to get traffic citations for failing to yield, turning improperly, and running red lights and stop signs, an indication of decreased driving ability. Car accidents are more dangerous for seniors than for younger people. A person 65 or older who is involved in a car accident is more likely to be seriously hurt, more likely to require hospitalization, and more likely to die than younger people involved in the same crash. In particular, fatal crash rates rise sharply after a driver has reached the age of 70 (Safe Senior Citizen Driving, 2004).

Obviously, safe driving is an important issue for our country's older adults. Everyone ages differently, so some people are perfectly capable of continuing to drive in their 70s, 80s, and beyond. Many elders, however, are at higher risk for road accidents. A few of the factors that contribute to increased risk are:

- Loss of hearing acuity
- Loss of visual acuity
- Chronic disease and physical impairment
- Medications

Driving symbolizes autonomy, control, competence, self-reliance, freedom, and belonging to the mainstream of society, so most older persons alter their driving when their abilities decline. They may drive only during daylight hours, avoid heavy traffic times, limit the geographic area in which they drive, or limit driving to less complicated roadways. Some couples begin driving in tandem with the passenger acting as copilot. Sometimes after the death of a spouse, family members notice that "for the first time, Dad is having problems with driving." What they may not realize is that Dad had problems with driving before his wife died, but she had served as his eyes and ears when he was behind the wheel.

Families face a difficult time when an older relative shows signs of unsafe driving. They may be both worried about safety and reluctant to raise concerns with their family member or to take action. The issue is even more complicated when the older person is cognitively impaired and does not perceive his or her deterioration and potential driving risk. Studies show that persons with Alzheimer's disease are likely to rate themselves as highly capable of driving when they are not.

Sometimes a family member may rationalize that "Mom only drives short distances in the neighborhood" or may think "I just can't ask Dad not to drive. The car is too important to him." Some families are continually faced with a cognitively impaired person who cannot remember from day to day that he or she cannot drive and insists on driving.

Families may need assistance in assessing a person's driving ability and how to best carry out a recommendation that their relative should limit or discontinue driving. Health care professionals play a critical role in discussing the issue of driving with older persons. Some older persons view health care professionals as more objective than the family, and thus are more willing to listen to their advice and recommendations. When asked in focus groups who should talk to them about driving, older persons responded that the physician should, since "when the doctor says you can't drive anymore, that's definite" (Persson, 1993). Many participants in focus groups indicated that family advice alone would not influence their decision to quit driving.

A written prescription from a physician or other health care professional that simply states "no driving" may remind the cognitively impaired person and divert blame from the family. Families also may need information about how to make a car inoperable for the cognitively impaired person.

If family members will be addressing the issue of driving with an older relative, the nurse could suggest they first check some of the resources in Table 6-2.

Family Caregiving

Providing care to frail, dependent older adults is increasingly common due to the rapidly aging population. Approximately 75% of family caregiving is still provided by women. Nearly one fourth of caregivers are spouses. Approximately one third of family caregivers are age 65 or older (National Alliance for Caregiving, 1997).

Caregiving may evolve gradually as a family member becomes frail and needs more assistance, or it can begin suddenly as the result of a stroke or accident. A family may adjust better to the demands of caregiving when a relative's need for

TABLE 6-2 Online Resources for Seniors Who Drive

PROGRAM	URL	FEATURES
AARP Driver Safety	www.aarp.com	AARP Driver Safety courses designed for older drivers, to help them hone their skills and avoid accidents and traffic violations. Features information on classes and on senior driving in general, including FAQs, driving IQ test, and close call test.
Senior Drivers	www.SeniorDrivers.org	Features videos, pictures, and text presentations to help seniors learn to drive more safely. Topics include exercising for driving safety, adjusting your car for driving safety, handling common and difficult driving situations, and handling emergencies.
Elderly Driving	www.luhs.org	(Loyola University Health System) Explains risks, statistics, and suggestions for older drivers.
Driving and the Elderly	www.ahealthyme.com	(Blue Cross of Massachusetts) "How do I know if I should stop driving?"
Physician's Guide to Assessing and Counseling Older Drivers	www.ama-assn.org	New 226-page guide includes checklists for vision and motor skills to assists physicians in evaluating the ability of their older patients to operate a motor vehicle safely.

Research

SAMPLE/SETTING

The sample consisted of 360 participants from nine randomly selected adult day health care (ADHC) sites of the New York State medical model ADHC programs, day care staff at the nine sites, and 246 primary informal caregivers of the day care clients.

METHODS

Data reflecting disturbing daytime behaviors was obtained from three sources: (1) direct observations of day care participants, (2) structured telephone interviews with each participant's primary informal caregiver, and (3) assessments by key day care staff. Item-level data and latent class estimates were used to examine the prevalence of disturbed behavior and the degree of disturbance as reported by the three sources.

FINDINGS

Because of the limited observation time, direct observation yielded very low prevalence of behavioral problems. There were no statistically significant differences between family and staff reports. Using family caregiver estimates, about 11% of ADHC clients were estimated to engage in severely disordered behavior, 16% in verbal-vocal agitation (e.g., repetitive questioning, complaining, demanding, argumentative behavior), 12% in affective disorders (e.g., seeking reassurance, depression, crying), 15% in cognitive or psychotic disorders, and 6.2% in asocial behavior. These varied only 2% to 4% from staff estimates.

Families reported that the most disturbing behaviors for them were repetitive questioning (13%), complaining (11%), demanding (11%), and depression or sadness (11%). Staff found nonparticipation and refusal to cooperate most disturbing (15%). Families found misplacing and losing objects more disturbing (9%) than did staff (3%).

IMPLICATIONS

Difficulty in managing disturbed behavior is a common stressor leading to staff burnout and to families placing older family members in care facilities. It is important for nurses to assess what behaviors family caregivers identify as problematic and to provide caregivers with the information and skills that will increase their capability and confidence to cope with difficult behaviors.

To avoid burnout, it is equally important for nurses, especially those working with persons who have Alzheimer's disease and related disorders, to know how to reduce the potential for disturbing behavior and to best manage disruptive behaviors when they occur. These interventions apply regardless of the setting in which a nurse is working with older clients and their families.

Teresi JA et al: Prevalence of behavior disorder and disturbance to family and staff in a sample of adult day health care clients, *Gerontologist* 37(5):629, 1997.

support gradually increases rather than when the person's functional ability declines rapidly.

A family member with a dementing illness such as Alzheimer's may not only require increasing assistance and supervision as the disease progresses, but also will become increasingly impaired in language, reasoning ability, memory, and social behavior (Schmall, 1996). Although a person who is physically ill but mentally intact can show appreciation to the caregiver, "thank you" is a phrase not generally used by the cognitively impaired person. This may lead to additional stress on the caregiver, who feels unappreciated (see Research box).

Losing the person that family members have always known is one of the most difficult aspects of coping with a progressive, dementing illness. As one woman said, "I've already watched the death of my husband. Now I'm watching the death of the disease." Another stated, "The personality that was my husband's is no longer present. I feel as though I am tending the shell of who he was—that is, his body. That is all that remains."

More and more families are faced with long-distance caregiving. They may find themselves driving or flying back and forth to repeated crises, spending long weekends "getting things in order," or "constantly checking on Mom and Dad." Such long-distance managing not only takes time and money but can be emotionally and physically exhausting as well. Trying to connect with and coordinate services from a distance can be frustrating, especially if older persons cancel the arrangements made by their families.

Care managers, many of whom are nurses, can be particularly helpful for long-distance caregivers. A care manager can evaluate an older person's situation and needs, establish an interface with health care providers and arrange for needed services, monitor the older person's status and compliance with treatment plans, provide on-the-spot crisis management, and keep the family informed about progress and changes in the older person's condition and situation. Care management services are offered by local Area Agencies on Aging (AAAs), hospitals, and private agencies and practitioners. AAAs can connect families with publicly funded care management services.

Placing the family member in a long-term care facility may merely change the kind of stress felt by the caregiver rather than alleviating it. The caregiver may feel a sense of failure—even when placement is the best decision. Stress also may result from difficult visits, travel to and from the care facility, worry about the quality of the care, family conflicts regarding placement, and the cost of the care. Some family members continue to do tasks in care facilities that they performed when providing care at home (e.g., providing assistance with eating, walking, and personal care).

Challenges and Opportunities of Caregiving. Few families are prepared to cope with the physical, financial, and emotional costs of caregiving. Most sons and daughters have not anticipated the possible need to provide care to their aging parent. Caregivers may become frustrated and exhausted because of unrealistic expectations or lack of knowledge and time. When caregiving is combined with other family responsibilities, the caregiver may feel that there is insufficient time in the day to complete all the tasks.

The cost of caregiving can place a burden on the finances of many families. It is less expensive to provide care at home; the annual cost to care for an adult dementia patient at home is $18,000, whereas in a long-term care facility it is $42,000 annually (Plowfield, Raymond, and Blevins, 2000).

If the caregiver is employed, work relationships may be compromised. The caregiver may be interrupted often at work, or may need to miss work completely. The employer may think that the caregiver is not "giving 100%" to his or her job. It is estimated that $26 billion in lost productivity can be attributed to family caregiving for older adults (Plowfield, Raymond, and Blevins, 2000). Adult day care is one alternative available to the working caregiver; however, programs are limited in number, availability, and hours and are often costly.

Chronic stress is another challenge to family caregivers. The family's normal routine may be disrupted. If the family providing care is from another locality, the time commitment of coordinating services and care providers can disrupt the family routine. Many families expect the daughter (either the oldest or the one living closest) to be the caregiver, regardless of her other commitments to her household or employer.

Many adult caregivers express frustration regarding the inequality of the contributions by their siblings. The siblings providing the majority of the care may resent those who are perceived to do less, while those who do less may feel guilt or frustration that their suggestions or offerings of help are rejected.

Caregiving can also be regarded as a beneficial opportunity. Close-knit families may view the caregiving situation as a way to demonstrate love and commitment. Frail older persons in this situation are reportedly less depressed and more satisfied with their care. Bonds between grandparents and grandchildren can be strengthened, along with other family relationships. Depending on the situation, the younger family may move in with their older relative, and as a result may receive room and board, child care, or financial assistance while they help out with the household chores.

Long-Distance vs. Nearby Family. Conflict can arise between family members who live near an older person and those who live at a distance because of their different perspectives (Schmall and Stiehl, 1998). To the family member who lives at a distance and sees the older person for only a few days at a time, the care needs may not seem as great as they do to the family member who has daily responsibility. In addition, the person may "perk up" in response to a visit by a rarely seen family member and may not display the symptoms and difficult behavior that he or she exhibited before the visit. Some older persons "dump" on one family member and show a cheerful side to another. Others take out feelings of frustration and loss on those providing day-to-day support and talk in glowing terms about sons and daughters who live at a distance.

Family members who are unable to visit regularly sometimes are shocked at the deterioration in their older relative. They may become upset because they have not been told "just how bad Mom or Dad is." However, they may have only two points of reference: the last time they saw their older relative (which may have been several months or a year earlier) and now. On the other hand, when changes have occurred gradually, family members who have regular contact with the person often are not aware of the degree of change because they have adjusted gradually.

Family conflict can occur because of these different experiences. The nurse often can help family members understand the reasons for different perceptions. It also may be helpful to remind distant family members not to let apparent differences in behavior between what they see and what the local caregiver has said discredit the caregiver. They also need to know that local caregivers often have to compromise with the older person and accept imperfect solutions to problems.

INTERVENTIONS TO SUPPORT FAMILY CAREGIVERS

Education

The number one need of many families is for information and referral (Schmall, 1995). Yet families frequently report that they were provided little or no information at the time a diagnosis was made, or that they were so overwhelmed they were not able to absorb the information that was shared (Aneshensel et al, 1995). It is important that health care professionals ask the family what they *want* to know, as well as providing them with information they *need* to know (Table 6-3).

One advantage of education—whether provided one-on-one or in group settings—over other intervention strategies is its nonintrusive nature. Many people who would not attend a support group or seek counseling may attend a program labeled "education." An educational program also can be a springboard for a person to seek other intervention programs. As one woman said:

> I avoided going to a support group because I didn't want to air my "dirty laundry." It was not until after I attended an educational program that I realized my concerns and fears were not abnormal. It was then I felt more comfortable talking to others and joining the support group.

The need for information may be even more critical for family members who provide care to persons with dementia, disruptive behaviors, or personal care dependencies because of higher stress in these caregiving situations (Office of Technology Assessment, 1987). For example, caregivers need information early on about the nature of a dementing illness, the limitations it causes, how it may affect the relationship between the caregiver and the care receiver, and strategies for coping. Although a caregiver's needs for information are diverse, they fall into six general categories (Schmall, 1994):

1. **Understanding the family member's medical condition.** Caregivers need information about the progres-

TABLE 6-3 Nursing Interventions for Family Caregivers

EDUCATION	TOPICS TO COVER
• Support group • Classes • Written information	• Normal aging • Disease processes (e.g., dementia, hypertension, depression) • Future progression of health needs • Difficult behaviors
Community Resources • Awareness of what is available • Family uses resources	• Adequate advance directives and guardianship plans • Living arrangements (adult day care, long-term care, in-home support) • Family resources (support groups, associations) • Need for state services (financial assistance) • Written list of resources and services with contact information
Assess Needs • Caregiver needs • Elderly person's needs	Nurse and family should meet together • Meeting in neutral territory • Be consistent in information given to the family • Give a written report • Confront all difficult issues
Satisfaction • Family and caregiver • Elderly person	• Family should have contact information for follow-up • Understand roles (caregiver, nurse) • Offer problem-solving assistance • Offer ongoing support • Family should complete a satisfaction report

From Plowfield LA, Raymond JE, Blevins C: Wholism for aging families: meeting needs of caregivers, *Holistic Nurs Pract* (14)4:51, 2000.

sion, signs, symptoms, and outcomes of medical conditions; common medical treatments; a condition's impact on an older adult's functional abilities; and implications for the caregiver and family. It is important to dispel any myths, misinformation, and unrealistic expectations. For example, when caregivers do not understand behavior caused by a dementia, they often view the person's behavior as intentional.

2. **Improving coping skills.** Coping skills may include stress management, social network–building skills, behavioral management skills, problem-solving skills, and the ability to perform specific tasks of caregiving—such as managing incontinence, feeding a person with swallowing difficulties, or meeting an older adult's emotional needs.
3. **Dealing with family issues.** Family issues often involve getting support from other family members, identifying how much and what type of help family members can give, and dealing with conflicting feelings toward family members who do not help. Decisions about older adult care and caregiving generally affect not only caregivers and care receivers but also other family members. Anger and family dissension can occur when caregivers do not attend to the thoughts and feelings of family members.
4. **Communicating effectively with older persons.** Family members often need to know how to effectively communicate their concerns to older persons who are competent, as well as how to communicate with those who are unable to understand or communicate. Communicating effectively with cognitively impaired persons often requires learning communication skills contrary to those learned over a lifetime; yet using appropriate techniques can reduce stress for everyone. Family caregivers who interacted in encouraging and supportive ways with their family member with dementia had lower levels of stress than family caregivers who used an authoritarian or reasoning style (Niederehe and Funk, 1987). The benefits of such information are reflected in the following adult son's comments:

   > The hardest thing about dealing with Alzheimer's disease is learning to relate in new ways and accepting my Dad as he is today. What a difference it made for me when I learned in the caregiver class to "step into my Dad's world," rather than keep asking him questions about things he simply could not remember. Our times together are now much more enjoyable for the both of us.

5. **Using community services.** Many caregivers need information about the range of community services, the types of help that are available, how to access services, and care facility options.
6. **Long-term planning.** This includes making legal and financial plans and considering changes in the current caregiving situation, including possible nursing facility placement.

Two major goals of caregiver education should be to (1) empower caregivers and (2) increase caregiver confidence and competence (Schmall, 1995). Feeling powerless can have a significant impact on a caregiver's physical and emotional health. Although the factors that affect feelings of powerlessness are complex and vary from person to person, it is helpful if health care professionals use approaches that do the following (Schmall, 1994):

- **Help caregivers set realistic goals and expectations.** Failing to achieve goals reinforces feelings of powerlessness. Achieving goals increases morale. A caregiver whose goal is to "make Mother happy" is less likely to experience "success" than a caregiver whose goal is to plan one enjoyable activity each week with her mother.
- **Provide caregivers with needed skills.** Being able to do the tasks that need to be done, get needed support, or access community resources enhances feelings of being in control.
- **Enhance caregivers' decision-making skills.** This includes sharing information about options and their potential consequences for older persons, caregivers, and other family members.
- **Help caregivers solve problems.** The ability to solve problems in managing care reduces feelings of powerlessness and stress. Since personal perceptions affect a person's approach to problem solving, it is important to assess a caregiver's perceptions of problems and explore reframing as a coping technique. Reframing is looking at things in a different way—for example, finding something positive in a difficult situation (Schmall, Cleland, and Sturdevant, 1999). It can be particularly helpful when the actual situation cannot be changed. For example, a nurse might help a caregiver reframe the behavior of her father with Alzheimer's disease from a view of "Dad is purposefully behaving that way to get to me" to "Dad's behavior is part of the disease."

People are more likely to do something if they believe they will be able to perform it successfully. They also have to believe that a skill or action will make a positive difference; otherwise, they probably will not adopt it (Stiehl and Bessey, 1993). Therefore one of the goals of education should be to provide caregivers with the confidence that they can do a task or take an action. This means it is critical to give caregivers an opportunity to practice skills in a learning environment that is nonthreatening and psychologically safe.

Skill building is enhanced when caregivers have the opportunity to practice skills in an educational setting and receive feedback; to apply skills in the home environment; and to then return to discuss how well the techniques worked, the problems that were encountered, and what they might do differently the next time in applying the skills.

It is important to discuss the barriers caregivers may confront in the real world and ways to overcome these barriers. For example, professionals often talk about the importance of caregivers setting limits, but they do not always prepare caregivers for the possible consequences of doing so. For instance, an older person's manipulative behavior may worsen for a time after a caregiver begins setting limits, particularly if in the past such behavior generally resulted in the older person getting what he or she wanted.

Family members also need to know that at times they may have to step back and wait until a crisis occurs before they can act (e.g., when a mentally intact older family member refuses to go to a physician or refuses to stop drinking despite attempts at intervention). In such situations, however, family members often feel they have failed. They may need help to recognize when "failures" are the result of a challenging situation and not their performance.

Sharing printed information (e.g., handouts the nurse has prepared, pamphlets, articles) and videotapes is another important way to provide education. The value of bibliotherapy (literally, this means healing through books, but it also refers to materials in other media, including pamphlets, audiotapes, and videotapes) is recognized in chemical dependency treatment. According to Toft (1993), "A book or tape carries the voice of a human being; reading, listening, or watching is a form of meeting. Bibliotherapy is valuable for people learning new behaviors. It gives them the opportunity to reflect and the tools to turn that reflection into action."

Bibliotherapy may be equally valuable for some caregivers. Fortinsky and Hathaway (1990) found that active and former caregivers of family members with Alzheimer's disease rated written materials about the disease process as their most important need at the time of diagnosis. The comments of caregivers also indicate the value of printed materials:

- "*The 36-Hour Day* is my 'Bible' in dealing with my husband's illness. When I am at a loss about what to do, I turn to it. It has gotten me through many tough times."
- "In reading the Oregon State University Extension publication *Depression in Later Life,* my brother and I realized we should not consider it normal for Dad to be depressed just because he is 73. We followed the advice about talking with Dad about the physical changes we saw in him rather than talking with him about 'being depressed.' It worked. . . . I thought we'd never get him to see a doctor."
- "I learned a lot of crucial information from materials the Alzheimer's Association sent to me."

Adults also learn independently. Workbooks can provide caregivers with a step-by-step guide for taking action. *The Carebook: A Workbook for Caregiver Peace of Mind* (Beedle, 1997) gives caregivers a step-by-step guide for preparing substitute caregivers. Information and forms in *Organizing Your Family Records* and *Do You Know Your Valuable Papers?* can help families talk with aging parents about financial records and the organization and storage of important documents (Gregerson, 1993).

Because people's time often is limited, Toft (1993) suggests that educational materials be short and to the point, solution focused, and designed to empower people. Print materials provided to caregivers, when shared with other family members, can help create a common base of information and understanding (Schmall, 1994). Sometimes other family members "listen" more readily to information in a handout developed by a professional than to the same information shared verbally by caregivers. Printed materials are beneficial for another reason. It is difficult for people who are anxious or in crisis to hear and remember everything that is said. Written information gives them a reference for later use.

Another resource for families is the Internet. The Alzheimer's Association and other health and caregiving organizations offer a variety of helpful information through their websites. If families do not have access to the Internet, encourage them to ask the local library to help locate appropriate websites.

Respite Programs

Studies suggest that family members are better able to tolerate long-term caregiving if they obtain respite—that is, "relief" or "time off" from caregiving responsibilities. Without breaks, the stresses inherent to caregiving can jeopardize the physical and mental health of caregivers and can even lead to neglect or abuse of care receivers (Schmall, Cleland, and Sturdevant, 1999; Zarit and Zarit, 1998).

Although the primary intended beneficiaries of respite services are caregivers, care receivers also benefit. In many cases, respite care providers may be the only source of outside-the-family socialization for care receivers. Care receivers also benefit from caregivers being more "refreshed" after a break in caregiving.

Respite services may be provided in-home or out-of-home and for a few hours, a day, overnight, a weekend, or longer. In-home respite care can include companion sitter programs or the temporary use of homemaker or home health services. Out-of-home respite services include adult day programs or short stays in adult foster care homes, long-term care facilities, or hospitals.

Respite services often are underused by caregivers. Barriers to access and use of services include (Schmall, 1993):

- **Lack of awareness.** Often, families are not aware of the availability of respite services or of program eligibility, or they are not familiar with the provider agency.
- **Apprehension.** With in-home respite services caregivers may be apprehensive about leaving a family member with a "stranger" or nonprofessional.
- **Caregiver attitudes.** Some caregivers think "I can care (or should be able to care) for my family member myself" or "No one can care for my family member like I can." Others feel guilty and selfish to leave ill family members in the care of someone else so that they can meet their own needs.
- **Timing.** Caregivers often view respite services as "a last resort." They seek help much too late—when they are in crisis, or a family member is severely debilitated and requires care beyond what a program can provide.

- **Finances.** The cost of respite care, or the anticipation of future expenses, is another reason some caregivers may be unwilling to use or delay using such programs. Others are unwilling to pay for a program they view as a "babysitting service."
- **Care receiver resistance.** Negative reactions by care receivers, such as resentment toward someone coming into the house or a caregiver's leaving, may keep caregivers from using respite programs.
- **Energy required to use the program.** The time and energy required to prepare and transport care receivers can limit use of adult day programs.
- **Program inflexibility and bureaucracy.** Program inflexibility may contribute to caregivers' low usage of respite care. System barriers reported by caregivers include (1) services not being available when most wanted or needed, such as during weekends or in the evenings; (2) services accommodating only older persons with a narrow band of need; (3) lack of responsiveness of the service system to changing conditions of care receivers; (4) system not allowing caregivers to have one respite worker with whom they can relate over time; and (5) the necessity of making several calls to arrange for respite care (Malone-Beach, Zarit, and Spore, 1992).

These are issues the nurse may need to address when working with a caregiver who hesitates or refuses to use a respite program. It is important to first identify the reasons a caregiver is reluctant to use a program, then work with the caregiver to reduce or eliminate the identified barriers.

Caregivers who delay using respite care until a crisis or until they are "burnt out" are less likely to benefit from it because it is "too little . . . too late" (Deimling, 1989). Respite care is most beneficial when a caregiver begins to use it early in caregiving to *prevent* physical and mental exhaustion rather than to treat it. Dunn (1987) suggests that one reason respite may be viewed as a "service of last resort" is that the message often given to caregivers is "respite is a service when you are having trouble coping or the condition of your loved one is progressing to the point where placement may be necessary."

In general, female caregivers appear to have more difficulty using respite and adult day programs. Because they have been socialized as nurturers and caregivers, women may buy into the view that "caregiving is women's work" and may believe caregiving is something they *should* do. As a result, they may be more reluctant to let go of the caregiver role and to accept outside help. Men, on the other hand, may feel less secure in the caregiver role and may perceive that they lack the necessary skills to take care of someone else. Thus they tend to be more willing to use services.

The nurse should help caregivers recognize that caregiving is a job. Just as employees benefit from regular breaks and vacations, caregivers benefit from a "break" in the job. The nurse should emphasize that the need for respite care begins with the onset of caregiving.

The message a nurse conveys about respite to caregivers may be important. Although respite programs are designed primarily to benefit the caregiver, some caregivers are reluctant to take advantage of services for themselves. One study (Beisecker and Wright, 1991) found that caregivers who perceived adult day care as primarily benefiting themselves were less likely to use the service than caregivers who perceived adult day care as primarily benefiting care receivers:

> Caregivers generally had more difficulty accepting assistance if the focus was on their needs or if the service was perceived as merely "babysitting.". . . Some caregivers indicated they could more readily accept a service if it focused on the client and not them. Many caregivers did not see a connection between their own physical and psychological well-being and being able to continue with caregiving (Malone-Beach, Zarit, and Spore, 1992).

Therefore resistance to respite and day care programs may decrease if the nurse emphasizes how a program can benefit care receivers.

Lawton, Brody, and Saperstein (1989) suggest additional ways to increase the appeal of respite care to caregivers: (1) portray respite as a program that is helpful to anyone, even the most successful of caregivers; (2) emphasize how respite helps to maintain the positive aspects of caregiving; and (3) provide reassurance that caregivers deserve time away from caregiving, and that they are not deserting their family members by taking such breaks in caregiving. They state that "these appeals affirm the basic strengths of the caregiver, yet they will not be lost on the overworked or depressed caregiver."

It is generally assumed that respite is inherently beneficial to caregivers. However, different uses of respite time may lead to different outcomes (Wright, Lund, and Caserta, 1990). Caregivers who use respite time primarily for discretionary activities such as socializing, rest, and exercise experience more favorable outcomes than caregivers who spend the time primarily in obligatory activities such as doing housework, performing other domestic chores, or providing care to another person. As a nurse, it may be worthwhile to discuss with caregivers how they plan to use respite time and encourage caregivers to engage in discretionary activities that they enjoy.

Even when formal respite services are not available, the nurse plays a vital role in encouraging caregivers to take breaks in caregiving and helping them identify and overcome barriers to obtaining respite. Members of a caregiver's informal support system may be able to provide respite when formal services are unavailable or inaccessible. Some caregivers need help to reach out and ask for assistance, particularly if they view asking for help as a sign of weakness, helplessness, inadequacy, or failure. A written "prescription for respite" by a health care provider for certain hours of respite per week or month may provide the authority a caregiver needs to begin taking breaks from the demands of caregiving (Box 6-3).

BOX 6-3 Video Respite: an Innovative Caregiver Resource

"I can't seem to find any time for myself. I'm suffocating."

"I never have time alone, not even in my own home. I can't even take a bath, fix dinner, or make a phone call without interruption. I have no privacy."

"I'm tired of my mother following me around and asking questions constantly, like a broken record. I need some time and space to breathe."

Such comments are common from caregivers of persons with dementia. One of their greatest needs is for regular breaks from caregiving. Although adult day care and respite programs provide family caregivers with much needed time away from the demands of caregiving, they often need 15-minute or half-hour breaks to take a short rest, to have time alone, to attend to personal matters, to make telephone calls, or to do household chores without interruption. *Video Respite,* developed by researchers at the University of Utah Gerontology Center after 10 years of research on caregiving, is a unique, innovative approach to making it possible for caregivers to get these brief "breaks" in caregiving without leaving home.

Video Respite consists of a series of videotapes simulating a personal and friendly visit. Each video actively engages persons who have moderate to advanced memory and cognitive impairments in an enjoyable and meaningful interaction. As the memory-impaired individual "interacts" with the person on the videotape, a caregiver can take some time for himself or herself.

Video Respite currently includes thirteen video programs, ranging from 25 to 59 minutes in length. Each captures and maintains the attention of persons with dementia through the recollection of pleasant memories and music and involvement in singing and in doing simple hand, arm, and leg movements. Although some persons may not be able to do all of the physical exercises, the videotapes do hold the attention of memory-impaired persons, as evidenced by their participatory actions such as toe-tapping. Brief descriptions of the videotapes follow:

Gonna Do a Little Music. While playing the guitar and autoharp, Marianne engages the viewer in singing familiar songs. She discusses memories related to love, music lessons, family gatherings, and childhood friends.

Remembering When. This tape includes memories of school days—for example, songs and routines such reciting the Pledge of Allegiance—city and country life, and a brief recollection of the Roaring Twenties. Kyle, a toddler, visits.

A Yankee Doodle Dandy Time. Becky recalls and prepares for a Fourth of July celebration. Becky's cat joins her in recollections about the American flag, marching bands, and parades.

Movement, Music & Memories. Cathy encourages viewers to stretch, walk, and march in place through the use of favorite songs. This tape also includes a visit by a boy playing kickball and a lamb.

Sharing Christmas Cheer. George discusses the traditions of Christmas trees, gifts, and stockings, and many familiar carols are sung.

Sharing Favorite Things. Joyce discusses pleasant memories of growing up. There are visits by a dog and a 1-year-old baby to whom the viewer is invited to sing "Happy Birthday."

Those Good Ole School Days. This tape involves recollections of early school days—long walks to school, games, trips to the candy store—and the singing of familiar school-related songs.

Two of the videos were developed to be more gender-specific:

Ladies...Let's Chat. Diane chats about topics from family gatherings and meal preparation to dressing up with hats and courtship days. Her two grandchildren visit.

Lunchbreak with Tony. On his work break, Tony discusses work days, jobs, co-workers, baseball, first cars, and first loves. Tony's dog, Sparky, visits.

Four videotapes are more culture specific:

Favorite Canadian Memories. Dawn, her baby, and others share early memories of growing up in Canada, including Expo '67, ice skating, and hockey nights. Dawn's brother, dressed in a hockey uniform, visits.

A Kibitz with David. David, a Jewish man, recalls weddings, Passover, Chanukah, and other holiday celebrations. David's wife and children help light the Shabbos candles and sing favorite Yiddish songs.

Celebrating African-American Culture. This is a look at the celebrations and personal memories of African Americans. It includes "good old home cooking" and singing traditional songs.

A Visit with Maria. Recorded in Spanish, Maria invites viewers to sing along with old favorite songs and share memories of childhood days and festivals.

It is exciting to observe a person with Alzheimer's disease "converse" with Marianne, Joyce, Tony, and others on the videotapes and, even more important, feel good about his or her "visit." Strengths of these videos for the person with Alzheimer's disease include:

A personalized approach. The people on the videos are friendly and present themselves and the content in such a way that it feels as though the viewer is being talked to directly.

An opportunity for positive interaction. Questions, pauses, and feedback from "the visitor" encourage involvement and conversation from the memory-impaired person.

A focus on long-term memory. Through familiar images and childhood songs, the videos capture the attention and trigger long-term memories for persons with dementia. The objects, people, events, and early life experiences that are discussed are familiar to most of today's older persons.

BOX 6-3 Video Respite: an Innovative Caregiver Resource—cont'd

A way to help the person "feel good." The "visitors" give a lot of positive feedback. For example, in one video, viewers hear comments such as "You did a great job," "That was great," "You have wonderful eyes," "Do whatever feels best to you. If you want to just sing or hum along, that's okay," and "Thank you for spending this time with me. You have given me joy today."

A slow pace and visually uncluttered screen. The slower pace gives persons with memory impairment the necessary time to understand and respond to information. The visual simplicity helps to keep the viewer focused and reduces distraction. The faster pace and content of most television programs are not optimum for sustaining the attention of most persons with Alzheimer's disease.

Studies conducted by University of Utah researchers also show that the videos can be useful in calming the person who is agitated. One caregiver stated:

When Herb is agitated and I'm at my wit's end is when I need the tape the most, and I forget to use it. And then I'll call my son, and he'll say, "Put the tape in first. If that doesn't work, then I'll be over." But it always works. He's not attentive to TV, but he is to the tape.

Because of the loss of recent memory with Alzheimer's disease, the *Video Respite* tapes can be used again and again. Another caregiver reported:

This kept Mother entertained like nothing else has for years. I could use it every day, or back-to-back, because it's like a new tape each time. If she is depressed or irritable, it will get her out of it. She won't watch TV, but she is glued to the tape.

Because *Video Respite* tapes engage the person with Alzheimer's disease, caregivers can get short breaks in caregiving whenever needed. For a caregiver, 30 to 50 minutes of uninterrupted time can be significant. The tapes are also: (1) quick, convenient, and easy for a caregiver to incorporate into the daily routine; (2) portable, so that they can be used in many different settings or places; and (3) appropriate for repeated use. The videos also may help to give caregivers who feel helpless a greater sense of control. As one caregiver said, "The videos help me to feel as though I am doing something positive for Mother."

Considerable research and evaluation, including a 2-year grant from the national Alzheimer's Association, went into the development of these *Video Respite* tapes. Tests of *Video Respite* in nursing facilities, special care units, and adult day care programs also show favorable results.

Video Respite is not a panacea or a substitute for a caregiver or other services; however, it does offer considerable promise in providing caregivers with an opportunity for respite time.

From Innovative Caregiving Resources, PO Box 17809, Salt Lake City, Utah 84117-0809.

Support Groups

In many communities, caregiver support groups have developed. Some support groups are oriented to specific diseases such as cancer, Parkinson's disease, lung disease, stroke, or Alzheimer's disease and related dementia. Others are for family caregivers in general.

A support group can be a place where caregivers get advice, gain knowledge about their older relatives' medical conditions and problems, share experiences and feelings, develop new coping strategies, and learn about community resources and care alternatives. A support group may help normalize a caregiver's experience. Discovering that they are not alone can provide much-needed emotional relief to some caregivers. For the isolated caregiver deprived of intimacy and support from the care receiver, a support group also may provide an acceptable outlet for socializing. Although many caregivers benefit from support groups, they are not for everyone.

Research on caregiver support groups has several limitations; however, findings to date suggest the following (Gallagher-Thompson, 1994; Zarit, 1994):

- Levels of caregiver burden may be more influenced by changes in a person's caregiving situation than by support group participation.
- A support group with a focused agenda, such as dealing with feelings of anger or depression, may have more measurable benefits than a broadly focused support group.
- Some caregivers may benefit most from an initial period of counseling in which their specific concerns are addressed, followed by participation in a support group.
- Support groups may be most fruitful when tailored for specific groups of caregivers. The needs of male caregivers may differ from those of female caregivers; the needs of spouses may differ from those of adult children; and the needs of newly diagnosed families may differ from those of families dealing with late-stage chronic illness.

Family Meetings

Although one family member is generally responsible for caregiving, other family members are important in providing support. However, each family member may have a different idea about what the problem is or how to handle it. For example, one brother might not want a parent's resources—his potential inheritance—spent for in-home care; he may prefer that the family provide the needed care. Another brother may believe "Mom's money is there to spend on her" and prefer to purchase services. Beliefs about what is best often differ, creating family dissension. One person may be adamant that the older person should be kept at home at all costs; another may think a care facility is the best setting. Intense conflicts can result.

Unless differences are discussed and resolved, disagreements among family members usually magnify. The family meeting is one strategy for deciding how to share caregiving responsibilities and for reaching a consensus about needs, problems, and decisions (Schmall, Cleland, and Sturdevant, 1999).

A family meeting should be held as early as possible after the need for caregiving arises. Everyone who is concerned or who may be affected by decisions should be involved, including the older person (if possible) for whom plans are being made. Calling distant family members to get their input and keeping them informed can help them feel involved in the decision making. A family member should not be excluded because of distance, personality, family history, or limited resources. It is just as important to invite the difficult, argumentative family member or the one who seldom visits as it is to involve those who are supportive. Such involvement ensures greater success and support for any plans that are developed and can help prevent later undermining of decisions.

Sometimes, families find it helpful to hold a two-step meeting. The first meeting is held without the older person to discuss ideas and feelings, raise concerns, and identify needed information. The purpose is not to make the decision or to "gang up" on the older person. A second meeting is then held in which the older person is actively involved in identifying and evaluating options and making decisions.

A family meeting is not always easy. It is most difficult for family members who have never discussed emotion-laden concerns, who hold differing values and outlooks in regard to the situation, or who have a history of poor relationships and conflict. A family in conflict may become angry and get sidetracked from current issues and the decisions that need to be made. Old resentments and conflicts that have been dormant since childhood can reemerge with regard to relationships, family roles, expectations, the authority to make decisions, and even inheritance. A family meeting often is even more important in these situations.

If family conflicts or hidden resentments prevent rational discussion, it often helps to have a health care professional skilled in working with older adults and their families facilitate the family meeting. The professional—whether a nurse, social worker, member of the clergy, or counselor—should be well versed in aging-related issues and family dynamics, and have group facilitation skills. The mere presence of an "outsider" often keeps the atmosphere calm and the discussion focused and objective. An objective third party also can help move the family past emotions to common interests and can handle many difficult situations. Some practitioners and agencies offer family consultation services that include facilitation of family meetings.

A family meeting is more likely to be successful if the following are considered (Schmall and Stiehl, 1998):

- Hold the family meeting in a neutral setting. However, a family meeting in the older person's home may help give him or her a greater sense of control, especially if the person is feeling a loss of control over his or her life.
- Create a feeling of support and confidentiality.
- Acknowledge that everyone has a different relationship with each other and that current life circumstances vary. These factors need to be respected and considered as decisions are discussed and made.
- Have each family member address the problem from his or her perspective. This increases commitment to the process and contributes to defining "the problem" and reaching agreement on and possible solutions.
- Give everyone the opportunity to express feelings, voice preferences, and offer suggestions without being criticized.
- Keep the family meeting focused on current concerns rather than on other issues, past conflicts, personalities, or resentments.
- Focus on the positive things family members do, or are willing and able to do, and encourage everyone to be honest about their limitations. Sharing information about other responsibilities can help others understand the reasons support might be limited.
- Prepare a written plan about decisions made, what each person will do, and when he or she will do it. A written plan can prevent later disagreements.

WORKING WITH FAMILIES OF OLDER ADULTS: CONSIDERATIONS AND STRATEGIES

Identify Who Is the Client and Who Is the Family

Critical questions to ask when working with older adults include: Who is the client? Is it just the older person? Should the older person's family also be considered the "client"?

Although the older person is generally identified as the client, sometimes it is appropriate to consider the family as the client as well. Family members are often intimately involved in the decisions to be made, affected by potential decisions, or actively involved in caregiving for the older person. If only the needs of the older person are considered and not the needs and situation of the family, the care plan may have less chance for success, particularly if family members will be responsible for carrying it out.

Another significant question to ask is, "Who is family, as defined by the older person?" The definition of family needs to be broadened beyond blood relatives to include other persons who are significant in the older person's life (Schmall, 1995). Many older persons are connected to others by love and friendship and function as a family to each other. These relationships often extend into caregiving. The following are examples of such "families" (Schmall, 1994):

- Red, who divorced in his early 70s, never had children. His only blood relatives were his nieces, nephews, and older adult sisters, all of whom lived hundreds of miles away. During the last 12 years of his life, nearly all support was provided by a person Red referred to as "my adopted granddaughter." When medical crises occurred and care arrangements were needed, Red looked to his "granddaughter" to make the necessary arrangements.

- Florence's son divorced his first wife, Jane, and remarried. The divorce, however, did not end the relationship between Florence and Jane. Florence continued to view Jane as "the daughter I never had," not as her "ex–daughter-in-law." When Florence became frail, she did not turn to her sons or the current daughters-in-law for help; she turned to Jane for both day-to-day assistance and emotional support.
- Elizabeth and Mary had lived together as a couple for 30 years when Elizabeth developed cancer. Although Elizabeth's "blood relatives" were supportive during the downhill course of the disease, Mary was the primary caregiver, the person Elizabeth consulted when she faced medical decisions, and the one who made decisions when Elizabeth was no longer able to do so.

In created but not legally recognized families, it may be important to help individuals take steps—such as completing an advance medical directive (AMD), power of attorney for health care, or durable power of attorney for financial decisions—to ensure that the relationships continue into caregiving, especially if one person loses the capacity to make decisions. As Mary stated, "Elizabeth's giving me power of attorney for health care ensured that our relationship could continue as it had been for 30 years. We knew another couple who were in a similar situation, and the [blood] relatives stepped in and took over control, disregarding the relationship Jim and Bill had for 20 years."

In the health care setting, it may be important to reevaluate the definition of family. If "blood relatives only allowed in intensive care" and other rules are followed, some older persons may be deprived of their most significant sources of support.

Other important questions for the nurse to ask are, "Who is the decision maker?" and "Who owns the care plan?" The nurse's primary role is to empower older persons and their families. This means giving the information, guidelines, options, and skills that will enable them to make the best decisions possible and to better manage a medical condition or their situation. However, it is easy to become frustrated and angry—and eventually experience burnout—if older persons or families choose a course of action that the nurse feels is not the best. Remember, nurses have not failed when an older person or family selects an option different from the nurse's recommendation. Depending on the situation, the primary responsibility for implementation lies with the older person or the family.

Assess the Family

There are no easy answers when an older person's life situation or physical or mental status changes. What may be the best answer for one older person and his or her family may be inappropriate for another family whose situation seems exactly the same.

Each older person and family system is different. It can be just as important to understand the family's history, current life circumstances, and needs as it is to know about an older person's needs and level of functioning. A family's willingness to provide care, for example, says nothing about their actual ability to do so. Sometimes the care an older person needs exceeds that which an individual or family can provide, and the caregiver becomes the "hidden client." As one adult daughter stated, "My father was the person with Alzheimer's disease, but his illness also killed my mother." Failing to evaluate the ability of family members to provide caregiving is a disservice to older clients.

Information from a family assessment can result in more effective older adult care planning and decision making. Another benefit of assessing how well a caregiver is doing is that it validates a person's caregiving efforts and sends a message that the nurse is concerned about the caregiver's well-being, as well as the older adult's health.

There are many tools for assessing family functioning and the level of caregiving burden (Zarit and Zarit, 1998). Depending on the family, the older adult, and the decisions to be made, the following may be among the important factors to consider in conducting a family assessment.

Past Relationships. Lifetime relationships can influence the family's ability to plan, to make decisions together, and to provide support. Remember, every adult child has a different history with an aging parent, even if they shared the same family events. Families with a history of alcoholism, poor relationships, or abusive behavior cannot always be expected to provide the assistance an older person needs.

Consider the degree of emotional intensity—the closeness, affection, and openness—in the relationships among family members. Parental or spousal disability sometimes threatens a person's identity or the level of emotional relationship that has been established. For example, some married couples, parents, and children have been emotionally distant for many years. Some spouses have shared the same household but lived separate lives. Some adult children have maintained emotional distance from a parent by living and working at a geographic distance. People in these situations may be reluctant to enter the care system or may have more difficulty with caregiving. It may be unrealistic to expect such family members to meet the emotional needs of the older person; they may feel more comfortable with meeting a person's instrumental needs—that is, doing tasks.

Family Dynamics. Family dynamics are the ways family members interact with one another, including their communication patterns, family alliances, and symbiotic relationships. What are family members' views about how decisions should be made? How do they view the older adult's role in decisions about his or her life? To what degree are family members paternalistic—that is, expecting the older person to submit to their decisions or a health care professional's recommendations?

Roles. It can be useful to know whether individual family members have distinctive roles. If so, what role or roles does each person have? What expectations are held by the person fulfilling the role and by other family members? Do any of the roles generate conflict for the people who bear them? For example, family members may have always assumed that if a parent needed care, a particular daughter would provide the care because she is the oldest, lives the closest, is a nurse, or has always taken care of everyone who needed help. The daughter also may have viewed caregiving as her role. However, this "assigned" role may or may not be realistic, given the daughter's current life situation or the parent's needs. Sometimes, an older person or a family member may not make a decision until the "decision maker" in the family is consulted. The importance of considering who plays which roles is exemplified by this daughter's comments:

> I lived in the same town as my Dad, so when he needed help, I was the one who provided it on a daily basis. Dad expected me to help because I was his daughter. But, when it came to making decisions, my opinions never counted with him. His son's opinions, however, mattered, and he would listen to them. I think his basic view throughout his life was "women are there to serve men" and "men are by far more knowledgeable than women." It didn't matter that I had a college education, and my brother didn't.

A survey by the Benjamin Rose Institute found that it is not unusual for an older person and his or her case manager to have different perceptions about who is the primary informal caregiver to the older person (Noelker, 1994). Knowing who does what for the older person makes for more effective planning.

Old family roles can also come to the foreground when brothers and sisters are brought together to address the care needs of a parent. One daughter stated:

> I lived in the same community as my parents, so when they became ill, I did everything that needed to be done and arranged for support services. Both of my sisters lived hundreds of miles away. Although I am a competent business woman, it seemed that when both of my sisters, who are older, came home, I immediately became the "baby of the family" again.

The roles of family members vary. Examples of potential roles include the prime mover, the person who gets things done in the family; the scapegoat, the person who becomes the focus of attention when problems arise; the decision maker, a role that may vary depending on whether the decision to be made regards finances, living arrangements, or health care; the peacemaker, who always tries to create peace when there is family dissension; the pot-stirrer, the person who seems to keep things "stirred up" in the family; the black sheep; the burden bearer; the favorite child; the model child; and the escapee, who disappears when there are tough decisions to be made or work to be done.

It can be helpful to identify how family roles—especially those of the older person—are affected as a result of the older adult's increased frailty. What are the perceptions of family members regarding the role of the older person? Do any adult children perceive that their role is now to "parent their parent"?

Sometimes people talk about "role reversal." Although a family member may take on "parentlike" responsibilities, in the emotional sense a parent is still a parent and a spouse is still a spouse, no matter how dependent a person has become. Decades of adult experiences cannot be repressed. If family members think of an older family member as a child, they are more likely to treat that person in childlike ways and, in return, get childlike behavior.

Consider the older adult's view of his or her role with respect to the rest of the family. For example, does the older person believe he or she is still a contributing family member, or does he or she feel a loss of role? Does the person think he or she is entitled to care from family members, for example, "just because I am your parent?" Paulette tells her story:

> I could see Dad deteriorating. When Dad could no longer live alone at home, he refused to consider anyone but "his daughter helping him." When the time came that Dad had to move from his home, he said to me adamantly, "Your mother took care of her mother and my father until they died," implying that I also should do the same with him. To Dad, "taking care of" meant he would live in our home. He felt that this is "what daughters are supposed to do."

Loyalties and Obligations. This refers to interpersonal allegiances. Family members often struggle with two questions: (1) What should be my primary priority—meeting the needs of my aging family member? My spouse and children? My career? and (2) How much do I owe to whom? Caregivers who have not been able to deal with these questions may find themselves stressed by trying to do too much. They may feel guilty because they feel they are not doing enough.

Sometimes family members, in looking at older adult care issues, also weigh how much various family members "owe" to the person who needs assistance. Is any particular family member viewed as being more obligated or more indebted to providing care because of how much the older person has given him or her in the past? In other words, which family members are viewed as "creditors" and which as "debtors," and to whom do they owe? For example:

> Sue did not feel obligated to provide hands-on care to her mother. She thought that "Mother never did anything to help me. All I got from her was criticism—about everything!" On the other hand, Louise (Sue's younger sister) said, "Mother has always been there for me. I don't know what I would have done after my divorce if Mom hadn't opened her doors to me and my three children for

those 2 years." Sue also believed Louise "owed" their mother more than she did.

It is important to be aware that levels of stress tend to be higher for the person who provides caregiving only out of a sense of obligation.

Dependence and Independence. Some families accept and adjust more easily than other families to the increased dependence of a family member. Answers to the following questions can help determine how well family members are dealing with or will deal with increased frailty in an older family member:

- What are the attitudes and expectations of family members, including the older person, about dependency?
- Has the family experienced a shift in who is dependent? If so, what is the response of individual family members to this shift?
- Are any family members threatened by the increased dependence of the older person?
- Is the older person giving family members mixed messages about how independent or dependent he or she is?
- Do family members perceive the dependency needs of the person realistically? Is anyone denying, minimizing, or exaggerating the dependence? Is anyone overprotecting or forcing dependency?

Providing caregiving to a family member can be more difficult if the caregiver has been the dependent person in the relationship. The care receiver also may resent the caregiver exercising more control.

Caregiver Stress. It is critical to assess the nature and extent of caregiver stress. In addition to identifying actual stressors—which may or may not be a direct result of caregiving—the nurse must assess their significance to the caregiver. The meaning a caregiver gives to a stressor is a stronger predictor of its impact than the actual stressor (Zarit, 1994). Other useful areas to assess are a caregiver's style of coping; the caregiver's support system; the caregiver's evaluation of the adequacy of his or her support system; the care needs of the older person, including behavioral and emotional problems, and the caregiver's perception of those care needs; and financial resources.

Just as an older adult's situation can change and require reassessment, so can a family's situation and a caregiver's ability to provide care. As Gallo, Reichel, and Anderson (1988) found:

> The assessment of family functioning is not a static determination. The strength of the support for the elder needs to be periodically reevaluated. Change in the elder's condition may compel a fresh look at caregiving roles and stresses. The spouse may be able to manage a demented elder until the tasks of caregiving become too physically demanding because of the development of incontinence by the patient. Changes within the family may necessitate a restructuring of social support. A new job may take a child away from an elderly parent. The death or illness of a spouse may leave an elder stranded. New sources of assistance may need to be rallied in order to provide adequate care for the family member.

Encourage Families To Plan in Advance of Need

Families tend not to discuss age-related issues until faced with a crisis (Noelker, 1994; Schmall, Cleland, and Sturdevant, 1999). As a result, many adult children are often unaware of parental preferences, views about care arrangements, or the existence and location of important documents.

Planning requires anticipating negative situations—dependency, disability, incapacity, and death—and exploring solutions to uncertain, hard-to-face problems (Schmall, Cleland, and Sturdevant, 1999). Discussing such subjects can be uncomfortable for all family members. For some people, talking about potential incapacity and inability to manage finances is more difficult than talking about death.

A critical time for discussion is when a family member shows signs of deterioration or has been diagnosed with a degenerative disease such as Alzheimer's. Waiting for a situation to worsen reduces the options. Although planning does not prevent all problems, it does prepare families to act more effectively if a crisis occurs. Planning can also:

- Help avoid crisis decision making and make decisions easier in difficult times
- Reduce emotional and financial upheaval later
- Ensure that the older person's lifestyle, personal philosophies, and choices are known should a time come when the person is unable to participate in making decisions
- Decrease the possibility that the family will have to take more intrusive, restrictive actions such as petitioning the court for guardianship or conservatorship if their older family member becomes incapacitated
- Reduce disagreements and misunderstandings among family members

Families may find the following suggestions helpful in opening up discussion with a reluctant older family member (LaBuda and Schmall, 1998; Schmall, Cleland, and Sturdevant, 1999).

Look for Natural Opportunities To Talk. A natural opportunity might be a life event, such as when a friend or another family member experiences a health crisis, is diagnosed with Alzheimer's disease, or moves into a care facility; a situation reported in the media, such as a person dying without a will; or when the older person is recovering from an illness. If a parent says, "When I die . . . ," family members should listen and encourage the expression of feelings. Too often, families discourage discussion by saying things like, "Don't be so morbid," "You'll probably outlive all of us," or "We have lots of time to talk about such things."

Talk about "What Ifs." A family member might say, "If a time came when you could no longer make decisions about your own health care, who would you want to make decisions for you?" or "If you could no longer care for yourself at home, even with the help of community services, what would you want to happen?"

Share Personal Preferences and Plans in the Event of One's Own Illness or Death. It is important for adult children to remember that incapacity is not always a function of getting older. Some parents are more open to discussion when their adult children also have planned for future possibilities—for example, prepared a will, an AMD, or a durable power of attorney.

Express Good Intentions and a Willingness To Listen. The objective is to set the right tone for discussion. A loving, caring approach moves a discussion farther than an "I know what's best for you" attitude. A paternalistic approach is likely to create resistance.

An appropriate role for the nurse is to educate older clients about the benefits of planning and the importance of making plans while their capacities are intact. A positive approach is to emphasize that making plans in advance of need can give people greater control and provide greater assurance that their preferences will be known and honored.

Help Family Members Communicate Their Concerns Honestly and Positively. Open, honest communication helps build and maintain relationships, but such communication is not easy if family communication has been about "game playing." Adult sons or daughters may say only what they think a parent wants to hear or what they think will not upset a parent. However, this tends to create mistrust and wastes energy as family members "walk on eggshells" around each other.

Family members often express concerns using "you" messages; that is, telling the person what to do or not to do. An example of such a message is, "Mother, you are no longer safe living in your home. It's time for you to move into a retirement facility." The worst "you" message is a threat: "If you don't . . . then I will . . . ." "You" messages sound dictatorial, create defensiveness and resistance, and close off communication.

An older person is more likely to listen to family members who express their concern about an issue, rather than family members who talk as if it is the older person who has the problem. The nurse can suggest they use "I" messages. With a good "I" message, a person states his or her feeling, describes the specific behavior or situation of concern, and gives a concrete reason for the concern. "I" messages are specific rather than general and focus attention on problems, not personalities. An example of an "I" message is, "Mom, because of your recent fall, I'm concerned about your safety living in this house. I'm afraid you might fall again, and the next time, you might not be found for several hours or longer. Can we talk about my concern?"

The words "I am concerned about . . ." sound quite different to a person than "You should . . . ." When done correctly, "I" messages come across as "speaking from the heart." "I" messages also communicate that the person bringing up the issue or concern recognizes that what is being said is his or her belief; this leaves room for other perceptions. It also is more difficult for another person to argue with an "I" message because the speaker merely shared his or her feelings.

Adequately expressing one's concerns to an older family member is only one part of effective communication. Family members also may need help to listen actively and to empathize; that is, to understand the feelings and emotional needs of the older person. Sometimes, when family members think an older person needs to make a change—for example, move to a group-living situation or give up driving—they focus only on the change as being "for the best" and fail to acknowledge the older person's losses and feelings. The older person may experience a wide range of feelings: fear, anger, grief, helplessness, frustration, and relief. It is easier for many older persons to talk openly about their situations, concerns, and feelings if the family member listens, acknowledges, and accepts these feelings.

It is helpful if family members try to imagine how a situation looks and feels from the perspective of the older person. The nurse should encourage adult children to ask themselves, "How would I feel if I were in Dad's shoes?" Older persons who sense empathy and understanding are more willing to listen to concerns expressed by family members.

Additional communication techniques to help caregivers communicate more effectively can be found in *Taking Care of You: Powerful Tools for Caregiving* (Schmall, Cleland, and Sturdevant, 1999).

Involve the Older Person in Decision Making

Too often, the older person, especially if he or she is frail, is excluded from decisions being made about his or her own life. Family members may fail to tell the person what is happening or about the decisions under consideration. A person who is excluded from decision making is more likely to become angry, demanding, helpless, or withdrawn. Plans also are more likely to backfire.

Involvement in decision making provides greater assurance that a person will accept and adapt to a change, even if the change is not the person's preferred choice. A person who is railroaded into a new situation usually adjusts poorly. For example, studies find that nursing facility residents who are involved in the entry decision feel more in control of their lives, report higher levels of well-being, and are more likely to adjust than those who are forced to make the move (Noelker, 1994; Schmall, 1993).

Change produces anxiety, but not being involved in decisions about a potential change creates even more anxiety and an atmosphere of distrust. Even a person who cannot actively participate in making or carrying out decisions should still be informed about alternatives and plans that are being made.

Only in a few extreme cases, such as when people are afflicted with advanced Alzheimer's disease or suffering from a massive stroke, are they unable to make decisions. It is critical for a family to understand that an older family member with a memory impairment may be unable to remember discussions or agreements made. Yet the person often feels a sense of being involved in what is happening. One son stated:

> Talking to a parent about a potential move is good advice even if it does not always work out. I talked to my mother many times concerning her condition (in response to her own concerns) and we agreed on the appropriate plan. She could not remember even 30 minutes. . . ." It is well to understand that even when everything has been done with love and careful consideration, the loved one may not understand and may be unhappy. However, it is still a good idea to discuss the plan so that the family will have a feeling of doing what is right (Schmall, 1993).

Families usually must take greater control in making and carrying out decisions regarding older relatives with Alzheimer's disease or other dementia. It is unrealistic to expect the person with the disease to be able to do so. However, the older person may express anger, hostility, and rejection toward family members. A nurse should prepare family members for such reactions and help them understand that these feelings really are the result of the "pain of the situation." One person wrote about her difficult situation:

> My grandmother and I had always been close. As a result of a series of small strokes, changes occurred, which included her driving down streets in the wrong lanes. We tried talking with my grandmother about her unsafe driving, but to no avail. Finally, I had to remove her car from the premises. We talked with her about the reasons she could no longer drive and made plans for meeting her transportation needs. For weeks, my grandmother was angry and accused me of stealing her car. Of course, it hurt, but I also realized that it probably felt to my grandmother as though her car had been stolen, and because of the disease process (and her lifelong personality), it was unrealistic for me to expect her to fully comprehend the true situation.

Health care providers also need to avoid taking a paternalistic approach—that is, communicating primarily with the family about an older person's condition, care plans, and the decisions to be made even though the older person is present and capable of participating in and making decisions. As Noelker (1994) stated, "Regardless of whether the intent is to avoid fatiguing or troubling the older person, obtain the most complete and accurate information, or complete the process as quickly as possible, this approach serves to undermine the older person's sense of control and esteem."

Validate Feelings

Families experience many emotions when faced with difficult decisions and caregiving. These emotions may include grief, frustration, anger, resentment, embarrassment, or guilt. At times caregivers may wish that care receivers would die. The increasing frailty of an older family member can become a daily reminder of that person's mortality—and a caregiver's own mortality.

Family members may also need to adjust their perception of the ill person, and this can be emotionally painful. It may not be easy to accept that "my husband is no longer the strong and powerful man he once was," or "my mother who crocheted beautifully now no longer recognizes what to do with a crochet hook." It is particularly painful when a family member is no longer recognized by the person with Alzheimer's disease or a related disorder. In *The Loss of Self*, Eisdorfer and Cohen (1987) discuss the importance of caregivers "setting emotional distance"—that is, creating some detachment by viewing the family member as a person with a disease over which neither the person nor the caregiver has any control, while at the same time maintaining a closeness to the person.

Because feelings, beliefs, and attitudes influence behavior, it is important to address the belief systems and feelings of family members. When feelings are not dealt with, decisions are more likely to be made on the basis of guilt, promises, and "should's and should not's," rather than on the circumstances and what is best for everyone.

Feelings are validated by bringing them up for discussion and acknowledging their commonality. A nurse should emphasize that feelings are neither good nor bad; it is how family members act on their feelings that makes a difference.

Address Feelings of Guilt

It is important to deal with feelings of guilt family members may have. Guilt reduces objectivity and the ability to make decisions that are best for everyone. In addition, decisions made on the basis of guilt are likely to create feelings of resentment. For example, family members who feel guilty about moving a relative into a care facility are more likely to be critical of staff, overprotective of their older relative, or reluctant to visit.

Feelings of guilt generally result from the feeling that one has broken a "rule." Most guilt "rules" are black-and-white, inflexible, and impossible to conform to completely. Examples of rules include:

- "A good daughter provides care to an ailing parent."
- "You should always keep a promise."
- "I vowed we would be together for better or for worse."
- "A son doesn't tell his father what to do."
- "A loving person would never put a family member in a nursing facility."

Telling people they have no reason to feel guilty generally does not lessen the feelings of guilt. It is more desirable to help people (1) identify and examine the rules that are causing the guilt feelings; (2) evaluate the impact of that rule (a critical question to ask is, "Does the rule work to the detriment of anyone—yourself, the person receiving care, or other family members?"); and (3) rewrite the rule, often with qualifiers, to make it more realistic and appropriate to the current situation.

If a promise is the source of guilt feelings, explore with the person the conditions under which the promise was made and the current situation. Usually the conditions are quite different. Comparing "what was" with "what is" can often help a family member look more objectively at the current situation.

Emphasize Goodness of Intent of Actions

Sometimes a family member may say, "I wish I had known this information earlier. I would have done things differently." In most cases families are trying to make good decisions and do what is best. Actions are generally based on good intentions. For example, after a workshop, one woman wrote:

> A year ago, we moved Mother from Texas to Oregon. She had lived in the small Texan community all of her life, and of course, everyone knew Mom. I now realize why the move has been so difficult for Mom and that she probably would have been less lonely living in Texas, even though it would have meant moving her into a care facility. I came to the workshop feeling guilty, and I could have left the workshop feeling an even heavier load of guilt except that [the nurse] emphasized the goodness of intent behind actions. For me, this was to give Mom the help she needed, to keep Mom out of a nursing facility and in a home environment, and to add the "pleasure of family" to her life.

In working with families, it is important to start with the premise that most families are doing their best. Then a nurse can help them to discuss and reinforce the "goodness of intent" underlying their actions when the actual action taken may turn out not to be the best choice.

Recognize Your Role As Permission Giver

Because health care professionals are often looked to as "experts," their messages can carry a lot of power and authority with families. The following are 10 important messages that can be helpful for nurses to share, as appropriate, with family caregivers (Schmall, 1997):

1. **Take care of yourself.** Providing care to an older family member at the expense of the caregiver's own health or relationships with spouse or children does not benefit anyone, including the person who needs care. Although a caregiver may be unable to mitigate the impact of an illness on the older person, it is critical that the caregiver does not allow a family member's illness to destroy him or her or other family members.
2. **Maintain contact with friends and involvement in outside activities.** This is critical to caregiver well-being. Studies show that caregivers who sacrifice themselves in the care of others and remove pleasurable events from their lives can become emotionally exhausted, depressed, and physically ill. Caregivers should ask, "What happens if my family member enters a care facility or dies? Will I have been so wrapped up in caregiving that I will be 'used up' and without a life separate from caregiving?"
3. **Caregiving to adults is more stressful than child-rearing.** With a baby, a person looks forward to the child's increasing independence. But with older adult caregiving, the prognosis is generally for decline and increasing dependence, not recovery. In addition, it is generally difficult to predict how long caregiving will be needed.
4. **It is all right not to love (or like) the older person who needs care.** Not all older family members have been lovable or likable. It is important for caregivers to take into consideration personalities and past relationships as they consider their level of involvement in caregiving.
5. **Asking for help is a sign of strength.** Asking for help is not a sign of weakness, inadequacy, or failure. Knowing the limits and reaching out for assistance before a caregiver is beyond them is characteristic of a strong individual and family. It also helps to ensure high-quality care for the care receiver.
6. **Caregivers have a right to set limits and to say no.** Trying to do it all or to do it alone only makes caregivers physically and emotionally exhausted.
7. **Begin taking regular breaks early in caregiving—it is not selfish.** Breaks from the demands of caregiving are a must. They are as important to health as diet, rest, and exercise. Respite benefits the care receiver as well as the caregiver—caregivers are likely to be more loving and less exhausted. Caregivers should ask, "If my health deteriorates or I die, what will happen to my family member?" If caregivers wait until they are "burnt out," these breaks will not be enough.
8. **Make caregiving decisions based on the needs of everyone involved.** Decisions should not be made only on the basis of the needs and desires of the older person.
9. **Moving a family member into a care facility can be the most loving step to take.** It does not mean an end to a caring relationship. Being a manager and coordinator of a family member's care is just as important

as providing hands-on care. When a caregiver is no longer devoting time to meeting the person's physical and safety needs, he or she will be better able to meet the person's emotional and social needs. Having these needs met adds immensely to a person's quality of life.

10. **Caregivers should focus on what they have done well—and forgive themselves.** Too often, caregivers focus only on what they have not done or have done poorly. They should remind themselves of the many things they have done well. They should ask, "What are my personal strengths? How have I made a difference for my family member? What have I done that I feel good about?" Not everything will be as caregivers would like. At times caregivers will wish they had done things differently. They are only human. If they make a mistake, they should admit it, learn from it, and then go on.

Although family members and friends may have given these messages, many caregivers do not take such messages to heart until they hear them from a health care professional.

Recommend a Decision-Making Model to Families

Many times, families find it helpful to have a model to follow as they make decisions or solve problems. Fig. 6-2 depicts one six-step model (Schmall, Cleland, and Sturdevant, 1999).

Gather Information. The goal is for the family to make an informed decision; therefore the first step is for them to clearly identify the issue and to gather pertinent information. Families are often so concerned about making a decision or handling a difficult situation that questions which could provide a better base for decision making go unasked and unanswered. A professional assessment of the older person's health and level of function also may be needed.

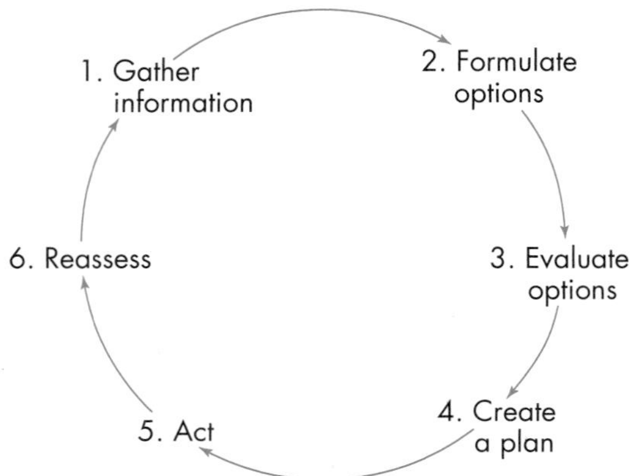

Fig. 6-2 Making a decision. (From Schmall V, Cleland M, Sturdevant M: *Taking care of you: powerful tools for caregiving*, ed 1, Portland, Ore, 1999, Legacy Health Systems.)

Formulate Options. Once the issue has been identified, the nurse should help the family see all possible options for resolving it. This involves considering the resources of the older person, the family, and the community.

This should be the brainstorming portion of decision making. By generating a variety of possible options, families increase the chances of a successful outcome. In addition, keeping the decision separate from the possible options or solutions tends to take pressure away from people defending positions.

Evaluate Options. After all options have been identified, the next step is for the family to assess the advantages and limitations of each option. It is helpful to first identify criteria or standards by which potential options will be evaluated. These can include financial constraints and personal preferences.

Agreeing on the criteria makes it easier to identify the best of the options. A good guideline to follow is, "Be easy on people; be tough on issues." Keeping the focus on the issue, not the positions people take, increases effective decision making. Nurses can help families identify potential consequences of various options.

It is critical that family members be open and honest about their abilities to fulfill any responsibilities associated with an identified alternative. Honest communication helps prevent unrealistic expectations and keeps people from feeling overwhelmed or burdened.

Create a Plan. Sometimes this is the most difficult aspect of decision making, especially if there does not seem to be a single best choice. However, identifying and evaluating all possible alternatives helps families avoid unsatisfactory decisions that may be regretted later. Also, families sometimes think that there is simply no good choice and that they must select "the best of the worst." It is important for the professional to recognize that a plan developed by one family may be quite different from a plan developed by another family whose "problem" appears to be the same.

Some families find that writing down the plan and indicating who has agreed to do which tasks by when can reduce disagreements. A written plan also can be useful later when the plan is reevaluated.

Act on the Plan. The fifth step in decision making is to put the plan into action. As with any decision, a plan should not be considered as "final and forever" because situations do change. If possible, it can be helpful to establish a trial period, approaching the decision from the perspective of "This seems like the best decision for now. Let's give it a try for 1 month, then evaluate the situation and how well our plan is working." This can be difficult to do, especially if the family wants closure to a difficult situation. However, flexibility is a key to high-quality decision making.

Reassess. It is important that the family makes plans for assessing the outcomes of the decision by asking, "How well is the plan working?" and then adjusting the plan as necessary.

Decision making is seldom easy. It is influenced by many factors, such as the specific decision being faced, the personalities of family members, the quality of family relationships and communication, whether the older person is mentally intact and capable of full participation in making the decision, whether decisions are being made in advance of need or at a time of crisis, and whether family members are living nearby or at a great distance. However, a model for decision making can provide families with a method for approaching decisions (see Fig. 6-2).

Home Care

1. Collaborate with social workers to identify community resources for assisting caregivers and homebound older adults.
2. Assist family members in discussing AMDs with homebound older adults.
3. Communicate homebound older adults' needs and progress to long-distance family members.
4. Refer caregivers to support groups to help ease burden of caring for homebound older adults with chronic illnesses.
5. Refer to a respite program so caregivers can obtain "time out" from caregiving responsibilities.
6. Collaborate with social workers when conducting family meetings aimed at reducing conflict that may occur from the stress of caring for homebound older adults.
7. Validate family members' and homebound older adults' feelings by bringing them up for discussion and acknowledging them.

SUMMARY

Providing high-quality care to older adults requires recognizing the family's role and assessing and responding to the needs of family members, particularly the caregivers. Family members should be considered as a part of the care team, not as outsiders. The nurse should invite families to share the knowledge they have gained through caregiving, particularly when placing an older relative in a care setting.

It is also important to be nonjudgmental and to remember that each family has its own history and values. Nurses need to be aware of their own values regarding what constitutes a family and their feelings about family behavior and relationships. It is important that nurses not allow personal values to prevent them from working effectively with families whose values or relationships with each other may be different. Nurses should not label such families as "dysfunctional." It is necessary to identify the strengths within each family and to build on those strengths, while at the same time recognizing the family's limitations in providing support and caregiving.

Key Points

- Families are significant in the lives of older persons and provide 80% of the support to older adults.
- Common dilemmas and decisions families face in later life involve changes in living arrangements, nursing facility placement, financial and legal issues, end-of-life medical treatments, the safety of an older family member's driving, and caregiving.
- Moving an older family member to a nursing facility is a difficult decision for most families.
- When working with older adults it is as important to address the family's needs as to focus on the older person's needs. If only the older person's needs are considered, a care plan is less likely to be successful, particularly if the family is responsible for implementing it.
- Caregiving tends to be more stressful if the care receiver has a dementing illness, behavioral problem, or emotional disturbance than if a care receiver is only physically disabled.
- The meaning a caregiver ascribes to a stressor is a stronger predictor of its impact than the actual stressor.
- Family caregivers often experience restriction of personal activities and social life, emotional strain, competing demands, role conflict, and financial stress. They may need to adjust their expectations in regard to their ill family member, themselves as caregivers, and their stage of life.
- Caregiving for frail older adults differs from providing care to children.
- Education—whether provided one-on-one or in a group setting—should be designed to empower caregivers and to increase their confidence and competence in problem solving, decision making, and applying skills.
- Respite is most effective when a caregiver begins to use it early to prevent physical and emotional exhaustion rather than to treat it.
- The family meeting is one strategy for a family to use to decide how to share caregiving responsibilities and to reach a consensus about problems, needs, and decisions.
- *Family* is more than relationships determined by blood and marital ties.
- Factors to consider in conducting a family assessment include a history of relationships, family dynamics, family roles, the impact of increased dependence of an older person on all family members, the family's ability to provide the needed care, and the nature and degree of caregiver stress.
- Strategies and considerations for nurses in working with families of older adults include:
  —Identifying who is the client and who is family
  —Conducting an assessment of the family as well as the older person
  —Encouraging families to plan in advance of need

—Helping families communicate their concerns to older relatives honestly and in positive ways
—Involving the older person in decisions to be made about his or her life
—Validating the feelings and experiences of family members
—Addressing feelings of guilt
—Emphasizing the goodness of intent of actions
—Recognizing the nurse's role as "permission giver"
—Recommending a decision-making model

- The nurse should try to "step into the shoes" of family members. Nurses who look at the situation from the perspective of a family member can increase their understanding of "where a person is coming from," and thus improve their insight and sensitivity.

Critical Thinking Exercises

1. Think about your own family relationships. What individual and family values might influence your care of an older adult and his or her family members? How might your current perceptions change over the next decade?
2. An 82-year-old woman is recovering from pneumonia. She has Alzheimer's disease and has become increasingly hostile and unmanageable in the home setting. Her 65-year-old daughter is distraught about the idea of placing her mother in a long-term care facility but feels she is not able to care for her. What is your role as nurse in this situation?

REFERENCES

Aneshensel CS et al: *Profiles in caregiving: the unexpected career,* New York, 1995, Academic Press.

Baldwin K, Shaul M: When your patient can no longer live independently: a guide to supporting the patient and family, *J Gerontol Nurs* 27(11):10, 2001.

Beedle J: *The carebook: a workbook for caregiver peace of mind,* Portland, Ore, 1997, Ladybug Press.

Beisecker A, Wright L: *Benefits and barriers to use of ADC: perceptions of family caregivers of individuals with Alzheimer's disease,* paper presented at the annual meeting of the Gerontological Society of America, San Francisco, Nov 1991.

Costa DL: *Becoming oldest-old: evidence from historical U.S. data,* Chestnut Hill, Mass, 2003, Center for Retirement Research at Boston College.

Deimling GT: The respite experience, *Benjamin Rose Inst Bul,* 3rd quarter:1, 1989.

Doty P, Jackson ME, Crown W: The impact of female caregivers' employment and status on patterns of formal and informal eldercare, *Gerontologist* 38(3):331, 1998.

Dunn L: Respite: preventing burnout, *Advice Adults Aging Parents* 2(6):2, 1987.

Eisdorfer C, Cohen D: *The loss of self,* New York, 1987, Penguin.

Fink SV, Picot SF: Nursing home placement decisions and post-placement experiences of African-American and European-American caregivers, *J Gerontol Nurs* 21(12):35, 1995.

Fortinsky RH, Hathaway TJ: Information and service needs among active and former family caregivers of persons with Alzheimer's disease, *Gerontologist* 30(5):604, 1990.

Gallagher-Thompson D: Direct services and interventions for caregivers. In Cantor MH, editor: *Family caregiving: an agenda for the future,* San Francisco, 1994, American Society on Aging.

Gallo JJ, Reichel W, Anderson L: *Handbook of geriatric assessment,* Rockville, Md, 1988, Aspen Publishers.

Goetting MA, Schmall VL: Talking with aging parents about finances, *J Home Econ* 85(1):42, 1993.

Greenwell L, Bengston VL: Geographic distance and contact between middle-aged children and their parents: the effects of social class over 20 years, *J Gerontol Soc Sci* 52B(1):S13, 1997.

Gregerson D: *Organizing your family records,* EC 1302, Corvallis, Ore, 1993, Oregon State University Extension Service.

Hughes R: *The demographics of divorce—United States and Missouri,* retrieved June 18, 2004, from http://missourifamilies.org/features/divorcearticles/divorcefeature17.htm.

Kinsella K, Velkoff VA: *An aging world,* Washington, DC, 2001, US Department of Health and Human Services, US Department of Commerce, National Institutes of Health, National Institute on Aging, US Census Bureau.

LaBuda D, Schmall V: *Home sweet home: how to help older adults live independently,* Appleton, Wis, 1998, Aid Association for Lutherans.

Lawton MP, Brody EM, Saperstein A: Respite care for Alzheimer's families: research findings and their relevance to providers, *Am J Alzheimer's Care Rel Disord Res,* Nov-Dec 1989.

Malone-Beach EE, Zarit SH, Spore DL: Caregivers' perceptions of case management and community-based services: barriers to service use, *J Appl Gerontol* 11(2):145, 1992.

National Alliance for Caregiving: *Family caregiver fact sheet,* Bethesda, Md, 1997, National Alliance for Caregiving.

Neal MB, Ingersoll-Dayton B, Starrels ME: Gender and relationship differences in caregiving patterns and consequences among employed caregivers, *Gerontologist* 37(6):804, 1997.

Niederehe G, Funk J: *Family interaction with dementia patients: caregiver styles and their correlates,* paper presented at the 95th annual convention of the American Psychological Association, New York, 1987.

Noelker LS: The interface between health and social services and family caregivers. In Cantor MH, editor: *Family caregiving: an agenda for the future,* San Francisco, 1994, American Society on Aging.

Norton SA, Talerico KA: Facilitating end-of-life decision making: strategies for communicating and assessing, *J Gerontol Nurs* 26(9):6, 2000.

Office of Technology Assessment: *Losing a million minds: confronting the tragedy of Alzheimer's disease and other dementias,* OTA-BA-323, Washington, DC, 1987, US Government Printing Office.

Oregon Health Care Decisions: *Making health care decisions when you can't speak for yourself,* Portland, Ore, 1995, Oregon Health Decisions.

Partners Program: best nursing practices in care for older adults, New York, 2003, John A. Hartford Foundation Institute for Geriatric Nursing.

Persson D: The elderly driver: deciding when to stop, *Gerontologist* 33(1):88, 1993.

Plowfield LA, Raymond JE, Blevins C: Wholism for aging families: meeting needs of caregivers, *Holistic Nurs Pract* 14(4):51, 2000.

Safe Senior Citizen Driving: *Seniors on the road,* retrieved June 14, 2004, from http://www.helpguide.org/aging/senior_citizen_driving.htm.

Schmall V: Ten caregiver tips, *Columbia-Willamette Alzheimer's Assoc Newsletter* 15(4):7, Fall 1997.

Schmall V: Dealing with Alzheimer's disease: caregiver issues, *Consultant Pharmacist* 11:22, 1996.

Schmall V: Family caregiver education and training: enhancing self-efficacy, *J Case Manage* 4(4):35, 1995.

Schmall V: Family caregiving: a training and education perspective. In Cantor MH, editor: *Family caregiving: an agenda for the future,* San Francisco, 1994, American Society on Aging.

Schmall V: *Choosing when there is no choice: the nursing home decision,* Alexandria, Va, 1993, American College of Health Care Administrators.

Schmall V, Cleland M, Sturdevant M: *Taking care of you: powerful tools for caregiving,* ed 1, Portland, Ore, 1999, Legacy Health Systems.

Schmall V, Nay T: *Helping your older family member handle finances,* Corvallis, Ore, 1993, Oregon State University Extension Service.

Schmall V, Staton M, Weaver D: *Families and aging: dilemmas and decisions—an educational board game,* Corvallis, Ore, 1995, Oregon State University Extension Service.

Schmall V, Stiehl R: *Coping with caregiving: how to manage stress when caring for elderly relatives,* Pacific Northwest Extension Publication, PNW 315, Corvallis, Ore, 1998, Oregon State University Extension Service.

Schmall V, Stiehl R: *Living arrangements in later life,* Pacific Northwest Extension Publication, PNW 318, Corvallis, Ore, 1994, Oregon State University Extension Service.

Schmall V, Webb LC: Respite and adult day care for rural elders. In Krout JA, editor: *Providing community based services to the rural elderly: research and practice,* Thousand Oaks, Calif, 1993, Sage Publications.

Stiehl R, Bessey B: *Managing learning in high performance organizations,* Corvallis, Ore, 1993, Learning Organization.

Teresi JA: Prevalence of behavior disorder and disturbance to family and staff in a sample of adult day healthcare clients, *Gerontologist* (37)5:629, 1997.

Toft D: Bibliotherapy: always a key component of recovery, *Hazelden News Professional Update* 1-3, Jan 1993.

Wright AD, Lund DA, Caserta M: *The use of respite services by caregivers of dementia patients: an analysis of time-use strategies,* poster presentation by National Council on Family Relations, Seattle, Nov 1990.

Zarit SH: Research perspectives on family caregiving. In Cantor MH, editor: *Family caregiving: an agenda for the future,* San Francisco, 1994, American Society on Aging.

Zarit SH, Zarit JM: *Mental disorders in older adults,* New York, 1998, Guilford Press.

7 Socioeconomic and Environmental Influences

SUE E. MEINER, EdD, APRN, BC, GNP

Learning Objectives

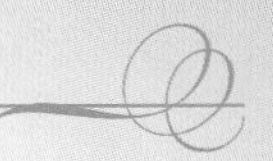

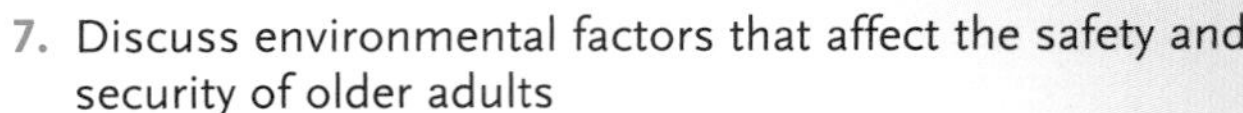

On completion of this chapter, the reader will be able to:

1. Identify the major socioeconomic and environmental factors that influence the health of older adults.
2. Explain the importance of age cohorts in understanding older adults.
3. Describe the economic factors that influence the lives of older persons.
4. Distinguish between the Medicare and Medicaid programs.
5. Discuss the influence of support systems on the health and well-being of older adults.
6. Distinguish between a conservator, guardian, and durable power of attorney.
7. Discuss environmental factors that affect the safety and security of older adults
8. Compare and contrast the housing options available for older adults.
9. Compare the influences of income, education, and health status on quality of life.
10. Analyze the effect of criminal victimization on the lives of older adults.
11. Relate strategies for protecting older persons in the community from criminal victimization.
12. Assess the ability of older adults to be their own advocate.

We are all products not only of our genetic inheritance but also of our environment and our life experiences. Social status, economic conditions, and environment influence our health and our response to illness. This chapter discusses the socioeconomic and environmental conditions that influence the way older adults respond to the health care system.

Socioeconomic factors such as income, level of education, present health status, and availability of support systems all affect the way older adults perceive the health care system. Benefits and entitlements may influence the availability of high-quality health care. A small number of older adults may not be competent to manage their own health care; they need the protection of a conservator or guardian (see Chapter 3). Environmental factors such as geographic area, housing, perceived criminal victimization, and community resources make a difference in older adults' needs for health care. One of the strongest and most consistent predictors of illness and death is socioeconomic status (Krause, 1997). The environment also influences safety and well-being. Therefore it is imperative that health care professionals understand the socioeconomic and environmental status of older adults. Although, in some cases, illness can lead to poverty, more often poverty causes poor health by its connection with inadequate nutrition, substandard housing, exposure to environmental hazards, unhealthy lifestyles, and decreased access to and use of health care services.

In 2002 research found that the nation's health has continued to improve overall, in part because of the resources that have been devoted to health education, public health programs, health research, and health care. The United States spends more per capita than any other country on health care, and the rate of increase in spending is going up. Much of this spending is on health care that controls or reduces the impact of chronic diseases and conditions affecting an increasingly older population; notable examples are prescription drugs and cardiac operations. The older population also averaged more physician contacts than persons under age 65, with 11 contacts versus 5 contacts (US Census Bureau, 2004-2005).

Older adult health care consumers often depend on the health care professional for advocacy. To be an effective advocate, the nurse must understand the factors that shape the older consumer's perceptions of environment, socioeconomic status, and access to health care.

SOCIOECONOMIC FACTORS

Age Cohorts

Persons who share the experience of a particular event or time in history are grouped together in what is called a *cohort*. They shared certain experiences at similar stages of physical, psychologic, and social development that influenced the way they perceive the world. Therefore they develop attitudes and values that are similar (Cox, 1986; Richardson, 1996). By understanding cohorts, the nurse develops a greater understanding of older adults' value systems. For example, persons who reached maturity in the Depression learned the value of having a job and working hard to keep it. Generally, persons in this cohort have been loyal workers. They feel better if they are "doing their jobs." The nurse might increase compliance with a treatment regimen by referring to the need for compliance as an older adult's "job."

Cohort classifications include age, historical events, and geographic area of residence. Today's older Americans have shared many momentous experiences. The "Roaring Twenties," the Depression, and World War II made impressions on everyone who lived through those events, but especially on those who were young at the time. Values and pace of life, which vary between communities and regions of the country, influence the perceptions of the residents of different areas.

The age cohort that reached young adulthood in the post–World War II era benefited from a very productive time in American history. The late 1940s, 1950s, and 1960s were times of rapidly increasing earnings and heavy spending. Strong unions negotiated for better pension plans and medical benefits. This cohort became accustomed to contacting professionals for services, thereby becoming more conscious of preventive health care than previous generations. This group has become aware of wellness techniques and self-care strategies that improve health. Members of this cohort usually have at least a high school education and often have some form of higher education. Many pursued further educational opportunities. As a group, however, they experience a less cohesive family life. Many have moved from their home communities and have experienced divorce, remarriage, or other circumstances that complicate family support (Johnson, 1992).

The age cohort that matured just before and during World War II was strongly influenced by the war. Many persons gained identity and status by participating in the war. Those who served in the armed forces were shaped by their direct involvement, whereas most of those at home worked in the defense industry; experienced rationing of food, clothing, and fuel; and waited for the men and women in the service to come home. Life revolved around the war. Movies and music featured war themes, and rationing was a reminder that all resources were needed primarily for the war effort. Signs and billboards urged people to sign up or to purchase war bonds. Windows of houses displayed stars to honor family members who were serving or who had died in the war.

The work force was expanded to include more women, many of whom continued to work after the war. In 1940, 12 million women were working; by 1945, 19 million women were working (Wapner, Demick, and Redondo, 1990). Men and women serving in the armed forces became accustomed to regular physical and dental checkups, and they extended these practices to their families after the war. Many veterans took advantage of the G.I. Bill to pursue a college education, which would have unobtainable otherwise. With the help of veterans' benefits, they purchased houses for little or no money down. Having experienced the trauma of war, this group developed an appetite for the good things in life and willingly paid for them.

Today the oldest Americans are strongly influenced by having lived through the Great Depression of the 1930s. At the time, today's oldest older adults (ages 95 and older) were struggling to keep families together, and today's younger older adults were attempting to find work and start families. The struggles of those times have shaped the lives of older Americans over age 80.

Persons of this era are generally frugal and often do not spend money, even if they have it. The oldest older adults fear they will outlive their money, since they remember what it is like to have nothing. In addition, this age cohort did not have the experience of receiving regular health care. Visits to the doctor or dentist occurred only when absolutely necessary, with home remedies used as the first line of defense. Education often ended with the eighth grade so children could help support the family. A college education was rare.

During this era, families were close and supportive. However, the family was a closed unit, and personal matters remained within the family. Unhappy family situations, mental illness, family finances, and abusive situations were not usually discussed outside the family. Gender roles were well defined.

Many of today's conveniences, including antibiotics, were not available during the 1930s. The technology now used in health care settings, ranging from electronic thermometers to computed tomography and positron emission tomography scanners, represent a true technologic explosion to persons who have witnessed its development. Today's older adult cohort has survived many significant changes.

Income Sources

Income and income sources for older adults differ according to age. Although income generally decreases with age, net worth peaks among householders ages 65 to 69. However, even though net worth decreases with advancing age, it remains substantial in older age-groups (Table 7-1). For those with property and money to invest, this is primarily a result of home equity increases and investments producing a higher yield.

Social Security is the primary income source for Americans over age 65. This federal government package of protection provides benefits for retired individuals, survivors of participants, and the disabled. Funds for Social Security are derived from payroll taxes, and benefits are earned by accumulating credits based on annual income. A person can earn up to four credits a year by working and paying Social

Security taxes. In 1998 a person received one credit for each $700 in earnings up to a maximum of four credits a year. The number of credits needed to receive retirement benefits depends on the date of birth. Those born in 1929 or later need 40 credits (10 years of work). Those born before 1929 need fewer than 40 credits (e.g., 39 credits if born in 1928, 38 credits if born in 1927) (*Retirement,* 1997).

Retirement age in the United States is not mandatory but is usually age 65. A person can begin receiving Social Security retirement benefits as early as age 62. However, if a person begins receiving early benefits, monthly payments will be lower. Those born before 1938 are eligible for full Social Security benefits at age 65. However, beginning in 2003 the age at which full benefits are payable began increasing in gradual steps from 65 to 67 (Table 7-2). For those who wish to delay retirement, the benefit increases by a certain percentage depending on the year of birth. The yearly rate of increase varies from 3% for those born before 1924 to 8% for those born in 1943 or later (*Retirement,* 1997).

Social Security earnings must be limited, since the purpose of the program is to provide continuing income to a retired worker when traditional work income is cut off or reduced. Benefits are reduced if a person earns more than the exempt amount (Box 7-1). After age 70 there is no reduction in benefits. Only earnings from employment or self-employment are included. Income from savings, pensions, and investments do not count against benefits (*SSI,* 1993).

Very poor older adults depend on another federal government program. Supplemental Security Income (SSI) pays monthly checks to persons who are aged, disabled, or sight impaired, and who have few assets and minimum income. This program is also regulated by the Social Security Administration, but the money to provide benefits is from income tax sources rather than Social Security payroll taxes. Eligibility depends on income and assets. A single person received $494 per month, and a couple received $741 per month in 1998. Some states add money to this basic rate (*Understanding the Benefits,* 1998).

TABLE 7-1 Family Net Worth—Mean and Median of Net Worth by Selected Characteristics: 1995

CHARACTERISTIC	PERCENT OF FAMILIES	NET WORTH (IN THOUSANDS) MEAN	MEDIAN
All ages	100%	$205.9	$56.4
Under 35 years old	27.2%	47.2	11.4
35 to 44 years old	23.4%	144.5	48.5
45 to 54 years old	14.4%	277.8	90.5
55 to 64 years old	13.9%	356.2	110.8
65 to 74 years old	12.0%	331.6	104.1
75 years and older	9.0%	276.0	95.0

From US Census Bureau: *Statistical abstract of the United States: 1997,* ed 117, Washington, DC, 1997, US Government Printing Office.

TABLE 7-2 Age to Receive Full Social Security Benefits

YEAR OF BIRTH	FULL RETIREMENT AGE
1937 or earlier	65
1938	65 and 2 months
1939	65 and 4 months
1940	65 and 6 months
1941	65 and 8 months
1942	65 and 10 months
1943-1954	66
1955	66 and 2 months
1956	66 and 4 months
1957	66 and 6 months
1958	66 and 8 months
1959	66 and 10 months
1960 or later	67

From *Understanding the benefits,* Baltimore, 1998, US Department of Health and Human Services, Social Security Administration.

Ages 55 to 64. Those in the preretirement age cohort of 55 to 64 are generally in their peak earning years. Most are married, but few have children under age 18 still residing in the family home. The heavy expenses of child rearing are over, and homeowners have completely or nearly paid for their homes. This age cohort tends to have an increased disposable income yet is acutely aware of impending retirement; thus saving and investing are priorities.

Income sources for this age-group are diverse. Most members of the group are still working; thus wage and salary earnings are substantial. Households often have two incomes, since more women in this age-group work. However, the

BOX 7-1 Social Security Earnings Limits

Social Security beneficiaries under age 70 receive full benefits as long as their earnings are under the limits indicated below. Figures are for 1998.

Ages 70 or older—No limit on earnings

Ages 65 to 69—$14,500; for every $3 over the limit, $1 is withheld from benefits

Under age 65—$9,120; for every $2 over the limit, $1 is withheld from benefits

Disabled individual—$500 per month

From *Social Security Update 1998,* Baltimore, 1998, US Department of Health and Human Services, Social Security Administration.

number of men in this age-group participating in the labor force has fallen dramatically since 1970. Those who are displaced from their jobs before the age of 60 experience a loss in earnings of 39%, and the rate of health insurance coverage is 16% lower than for those who are employed (Couch, 1998). Many retire early (between ages 60 and 65), and those who do so tend to have strong pension packages. For those over age 62, Social Security may provide part of their income. Interest and investment dividends contribute to income, but the income from these sources is usually insignificant (Wapner, Demick, and Redondo, 1990).

Persons in this age-group are generally healthy and have resources to maintain housing. The average annual income of families ages 55 to 64 is approximately over $48,000. This group has been vested in pension plans most of their working lives, and because of higher earnings, they have contributed more to Social Security than older age-groups. Many held jobs with disability benefits, which now may be contributing to income. Those who served in the armed forces may be eligible for veterans' benefits.

Ages 65 to 74. Retirement ordinarily causes income to decrease by about 35% or more. The median income before taxes for households ages 65 to 74 is $27,000, which is approximately $11,000 less than the median income of households in the 55 to 64 age bracket (US Census Bureau, 2004-2005). This reduction in income is often offset by reduced expenditures associated with working, such as transportation, clothing, and meals (Table 7-3). In this age-group 19% of household heads continue to work. However, only half of those wage earners bring home more than $12,500 per year (US Census Bureau, 2004). The work is generally part time, so the portion of household income from wages and salary is reduced.

Of the persons in this age-group, 95% receive Social Security income. Almost half of the households in this group have income from pensions. For those who have investments, earnings from this source are about twice the investment earnings of younger retirees or preretirees. Only about 4% receive disability payments, since jobs offering disability benefits were rare until recently (US Census Bureau, 2004-2005).

Today this age-group includes many veterans from World War II. In 1994 there were close to 8.6 million veterans ages 65 or older. About 4% were women (US Census Bureau, 2004-2005). Veterans' benefits are important to this age-group because of the increased risk of chronic disease and other acute health problems. Eligibility for veterans' benefits is based on military service, service-related disability, and income. Benefits are considered on an individual basis (*Federal benefits for veterans and dependents,* 1993) (Box 7-2). Although benefits such as Medicare, food stamps, and housing assistance are not often thought of as income, they are factors used when assessing the poverty status of older adults in the United States.

TABLE 7-3 Average Annual Income and Expenditures of All Consumer Units (in Dollars): 1995

CHARACTERISTIC	ALL UNITS	55 TO 64 YEARS OLD	65 YEARS AND OLDER
Income before taxes	40,611	45,264	28,301
Total expenditures	32,277	32,604	22,265
Food: total	4,505	4,539	3,388
At home	2,803	2,832	2,367
Away from home	1,702	1,707	1,021
Housing: total	10,466	10,291	7,590
Shelter	5,932	5,358	3,668
Fuel, utilities, public services	2,193	2,442	1,982
Household operations and furnishings	2,341	2,491	1,940
Apparel and services	1,704	1,833	876
Transportation	6,016	5,726	3,377
Health care	1,732	1,909	2,647
Insurance and pensions	2,967	3,211	802
Entertainment	1,612	1,577	929
Personal care products	403	407	326
Reading and education	634	680	294
Miscellaneous	1,035	1,262	742
Cash contributions	925	1,043	1,101
Personal taxes	3,055	3,128	1,083

From US Census Bureau: *Statistical abstract of the United States: 1997,* ed 117, Washington, DC, 1997, US Government Printing Office.

Ages 75 to 84. After age 75, women outnumber men in American society. Many persons in this age-group live alone, which affects their average household income. Most women in this age-group did not work outside the home, so their incomes depend on their spouses' pensions or Social Security benefits. Surviving spouses with no work experience receive about two thirds of the overall income earned before the death of their spouses (Wapner, Demick, and Redondo, 1990).

When persons in this age-group were working, salaries and wages were much lower; thus they contributed less to Social Security. Pensions were less generous or nonexistent.

BOX 7-2 Veterans' Benefits

Benefits for eligible veterans include:

- Disability compensation
- Pension
- Education and training
- Home loan guaranties
- Life insurance
- Burial benefits
- Health care benefits

These factors combine to reduce the income range of most persons in this age-group.

Since few persons in this age-group are employed and most who still work are self-employed, wages and salaries are a small income factor. Social Security is the most important factor. Pensions are available to fewer persons, and those who receive pensions receive less than younger age-groups. Income from investments increases slightly (Wapner, Demick, and Redondo, 1990).

As health problems increase with age, so do expenses for prescriptions and assistive devices such as eyeglasses, hearing aids, and dentures. The quality of housing deteriorates as the houses age and less money is available for maintenance. Decreased strength and endurance reduce the ability to conduct household chores. Income is reduced as expenses increase.

Ages 85 and Older. This group is the fastest growing segment of our population (Table 7-4). Although the life span of Americans has been prolonged by medical and social advances, this age cohort is at risk for an increase in chronic disease, resulting in decreased ability to perform activities of daily living (ADLs) and increased expenses for assistance, assistive devices, and medication (US Census Bureau, 2004-2005; Van Nostrand, Furner, and Suzman, 1993).

TABLE 7-4 Population 65 Years Old and Older by Gender and Age-group: 1980 to 1996

	PERCENT DISTRIBUTION		
GENDER AND AGE-GROUP	1980	1990	1996
ALL PERSON			
65 years and older	100	100	100
65 to 69 years old	34	32	29
70 to 74 years old	27	26	26
75 to 79 years old	19	20	20
80 to 84 years old	12	13	14
85 years and older	9	10	11
MEN			
65 years and older	100	100	100
65 to 69 years old	38	36	33
70 to 74 years old	28	27	28
75 to 79 years old	18	19	20
80 to 84 years old	10	11	12
85 years and older	7	7	8
WOMEN			
65 years and older	100	100	100
65 to 69 years old	32	30	27
70 to 74 years old	26	25	25
75 to 79 years old	19	20	20
80 to 84 years old	13	14	15
85 years and older	10	12	14

From US Census Bureau: *Statistical abstract of the United States: 1997,* ed 117, Washington, DC, 1997, US Government Printing Office.

This group has the lowest average annual income level (under $15,000) of all older Americans (US Census Bureau, 2004). Social Security is the primary income source, although fewer members of this group are covered by Social Security. Pension and investment income is less than for younger groups, whereas SSI is increased. More members of this age-group receive assistance from family, but the amount is small and often sporadic. Few receive wages or salary.

The 85 and older group is more likely to need assistance with ADLs. They are also more likely to need institutional and home care (US Census Bureau, 2004; Van Nostrand, Furner, and Suzman, 1993). Dependence on medication and assistive devices increases.

If persons in this age-group live independently, their housing is likely to be old and in need of repairs and maintenance (Mack et al, 1997). Adaptations to compensate for decreasing abilities help older adults remain in their homes, but these changes can be costly. Some older adults choose to move in with family or to facilities that offer assistance.

The nation's political climate or financial stability can affect the sources of income of older adults at any time. Decreased interest earnings, for example, affect those with money market investments or certificates of deposit; stock market fluctuations affect the value of stock portfolios and mutual funds; and the political climate affects the type and amount of taxes paid. Social Security and SSI are indexed for inflation. As Atchley (1992) states, "Ironically, while low income people often have inadequate funds, the amount they do receive is more secure against economic shifts than the incomes of those in higher earning brackets" (see Cultural Awareness box).

Poverty

In 1996 almost one fifth (18.4%) of those ages 65 and older were classified as poor or near-poor, with income between the poverty level and 125% of this level (American Association of Retired Persons (AARP), 1997). One of every 11 (9.4%) older white adults are poor, compared with one fourth (25.3%) of older black adults and one fourth (24.4%) of older Hispanic adults. The poverty rate for older women is 13.6%, whereas the rate for older men is 6.8%. Almost half (47.5%) of older black women who live alone are poor. The poverty rate is also high for those who live in metropolitan areas or the South, have not completed high school, or are too ill or disabled to work (AARP, 1997; US Census Bureau, 2004). When the income of older adults is calculated, government benefits such as Medicare, food stamps, and subsidized housing are considered part of the income.

Older black and Hispanic adults are more vulnerable to poverty than are whites. Many are more likely to have held low-paying jobs with few or no benefits. They are less educated (Table 7-5) than whites (US Census Bureau, 2004).

Inadequate income may affect the quality of life for older adults. For example, basics such as housing and diet may

Cultural Awareness

CULTURAL DIFFERENCES IN THE HEALTH PRACTICES OF ECONOMICALLY DISADVANTAGED OLDER ADULTS

Gender and ethnic differences in personal health practices were examined with a sample of 1021 Medicaid recipients ages 65 and older. Six health practices were studied, including never smoking cigarettes, not currently smoking cigarettes, limiting consumption of alcoholic beverages, exercising regularly, maintaining desirable weight for height, and maintaining adequate social networks.

Although gender differences were noted with respect to all the health practices examined, neither men nor women consistently adhered to desirable health practices. Women were more likely than men to refrain from smoking and drinking, risk factors that have been linked to major health consequences. Ethnicity was also a factor in all the health practices examined. Hispanic and black older adults were very similar to whites, whereas Asian/Pacific Islander older adults generally adhered to more desirable health practices than did whites, blacks, or Hispanics. Hispanics ages 75 and older were twice as likely as whites to engage in physical exercise. Older blacks were only half as likely to maintain recommended body weights as whites. Generally, Asian/Pacific Islanders ages 65 to 74 engaged in more desirable health practices than did whites—not smoking, limiting drinking, and getting regular exercise. The implications of these findings could benefit health promotion programs for low-income older adults.

Modified from Lubben JE, Weiler PG, Chi I: Gender and ethnic differences in the health practices of the elderly poor, *J Clin Epidemiol* 42(8):725, 1989.Modified from Supportive Care Services Committee: *City of Hope patient handbook for cancer pain management*, Duarte, Calif, 1994, City of Hope National Medical Center.

be inadequate. An aging wardrobe and lack of transportation may cause the older adult to avoid social contact, leading to isolation. Older adults may delay seeking medical help or may not follow through with the prescribed treatment or medications because of limited income. Eyeglasses, hearing aids, and dental work may become unaffordable luxuries. Identifying an older client's income level enables the nurse to direct the client to agencies and services that are available to those with limited resources (Fig. 7-1).

Education

Education has been shown to have a strong relationship to health risk factors (Brown, 1995). The level of education influences earning ability, information absorption, problem-solving ability, value systems, and lifestyle behaviors. The more educated person often has greater access to wellness programs and preventive health options (Land et al, 1994).

The education level of the older population has been steadily increasing, reflecting increased mandatory education and better educational opportunities in the last 50 years. The percentage of individuals who completed high school varies by race and ethnic origin. In 1995, 67% of older white adults had completed high school, compared with 37% of black Americans and 30% of Hispanics (AARP, 1997; US Census Bureau, 1996).

Many older adults are continuing their education in their later years. In 1994-1995, 15% of those over age 65 participated in adult education courses (US Census Bureau, 1996). Some are completing high school or taking college courses. High school equivalency programs and reduced college tuition foster this trend. Others take advantage of continuing education programs such as Elderhostel to explore subjects of interest. The Elderhostel program offers opportunities for persons over age 60 and their spouses to attend courses on specific topics, often held in 1-week segments on college campuses throughout the world. Low costs, made possible by volunteer professional instructors, on-campus housing, and other cost-saving factors, make the programs available to many.

Seeking educational opportunities in later life has many benefits for older adults. Of those enrolled in adult education, 86% give personal or social reasons for participating. Lifelong learning promotes intellectual growth, increases self-esteem, and enhances socialization. Older adults have an opportunity to stimulate creativity and to remain alert and involved with the world (Clough, 1992; Penning and Wasyliw, 1992). Erikson's seventh stage of development stresses the importance of generativity versus stagnation to the individual's sense of achievement and fulfillment in life (Cox, 1986). Education provides an opportunity to avoid stagnation and isolation, and adds to the enjoyment of later life (Box 7-3).

TABLE 7-5 Educational Attainment of Older Adults by Age: 1996

	PERCENTAGE OF POPULATION—HIGHEST LEVEL			
AGE	HIGH SCHOOL GRADUATE	ASSOCIATE'S DEGREE	BACHELOR'S DEGREE	ADVANCED DEGREE
55 to 64 years old	37	5.4	11.8	8.4
65 to 74 years old	36.3	3.6	9.3	5.6
75 years and older	30.8	3.1	8.3	4.3

From US Census Bureau, *Statistical abstract of the United States: 1997*, ed 117, Washington, DC, 1997, US Government Printing Office.

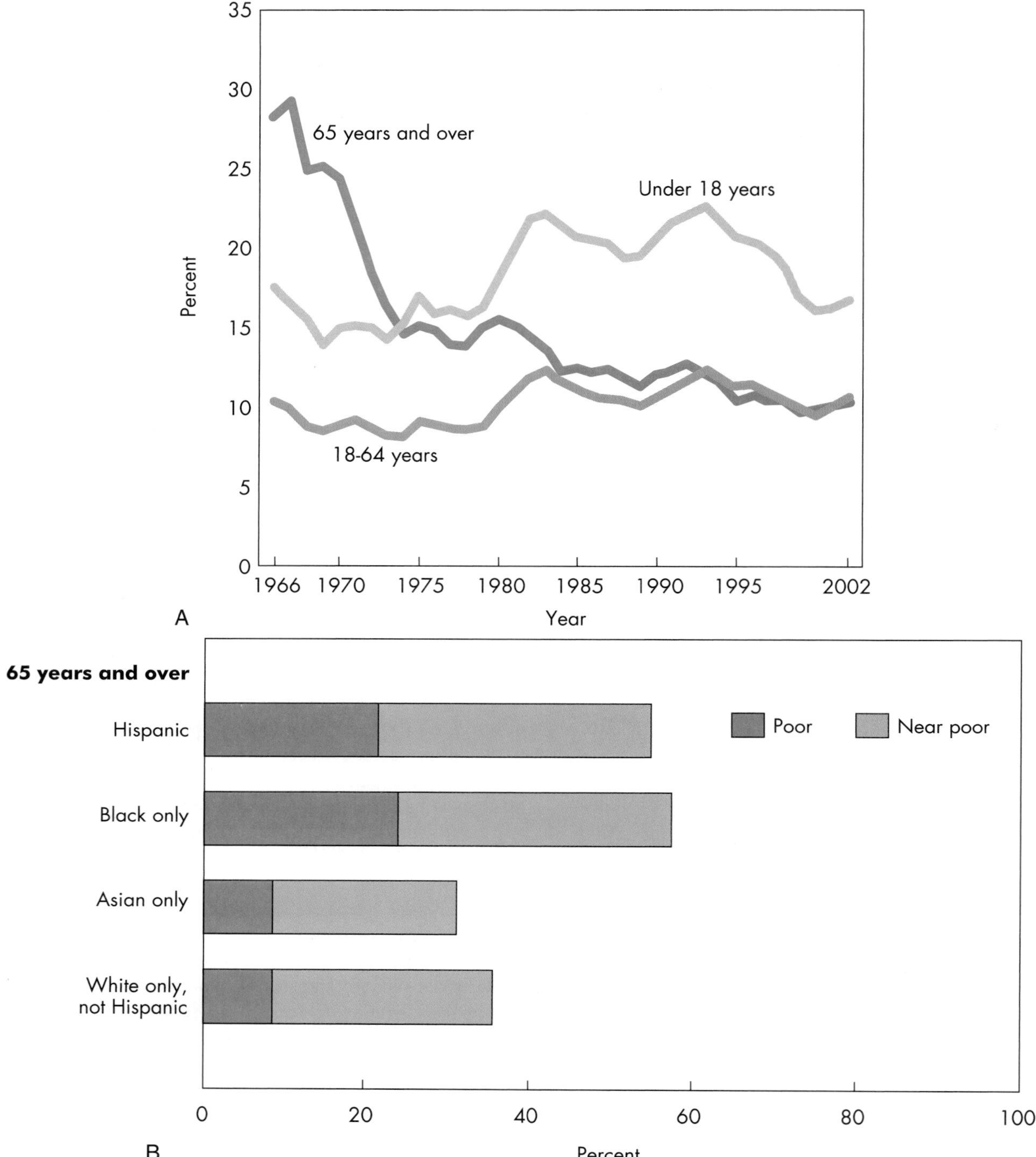

Fig. 7-1 **A,** Poverty rates by age: United States, 1966-2002. **B,** Low-income population by age, race, and Hispanic origin: United States, 1950-2050. NOTES: Poor is defined as family income less than 100% of the poverty level, and near poor as 100% to 199% of the poverty level. Persons of Hispanic origin may be of any race. Black and Asian races include persons of Hispanic and non-Hispanic origin. (From US Census Bureau, Current Population Survey, 2003.)

BOX 7-3 Client Teaching Strategies

Older adults often have short-term memory deficits or limited vision or hearing abilities that affect teaching. To improve comprehension and compliance, consider the following suggestions:

- Provide a comfortable environment with adequate lighting and minimal distractions.
- Repeat important information at least three times.
- Present information in several forms: written material, discussion, video and audio tape, and photos and pictures.
- With written material, use large print and clear black letters on a contrasting background.
- Speak at a moderate pace and volume with a low tone of voice. Check for understanding by asking the patient to explain in his or her own words.
- Use appropriate gestures to enhance understanding.
- Check back later to assess understanding.

Health Status

The health status of older adults influences their socioeconomic status. Persons over age 65 have an average of two chronic conditions (Lorig, 1993). The most common chronic problems in 1994 were arthritis (50%), followed by hypertension (36%), heart disease (32%), hearing impairments (29%), cataracts (17%), orthopedic impairments (16%), sinusitis (15%), and diabetes (10%) (US Census Bureau, 2004). The influence health problems exert often depends on the older person's perception of the problem. Among noninstitutionalized persons, 74.3% of those ages 65 to 74 consider their health to be good, very good, or excellent compared with others their age, as do 66.8% of those 75 and over (US Census Bureau, 1996). Some approach health problems with an attitude of acceptance, whereas others find that chronic problems require considerable energy, and they spend extensive time and resources to find ways to cope or adapt (Burke and Flaherty, 1993).

Functional status is affected by chronic conditions. The Centers for Disease Control and Prevention (CDC) reports in *Healthy Aging for Older Americans* (2004) that functional status is important because it serves as an indicator of an older adult's ability to remain independent in the community. Functional ability is measured by the individual's ability to perform ADLs and instrumental activities of daily living (IADLs). ADLs include six personal care activities: eating, toileting, bathing, transferring, dressing, and continence. The term *IADLs* refers to the following home-management activities: preparing meals, shopping, managing money, using the telephone, doing light housework, doing laundry, using transportation, and taking medications appropriately. Data concerning the ability to perform ADLs and IADLs were gathered through the National Health Interview Survey. For more information on chronic conditions and their impact, see Chapter 17.

Nurses can work with older adults to prolong independence by encouraging self-management of chronic conditions. Self-management is defined as learning and practicing the skills necessary to carry on an active and emotionally satisfying life in the face of a chronic condition (Lubkin and Larsen, 2002). Education and support help older adults make informed choices, practice good health behaviors, and take responsibility for the care of a chronic condition.

The amount of money available for food, shelter, clothing, and recreation can be greatly affected by the cost of medication, health care equipment, glasses, hearing aids, dental care, medical care, home care assistance, and nursing facility care, some of which may not be covered by insurance programs. In addition, the insurance premiums themselves may cause financial distress. Restricted finances can affect the safety of the environment, nutritional status, and social opportunities, which can result in an altered quality of life.

By making older adults aware of programs such as equipment loan programs, as well as optical, auditory, and dental assistance programs, the nurse can help them receive services necessary to maintain health status and thus to maximize quality of life even though finances are restricted.

Insurance Coverage

Older Americans should review their insurance coverage often to see if the coverage they have is necessary, appropriate, and adequate. Residential insurance purchased several years ago may be inadequate today. For example, home insurance should cover at least 80% of the replacement cost; however, many older adult homeowners are insured for the assessed value of the home when it was purchased. Content and liability coverage may also be inadequate. Older homeowners may be unaware that policies are outdated, or they may not be able to afford the premiums an update would require. An insurance checkup would reveal inadequacies. Older adults may wish to investigate several insurance companies to find the best coverage for the least cost. AARP publishes information related to insurance needs (AARP, 2005).

Many older adults have automobiles that have reached maximum depreciation. These automobile owners may still be carrying full coverage when all they need is liability insurance. They may also be able to save money by investigating senior discounts, choosing higher deductibles, and comparing premiums from several companies. Completion of a defensive driving course such as the AARP Driver Safety (2005) program may help older adults qualify for lower insurance rates.

Life insurance is valuable when providing for dependents. In old age the primary reason for life insurance is to cover burial expenses. A single-term policy would accomplish this purpose. Many older adults can substantially reduce life insurance coverage. Proceeds from those policies and premium payments that are no longer due may be redirected for greater benefit.

Health insurance is a necessity for older adults because medical problems—and therefore medical expenses—increase with age. As persons age, they visit the doctor more often (US Census Bureau, 2004). Older adults spend more time in the hospital—an average of 6.8 days—compared with the average of 4.5 days spent by those under age 65 (AARP, 1997; US Census Bureau, 2004). They also require more long-term care. Those persons ages 65 to 74 represent only 12.5% of the long-term care population, whereas older adults ages 75 to 84 make up 57.7% of that population, and those over age 85 are 22% of that population (Van Nostrand, Furner, and Suzman, 1993).

Prescription drug and other assistance programs began in 2004. Eligibility for the Medicare-approved drug discount card requires that the person have Medicare Part A and /or Part B and are not receiving outpatient prescription drug benefits through Medicaid. Some state pharmacy assistance programs that are not Medicaid can still support eligibility for the drug card program. The savings can be between 11% and 18% on many brand-name drugs and even more on generic drugs. This benefit is available regardless of income level. The cost is currently $30 annually for a drug card. If the older adult has limited income, the annual enrollment fee can be waived, and an additional $600 credit could be available (Medicare, 2005).

Medicare is a federal health insurance program for persons over age 65 or persons of any age who are disabled or have permanent kidney failure. Medicare has two parts: hospital insurance and medical insurance.

Part A, the hospital insurance, helps pay for inpatient hospital care and some follow-up care such as a skilled nursing facility, home health services, and hospice care. A person is eligible for Medicare Hospital Insurance if he or she is age 65 or older and (1) is eligible for any type of monthly Social Security benefit or railroad retirement system benefit, or (2) is retired from or the spouse of a person who was employed in a Medicare-covered government position (*The Medicare 1998 Handbook*, 1998).

Part A is financed through part of the Social Security tax. Most Medicare recipients pay a supplemental premium that is deducted from monthly Social Security payments. In addition, they pay an annual deductible on hospital and skilled nursing care benefits.

Part B, the medical insurance, helps pay for (*The Medicare 1998 Handbook*, 1998):

- Physician services
- Outpatient hospital services and home health visits
- Vision services provided by a qualified optometrist (excluding the cost of glasses)
- Physical therapy
- Inpatient treatment of mental illness
- Outpatient rehabilitation
- Diagnostic x-ray, laboratory, and other tests
- Blood for transfusions
- X-ray therapy
- Surgical dressings, splints, and casts
- Necessary ambulance services
- Rental or purchase of durable medical equipment used in the home
- Colostomy bags and supplies
- Braces for limbs, back, or neck
- Artificial limbs or eyes
- Pneumonia vaccine

Part B is financed by monthly premiums. In 2005 the monthly premium is $78.20 for most beneficiaries with an annual deductible of $100 and a patient coinsurance payment of 20% of the Medicare-approved amount (*www.medicare.gov*, 2005).

Medicare covers long-term care only in skilled care facilities and only under specific situations. Long-term care that is not covered by Medicare can deplete a person's savings in a very short time. Therefore some persons purchase long-term care insurance. Most policies offer a specific coverage amount per day for a specific time (e.g., $60 per day for 3 years). Some also cover in-home care. Premiums depend on the extent of the benefits and the age and health of the purchaser.

Medicare rules and benefits change often. In 1998 Medicare+Choice was introduced as a result of the Balanced Budget Act of 1997. The Medicare+Choice program offers beneficiaries a variety of health care delivery models, including coordinated care plans such as health maintenance organizations, preferred provider organizations, provider-sponsored organizations, and medical savings accounts. As of 1999 the beneficiary has the opportunity to annually choose between Medicare+Choice and traditional Medicare (Balanced Budget Act of 1997).

Many older adults do not understand Medicare and are often confused by the paperwork, billing, and notices they receive regarding claims. They are encouraged to contact the Social Security Administration or the insurance departments of their local medical facilities if they have questions.

Those older adults who are still working may continue to be covered by their employers' health insurance plans. A retiree is sometimes covered by a former employer's health plan. In that case the employer's insurance supplements the Medicare insurance. Many insurance companies offer supplemental insurance for those not covered by present or former employers. These are referred to as Medigap policies. Persons shopping for Medigap insurance should look for insurance that meets their specific needs at the most reasonable cost.

Medicaid is a state-administered program designed for persons with very low incomes. It uses federal funds and covers certain medical expenses not covered by Medicare. Each state has different coverage and requirements.

Some insurance companies offer policies that cover one specific disease, such as cancer. These policies might be appropriate for someone who is at high risk for that specific disease, but generally are not cost effective.

AARP has several publications that explain insurance policies in a language that most people can understand. Some of the publications are free; others are available at a minimum cost. The Social Security Administration publishes free pamphlets, updated annually, that explain Medicare. Insurance trade associations such as the Health Insurance Association of America, the Insurance Information Institute, and the American Council of Life Insurance publish a variety of free educational materials to help people understand insurance. Each state has an insurance department that can provide specific information for insurance in that state (Fig. 7-2).

Support Systems

Throughout life people make new acquaintances, develop friendships, and form family circles. People identify with schools, churches or synagogues, clubs, neighborhoods, and towns. These are the places and people they turn to when they need advice or help, want to celebrate, or are grieving. With age a person loses some of these support systems. Family and friends move away or die, and organizations and neighborhoods change. Changing work roles and financial status may require changes in the groups with whom a person associates. To cope with losses of family members, friends, health, and independence, individuals need a large social network. In a study of poor, frail older adults, Mor-Barak, Miller, and Syme (1991) found that social networks act as buffers against the harmful effects that major life events have on the health of older adults; that is, social networks can relieve the harmful consequences of life events on health. Neal Krause (1997) found that anticipated support is associated with lower mortality risk in the upper social clasees.

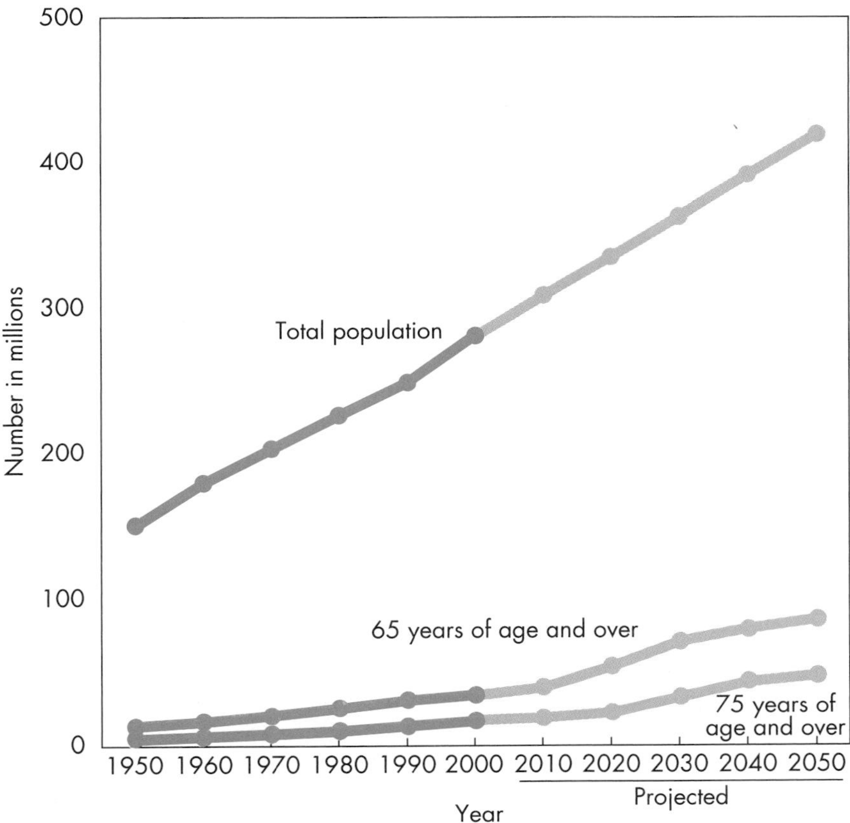

Fig. 7-2 Total population, population 65 years and over, and 75 years and over: United States, 1950-2050. (From US Census Bureau, Current Population Survey, 2003.)

They are more likely to believe that others will help if the need arises.

Marital status affects older persons in several ways. A married person is likely to live in a household with more income than an older adult who lives alone. Nutritional status is likely to be better for the married person than for the person living alone. Men benefit most from marriage. They do not cultivate the close friendships that women do outside the marriage, so the spouse is a vital friend and supporter. In a study of how age and gender affect the perception of quality of support, Lynch (1998) found that men appear to perceive spousal support as the most positive, whereas women seem to perceive the support received from children as the most positive. Traditionally, men do not engage in cooking, cleaning house, mending clothes, and doing the laundry, and thus miss these services when they lose their spouses. There are also more older women than older men, so many men marry again. In 1995 about 77% of men over age 65 were living with their spouse (AARP, 1997; US Census Bureau, 1996). Because there is a greater chance of a woman outliving her spouse, more older women live alone. In 1995 only about 48% of women over age 65 lived with their spouse.

An older adult man sees his role in marriage as the provider and protector. A woman feels responsible for her family's comfort and happiness. These roles may be blurred in older marriages as disease and disability increase, forcing role changes. When the older adult loses his or her traditional role, self-esteem and satisfaction with life may be affected.

Children continue to provide support to their older parents. About two thirds of older adults in the United States live within 30 minutes of a child. Many visit at least weekly with children, and most talk on the phone at least once a week with a child. Female children are more likely to assist with hands-on care, whereas male children are more likely to provide business and financial support (Miller and Montgomery, 1990; US Census Bureau, 1996). Although many families are separated by miles, children are concerned about their parents and attempt to arrange needed services for them. Area Agencies on Aging (AAAs), local social service organizations, and private care managers are some of the resources available.

Often older adult siblings draw closer and may live together, providing support for each other as they grow older. Many older adults develop extended families of younger neighbors or fellow church members. These extended families provide both emotional and practical support.

The financial status of older adults can affect their support systems. Older adults tend to feel an obligation to return favors. If someone does something for them, they want to be able to reciprocate. If they are financially unable to do this, they might withdraw so as not to be put in an embarrassing position. In addition, the inability to afford adequate clothing or to maintain clean clothing can cause others to avoid them.

The emotional status of older adults can also affect the support systems. It may be difficult for friends and family of depressed or negative older persons to maintain contact with them because of the behaviors exhibited. A complete health history and physical examination should be conducted to rule out physical causes of emotional problems. Peer counseling, support groups, or professional assistance from mental health professionals, clergy, or a community nursing service may help them express feelings and concerns. Close friends may be able to help the person find the positive aspects of life. Spirituality and religious practice provide positive support for older adults. Participation in religious community events helps eliminate feelings of isolation and diminishes depression. Many older adults use song, prayer, or meditation to express feelings. For many, faith is an effective coping mechanism and provides hope and support through illness and loss (Cramer, 1994; Forbes, 1994; Koenig and Weaver, 1998).

Benefits and Entitlements

In addition to Social Security, SSI, Medicare, and Medicaid, older Americans are eligible for a variety of other benefits and entitlements that affect their socioeconomic status. Entitlement programs require that the beneficiary meet certain guidelines of income or disability, whereas other benefits, such as senior discounts, may be enjoyed by all older Americans.

Subsidized housing is available in almost every community in the nation. Most are supervised by the U.S. Department of Housing and Urban Development with one major program under the authority of the Farmers Home Administration of the U.S. Department of Agriculture. Once a person establishes eligibility, he or she may locate suitable housing in existing rental buildings or public housing developments. The housing authority then contracts with the building owner for rent payments on the unit, or the renter pays a portion of the rent and the housing authority pays the rest. Eligibility standards differ for each program. An individual's income, assets, and expenses are all considered in determining eligibility.

Another entitlement program available to older adults is food stamps. Food stamp programs are usually administered by a state's Department of Health and Human Services. Eligibility and the amount of food stamps a family may receive are based on family size, available income, and other resources. Nutritious meals are available at congregate meal sites throughout the country. A small donation is requested for each meal. If older adults are homebound, arrangements can usually be made to have a meal delivered.

Energy assistance is also available. This program is administered differently in each community. Information on the program can be obtained at the local senior center or utility company. Again, income requirements must be met.

In 2003 there were 12,065,000 military veterans over age 60 in the United States (US Census Bureau, 2004-2005). Many of these veterans are eligible for veterans' benefits. The benefit used most often is access to Veterans Administration (VA) health care. As the population has aged, the large number of veterans from World War II has put a strain on the VA health care facilities. As a result, the VA has tightened the rules, making it more difficult to qualify for care. Veterans who require health care because of a war-related injury or disease are given priority. Those needing long-term care are now being referred back to their communities for that care (*Federal benefits for veterans and dependents,* 1993).

Local AAAs provide several services for older adults. AAAs were created in 1973 as an amendment to the Older Americans Act. The purpose of the agencies is to plan and implement social service programs at the local level. Benefits available through these agencies include:

- Nutrition services through congregate meal sites and home-delivered meals
- Recreational opportunities
- Chore service
- Legal assistance
- Transportation
- Information and referral

It is not the purpose of the AAAs to duplicate services of other agencies. In fact, these agencies try to encourage community-based services. However, if a service is not available, the AAA attempts to provide it (Fig. 7-3).

Conservators and Guardians

When older adults are unable to handle their own financial affairs, a conservator may be appointed. This does not necessarily indicate that older persons are incompetent. For example, if a person is visually impaired, he or she may voluntarily select a conservator. However, if an older person is incompetent, the court selects the conservator. In either case the conservator is legally appointed and court supervised (see Chapter 3).

A guardian may be appointed to handle decisions not related to financial matters. The guardian makes decisions about housing, health care, and other similar matters. This may be the same person as the conservator or a different person.

A guardian or conservator may affect a person's socioeconomic status. By handling his or her assets wisely, a conservator may help an older person remain at least financially independent for longer than he or she could have otherwise. By supervising housing and health matters, the knowledgeable guardian may assist the older person to function at the highest possible level (Box 7-4).

ENVIRONMENTAL INFLUENCES

Environment contributes to a person's perception of life. Although the environment might not be noticeable unless it is uncomfortable, it does significantly affect emotional and physical health and well-being. Environment can be described as hot or cold, dark or light, hard or soft, safe or dangerous. Environmental factors such as adequate shelter, safety, and comfort contribute to a person's ability to function well. These factors take on added importance to older adults with decreased functional ability. Geographic location, transportation, housing, and safety issues as they relate to the environment of the older person are discussed in the following sections.

Geographic Location of Residence

Geographic factors influence individuals differently. Climate is important to older adults because they are susceptible to temperature extremes. Those who live in cold climates need adequate heat and clothing; those in temperate areas need cooling systems during warm seasons. Because older adults are concerned about accidental injuries, weather extremes such as snow and ice can contribute to isolation.

Whether a person lives in an urban or rural location can affect access to services, availability of support systems, and safety perceptions. Urban neighborhoods tend to be older and subject to change because of suburban migration. The notion of a friendly and convenient neighborhood in larger urban areas is rapidly declining. Such changing neighborhoods may affect the socialization of older adults because of the foreign and frightening atmosphere created. The majority of older Americans have lived in the same geographic area for more than 30 years and are not planning to move.

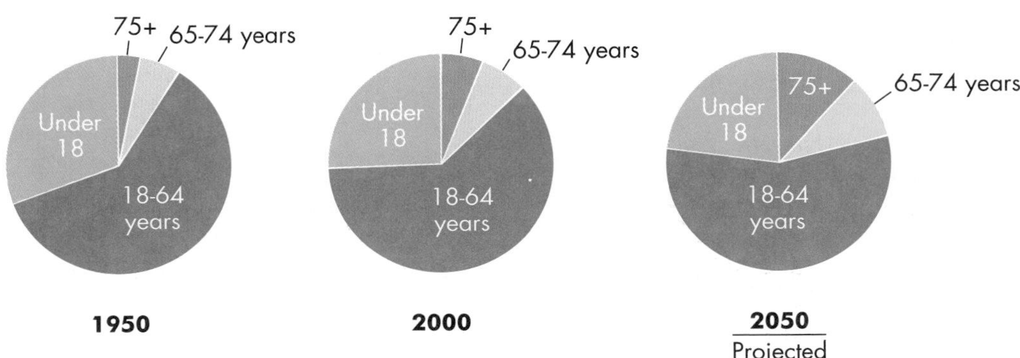

Fig. 7-3 Percent of population in four age-groups: United States, 1950, 2000, and 2050. (From US Census Bureau, Current Population Survey, 2003.)

BOX 7-4 Definitions

Conservator—A *conservator* manages an older person's financial resources. An annual report must be filed with the court detailing how the funds were spent on the person's behalf.

Guardian—A *guardian* is appointed to make personal care decisions for the disabled individual. Personal care includes medical treatment and other decisions promoting comfort, safety, and health. The guardian must file an annual report with the court on the individual's condition.

Durable power of attorney—A *durable power of attorney* is a document by which one person (the principal) gives legal authority to another (the agent or attorney-in-fact) to act on behalf of the principal. It is called *durable* because it continues to be effective even after the principal has lost capacity as a result of illness or injury. The two types of durable power of attorney are:

- **Durable power of attorney for financial matters**—This authority to handle financial affairs can be as broad or limited as the parties agree upon.
- **Durable power of attorney for health care decisions**—The agent or attorney-in-fact is not required to report actions on behalf of the principal to the court.

From American Association of Retired Persons: *A matter of choice,* Washington, DC, 1991, The Association. In Hamilton A, editor: *Legal guide for senior citizens,* Topeka, Kan, 1991, Kansas Department on Aging.

Older adults residing in rural areas have different problems. Geographic isolation may result from long distances between contacts and services, and inadequate transportation services. However, the social supports obtained through churches, friends, and neighbors can be strong and reliable. Although a larger percentage of older adults in rural areas own their own homes compared with those in metropolitan areas, they occupy a disproportionate share of the nation's substandard housing. Also, there are fewer formal services available for rural older adults (Coward, 1993).

Transportation

To many older adults an automobile is a symbol of independence. In some areas an automobile is necessary for transportation to shopping areas, medical facilities, and social centers. Using data from the Public Use Microdata Sample, Cutler and Coward (1992) found that 76% of older adults live in households where personal transportation is available. However, the data do not indicate whether the older adults actually use available vehicles. Advancing age, being a woman, and residing in inner cities were associated with a greater likelihood of lack of transportation.

Low-cost transportation is an objective of the Older Americans Act and is the responsibility of the Administration on Aging. Each AAA is charged with ensuring that transportation is available in its area. Obstacles preventing public transportation use include cost, scheduling, distance from home, availability in rural areas, lack of awareness of the service, and reluctance of some older adults to use public transportation.

Research

SAMPLE/SETTING

Data were collected from 34 men and 69 women living in their own house or apartment. The mean age for men was 73 years, 7 months, and for women 73 years, 1 month.

METHODS

Interviews were conducted in the participants' residences using open-ended questions. Responses were recorded on response sheets and tape recorded for later reference.

FINDINGS

Older adults viewed factors such as finances, health, family support, a sense of identity, and a feeling of independence as contributing to their ability to continue living in the community. They viewed threats to continued independent living as both (1) factors connected to losses and maintenance of capability and (2) impediments to further growth of their personal well-being.

IMPLICATIONS

Community care enables older adults to remain living in the community. Older adults must be committed to facilitating their own living arrangements by becoming active participants in the evaluation and planning of their community care. The concept of community care must not be limited to health; many aspects of an older adult's social and economic status affect independence and quality of life.

Mack R et al: Perceived risks to independent living: the views of older community-dwelling adults, *Gerontologist* 37(6):729, 1997.

Housing

Home is a true reflection of the individual, and for the older person it signifies independence. Emotional and physical health are affected by where a person lives (see Research box).

After World War II, home ownership was encouraged by offers of insured mortgages and deductions of property taxes and mortgage interest to stimulate the postwar economy. Therefore home ownership was a goal many in the older generation sought to achieve (Burke and Flaherty, 1993). The home is often the major asset and, in fact, may be the only asset. It may be the house in which an older person was born and reared, then raised his or her own children. More often, a young married couple bought the house, raised the family in that same house, then continued to live there as a couple or after the death of a spouse.

The availability of features that support older adults' abilities to function in their homes is often a concern. Most homes occupied by older adults were designed for younger, more active individuals. Many older Americans have performed a home modification to adopt the environment to specific needs, whereas many others still need modification to their houses. For those who wish to remain in their homes but need funds for maintenance and repairs or even extra income, home equity conversion, also known as reverse mortgage, might be an alternative. The home owner arranges for regular payments from a bank in exchange for the future transfer of the property to the bank.

Older adults who rent face the problem of locating affordable rental property. Once it is located, increases in rental cost can outpace older adults' fixed income. The tenant–property manager relationship can change as the property management changes hands. As with home owners, the building's structure and appliances may be inadequate to support independent functioning.

In urban areas some older adults live in single-room–occupancy (SRO) hotels. SRO hotels offer single, sparsely furnished rooms with limited cooking facilities and communal bathrooms. Tenants are traditionally single persons with limited incomes, mental illness, or substance abuse problems. Typically, they have few contacts with other tenants and no family to provide support. An increasing incidence of chronic disease and disability can keep individuals from leaving their rooms and can further restrict the person's living environment. This can affect tenants' physical and mental health by isolating them and preventing access to services.

Safety can be a problem in all these living arrangements. Aging furnaces and appliances; worn linoleum or carpeting; poor lighting; unprotected stairs; lack of smoke alarms and assistive grab bars; and aging, sagging, or broken furniture all pose hazards for older adults (see Chapter 12).

For those who decide to give up their homes, there are several options (Fig. 7-4). Independent housing options may include mobile homes, condominiums, and cooperatives.

Increasingly older adults are sharing houses. They may move in with family into a single room, an accessory apartment, or a portable housing unit on the family property. Others team up with a group of older adults to buy or rent a house. Typically in this situation each person has a private room, and they share the living, dining, and kitchen areas. Chores are also shared, and in some instances, a house-

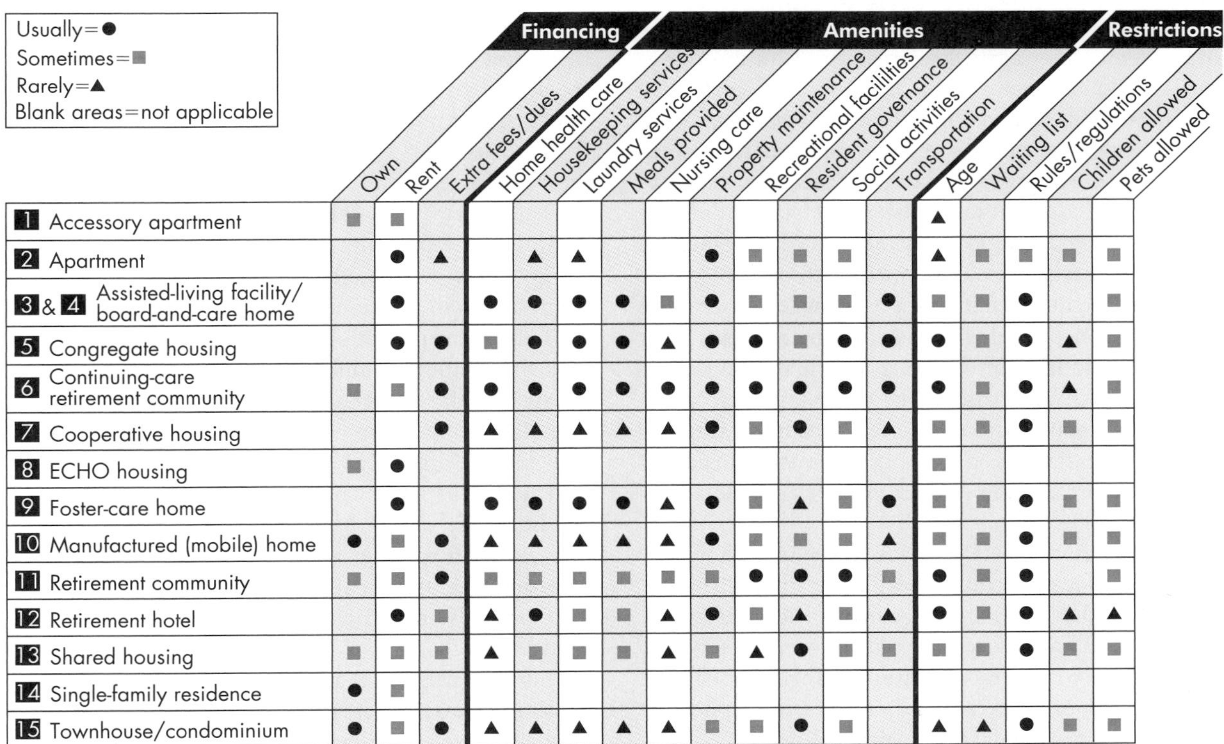

Usually=●
Sometimes=■
Rarely=▲
Blank areas=not applicable

	Financing			Amenities										Restrictions				
	Own	Rent	Extra fees/dues	Home health care	Housekeeping services	Laundry services	Meals provided	Nursing care	Property maintenance	Recreational facilities	Resident governance	Social activities	Transportation	Age	Waiting list	Rules/regulations	Children allowed	Pets allowed
1 Accessory apartment	■	■												▲				
2 Apartment		●	▲		▲	▲			●	■	■	■		▲	■	■	■	■
3 & 4 Assisted-living facility/ board-and-care home		●		●	●	●	●	■	●	■	■	■	●	■	■	●		■
5 Congregate housing		●	●	■	●	●	●	▲	●	●	■	●	●	●	■	●	▲	■
6 Continuing-care retirement community	■	■	●	●	●	●	●	●	●	●	●	●	●	●	■	●	▲	■
7 Cooperative housing			●	▲	▲	▲	▲	▲	●	■	●	■	▲	■	■	●	■	■
8 ECHO housing	■	●												■				
9 Foster-care home		●		●	●	●	●	▲	●	■	▲	■	●	■	■	●	■	■
10 Manufactured (mobile) home	●	■	●	▲	▲	▲	▲	▲	●	■	■	■	▲	■	■	●	■	■
11 Retirement community	■	■	●	■	■	■	■	■	■	●	●	●	■	●	■	●		■
12 Retirement hotel		●	■	▲	●	■	■	▲	●	■	▲	■	▲	●	■	●	▲	▲
13 Shared housing	■	■	■	▲	■	■	■	▲	■	▲	●	■	■	■	■	●	■	■
14 Single-family residence	●	■																
15 Townhouse/condominium	●	■	●	▲	▲	▲	▲	▲	■	■	●	■		▲	▲	●	■	■

Fig. 7-4 Which living arrangement is for you? (From Porcino J: Designs for living, *Modern Maturity* 36[2]:32, 1993.)

keeper or manager for the house is hired. Some older adults take in boarders to help with expenses and household chores. The boarder is often a younger person who can do the "heavy" housework.

Home matching programs are gaining in popularity. These agencies locate and match persons who can share a home. Through interviews and screenings conducted by the agency, applicants are able to locate a compatible housemate. With home sharing, common areas of the house such as the kitchen and living room are always available to use. But personal space such as bedroom and bath are private. Home sharing is not for everyone. For more information, go to www.aarp.org/life/housingchoices/Articles/a2004-02-26-housesharing.html.

A growing number of older adults are living a mobile life. These are usually the young-old who live in warmer climates in the winter and cooler climates in the summer. They may own a home in one area and rent in another, or they may use a recreational vehicle as a second home. The real nomads are those who travel all year from place to place in recreational vehicles. As these older adults age and begin to have health problems, they often return to their home communities where long-established support systems of family and friends are available.

Retirement communities appeal to some. In a survey of older Americans, 10% of respondents lived in retirement housing (US Census Bureau, 2004). These communities may have facilities for independent persons only, or they may include a variety of housing alternatives for those with various levels of dependency. Separate housing units for independent residents, congregate apartment units for those who need meals or housekeeping help, and nursing facilities for those who need more care may be found in a continuing care community. Residents may move from one level to another as their needs change. Most such communities require a substantial entrance fee in addition to monthly charges. Benefits include activity programs and assistance with housekeeping and chores. Transportation is often included.

For those who require increasing assistance but are still able to function independently, assisted living facilities are a viable option. These facilities have separate living units with common dining facilities and social rooms. Meals, transportation, housekeeping, and some laundry services are provided. Most have activity programs and encourage residents to socialize. Staff are present around the clock should a resident need help.

Board and care homes, also known as sheltered housing, provide a home to a small number of older adults. Services provided vary widely. Basic rent usually includes room, board, laundry, and housekeeping. Some offer other services, such as assistance with personal care, for an additional fee. Board and care homes try to create a homelike atmosphere by remaining small and friendly (Wolinsky et al, 1992).

Nursing care facilities are another housing option for persons who are no longer able to function independently. Residents of nursing care facilities depend on assistance with ADLs for survival. The resident occupies a single room or shares a room with one or more persons. The facility is staffed 24 hours a day with nursing professionals and trained personnel who can provide needed assistance. The services on the premises generally include meals, personal laundry services, and a hair salon. Activity programming is provided to meet the needs of individual residents. Rehabilitation services are available as required by the residents.

In any assistive facility, it should be noted that residents are renting their room or part of their room, and to them, it is home. It should be arranged as residents wish and furnished with as many personal possessions as possible to provide a sense of historical continuity, belonging, identity, and comfort (Johnson, 1996). Staff should be encouraged to treat residents in a courteous and respectful manner, as if they were visitors. For example, a person would not go to a friend's house and turn on the television or rearrange the furniture without permission. By recognizing the importance of older adults' personal space, staff members reaffirm older adults' rights and enhance their sense of dignity.

When older persons change environments, there are dangers of translocation crises resulting from relocation stress. Moving to any new setting is often associated with loss. Older persons may move because of a loss of spouse, health, home, or functional independence. Depression, withdrawal, confusion, increased dependency, lowered life satisfaction, and increased health problems may result from a move, especially if older adults are not prepared or the move is abrupt. If older persons make the decision to move after careful consideration over time, they are familiar with the new environment, and they are able to take cherished possessions with them, they can make the move with minimum stress. Preadmission and ongoing assessments of residents and their spouses and family can ease the adjustment (Rosenkoetter, 1996). When the move is precipitous, with little or no input from the older adults, the move may have negative effects on health and possibly increase mortality (Johnson, 1996; Manion and Rantz, 1995).

There is a segment of the older population that is homeless. Data about homelessness are difficult to quantify because of the nature of the problem. Older adults in the homeless population are defined as those over 50 because they tend to look and act 10 to 20 years older (DeMallie et al, 1997). Estimates of the number of older adults among the homeless range from 1 in 16 to 1 in 4. Women are increasing in number among homeless older adults. Most have some source of income (Social Security or SSI), but it is usually insufficient to obtain adequate housing. Approximately 30% of homeless older adults have mental illness or dementia. Many may also suffer from chronic illness and visual and hearing problems. Impaired judgment may lead to financial mismanagement, eviction, or exploitation of property by others, leading to a loss of residence. Locating a new residence is difficult because of

Research

SAMPLE/SETTING

The sample included 201 homeless women ages 50 and over. The sampling was stratified into four overlapping sectors: (1) persons using eight public shelters that housed homeless women; (2) women using five homeless shelters operated by religious or voluntary agencies; (3) women using four drop-in centers; and (4) women using various public areas such as parks and bus, ferry, and train terminals. Interviews were conducted over a 2-year period. The mean age of the sample was 59 years; 51% were black, 34% were white, 10% were Hispanic, and 5% were other racial groups.

METHODS

Interviews were conducted using two instruments: audiotapes and videotapes. The interviews took approximately 2 hours.

FINDINGS

Of the variables examined, only two variables—perceived support and number of community facilities attended—were significant predictors of being domiciled on follow-up. Three additional variables—absence of psychosis, a lifetime history of less than 1 year of homelessness, and number of entitlements—attained near-significance. However, what is most striking was the apparent lack of suitable housing options for older homeless women as evidenced by the high percentage of women who received no housing offers and the large number who rejected offers that were made. This was also reflected in a survey of directors of homeless programs.

IMPLICATIONS

Older homeless women may require more intensive case management to assist in the process of leaving shelters and finding suitable housing. The nurse who becomes aware that a client is homeless should collaborate with the case management team to help find suitable housing.

Cohen C: Predictors of becoming redomiciled among older homeless women, *Gerontologist* 37(1)67, 1997.

limited income, mental and physical health problems, and a lack of information about affordable housing (Cohen, 1997) (see Research box).

Homeless older adults require interventions that can connect them with needed services. Medical and mental assessments, emergency shelter, and long-term supervision may be required. In a study by Harris and Williams (1991), homeless men identified needs such as clean water, healthful food, adequate rest and exercise, medications and health care, adequate clothing, a safe place to stay at night, and money and facilities for bathing and washing clothes.

Whatever the housing status of the older person, it must be remembered that each person has a right to determine where to live unless he or she is proven incompetent. Nurses, as health care professionals, must respect that right and work with the person to maintain as much independence and dignity as possible.

AARP provides many books on housing options, adaptations, and safety. Many are free or available at minimum cost. The federal government also provides materials on housing options through the Consumer Information Center.

Criminal Victimization

Data sources such as the U.S. Department of Justice, the Law Enforcement Assistance Administration, and the findings of "victim surveys" over the last 30 years show that there is a higher victimization rate among older adults in connection with assault, robbery, rape, theft, and burglary than in the younger population (US Department of Justice, 1994) (Box 7-5). Older adults appear to be particularly susceptible to crimes motivated by economic gain. Older adults are more likely to be injured in a violent crime. Among violent crime victims ages 65 or older, 9% suffer serious injuries like broken bones and loss of consciousness. When injured, almost half the older victims receive medical care in a hospital (US Department of Justice, 1994) (Box 7-6).

Whatever the actual risk, it is the perception of risk by older adults that affects their lifestyles (Fattah and Sacco, 1989). Declining health and limited finances contribute to feelings of vulnerability. As a result, older persons may withdraw behind locked doors, becoming isolated. They may rarely leave home and may even refuse to permit services within the home. Such self-imposed social isolation has a negative effect on older adults' overall health and well-being.

Older adults are often victims of fraud and scams. Just how often is not known because older adults may not realize they have been victimized or may be too embarrassed to admit to victimization. After accounting for women being a higher proportion of the older population, they are abused at a higher rate than men. The nation's oldest elders (80 years and above) are abused and neglected at two to three times their proportion of the elderly population (Box 7-7).

In nearly 90% of elder abuse and neglect cases with a known perpetrator, it is a family member such as an adult child or a spouse (National Center on Elder Abuse, 1998).

Older adults become victims for several reasons (Box 7-8). They are perceived as vulnerable. The ageist views of society often portray older adults as weak and gullible; older adults may even see themselves this way.

Older adults are highly visible. Appearance advertises age. Predictability of daily routines and movements make older adults more vulnerable to criminals. They tend to rely on public transportation, and if they live in undesirable urban areas, they are vulnerable when walking to and from that transportation.

The level of dependency is an indicator for victimization. The more dependent an individual is, the greater the risk of

BOX 7-5 Types of Crimes Committed Against Older Adults

The types of crimes most often committed against older adults include:

Larceny or theft—Noncontact crime resulting in loss of property
Robbery—Taking of property by force or threat of force
Burglary—Taking of property by being in the victim's residence, place of business, or automobile without authorization
Auto theft—Taking of vehicle with intent to keep it
Assault—Verbal communication (such as a threat) that makes the victim reasonably apprehensive of physical harm
Battery—Physically harming the victim
Fraud—Intentional deception to cause a person to give up property or some lawful right
Abuse or neglect—Willful or negligent acts of caregivers resulting in physical or emotional harm to the older adult

From Ferraro K, LaGrange R: Are older people most afraid of crime? Reconsidering age differences in fear of victimization, *J Gerontol* 47(5):S233, 1992; USDHHS-AOA: *National elder abuse incident study,* National Center on Elder Abuse, 1998, http://www.ojp.usdoj.gov/ovc/assist/nvaa2000/Academy/Chapter 14.htm.

BOX 7-6 Older Adult Crime Victims

- Older men generally have higher victimization rates than older women. However, older women have higher rates of personal larceny with contact, such as purse snatching.
- Older adults, ages 65 to 74, have higher rates of victimization than those ages 75 or older.
- Older blacks are more likely than older whites to be crime victims. However, rates of personal larceny that do not involve contact between the victim and offender are greater for whites.
- Older adults with the lowest incomes experience higher violence rates than those with higher family incomes. Older adults with the highest family income have the highest rates of personal theft or household crime.
- Older persons who are either separated or divorced (from among all marital statuses) have the highest rates of victimization for all types of crime.
- Older residents in cities have the highest rates of victimization for all types of crime, compared with suburban or rural older adults.
- Older renters are more likely than owners to experience both violence and personal theft. However, older homeowners are more likely than renters to be victims of household crime.

From US Department of Justice: *Elderly crime victims: national crime victimization survey,* Annapolis Junction, Md, 1994, Bureau of Justice Statistics Clearinghouse.

BOX 7-7 Consumer Frauds Most Perpetrated Against Older Adults

- **Health and medical frauds**—Quackery or merchandising of drugs, health aids, or insurance
- **Mail order frauds**—Merchandising through the mail that includes false or misleading information about the product
- **Income creation and investment frauds**—Get-rich-quick schemes such as pyramid selling, work-at-home scams, the sale of fraudulent franchises, and real estate investment opportunities
- **Social psychologic frauds**—Merchandising of products and services that exploit fears by promising solutions to problems and loneliness
- **Con games**—Schemes such as the "pigeon drop," the vacation lure, the bank swindle, or the oil well investment; usually perpetrated by professional con operators
- **Telemarketing scams**—Sweepstakes or contests that require payment in advance to enter or claim a prize, with payment usually by credit card; merchandising that pressures people to buy without being sent written information about the products or services they are being sold

victimization. Some older adults have a diminished sense of sight or hearing. They may be unable to see well enough to recognize danger in the immediate area or to read contracts. They may not hear well enough to understand what is being said and may not ask for clarification. Loss of physical strength reduces the ability to fight back. If there is a loss of

BOX 7-8 Reasons Older Adults Are Fraud Victims

1. Older adults are often lonely and isolated. They are more likely to be at home and therefore available to both door-to-door and phone scams. They welcome con artists who are willing to spend time visiting.
2. Older adults have fewer resources to turn to for advice. They may be reluctant to "bother" friends, family, or professionals.
3. Older adults may be more susceptible to con artists who are polite, who appear knowledgeable, or who represent authority.
4. Older adults often have concerns about maintaining a comfortable lifestyle on a fixed income, affording good medical and long-term care, and providing for spouse and children.
5. Chronic illness leads many older adults to consider medical remedies offered by health fraud promoters.
6. Many older adults believe it is impolite to hang up on a caller or turn someone away at the door.

cognitive ability, older adults are less able to reason rationally and are therefore vulnerable to fraud and abuse.

Con artists commonly prey on older adults. A study funded by AARP categorized one third of those over age 75 as "highly vulnerable" to fraud, compared with 24% among those ages 65 to 75 and 7% of those younger than 65 (*Elderly on mailing lists*, 1994). Loneliness and a life of trusting others leave older adults vulnerable. Door-to-door con artists use friendliness to gain the trust of the older person. They visit for as long as it takes to accomplish their goal. They rely on older adults' fears related to safety and health to sell their products. They convince older adults that the roof needs repair, the driveway needs sealing, or a burglar alarm system should be installed. Other older adults respond to appeals and advertising seen on the television, in the Sunday supplements of newspapers, or in the mail. They may order products that turn out to be different from what was advertised; for example, a "solar clothes dryer" for $39.99 that ended up being a clothesline and clothespins (Bekey, 1991). Illegal telemarketing is increasingly claiming older victims.

Older adults who have been victimized are likely to be confused, disoriented, fearful, or angry. When trying to assist older adult victims, the nurse should give the impression of nonhostile authority. Firm direction should be tempered with empathy. It is important to listen carefully to victims. This conveys an attitude of empathy and respect and helps the victims sort out the facts. The nurse must remain calm and reassure them that help will be provided throughout this crisis.

At times the nurse may need to allow time for victims to regain composure. One way to accomplish this is to distract them by asking for demographic information. Inquire about address, phone number, family, and other support systems to help calm older adults.

Follow-up procedures such as referral to a social service agency or victim support group, or a phone call to let a victim know how the case is progressing, help victims know that the professional cares. However, precautions must be taken to avoid encouraging excessive dependency.

Community resources for crime victims vary from one area to another. In some communities, victim and witness assistance programs can offer short-term immediate help. Support groups may help victims work through feelings of anger and fear. Volunteer action programs, such as a neighborhood watch, aid in prevention and also help older adults feel safer. The AAA is a good resource for information about assistance programs for older persons. Local law enforcement agencies are also available for help.

Every state has an older adult abuse law that includes methods for reporting suspected abuse (see Chapter 3). Most state laws define abuse and provide a system of investigation. Many states maintain a registry of reports on suspected abuse. Some states mandate professionals working with older adults to report suspected abuse. In other states, reporting is voluntary. The local Department of Social Services or AAA can provide information on reporting requirements.

It is important for older adults to feel control over their environment and have a voice in the community. Educational programs help older adults identify potential crime situations and ways to protect themselves. Law enforcement organizations and AARP are establishing local senior advisory groups to assist sheriff and police departments in understanding senior community needs. Such groups are also identifying and recommending programs, as well as assisting in planning and integrating law enforcement concerns with other social service needs throughout the community (Miller, 1992). Older adults who take responsibility for their own environment feel in control, and that attitude is recognized by those who would victimize older adults.

ADVOCACY

Older adults as a group are good advocates for their own special needs and interests. They write to legislators, consumer protection groups, government agencies, and other groups that control issues affecting older adults. By advocating for themselves, older adults are taking charge of their environment, their resources, their mental and physical health, and the future of all older adults. Older adults know from experience that they can make a difference.

Some older adults, however, are not able to plead their case. For example, older women were not taught to be assertive and to stand up for themselves. The physically or mentally disabled, the undereducated, minority groups, those who do not speak the local language, and the financially disadvantaged all need assistance to take advantage of services and programs that may benefit them.

Advocacy is basic to professional nursing because it seeks to protect the human rights of clients within the health care system (Segesten and Fagring, 1996). Advocacy is an ongoing process as opposed to a single isolated event. As a moral concept, advocacy requires the nurse to speak up for the client's rights and choices, to help the client clarify his or her decision, and to protect the client's privacy and autonomy in decision making (Hamic, 2000).

The nurse is often the best person to initiate and provide that assistance. The nurse is trained to listen and assess, is aware of aging physiology and psychology, is familiar with community resources, and is motivated to serve older adults. The nurse may be the one member of the formal support group with the most complete information about older adults.

By listening to and consulting with older adults, the nurse develops an understanding of the values and perceptions that guide older adults' thoughts and feelings about life. The nurse forms partnerships with older adults to defend and promote their rights.

The nurse advocate determines what older adults want, then helps find ways to satisfy those desires. If staying at home is important to an older adult, the nurse can assist in enabling the person to stay home. By involving older persons in the planning from the start, the nurse establishes partnerships that strengthen older adults' self-esteem, promote dignity, and enhance satisfaction with life.

Within the hospital or nursing facility the nurse can advocate for older adults by clearly documenting their concerns and problems and any nursing care approaches. The nurse is in a key position to advocate for older adults by bringing problems to the attention of the physician, social services department, or administrator as appropriate. In cases where client competency is questioned, it may be appropriate for the nurse to encourage the client to obtain legal counsel or to insist on comprehensive evaluations by a qualified geriatric specialist to determine the cause of symptoms.

Whatever the setting, the nurse's advocacy for older adults is important to ensure the older adults of continuing to control their lives. There are many organizations in the United States that advocate for older adults (Box 7-9). Local and regional organizations also advocate for older adults, including state Departments of Aging and the local AAA.

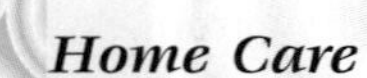

Home Care

SOCIOECONOMIC INFLUENCES

- Assess older adults' outside sources of income. Many supplemental policies cover excess costs that Medicare does not cover, thus ensuring more equipment and supplies for older adults.
- The goal of home care is to restore older adults' independence by teaching self-management of chronic conditions.
- Use social workers to identify community resources for financial assistance for homebound older adults.
- Arrange for meals to be delivered to homebound older adults if necessary.
- Contact the Area Agency on Aging for referral to employment and legal services and social opportunities for older adults.

ENVIRONMENTAL INFLUENCES

- Many meal delivery services provide food that has been prepared and frozen. Assess the functional ability and environment of older adults to ensure they can prepare the food that has been delivered (e.g., make certain they have a stove or microwave and electricity).
- Use a social worker to identify community resources for housing options for homebound older adults with multiple problems.
- Refer to the Area Agency on Aging for resources for home repair and transportation.
- Assess for signs of older adult abuse that may be manifested by consumer frauds. Report any suspicion of consumer fraud.
- Reduce potential for consumer fraud by decreasing social isolation in homebound older adults.

BOX 7-9 Advocacy Organizations for Older Adults*

- AARP
- Alzheimer's Disease and Related Disorders Association
- American Health Care Association (Nursing Homes)
- American Society on Aging
- Gerontological Society of America
- Gray Panthers
- Hispanic Council on Aging
- National Association of Professional Geriatric Care Managers
- National Association of Social Workers
- National Council on Aging
- National Gerontological Nursing Association
- Older Women's League (OWL)

*For addresses and phone numbers, see Appendix 7A.

SUMMARY

Older adults' perceptions of the health care system in its entirety are influenced by experience. The nurse needs a sound understanding of the major historical events that have influenced the perceptions of today's older adult clients so as to understand their response to health care issues.

Recent and present socioeconomic issues, including income sources, prosperity or poverty, education level, health status, and formal and informal support systems, all affect the ability of older adults to comprehend and comply with health care regimens.

Older adults and their families may not be aware of community resources. The nurse should be aware of housing options, nutrition programs, transportation opportunities, respite programs, and legal assistance programs that are available in the community.

By understanding the eligibility requirements for benefits and entitlements, the nurse can assist older adults in receiving optimum services. By understanding the necessity for and the availability of durable power of attorney, conservatorship, or guardianship, the nurse can help older adults and their families cope with diminishing abilities.

The sensitive nurse understands the concerns of older adults, and supports and reassures them. The nurse can also encourage the older adults' informal support systems of friends and family. Often, the nurse can coordinate the formal and informal support systems for maximum positive effect on the health and well-being of older adults.

Advocates for older persons, whether they are the older adults themselves or professionals in the field of aging, can help make socioeconomic and environmental factors a positive rather than a negative influence on older adults.

To provide maximum benefits to aging health care consumers, the nurse must understand the factors that influence their perceptions of their health. To work with older adults successfully, the nurse must understand not only where they are but also where they have been.

Key Points

- Socioeconomic factors such as income level, income sources, insurance coverage, benefits and entitlements, and education level influence older adults' perceptions of their health and approach to health care.
- Environmental factors such as geographic location, housing, transportation, and perception of safety influence the availability of services, as well as older adults' knowledge and use of those services.
- The strength of the formal and informal support systems, including community services, medical care, spiritual resources, and family and friends, may affect the maintenance of independence for older adults.
- Experience has a strong influence on shaping value systems, coping skills, and perceptions. It is important to understand the events that occurred early in older adults' lives to understand their values and perceptions.
- Education has a strong positive influence on economic well-being and on health status. Education prepares persons to make positive decisions that contribute to a higher perceived quality of life.
- Medicare is a federal program that provides health insurance for older adults. It consists of two parts: Part A is hospital insurance that helps pay for inpatient care and some follow-up care, and Part B is medical insurance that helps pay for physician services and some outpatient services.
- Medicaid is a state-administered program that uses federal funds to provide some medical expenses not covered by Medicare. Each state has different coverage and requirements. Medicaid is designed for persons with very low incomes and minimal assets.
- Older adults who are no longer able to handle their affairs or make decisions about their lives may benefit from a conservator, guardian, or durable power of attorney. A conservator manages financial resources, a guardian makes personal decisions, and a durable power of attorney is a document that names an agent to act on behalf of a person for a specific function, such as in making financial or health care decisions.
- The condition of homes and furnishings, the composition of neighborhoods, and the availability and type of transportation affect the security and safety of older adults. Aging and outdated homes and appliances, worn furniture, and unreliable transportation can lead to accidents and injury. Deteriorating neighborhoods with changing populations may foster feelings of insecurity in older adults.
- Most communities in America have a variety of housing options to meet the needs of older adults, including single family residences, apartments, congregate housing, shared housing, retirement communities, assisted living facilities, and nursing facilities. Each option provides a different level of service to help older adults maintain maximum independence.
- Perceived victimization in older adults may result in increased suspicion and eventual withdrawal and isolation, which can have negative effects on health and well-being.
- A strong support system helps protect older adults from criminal victimization. Professional service providers, friends, and family may monitor older adults' environments and offer guidance when necessary. Community programs such as neighborhood watch programs and educational programs on victimization help older adults actively participate in crime prevention.
- Through advocacy, nurses can protect the dignity of older adults and improve their quality of life.

Critical Thinking Exercises

1. A 67-year-old chronically ill woman has few financial resources, no formal education, and only one child who can assist her. Her son is married, has five children, and has a job that barely manages to support him and his family. Speculate how the woman's situation may affect her perception of her health care. In what ways can the nurse intervene to assist her?
2. A 75-year-old man is a retired banker whose wife died several years ago. He is able to perform all ADLs but needs help with meal preparation and transportation. He lives in a deteriorating neighborhood and no longer feels safe. He does not want to live with family members or completely give up his independence. What housing options would be appropriate for him? What advantages would such housing options offer over living alone?

References

American Association of Retired Persons: Checklist, 2005, website: http://www.aarp.org/benefits/articles/a2002-05-30-benefits_discount_checklist.html.

American Association of Retired Persons: *Driver safety program,* 2005, website: http://www.aarp.org/lite/drive/.

American Association of Retired Persons: *A profile of older Americans,* Washington, DC, 1997, The Association.

American Association of Retired Persons: *Understanding senior housing for the 1990s,* Washington, DC, 1993, The Association.

Atchley RC: The myth of fixed income, *Aging Today* 3(5):0, 1992.

Balanced Budget Act of 1997, Pub. Law No. 105-33, § 1851(a), 1997.

Bekey M: Dial S-W-I-N-D-L-E, *Modern Maturity* 34(2):31, 1991.

Brown V: The effects of poverty environments on elders' subjective well-being: a conceptual model, *Gerontologist* 35(4):541-548, 1995.

Burke M, Flaherty MJ: Coping strategies and health status of elderly arthritic women, *J Adv Nurs* 18:7, 1993.

Centers for Disease Control and Prevention (CDC): *Healthy aging for older adults,* Atlanta, Ga, 2004, The Agency.

Clough B: Broadening perspectives on learning activities in later life, *Educ Gerontol* 18(5):447, 1992.

Cohen C: Predictors of becoming redomiciled among older homeless women, *Gerontologist* 37(1):67, 1997.

Couch K: Late life job displacement, *Gerontologist* 38(1):7, 1998.

Coward R: Double jeopardy—aging beyond the country myth, *Aging Today* 14(5):7, 1993.

Cox H: *Later life,* Englewood Cliffs, NJ, 1986, Prentice Hall.

Cramer D: Religion and spirituality: key elements to health promotion among older adults, *Perspect Health Prom Aging* 9(3), 1994.

Cutler S, Coward R: Availability of personal transportation in households of elders: age, gender, and residence differences, *Gerontologist* 32(1):77, 1992.

DeMallie D et al: Psychiatric disorders among the homeless: a comparison of older and younger groups, *Gerontologist* 37(1):61, 1997.

Elderly on mailing lists, *Elder Law Issues* 2(17), 1994.

Fattah E, Sacco V: *Crime and victimization of the elderly,* New York, 1989, Springer-Verlag.

Federal benefits for veterans and dependents, Washington, DC, 1993, Office of Public Affairs.

Forbes E: Spirituality, aging, and the community-dwelling caregiver and care recipient, *Geriatric Nurs* 15(6)297-301, 1994.

Hamic AB: What is happening to advocacy? *Nursing Outlook* 48(3):103, 2000.

Harris JL, Williams LK: Universal self-care requisites as identified by homeless elderly men, *J Gerontol Nurs* 17(6):39, 1991.

Johnson C: Divorced and reconstituted families: effects on the older generation, *Generations* 17(3):17, 1992.

Johnson R: The meaning of relocation among elderly religious sisters, *Western J Nurs Res* 18(2):172, 1996.

Koenig H, Weaver A: Religion provides counseling tool, *Aging Today,* pp 9-10, Mar-Apr, 1998.

Krause N: Received support, anticipated support, social class, and mortality, *Res Aging* 19(4):387, 1997.

Land K et al: Estimating increment-decrement life tables with multiple covariates for panel data: the case of active life expectancy, *Demography* 31(2):297, 1994.

Lorig K: Self-management of chronic illness: a model for the future, *Generations* 17(3):11, 1993.

Lubkin IM, Larsen PD: *Chronic illness: impact and interventions,* ed 5, Sudbury, Mass, 2002, Jones and Bartlett.

Lynch S: Who supports who? How age and gender affect the perceived quality of support from family and friends, *Gerontologist* 38(2):231-238, 1998.

Mack R et al: Perceived risks to independent living: the views of older, community-dwelling adults, *Gerontologist* 37(6):729, 1997.

Manion P, Rantz M: Relocation stress syndrome: a comprehensive plan for long-term care admissions, *Geriatr Nurs* 16(3):108, 1995.

The Medicare 1998 Handbook, Baltimore, 1998, US Department of Health and Human Services, Health Care Financing Administration, website: www.medicare.gov/MedicareEligibility/home.asp?Q.

Miller B, Montgomery A: Family caregivers and limitations in social activities, *Res Aging* 12(1):72, 1990.

Miller W: The graying of America and its implications for policing, *Police Chief* 59:56, 1992.

Mor-Barak ME, Miller LS, Syme LS: Social networks, life events, and health of the poor, frail elderly: a longitudinal study of the buffering versus the direct effect, *Fam Commun Health* 14(2):1, 1991.

Penning M, Wasyliw D: Homebound learning opportunities: reaching out to older shut-ins and their caregivers, *Gerontologist* 32(5):704, 1992.

Retirement, Baltimore, 1997, US Department of Health and Human Services, Social Security Administration.

Richardson J: The cohort factor—as important as diversity, *Aging Today,* Nov-Dec 1996.

Rosenkoetter M: Changing life patterns of the resident in long-term care and the community-residing spouse, *Geriatr Nurs* 17(6):267, 1996.

Segesten K, Fagring A: Patient advocacy—an essential part of quality nursing care, *Int Nurs Rev* 43(5):142, 1996.

SSI, Baltimore, 1993, US Department of Health and Human Services, Social Security Administration.

Understanding the benefits, Baltimore, 1998, US Department of Health and Human Services, Social Security Administration.

US Census Bureau: *Statistical abstract of the United States, 2004-2005,* http://www.census.gov/prod/www/statistical-abstract-04.html.

US Census Bureau: *65+ in the United States: current population reports, special studies,* Washington, DC, 1996, US Government Printing Office.

US Department of Justice: *Elderly crime victims: National Crime Victimization Survey,* Annapolis Junction, Md, 1994, Bureau of Justice Statistics Clearinghouse.

Van Nostrand JF, Furner SE, Suzman R, editors: Health data on older Americans: United States, 1992, National Center for Health Statistics, *Vital Health Stat* 3(27):26, 1993.

Wapner S, Demick J, Redondo JP: Cherished possessions and adaptations of older people to nursing homes, *Int J Aging Human Dev* 31(3):219, 1990.

Wolinsky F et al: The risk of nursing home placement and subsequent death among older adults, *J Gerontol* 47(4):S173, 1992.

APPENDIX 7A

Resources

ORGANIZATIONS OF OLDER ADULTS

AARP
601 E Street NW
Washington, DC 20049
(202) 434-2277

Gray Panthers
2025 Pennsylvania Ave. NW
Suite 821
Washington, DC 20006
(202) 466-3132

Older Women's League (OWL)
666 11th Street NW
Washington, DC 20001
(202) 783-6686

ORGANIZATIONS OF PROFESSIONALS WORKING IN THE FIELD OF AGING

American Health Care Association
1201 L Street NW
Washington, DC 20005-4014
(202) 842-4444

Gerontological Society of America
1275 K Street NW
Suite 350
Washington, DC 20005-4006
(202) 842-1275

Hispanic Council on Aging
2713 Ontario Road NW
Washington, DC 20009
(202) 265-1288

National Association of Professional Geriatric Care Managers
1604 North Country Club Road
Tucson, AZ 85716-3102
(520) 881-8008

National Association of Social Workers
750 First Street NE
Washington, DC 20002
(202) 408-8600

National Gerontological Nursing Association
7250 Parkway Drive
Suite 510
Hanover, MD 21076
(800) 723-0560

ORGANIZATIONS OF BOTH PROFESSIONALS AND OLDER ADULTS

Alzheimer's Disease and Related Disorders Association
919 North Michigan Avenue
Chicago, IL 60611-1676
(312) 335-8700

American Society on Aging
833 Market Street
Suite 511
San Francisco, CA 94103-1824
(415) 882-2910

National Council on Aging (includes National Institute of Senior Citizens and National Institute on Adult Day Care)
409 Third Street SW
Suite 200
Washington, DC 20024

8 Health Promotion and Illness/Disability Prevention

BARBARA RESNICK, PhD, CRNP, FAAN, FAANP

Learning Objectives

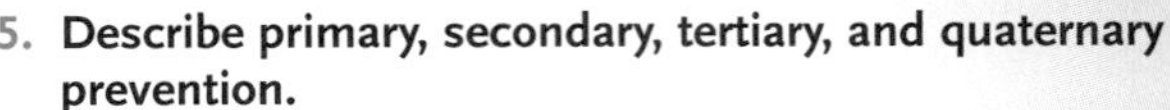

On completion of this chapter, the reader will be able to:

1. **Define health promotion, health protection, and disease prevention.**
2. **Identify models of health promotion and wellness.**
3. **Describe health care provider barriers to health promotion activities.**
4. **Describe client barriers to health promotion activities.**
5. **Describe primary, secondary, tertiary, and quaternary prevention.**
6. **Plan strategies for nursing's role in health promotion and public policy.**
7. **Develop approaches to support the empowerment of older adults.**

ESSENTIALS OF HEALTH PROMOTION FOR AGING ADULTS

The purpose of health promotion and disease prevention is to reduce the potential years of life lost in premature mortality and ensure a higher quality of remaining life. As Americans live longer, health promotion activities are all the more important because these individuals will have more years to benefit from preventive services. Health promotion and disease prevention activities include primary prevention, or the prevention of disease before it occurs, and secondary prevention, which is the detection of disease at an early stage. Some evidence suggests that seniors benefit just as much from primary and secondary health promotion activities as those who are middle-aged (Kim, June, and Song, 2003). Exercise, and reducing cholesterol levels, improves overall health status and physical fitness, including aerobic power, strength, balance, and flexibility, and helps prevent acute medical problems such as fractures, myocardial infarctions, and cerebrovascular accidents (Clarfield, 2002; Takeshima et al, 2002). Screening with mammography, a Pap test, digital examination for monitoring prostate size, and yearly evaluation of stool specimens for occult blood can help reduce mortality and morbidity among older adults (Sherman, Abel, and Tavakoli, 1996). Despite the positive outcomes of primary and secondary health promotion activities, only a small percentage of older adults actively engage in these activities. This is particularly true of the old-old age group (ages 90 and greater).

A number of variables have been found to affect older adults' participation in primary and secondary health promoting activities: (1) socioeconomic factors (Daly, 2000); (2) beliefs and attitudes (Leveille et al, 1999); (3) encouragement by a health care provider (Resnick, 2000; Resnick, 2002); (4) specific motivation based on self-efficacy and outcome expectations as defined by the theory of self-efficacy (discussed later) (Resnick, 2000); and (5) access to resources. Of these, self-efficacy and outcome expectations, as described in the theory of self-efficacy, have been shown to have the greatest influence on changing behavior and helping older adults engage in healthy behaviors (King, Rejeski, and Buchner, 1998).

Terminology

Health promotion is the science and art of helping people change their lifestyle to move toward a state of optimum health. *Optimum health* is defined as a balance of physical, emotional, social, spiritual, and intellectual health (Green and Kreuter, 1991). The promotion of health provides the pathway or process to achieve this balance. Box 8-1 lists areas of health promotion most relevant for older adults. A distinction should be made between health promotion and disease prevention. Health promotion addresses individual responsibility, whereas preventive services can be fulfilled by health providers (US Department of Health and Human Services, 2000). Disease prevention focuses on protecting as many people as possible from the harmful consequences of a threat to health (e.g., through immunizations).

Primary prevention is defined as measures provided to individuals to prevent the onset of a targeted condition

BOX 8-1 Areas of Health Promotion Most Relevant for Older Adult's Physical Fitness

- Smoking control
- Mind-body health
- Spiritual health
- Medical self-care
- Environmental health
- Nutrition
- Social health
- Weight maintenance
- Optimum nutritional status

(US Preventative Services Task Forces, 1996). Specifically, primary prevention measures include activities that help prevent a given health care problem. Examples include passive and active immunization against disease, health-protecting education and counseling, promotion of the use of automobile passenger restraints, and fall prevention programs. Since successful primary prevention helps avoid the suffering, cost, and burden associated with injury or disease, it is typically considered the most cost-effective form of health care.

Secondary prevention is defined as those activities which identify and treat asymptomatic persons who have already developed risk factors or preclinical disease but in whom the condition is not clinically apparent (US Preventative Services Task Forces, 1996). These activities are focused on early case finding of asymptomatic disease that occurs commonly and has significant risk for negative outcome without treatment. Screening tests for cancer are examples of secondary prevention activities. With early case finding, the natural history of the disease, or how the course of an illness unfolds over time without treatment, can often be altered to maximize well-being and minimize suffering.

Tertiary prevention is defined as activities that involve the care of established disease, with attempts made to restore the person to highest function, minimize the negative effects of disease, and prevent disease-related complications.

Quaternary prevention involves limiting disability caused by chronic symptoms while encouraging efforts to maintain functional ability or reduce any loss of function through adaptation. For additional information regarding quaternary measures of prevention, see the specific disorders in Part VI and Chapter 17.

MODELS OF HEALTH PROMOTION

This section provides a brief overview of four models of health promotion. The models selected represent different focus areas or constituents of health promotion programs.

The first is the ONPRIME Model, whose acronym stands for **o**rganizing, **n**eeds resources assessment, **p**riority setting, **r**esearch, **i**ntervention, **m**onitoring, and **e**valuation. This is intended as an instructional model aimed at change technology within health promotion programs, agencies, and organizations. The change technology focuses on behavior modification to achieve national goals of improved health across the life span.

The second example is the Health Belief Model, developed to determine the likelihood of an individual's participation in health promotion, health protection, and disease prevention services. Three basic components of this model are (1) the individual's perception of his or her susceptibility to and the severity of an illness or disease; (2) modifying factors such as knowledge of the disease, various personal psychosocial and demographic variables, and cues or triggers to action; and (3) a cost/benefit ratio that is acceptable to the individual (Rosenstock, 1974).

The PRECEDE/PROCEED Model, the third example, is complex and incorporates community involvement in most aspects of its direction. It is firmly based on multidisciplinary scientific designs and studies from epidemiology, education, and psychosocial sciences. The PRECEDE phase (which stands for **p**redisposing, **r**einforcing, and **e**nabling **c**onstructs in **e**ducation/environmental **d**iagnosis and **e**valuation) examines life quality, health goals, and health problems. The PROCEED phase (which stands for **p**olicy, **r**egulatory, and **o**rganizational **c**onstructs in **e**ducational and **e**nvironmental **d**evelopment) examines implementation and evaluation (Green and Kreuter, 1991; Lancaster, Onega, and Forness, 1992; National Institute of Nursing Research, 1995). This model is particularly useful in planning health education programs.

The fourth and final model is the Health Promotion Model. This model presumes an active role by the participant in developing and deciding the context in which health behaviors will be modified. Three basic categories are older adults' characteristics and life experiences, their perceived personal decision making (self-efficacy), and the effect of the plan of action on health-promoting behaviors (Pender, 1996).

To fully understand these relatively complex models, additional reading is recommended. The reference list at the end of this chapter provides full citations for students wishing to learn more about each model that is briefly overviewed in this section.

The use of a model in the study, research, or practice of nursing provides a foundation and direction for the planning of one or more interventions. Note that the terms *conceptual model* and *functional model* are not interchangeable. A conceptual model is synonymous with a conceptual framework and is generally defined as a meaningful configuration of concepts that can be abstract or general (Fawcett, 1995). A functional model is a construct that can provide an organizational plan using a systematic process designed for testing by other members of the profession. It is a blueprint based on the author's ideas and research.

BARRIERS TO HEALTH PROMOTION AND DISEASE PREVENTION

According to the Centers for Disease Control and Prevention (CDC), in a report published using 1997 statistics (CDC, 1998), the seeking and delivery of health promotion or clinical preventive services among older adults is less than satisfactory. For example, the vaccination rate of adults over age 65 against pneumococcal infections did not meet minimum expectations in any state. Of the 26,469 persons over age 65 included in the survey, only 45.4% reported ever receiving pneumococcal vaccine. A continued public health effort will be put forth to encourage pneumococcal vaccination among older adults. The next wave of statistics gathered on this health promotion effort will, we hope, demonstrate an increase in pneumococcal immunization.

Health Care Professionals' Barriers to Health Promotion

Barriers to the provision of information about health promotion and disease prevention result in part from health care professionals' uncertainty about what services to offer, who to offer them to, and the frequency of follow-up programs. In particular, there are no clear and consistent guidelines as to what should be offered to an older adult with regards to secondary prevention activities. Walter and Covinsky (2001) recommend a framework that includes consideration of life expectancy, risk of cancer death and screening outcomes, consideration of the harm of screening, and patient values and preferences to help make these decisions, but this is not always done. Moreover, the beliefs and attitudes of health care professionals likely affect what is offered to older individuals. Another barrier is the lack of an organized system to facilitate the delivery of screening services (Griffith and Rahman, 1994).

Older Adults' Barriers to Health Promotion

A number of variables affect older adults' willingness to engage in specific primary and secondary health promoting activities. These include socioeconomic factors (Lewis and Asch, 1999; Messecar, 2000), beliefs and attitudes of both patients and providers (Clarfield, 2002), encouragement by a health care provider (Sims et al, 2000), specific motivation based on efficacy beliefs (Resnick, 2002), and access to resources (Gallant and Dorn, 2001). Age, number of chronic illnesses, mental and physical health, marital status, and cognitive status have all been associated with participation in health promotion activities (Gallant and Dorn, 2001; Kim et al, 1998; Messecar, 2000; Resnick, 2000). Generally, individuals who are younger, married, have fewer health problems, and have better cognitive status are more likely to participate in primary and secondary health-promoting activities (Kim et al, 1998; Messecar, 2000; Resnick, 2000). These findings, however, are not consistent. Specifically Gallant and Dorn (2001) reported that the factors influencing health behaviors varied by behavior, gender, and race. Therefore it seems that there may be sample-specific differences with regard to what factors influence health promotion behaviors.

Client barriers unrelated to health beliefs can include lack of transportation and financial limitations. Transportation is not readily available to many urban and rural older adults, or it is cost prohibitive (see Chapter 7). In addition, older adults incur the cost of many preventive services, since Medicare does not cover them all (Table 8-1). This can be hard on the fixed, limited income of many older adults.

Ethnic and cultural factors can have a negative effect on health care–seeking behaviors. The cultural diversity issue is complex and varies from one location to another throughout the United States (see Chapter 5). The diversity among communities has not been adequately considered by health policymakers. This creates barriers to programs; for example, requiring older adults to forfeit personal and family privacy to obtain individual services. In some cultures a fear of reporting health screening results that could serve as the impetus for additional protective or preventive services limits program development. Another problem in culturally diverse areas is a lack of coordination of preventive health services because of the differing ideas and

TABLE 8-1 Secondary Prevention: Medicare Reimbursement

SCREENING PROCEDURE	MEDICARE GUIDELINES FOR REIMBURSEMENT
Mammogram	Women older than 40 years of age are covered for one screening every 12 months. The usual Part B deductible is waived. Coverage includes the radiologic procedure and physician's interpretation.
Pap smears and pelvic examinations	Pap smears and screening pelvic examinations (also included are clinical breast examinations) are covered at 3-year intervals. Annual examinations are covered for women identified as high risk. The usual Part B deductible is waived.
Colorectal screening	Annual fecal occult blood test for those older than 50 years of age Flexible sigmoidoscopy every 4 years for those older than 50 years of age Colonoscopy every 2 years for those at high risk Screening barium enemas every 4 years for those older than 50 years of age (not high risk) and every 2 years for those who are high risk

beliefs held by health policymakers concerning the delivery of services.

Older adults vary with regard to their willingness to engage in health-promoting activities. With age, they may have less interest in engaging in health promotion activities for the purpose of lengthening life, and greater interest in engaging in these activities only if they improve current quality of life (Resnick, 2000). It is useful, therefore, to use an individualized approach to health promotion with older adults (Resnick, 2003).

HEALTH PROTECTION

Health protection is a classification of the *Healthy People 2010* project established by the U.S. Department of Health and Human Services (2000). *Healthy People 2010* provides our country with a wide range of public health opportunities that exist in the first decade of the 21st century. With 467 objectives in 28 focus areas, the project is directed toward two major goals: increase quality and years of healthy life, and eliminate health disparities.

The underlying premise of *Healthy People 2010* is that the health of the individual is almost inseparable from the health of the larger community, and that the health of every community in every state determines the overall health status of the country. That is why the vision for *Healthy People 2010* is "Healthy People in Healthy Communities." Many objectives focus on interventions designed to reduce or eliminate illness, disability, and premature death among individuals and communities. Others focus on broader issues, such as improving access to high-quality health care, strengthening public health services, and improving the availability and dissemination of health-related information. Each objective has a target for specific improvements to be achieved by the year 2010.

DISEASE PREVENTION

Primary Preventive Measures

The American College of Physicians (1994) developed guidelines to identify health behaviors of patients with known health risks and to provide specific preventive interventions. Primary prevention for older adults includes immunization programs, counseling for smoking cessation or alcohol limitation, nutritional support for weight conditions, moderate exercise for fitness, safety factors in and around the home, stress management, and appropriate use of medications. Other groups such as the American Geriatrics Society (1996) and the American Heart Association (2002) have recommendations and guidelines as well. Overall guidelines for primary prevention are reviewed in Table 8-2.

Generally, immunizations are strongly recommended for older adults and include an annual influenza vaccination in the

TABLE 8-2 Guidelines for Primary and Secondary Health Promotion Activities for Older Adults

HEALTH PROMOTION ACTIVITY	RECOMMENDATION	SUPPORTIVE EVIDENCE
Mammogram	Annually starting at age 40 and continue q 1 to 3 years until ages 70-85	Based on randomized trials; evidence for age to stop screening not well established
Pelvic examination/cervical smear	Every 1-3 years after 2-3 negative annual examinations; can decrease or discontinue after ages 65-70	Based on randomized trials; evidence for age to stop screening not well established
Fecal occult blood test	Annually after the age of 50	Evidence from nonrandomized or retrospective studies; fair evidence to support recommendation
Prostate examination	Annually after age 50 if life expectancy is at least 10 years	Based on expert opinions or other considerations; limited evidence to support recommendation
Exercise	Encourage aerobic and resistance exercise as tolerated; ideally 30 minutes of moderate exercise daily	Based on randomized trials
Low-cholesterol diet	Keep daily fat intake at less than 35% of total calories, and saturated fat and trans fatty acid intake at less than 7% of calories	Guidelines not well established
Alcohol intake	Moderate alcohol use, defined as 1 drink daily that does not exceed 1.5 ounces (45 ml) of liquor, 5 ounces (180 ml) of wine, or a standard can of beer (National Institute on Alcohol Abuse and Alcoholism, 2001)	Guidelines/safety not well established

early autumn of each year and a regular tetanus vaccination every 10 years. All older adults should receive a pneumococcal vaccination at or immediately following the 65th birthday, with an additional vaccination after 6 years or more for high-risk persons. Adults with high-risk status include those living in institutions and those with chronic medical conditions such as heart or lung disease, diabetes mellitus, cancer, or debilitation. It should be noted, however, that the CDC does not recommend routine revaccination of immunocompetent older adults; persons ages 65 and older should only be administered a second vaccination if they received the vaccine more than 5 years previously and were under age 65 at the time of primary vaccination. The second pneumococcal immunization or booster vaccination is still under investigation by research centers to determine the benefit of an additional immunization against pneumococcal pneumonia in independent, well older adults (Communicable Disease Control, 2002).

Smoking cessation can increase life expectancy and improve the quality of the remaining life span. Alcohol consumption risks include accidents while driving a motor vehicle or riding lawn mower and other types of injuries sustained in the home. Falls with fractures are frequently the result of intoxication in the home. If alcohol or inconsistent use of seat belts is not the cause of a motor vehicle accident, uncorrected vision deficits or ophthalmologic disease may be suspected.

Another risk factor for older adults is polypharmacy (see Chapter 22). Polypharmacy is the use of large quantities of different drugs to relieve symptoms of health deviation or symptoms resulting from drug therapy (Patel, 2003). Polypharmacy is compounded by the use of generic drugs or the substitution of over-the-counter drugs that are less potent than their prescription counterparts (Nixon, 2003). The nurse needs to completely review all medications taken routinely, randomly, by prescription, from friends, and over-the-counter by older adults. The list of medications should be reviewed for interactions, contraindications, and overmedication or overdosing.

Secondary Preventive Measures

Activities in secondary prevention consist primarily of detection of occult disease in early asymptomatic states. Common points of reference are the control of hypertension and the detection and treatment of cancers. For additional information regarding secondary measures of prevention, see the specific disorders in Part 4.

Annual screening recommendations for older adults include rectal examination with stool specimen for guaiac, prostate and breast examination, mammogram, oral cavity examination, and vision examination. Some authorities recommend annual laboratory screening examinations for thyroid function, liver function, and kidney function, as well as complete blood count, urinalysis, and total cholesterol (Table 8-3). The benefits of screening should outweigh the risks involved. Referral for treatment should be readily available. The cost effectiveness of screening tests needs to take into account the incidence of the disease being screened (Table 8-4).

TABLE 8-3 Preventive Screening Recommendations

TEST	FREQUENCY
Blood pressure	Annually
Hearing	Annually
Vision	Annually
Glaucoma	Annually
Mammogram	Annually
Dental or oral examination	Annually
Pap smear	Annually
Clinical breast examination	Annually
Prostate examination	Annually
Cholesterol screening	As clinically indicated
Prostate-specific antigen	As clinically indicated
Stool for occult blood	As clinically indicated
Thyroid function tests	As clinically indicated
Blood/urine sugar	As clinically indicated

Adapted from Ham RM, Sloane PD: *Primary care geriatrics: a case-based approach,* ed 3, St Louis, Mosby, 1997.

TABLE 8-4 Advantages and Disadvantages to Health Promotion Activities: Focus of Both Formal and Informal Teaching Intervention

ACTIVITY	ADVANTAGES	DISADVANTAGES
Alcohol use	Social benefit Protective effect on heart disease Increases high-density lipoprotein (HDL) cholesterol Decreased mortality after heart attack Decreased risk of congestive heart failure	Health complications: gastrointestinal, cardiac, dermatologic, cognitive and neurologic, impairment of nutritional state Risk of depression Risk of falls Drug interactions
Cervical smear	Increased risk for cervical cancer occurs with age and can result in unpleasant symptoms (foul-smelling discharge) if untreated.	Cervical cancer develops slowly and is unlikely to be the cause of death in those 90 years of age or older.

Continued

TABLE 8-4 Advantages and Disadvantages to Health Promotion Activities: Focus of Both Formal and Informal Teaching Intervention—cont'd

ACTIVITY	ADVANTAGES	DISADVANTAGES
Cervical smear—cont'd	Older women may not have had regular cervical smear tests done and may want this early screening. Only pursue if woman is willing to undergo treatment if disease is identified.	There is less risk if the patient is not sexually active. Testing is difficult and uncomfortable in older women, particularly those who are no longer (or never were) sexually active.
Mammogram	Increased risk for breast cancer occurs with age. If detected, these tumors are generally estrogen-receptor positive and treatable. Only pursue if woman is willing to undergo treatment if disease is identified.	New-onset breast cancer is not likely to cause death in those 90 years of age and older. Tumors in older women tend to be slow growing. There is discomfort associated with mammogram. There is stress and anxiety over investigations. If treated (e.g., through lumpectomy/radiation or hormones/tamoxifen), there are multiple complications of treatment.
Prostate	Increased risk for prostate cancer occurs with age. Only pursue if man is willing to undergo treatment if disease is identified.	Controversy persists with regard to effectiveness of treatment options and usefulness of treatment.
Fecal occult blood testing (FOBT)	Early detection of a growth that could cause the older adult discomfort and affect quality of life if left untreated. Easily performed with no discomfort to patient. FOBT has better predictive value in older adults than in the young adult population.	False positives that can result in additional testing and anxiety for patient.
Diet monitoring	Decreasing cholesterol with dieting reduces morbidity and mortality from cardiovascular disease. Focus should be on eating a healthy diet low in fat and high in fruits, vegetables, and grains, which can facilitate maintenance of ideal weight.	Restriction in diet may affect quality of life. Restricted diets can result in weight loss and failure to thrive. The impact of strict dietary restrictions are not well substantiated in those over 90 years of age.
Reducing nicotine	Smoking is associated with increased risk of sudden cardiac death, and myocardial infarction. Financial incentive May decrease peripheral vascular problems and chronic obstructive pulmonary disease, and may prevent further lung disease.	None
Exercise	Positive physical health benefits Positive mental health benefits Decreased fatigue Decreased pain Maintain weight Maintain physical function	None

Tertiary Preventive Measures

Tertiary level activities aim to prevent progression of symptoms. A good example of tertiary prevention is rehabilitation. Common conditions encountered by older adults that require tertiary care include arthritis, osteoporosis, stroke, Parkinson's disease, and urinary or fecal incontinence. For additional information regarding tertiary measures of prevention, see the specific disorders in Part 6.

THE NURSE'S ROLE IN HEALTH PROMOTION AND DISEASE PREVENTION

Nursing education is a dynamic process in which nurses are involved throughout their career. Knowledge concerning health care issues, practices, and innovations is ever changing. This evolution of science and technology must be tempered by the art of caring. Nursing as a caring profession is in a unique position to make human changes through self-development and the active sharing of information with individuals and the lay community.

Requisite Knowledge

The knowledge needed for health promotion and disease prevention activities includes an understanding of basic human needs, human behavior, human growth and development, ethnic and cultural diversity in aging, economic patterns, basics of political action, and, most important, behavior change and the challenges associated with behavior change among adults. Moreover, the nurse must have a comprehensive understanding of health policy and the impact of advocacy in obtaining needed care for older individuals. Specifically, knowing what services are covered under Medicare for older adults, and understanding and participating in advocacy for appropriate services, is essential to providing optimum nursing care.

Health promotion activities on behalf of older adults can be at local, regional, or national levels of action. At the local level, case finding is an initial step toward individualizing the needs unique to the older adults in a single community. Case finding can be initiated through the case managers in acute care facilities, Area Agencies on Aging, community centers for older adults, church groups, local AARP chapters, or the local health department. Additionally, nurses can volunteer for speakers' bureau opportunities to spread information regarding illness prevention and health promotion (see Research box).

Research

SAMPLE/SETTING

This study explored the factors that influence health promotion behaviors and described the impact of an individualized approach to decision making with regard to health promotion activities in a group of older adults living in a continuing care retirement community.

The study included a total of 134 residents. The majority of the individuals were white, unmarried, and female.

METHODS

Residents were invited, either during a face-to-face encounter or over the telephone, to participate during the annual administration of influenza vaccines. Baseline interviews were done in autumn 2000, and follow-up interviews were done in autumn 2001. All interviews were completed by graduate-level nursing students (i.e., master's or doctoral students). During the interviews participants were asked whether they had had (1) a recent mammogram (within the past one or two years); (2) a recent cervical smear test (within the past one or two years); (3) an annual prostate examination; (4) a recent testing of stools for occult blood (within the past year); and (5) a recent skin evaluation (within the past year). Participants were also asked about exercise behavior, smoking and alcohol use, and adherence to a low-cholesterol diet.

Over the course of the year from baseline to follow-up testing, the geriatric nurse practitioner in the facility provided both formal and informal education about health promotion activities. For example, during one of the monthly health talks, which were attended by 50 residents, the focus was on primary prevention and the advantages and disadvantages of engaging in healthy behaviors such as exercise, diet, smoking cessation, and moderation in alcohol use. Another monthly health talk addressed the advantages and disadvantages of cancer screening for older adults. In addition, this information was provided in the resident newsletter and reinforced during one-on-one interactions with residents. That is, residents were encouraged to come and talk with the nurse practitioner about health promotion behaviors and helped to make decisions about participation in specific activities based on their current situation.

FINDINGS

With regard to primary prevention there was a statistically significant decrease in the percentages of individuals willing to participate in dietary restrictions ($p = 0.012$). There was no statistically significant difference in any of the other health behaviors over the course of the year. Specifically, there was no change in nicotine use ($p = 0.34$), alcohol use ($p = 0.12$), or regular exercise ($p = 0.36$). Likewise there was no statistically significant change in participation in secondary prevention activities. There was no change in screening for skin lesions ($p = 0.12$), stool tests for occult blood ($p = 0.07$), mammograms ($p = 0.69$), cervical smears tests ($p = 0.12$), or prostate examinations ($p = 0.72$). There were, however, positive trends with regard to increase in exercise, decrease in alcohol and nicotine use, and a slight increase in all cancer screenings.

IMPLICATIONS

The results of this study did not support a statistically significant change following exposure to individualized care practices. However, there was a decrease in the percentage of individuals who drank alcohol or smoked, an increase in those who exercised regularly, and a decrease in those who were interested in going for cancer screenings. These changes suggest that, when encouraged to consider the advantages and disadvantages of health promotion activities, older adults may be more willing to engage in those activities that have a direct and immediate benefit. However, they are not as willing to go for testing and screening of diseases that may have less impact on their daily lives.

Resnick B: Health promotion practices of older adults: testing an individualized approach, *J Clin Nurs* 12(1):46, 2003.

Regionally, involvement can begin by contacting the state department on aging regarding rules and regulations for care for older adults. Another way to get involved is to attend and interact at state legislature meetings and hearings. Some states have set aside an annual nurse lobby day in the state capitol. Meetings with legislators can provide an opportunity for the nurse to express opinions related to health care issues.

At the national level, action can begin with personal education involving public policy. This education can include (1) becoming aware of current and changing social policy; (2) studying the facts and the opinions of leaders on all sides of an issue; (3) speaking to civic groups, political party groups, and senior citizen groups; (4) testifying before the legislature as an advocate for healthy aging; (5) being informed on the issues and knowing social and political hot buttons; (6) putting the best foot forward with lobbying; (7) studying issues and techniques of negotiation and compromise; and (8) actively supporting the role of the advanced practice nurse working with physicians as a primary provider of health care.

Assessment

When assessing an individual, the nurse must look at potential health hazards to identify risk factors for illness or injury. Contributing risk factors can include habits, lifestyle patterns, personal and family medical history, and environmental conditions. An example of an environmental risk factor is the presence of clutter, poor lighting, and poor footwear, which puts the older person at risk for falling.

Assessment for health promotion and disease prevention begins with collecting data about the person. The assessment must be developed in a comprehensive manner (see Chapter 4). Subjective data can be obtained through the health history. Objective data can be obtained through a complete physical examination. To obtain a complete, nursing-focused assessment, the nurse must have an understanding of functional health patterns of aging. Eleven of the basic functional health patterns of older adults that are important to assess are:

- Self-perception/self-concept pattern
- Roles/relationships pattern
- Health perception/health management pattern
- Nutritional/metabolic pattern
- Coping/stress-tolerance pattern
- Cognitive/perceptual pattern
- Value/belief pattern
- Activity/exercise pattern
- Rest/sleep pattern
- Sexuality/reproductive pattern
- Elimination pattern

The following discussion expands on these identified functional health patterns, which are based on Gordon's typology of 11 functional health patterns (1997). Each pattern presented includes a description and subjective and objective assessments. Within each of these patterns, the nurse needs to identify the aging adult's knowledge of health promotion, ability to manage health-promoting activities, and value given to activities of health promotion.

Self-Perception/Self-Concept Pattern

Description: This pattern encompasses a sense of personal identity; body language, attitudes, and view of self in cognitive, physical, and affective realms; and expressions of sense of worth and emotional state. Perceptions of self should be explored with direct questions, asked with sensitivity. Emotional patterns can be identified during this exploration of perceptual patterns.

Subjective: Determine the client's feelings about his or her competencies and limitations, withdrawal from previous activities, self-destructive actions, excessive grieving, and increased dependency on others. Assess changes in eating, sleeping, and physical activity patterns. Explore the person's perception of his or her identity, self-worth, self-perception, body image, abilities, successes, and failures.

Objective: Identify verbal and nonverbal cues related to the above subjective data. Verbal cues elicit feelings about self (strengths and limitations), and nonverbal cues include a change in personal appearance. Using tools for assessing anxiety and depression is helpful.

Roles/Relationships Pattern

Description: This pattern encompasses the achievement of expected developmental tasks. Basic needs for communication and interactions with other people, as well as meaningful communications and satisfaction in relationships with others, are examined.

Subjective: Determine family structure, history of relationships, and social interactions with friends and acquaintances. Assess the perceived reasons for unsatisfactory relationships, and identify attempts to change patterns and outcomes.

Objective: Examine the family dynamics of interdependent, dependent, and independent practices among members.

Health Perception/Health Management Pattern

Description: This pattern encompasses the perceived level of health and current management of any health problems. Determine health maintenance behaviors and the importance the older adult places on these behaviors.

Subjective: Determine the level of understanding of any treatments or therapy required for management of health deficits or activities; include assessment of performance of activities of daily living (ADLs) and/or instrumental activities of daily living (IADLs).

Objective: Observe for cues that indicate effective management of deficits, including the physical environment in which the client resides. Assessment should include information about prior health promotion activities (e.g., mammography, vaccinations) and management during sickness and wellness.

Nutritional/Metabolic Pattern

Description: This pattern encompasses evaluation of dietary and other nutrition-related indicators.

Subjective: Determine the older adult's description, patterns, and perception of food and fluid intake and adequacy for maintaining a healthy body mass index. It may not be realistic to obtain an accurate 24-hour food and fluid recall; however, the nurse could possibly get information on how meals are prepared, who prepares them, and approximately how much is eaten during a typical day. Identify any recent weight loss or gain, and identify food intolerances, fluid intake, and gastrointestinal symptoms.

Objective: Observe general appearance and various body system indicators of nutritional status. Note height, weight, and fit of clothes. If possible, observe the older adult eating a meal.

Coping/Stress-Tolerance Pattern

Description: This pattern encompasses the client's reserve and capacity to resist challenges to self-integrity, and his or her ability to manage difficult situations. The ability to successfully tolerate stress through personal coping behaviors is important to incorporate into any health promotion plan. Of equal importance is the identification of the person's support systems.

Subjective: Assess ways to handle big and little problems that occur in everyday life. Determine the past and current amount of stress present in the older adult's life. Discuss any recent losses and the methods used to deal with those specific situations. Identify any stress-reducing activities that are practiced and the usual results obtained.

Objective: Observe for the use of coping skills and stress-reducing techniques, and note their effectiveness.

Cognitive/Perceptual Pattern

Description: This pattern encompasses self-management of pain, presence of communication difficulties, and deficits in sensory function. Modes include vision, hearing, taste, smell, touch, and compensatory assistive devices used when a deficit exists.

Subjective: Inquire about difficulties with sensory function and communication, as well as the assessment of any cognitive changes.

Objective: Assess usual patterns of communication, and note the client's ability to comprehend. Also note the ability to read, hear the spoken word, smell, and distinguish tactile sensations and tastes. Administer mental status examination.

Value/Belief Pattern

Description: This pattern encompasses elements of spiritual well-being that the older adult perceives as important for a satisfactory daily living experience and the philosophic system that helps him or her function within society.

Subjective: Identify the older adult's values and beliefs about spirituality, with a special emphasis on how this influences health promotion behaviors.

Objective: Determine what is important in the older adult's life to support coping strategies. Note any references made to spirituality or religious affiliation and practices, as well as choices and decisions that are determined by values, beliefs, and spiritual practices.

Activity/Exercise Pattern

Description: This pattern encompasses information related to health promotion that encourages the older adult to achieve the recommended 30 minutes daily of physical activity on most days of the week.

Subjective: Screen for safety related to exercise and physical activity, using screening measures such as the Physical Activity Readiness Questionnaire (PAR-Q). Self-screening tools such as the PAR-Q and the PAR-Q & You (Canadian Society for Exercise Physiology, 2002) were developed to efficiently prescreen individuals before initiating an exercise program. The PAR-Q identified individuals who were considered high risk for moderate to vigorous levels of physical activity and recommended that these individuals be seen by a health care provider for further evaluation. Since the PAR-Q was initially developed for adults, its wording was revised to be more appropriate for older adults (Cardinal and Cardinal, 1994). In addition, assess daily routines and activities, including patterns of exercise, leisure habits, recreation, and hobbies; and inquire about any limitations or changes in these patterns. Identify IADLs that are practiced with or without difficulty. Inquire about the older adult's typical day. Assess for fear of falling and fall potential, and conduct a fall history.

Objective: Obtain vital signs and conduct cardiopulmonary and musculoskeletal system assessments. Assess self-care ability by observing and/or asking the client about self-care activities such as bathing, dressing, toileting, and feeding, if possible. Note the use of adaptive tools or equipment.

Rest/Sleep Pattern

Description: This pattern encompasses the sleep and rest patterns over a 24-hour period and their effect on function. Assess rest and sleep patterns of the older adult for usual pacing of activities with consistent energy reserves that do not require immediate rest.

Subjective: Assess usual sleep patterns, including bedtime and arousal time, quality of sleep, sleep environment, and distribution of sleep hours within a 24-hour period. Inquire about episodes of insomnia and deterrents to sleep such as pain; anxiety; depression; use of pharmacologic agents such as caffeine, over-the-counter agents that may cause arousal, alcohol, and prescribed medications such as some treatments for depression; lack of exercise; and inappropriate sleep hygiene. Identify time and circumstance for regular rest periods. Record any activities associated with a rest period.

Objective: Have client keep a sleep diary that includes naps and rest periods. If possible, observe daily activities and note the effects of sleep disturbance on functional ability.

Sexuality/Reproductive Pattern

Description: This pattern encompasses the older adult's behavioral expressions of sexual identity.

Subjective: Assess client's satisfaction or dissatisfaction with current circumstances related to sexual function and intimacy, including perceived satisfaction or dissatisfaction with sexuality or sexual experiences.

Objective: Discuss current sexual relationship. When none is present, elicit the meaning this has for the client's overall emotional and physical well-being.

Elimination Pattern

Description: This pattern encompasses bowel and bladder excretory functions.

Subjective: Assess lifelong elimination habits and excretory self-care routines. Inquire about client's perceptions of normal bowel and bladder function, and explore specifically for recent changes in usual bowel and bladder function. Assess for the impact of elimination patterns, and ability to control elimination, on quality of life.

Objective: Perform abdominal and rectal examination; external genitalia and pelvic examination may be indicated. Note daily intake of food, particularly amount of dietary fiber, and assess total fluid intake over a 24-hour period.

A nurse's approach to completing thorough functional health assessments of older adults must be positive and reassuring. Permitting older adults to be active participants in this process is important to the success of gaining insight into their needs (see Research box).

> **Research**
>
> **SAMPLE/SETTING**
>
> Independent, community-dwelling older adults ages 57 to 83 (28 subjects)
>
> **METHODS**
>
> Key-informant criterion and critical case approach through a questionnaire based on a self-care wellness model
>
> **FINDINGS**
>
> Age was not related to differences in healthy behaviors. Many informants reported no digestive or sleep difficulties. All were active, regularly kept in touch with family and friends, thought their environment was safe, and managed stress well. All but one attributed their quality of life and zest for living to remaining active, eating healthy food, exercising, pacing themselves, doing preferred activities, and maintaining their spiritual beliefs.
>
> **IMPLICATIONS**
>
> Participant statements of actions can provide inspiration for less active seniors and a beginning framework for nurses for understanding and supporting wellness self-care behaviors in older adults.
>
> Clark CC: Wellness self-care by healthy older adults, *Image: J Nurs Scholarship* 30(4):351, 1998.

Planning

The role of nursing in promoting health among older adults relies on organized planning. The planning can begin by exploring older adults' personal ideas and beliefs concerning health needs. Reading current literature provided by the U.S. Department of Health and Human Services, National Institutes of Health, National Institute on Aging, or the CDC will keep the nurse aware of the latest specific health promotion recommendations. Internet addresses for these and other information centers are located at the end of this chapter.

Keeping well versed on current health policy information will safeguard client rights. Then the nurse can inform older adults of significant policy changes as soon as they are made at the highest (federal) level. Often the dissemination of health policy is slow, and news reaches the recipient long after the fact. When policies are retroactive or are to be enforced on a certain date, passing the information on to older adults can be crucial to their health and well-being.

Planning involves understanding and use of behavior change and behavior change theories, such as the theory of self-efficacy. The theory of self-efficacy states that the stronger the individual's belief that he or she can perform a behavior, and the stronger his or her belief in a positive benefit to performing the behavior, the more likely he or she is to engage in the given activity. Recommendations to facilitate behavior change are shown in Table 8-5.

Implementation

Implementation can begin by adopting a proactive stance toward an action plan for health promotion of the older individual. Seeking activities, locations, and means for disseminating health promotion information to a group of older adults in an example of implementing a proactive stance. Proactive activities can have benefits and liabilities. The benefits include an early approach to a problem that has not been acted on previously. Annual health promotion screenings can be incorporated into programs that provide vaccinations for older adults and can include screenings for bowel cancer, diabetes, osteoporosis, and macular degeneration (Resnick and Andrews, 2002). Likewise, monthly health talks provided in senior centers, senior housing sites, or continuing care retirement communities can be a useful way to repeatedly advocate and educate about health promotion activities such as exercise, prevention of osteoporosis, or safe medication use.

Evaluation

Evaluation involves determining the effectiveness of your care plan. Was the client able to achieve the mutually established goals? The nurse should consider why these goals

TABLE 8-5 Interventions to Motivate Individuals to Change Behavior

FACTORS	INTERVENTIONS TO IMPROVE MOTIVATION TO PERFORM FUNCTIONAL ACTIVITIES
Efficacy beliefs	Interventions to strengthen efficacy beliefs: 1. Use verbal encouragement of capability to perform. 2. Expose older adult to role models (similar others who successfully perform the activity). 3. Decrease unpleasant sensations associated with the activity. 4. Encourage actual performance/practice of the activity.
Unpleasant physical sensations (pain, fear)	1. Facilitate appropriate use of pain medications to relieve discomfort. 2. Use alternative measures such as heat or ice to relieve pain associated with the activity. 3. Use cognitive therapy: • Explore thoughts and feelings related to sensations. • Help patient develop a more realistic attitude to the pain (e.g., pain will not cause further bone damage). • Use relaxation and distraction techniques. • Use graded exposure to overcome fear of falling.
Individualized care	1. Demonstrate kindness and caring to patient. 2. Use humor. 3. Use positive reinforcement after a desired behavior. 4. Recognize individual needs and differences such as providing a rest period or favorite snack.
Spirituality	1. Explore the influence of spirituality and traditional religion and, as appropriate, encourage patient to participate in this. 2. Physically be with the older adult and listen. 3. Use life review. 4. Encourage spiritual experiences: pets, children, journal keeping, reading, friends, prayer.
Social support	1. Evaluate the presence and adequacy of social network. 2. Teach significant other(s) to verbally encourage or reinforce desired behavior. 3. Use social supports as a source of goal identification.
Goal identification	1. Develop appropriate, realistic goals with older adult. 2. Set goals that can be met in a short time frame—daily or weekly. 3. Set goals that are challenging but attainable. 4. Set goals that are clear and specific.

were or were not achieved and negotiate with the client to establish appropriate and realistic revised goals and realistic steps to achieve them.

SUPPORTING GERIATRIC EMPOWERMENT

Nurses can provide a bridge between the theory of health promotion and the implementation of health promotion, health protection, and preventive services. The active participation of nurses in encouraging older adults to set goals aimed at maintaining function and independence long into their ninth decade of life is essential. Nurses can participate in collaborative interactions with other health care professionals and older adults through advocacy programs (see Research box).

Learning about community resources, and local, state, and federal programs that can provide information or services to older adults, and then disseminating the information to older adults in a variety of settings are legitimate nursing roles. Health promotion programs and activities can be provided to individuals, small groups, and larger groups where older adults congregate. Many retirement centers, assisted living facilities, church groups and organizations, Salvation Army centers, and senior citizen centers look for speakers on a variety of health subjects. In most cases the managers of these facilities welcome nursing students or registered nurse volunteers to present health promotion or disease prevention programs on a regular basis. Empowering older adults requires initiative, organization, and knowledge of the major areas of health promotion relevant to this population.

Nurses should ideally use an individualized approach to health promotion when working with older individuals. This approach focuses on providing appropriate education both formally in health promotion classes and informally during health care visits. The education should provide current recommendations for health promotion activities (e.g., when to get a mammogram) and help older clients decide what health behaviors they want to engage in. This type of individualized approach has the advantage of being cost effective in that screening is not performed if the individual does not have

> **Research**
>
> **SAMPLE/SETTING**
>
> Convenience; 10 advance directive documents from various sources
>
> **METHODS**
>
> Advance directive documents were electronically scanned in 1994, then evaluated using three readability formulas: Flesch-Kincaid Grade Level, Flesch Reading Score, and Gunning's Fog Index.
>
> **FINDINGS**
>
> The average readability of the 10 documents, using school grade levels as a known factor, was Gunning's Fog Index at an 18.2 grade level, Flesch-Kincaid Grade Level at an 11.3 grade level, and Flesch Reading Score at 43.2 (a score of 30 to 50 indicates a difficult reading level).
>
> **IMPLICATIONS**
>
> The reading levels were determined to be significantly above the recommended reading level for clients. Understanding is essential before signing any document, especially one that can have a profound effect on end-of-life decisions and care. Older adults are frequently required to complete advance directives. Gerontologic nurses are in a unique position to advocate for older adults to ensure such important documents are understandable.
>
> Ott BB, Hardie TL: Readability of advance directive documents, *Image: J Nurs Scholarship* 29(1):53, 1997.

any intention of pursuing abnormal results; plus, individualized health promotion increases adherence to positive health behaviors such as smoking cessation and exercise.

SUMMARY

This chapter discussed the practices of health promotion, health protection, and disease prevention in the older adult population. Several models of health promotion were presented. The first is a community change model identified by the acronym ONPRIME. The second, the Health Belief Model, is an example of a model used to determine the likelihood of one's participation in a health promotion program. The third model is the PRECEDE/PROCEED Model. This multidisciplinary model is aimed at communities. The Health Promotion Model presumes a collaborative effort by the participant and the health care professionals involved.

Barriers to participation in health promotion activities are complex issues involving both provider and participant. Reluctance on the part of the health care professional is compounded by the lack of coordination of preventive services. Barriers to health promotion and disease prevention programs by older adults were addressed in terms of past health care experiences, health beliefs, and factors not related to health, including lack of transportation and financial burdens. The issue of ethnic and cultural diversity and the resulting ineffectual coordination of services were discussed. The goals identified in the *Healthy People 2010* initiative in regard to health protection were presented.

Primary, secondary, tertiary, and quaternary prevention measures of disease prevention were discussed. Primary prevention includes immunizations and counseling programs. Prevention counseling is aimed at healthful living through cessation of smoking, limitation of alcohol consumption, physical fitness, weight management, and stress management. Other areas of concern include safety issues around the home and safe and appropriate medication use. Secondary prevention focuses on detection and early treatment of disease. Tertiary prevention involves eliminating or slowing the progression of symptoms, while quaternary prevention deals with limiting disabilities brought on by chronic conditions. Chronic illnesses do not need to be detrimental to functional abilities.

The nurses' role in health promotion and protection or prevention of disease can be based on a framework of functional health patterns. Data about these health patterns are best obtained by completing a comprehensive nursing assessment of each of the areas of function using positive and reassuring communication.

Using the nursing process to assess, plan action through goal setting, and implement a plan for health promotion, behavior change related to health care activities, or disease prevention, followed by evaluation, is necessary to achieve the best results. Suggested health promotion activities that focus on several levels of involvement are available to nurses who wish to become involved in social policy or political action. Involvement in a proactive movement to increased health promotion is possible at local, regional, and national levels. The use of an individualized approach and the empowerment of older adults to make their own health care decisions will help them achieve their optimum level of health, function, and quality of life.

Key Points

- Health promotion, health protection, and disease prevention became a national goal with the Healthy People 2010 initiative.
- Models of health promotion are available to guide the change process in establishing a local, regional, or national effort.
- Psychosocial factors, health beliefs, transportation, finance, ethnic and cultural influences, and a sense of futility can be barriers to health promotion.
- Health protection targets five areas: unintentional injuries, occupational health and safety, environmental issues, food and drug safety, and oral health.
- Primary prevention focuses on immunizations and health screening activities.

- Secondary prevention focuses on detection of occult disease.
- Tertiary prevention focuses on preventing the progression of symptoms while facilitating rehabilitation.
- Quaternary prevention deals with limiting disability caused by chronic disease.
- The nurses' role in health promotion begins with a complete health assessment using the functional health patterns framework; this should incorporate an individualized approach for each client.
- Using the nursing process in health promotion activities provides a sound foundation for success.
- Involvement in health promotion activities can be at the local, regional, and national levels.
- Using an individualized approach and empowering older adults to determine the level of health promotion and primary, secondary, tertiary, and quaternary prevention activities to achieve their optimum quality of life.

Critical Thinking Exercises

1. A 76-year-old woman brings her 95-year-old mother into the ambulatory clinic. The mother is deaf and motions for her daughter to talk for her. The daughter gives an account of the mother's health condition. While the health history of the mother is being given, the nurse notices several skin lesions on the daughter's lower arms. The daughter is overweight, seems out of breath, and is perspiring heavily although the room temperature is 76° F. What actions would you suggest the nurse take with the daughter? If an action is taken, when is the appropriate time to do so?
2. Several nurses have volunteered to give flu shots to older adults at a senior center. When the line to receive the injections slows down, one nurse notices a table of four older women playing cards. None of the women has approached the flu shot registration table. What actions, if any, are appropriate for the volunteer nurses in this situation? Does the fact that the nurses are volunteers change any potential course of action?

References

American College of Physicians Task Force on Adult Immunization and Infectious Disease Society of America: *Guide to adult immunization,* Philadelphia, 1994, The College.

American Geriatrics Society: *AGS position statement prevention and treatment of influenza in the elderly,* New York, 1996, The Society.

American Heart Association: AHA scientific statement: AHA guidelines for primary prevention of cardiovascular disease and stroke: 2002 update, No. 71-0226, *Circulation* 106:388, 2002.

Canadian Society for Exercise Physiology: *PAR-Q and you, physical activity readiness questionnaire—Par* Q (revised 2002), Gloucester, Ontario, website: *www.cooperinst.org/images/par_q.pdf,* last accessed March, 2005.

Cardinal B, Cardinal M: Preparticipation physical activity screening within a racially diverse, older adult sample: comparison of the original and revised physical activity readiness questionnaires, *Res Q Exercise Sport* 71(3):302, 1994.

Centers for Disease Control and Prevention: Influenza and pneumococcal vaccination levels among adults aged 65 or over in the United States 1998, *JAMA* 280(21):1818, 1998.

Clarfield AM: Teaching public health related to the elderly, *Public Health Rev* 30(1-4):271, 2002.

Communicable Disease Control: Statement of recommended use of pneumococcal vaccine, *Canada Communicable Disease Report,* vol 28, ACS 2, Jan 15, 2002.

Daly M: Health promotion and disease prevention. In Adelman AM, Daly MP, editors: *20 common problems in geriatrics,* New York, 2000, McGraw Hill.

Fawcett J: *Analysis and evaluation of conceptual models of nursing,* ed 3, Philadelphia, 1995, FA Davis.

Gallant M, Dorn G: Gender and race differences in the predictors of daily health practices among older adults, *Health Educ Res* 16(1):21, 2001.

Goldberg T: Preventive medicine and screening in older adults, website: http://members.aol.com/tgoldberg/prevrecs.htm, accessed Sept 2001.

Gordon M: *Nursing diagnosis: process and application,* ed 4, St Louis, 1997, Mosby.

Green L, Kreuter M: *Health promotion planning: an educational and environmental approach,* ed 2, Mountain View, Calif, 1991, Mayfield.

Griffith H, Rahman M: Implementing the put prevention into practice program, *Nurse Pract* 19(10):12, 1994.

Kim J et al: Racial differences in health status and health behaviors of older adults, *Nurs Res* 47(4):243-250, 1998.

Kim CG, June KJ, Song R: Effects of a health-promotion program on cardiovascular risk factors, health behaviors, and life satisfaction in institutionalized elderly women, *Int J Nurs Studies* 40(4):375, 2003.

King A, Rejeski J, Buchner D: Physical activity interventions targeting older adults: a critical review and recommendations, *Am J Prevent Med* 15:316, 1998.

Lancaster J, Onega L, Forness D: Educational theories, models, and principles applied to community health in nursing. In Stanhope M, Lancaster J, editors: *Community health nursing: process and practice for promoting health,* ed 3, St Louis, 1992, Mosby.

Leveille S et al: Aging successfully until death in old age: opportunities for increasing active life expectancy, *Am J Epidemiol* 149(7):654, 1999.

Lewis JD, Asch DA: Barriers to office-based screening sigmoidoscopy: does reimbursement cover costs? *Ann Intern Med* 130:525-530, 1999.

McCarthy E et al: Mammography use, breast cancer stage at diagnosis, and survival among older women, *J Am Geriatrics Soc* 48:1226, 2000.

Messecar DC: Mammography screening for older women with and without cognitive impairment, *J Gerontol Nurs* 26(4):14-24, 2000.

National Institute on Alcohol Abuse and Alcoholism: NIH Publication No. 96-4153, Bethesda, Md, 2001, National Institutes of Health.

National Institute of Nursing Research: *Community-based health care: nursing strategies,* Bethesda, Md, 1995, National Institutes of Health.

Nixon RG: Geriatrics and their meds: problems and perils, *Emerg Med Serv* 32(2):35, 2003.

Patel RB. Polypharmacy and the elderly, *J Infusion Nurs* 26(3):166, 2003.

Pender NJ: *Health promotion in nursing practice,* ed 3, Norwalk, Conn, 1996, Appleton & Lange.

Resnick B: Health promotion practices of older adults: testing an individualized approach, *J Clin Nurs* 12(1):46, 2003.

Resnick B: The impact of self-efficacy and outcome expectations on functional status in older adults, *Top Geriatric Rehab* 17(4):1, 2002.

Resnick B: Health promotion practices of the older adult, *Pub Health Nurs* 17(3):160, 2000.

Resnick B, Andrews C: End-of-life treatment preferences among older adults: a nurse practitioner initiated intervention, *J Am Acad Nurse Pract* 14(11):517, 2002.

Rosenstock IM: Historical origins of the Health Belief Model. In Becker MH, editor: *The Health Belief Model and personal health behavior*, Thorofare, NJ, 1974, Slack.

Sherman J, Abel E, Tavakoli A: Demographic predictors of clinical breast examination, mammography, and Pap test screening among older women, *J Am Acad Nurse Pract* 8(5):231-236, 1996.

Sims J et al: Health promotion and older people: the role of the general practitioners in Australia in promoting healthy aging, *Aust NZJ Public Health* 24(4)356-359, 2000.

Takeshima N et al: Water-based exercise improves health-related aspects of fitness in older women, *Med Sci Sports Exercise* 34(3):544, 2002.

US Department of Health and Human Services: *Healthy people 2010: understanding and improving health*, ed 2, Washington, DC, 2000, US Government Printing Office.

US Preventative Services Task Forces' Guide to Clinical Preventive Services, ed 2, Washington, DC, 1996, US Government Printing Office.

Walter L, Covinsky K: Cancer screening in elderly patients: a framework for individualized decision making, *JAMA* 285(21):2750, 2001.

Internet Addresses

AARP: www.aarp.org

Administration on Aging: http://www.aoa.gov

Alliance for Aging Research: *http://www.agingresearch.org*

Americangeriatrics.org/products/positionpapers/

American Society on Aging: http://www.asaging.org

BenefitsCheckUp: http://www.benefitscheckup.org

Centers for Disease Control and Prevention: http://www.cdc.gov

Healthy People 2010 documents online: http://www.health.gov/healthy-people/, or call (800) 367-4725

Information on Wellness Activities: http://www.wellmedia.com

National Council on the Aging: http://www.ncoa.org

National Health Information Center: http://www.health.gov/nhic/

National Institute on Aging: http://www.nih.gov/nia/

National Institutes of Health: http://www.nih.gov

Partnership for Prevention: http://www.prevent.org/publications/Active_Aging.pdf

U.S. Department of Health and Human Services: http://www.os.dhhs.gov

9 Health Care Delivery Settings

SUE E. MEINER, EdD, APRN, BC, GNP

Learning Objectives

On completion of this chapter, the reader will be able to:

1. Describe acute care hospital use patterns in the older adult population.
2. Describe a functional model of nursing care.
3. Identify risks associated with hospitalization of older adults.
4. Identify ways to modify the physical and social environment to improve care for hospitalized older adults.
5. Identify special considerations in caring for critically ill older adults and older adults suffering from trauma.
6. Describe two nursing interventions for each of the three conditions that make up the geriatric triad.
7. List adaptations that can be made to facilitate learning in older adults.
8. Describe a profile of a "typical" noninstitutionalized older adult, including common diagnoses and functional limitations.
9. Distinguish the categories and types of home care organizations in existence.
10. Explain the benefits of home care.
11. Analyze the effect of the recent changes instituted by Medicare on home health agencies and home health clients.
12. Discuss the philosophy of hospice care and how it differs from traditional home health care.
13. List five common factors associated with institutionalization.
14. Identify differences between the medical and psychosocial models of care for institutional long-term care.
15. Summarize key aspects of resident rights as they relate to the nursing facility.
16. List assessment components included in the minimum data set of the Resident Assessment Instrument.
17. Describe common clinical management programs in the nursing facility for skin problems, incontinence, nutritional problems, infection control, and mental health.
18. Differentiate types of nursing care delivery systems found in the nursing facility.
19. Describe assisted living, special care units, and subacute care units as specialty care settings of the nursing facility.

This chapter focuses on care of the older adult in acute care, home and community health, and long-term care settings. Among subsets of these delivery settings are housing options, hospice care, and delivery systems such as functional nursing, team nursing, and primary team nursing. Long-term care settings can be categorized on a continuum according to care and services required by the residents served.

With the steady growth in the number of older adults in this country, it is now estimated that most of a nurse's career is spent working with older adults, and almost all nurses will care for older adults in the acute care setting at some time. Older adults are a diverse, heterogeneous group in terms of age, life experiences, the aging process, health habits, attitudes, and response to illnesses. Nurses need to have specialized knowledge, skills, and abilities to care for older adults during hospitalization.

The discussion of home and community nursing for older adults includes topics regarding health care needs of community-living older adults, community-based services, and the role of home health agencies and hospice nurses in community-based care for this population.

The nursing home is the dominant setting in which long-term care is provided for people who require regular or continuous skilled nursing care. Nursing facility, nursing center, and health care center are other names. Before 1987 the nursing home was commonly referred to as either a skilled nursing facility (SNF) or an intermediate care facility. With the passage of the Omnibus Budget Reconciliation Act of 1987 (OBRA), distinctions between a SNF and an intermediate care facility were no longer meaningful. The term *nursing facility* replaced both these terms. In this chapter, long-term care will refer to the nursing facility.

Each of these settings will be presented in sequence.

CHARACTERISTICS OF OLDER ADULTS IN ACUTE CARE

The over-85 group is the fastest growing segment of the U.S. population. The most common diagnosis-related groups (DRGs) in hospitalized older adults include heart failure, pneumonia, cerebrovascular disorders, angina, psychoses, major joint procedures, digestive disorders, nutritional and metabolic disorders, cardiac arrhythmias and conduction disorders, and bronchitis and asthma (Powell, 1996). The major causes of death in those over 65 are heart disease, cancer, stroke, chronic obstructive pulmonary disease (COPD), pneumonia, and influenza (National Center for Health Statistics, 2003).

Chronic conditions is a general term that includes chronic illness and impairments, with an individual's level of disability typically categorized based on the amount of assistance required in both basic activities of daily living (ADLs) and instrumental activities of daily living (IADLs). Arthritis, hypertension, and heart disease are the most prevalent chronic diseases, as well as the leading causes of disability, in older adults. The exacerbation of a chronic illness may precipitate hospitalization, and the complications that may occur profoundly affect the progress of a hospitalized patient. Because the acute event for which an older patient is hospitalized is frequently superimposed on a chronic condition or disease, this older age-group is increasingly influencing the acute care environment and the professional caregiver skills required in this setting.

CHARACTERISTICS OF THE ACUTE CARE ENVIRONMENT

Caregivers are challenged to attend to the diverse needs of each individual admitted to the acute care setting. The older adult is not likely to be admitted to the hospital until a high level of acuity or complexity exists. The intensity of care required for the typically emergent condition for which an older adult was admitted, compounded by the normal aging process, chronic illness, and impaired functional status, requires astute care planning and case management on the part of the health care team. The health care team's success in providing this care is influenced by the philosophy of care, awareness of the risks of hospitalization, and safety features of the acute care environment.

Philosophy of Care

Rapidly rising costs and concerns over quality in acute care have fostered a climate in which the value and efficacy of hospitalization have come under increasing scrutiny. With an increasing number of aged hospitalized patients, the technologic and mechanistic orientation toward care is being recognized as obscuring those activities aimed at improving function of the chronically, physically, and mentally disabled. Effective caregiving practices can enable older persons to maintain or improve their independence and to return to their preferred setting at discharge. However, in the hospital setting health care professionals can become so involved in addressing the acute condition they fail to appreciate the underlying problems and how these too influence the patient's health and recovery.

The hospital is a highly technologic system that is in a good position to address both chronic and acute problems. The focus needs to be not only on the restoration of health but also on the promotion and preservation of health. High technology ("high tech") is a common and prominent orientation for acute care settings. The high value placed on technology fosters a task orientation that may detract from the holistic focus required for the care of older adults. A balance between "high tech" and "high touch" is required to ensure effective care and a high level of functional status for older adult patients.

Acute care centers have traditionally provided care within a medical model with the focus on diagnosis and treatment, rather than on a functional model, which more broadly integrates all aspects of care. With older adults, particularly those hospitalized because of an exacerbation of a chronic illness, focusing on a functional model helps address concerns related to both their medical and functional stability. The biomedical model practiced in the hospital needs to be expanded to include this functional model, in which the main goal may not be curing the disease, but managing the disease, with a focus on self-care and symptom management strategies.

Risks of Hospitalization

Adverse Drug Reactions. *Polypharmacy* (taking five or more drugs during the same period) is a common cause of iatrogenic illness (Kane, Ouslander, and Abrass, 1994). Hospitalized patients are often admitted with a large number of prescribed, over-the-counter, and homeopathic drugs in their bodies; when given additional medications during their hospital stay, they have a heightened risk for an adverse drug reaction.

Conversely, adverse drug reactions frequently precipitate hospitalizations and, though often unreported, are among the most common iatrogenic events in the acute care setting. The hospital staff needs to get an accurate drug history of a patient; be aware of pharmacokinetic and pharmacodynamic changes related to aging; and have a working understanding of drug-disease, drug-drug, and drug-food interactions in older adults (Fletcher, 1995). Nurses who are on the front lines should be particularly aware of drugs that may be high risk when used in older adults and carefully monitor patients taking them for signs and symptoms of toxicity (DeMaagd, 1997).

Falls. Studies indicate that up to 84% of all adverse inpatient incidents are related to falls, and patients ages 65 and older experience the most falls, with approximately 10% falling more than once during their hospital stay (Wilson, 1998). Risk factors for hospital falls include both intrinsic and extrinsic factors. Intrinsic factors include age-related physiologic changes and diseases, as well as medications that affect cognition and balance. Extrinsic factors include environmental hazards such as cluttered hospital rooms, wheels on beds and chairs, and beds higher than what an older adult usually has at home. Fall rates appear to be highest during the first week of hospitalization (possibly because of the acute illness and environmental unfamiliarity) and then again during the third week of the hospital stay (possibly because of a combination of deconditioning and remobilization efforts before an impending discharge) (Tideiksaar, 1993) (see Chapter 12).

Infection. Older adults are generally more vulnerable to infections because of physiologic changes in the immune system and underlying chronic disease (see Chapter 17). The nosocomial (hospital-acquired) infection rate for hospitalized patients in general is approximately 5%, with the greatest incidence in the older patient population (*Merck manual of geriatrics*, 2000). This may be a low estimate, because the atypical presentation of older adults with infections makes infections more difficult to diagnose. The respiratory and urinary tracts are the most common sites of infection. Urinary tract infections (UTIs) occur frequently, although bacteriuria in an older adult is often asymptomatic. Subclinical infection and inflammation can occur with presenting symptoms such as acute confusion, functional capacity deterioration, anorexia, or nausea, rather than the classic symptoms of fever and dysuria (Taylor, 1998). Urinary catheterization, which is often necessary when an older patient is acutely ill, often causes bacteriuria, and catheter-associated bacteriuria is a significant cause of death secondary to bacteremia (Ackermann and Monroe, 1996). Nosocomial pneumonia is twice as likely to occur in older patients as in younger ones (Hanson, Weber, and Rutala, 1992), and the absence of typical signs and symptoms often leads to a delay in diagnosis and treatment in older adults.

Other common sites of infection in hospitalized older adults include skin and soft tissue, wounds, and the gastrointestinal tract and blood. Increasing age has also been shown to be a risk factor for colonization and infection with antibiotic-resistant strains of organisms (Terpenning et al, 1994), such as methicillin-resistant *Staphylococcus aureus* (MRSA) and vancomycin-resistant enterococcus. Control of the spread of resistant strains of organisms continues to be a problem in institutional settings. Adhering to basic principles of infection control is critical for nurses. Hand washing, disinfection of the environment, and appropriate precautions taken with those infected or colonized with resistant strains are essential. Paying special attention to older patients and addressing their needs as they relate to adequate nutrition, the importance of avoiding instrumentation, and the prevention of skin trauma are also supportive.

Hazards of Immobility. Once older adults are hospitalized, immobilization through enforced bedrest or restraint often results in functional disability. Immobilized patients are vulnerable to rapid loss of muscle strength, reductions in orthostatic competence, urinary incontinence or retention, fecal impaction, atelectasis and pneumonia, acute confusion, depression, skin breakdown, and many other complications (Kane, Ouslander, and Abrass, 1994). The occurrence of iatrogenic illnesses often represents a vicious circle, referred to as the *cascade effect*, in which one problem increases the person's vulnerability to another one. Gerontologic nurses must be leaders in advocating more appropriate care and treatment of hospitalized older adults to prevent or at least reduce the occurrence of iatrogenic illness.

Safety Features

Older adults have a decreased ability to negotiate within and adapt to an unfamiliar environment. Multiple stimuli, such as contact with many departments and personnel or multiple room changes, can prompt confusion and exhaustion, as well as result in the loss of crucial personal items necessary for maximum functioning, such as hearing aids, prostheses, dentures, and eyeglasses.

The environment can be modified in many ways for older adult patients (Box 9-1). Some modifications require additional resources, but some changes can result from observations and require minimum creativity on the part of the nursing staff.

NURSING IN THE ACUTE CARE SETTING

The nursing staff in the hospital provides the lion's share of the health care delivered there. Nurses are considered an integral part of the health care team and frequently provide leadership to this team. Those with gerontologic nursing skills can be instrumental in ensuring that high-quality, cost-effective health care is provided to hospitalized older patients; they can also help equip older patients and their families with the necessary self-care skills at discharge. The quality of the nursing care provided is influenced by the philosophy of nursing, the gerontologic nursing–specific competency and expertise of the nursing staff, and the various aspects of the gerontologic nursing role that are implemented in acute care.

Gerontologic Nursing–Specific Competency and Expertise

Developing gerontologic nursing competency helps the nursing staff customize the care provided to patients ages 65 and older. It enhances the nurse's job performance and the quality of care delivered. The Joint Commission on Accreditation of Healthcare Organizations (JCAHO) (1998) requires documentation that all staff members (e.g., nurses, unlicensed assistive personnel, phlebotomists, physical therapists) have a documented competency assessment that includes the special needs and behaviors of the specific patient age-groups (e.g., geriatric, pediatric, adolescent) that are being cared for in the assigned area. JCAHO further requires that this be done on initial employment and then periodically reviewed.

A priority at the beginning of every hospitalization is the assessment of the older adult's baseline functional status in order to develop an individual care plan within the acute care

BOX 9-1 Environmental Modifications

- Stabilized furnishings (e.g., removing or locking wheels)
- "Blue" fluorescent lighting
- Nightlights
- Extra lighting in bathrooms
- Consistent lighting intensity
- Light switches that glow
- Solid-color designs for floors (i.e., avoidance of patterns)
- Nonskid, nonglare floor wax
- Carpeting with uncut, low pile and padding underneath
- Contrasting color to identify boundaries between floor and wall
- Nonglossy wall surfaces
- Polarized window glass to decrease glare
- Nonglare glass over pictures; avoidance of abstract designs
- Rounded handrails for easy grasp in all areas where walking occurs; use of high-contrast colors in these areas
- Levers for doors and dressers instead of knobs
- Large-numbered, white-on-black (or black-on-white) clocks with nonglare glass
- Large-print calendars within patient's line of vision
- Telephones with large numbers
- Cases for glasses and prostheses attached to bedside and within reach
- Amplified and hearing aid–compatible phones
- Pocket talker
- Beds that lower to a height that enables patient to sit on edge with both feet on the floor
- Use of no side rails or half-rails to deter climbing over rails
- Bed or chair exit alarms
- Chairs with armrests
- Portable elevated toilet seats
- Grab bars in shower and around toilet

Modified from Morath J, Fulton J: Acute care of elders. In Burnside I: *Nursing and the aged,* ed 3, New York, 1988, McGraw-Hill; and Tideiksaar R: Environmental modifications. In *Falls in older persons: prevention and management in hospitals and nursing homes,* Boulder, Colo, 1993, Tactilitics.

BOX 9-2 Functional Assessment Tools

Barthel Index—Measures 15 self-care and mobility functions; used commonly in rehabilitation; range is 0 (total dependence) to 100 (maximum independence); a score of 40 or less indicates severe level of dependence (Granger, Albrecht, and Hamilton, 1979)

Functional Assessment Inventory (FAI)—A shortened form of the Older Americans Resources and Services Multidimensional Functional Assessment Questionnaire (OARS-MFAQ); measures five areas, including physical health, ADLs, mental health, social resources, and financial resources (Pfeiffer, 1982)

Instrumental Activities of Daily Living (IADLs)—Measures more complex activities, such as home management skills, management of finances, and transportation (Lawton and Brody, 1969)

Katz Index for ADLs—Measures six different ADL functions and is scored by performance vs. ability; 1 point given for each dependent task and 1 for each independent task (Katz et al, 1963)

PULSES Profile—Used in rehabilitation settings; measures functional performance in mobility, self-care ability, medical status, and psychosocial functions; items scored on a 4-point scale from independent to dependent; overall scores range from 6 (most independent) to 24 (most dependent) (Granger, Albrecht, and Hamilton, 1979)

Rapid Disability Scale-2—Measures 18 areas incorporating ADLs, IADLs, degree of disabilities, and degree of special problems (e.g., depression, confusion) (Linn and Linn, 1982)

environment (St. Pierre, 1998) (Box 9-2). Systematic functional assessment in the acute care setting also provides a benchmark of a patient's progress as he or she moves along the continuum of care, and it promotes systematic communication of the patient's health status between health care settings (Kresevic et al, 1997). The uniqueness of assessment in the acute care setting includes recognition that older adults are in an unfamiliar environment, which is not conducive to optimizing function at a time when reserves and homeostatic needs are compromised by acute illness. Many common assessment tools for ADLs and mental status include areas of function that may not be easily assessed at the time of admission or may not be as significant at that time (i.e., orientation when a calendar is not present in the room and when daily routines are disrupted). The primary goal of the acute care nurse is to maximize the older patient's independence by enhancing function. Functional strengths and weaknesses need to be identified. Then the care plan must provide for interventions that build on identified strengths and help the patient overcome identified weaknesses (see Chapter 4). Function integrates all aspects of the patient's condition; any change in functional status in an older adult should be interpreted as a classic sign of illness or as a complication. By knowing an older patient's baseline function, the nurse can assess new-onset signs or symptoms before they trigger a downward spiral of dependency and permanent impairment.

Gerontologic nursing expertise is particularly needed in the acute care setting to guide the nursing staff in understanding the unique needs of older patients and enhancing the staff's skill in managing common geriatric syndromes (Francis, Fletcher, and Simon, 1998; St. Pierre, 1998). The advanced practice nurse in gerontologic nursing functions in the role of clinician, educator, consultant, and researcher. A growing number of acute care settings are recruiting and hiring gerontologic advanced practice nurses. Gerontologic nurse practitioners are also being employed to assist with the day-to-day assessment and management of patients in the acute care setting. Some studies demonstrate a significant decrease in the length of stay when patients are comanaged by a nurse practitioner and an attending physician (Miller, 1997). The advanced practice nurse can be instrumental in developing and implementing protocols for managing common geriatric syndromes like those defined in the geriatric triad.

The geriatric triad includes falls, changes in cognitive status, and incontinence (Wells, 1992). These three conditions need special attention during hospitalization. Falls are common throughout life. Of significance for older adults is the fact that falls can be a classic sign of illness; an older adult in the acute care setting is often at high risk for falls and consequent injuries. Strange environment, confusion, medications, immobility, urinary urgency, and age-related sensory changes all contribute to this increased risk. Falls resulting in injury can be minimized by gait training and strengthening exercises, appropriate nutrition, careful monitoring of medications, supervised toileting, environmental modifications, proper footwear, and control of orthostatic hypotension (Brady et al, 1993). Bed and leg alarms to provide warnings of patient movement and thereby minimize falls are being tried in many institutions (see Chapter 12) (see Emergency Treatment box).

Critical Care and Trauma Care

Older adults admitted to the hospital in general are critically ill, and effective nursing care requires an understanding of their impaired homeostatic mechanisms, their body systems' diminished reserve capacity, and their impaired immunologic response. The homeostatic mechanisms are altered with age so that the abilities to generate a fever, to respond to alterations in tissue integrity, and to sense pain may be very different from those manifested by young or middle-age adults in critical care (Walker, 1992). The atypical and subtle nature of disease presentation becomes even more important in the ICU where the patient is often less able to articulate discomfort and new problems can arise quickly. The nurse must be aware that the most common presenting symptom of sepsis in older patients is acute mental status change (Stanley, 1996). Astute observation for delirium is essential to aggressively manage its underlying cause (see Chapter 29). Delirium in this setting in the past was referred to as "ICU psychosis" and was thought to be due to sensory overload or sensory deprivation. The causes are now recognized as multifactoral and, in this environment, are often secondary to acute illness, drugs, and environment. Critically ill individuals are at particular risk for delirium because of impaired physical and mental defenses (St. Pierre, 1996) (Table 9-1).

Two additional issues for critical care of older adults are prevention of nutritional compromise and recognition of adverse drug reactions. Up to 65% of hospitalized older adults are malnourished on admission or acquire nutritional deficits while hospitalized (Sullivan and Lipschitz, 1997). In the critical care setting, patients are sicker, with ever-changing metabolic requirements that necessitate daily nutritional monitoring. Clinical recognition of the pharmacokinetic and pharmacodynamic changes associated with aging is most important in the critical care setting, where more drugs are used to combat more problems (see Chapter 22). Drugs given in the critical care context can be lifesaving and life threatening at the same time (Planchock and Slay, 1996).

The most common traumatic injuries (see Chapter 12) experienced by those over age 65 are a result of falls, automobile accidents, and burns. Older adults suffer injuries of equivalent severity to those of younger persons; however, the consequences are more severe (Robbins and Courts, 1997). It is essential to obtain a thorough history of an injury from the patient and his or her family, including the circumstances surrounding the event and the events leading up to the injury. Health care professionals in the field need to realize that older adults do not tolerate hypoperfusion long and can quickly go into cardiogenic shock and multisystem organ failure. Early hemodynamic monitoring is required. The vital signs of an older adult might be restored to normal, yet the person might still be in cardiogenic shock (Mandavia and Newton, 1998). As much as volume depletion is a concern, so is volume overload in patients with limited cardiac and renal reserve. Insertion of a catheter does increase the risk of infection in older adults but is often justified for its monitoring value (Robbins and Courts, 1997).

Thermoregulatory mechanisms become impaired as a person ages, and older adults with trauma are particularly vulnerable. Care should be taken to reduce heat loss by using warm intravenous solutions, warm blankets, and proper

EMERGENCY TREATMENT

FALLS

- Reassure patient and family.
- Examine for presence of injury.
- Assess for injury and call attending physician to assess physical injury.
- Advocate for adequate assessment to include methods designed to identify covert or symptomless consequences of the fall (e.g., computed tomography scan, radiograph).
- Explore the cause of the fall with the health care team by reviewing the patient's history, including any history of falls and any intrinsic or extrinsic factors that may be related to the fall.
- Document the incident and its precipitating factors, along with a plan to prevent future falls.
- Implement a fall prevention program.

TABLE 9-1 Changes in Cognitive Status

	DELIRIUM	DEMENTIA	DEPRESSION
Onset	Sudden and acute	Insidious, subtle, gradual; difficult to pinpoint	Can be sudden or gradual, depending on course; can pinpoint date
Duration	Brief; often clears within 1 month or when underlying disorder is resolved	2 to 20 years	Weeks to years; variable
Awareness	Clouded state of consciousness; disoriented	Alert and aware	Directed inward; self-absorbed
Mood/behavior	Easily distracted; incoherent speech; difficulty with attention and concentration; hallucinations and illusions; disturbed sleep-wake cycle; increased or decreased psychomotor activity; fluctuation of symptoms: lucid at times; often worse at night	Personality changes; emotionally labile; may become easily agitated, with catastrophic reactions	Often aware of cognitive problems; apathetic, with feelings of hopelessness or worthlessness; vague somatic complaints
Task performance	Often unable to carry out tasks; difficulty following directions	Tries hard to carry out activities; gradual loss of abilities	Able, but makes little effort
Mental function	Disorganized thinking; fluctuating impairments in memory, coherence, orientation, and perception	Impairments in memory, abstract thinking, judgment, and language; loss of common knowledge	Selective memory loss: "I don't know" answers on cognitive tests

environmental control. The degree of long-term recovery of older adults who survive injury is variable, and aggressive rehabilitation and social supports are important factors in recovery. Research supports the fact that older adults are at greater risk for complications and higher mortality even when injuries are not severe (Robb, 1991).

Special Care-Related Issues

In addition to ensuring safe and restorative care in the acute care setting, the health care team is responsible for a number of other older adult care issues, including those related to learning needs, decision making and self-care, and ethical and legal concerns.

Supporting and facilitating self-care behaviors for older patients and their families are responsibilities of the health care team, but such activities are most often implemented and coordinated by the nurse. Adaptations can be made to support and facilitate learning in older adults via the sensory, motor, and cognitive systems (Box 9-3). Assessment of sensory and cognitive status is the first step in determining if adaptations are needed. Sensory and cognitive changes require a multisensory approach. Teaching strategies should be individualized and need to include multiple sensory stimuli: seeing, hearing, touching, and smelling. Also important may be the presence of family members or other home caregivers during the teaching process to prepare them to reinforce information needs once a patient is home (Box 9-4).

Motivation and rewards to enhance learning and compliance with needed self-care are specific to each individual. Compliance with new health care regimens can be promoted by clearly identifying benefits of behaviors that are of value to the patient, reinforcing information through support systems, and involving significant others in the learning process. Older adults are much more capable of using previous experiences to problem solve than are younger persons. The nurse should teach what is *immediately applicable* to the life of an older adult. Decreasing the risk of a heart attack may not be nearly as important as increasing function so that the older adult can go to church or spend time with family. The content of teaching should address not only the care of a given disease but also the maintenance of functional status. The nurse should also document teaching and referrals, and prepare the patient for possible setbacks (Dellasega et al, 1994).

HOME CARE AND HOSPICE

Community-based service providers are challenged to develop affordable and appropriate programs to assist older adults to remain in the home while maintaining a good quality of life. Community-based services for older adults include

BOX 9-3 Adaptations for Older Learners

GENERAL TIPS

- Ensure the person is free of pain, hunger, thirst, and cold, and has voided; attend to physical needs.
- Assess sensory and cognitive functions.
- Physically offer fluids during session.
- Provide for toileting breaks.
- Set mutual long-term goals, with short-term goals to reach these.
- Encourage family participation.
- Break down psychomotor skills step by step.
- Problem solve any barriers.
- Provide variety; use diverse teaching methods.

TIPS TO ACCOMMODATE VISUAL CHANGES

- Make certain the patient's eyeglasses are clean and on.
- Use 14- to 16-point type on all reading materials.
- Use serif lettering.
- Use double or triple spacing between lines.
- Use nonglossy, off-white paper with black letters for high contrast.
- Avoid blues, greens, and violets to differentiate print or pictures from print.
- Use sheer curtains or polarized glass to minimize window glare.
- To minimize glare, avoid having the patient face a sunny window.
- Use halogen lights; focus light, aimed from behind the patient, directly on the object to be viewed.
- Use contrasting colors to help differentiate depth.

TIPS TO ACCOMMODATE HEARING CHANGES

- Minimize all background noise (e.g., turn off radio or television, close door).
- If person has hearing aids, make sure they are on and working.
- Sit face-to-face to facilitate lip reading.
- Speak normally, or lower the pitch of your voice.
- Use pictures, models, or written key words to reinforce verbal teaching.
- Select videos or slides or tape presentations that use speakers with deeper voices.
- Demonstrate tasks.

TIPS TO ACCOMMODATE COGNITIVE CHANGES

- Slow the pace and allow extra time for the person to respond.
- Schedule short sessions that present one topic at a time.
- Give only relevant information.
- Use examples or analogies related to life experiences.
- Give concrete, rather than abstract, information.
- Repeat key words often.
- Reinforce with printed materials.
- Whenever possible, use materials that the person can feel, touch, and manipulate.

Modified from Weinrich SP, Boyd M, Nussbaum J: Continuing education: adapting strategies to teach the elderly, *J Gerontol Nurs* 15(11):17, 1989; and Weinrich SP, Boyd M: Education in the elderly: adapting and evaluating teaching tools, *J Gerontol Nurs* 18(1):15, 1992.

an array of services targeted to help older adults remain at home. Home health care, community-based alternative programs, respite care, adult day care programs, senior citizen centers, homemaker programs, home-delivered meals, and transportation are a few of the services offered in different communities (Box 9-5). In some areas churches and neighborhoods have organized volunteer programs to help meet the needs of older adults who rarely leave home. Some of these programs rely on paid nurses and volunteers from the community.

To identify the needs of the older population, nurses in the community must have sharp assessment skills and knowledge of normal aging changes, chronic illnesses, and the effects of illnesses and treatments on older adults. They must also be aware of available community resources. Home health remains one way to help the older adult who has a physical or cognitive impairment stay in the home. Because of changes in reimbursement for federal programs that provide services for older adults and limited funds for state programs, home health nurses are challenged to use interventions that are both effective and cost-efficient.

FACTORS AFFECTING THE HEALTH CARE NEEDS OF NONINSTITUTIONALIZED OLDER ADULTS

Functional Status

Functional status is a term used to describe an individual's ability to perform the normal, expected, or required activities for self-care. It is a determinant of well-being and a measure of independence in older adults. Functional measures are much more useful in describing the service needs of older adults living in the community than are measures of acute and chronic illness. Because of their ability to predict service needs, functional measures are used to determine eligibility for many state-funded and federally funded community-based, long-term care programs. Physicians frequently order physical or occupational therapy as part of home health when there is a functional deficit (Sehya and Williams, 1999).

Functional status is often the key to whether an older adult needs home health care or a home health client is to be recertified for home care services. The use of adaptive equipment,

BOX 9-4 Case Study

An 86-year-old man has just been admitted with dehydration. He is not a good historian because of acute confusion. However, his family indicates that he is an active, independent man who recently participated in the Senior Olympics. The nurse instructs him not to get out of bed by himself because he is old and frail. He has to void and calls for the nurse, but he cannot wait, so he walks to the bathroom and falls. To protect him from further falls, he is put in a vest restraint. He already has a reddened area over his sacrum. He then needs to void again but cannot, so he wets the bed. The patient is now restrained and has an incontinent brief in place. Symptoms of depression and loss of appetite soon become evident. A feeding tube is inserted. The confusion gradually becomes more apparent; the patient pulls at his various tubes, prompting the nurse to apply wrist restraints. The patient's whole life has become a hospital bed. The cognitive impairments and the ever-changing environment prompt yelling out (from fear and anger). A chemical restraint is then applied in the form of a medication to reduce the agitation.

At what point in this case could the nurse have applied different interventions? What alternative interventions could have been attempted? What possible outcomes could have been achieved with these alternate interventions?

BOX 9-5 Services for Older Individuals

ACCESS SERVICES

- Case management
- Information and referral
- Transportation

COMMUNITY-BASED SERVICES

- Adult day care
- Congregate nutrition programs
- Elder abuse/protective services
- Health screening/wellness promotion services
- Housing services
- Institutional respite care
- Legal assistance
- Multipurpose senior centers
- Psychologic counseling
- Retirement planning

IN-HOME SERVICES

- Home-delivered meals
- Home health services
- Home hospice care
- Homemaker services
- Home maintenance and repair or chore services
- In-home respite care
- Personal emergency response systems
- Telephone monitoring and friendly visitors

as well as barriers to the client's function, should be noted. While assessing the client's functional status, the home health nurse considers the client's cognitive status, respiratory and cardiovascular status, and skin integrity. Deficits in these areas could impair the client's ability to perform ADLs and IADLs safely. The client's perception of self-care is also important because he or she could believe that no assistance is required when, in fact, a deficit exists (Neal, 1998).

For older adults, adapting to functional limitations is crucial to maintaining independence. The outcomes of severe functional impairments are costly options (e.g., institutionalization). The home health nurse is in a key position to assess for functional impairments. Early detection of limitations can lead to interventions that help preserve function and avoid more severe disability (Treml, 1996).

Cognitive Function

Cognitive impairment, which often affects an individual's functional status, is another eligibility criterion used by various community programs. Cognitive status is assessed on admission and again with every skilled nursing visit. Other disciplines are also responsible for reporting a change in cognition to the nurse or case manager in home health. A change in cognitive status frequently signals a change in another body system (see Chapter 29). The home health nurse must establish a baseline assessment and be alert to deviations. Cognitive impairments can be reversible or irreversible, and home health personnel are in a key position to detect any changes.

Cognitive impairments are associated with functional limitations. For example, individuals with deficits in memory, language, abstract thinking, and judgment have great difficulty executing ADLs or IADLs (e.g., shopping, paying bills, preparing meals, and personal care tasks) even though they may have no *physical* impairments or disabilities. Cognitively impaired individuals often need supervision and cueing, rather than physical assistance, to perform ADLs and IADLs.

Although cognitive impairment alone does not meet the criteria for home health care services covered by Medicare, many states provide services for individuals with Alzheimer's disease and related dementias through Medicaid and Medicare waiver programs. Medicare covers skilled nursing visits when (1) the skill is necessary to maintain the client's health, (2) the cognitive impairment interferes with the client's ability to perform the skill, and (3) there is no caregiver present or able to perform the skill. An older adult who requires daily insulin injections but is unable to draw up or administer the insulin because of a cognitive impairment is an example of someone who qualifies for home health care.

Housing Options for Older Adults

Although most older adults prefer to live independently, it is not always possible or appropriate; financial status, functional status, and physical health may dictate consideration of alternative housing options that provide a more protective and supportive environment. Table 9-2 describes the most common housing options for older adults. Each option has its advantages and disadvantages. The decision about which option is most appropriate depends on such factors as the amount and type of assistance an older person requires, financial resources, geographic mobility, preferences for privacy and social contact, and the types of housing available. AARP

TABLE 9-2 Housing Options for Older Adults

TYPE OF HOUSING	DESCRIPTION OF HOUSING
Accessory apartment	This is a self-contained apartment unit within a house that allows an individual to live independently without living alone. It generates additional income for older homeowners and allows older renters to live near relatives or friends and remain in a familiar community.
Assisted living facility (also called board and care home; personal care home; or sheltered care, residential care, or domiciliary care facility)	This is a rental housing arrangement that provides room, meals, utilities, and laundry and housekeeping services for a group of residents. Such facilities offer a homelike atmosphere in which residents share meals and have opportunities to interact. What distinguishes these facilities from simple boarding homes is that they provide protective oversight and regular contact with staff members. Some facilities offer additional services such as nonmedical personal care (e.g., bathing, grooming) and social and recreational activities. In many states these facilities operate without specific regulation or licensure; therefore quality of service may vary greatly.
Congregate housing	Congregate housing was authorized in 1970 by the Housing and Urban Development Act. It is a group-living arrangement, usually an apartment complex, that provides tenants with private living units (including kitchen facilities), housekeeping services, and meals served in a central dining room. It is different from board and care facilities in that it provides professional staff such as social workers, nutritionists, and activity therapists who organize social services and activities.
Elder Cottage Housing Opportunity (ECHO)	This is a small, self-contained portable unit that can be placed in the backyard or at the side of a single-family dwelling. The idea was developed in Australia (where it is called a "granny flat") to allow older adults to live near family and friends but still retain privacy and independence. ECHO units are distinct from mobile homes in that they are barrier-free and energy-efficient units specifically designed for older or disabled persons.
Foster home care	Foster care for adults is similar in concept to foster care for children. It is a social service administered by the state that places an older person who needs some protective oversight or assistance with personal care in a family environment. Foster families receive a stipend to provide board and care, and older clients have a chance to participate in family and community activities. Adult foster care is appropriate for older adults who cannot live independently but do not want or need institutional care.
Home sharing	Home sharing involves two or more unrelated people living together in a house or apartment. It may involve an older person and a younger person or two or more older people living together. The participants may share all living expenses, share rent only, or exchange services for rent. For the older homeowner, renting out a bedroom generates revenue that may make it possible to afford taxes and home expenses. Home sharing is viewed by many older adults as a practical alternative to moving in with adult children. Some communities provide house-matching programs, usually sponsored by local senior centers or Area Agency on Aging.
Life care or continuing care retirement community (CCRC)	This is a facility designed to support the concept of "aging in place." It provides a continuum of living arrangements and care—from assistance with household chores to nursing facility care—all within a single retirement community. Residents live independently in apartments or houses and contract with the community for health and social services as needed. If a resident's need for health and nursing care prohibits independent living, the individual can move from a residential unit to the community's health care unit or nursing facility. In addition to providing shelter, meals, and health care, a CCRC provides a variety of services and activities (e.g., religious services, adult education classes, library, trips, recreational and social programs). The key attribute of a CCRC is that it guarantees a lifetime commitment to care of an individual as long as the person remains in the retirement community. The major disadvantage of a CCRC is that it can be expensive; most CCRCs require a nonrefundable entrance fee and charge a monthly assessment, which may increase.

Modified from American Association of Retired Persons (AARP): *Tomorrow's choices,* Washington, DC, 1988, The Association; AARP: *Your home, your choice,* Washington, DC, 1984, The Association; and AARP: *Staying at home: a guide to long-term care and housing,* Washington, DC, 1992, The Association.

has several publications that describe each of these options in greater detail, including issues to consider when evaluating each option.

COMMUNITY-BASED SERVICES

Use of Community- and Home-Based Services by Older Adults

Assessment of functional status aids in determining the type of services an older adult needs to remain in his or her home. A low score on a functional status test does not necessarily indicate the need for institutionalization, but it means that the older adult needs assistance with specific activities (Moody, 1998). The type of services needed, the availability of the services, the cost of the services, and the requirements to qualify for the services can be determined by a home health agency.

Community services can be categorized into formal and informal services. Home health care is a short-term, formal service that provides assessment, observation, teaching, certain technical skills, and personal care. A client may receive home health care for a limited time and for a specific diagnosis. Homemaker services are another formal service. To qualify for most homemaker services, the older person must demonstrate a financial requirement and specified need for service. Informal services include senior citizen centers, adult day care services, nutrition services, transportation services, and telephone monitoring services. Community resources, formal and informal, must meet the client's needs (see Cultural Awareness box).

Because of fragmentation, noninstitutional long-term care depends on coordination of efforts between informal and formal care providers. In some instances families function as case managers, ensuring that resources and services are provided appropriately. In other situations case management services are provided by formal organizations, such as home health care agencies or managed care agencies. Nurses who work in the community and in home health care play a key role in coordinating formal and informal services. These nurses must be familiar with community resources and should assist older individuals and their families to access these resources. Home health nurses have a particular responsibility to assess older adults who are receiving home health services and to determine how their individual needs can best be met. The home health nurse identifies appropriate community resources, initiates the referral process, develops a care plan, coordinates services, evaluates the services, and determines if there is a need for additional services (Humphrey and Milone-Nuzzo, 1996).

Cultural Awareness

COMMUNITY-BASED LONG-TERM CARE FOR LATINO OLDER ADULTS

The number of Latinos older than 65 is projected to increase 500% by the year 2030. In a national survey of 2299 Latinos (of any Hispanic ancestry, but predominantly Mexican Americans and Puerto Rican Americans) ages 65 and older, Wallace and Lew-Ting (1992) found that Latinos have higher rates of disability than their white counterparts and a greater need for community-based long-term care.

Two major factors influence the interest and ability of Latino families to seek formal long-term care: cultural influences and structural influences. *Cultural influences* include the belief systems and preferences that cause certain patterns of health care use. Because long-term care often involves nontechnical assistance that can be provided by family members, Latino older adults tend to use nursing facilities less often as family members make sacrifices to help older relatives. More acculturated families provide lower levels of care and less informal support for older adults than less acculturated ones.

Structural influences include the way the health care system and other social institutions are organized and operated. They may present both incentives and barriers to the use of health services. Given the importance of income and insurance in determining long-term care use, there is a major gap in the health insurance status of Latino older adults. In the general population, one third of Latinos are uninsured, compared with 13% of whites and 19% of blacks. This is largely because Latinos are concentrated in industries that do not offer insurance, such as personal services and construction, and because they tend to live in states with stringent Medicaid eligibility criteria, such as Texas and Florida. As a result, serious illness in the family is considered a financial problem almost twice as often among Latinos as other whites (39% versus 19%).

Research reveals that the need for in-home health services for older Latinos is substantial. Mexican American older adults are less likely than the average Latino to use in-home health services despite similar levels of need. Nurses should not assume that Latino families are taking care of their disabled older members simply because of a cultural preference. Nurses should provide information and advice on the use of in-home health services when an older Latino client is physically disabled.

From Wallace S, Lew-Ting C: Getting by at home: community-based long-term care of Latino elders, *West J Med* 157:337-344, 1992. Adapted and reproduced with permission from the BMJ Medical group.

Profile of Community- and Home-Based Services

Area Agencies on Aging. The major goal of the Older Americans Act (OAA) of 1965 was to remove barriers to independent living for older individuals and to ensure the availability of appropriate services for those in need. Through Title III, the Administration on Aging and state and community programs were designed to meet the needs of older adults, especially those at risk for loss of independence. The OAA established a national network of federal, state, and area

Agencies on Aging (AAAs), which are responsible for providing a range of community services for older adults. States are divided into areas for planning and service administration. The OAA requires that each AAA designate community "focal points" as places where anyone in the community can receive information, services, and access to all of a community's resources for older adults. Multipurpose senior citizen centers often serve as these focal points, but community centers, churches, hospitals, and town halls may also be designated as focal points. The types of services provided through the OAA and AAAs include information and referral for medical and legal advice; psychologic counseling; preretirement and postretirement planning; programs to prevent abuse, neglect, and exploitation; programs to enrich life through educational and social activities; health screening and wellness promotion services; and nutrition services (Greenberg, 1995).

Multipurpose Senior Centers. Senior centers are community facilities that provide a broad range of services to older adults in the community. These services include (1) health screening; (2) health promotion and wellness programs; (3) social, educational, and recreational activities; (4) congregate meals; and (5) information and referral services for older individuals and their families. Senior centers are used primarily by relatively active and independent older adults, since such centers do not provide nursing and custodial care services. Older adults who require these types of services would benefit from attending an adult day care program. Funding for senior centers is provided primarily through the OAA and agencies such as the United Way.

Adult Day Care Services. Adult day care services provide a variety of health and social services to older adults who live alone or with their families in the community. Most people who use adult day care services are physically frail and/or cognitively impaired and require supervision or assistance with ADLs. Adult day care programs help delay institutionalization for older adults who require some supervision but do not need continuous care. This allows family members to maintain their lifestyles and employment and still provide home care for their older relative.

The majority of adult day care services operate 5 days a week during typical business hours. Charges vary with each facility, from per week to per day to per half-day. Adult day care services vary considerably in terms of eligibility criteria and the types of services provided. Key services may include transportation to and from the facility, assistance with personal care, nursing and therapeutic services, meals, and recreational activities.

Adult day care services are not federally regulated but may be licensed or certified by the state. Certification is required to receive federal funding such as Medicaid and OAA funding. Other funding sources include private pay, foundations, and long-term care insurance. Medicaid is a major funding source for most of these programs; however, participants usually pay part of the fee. Some facilities may accept only private pay or long-term-care insurance. Other private sources of funding include religious organizations, businesses, and the United Way.

Some programs accept only clients with dementia. It is difficult to combine clients with dementia and clients who have no cognitive impairment. This situation requires extra staff and usually a larger facility with separate areas for the two different groups. Staff in these programs are trained to work with persons with dementia.

Respite Care. Respite care provides short-term relief or time off for persons providing home care to ill, disabled, or frail older adults. Adult day care services are a form of respite provided outside the home. Respite care is often provided at home or in institutional settings such as specially designated hospital or nursing facility units. Respite staff include health professionals, trained volunteers, and personal care attendants. In-home and institutional respite may be provided on a regular schedule (e.g., 4 hours a week) or for longer time intervals (e.g., 1 week, a weekend, on an intermittent basis). Private pay and state programs that target lower income families are the two main funding sources for respite care.

Homemaker Services. Homemaker services include such things as housecleaning, laundry, food shopping, meal preparation, and running errands. Fees vary according to the type and frequency of services provided and are usually not covered by Medicare or Medicaid. These services are offered through home health agencies, AAAs, the Department of Health and Human Services, and private companies and organizations that provide other services to older adults. Prices vary with the type of agency offering the homemaker services. In most states no licensing or certification is required for the individual providing the care. Background checks and letters of recommendations are often the only qualifications for the positions.

Nutrition Services. Nutrition services provide older adults with inexpensive, nutritious meals at home or in group settings. Home-delivery programs such as Meals-on-Wheels deliver hot meals to the home once or twice a day, 5 days a week, and can accommodate special diets. Some Meals-on-Wheels programs sell nutritional supplements at reduced rates to older adults who cannot leave the home. Congregate meal sites provide meals in group settings such as senior centers, churches, synagogues, schools, and senior housing. The advantage of congregate meal sites is that they provide social opportunities for older adults who are otherwise socially isolated. Most nutrition programs charge a minimum fee or ask for donations. Another advantage of home-delivered meals is that the volunteer delivering the meal is able to check on the older adult daily and report any problems to the supervisor. In some instances a Meals-on-Wheels volunteer has been the first person to discover an older adult who fell in the home and was unable to seek assistance.

Transportation Services. Many communities provide transportation services for disabled older adults through public or private agencies. The transportation may be handled by volunteer drivers in cars or by a bus, taxi, train, or a public van equipped to accommodate wheelchairs. The fee for such transportation services is usually minimum and is often based on a sliding scale. In addition, many facilities that serve older adults (e.g., adult day care services, senior centers, health facilities) have their own transportation services.

Telephone Monitoring and Friendly Visitors. Telephone monitoring programs provide regular phone contact (usually daily) to older persons who live alone or are alone during the day. The phone calls provide social contact, as well as a check for those who are concerned about their health and safety. Friendly visitors make home visits for the purpose of companionship, assistance with correspondence, and needs assessment. Telephone monitoring staff and friendly visitors are volunteers who work through local community organizations such as churches, synagogues, senior centers, and social service agencies. Even if older adults live in areas where these formal services are not available, nurses can encourage informal telephone monitoring and visiting by family members, friends, and neighbors. There are also telephone services that will call individuals to remind them to take their medications. These services are usually offered for a monthly fee.

Personal Emergency Response Systems. Personal emergency response systems (PERSs) are home monitoring systems that allow older persons to obtain immediate assistance in emergent situations, such as after a fall or when suffering life-threatening symptoms. A PERS consists of a small device worn on the body that, when triggered, will send an alarm to a central monitoring station. The central monitoring station then contacts predesignated persons or the police, who respond to the emergency. A PERS can be purchased or leased for a monthly fee. Because these devices are relatively expensive, they are not a practical alternative for older adults in lower income brackets. They are not recommended for persons with dementia because resetting the device is too difficult and the device may be triggered too often for nonemergencies.

HOME HEALTH CARE

Home care consists of multiple health and social services delivered to recovering, chronically ill, or disabled individuals of all ages in their place of residence. There are three main categories of home care providers, known as *home care organizations* (National Association for Home Care [NAHC], 1999). Medicare-certified agencies include hospice and freestanding and facility-based home health agencies.

Home health services are covered by Medicare, Medicaid, private insurance, managed care plans, and private pay. Persons of all ages are eligible for home health services. Criteria for services vary based on the type of insurance. The majority of home health care recipients are ages 65 and older. Medicare, the primary payer source for home health services, requires the home health client to (1) have a skilled care need, (2) be homebound, (3) be unable to perform the skilled care alone and have no one in the home to provide care, and (4) require only intermittent care. If a caregiver is present, he or she must be unwilling or unable to provide the care needed by the registered nurse (RN). Being homebound means that the home health client has a physical reason (e.g., being bedridden) or medical condition that limits his or her ability to leave home. The use of assistive devices or a wheelchair alone does not qualify an individual for the homebound status. The home health client is allowed to leave home for medical reasons, but it must be an *effort* to do so. In other words, if the client could get to a physician's office to receive care on a regular basis, Medicare would deny the home health services. The client must also have a physician's written plan of treatment for the service specifying the frequency and duration of care provided.

Medicare establishes specific criteria for Medicare coverage by the physician, home health agency, disciplines providing care, and other entities (e.g., medical supply companies) that provide goods or services to the client. The purpose of eligibility criteria is to ensure that Medicare dollars are being spent in the most cost-effective manner. Other payer sources (e.g., health maintenance organizations [HMOs], private insurance) use Medicare criteria as a guideline for eligibility but have the flexibility to vary the criteria with individual circumstances (Rosenzweig, 1995).

Medicaid is delivered by each state and has its own criteria for reimbursement. This program can choose to pay however needs are best met. Other funding sources of home health include social service block grants, OAA funds, and general state revenues. The dollar amount spent on home health by sources other than Medicare and Medicaid varies with each state. The Veterans Administration, the Civilian Health and Medical Program of the Uniformed Services (CHAMPUS), and the Civilian Health and Medical Program of the Department of Veteran's Affairs (CHAMPVA) have their own coverage guidelines and payment methods for home health, and each covers different home health services (Rosenzweig, 1995).

Managed care companies have various methods for approving services related to home health care. The admission assessment is usually approved first. Then, based on the diagnosis, the functional status of the home health client, and the ability of the caregiver to provide help, the company assigns further home health visits. Other companies approve a specified number of visits based on the diagnosis and information from the referring physician. The home health agency stays in close communication with the managed care company to report progress and request any changes in the original care plan.

Home Health Agency

The predominant and most familiar provider of home care is the home health agency. Home health agencies have as their primary function the treatment or rehabilitation of clients through the intervention of skilled nurses or therapists. Clients admitted to a home health agency must be under a physician's supervision, and services must be provided in accordance with a physician's signed order. Home health agencies can provide a different combination of services. Skilled nursing and physical therapy can stand alone, meaning either the skilled nurse or physical therapist can serve as case manager. Speech therapists, occupational therapists, and medical social workers are not allowed to admit clients to home health care but must work with a skilled nurse or physical therapist. In addition, many agencies offer nutritional services on a limited basis. Agencies may also provide disposable medical supplies as appropriate to the diagnosis and treatment plan for a client.

Proprietary Agencies

A proprietary, or for-profit, home care agency is designed to make money for its owners. Until 1982, proprietary home care agencies were not allowed to participate in Medicare. This was changed in response to a concern that there were not enough home care services available to meet the demand. As a result, the Omnibus Budget Reconciliation Act of 1982 allowed proprietary home care agencies to become Medicare-certified, but they were not allowed to make a profit on the Medicare portion of their business. Owners of a for-profit entity are stockholders in the corporation.

Facility-Based Agencies

A facility-based home care agency is a department or component of an organization. It can be a part of a SNF or rehabilitation center, or it can be hospital based. The vast majority of agencies are hospital based, meaning that they function as a department of the hospital. These agencies may or may not share clinical, financial, or management services with the hospital.

The first hospital-based home care agency was established in 1947. Its programs offered nursing care and housekeeping and chore duties. In 1958 radiology services, nutritional services, and physical therapy were offered. With the enactment of Medicare and Medicaid in 1966, nurses were able to offer more home care to the sick and disabled (Allender, 1998). Hospital-based home care agencies were few in number until the enactment of Medicare reform (OBRA in 1987), when hospitals began to be paid for clients on Medicare on the basis of DRGs. With shorter lengths of stay, hospitals established home care agencies or affiliated with existing home care agencies to provide options for clients who were going home with existing health care needs.

What determines a facility-based home care agency from the Medicare program's point of view is whether it receives an allocation of the institution's corporate overhead. A facility-based home care agency, according to the JCAHO (1998), shows evidence of an organizational and functional relationship between the home care agency and the facility or public representation of the home care agency as a service of the facility.

Visiting Nurse Associations

A visiting nurse association (VNA) or community nursing service is a community-based home care agency with a governing board consisting of community representatives. Because of the commitment to provide home care services to a defined community and a not-for-profit status, VNAs are often recipients of United Way or Community Givers funds.

Benefits of Home Care

In survey after survey, older Americans choose "home" as their treatment place of choice. Because of changes in technology, equipment is smaller, easier to manage, and less expensive. As a result, individuals who at one time could be treated only in the hospital can now be managed at home. Family, friends, and even clients themselves can be taught to manage enteral and parenteral feedings, central lines, pain control, antibiotic therapy, and urinary catheters with a minimum of assistance.

Among those older adults who can benefit from home care services are individuals who:

- Have chronic medical conditions with exacerbations, such as congestive heart failure, COPD, unstable diabetes, kidney and liver disease with subsequent transplantation, or recent strokes
- Have chronic mental illnesses, such as depression, schizophrenia, and other psychoses
- Need assistance with medical regimens to prevent readmission to an acute care facility
- Need continued treatment after discharge from a hospital or nursing facility (e.g., wound care, intravenous therapy, physical therapy)
- Require short-term assistance at home after same-day or outpatient surgery, are terminally ill and want to die, or have families that want them to die with dignity in the comfort of their own homes

Home care is less expensive than hospitalization in most cases. For example, considerable savings can be achieved through the use of home care services with infusion therapy vendor support. Although home care services are being used because of financial considerations, there are also sound medical and humane reasons for treatment to take place in a person's home. There is evidence that people recover faster at home than in institutions, and nosocomial infections from exposure to multiple infectious processes are minimized in a person's home (see Research box).

CONTINUITY OF CARE

Enhancement of the continuum of care from hospital to home is a goal shared by both hospital and home care personnel. Continuity of care involves assisting older adults to remain in the home and avoid institutionalization by having available resources that are responsive to their needs (Moody, 1998). To ensure that a continuum of care exists from hospital to home, health care providers should follow the Plan, Do, Check, Act Cycle (Box 9-6).

Box 9-7 lists client characteristics that should suggest further evaluation for a home care referral. These characteristics alone do not warrant the need for home health care, but in combination with one another or with a new diagnosis that requires monitoring, they provide an excellent guideline to determine the need for services. The assessment can be done as a prehospitalization screening, at the time of admission to the hospital, after a client's condition has changed, or as a client is being discharged. What really matters is that the client be assessed for home care needs before he or she leaves the hospital.

Ideally, a client is screened for home care needs at the time of admission to a hospital to ensure adequate time to plan for continuity of care. In most instances, unless a client is already known to a home care agency, discharge planning occurs late in the hospital stay. As hospital lengths of stay become increasingly shorter, the time available to plan adequately for a client's postdischarge care is limited. Home care agencies and hospital discharge planners or case managers need to develop a good working relationship to ensure that clients going home have a plan that picks up where the hospital plan leaves off. To ensure a smooth transition, members of all disciplines who were caring for a client in the hospital—nurses, physicians, physical therapists, social workers, and others—should provide qualitative and quantitative

Research

SAMPLE/SETTING

The sample included 16 home health nurses from agencies in various regions of Massachusetts. The nurses had an average of 12 years of home health care experience. Education of the participants varied from diplomas to master's degrees.

METHODS

All participants met over one summer and participated in six group interviews. The groups ranged in size from two to five. Data were collected until saturation was reached. The participants were asked to (1) identify positive and negative changes in the health care system; (2) identify changes in the client population, with subcategories of (a) client-increased acuity and need, and (b) new categories of clients; and (3) respond to the following subcategories: (a) new focus in client care; (b) increasing stress, frustration, and responsibility; (c) pride in role; (d) home health care, last positive place to practice; and (e) acceptance and resilience.

FINDINGS

The home health nurses described change as constant and inevitable. Positive aspects of change included a growth in the type and quality of community-based services, improved system of communication among disciplines, and access of home care agencies to previously unavailable hospital staff. Negative aspects of change included system complexity, competition for survival, and demands from Medicare and other payers for reimbursement. All the nurses agreed that client acuity had increased. Shorter hospital stays were the primary reason cited for this increase. Clients received less discharge teaching, which placed the responsibility on the home health nurse. New focuses in home health include mental health diagnoses, an increase in persons with AIDS, clients who have outpatient surgery, and newly diagnosed clients with diabetes who have not received previous teaching. Responses to changes by home health nurses included (1) starting discharge teaching earlier, (2) focusing on client empowerment, and (3) changing the way approval for reimbursement is obtained. Obtaining reimbursement was identified as one of the main stressors for home health nurses. Managed care restrictions on costs have also contributed to their stress. Many nurses think that managed care companies do not understand the needs of home health clients, especially those of older adults.

Despite the negative results from recent changes, nurses take pride in their management, advocacy, and client skills. Being in charge of total client care instills a certain pride in a home health nurse. This pride is also a result of the expanding role of home health. Home health nurses have more responsibilities and autonomy today. Rewards include successfully discharging an older adult to self-care. The last theme addressed was acceptance and resilience. Acceptance is the acknowledgment of changes and the willingness to work with them. Resilience is the ability to cope successfully with the changes. Both of these are necessary in today's home health system.

IMPLICATIONS

There is a definite need to address changes in home health. Agencies need to help nurses adapt to changes and develop policies and procedures to deal with these changes. Nurses need to be involved at all levels where changes occur—local, state, and federal. Nurses who wish to remain in home health must be advocates for their clients so that the quality of care will not be compromised. Orientation programs must include change theory, and management must understand stress and coping related to change.

Ellenbecker CH, Warren K: Nursing practice and patient care in a changing environment, *Home Health Nurs* 16(8):531, 1998.

BOX 9-6 Plan, Do, Check, Act Cycle

PLAN
- Gather data on admission.
- Identify goals for discharge.
- Identify specific functional problems.
- Validate that a problem exists.
- Structure problems by delineating components.

DO
- Gather information about resources.
- Select all possible options.
- Identify measurable objectives in terms of the client's functional problems.
- Analyze each option for capacity to fulfill objectives.
- Identify advantages and disadvantages.

CHECK
- Compare alternatives for probability of fulfilling discharge objectives.
- Project results of alternatives.
- Explore alternatives with the client and family.
- Choose among alternatives.

ACT
- Develop the discharge plan.
- Implement the plan.
- Evaluate and follow up on the plan.
- Revise the plan as indicated.
- Update the resource file.

BOX 9-7 High-Risk Client Indicators for Home Care Services

- Unexpected readmission to the hospital within 15 to 30 days
- Frequent readmissions
- Alteration of health care problem or management
- Changes in mental status
- Frequent readmissions
- Noncompliant behavior before or during hospitalization
- Terminal or preterminal condition
- Seen in the hospital by physical, occupational, or speech therapist
- After amputation
- After hip or knee replacement
- New assistive devices
- Foley catheter, ileal conduit, suprapubic catheter, and/or incontinence
- Complex health management regimen
- Enteral or parenteral feedings
- Ostomies or tubes of any kind
- Draining wounds
- After wound débridement or irrigation and débridement for decubitus
- Pain management
- Intravenous antibiotics
- Peripherally inserted central catheter
- Intravenous chemotherapy
- Multiple medications or a major medication change
- Ventilator dependence
- Low–air loss bed or other complex medical equipment

information about the client's disposition at discharge. The same principles apply to the discharge process from SNFs or rehabilitation facilities.

In most cases a social worker is responsible for notifying the home health agency of a client's discharge. The home health agency requests information needed to ensure a smooth transition from the facility to home. In addition to demographics, necessary information includes:

- Identification of the physician who will sign the home care orders
- Orders for home health care treatments (e.g., wound care, intravenous therapy, physical therapy, occupational therapy, speech therapy)
- A description of a client's knowledge about the disease and the treatment
- A summary of a client's independence with skills
- Quantitative measures of range of motion and client response to treatment modalities
- Known social situations that could complicate or hinder the home treatment plan
- A list of supplies and medications going home with a client
- Expectations for rehospitalization or follow-up clinic visits
- Anything that would enhance a timely and efficient response from a home care agency

Role of the Home Care Agency

Admission to the home care agency begins with the referral intake. Referrals are called in to the home care agency, then the agency confirms home care benefits; schedules the admission visit consistent with the expectation of the discharge planner, physician, or client; and communicates the referral information to the nurse who will be admitting the client into service. The client must be admitted within 24 hours of discharge according to Medicare regulations.

Nurses are assigned to clients in various ways. Some assignments are made according to (1) geographic areas, (2) the client's special needs, or (3) the nurse's specialty. Examples of specialties include infusion therapy, psychiatric nursing, and cardiovascular nursing.

IMPLEMENTING THE PLAN OF TREATMENT

The Nurse's Role

The nurse conducts the initial evaluation visit after a client is referred for home care. During the initial visit and throughout subsequent visits, the nurse assesses the client's physical, functional, emotional, socioeconomic, and environmental well-being. Nurses initiate the care plan and make revisions as appropriate throughout the length of stay in home care.

Other activities requiring the specialized skill of RNs include:

- Health and self-care teaching
- Coordination and case management of complex care needs
- Medication administration (e.g., intramuscular, subcutaneous) and teaching about all medications
- Wound and decubitus care
- Urinary catheter care and teaching
- Ostomy care and teaching
- Postsurgical care
- Care of the terminally ill client

Additional activities provided by some home care nurses are:

- Case management
- Intravenous therapy, enteral and parenteral nutrition, and chemotherapy
- Psychiatric nursing care

Characteristics of a Home Care Nurse. Home health nursing is a subspecialty of community health nursing. It is community based in that the focus is the client and family, not an aggregate population. The American Nurses Association (ANA) has endorsed practice standards for home health nurses. As with other specialties, the standards address theory, research, ethics, and professional development. *The Statement on the Scope of Home Health Nursing Practice,* published by the ANA (1999), presents the conceptual model for home health nursing. The model depicts the holistic practice of the home health nurse. The American Nurses Credentialing Center certifies home health nurses. Requirements include a bachelor's degree in nursing, being licensed as an active RN in the United States, at least 2 years of practice as an RN, current practice of at least 8 hours a week in home health, and 2000 hours in home health nursing during the past 2 years. Once these requirements are met, the RN may sit for the certification examination (McEwen, 1998).

Nurses who work in home care require a diverse set of skills and abilities. Most home care agencies require a nurse to have a minimum of 2 years of hospital experience before working as a home health nurse. Working in home care requires knowledge of acute and chronic disease processes and how they affect older adults. Knowledge of gerontology, pharmacokinetics in older adults, rehabilitation nursing, and principles and presentation of disease processes in older adults are some areas in which home care nurses need to be competent. The home care nurse also needs to know adult learning principles and interpersonal communication techniques, and he or she must be aware of cultural differences and how they affect health and health care.

The home care nurse coordinates care with all disciplines involved with the case and reports findings, changes, and recommendations to the primary physician. The home care nurse also works cooperatively with community resources and governmental agencies if a situation warrants. The nurse, often the sole health care provider who visits a client's home, knows that observations made must be acted on immediately and that the instruction provided must last until the next visit. If emergency hospitalization is required, the nurse coordinates it with the family, the physician, the hospital, and emergency services.

Home care nurses need to be conscious of their own safety. Some neighborhoods are dangerous, and visits sometimes need to be made in the evening or night. The home health nurse should never go into a situation that might be physically threatening or dangerous. He or she must be self-reliant, self-assured, and comfortable in providing care in the client's locale. Taking precautions at all times, not just in potentially dangerous neighborhoods, will ensure the nurse's safety.

Role of the Home Health Aide

In 1998 there were 124,248 home health aides (HHAs) in Medicare-certified agencies. HHAs are the second largest group of employees in home care (NAHC, 1999). Under the direction of an RN, HHAs assist clients with intermittent personal care services (e.g., ADLs, hygiene), take vital signs, perform simple duties (e.g., nonsterile dressing changes, Foley catheter care), assist with medications that are normally self-administered, and report changes in clients' conditions or needs. The HHA is a nonprofessional caregiver who has completed a course of study and been certified by an appropriate agency. In addition, an HHA is required to complete at least 12 hours of in-service training each year of employment. The HHA must demonstrate competency in certain required skills and subjects taught in in-service training at least once a year (Apple and Truscott, 1995).

Since the HHA sees the client more often than caregivers from the other disciplines do, he or she is one of the most important members of the home care team. The client feels comfortable with the aide and often shares concerns that the nurse or therapist cannot elicit. The RN supervises the HHA on a bimonthly basis (Apple and Truscott, 1995).

Home health agencies also employ personal care attendants (PCAs). PCAs are generally hired for private duty cases in which only a sitter is required (as opposed to someone who provides personal or skilled care). No formal or informal training is required, but individual agencies may provide orientation and some training. Duties performed by PCAs may include, but are not limited to, the following:

- Preparing light meals
- Helping the client to the bathroom
- Assisting with dressing and ambulation
- Light housekeeping

OASIS

OASIS is an assessment tool that is integrated into an agency's assessment form. It is used to monitor outcomes of home care. OASIS is mandated by the Centers for Medicare and Medicaid Services (CMS) for all adult clients except maternity clients. Its purpose is to improve performance through a new approach called outcome-based quality improvement (Steinbach and Zuber, 1997). OASIS was developed to help shape the future direction of Medicare reimbursement and the future of home health.

OASIS data are reported to regulatory bodies at least every 30 days. The completion and reporting of OASIS data are part of the conditions of participation for the Medicare program (Mikos and Koch, 1999). OASIS is intended to eliminate the process requirements of CMS and providers and to focus on outcomes of care, such as satisfaction and improved client outcomes. OASIS data are completed on admission, discharge, interruption of services, and resumption of services. Surveyors who monitor agencies use the data for on-site reviews. They compare the data on OASIS to a client when visiting the client in the home.

HOSPICE

Dying is the final phase in the trajectory of a chronic illness. Terminal illnesses such as cancer and acquired immunodeficiency syndrome (AIDS) remain incurable. However, because of pharmacologic and technologic advances in treatments, cancer and AIDS are now considered chronic illnesses. Many chronically ill persons choose to remain in their homes during the last phase of their illness to prepare for their death in familiar surroundings, together with family and friends. Hospice provides care and services to terminally ill persons and their families that enable individuals to die in facilities or at home.

Hospice Philosophy

Hospice is a special kind of medically directed compassionate care for dying individuals and their families. It is a concept of care, not a particular place or building. The care is designed to address the physical, emotional, psychologic, and spiritual needs of dying persons and to provide support services for their families during both the dying and bereavement processes. The goal of hospice is to provide comfort care, not cure. Individuals with incurable or irreversible diseases that do not respond to treatment may choose hospice care. In addition, when a person and family have decided to stop pursuing aggressive medical treatment, hospice is an appropriate choice.

Hospice and Palliative Care. A clarification of terms commonly used in the end-of-life literature and clinical practice is necessary. In the United States the terms *hospice* and *palliative care* are frequently used. Palliative care is the broader concept; it is therapy aimed at relieving or reducing the intensity of uncomfortable symptoms, not aimed at producing a cure. Hospice is a specific type of palliative care. Because of reimbursement policies such as the Medicare hospice benefit (discussed later in this chapter), American hospices are mandated to include specific services and are subject to the eligibility requirements that clients have a terminal diagnosis and 6-month prognosis. Palliative and hospice care both have the goal of comfort, not cure. However, palliative care is provided in settings outside a hospice program and currently is not subject to the same regulations as are hospice programs.

In Canada the term *palliative care* is pervasive, and *hospice* usually refers to a particular agency or program. Many of the palliative care journals are international and originate in Canada, the United Kingdom, and the United States. Therefore it is critical to understand the meaning of the terms as used in the literature about end-of-life care in the respective country of origin. In addition, the health care delivery systems and the private versus governmental insurance programs also differ among the countries. Canadian and British terminally ill persons, families, and health care providers do not have the constraints of the 6-month prognosis required by the U.S. system.

A widely accepted definition of palliative care, developed by the World Health Organization (WHO), reads, in part:

> Palliative care is the active total care of clients whose disease is not responsive to curative treatment. Control of pain, of other symptoms, and of psychological, social, and spiritual problems is paramount. The goal of palliative care is achievement of the best possible quality of life for clients and families. It affirms life and regards dying as a normal process. Palliative care neither hastens nor postpones death. It emphasizes relief of pain and other distressing symptoms, integrates the physical, psychological, and spiritual aspects of client care, and offers a support system to help the family cope during the client's illness and in their own bereavement (WHO, 1990).

Since the 1990s tremendous interest in palliative care and end-of-life issues has evolved throughout the world. Palliative medicine is a recognized medical specialty in the United Kingdom and Canada. In the United States numerous initiatives, federal funding, and financial support from private foundations are available for research and innovative programs regarding end-of-life issues. As the research-based knowledge continues to grow, interventions to achieve the outcomes of high-quality end-of-life care for all can become a reality.

Hospice Services

There are approximately 1700 hospices in the United States. Those that are Medicare-certified number 1110 (National Association for Home Care, 2000). Services provided by a comprehensive hospice program include physician services, nursing care, medical social work, counseling services and spiritual care, certified nursing assistant services, additional therapies as needed (e.g., physical, occupational, and speech therapy), inpatient care related to difficulty in managing symptoms, medications, supplies, equipment, volunteers, respite services, continuous care in times of crisis, and bereavement services. These services constitute a basic level of hospice care established through the development of the National Hospice Organization's (NHO's) *Standards of a Hospice Program of Care* and the federally mandated operating standards for Medicare certification for hospice programs (Lattanzi-Licht, Mahoney, and Miller, 1998).

Hospice services are provided by an interdisciplinary team consisting of the client's own physician, hospice physicians, nurses, HHAs, medical social workers, chaplains, bereavement coordinators, and volunteers. Team members use their skills and expertise to meet the needs of dying persons and their families. These needs may include teaching family and friends how to administer medications, helping dying persons maintain as much mobility and activity as possible, and listening and responding to a dying person's needs. Help from the hospice team is available 24 hours a day. One member of the team is always on call and will make home visits as needed. However, the dying person and his or her family direct the care and are directly involved in the decision-making processes.

Hospice professionals anticipate problems and concerns, including preparing a family for the loss of a dying person. After the death, various types of bereavement services are available: individual and family counseling, bereavement volunteer visits, support groups, and grief classes. The bereaved family members choose whether and to what degree they would like to participate in any of the activities and services provided.

Historically, the majority of hospice programs in the United States follow the home care model. This means that the interdisciplinary team provides routine hospice care in a terminally ill person's own home. In contrast to traditional home health care, it is not necessary for a terminally ill person to be homebound or to have a skilled nursing need. A family member or friend is usually designated as the primary family caregiver. Family members provide the 24-hour care of the dying person, and the hospice team consults and supports the family in their commitment to care for the hospice client. However, the creativity and innovation of the hospice team enables many dying individuals to remain in their homes without family caregivers.

Based on the needs of a dying person and his or her family, other levels of care are also available. Inpatient care is available when the client experiences acute or severe pain or symptom management problems. Inpatient respite care provides family caregivers with release time from the daily care of the client. This type of respite care is usually limited to 5 consecutive days. Continuous care is reserved for times of crisis. This service is provided in the client's home by nurses and HHAs. It allows up to 24-hour care.

Medicare Benefit

Hospice services are a fully covered Medicare benefit. Anyone covered by Medicare Part A is eligible for hospice care. The following three conditions must be met to qualify for the Medicare hospice benefit. First, a terminally ill person's physician and the hospice medical director must certify that the client is terminally ill and has a life expectancy of 6 months or less. Second, a client must choose to receive care from a hospice instead of receiving standard Medicare benefits. Third, care must be provided by a Medicare-certified hospice program. The Medicare benefit pays for two 90-day periods of hospice care and an unlimited number of 60-day periods, if the client is reassessed and recertified as terminally ill at the beginning of each period. Hospice clients may change their minds at any time, discontinue hospice care, and return to the cure-oriented care covered by standard Medicare benefits (NHO, 1998b).

The Medicare hospice benefit covers pain- and symptom-control medications for a terminal illness. However, under Medicare regulations, a hospice may charge 5% of pharmacy services (Stephenson, 1998). In choosing a hospice, clients or their families must determine the hospice program's policies on medication charges. (This regulation also applies to respite services.) Durable medical equipment needed to care for a client in the home is also covered. The Medicare hospice benefit does not pay for treatment or services unrelated to the terminal illness. Attending physician charges continue to be reimbursed in part through Medicare Part B coverage. The standard Medicare benefit program continues to pay covered costs necessary to treat unrelated conditions that the hospice client may have concurrently with the terminal diagnosis (NHO, 1998b).

HMOs are not required by law to provide hospice services. However, most HMOs do provide these end-of-life services. In addition, HMOs that receive Medicare funding are required to inform their members who are Medicare beneficiaries of Medicare-certified hospice programs located in their geographic area. If such a person chooses hospice care, he or she does not need to leave the HMO and will continue to receive HMO benefits not covered by Medicare (NHO, 1998b). Most private insurance companies and Medicaid also provide hospice benefits.

Location of Care

In the United States hospice care is primarily provided in the home. However, other sites include hospital-based units, freestanding independent facilities, and long-term care facilities (nursing facilities). The use of these facilities is based on the needs of a dying client and his or her family and on the type of services offered in the client's geographic area.

The hospice team recognizes that circumstances change. For example, a dying person and his or her family may initially choose to care for the dying person at home with the support of hospice. Later, the primary caregiver may become exhausted or sick and be unable to provide that care any longer. The hospice team will assist the family in choosing an alternative to home-based hospice care. The transition between locations of care should be seamless with the assistance of the hospice team.

OVERVIEW OF LONG-TERM CARE

Definition

Long-term care has several meanings in the gerontologic nursing literature. The phrase is most accurately used to describe a collection of health, personal, and social services provided over a prolonged period to people who have lost or never acquired functional capacity (Kane and Kane, 1987). Recipients of long-term care services typically include older adults but may also include developmentally disabled persons, persons permanently impaired from traumatic injuries, and chronically ill younger persons. Services range from supportive care to very complex care. Long-term care settings can be categorized on a continuum according to the complexity of care provided and the amount of skilled care and services required by the residents served. Settings go from more structured to less structured as one moves from the institutional setting to community-based programs to the home setting. Table 9-3 illustrates this continuum of long-term care service settings.

Persons living in nursing facilities are called *residents.* The facility is their permanent or temporary home. Some residents require nursing care until death. Other residents are admitted from an acute care hospital. They stay for a short time to recover from an acute illness, injury, or surgery and then return home. Medical, nursing, dietary, recreational, rehabilitative, social, and spiritual care is usually provided. All nursing facilities must function under the federal regulations set forth by OBRA. Some facilities are also accredited by the JCAHO.

TABLE 9-3 Continuum of Settings in Which Long-Term Care Is Provided

INSTITUTIONAL	COMMUNITY	HOME
Nursing facility	Adult day care center	Home health nursing
Group home	Senior center	Home health rehabilitative services
Board and care facility	Congregate meal programs	Homemaker
Assisted living	Hospice	Home-delivered meals
Continuing care retirement communities		Adaptive devices to home environment
Hospice		Hospice

Factors Associated With Institutionalization

As life expectancy and the size of the older adult population increase, the risk of a person entering a nursing facility at some point also grows. See Fig. 9-1 for a state-by-state average of the nursing home resident population in 2000.

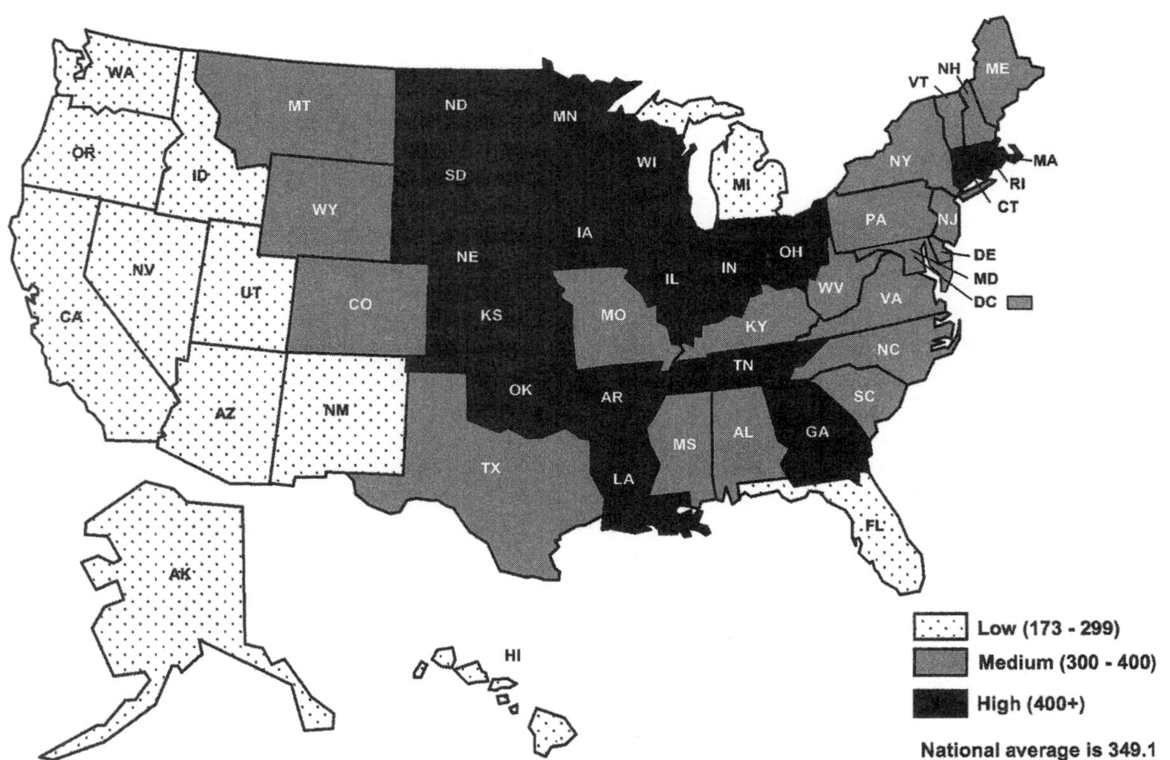

Fig. 9-1 Nursing home resident rate by state, 2000. (From the National Center for Health Statistics, 2003.)

Personal factors associated with institutionalization include advanced age; physical disability; mental impairment; white race; living without a spouse; and the presence of chronic medical conditions, such as heart disease, arthritis, hypertension, and diabetes (Jette et al, 1992; Millsap, 1995) (see Cultural Awareness box). Factors contributing to the need for institutionalization can be categorized according to characteristics of the person, characteristics of the person's support system, and the community resources available to the person (Box 9-8).

According to a 1997 report by the National Center for Health Statistics (U.S. Department of Health and Human Services, 1997a, 1997b), many older persons receive long-term care services in the home from relatives and friends and in small group settings with intermediate levels of care. Despite an older person's preference to stay at home, admission to a nursing facility becomes necessary when the person's physical and mental capabilities deteriorate to a point where adequate family and community resources are no longer available. The total number of men and women over the age of 65 has risen (National Center for Health Statistics, 2003), although the number of nursing home residents per 1000 older adults has dropped. This trend was noted between 1985 and 1999 (Figs. 9-2 and 9-3).

Medical and Psychosocial Models of Care

Nursing facilities evolved from the acute care hospital system and the medical model (Lidz and Arnold, 1995). Like hospitals, nursing facilities were designed around the departments and professionals rather than the consumers they served. Although the organization of nursing facilities tends to be hierarchic and bureaucratic, alternative methods of staffing are being developed and implemented (Goldman, 1998). This emphasis is on using more licensed nursing personnel and forming primary nursing and case manager roles. Within these more recently introduced models, graduates with a bachelor of science in nursing will have many opportunities to fill midlevel management roles and thus have the opportunity to effect positive changes in long-term care.

The medical model places residents in a sick role and in need of physician-directed help. Compliance with the medical regimen is emphasized. Residents are expected to comply with staff and medical decisions rather than actively participate in determining them (Lidz and Arnold, 1995). But one of the changes mandated by OBRA is an emphasis on the social and psychologic health of nursing facility residents, in addition to the traditional medical concerns. Residents' subjective evaluations of their quality of life need to be solicited and valued. Psychosocial models of care emphasize resident decision making and the exercise of personal choice. The ideal long-term care facility is a combination of both medical and social models, not exclusively one and the other (Box 9-9).

Sometimes nursing facility personnel do not fully understand resident rights. Creative strategies are necessary to enhance a resident's perception of autonomy. The baccalaureate-prepared nurse is in a wonderful position to combine his or her knowledge of medicine, nursing, psychology, and sociology into a model that truly provides individualized care to each resident in the nursing facility.

BOX 9-8 Factors Affecting the Need for Nursing Home Admission

CHARACTERISTICS OF THE INDIVIDUAL

- Age, sex, and race
- Marital status
- Living arrangements
- Degree of mobility
- Ability to perform basic ADLs and IADLs
- Urinary incontinence
- Behavior problems
- Mental status
- Memory and cognitive impairment
- Mood disturbance
- Tendency to fall
- Clinical prognosis
- Income
- Payment eligibility
- Need for special services

CHARACTERISTICS OF THE SUPPORT SYSTEM

- Family capability
  —Age and health of spouse (if married)
  —Presence of responsible relative (usually an adult child)
  —Family structure of responsible relative
  —Employment status of responsible relative
- Physician availability
- Amount of care currently received from family and others

COMMUNITY RESOURCES

- Formal community resources
- Informal support systems
- Presence of long-term care institutions
- Characteristics of long-term care institutions

From Ouslander J, Osterweil D, Morley J: *Medical care in the nursing home*, New York, 1991, McGraw-Hill.

Cultural Awareness

CULTURAL DIVERSITY IN NURSING FACILITIES

Historically, a higher percentage of older adults from culturally diverse backgrounds has been cared for in home environments compared with those who are white. Among the over-85 age-group residing in nursing facilities, 23% are white, 10% are Hispanic, and 10% are Asian/Pacific Islander in heritage (Wray, 1992; Yeatts, Crow, Folts, 1992).

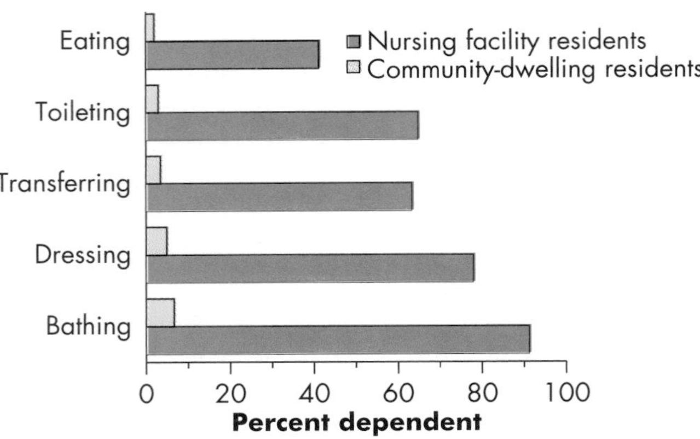

Fig. 9-2 Ability to perform basic ADLs among nursing facility residents and community-dwelling older adults. (From Ouslander J, Osterwell D, Moreley J: *Medical care in the nursing home,* New York, 1991, McGraw-Hill.)

CLINICAL ASPECTS OF THE NURSING FACILITY

Resident Rights

One of the accomplishments of the Institute of Medicine's 1986 Committee on Nursing Home Regulation report was to lay the foundation for greater regulatory support of resident rights in the nursing facility. Emphasis on resident rights was directly related to a revised view that residents really did have the right to autonomy and to be active participants and decision makers in their care and life in the institutional setting.

Resident rights that are unique to the nursing facility are to be promoted in several ways. These include (Gamroth, Semradek, and Tornquist, 1995):

- Establishment and maintenance of a resident council
- Public display of posters listing resident rights
- Public display of local ombudsman program information
- Public display of annual state inspection results
- Aggressive attempts to provide opportunities for residents to exercise their right to vote during public elections
- Provision of opportunities for competent residents to self-administer medications
- An informed consent process for the use of side rails and chemical and physical restraints
- An informed consent process for the withdrawal or withholding of life-sustaining treatments
- A grievance process whereby residents and families can challenge the care that is given

All departments within the nursing facility, including social services, activities, nursing, dietary, and maintenance, must share responsibility for ensuring the enforcement of these resident rights. Ideally, this effort will be the operational philosophy for all nursing facilities.

Regulatory enforcement focuses strongly on resident safety without always considering a resident's individual right to be autonomous and make a conscious decision to place himself or herself at risk (e.g., for falling) in order to retain some degree of independence. Each situation must be

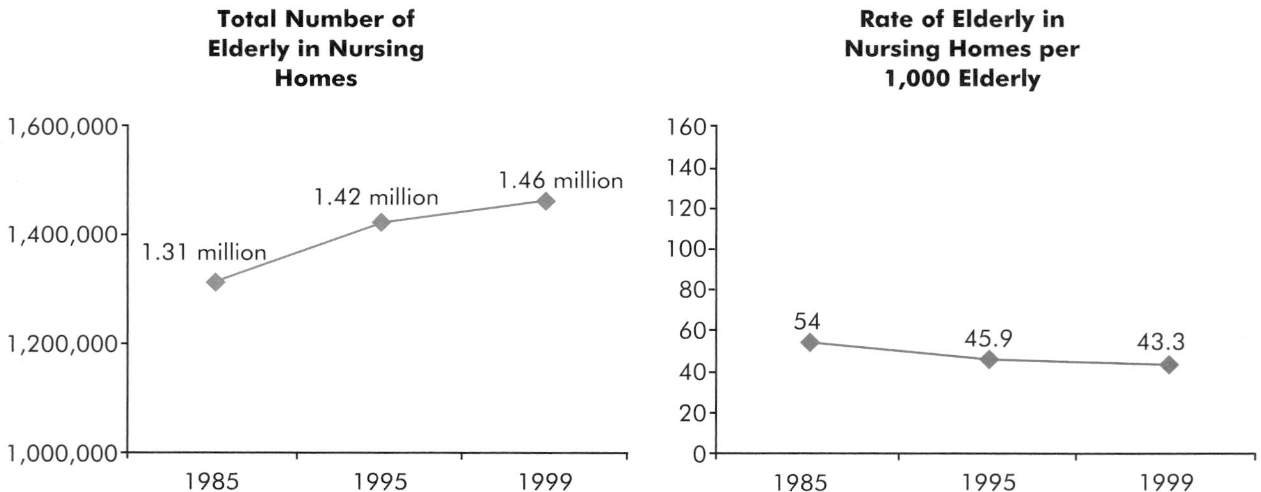

Fig. 9-3 Change in nursing home institutionalization rate for the elderly, 1985-1999. (From the National Center for Health Statisitics, 2001.)

BOX 9-9 Major Regulatory Level A Requirements Defined by OBRA '87

- Resident rights
- Admission, transfer, and discharge rights
- Resident behavior and facility practices
- Quality of life
- Resident assessment
- Quality of care
- Nursing services
- Dietary services
- Physician services
- Specialized rehabilitative services
- Dental services
- Pharmacy services
- Infection control
- Physical environment
- Administration

evaluated individually, and the legalities can be complicated (Applebaum, 1998).

Resident Assessment

Interdisciplinary functional assessment of residents is the cornerstone of clinical practice in this setting. OBRA prescribed the method of resident assessment and care plan development in an instrument known as the Resident Assessment Instrument (RAI) Version 2.0. The RAI consists of three parts: the minimum data set (MDS), the resident assessment protocols (RAPs), and the utilization guidelines specified in the State Operations Manual transmittal no. 272 (Heath Care Financing Adminstration [HCFA], 1995).

The MDS is a tool that includes a comprehensive assessment of residents. Tool categories include resident background information; cognitive, communication and hearing, and vision patterns; physical functioning and structural problems; mood, behavior, and activity pursuit patterns; psychosocial well-being; bowel and bladder continence; health conditions; disease diagnoses; oral, nutritional, and dental status; skin condition; medication use; and special treatments and procedures. It is meant to provide a total picture of a resident. This resident profile is used to develop an individualized, comprehensive care plan for each resident.

Deadlines for completion of each tool section, as well as care-planning decisions emanating from the assessment process, are prescribed by regulation. Box 9-10 lists the 18 problem areas that need to be addressed in the care-planning process. The outcome of the interdisciplinary team's clinical decision making related to the 18 problem areas as it feeds into care plan development is explicitly described in the RAP summary.

The specific method used to complete the RAI varies from facility to facility. Some facilities assign one nurse to complete all documentation related to the RAI; others distribute this responsibility among all the nurses. The RAI is completed for each resident on admission, annually, when a significant change of condition occurs (as defined by the CMS manual), and quarterly, using a one-page abbreviated version of the RAI. For persons admitted for skilled care under Medicare Part A, the MDS and RAI are completed at 5 or 14 days, 30 days, 60 days, 90 days, and with any significant change.

BOX 9-10 Problem Areas of the Resident Assessment Protocol Summary

- Delirium
- Cognitive loss and dementia
- Visual function
- Communication
- ADL functional and rehabilitation potential
- Urinary incontinence and indwelling catheter
- Psychosocial well-being
- Mood state
- Behavioral symptoms
- Activities
- Falls
- Nutritional status
- Feeding tubes
- Dehydration and fluid maintenance
- Oral and dental care
- Pressure ulcers
- Psychotropic drug use
- Physical restraints

Both licensed vocational or practical nurses and RNs may contribute to the RAI. However, only an RN can sign the document and function as the RN assessment coordinator (RAC). The RAC signs and certifies the completion of the assessment, not the accuracy of the assessment data (HCFA, 1995). Contributions to the RAI are also made by the dietary supervisor, social worker, recreational therapist, medical records clerk, and physical and occupational therapists.

The overall goal of the RAI is to provide an ongoing, comprehensive assessment of a resident, emphasizing functional ability and both a physical and a psychosocial profile. It is also a key component in the development of a national database for long-term care.

Skin Care

Skin and nail care programs are important to a resident's overall health and quality of life. Skin care programs in the nursing facility are focused on prevention and treatment of skin problems. Preventive strategies include prevention of pressure ulcers, skin tears, and dry skin or xerosis.

Other skin-related problems commonly occurring and treated in this setting include MRSA infections, circulatory ulcers, dermatitis and eczema, herpes zoster, scabies, pediculosis, bullous pemphigoid, and skin tumors. The prevention of skin tears, pressure ulcers, and circulatory ulcers is an ongoing challenge for the staff in nursing facilities. The development of pressure ulcers during a person's stay in a nursing facility is considered an indicator of poor quality of care, although research and current knowledge of pressure ulcer etiology does not support this view as totally accurate. The facility must identify residents at risk for pressure ulcers. Aggressive and appropriate preventive measures are initiated to address each resident's specific and unique risk factors (see Chapter 30).

Most nursing facilities have a structured skin care program that is coordinated by an RN and involves all nursing department staff plus a physical therapist, occupational therapist, and dietitian. On admission, a resident's skin is thoroughly assessed. Individual risk for developing pressure ulcers is established, and preventive interventions are initiated as appropriate. These may include some type of special bed mattress, heel protectors, positioning devices, vitamin and nutritional supplements, skin lubricants, and a schedule for repositioning the resident in beds and chairs. The CNA plays a key role in providing effective preventive skin care by assisting the resident in routine bathing, toileting, and maintenance of schedules for turning and repositioning. The individualized care plan, developed by the interdisciplinary team, provides specific instructions concerning the preventive treatment measures for each resident.

Based on the physical examination, as well as RAI data, a care plan is initiated. Individual states have varying regulations concerning the required frequency of the nurse's clinical staging and routine assessment of pressure ulcers. Most facilities require at least weekly monitoring by an RN. The nurse measures and stages the ulcers and evaluates the efficacy of the treatment plan. The director of nursing may also work with the medical director or individual physicians practicing in the facility to coordinate and standardize treatments for various stages of pressure ulcers. Another alternative is to intervene in skin problems on a case-by-case basis according to the preference of the resident's attending physician.

Facilities may have sustained relationships with companies that manufacture specialized beds for residents with stage III or IV pressure ulcers. Often the company provides a nurse consultant as a clinical resource to the facility. The nurse functioning as the skin care program coordinator might meet routinely with the consultant. The two nurses often work collaboratively, along with the dietitian and physical therapist, to treat skin problems. Consistently following a treatment plan is essential for positive outcomes.

Incontinence

As functional dependence increases, the prevalence of incontinence increases. This common health problem has financial, physical, and psychosocial consequences, and incontinence is a common reason for placing a person in a nursing facility.

Caring for an incontinent resident is expensive; it requires more nursing time and frequent linen and clothing changes. Physical consequences of incontinence include skin breakdown, UTI, and an increased risk of falling and consequent hip fracture (Case-Gamble, 1995). Urinary incontinence is one of the most psychologically distressing health problems faced by older adults. It may lead to depression, decreased self-esteem, and social isolation (Case-Gamble, 1995).

One of the features of OBRA was the inclusion of specific standards and recommendations for the assessment and treatment of urinary incontinence. Clinical programs in nursing facilities are directed at prevention, treatment, and management of incontinence. Prevention is aimed at reducing the risk of developing urinary incontinence among at-risk residents of nursing facilities. Preventive measures include assessment of individual patterns of elimination so that anticipatory assistance with toileting may be provided, aggressive staff response to residents' requests for assistance in toileting, and arrangement of the physical environment to minimize the physical effort involved in getting to the bathroom.

Treatment programs are resident oriented and focus on creating changes in the function of the lower urinary tract. Interventions include surgery, pharmacologic interventions, bladder training, pelvic muscle exercises, and biofeedback procedures (Ouslander and Schnelle, 1993). It is important to identify those residents who can benefit from these therapies.

Management programs for urinary incontinence are the dominant form of intervention in the nursing facility. Some residents benefit from programs that involve behavioral approaches such as scheduled toileting, habit training, and prompted voiding. These approaches focus on changing the behavior of the caregiver and the resident to minimize the incontinence. But residents with dementia and other cognitive impairments may not benefit from these interventions; the use of incontinence pads and protective undergarments are necessary for these individuals. External condom catheters can be helpful for men.

Intermittent self-catheterization may be appropriate for residents who are cognitively intact and have adequate manual dexterity. Long-term, indwelling catheterization is indicated for residents who cannot empty their bladders and have not responded to other treatments. Residents who are terminally ill and those with skin breakdown may also benefit from indwelling catheterization. Indwelling catheterization is used only after other interventions have failed.

Effective management of urinary incontinence involves a well-coordinated and sustained effort between licensed nursing staff, certified nursing assistants, and activities staff. The nurse must play a key role in managing incontinence and preventing complications; management and treatment must be directed at the cause of incontinence (see Chapter 28).

Nutrition

Nutritional deficiencies contribute to adverse clinical outcomes in nursing facility residents. Protein-calorie undernutrition results from two broad categories of factors: those causing inadequate intake and those causing increased nutritional requirements (Abbasi et al, 1993) (see Chapter 10).

Inadequate intake in well adults results from eating functions altered by the normal aging process of the gastrointestinal tract, as described in Chapter 26. Other contributing factors include loss of manual dexterity, pain, dementing illnesses, certain mediations, and chronic medical disorders. Culture, religion, and personal choice also affect how and what a person eats. A resident's appetite is affected by personal comfort and unpleasant odors, sights, and sounds. Meeting a resident's nutritional needs requires involvement of the entire health care team. The physician, dietitian, nurse, speech/language pathologist, occupational therapist, social worker, and nursing assistant all play roles in the assessment of individual needs, care planning, care plan implementation, and care plan evaluation. The resident is always included, and the resident's family may also provide important information.

Increased nutritional requirements may be a consequence of hyperactivity in some persons with dementing illnesses. Infectious illnesses, periods of recovery following surgical interventions that require tissue healing, and recovery from pressure ulcers place additional nutritional requirements on nursing facility residents.

Various clinical interventions are directed at the nutritional support of residents, including programs focused on maintaining adequate caloric intake and effective identification of residents requiring supplemental nutritional support.

Enhancement of the dining experience through improved aesthetics, improved dining room service, attractive food preparation, and increased sensitivity to the social nature of mealtimes are directed toward maintenance of adequate caloric intake. Other strategies related to this goal include increasing staff assistance for residents who need help with eating and improving staff techniques for providing assistance with eating. Sensitivity to dental needs and provision of the textures of foods most easily and safely consumed by each resident are additional strategies.

In nursing facilities the most common program for prompt identification of residents requiring supplemental nutritional support consists of routine weighing. Weights are taken daily, weekly, biweekly, or monthly, depending on the severity of weight loss or gain experienced by a resident. Interdisciplinary team members, including the nurse, restorative nursing assistant, dietitian, and speech/language pathologist, may meet routinely to review weight changes and develop interventions directed at supplemental nutritional support. In addition to the strategies already described, changes in therapeutic diets and the use of nutritional products (such as Ensure), vitamin supplements, and enteral nutrition products may be considered. Laboratory tests are often ordered to help monitor a resident's nutritional status.

Compliance with OBRA requires aggressive monitoring of the parameters of nutritional status, with attention focused on unplanned weight loss. The functional implications of reduced caloric intake are to be considered. Any unplanned weight loss of 5% or greater in 30 days or 10% or greater in 90 days is an indicator of poor quality of care. Any weight loss or weight gain must be carefully monitored. The reasons for the loss or gain and the interventions taken must be documented.

Medications

One of the basic services provided in nursing facilities is administration of medications through oral, intravenous, intramuscular, subcutaneous, and enteral routes. In the nursing facility the licensed nurse is often responsible for the administration, documentation, storage, ordering, cart stocking, and destruction of many medications. In some states, medication aides are used to administer medications. The RN is responsible for monitoring the medication's therapeutic effects, side effects, and any allergic reactions. The RN also monitors and evaluates the skills of medication aides on an ongoing basis. Because most nursing facilities do not have an onsite pharmacy, the nursing staff is responsible for medication-related functions that would be handled by the pharmacy staff in an acute care hospital.

Monitoring for the clinical manifestations of polypharmacy, the occurrence of adverse drug reactions, and the overuse of "as required" (prn) drug orders has increasingly been emphasized since the passage of OBRA. The pharmacist contributes to this monitoring effort in a monthly drug review of each resident's medical record, and the nurse has numerous structured opportunities to monitor for these clinical problems. These opportunities include routine interactions with residents while administering medications and assessment at quarterly care-planning conferences, monthly reviews of psychotropic drug regimens, and completion of the long form of the MDS (Meiner, 2004; Meiner, 1997; Williams, Thompson, and Brummel-Smith, 1993). Facilities must have policies and procedures to monitor for drug interactions and side effects.

The routine use of certain drugs, including long-acting benzodiazepines, hypnotics, sedatives, anxiolytics, and antipsychotics, has been curtailed since the passage of OBRA. Recommended drug dosages and indications for the use of such medications are given to federal and state survey teams to assist them in the survey and inspection process of each nursing facility (HCFA, 1994).

Residents have the right to participate in decisions about care and treatment. They must be informed of any changes in their medication regimens. Nurses must document their ongoing instruction to each resident (or the resident's legal representative) regarding the initiation of new drug therapy and changes in the dosages of medications. If a resident is cognitively intact, the opportunity to self-administer medications is to be provided (HCFA, 1994). Facilities must have and follow policies and procedures for identifying and following up on medication errors.

Rehabilitation

The provision of rehabilitation programs in nursing facilities has increased over the past 15 years. Factors contributing to this growth in rehabilitation include the OBRA regulatory mandate that facilities provide services directed at achieving the highest practicable level of physical, mental, and psychosocial well-being for residents; the growth of the subacute level of care, including nursing facility participation in managed care programs; and sustained political will to control the growth of health care expenditures (Gill, Howells, and Hoffman, 1993).

Rehabilitation teams in nursing facilities consist of the physician; physical therapists; occupational therapists; speech/language pathologists; and facility interdisciplinary team members, including the nurse, social services representative, activity coordinator, and clinical dietitian. Ideally the rehabilitation team is coordinated by a medical director with rehabilitation training and experience.

For facilities receiving funds from Medicare, managed care organizations, or private insurance groups, weekly rehabilitation meetings are held to review clinical cases. Residents and family members participate in these meetings to mutually set goals and review progress. Weekly meetings promote communication, effective discharge planning, and resident and family education.

Rehabilitation programs can be categorized into two groups. The more intensive rehabilitation programs are reimbursed through the Medicare Part A program, managed care organizations, or private insurance groups. Some of these intensive rehabilitation programs seek credentialing by JCAHO and the Commission for Accreditation of Rehabilitation Facilities (CARF) in order to be recognized as benchmark quality programs. Intensive rehabilitation includes daily or twice-daily therapy sessions involving two or more therapy specialties. These sessions are directed toward returning a resident to a prior level of function and to residence in the community. Endurance building, strengthening, ADL training, treatment of aphasia and dysphagia, cognitive testing and retraining, new disability adaptations training (e.g., after stroke or amputation), and training with new adaptive equipment are therapeutic components of these programs.

The less intensive rehabilitation programs that exist in nursing facilities are reimbursed through the Medicare Part B program or private payments, or they are part of the basic services offered by the nursing facility. These services include restorative nursing programs involving ambulation, ADLs, self-feeding, and range of motion. Such programs are provided by specially trained certified nursing assistants or facility nursing staff. These programs are established, revised, and supervised by the physical and occupational therapists and the speech/language pathologist. Program goals are focused on the maintenance of functional gains achieved during the more intensive rehabilitation program, regaining a level of function lost because of a short-term illness, and prevention of unnecessary loss of function.

Facilities must provide the required rehabilitation services or obtain them from an outside source. Needs of the individual resident are based on a comprehensive assessment. The goal is to help the resident maintain or regain the highest possible level of physical, mental, and psychosocial well-being.

Infection Control

The development and spread of infections are a major health and safety hazard in nursing facilities. A written program to protect residents, staff, and visitors from infection is required. Facility policies and procedures must include the use of standard precautions and transmission-based precautions, as outlined by the Centers for Disease Control and Prevention (CDC). They must also follow the Occupational Safety and Health Administration's (OSHA's) Bloodborne Pathogen Standard.

OBRA requires nursing facilities to have an infection control program designed to provide a safe, sanitary, and comfortable environment; its purpose is to help prevent the development and transmission of disease. Facilities must have policies and procedures for investigating, controlling, and preventing infections. Records of incidents and corrective action taken related to infections must be maintained. The infection control program should be able to identify new infections quickly. Special attention is given to residents at high risk for infection (e.g., those who are immobilized, have invasive devices or procedures, have pressure ulcers, have been recently discharged from the hospital, have decreased mental status, or are nutritionally compromised). The program must also include measures to prevent outbreaks of communicable diseases, including tuberculosis (TB), influenza, hepatitis, scabies, and MRSA. Preventive measures involve TB testing and screening programs for residents and staff. The facility must have procedures for following up on any positive results. Programs to make annual influenza vaccinations and pneumococcal pneumonia vaccinations available as appropriate are also in place.

According to OSHA, employees at risk for exposure to bloodborne pathogens must receive free information and training on employment and annually thereafter. Employers must make the hepatitis B vaccine available to employees within 10 working days of being hired. Personal protective equipment such as gloves, goggles, face shields, gowns, shoe covers, and surgical caps are available free to employees; they must also receive instructions on when and how to use this equipment.

An infection control committee consisting of staff members representing each department meets either monthly or quarterly to review data describing the prevalence and incidence rates of infection. This committee discusses any new or proposed revisions in policies and procedures. Typically, one nurse is designated as the infection control nurse and is responsible for coordinating surveillance, data-collecting activities, and ongoing educational sessions for the facility (Culley and Courtney, 1993). The infection control nurse is the facility's resource for information related to the infection control program. It is this person's responsibility to obtain and use current information from the CDC, OSHA, CMS, and state department of health to ensure that the facility's infection control program is effective and meets standards. The facility's medical director and consulting pharmacist also are valuable resources.

Every department and every employee has a responsibility to know and follow the policies and procedures outlined in the infection control program. Policies and procedures include handwashing; standard precautions; respiratory protection; the Bloodborne Pathogen Standard; linen handling; housekeeping; hazardous waste disposal; and proper use of disinfectants, antiseptics, and germicides.

Mental Health

General topics related to mental health and aging are described in Chapter 14. Among the aged and institutionalized population, mental health issues of particular concern include a variety of behavioral problems that may jeopardize the safety of the resident or other residents (e.g., wandering, kicking, hitting). Because the residents live in a community setting, behavioral problems are not just an issue for the affected resident. The aberrant behavior of one resident has an effect on other residents.

Residents manifesting behavioral problems commonly have dementing illnesses. More than 60% of nursing facility residents have some degree of cognitive deficit. These deficits frequently precipitate behaviors that are difficult to understand and ameliorate. The use of physical and chemical restraints has finally been restricted, and emphasis is now placed on using behavioral interventions and environmental modifications (see section on Special Care Units). Doors can have alarms to deter wandering, and exercise, music, massage, low-stimulation environments, lighting, and aromatherapy can be employed to decrease agitation.

Most important, nurses are learning ways to determine the causes of the disturbing behaviors by assessing for pain, hunger, infection, and inappropriate environmental stimulation. Psychotropic medications are to be used only as a last resort, and the side effects are to be carefully monitored. As research continues to identify the various types of dementia, it will become more and more important to specifically diagnose the type. All dementia is not Alzheimer's disease, and residents with other types of dementia may have negative and dangerous responses to psychotropic medications.

End-of-Life Care

The nurse working in a nursing facility is responsible for helping the entire health care team meet the physical, spiritual, and psychosocial needs of dying residents. Ministering to the residents' families is an important part of this care. Knowledge about a resident's culture and religious beliefs helps the team provide more effective and compassionate care. Some facilities provide hospice training for staff. Hospice programs may also provide care to residents in the nursing facility (see Chapter 20).

MANAGEMENT ASPECTS OF THE NURSING FACILITY

The Nursing Department

The nursing department is the largest department in the nursing facility. The director of nursing is responsible for managing the entire nursing staff. This consists of RNs, licensed vocational or practical nurses, certified nursing assistants, and, occasionally, gerontologic nurse practitioners. In some facilities, nurse managers (usually RNs) assist the director of nursing in managing and carrying out functions of the nursing department. Nurse managers may be responsible for a particular shift, a nursing unit, or specific nursing department functions, such as infection control, restorative nursing, total quality management (TQM), and nursing education. Some facilities use unit charge nurses. These are usually RNs, but in some areas they are licensed vocational or practical nurses. Some facilities employ nurse practitioners to provide clinical expertise and serve as a valuable resource for the nursing staff. Nurse practitioners often work closely with the medical director and the resident's primary care physician to manage the resident's day-to-day care. They may write orders for medications and treatment following collaborative practice protocols.

Of the RN work force, 8% work in long-term care facilities (Culley and Courtney, 1993). Certified nursing assistants are the largest employee group in the nursing departments and the facilities as a whole, making up 66% of the work force in the nursing facility (Schnelle et al, 1993).

Working in the nursing facility presents rewards, opportunities, and challenges for nurses. Rewards include the chance to establish long-term relationships with residents and family members and an opportunity to work in a setting that has a holistic orientation toward resident care. Nurses employed in nursing facilities have many opportunities to use their professional skills as clinicians, teachers, and managers. They are part of an interdisciplinary team that provides a broad spectrum of health care services. The nurse frequently takes a leadership role in developing policies and procedures, assessing resident care needs, developing and implementing care plans, and evaluating outcomes. Excellent assessment and critical thinking skills are very important. A qualified, creative nurse can advance from staff nurse to charge nurse to nurse manager. There are also opportunities to chair committees on topics such as TQM, infection control, restorative nursing, and pharmacy. Opportunities for professional growth continue to increase in this evolving, challenging area of health care. But nurses who choose long-term care as a career must be willing to function in a highly regulated industry. Funding for innovative programs and services is often limited, and in some geographic areas, salaries are lower than in acute care settings.

Nursing Care Delivery Systems

Several nursing care delivery systems are found in nursing facilities. This section discusses the pros and cons of the various delivery systems. Unfortunately, the system that is most likely to be in place is the one that is the least expensive. Federal regulations regarding staffing requirements for nursing facilities are broad and vague. They are not based on resident acuity and leave it up to individual facilities to determine whether it can provide the care required for any given resident. Few, if any, states have required staffing ratios that are more stringent than the federal requirements.

One nursing care delivery system is functional nursing. Jobs of licensed nurses and certified nursing assistants are determined according to work tasks. For example, there may be an MDS nurse, an admission nurse, a medication nurse, a treatment nurse, a restorative nursing assistant, and possibly a dining assistant. Certified nursing assistants may take groupings of rooms as an assignment for a variable period. A charge nurse functions as the first-line manager. This care delivery system is widely used because it can somewhat efficiently carry out basic care while maintaining only the minimum staffing levels required by regulations. However, if there is poor verbal communication between staff members and inadequate written documentation, many resident issues and care needs go unaddressed.

Team nursing is a more integrated care delivery system than functional nursing. The licensed nurse, working with a group of residents (usually 30 to 50), provides medications and treatments to residents, functions as charge nurse or first-line supervisor to the certified nursing assistants, and maintains the required documentation for the residents. The licensed nurse may change the resident group assignments on a scheduled basis, usually weekly or monthly. Certified nursing assistants may change every week or every month. There are several disadvantages to the team nursing system. Long-term continuity cannot be provided when certified nursing assistants and licensed nurses change group assignments so frequently. Staff don't form attachments to residents, and residents, particularly those with memory loss, often have difficulty coping with these changes (e.g., remembering new names and faces, adjusting to the expectations of new personnel) (Goldman, 1998). The other major disadvantage of this system is the burden placed on one licensed nurse to safely and efficiently provide medications and treatments to 50 residents, thoroughly assess episodic health problems, and meet documentation requirements.

A third delivery system is primary team nursing. This involves the combination of a licensed nurse and a certified nursing assistant working together to care for approximately 10 to 15 residents (McCainey, 1998). This team provides all nursing care, including admissions, assistance with ADLs, and administration of medications and treatments. The main disadvantage is there may be too few staff members to meet all resident needs and a risk of inadequate coverage when some staff are on break (Goldman, 1998).

Regardless of the care delivery system used, the RN practicing in the nursing facility is challenged to work effectively with licensed vocational or practical nurses and certified nursing assistants, incorporating them into a professional practice model. It is essential that the RN practicing in this setting have excellent supervisory and management skills. The leadership positions in the department of nursing are held by RNs; these positions include director of nursing services and, increasingly, director of staff development. The baccalaureate-level nurse is the best prepared to fill these positions and significantly affect the quality of care and the quality of life of many residents (see Research and Cultural Awareness boxes, p.203).

SPECIALTY CARE SETTINGS

Assisted Living Programs

Assisted living facilities are an increasingly attractive long-term care setting, placed between home care and the nursing facility in the continuum of long-term care (Dewey, 1994). Regulations are minimum, so there is great diversity in the types of service delivery models used, the types of services offered, and the setting within which assisted living is provided.

Assisted living settings are homelike and offer an array of services, including meals, assistance with bathing and dressing, social and recreational programs, personal laundry and housekeeping services, transportation, 24-hour security, an emergency call system, health checks, medication administration, and minor medical treatments (Kane and Wilson, 1993). Many services are purchased individually as needed by the resident.

The professional nurse can provide a broad and holistic array of services to residents in assisted living facilities. There are opportunities to incorporate both health promotion and illness care into the model. Resident education can delay admission to long-term care. The professional nurse will help coordinate the services provided by various departments, such as activities, social services, physical and occupational therapy, and housekeeping. As the need for assisted living facilities continues to grow, so will the opportunity for professional nurses to define their contributions and enhance the services offered to frail older adults.

Special Care Units

Since the 1980s the popularity of specialized units for persons with dementia has expanded. *Special care unit (SCU)* is

Research

SAMPLE/SETTING

The sample consisted of 586 people ages 60 and older from three Philadelphia-area large, nonprofit, religious-affiliated nursing facilities.

METHODS

Disturbing behaviors were determined from a behavior subscale of the Psychogeriatric Dependency Rating Scale. Physical characteristics of the environment were measured using room type and physical restraint intensity. Organizational climate was measured using staff mix. The psychosocial milieu was measured using nursing staff burnout scores, staff members' perceptions of the importance of restraints in the care of older persons, and the number of alternatives to restraints that staff members could list. Cognitive status was measured using the Folstein Mini-Mental State Examination (FMMSE). Mood was measured using the Cornell Scale for Depression.

FINDINGS

Scores for agitated psychomotor behavior accounted for most of the explained variance in disturbing behaviors. There were significant relationships between the occurrence of agitated psychomotor behavior, greater functional dependency of residents, lower mental status scores, and greater use of psychotropic drugs. There were also significant relationships between agitated psychomotor behavior, restraint use, and a staff mix with fewer licensed personnel.

IMPLICATIONS

When staffing ratios are developed, a higher ratio of licensed personnel may reduce the incidence of disturbing behaviors. Residents with disturbing behaviors require a broad base of professional skill and expertise that is best provided by professional-level nursing staff. Kolanowski A et al: Contextual factors associated with disturbing behaviors in institutionalized elders, *Nurs Res* 43(2):73, 1995.

the designation given to freestanding facilities or units within nursing facilities that specialize in the care of people with Alzheimer's disease and other types of dementing illnesses. Behavioral manifestations of dementia are managed in the environment without the use of chemical or physical restraints whenever possible.

It is advisable for SCUs to have objective, measurable criteria for admission. An objective discharge policy should also be in place. These admission and discharge criteria are helpful to both nursing staff and families who are reluctant to transfer residents to another care setting when a particular resident can no longer benefit from the specialized milieu of the SCU and no longer requires a secured unit. Admission criteria can also deter SCU placement for nondemented residents who have other behavioral problems.

Cultural Awareness

RESEARCH ON ATTITUDES TOWARD NURSING FACILITY RESIDENTS AMONG AIDES OF THREE CULTURAL GROUPS

In a study by Robinson (1994), the attitudes of 255 nursing facility aides from three cultural groups (African American, English-speaking Caribbean, and Haitian) toward older nursing facility clients were assessed. The sample was drawn from five nursing facilities in the metropolitan New York area. Aides from all three groups had positive attitudes toward the older adults in their care, with the English-speaking Caribbean group expressing the most positive attitudes. Results were interpreted as reflecting the cultural norms of the three groups, which included the infrequent placement of older persons in nursing facilities. Although the aides believed older adults were valuable and stated that they enjoyed their interactions with residents, they regarded the act of placing an older relative in a nursing facility as negative. The researchers concluded that these findings suggest a need for in-service workshops in cultural diversity for aides who serve clients from different cultures.

SCUs have physical environmental features that control stimuli and maximize safety, yet minimize environmental barriers to freedom of movement (e.g., door alarms, outside fencing to facilitate safe wandering). Program features emphasize nutrition (e.g., finger foods, portable foods), structured daily activities, family involvement, and special staff training in behavioral manifestations of dementia and communication with demented residents. An interdisciplinary team coordinates services and care.

Employment opportunities for the nurse in the SCU are similar to those in the traditional nursing facility. The SCU is a desirable work setting if the nurse has a particular interest in the health care needs of persons with Alzheimer's disease and other dementing illnesses that have behavioral manifestations. It is not a work setting that everyone can enjoy. Nurses who work with these special resident populations are in a position to provide valuable consultation regarding persons with Alzheimer's disease to nurses practicing in other settings, including hospitals, home care, and nursing facilities.

Subacute Care

Subacute care, a $1 billion business annually, has become an increasingly popular level of care (Burk, 1994). The growth of subacute care has been spurred by the belief that up to 40% of clients in acute medical or rehabilitation hospital units could be treated as effectively in less costly settings. With increased political awareness of the rising costs of the Medicare and Medicaid programs, the prospect of significant savings provided by subacute care is an attractive one.

Insurance companies are looking to less costly settings to provide patient care. It is estimated that subacute care could eventually replace almost 50% of current acute care hospital lengths of stay.

Subacute care is an industry category rather than a reimbursement or regulatory category. Professional organizations have developed guidelines for the clinical and business development of this level of care. Facilities with subacute care programs are able to obtain accreditation through JCAHO and CARF. These accreditations are granted to facilities with well-defined subacute programs. Care may be reimbursed through Medicare, HMO benefits, private payment, or Medicaid.

Persons in a subacute unit are stable and no longer acutely ill or requiring daily physician visits. They may require services such as rehabilitation, intravenous medication therapy, parenteral nutrition, complex respiratory care, and wound management.

The nursing facility has not traditionally been considered a setting in which aggressive rehabilitative services or acute care treatments such as intense rehabilitation, ventilator care, and intravenous infusion therapy are provided. Subacute care is a growing industry in which services such as these are offered to older persons, clients of managed care organizations, and clients whose private insurance company has contracted with a nursing facility to provide care. To care for such clients, the nursing staff requires a level of clinical skill beyond what is typically needed in the nursing facility. Staffing levels, particularly related to licensed nurses, are higher in response to the increased client acuity (Gill and Balsano, 1994). Physician involvement is also greatly increased.

INNOVATIONS IN THE NURSING FACILITY

Creativity in "Everyday" Nursing Facilities

All that is required to put a little life and love into any nursing facility is some creative thinking, a desire to make life better for residents, and adequate funding. As in similar endeavors, obtaining the financial resources can be the most difficult aspect of this process. However, the innovative nurse accepts this challenge and looks beyond the usual sources to obtain the necessary resources to develop and support new interventions.

Nursing facilities all over the country have acquired dogs, cats, and other animals that can live in the facility and serve as loving companions to the residents. More functionally capable residents can sometimes take primary responsibility for walking and feeding these pets. Aviaries containing tiny birds provide hours of enjoyment for many residents. Music therapy, touch therapy, and aromatherapy are among other innovative activities currently being used in nursing facilities. Indoor and outdoor gardening projects are therapeutic for many residents (Box 9-11).

Gerontologic Nurse Practitioners in the Nursing Facility

Over the past two decades, many studies have been conducted to evaluate the impact of the nurse practitioner on

BOX 9-11 Case Study

The following situation depicts how a team of home care providers, coupled with a determined client, can accomplish more than any one discipline working independently.

SITUATION

Mrs. T is a 68-year-old Polish housewife who suffered a left-sided cerebrovascular accident on February 25. Her hospitalization consisted of a stay in an acute care facility followed by an extensive stay in a rehabilitation setting. She was discharged to home with a referral to home care on May 1. On admission to home care, the nurse's assessment indicated that Mrs. T had right hemiparesis and aphasia. She had bowel and urinary incontinence with an indwelling Foley catheter. Her blood pressure was 152/94 mm HG; apical pulse was 74 beats per minute; respirations were 20 breaths per minute; and temperature was 98.0° F (36.6° C). These vital sign findings remained consistent throughout the initial stages of her home care program. She also complained of gastrointestinal pain. Her behavior was described as labile with periods of agitation, tearfulness, hyperventilation, and impulsiveness. Mrs. T required 24-hour supportive care with maximum assistance with ADLs. She wore a right short leg brace and a sling to prevent subluxation of her right arm. A wheelchair, hospital bed, and commode were ordered by the hospital discharge planner to aid in Mrs. T's care. She was given prescriptions for the following medications:

- Folic acid 1 mg orally (po) every day (qd)
- Colace 240 mg po, qd
- Dulcolax suppository $^{1}/_{2}$ to 1 rectally, every morning as needed (prn)
- Pepcid 40 mg po, every hour of sleep (qhs) prn
- Enteric-coated aspirin 325 mg po, qd
- Metamucil 1 tbsp po, qd, prn
- Milk of magnesia 2 tbsp po, prn
- Norvasc 5 mg po, qhs

Although Mrs. T had the support of two sons and her sister, the primary caregiver was her 70-year-old retired husband. Mr. T wanted his wife at home but had no experience or desire to assist with caregiving. This attitude made it more difficult for the home care team to develop and implement the care plan.

BOX 9-11 Case Study—cont'd

Because of the severe sequelae of the stroke, the following services were ordered:

- Nursing—one to three times a week to observe vital signs, ensure medication compliance, assess bowel and bladder function, change Foley catheter, and begin bowel training program
- Physical therapy—two or three times a week to decrease spasticity, increase range of motion, and increase endurance
- Speech pathology—two times a week to improve communication abilities
- Occupational therapy—two or three times a week to assess and reinforce ADLs
- Medical social work—two to four times a month to assist with community resources and possible placement in a nursing facility
- HHA service—three or four times a week to assist with personal care

Early in the home care program, it was determined that Mrs. T's labile behavior was interfering with her home rehabilitation program. She cried easily, became agitated, and hyperventilated when frustrated. When transferring or walking, she anticipated the next move before it was time to move, thereby increasing her risk for falls and injury. The hyperventilation interfered with therapy, so the treatment would have to stop until she became calm and ready to continue. After some discussion of this problematic behavior, the team determined that teaching Mrs. T to breathe slowly, deeply, and through pursed lips would diminish the hyperventilation. This technique was so successful that Mrs. T was able to recognize independently when she was beginning to hyperventilate and then stop herself. A psychiatric occupational therapist provided additional assistance to Mrs. T and the team to minimize the additional labile behaviors. During this time the primary nurse assisted Mrs. T with a bowel and bladder program and was able to remove the Foley catheter successfully. Bowel control was achieved through dietary changes and consistent use of the commode. Mrs. T's blood pressure was also under control, and her gastrointestinal upset was diminished by consistently eating breakfast.

The HHA worked with physical and occupational therapists to reinforce the exercises and safe transfer techniques. Since the aide was assisting with personal care, she was able to reinforce physical and occupational therapy exercises while assisting with transfers, walking, and bathing. The aide reported that Mrs. T wanted to use the bathtub and recommended that placement of the commode in the tub could allow Mrs. T to transfer safely to the commode and then into the tub. This observation and recommendation from the HHA greatly enhanced Mrs. T's progression with self-care activities.

Although team members worked on their individual treatment plans, they also shared observations and planned combined goals with Mrs. T. Her husband, however, distanced himself from the planning and indicated that he wanted to be only minimally involved with her treatment. He did, however, reiterate his commitment to have her at home and "try to make it work."

With the active involvement of all the team members, Mrs. T made significant progress toward independence. She progressed from using only the wheelchair to a hemiwalker and was ready to begin training with a four-prong cane. Then, on October 10, her husband died suddenly, having recently been diagnosed with pancreatic cancer. This unexpected event caused Mrs. T to become depressed and to regress. She made suicidal statements that alarmed several of the team members. The team requested the involvement of a psychiatric nurse to work with Mrs. T on the grieving process and to conduct a suicide risk assessment. Although it is usually necessary to have a psychiatrist involved when a psychiatric nurse makes visits, in this case the psychiatric nurse visited in place of the primary nurse and also provided medical and surgical nursing services. The psychiatric nurse made three visits, working with Mrs. T on the grieving process, planning for the upcoming holidays, and dealing with issues of altered body image brought on by the stroke. Mrs. T shared her concern that her grandchildren were afraid of her because of her stroke. At this point Mrs. T indicated that she was ready to continue her treatment, and she made no further allusion to suicide.

Since Mrs. T was now alone and the temporary assistance from her adult children was not a permanent solution, a referral was made to social work to help Mrs. T plan for her future living arrangements. A 24-hour, live-in homemaker was hired as a temporary measure until Mrs. T could decide if she wanted to move to a retirement community. In some respects the presence of the homemaker encouraged Mrs. T to make greater accomplishments, since she refused to allow the homemaker to do certain things in the kitchen and would not allow her to assist with personal care. Mrs. T also tackled stair climbing so she could get outside for walks.

At this time Mrs. T continues with her home exercise program. She has not made a decision about moving, so her live-in homemaker is still with her. She is completely independent in dressing, bathing, meal preparation, and ambulation. The team of home care personnel has conducted several case conferences regarding Mrs. T and her progress. This progress is the result of the dedication of a diverse team of home care workers and the desire of an individual to work hard and set her sights on goals that no one thought she could attain.

older adult residents of nursing facilities. Long-term care facilities that use gerontologic nurse practitioners are able to provide more timely care to acutely ill residents. The use of gerontologic nurse practitioners in collaboration with physicians has been shown to reduce emergency department transfers, hospital days, and subacute days (Burl et al, 1998). Several HMOs are using physician–nurse practitioner teams to provide primary care to nursing facility residents (Fama and Fox, 1997).

A nurse practitioner hired by a facility must have the full support of administration to have a real effect on care. He or she must be free to be an educational resource for staff without being required to participate in staff evaluations. The nurse practitioner must also have the full support of the facility medical director, who serves as a resource for the practitioner and sanctions his or her services and expertise.

Despite studies demonstrating the cost effectiveness of nurse practitioners in nursing facilities, few facilities currently employ them on a full-time basis. The major employment opportunities are with groups of physicians who carry a large nursing facility practice. These gerontologic nurse practitioners may go on rounds with the physician or see nursing facility residents independently on alternate months, with the physician seeing residents in the intervening months. Medicare reimburses both the physician and the nurse practitioner for this method of overseeing residents. In addition to seeing residents in the nursing facility, the practitioner may handle telephone calls from nursing facilities, triage problems, diagnose problems, and prescribe treatments and medications as needed.

THE FUTURE OF THE NURSING FACILITY

The future of the nursing facility is complicated and uncertain. Its destiny is intimately linked to public policy regarding health care reform, long-term care, and mechanisms of reimbursement. Certain aspects of this service setting are flourishing, including subacute care and SCUs for the cognitively impaired. Some industry analysts believe that the rapidly developing market of assisted living programs will radically change the face of the nursing facility over the next 10 years. It is speculated that the nursing facility will exist to provide care for severely cognitively and physically impaired residents.

Whatever happens, it is essential that the professional nurse play a dominant role in improving and transforming this practice setting. Nurses can better prepare themselves to play this role by becoming better educated in gerontologic nursing, nursing administration, health care regulation, and public policy related to long-term care.

Nurses need to be leaders in helping to shape the future of how and where long-term health care is provided. Being creative in a highly regulated industry is a significant challenge. Professional nurses who conceptualize their practice as including care for the whole person, principles of health promotion and disease prevention, and creative use of the organizational and social environment to achieve health outcomes will make a valuable contribution to society. Through such efforts by nurses and other like-minded professionals committed to achieving excellence, the nursing facility will be a place where people truly can live out their days with dignity, integrity, and a sense of personal autonomy.

SUMMARY

Although gerontologic nursing is a recognized specialty, most nurses working in a variety of practice settings today are working primarily with older adults. Nurses need to provide competent, evidence-based care. The growing number of certified basic and advanced practice gerontologic nurses will help in the endeavor, as will the inclusion of more gerontologic content in nursing school curricula. New acute care models will improve the care of hospitalized older adults, as will the development and dissemination of protocols that guide the assessment and treatment of commonly encountered geriatric syndromes.

Attitudes affect care delivery, and a nurse's respect and care for the special needs of older adults are essential. The diverse roles of acute care nurses working with older patients include those of practitioner, advocate, collaborator, educator, and case manager. In addition to ensuring safe and restorative health care in the hospital, the nurse must also address the learning needs, decision making, and ethical and legal issues involved in caring for older persons.

The health care needs of a growing, noninstitutionalized older adult population, coupled with rapid changes in today's health care delivery system, demand continued exploration of alternative services and delivery mechanisms that support the care of older persons in home and community settings. This chapter explored the current health care needs of community-residing older persons; community-based services; the role of family members and friends in providing informal care; and the role of home care agencies and home health nurses in community-based care for this population.

The need for programs and services aimed at supporting older persons and their caregivers in the community setting will continue to grow. Options for care must expand, and nontraditional alternatives must be developed for use by various health care personnel. The reimbursement structure is currently, and will clearly continue to be, challenged to accommodate these developments.

This chapter presented a variety of issues relevant to long-term care. Care of this type has evolved into the specialty care settings discussed. Clearly, the entire long-term care industry is not only one of the greatest challenges to society at large, but also to all health care professionals.

Recent attempts at regulating nursing facilities for the benefit of residents' overall health and well-being are an important yet modest step toward reform. The role of professional nurses in continuing to make positive changes within this setting must continue to be one of caring and innovative leadership).

Key Points

- Adults over age 65 account for 47% of the country's inpatient days; the average length of stay is 2 days longer than that of younger patients.
- The physical and social environment in which care occurs must be modified to facilitate maintenance of function and reduce the incidence of iatrogenic complications.
- Three conditions that require special attention during the hospitalization of older adults are falls, changes in cognitive status, and incontinence.
- New models of acute gerontologic nursing care have emerged that are demonstrating improvements in the quality of the nursing care provided to hospitalized patients.
- Increasing numbers of older adults are discharged from hospitals with significant needs related to medical care and functional impairments; therefore home health care for older adults is becoming more common and more complex.
- Older adults, family members, and health care providers, including gerontologic nurses, must learn about hospice care in order to make timely and appropriate referrals.
- Terminally ill older adults and their families are not maximizing the benefits of hospice care because of late referrals and misunderstanding of the Medicare hospice benefit.
- The Medicare hospice benefit covers (1) services and visits by all hospice staff, (2) durable medical equipment, (3) supplies needed for the plan of care, (4) medications related to the terminal diagnosis (may involve a small copayment at the discretion of the individual hospice), and (5) dietary supplements.
- Home care is often chosen as a preferred treatment site because people want to be home, home care is usually less expensive than hospitalization, and home care minimizes exposure to multiple infectious processes. In addition, technology has evolved to support complex treatments in the home.
- Assessment for home care should be done early in a client's hospital stay. Hospital discharge planners and home care managers must work together to ensure the continuity of care necessary for a timely and effective discharge.
- The home care nurse assesses the physical, functional, emotional, socioeconomic, and environmental well-being of clients. The nurse works in collaboration with all other members of the home care team whose services are needed to address the home care plan of treatment.
- Hospice nurses perform comprehensive, holistic assessments that are similar to those of home health nurses. In addition, the spiritual dimension is an important component of hospice care. In hospice the terminally ill person and the family are the unit of care. Therefore all assessments by members of the interdisciplinary hospice team address both as a unit.
- Residents in nursing facilities can be categorized according to their length of stay as short-term residents or long-term residents.
- Risk factors associated with institutionalization include advanced age, physical disability, mental impairment, white race, living without a spouse, and the presence of chronic medical conditions.
- The minimum data set (MDS) includes comprehensive and interdisciplinary assessment of residents.
- The registered nurse (RN) plays a key role in all clinical programs, including programs for skin care, management of incontinence, nutrition, infection control, and the promotion of mental health.
- Nursing care delivery systems in nursing facilities include functional nursing, team nursing, and primary team nursing.
- Assisted living programs, special care units (SCUs) for dementia, and subacute care units provide unique opportunities for RNs wishing to specialize in one aspect of the care provided in institutional settings.
- Recent innovations in the nursing facility involve self-governance programs for residents, nursing education programs, and the use of gerontologic nurse practitioners.

Critical Thinking Exercises

1. You have just admitted a 92-year-old woman to your nursing unit. How will you modify the hospital's physical and social environment to accommodate the needs of this patient? Why are such modifications necessary?
2. An 88-year-old man is being treated for a cardiac disorder. He is alert and interested in his care, but he has a hearing deficit. On teaching him about his cardiac medications, you notice that he often gets confused about the dosing schedules, names, and side effects of each medication. Offer several strategies to help him remain independent and maintain accurate medication schedules and monitoring.
3. A 90-year-old woman has been living with her 68-year-old daughter for 5 years. The daughter is suffering from complications of long-term diabetes and feels that she is no longer able to care for her mother. No other family members are willing to take the woman into their home. How would you go about determining the options available to the mother?
4. Symptom management is a critical part of hospice nursing care. What is meant by the statement, "Make pain assessment the fifth vital sign"? What are some strategies you can use in assessing the pain status of older adults?
5. What is OBRA, and what positive effects is it designed to make on the care of older adults residing in long-term care facilities?
6. A 90-year-old man has fractured his hip, and his recovery has been very slow. He has suffered occasional complications, but he is progressing. Why might long-term care be advantageous to him during his recovery?

References

Abbasi A et al: Nutritional problems in the nursing home population: opportunities for clinical interventions. In Rubenstein S, Wieland D, editors: *Improving care in the nursing home: comprehensive reviews of clinical research,* Newbury Park, Calif, 1993, Sage.

Ackermann RJ, Monroe PW: Bacteremic urinary tract infection in older people, *J Am Geriatr Soc* 44:927, 1996.

Allender J: *Community and home health nursing,* Philadelphia, 1998, JB Lippincott.

American Nurses Association: Scope of home health nursing practice, Publication No 9905HH, Washington, DC, 1999, American Nurses Publishing.

Apple R, Truscott S: Role of homemaker/home health aide in home care. In Morgan K, McClain S, editors: *Core curriculum for home health care nursing,* Gaithersburg, Md, 1995, Aspen.

Applebaum R: Long term care policy: lots of smoke, not many mirrors, and little progress, *Gerontologist* 38(11):135, 1998.

Brady R et al: Geriatric falls: prevention strategies for the staff, *J Gerontol Nurs* 19(9):26, 1993.

Burl JB et al: Geriatric nurse practitioners in long-term care: demonstration of effectiveness in managed care, *J Am Geratric Soc* 46(4):506-510, 1998.

Case-Gamble A: Urinary incontinence in the elderly. In Stanley M, Gauntlett Beare P, editors: *Gerontological nursing,* Philadelphia, 1995, FA Davis.

Culley J, Courtney J: Nursing in the long-term care facility. In Goldsmith S, editor: *Long-term care administration handbook,* Gaithersburg, Md, 1993, Aspen.

Dellasega C et al: Nursing process: teaching elderly clients, *J Gerontol Nurs* 20(1):31, 1994.

DeMaagd G: High-risk drugs in the elderly population, *Geriatr Nurs* 16(5):198-207, Sept-Oct 1995.

Dewey J: The shaping of an industry: will the assisted living boom lead to new regulation? *Provider* 20(11):39, 1994.

Fama T, Fox PD: Efforts to improve primary care delivery to nursing home residents, *J Am Geriatr Soc* 45:627, 1997.

Francis D, Fletcher K, Simon L: The geriatric resource nurse model of care. In Abraham I, Fulmer T, Milisen K: Advances in geriatric nursing, *Nurs Clin North Am* 33(3):481, 1998.

Gamroth L, Semradek J, Tornquist E: *Enhancing autonomy in long-term care: concepts and strategies,* New York, 1995, Springer.

Gill C, Howells J, Hoffman E: Rehabilitation in the nursing facility. In Rubenstein L, Wieland D, editors: *Improving care in the nursing home: comprehensive reviews of clinical research,* Newbury Park, Calif, 1993, Sage.

Gill H, Balsano A: The move toward subacute care, *Nurs Homes* 43(4):7, 1994.

Goldman B: Traditional staffing models in long-term care, *J Gerontol Nurs* 24(9):29-34, Sept 1998.

Granger CV, Albrecht GL, Hamilton BB: Outcome of comprehensive medical rehabilitation: measures of PULSES profile and Barthel index, *Arch Phys Med Rehab* 60:145, 1979.

Greenberg S: *Title III: state and community programs,* accessed in 1995 via website: http://www.aoa.dhhs.gov.

Groegar JS et al: Descriptive analysis of CCU in the US: patient characteristics and ICU utilization, *Crit Care Med* 21:279, 1993.

Hanson LC, Weber DJ, Rutala WA: Risk factors for nosocomial pneumonia in the elderly, *Am J Med* 92:161, 1992.

Health Care Financing Administration: *Resident assessment instrument training manual and resource guide,* Baltimore, 1995, The Administration.

Health Care Financing Administration: *Survey, certification and enforcement procedures,* Baltimore, 1994, The Administration.

Health Care Financing Administration: *Health Care Financing Rev* 21(3):231-273, 2000

Humphrey C, Milone-Nuzzo P: *Orientation to home care nursing,* Gaithersburg, Md, 1996, Aspen.

Institute of Medicine: *Improving the quality of care in nursing homes,* Washington, DC, 1986, National Academy Press.

Jette A et al: High-risk profiles for nursing home admissions, *Gerontologist* 32(5):634, 1992.

Joint Commission on Accreditation of Healthcare Organizations: *Accreditation manual for hospitals,* Oakbrook Terrace, Ill, 1998, The Commission.

Kane R, Kane R: *Long-term care: principles, programs, and policies,* New York, 1987, Springer.

Kane RL, Ouslander JG, Abrass IB: *Essentials of clinical geriatrics,* ed 3, New York, 1994, McGraw-Hill.

Kane R, Wilson K: *Assisted living in the United States: a new paradigm for residential care for frail older persons?* Washington, DC, 1993, American Association of Retired Persons.

Katz S et al: Studies of illness in the aged: the index for ADL: a standardized measure of biological and psychosocial function, *JAMA* 185:914, 1963.

Kresevic DM et al: Assessment of function: critically important to acute care of elders, *Geriatr Nurs,* Sept/Oct 1997.

Lattanzi-Licht M, Mahoney JJ, Miller GW: *The hospice choice: in pursuit of a peaceful death,* New York, 1998, Fireside.

Lidz C, Arnold R: The medical model and its effect on autonomy: a comparison of two long-term care settings. In Gamroth L, Semradek J, Tornquist E, editors: *Enhancing autonomy in long-term care: concepts and strategies,* New York, 1995, Springer.

Mandavia D, Newton K: *Geriatric trauma,* Emerg Med Clin North Am 16(1):257, 1998.

McCainey CA: The development of the empowered aide model: an intervention for long-term care staff who care for Alzheimer's residents, *J Gerontol Nurs* 24(1):17, 1998.

McEwen M: *Community-based nursing,* Philadelphia, 1998, WB Saunders.

Meiner SE: Polypharmacy at the end-of-life. In Matzo MO, Sherman DW, editors: *Quality nursing care for the older adult at the end of life,* St Louis, 2004, Mosby.

Meiner SE: Polypharmacy in the elderly: early intervention can prevent complications, *Adv Nurs Pract* 5(7):28-34, 1997.

Merck manual of geriatrics, ed 3, Whitehouse Station, NJ, 2000, Merck Research Laboratories.

Mikos CW, Koch LA: The legal considerations surrounding OASIS reporting requirements, *Caring* (18)3:20, 1999.

Miller SK: Impact of a gerontological nurse practitioner on the nursing home elderly in the acute care setting, *AACN Clin Issues* 8(4):609, 1997.

Millsap P: Nurses' role with the elderly in the long-term care setting. In Stanley M, Gauntlett Beare P, editors: *Gerontological nursing,* Philadelphia, 1995, FA Davis.

Moody H: *Aging,* ed 2, Thousand Oaks, Calif, 1998, Pine Forge Press.

National Association for Home Care: *Basic statistics about home care,* Washington, DC, 1999, The Association.

National Association for Home Care: *2000 NAHC Legislative blue print for action: hospices,* Washington, DC, 2000, The Association

National Center for Health Statistics: *Health, United States,* 2002, Hyattsville, Md, 2003, The Center.

National Hospice Organization: *Hospice under Medicare,* South Deerfield, Mass, 1998b, Channing L Bete Co.

Neal LJ: Functional assessment of the home health client, *Home Health Nurs* (16)10:670, 1998.

Ouslander J, Schnelle J: Assessment, treatment, and management of urinary incontinence in the nursing home. In Rubenstein L, Wieland D, editors: *Improving care in the nursing home: comprehensive reviews of clinical research,* Newbury Park, Calif, 1993, Sage.

Planchock NY, Slay LE: Pharmacokinetic and pharmacodynamic monitoring of the elderly in critical care, *Crit Care Nurs Clin North Am* 8(1):79, 1996.

Powell, SK: *Nursing case management: a practical guide to success in managed care,* Philadelphia, 1996, Lippincott-Raven.

Robb J: Trauma care. In Fulmer T, Walker M, editors: *Critical care nursing of the elderly,* New York, 1991, Springer.

Robbins LM, Courts NF: Care of the traumatized older adult, *Geriatr Nurs* 18(5):209, 1997.

Robert Wood Johnson Foundation: *Chronic care in America: a 21st century challenge,* Princeton, NJ, 1996, The Foundation.

Rosenzweig E: Trends in home care entitlements and benefits, *J Gerontol Soc Work* 24(3-4):9, 1995.

Sachs Group Newsletter, 1st quarter, Evanston, Ill, 1999.

Schnelle J et al: Managing nurse aides to promote quality of care in the nursing home. In Rubenstein L, Wieland D, editors: *Improving care in the nursing home: comprehensive reviews of clinical research,* Newbury Park, Calif, 1993, Sage.

Sehy YB, Williams M: Functional assessment. In Stone J, Wyman J, Salisbury S, editors: *Clinical gerontological nursing,* ed 2, Philadelphia, 1999, Saunders.

Sloan RW: Principles of drug therapy in geriatric patients, *Am Fam Phys* 45:2709, 1992.

St. Pierre J: Functional decline in hospitalized elders: preventive nursing measures, *AACN Clin Issues* 9(1):109, 1998.

St. Pierre J: Delirium in hospitalized elderly patients: off tract, *Crit Care Nurs Clin North Am* 8(1):53, 1996.

Stanley M: Sepsis in the elderly, *Crit Care Nurs Clin North Am* 8(1):1, 1996.

Steinbach P, Zuber RF: Tips for using OASIS now, *Home Health Nurs* 15(4):261, 1997.

Stephenson CA: Hospice services. In Hogstel MO, editor: *Community resources for older adults: a guide for case managers,* St Louis, 1998, Mosby.

Sullivan D, Lipschitz D: Evaluating and treating of nutritional problems in older patients, *Clin Geriatr Med* 13(4):753, 1997.

Taylor ME, Oppenheim BA: Hospital-acquired infections in elderly patients, *J Hosp Infect* 38:245-260, 1998.

Terpenning MS et al: Colonization and infection with antibiotic-resistant bacteria in a long term care facility, *J Am Geriatr Soc* 42:1062, 1994.

Tideiksaar R: *Falls in older persons: prevention and management in hospitals and nursing homes,* Boulder, Colo, 1993, Tactilitics.

Treml L: Basic mobility needs. In Emlet C et al, editors: *In-home assessments of older adults,* Gaithersburg, Md, 1996, Aspen.

US Department of Health and Human Services: *Advance Data* 280, Jan 23, 1997a.

US Department of Health and Human Services: *Advance Data* 289, July 2, 1997b.

Walker MK: The physiology of normal aging. In Fulmer T, Walker M, editors: *Critical care nursing of the elderly,* New York, 1992, Springer.

Wells T: Managing falls, incontinence, and cognitive impairment: nursing research. In Funk SG et al, editors: *Key aspects of elder care,* New York, 1992, Springer.

Williams B, Thompson J, Brummel-Smith K: Improving medication use in the nursing home. In Rubenstein L, Wieland D, editors: *Improving care in the nursing home: comprehensive reviews of clinical research,* Newbury Park, Calif, 1993, Sage.

Wilson EB: Preventing patient falls, *AACN Clin Issues* 9(1):100, 1998.

World Health Organization: *Cancer pain relief and palliative care,* Technical Report Series 804, Geneva, 1990, World Health Organization.

WEBSITES

Long-term care hospital information: www.cms.hhs.gov/providers/longterm/default.asp

Medicare information: www.medicare.gov

Medicare learning network: www.cms.hhs.gov/medlearn/ltchpps.asp

Medicare press release updating: www.cms.hhs.gov/media/press/release.asp

Medicare trustees reports: www.cms.hhs.gov/publications/trusteesreport

10 Nutrition

KATHLEEN M. ROURKE, PhD, RN, RD, CHES

Learning Objectives

On completion of this chapter, the reader will be able to:

1. Differentiate between the social, cultural, and emotional aspects of food and the physiologic aspects of nutrients and food.
2. Correlate the physiologic changes of aging with food intake patterns.
3. Differentiate between a nutritional screen and a nutritional assessment.
4. Identify the steps and core data collection elements for a nutritional assessment.
5. Describe the changes in nutritional requirements for aging persons.
6. Describe the role of therapeutic diets and nutritional support in nutritional therapies.
7. Identify major dietary guidelines and recommendations for healthy persons of all ages.

SOCIAL AND CULTURAL ASPECTS OF FOOD

Although at its core the role of food is simply that of providing energy and nutrients for bodily functions, few individuals view food from this perspective. Over the course of history, different types of foods have served as poisons, potions, or panaceas for health, potency, long life, and love. Hippocrates (460-377 BC), the "Father of Medicine," reflected his commitment to the importance of diet in a statement from the Hippocratic Oath: "I will apply dietetic measures for the benefit of the sick according to my ability and judgment; I will keep them from harm and injustice" (Tannahill, 1988). Cato the Elder (234-149 BC), a Roman statesman, ate large amounts of cabbage in the belief it had special healing properties. A later Roman scholar, Pliny the Elder (23-79 AD), ate the foot and snout of the hippopotamus to enhance sexual potency, whereas a Chinese physician of the sixth century BC prescribed certain foods for clients to stimulate the yin (female principle) and the yang (male principle) to keep a person healthy (Tannahill, 1988).

In present societies food and diet are manipulated to enhance athletic performance, carbohydrates are avoided to force the body into ketosis in an effort to burn fat for weight loss, and supplements are taken to replace the vitamins and minerals missing from the "fad diets" many Americans eat. Comfort foods are now a designated and popular category, particularly after September 11, 2001, when purchases of donuts and pastries increased significantly (Balon, 2002; *Comforted but unfattened*, 2002).

Food is much more than fuel for the body; food in our society is a social centerpiece, a source of comfort, and a symbol of celebration. Consider the monthly calendar:

- January: New Year's and Super Bowl
- February: Valentine's Day
- March: St. Patrick's Day
- April: Passover and Easter
- May: Mother's Day and Memorial Day
- June: Father's Day
- July: Fourth of July
- August: summer fairs
- September: Labor Day
- October: Halloween
- November: Thanksgiving
- December: holidays

In addition to these holidays, there are birthdays, anniversaries, and other personal holidays. Life, death, and everything in between is celebrated with food. Culturally, food is a symbol of heritage, land, and environment, and religiously food is abstained from, eaten only on certain days, and certainly blessed by a higher power for the energy it provides to the body. Religious practices also specify prohibited foods and beverages (see Cultural Awareness boxes).

Nutritional interventions that do not take into account the social, cultural, and emotional aspects of food are rarely effective because few individuals "eat to survive"; most of us "survive to eat." For the nurse, understanding the social, cultural, and emotional aspects of eating for a patient can be a great asset in working with nutrition and health issues. This is especially true in the geriatric population who hold strong ties to their culture, need social interaction to enhance functional status, and may be emotional labile when different foods are presented. For some, food can be a private and delicate point, which the health care practitioner must be sensitive to during conversation. The nurse is unlikely to influence

Cultural Awareness

SELECTED EXAMPLES OF CULTURAL MEANINGS IN FOOD

- Critical life force for survival
- Relief of hunger
- Peaceful coexistence
- Promotion of health and prevention of disease or illness
- Expression of caring for another
- Interpersonal closeness or distance
- Promotion of kinship and familial alliances
- Solidification of social ties
- Celebration of life events (e.g., birthday, marriage)
- Expression of gratitude or appreciation
- Recognition of achievement or accomplishment
- Business negotiations
- Information exchange
- Validation of social, cultural, or religious ceremonial functions
- Means to generate income
- Expression of affluence or social status

basic beliefs about foods and their religious significance and should attempt to make recommendations that are consistent with religious beliefs.

Overall, within the medical field and compared with fields like biochemistry, chemistry, and biology, the field of nutrition is a young science. Changes in nutrition and food policy occur frequently, confusing the consumer as well as the health care practitioner who is not solely focused on nutrition. Many new frontiers remain to be discovered. For instance, there is a major focus in research regarding the impact of nutrient substrates on disease prevention, immune system stimulation, and response to critical illness (Mendez et al, 1997; Schilling et al, 1996). Researchers studying this use of nutrients have coined the term *nutriceuticals* to imply the pharmaceutical effects of nutrients and nutrient substrates.

Nursing professionals should be encouraged to work with a dietitian, who is constantly updated on the latest nutritional applications for patient care. This collaborative relationship can optimize patient outcomes and enhance work efficiency for each practitioner. Both dietitian and nurse can thus bring

Cultural Awareness

DIETARY PRACTICES OF SELECTED RELIGIOUS GROUPS*

Prohibited Foods and Beverages

Hinduism
All meats

Islam
Pork and pork products
Animal shortenings
Alcoholic products (including extracts such as vanilla or lemon)
Marshmallows, gelatin, and other confections made with pork
NOTE: Fasting is common. Mandatory fasting in the daylight hours during months of Ramadan.

Judaism
Pork
Predatory fowl
Shellfish or scavenger fish (e.g., catfish, shrimp, escargot, lobster) (Fish with fins and scales are permissible.)
Mixing milk and meat dishes at same meal
Blood by ingestion (e.g., blood sausage, raw meat) (Blood by transfusion is acceptable.)
Notes

1. Only meat from cloven-hoofed animals that chew cud (e.g., cattle, sheep, goat, deer) is allowed. The animals must have been slaughtered observing rigid rules that result in minimal pain to the animal and maximum blood drainage.
2. Foods should be kosher (meaning "proper" or "fitting"), which is accomplished in one of two methods:
   a. Meat is soaked in cold water with coarse salt for a half hour and drained to deplete blood content. It is then thoroughly washed under cold, running water and drained again before cooking.
   b. Meat is first prepared by quick searing or cooking over an open flame, which permits liver to be eaten, since it cannot be prepared by the above method.
3. Meat and dairy products cannot be served at the same meal nor can they be cooked or served in the same set of dishes. Milk or milk products may be consumed just before a meal but not until 6 hours after eating a meal with meat products. Fish or eggs can be eaten with dairy products or meat meals.

Mormonism (Church of Jesus Christ of Latter-Day Saints)
Alcohol
Tobacco
Stimulants (including beverages containing caffeine, such as coffee, nonherbal teas, colas, and selected carbonated soft drinks)

Seventh-Day Adventist Church
Pork
Certain seafood, including shellfish
Fermented beverages
Notes

1. Optional vegetarianism includes (a) strict vegetarianism, (b) ovolacto vegetarianism, or (c) no pork or pork products, shellfish, or blood.
2. Snacking between meals is discouraged.

* These dietary practices are generalizations; not all of these religions will follow these guidelines.

a higher quality of health care to the patient and grow as practitioners. Allied health researchers and practitioners perceive dietary intake as one of the most significant, controllable tools for wellness, disease prevention, rehabilitation, and treatment or therapy for a wide range of disorders. It requires a total team approach and an appreciation for the social, cultural, and emotional aspects that food represents to the vast majority of the population to make changes in poor dietary choices.

DEMOGRAPHICS OF THE AGING POPULATION

The "graying of the American population" can be considered one of the most far-reaching medical and nutritional issues of the millennium. Medically this is a population that has served its country, worked hard, and now faces a health care system that views patients in terms of cost. Some of the individuals in this population are survivors of deadly bacterial diseases that plagued the world in the early 1900s. With the development of antibiotics and a growing pharmaceutical industry, these individuals who helped to automate this country are not only living longer but are hearty souls capable of overcoming many adversities.

Nutritionally the aging population comprises individuals who still know how to cook and believe in fresh foods, family meals, and cultural connections. Older adults are less comfortable with the fast-paced world in which food choices are being made, and they are not as comfortable with the "high tech" cooking gadgetry of the new millennium.

It is no secret that the aging population is growing. The 85 and older age cohort, which represented 3.4 million of the total population in 1993, is the fastest growing segment and makes up 10% of the older population. In the 120-year period between 1870 and 1990, individuals over age 65 grew from 1 million to 32 million. In 2030 those over 65 years of age are expected to represent at least 20% of the population (Stadler and Teaster, 2002). Chronic diseases are compromising health status at later states in life; these chronic diseases have repeated and direct correlates with dietary intake, exercise, stress management, and locus of control and include cardiovascular disease, cancer, stroke, osteoporosis, and diabetes. More often, the diagnoses of such diseases occur among the old-old (ages 85 and older), closer to the period of dying and death (the ninth and tenth decades of life).

Life expectancy has increased, but life span has not. Today's average life expectancy at birth is about 75.7 years, whereas life span is still considered to be 115 years, although a record of 122 years was set in March 1994 by a woman in France. The old-old will continue to be the fastest growing group, and it is predicted (by the U.S. Census Bureau) to be 8.6 million by 2030. By 2050 this group may be 25% of the 65 and older population (AARP, Administration on Aging, 2004).

The social and economic consequences of America growing older, coupled with lower birth and mortality rates, are vast, including a heavy demand on the health care industry. Nutrition, exercise, and engagement in other activities such as lifelong learning and education will increase and enhance the functional capacity of this generation of individuals and their families, as well as society (Stadler and Teaster, 2002).

PHYSIOLOGIC CHANGES IN AGING THAT AFFECT NUTRITIONAL STATUS

Aging produces physiologic changes; however, assumptions about the aged are often generalizations without merit. A distinction should be made between the healthy aging person and the aging person with acute or chronic disease. For the healthy aging person, exercise and the resulting maintenance of muscle mass are emerging in research as one of the greatest determinants of maintaining vitality (Cress et al, 1999). Loss of lean body mass, essentially loss of skeletal muscle, can lead to decreased strength and mobility, predisposing aging adults to falls and affecting (although minimally) metabolism. Exercise is effective in maintaining skeletal muscle mass, and it enhances functional status and fitness levels for aging adults by 10 to 20 years (Cress, 1999).

Functional impairment often leads to malnutrition. Older adults with functional impairments may have difficulty performing, or be unable to perform, activities of daily living (ADLs) related to eating. They may be unable to shop for groceries, prepare food, or eat. Conditions that result in shortness of breath, pain, or limited mobility affect an individual's ability and desire to eat. In addition, some medications alter sensory receptors, resulting in differences in taste or smell. For many of the elderly, foods that were once cherished and enjoyed as part of their culture now smell very different and are simply avoided. A report published by the AARP found that 23% of aging adults who live at home have health-related impairments in ADLs (AARP, 1994).

Physiologic changes that are common in older adults can lead to problems with nutrition. Organ function declines with age; this can affect digestion, metabolism, absorption of nutrients, and the ability to eliminate waste products via the kidneys (Keithley, 1996). The gastrointestinal system slows with age, resulting in less efficient absorption of nutrients (Zulkowski and Albrecht, 2003). Changes in the oral cavity include tooth loss or ill-fitting dentures, mouth dryness, and decreased esophageal motility. Satiety triggers are diminished in older adults, yet given the increased risk for skin breakdown and the likelihood of a compromised immune, circulatory, and respiratory system, the majority of the elderly populations have increased protein requirements (Zulkowski and Albrecht, 2003).

Delayed gastric emptying, hiatal herniation, and decreased secretion of gastric juices may cause bloating and discomfort. Changes in the pH of the gastrointestinal tract can lead to the malabsorption of B vitamins. Hepatic and renal reserves are decreased, making it harder to metabolize medications and alcohol and to conserve water or excrete nitrogenous wastes.

Thirst regulation is often affected, making dehydration a prime risk among older adults (see Research box).

Older adults are at risk of dehydration caused by a decreased intake of fluids, loss of sodium, and increased fluid losses. Physiologically, the decreased intake can be related to altered thirst; older adults may not feel thirsty even when hypovolemic and often do not compensate for fluid losses during illness. Confusion, depression, and dementia also contribute significantly to reduced food and fluid intake. Dehydration can take three main forms. Isotonic dehydration results from the loss of sodium and water, such as during a gastrointestinal illness. Hypertonic dehydration results when water losses exceed sodium losses. This type of dehydration is the most common and can occur from fever or limited fluid intake. Hypotonic dehydration can occur with diuretic use when sodium loss is higher than water loss (Weinberg and Minaker, 1995).

Research

SAMPLE SETTING

The subjects were individuals 65 years of age and older.

METHODS

The Medicare Provider Analysis and Review (MEDPAR) files maintained by HCFA were reviewed. The data from the files were used to calculate hospitalization rates, demographic characteristics, and associated diagnoses for patients who were admitted to the hospital during 1991. The contribution to mortality was also analyzed.

FINDINGS

Warren et al found that 6.7% of Medicare patients hospitalized had dehydration as a top five diagnosis and that Medicare reimbursed $446 million for hospital costs related to dehydration as a primary diagnosis. Older adults, men, and blacks were at the highest risk. Infection was the diagnosis most closely associated with hospitalizations for dehydration; this included respiratory illness, urinary system infection, gastroenteritis, and sepsis. Nearly 50% of the subjects died within 1 year of admission, and 17.4% died within 30 days of admission.

IMPLICATIONS

Dehydration in older adults is costly in terms of health and life, not to mention dollars. The old-old, ages 85 to 99 years, were six times more likely to be hospitalized for dehydration than their younger counterparts. The nurse should be alert to the risk of dehydration in older adults who develop infections. Interventions to educate older adults about the dangers of dehydration during respiratory illness, urinary tract infections, and gastroenteritis are of prime importance in home health care and public health education programs. The mortality rate for dehydration that requires hospital admission is significant.

Warren JL et al: The burden and outcomes associated with dehydration among US elderly, 1991, *Am J Pub Health* 84:1265, 1994.

PSYCHOSOCIAL AND SOCIOECONOMIC FACTORS RELATED TO MALNUTRITION

Poverty is a significant problem for older Americans, particularly as individual ages. The U.S. Census Bureau reports (2003) that 10.1% of adults ages 65 and older were below the poverty level. When individuals have a fixed income to cover housing, clothing, utilities, food, health care, medications, and other expenses, food may be sacrificed, especially as the percentage of income required for health care rises. It is estimated that 61% of women and 31% of men over the age of 65 live on annual incomes under $10,000. The cost of medication for the elderly has significantly compromised many already low-income budgets, forcing individuals to do without food or the medication (Zulkowski and Albrecht, 2003). Food may be limited first in quality as a transition to high-fat, high-carbohydrate convenience foods occurs, followed by a limitation in quantity.

Social isolation is another factor contributing to malnutrition. Older adults may skip meals completely when they live alone and have no one with whom to prepare and share meals. Grieving over the loss of a spouse or friends also affects diet quality and intake. Psychosocial factors, such as isolation and depression, and economic issues, such as poverty or the limitations of a fixed income, can affect food purchases and intake. Approximately 8% to 16% of older adults do not have access to a nutritious, culturally acceptable diet, and federal programs to combat hunger and malnutrition reach only about one third of the population they are intended to benefit. Many of those who receive home-delivered meals have two or three chronic health conditions, and 43% have been hospitalized within the previous year (Ponza, Ohls, and Millen, 1996). Meals-on-Wheels programs and congregate dining arrangements can bring meals and socialization opportunities to older adults who are at risk. Physiologic, psychosocial, and economic factors must be assessed by the nurse or dietitian during nutritional screening or a comprehensive nutritional assessment.

NUTRITIONAL SCREENING AND ASSESSMENT

Nutritional Screening

Nutritional screening is an abbreviated assessment of nutritional risk factors to determine which clients are in need of a more comprehensive assessment and nutritional interventions. A variety of tools have been developed to conduct nutritional screening. Perhaps the most widely used of these tools is the "Determine Your Nutritional Health" screening tool developed as part of the Nutrition Screening Initiative (NSI) (Fig. 10-1).

The Warning Signs of poor nutritional health are often overlooked. Use this checklist to find out if you or someone you know is at nutritional risk.

DETERMINE YOUR NUTRITIONAL HEALTH

Read the statements below. Circle the number in the yes column for those that apply to you or someone you know. For each yes answer, score the number in the box. Total your nutritional score.

	YES
I have an illness or condition that made me change the kind and/or amount of food I eat.	2
I eat fewer than 2 meals per day.	3
I eat few fruits or vegetables, or milk products.	2
I have 3 or more drinks of beer, liquor or wine almost every day.	2
I have tooth or mouth problems that make it hard for me to eat.	2
I don't always have enough money to buy the food I need.	4
I eat alone most of the time.	1
I take 3 or more different prescribed or over-the-counter drugs a day.	1
Without wanting to, I have lost or gained 10 pounds in the last 6 months.	2
I am not always physically able to shop, cook and/or feed myself.	2
TOTAL	

Total Your Nutritional Score. If it's —

0-2 **Good!** Recheck your nutritional score in 6 months.

3-5 **You are at moderate nutritional risk.** See what can be done to improve your eating habits and lifestyle. Your office on aging, senior nutrition program, senior citizens center or health department can help. Recheck your nutritional score in 3 months.

6 or more **You are at high nutritional risk.** Bring this checklist the next time you see your doctor, dietitian or other qualified health or social service professional. Talk with them about any problems you may have. Ask for help to improve your nutritional health.

These materials developed and distributed by the Nutrition Screening Initiative, a project of:

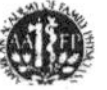
AMERICAN ACADEMY OF FAMILY PHYSICIANS

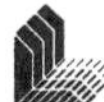
THE AMERICAN DIETETIC ASSOCIATION

NATIONAL COUNCIL ON THE AGING

Remember that warning signs suggest risk, but do not represent diagnosis of any condition. Turn the page to learn more about the Warning Signs of poor nutritional health.

Fig. 10-1 Determine Your Nutritional Health. (Reprinted with permission from the Nutrition Screening Initiative, a project of the American Academy of Family Physicians, the American Dietetic Association, and the National Council on the Aging, and funded in part by a grant from Ross Products Division, Abbott Laboratories Inc.)

The Nutrition Checklist is based on the Warning Signs described below. Use the word DETERMINE to remind you of the Warning Signs.

DISEASE

Any disease, illness or chronic condition which causes you to change the way you eat, or makes it hard for you to eat, puts your nutritional health at risk. Four out of five adults have chronic diseases that are affected by diet. Confusion or memory loss that keeps getting worse is estimated to affect one out of five or more of older adults. This can make it hard to remember what, when or if you've eaten. Feeling sad or depressed, which happens to about one in eight older adults, can cause big changes in appetite, digestion, energy level, weight and well-being.

EATING POORLY

Eating too little and eating too much both lead to poor health. Eating the same foods day after day or not eating fruit, vegetables, and milk products daily will also cause poor nutritional health. One in five adults skip meals daily. Only 13% of adults eat the minimum amount of fruit and vegetables needed. One in four older adults drink too much alcohol. Many health problems become worse if you drink more than one or two alcoholic beverages per day.

TOOTH LOSS/ MOUTH PAIN

A healthy mouth, teeth and gums are needed to eat. Missing, loose or rotten teeth or dentures which don't fit well or cause mouth sores make it hard to eat.

ECONOMIC HARDSHIP

As many as 40% of older Americans have incomes of less than $6,000 per year. Having less--or choosing to spend less--than $25-30 per week for food makes it very hard to get the foods you need to stay healthy.

REDUCED SOCIAL CONTACT

One-third of all older people live alone. Being with people daily has a positive effect on morale, well-being and eating.

MULTIPLE MEDICINES

Many older Americans must take medicines for health problems. Almost half of older Americans take multiple medicines daily. Growing old may change the way we respond to drugs. The more medicines you take, the greater the chance for side effects such as increased or decreased appetite, change in taste, constipation, weakness, drowsiness, diarrhea, nausea, and others. Vitamins or minerals when taken in large doses act like drugs and can cause harm. Alert your doctor to everything you take.

INVOLUNTARY WEIGHT LOSS/GAIN

Losing or gaining a lot of weight when you are not trying to do so is an important warning sign that must not be ignored. Being overweight or underweight also increases your chance of poor health.

NEEDS ASSISTANCE IN SELF CARE

Although most older people are able to eat, one of every five have trouble walking, shopping, buying and cooking food, especially as they get older.

ELDER YEARS ABOVE AGE 80

Most older people lead full and productive lives. But as age increases, risk of frailty and health problems increase. Checking your nutritional health regularly makes good sense.

The Nutrition Screening Initiative, 2626 Pennsylvania Avenue, NW, Suite 301, Washington, DC 20037

© The Nutrition Screening Initiative is funded in part by a grant from Ross Laboratories, a division of Abbott Laboratories.

A5944(1.00)/DECEMBER 1995

Fig. 10-1 cont'd, Determine Your Nutritional Health. (Reprinted with permission from the Nutrition Screening Initiative, a project of the American Academy of Family Physicians, the American Dietetic Association, and the National Council on the Aging, and funded in part by a grant from Ross Products Division, Abbott Laboratories Inc.)

The NSI (Dwyer, 1991), a 5-year, multifaceted national effort to promote routine nutrition screening, began in 1990 under the direction of the American Academy of Family Physicians, the American Dietetic Association, and the National Council on the Aging. As part of the initiative, a nutritional health checklist was developed to be used by older adults or caregivers to determine risk factors associated with nutrition and health. A score of 3 or more indicates moderate to high nutritional risk and triggers the need for a more comprehensive nutritional assessment. The Level II Screen is a tool for health care professionals to conduct a more in-depth assessment of nutritional status (Fig. 10-2).

The importance of nutritional screening is emphasized in the standards and guidelines developed by the Health Care Financing Administration (HCFA) (now the Centers for Medicaid and Medicare Services [CMS]) and the Joint Commission on Accreditation of Healthcare Organizations (JCAHO). The Outcome and Assessment Information Set (OASIS) implemented by CMS includes data elements relating to food intake and nutritional status (HCFA, 1998). This massive project is designed to collect and measure client care outcomes for home care clients. Nutrition-related outcomes for OASIS in home care include "improvement in eating and stabilization in light meal preparation." The focus of the OASIS project is to develop outcome measures that lead to performance improvement.

A variety of studies have shown that nutrition affects immune status and length of hospital stay (American Dietetic Association, 1995a; Bower 1995; Kudsk et al, 1996; Mendez et al, 1997). Outcome management attempts to identify critical interventions that produce a positive clinical outcome at lower cost. Because nutrition is an integral intervention in many diseases, disease state management programs or clinical pathways often incorporate nutritional interventions. Malnourished, hospitalized clients have more infections and other complications, which significantly increase the costs of hospitalization and care (Robinson, Goldstein, and Levine, 1987).

Standards developed by the JCAHO require nutrition screening of all hospitalized and home care clients who receive clinical services (JCAHO, 1998). The standards also require referral for a comprehensive assessment if the client is found to be at moderate to severe nutritional risk.

Nutritional Assessment

A nutritional assessment is a comprehensive evaluation of a client's nutritional status and typically includes data collection in each of the following areas: demographic and psychosocial data, medical history, dietary history, anthropometrics, medications and laboratory values, and a physical assessment. Nutritional assessment may be performed as a result of an identified risk on a nutritional screening or when the risk status is obvious without a preliminary screening. The American Society for Parenteral and Enteral Nutrition (ASPEN) published standards that identify nutritionally at-risk clients (Box 10-1) (ASPEN, 1995). ASPEN also identified the goals of a nutritional assessment as follows:

- Establish baseline subjective and objective nutrition parameters.
- Identify specific nutritional deficits.
- Determine nutritional risk factors.
- Establish nutritional needs.
- Identify medical and psychosocial factors that may influence the prescription and administration of nutrition support.

Diet History. In addition to a complete history and physical assessment, clients who are found to be at nutritional risk require a more specific evaluation of their dietary intake patterns. Information that is typically part of a diet history includes number of meals and snacks per day; chewing or swallowing difficulties; gastrointestinal problems or symptoms that affect eating; oral health and denture use; history of diseases or surgery; activity level; use of medications; appetite; need for assistance with meals and meal preparation; and food preferences, allergies, and aversions. A diet history may also include a food recall. For accuracy and relevancy, the food recall must include specific information about the type of food ingested, the preparation method, and an accurate estimate of the amount. The client should also be cautioned to select days for recording that are typical of his or her intake patterns. Clients should be instructed about how to estimate portion sizes and given samples from which to estimate their intake (4 oz of meat is the size of a pack of cards; a serving of vegetables is usually ½ cup). The purpose of the food recall is to estimate the average number of calories and amount of protein ingested daily, and to detect any food intake patterns, such as overuse of fried foods or lack of vegetables or fruit. Some clients may need assistance from another person, if available, to complete the food recall.

For a more detailed picture of a client's diet and food patterns, a 3- to 7-day food intake history is obtained. Clients are asked to keep a detailed record of everything they eat, the time at which they eat, and the amount of each type of food item that is consumed. In addition to recording eating habits, clients are also asked to record activities and feelings, which allows the health care professional to determine if there are emotional issues or activities that may either interfere with or enhance eating pleasure.

The final means of assessing dietary patterns is by looking at food frequency. Food frequency questionnaires allow a health care professional to assess a particular nutrient category, such as calcium intake, or the adequacy of an individual's entire diet. A food frequency questionnaire is completed either by a medical assistant or by the patient during his or her wait in a health professional's office. Food frequency questionnaires are recommended for new clients because they allow the practitioner to collect reasonable dietary data

Level II Screen

Complete the following screen by interviewing the client directly and/or by referring to the client chart. If you do not routinely perform all of the described tests or ask all of the listed questions, please consider including them but do not be concerned if the entire screen is not completed. Please try to conduct a minimal screen on as many older clients as possible, and please try to collect serial measurements, which are extremely valuable in monitoring nutritional status. Please refer to the manual for additional information.

Anthropometrics

Measure height to the nearest inch and weight to the nearest pound. Record the values below and mark them on the body mass index (BMI) scale to the right. Then use a straight edge (e.g., paper, ruler) to connect the two points and circle the spot where this straight line crosses the center line (body mass index). Record the number below. Healthy older adults should have a body mass index between 22 and 27; check the appropriate box to flag an abnormally high or low value.

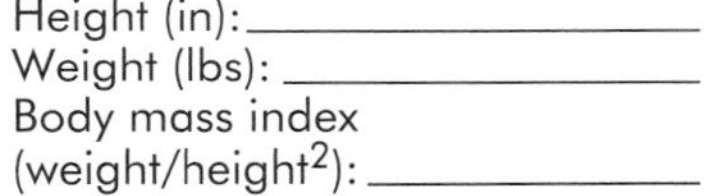

Height (in): ______________

Weight (lbs): ______________

Body mass index (weight/height^2): ______________

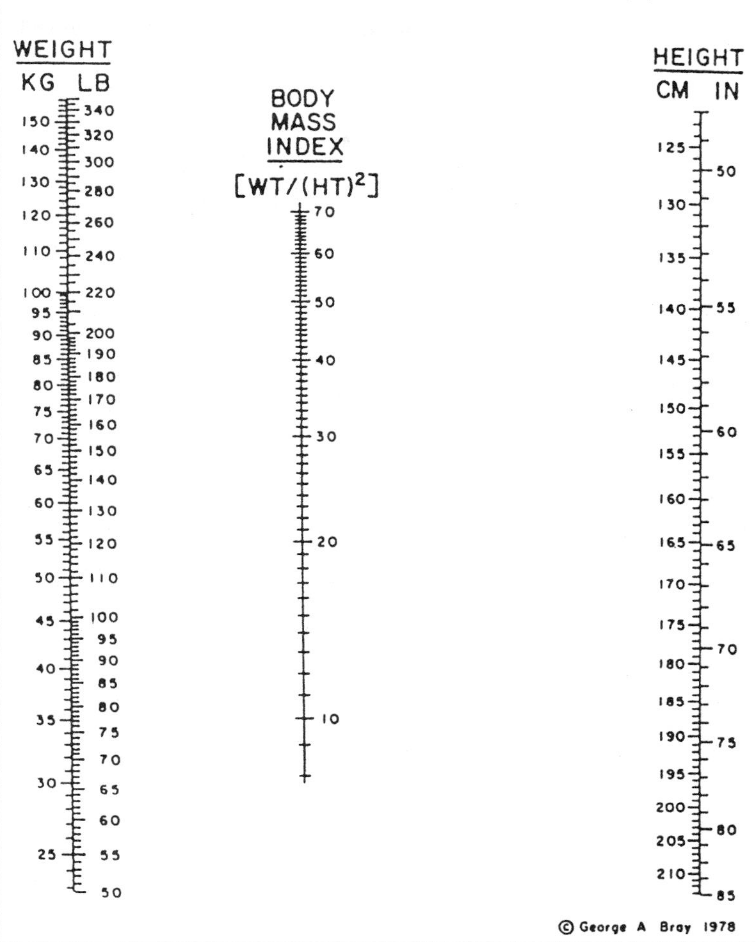

Please place a check by any statement regarding body mass index and recent weight loss that is true for the client.

- ☐ Body mass index <22
- ☐ Body mass index >27
- ☐ Has lost or gained 10 pounds (or more) of body weight in the past 6 months

Record the measurement of midarm circumference to the nearest 0.1 centimeter and of triceps skinfold to the nearest 2 millimeters.

Midarm circumference (cm): ______________

Triceps skinfold (mm): ______________

Midarm muscle circumference (cm): ______________

Refer to the table and check any abnormal values:

- ☐ Midarm muscle circumference <10%
- ☐ Triceps skinfold <10%
- ☐ Triceps skinfold >95%

Note: midarm circumference (cm) - {0.314 × triceps skinfold (mm)} = midarm *muscle* circumference (cm)

For the remaining sections, please place a check by any statements that are true for the client.

Laboratory Data

- ☐ Serum albumin below 3.5 g/dl
- ☐ Serum cholesterol below 160 mg/dl
- ☐ Serum cholesterol above 240 mg/dl

Drug Use

- ☐ Three or more prescription drugs, over-the-counter medications, and/or vitamin and mineral supplements daily

LEVEL II SCREEN

NAME:

DATE:

Fig. 10-2 Level II Screen. (Reprinted with permission from the Nutrition Screening Initiative, a project of the American Academy of Family Physicians, the American Dietetic Association, and the National Council on the Aging, and funded in part by a grant from Ross Products Division, Abbott Laboratories, Inc.)

Continued

Clinical Features

Presence of (check each that applies):

- ☐ Problems with mouth, teeth, or gums
- ☐ Difficulty chewing
- ☐ Difficulty swallowing
- ☐ Angular stomatitis
- ☐ Glossitis
- ☐ History of bone pain
- ☐ History of bone fractures
- ☐ Skin changes (e.g., dry, loose, nonspecific lesions, edema)

Percentile	Men 55-65 y	Men 65-75 y	Women 55-65 y	Women 65-75 y
Arm circumference (cm)				
10th	27.3	26.3	25.7	25.2
50th	31.7	30.7	30.3	29.9
95th	36.9	35.5	38.5	37.3
Arm muscle circumference (cm)				
10th	24.5	23.5	19.6	19.5
50th	27.8	26.8	22.5	22.5
95th	32.0	30.6	28.0	27.9
Triceps skinfold (mm)				
10th	6	6	16	14
50th	11	11	25	24
95th	22	22	38	36

From: Frisancho AR. New norms of upper limb fat and muscle areas for assessment of nutritional status. Am J Clin Nutr 1981; 34:2540-2545. © 1981 American Society for Clinical Nutrition.

Eating Habits

- ☐ Does not have enough food to eat each day
- ☐ Usually eats alone
- ☐ Does not eat anything on one or more days each month
- ☐ Has poor appetite
- ☐ Is on a special diet
- ☐ Eats vegetables two or fewer times daily
- ☐ Drinks milk or eats milk products once or not at all daily
- ☐ Eats fruit or drinks fruit juice once or not at all daily
- ☐ Eats breads, cereals, pasta, rice, or other grains five or fewer times daily
- ☐ Has more than one alcoholic drink per day (if a woman); more than two drinks per day (if a man)

Living Environment

- ☐ Lives on an income of less than $6000 per year (per individual in the household)
- ☐ Lives alone
- ☐ Is housebound
- ☐ Is concerned about home security
- ☐ Lives in a home with inadequate heating or cooling
- ☐ Does not have a stove and/or refrigerator
- ☐ Is unable or prefers not to spend money on food (<$25 to $30 per person spent on food each week)

Functional Status

Usually or always needs assistance with (check each that applies):

- ☐ Bathing
- ☐ Dressing
- ☐ Grooming
- ☐ Toileting
- ☐ Eating
- ☐ Walking or moving about
- ☐ Traveling (outside the home)
- ☐ Preparing food
- ☐ Shopping for food or other necessities

Mental/Cognitive Status

- ☐ Clinical evidence of impairment (e.g., Folstein<26)
- ☐ Clinical evidence of depressive illness (e.g., Beck Depression Inventory>15, Geriatric Depression Scale>5)

Clients in whom you have identified one or more major indicators of poor nutritional status require immediate medical attention; if minor indicators are found, ensure that they are known to a health professional or to the client's own physician. Clients who display risk factors of poor nutritional status should be referred to the appropriate health care or social service professional (e.g., dietitian, nurse, dentist, case manager).

Major Indicators

Significant weight loss over time
Significantly low or high weight-for-height
Significant reduction in serum albumin
Significant changes in functional status
Significant and inappropriate food intake
Significant reduction in midarm circumference
Significant increase or decrease in skinfold
Osteoporosis or osteomalacia
Folate or vitamin B_{12} deficiency

Minor Indicators

Concurrent syndromes
Alcoholism
Cognitive impairment
Chronic renal insufficiency
Multiple concurrent medications
Malabsorption syndromes

Symptoms
Anorexia, nausea, or dysphagia
Early satiety
Change in bowel habits
Fatigue or apathy
Memory loss

Physical signs
Poor oral or dental status
Dehydration
Poorly healing wounds
Loss of subcutaneous fat or muscle mass
Fluid retention

Laboratory tests
Reduced levels of serum albumin, transferrin, prealbumin, or ascorbic acid
Folate, iron, or zinc deficiency
Dehydration-related laboratory phenomena

Risk Factors

Inappropriate food intake
Poverty
Social isolation
Dependency or disability
Acute or chronic diseases or conditions
Chronic medication use
Advanced age

Fig. 10-2, cont'd Level II Screen.

BOX 10-1 Nutritionally At-Risk Clients

- Involuntary loss or gain of 10% or greater of usual body weight within 6 months, *or*
- Loss or gain of 5% of usual body weight in 1 month
- 20% over or under ideal body weight
- Presence of chronic disease or increased metabolic requirements
- Altered diets or diet schedules
- Inadequate nutrient intake for more than 7 days

Data from American Society of Parenteral and Enteral Nutrition, Board of Directors: Standards for nutrition support: hospitalized patients, *NCP* 10:208, 1995.

without compromising the patient's sense of privacy about food intake and diet.

Anthropometrics. Height and weight are the mainstays of anthropometric measurements. Ideally the client is weighed in the morning while wearing light clothing. Height is measured if possible. For clients who are unable to stand without assistance, height can be estimated by measuring the distance from the heel to the top of the knee (knee height) using a broad-bladed caliper. This measure can be used to estimate height using the following formula (*Nutritional assessment of the elderly through anthropometry*, 1988):

Knee Height as an Estimate of Stature

Stature for men $= (2.02 \times \text{knee height in cm}) - (0.04 \times \text{age}) + 64.19$

Stature for women $= (1.83 \times \text{knee height in cm}) - (0.24 \times \text{age}) + 84.88$

In comparing weight and height, the nurse can use instruments such as the Metropolitan Life Insurance Table of Weight for Height as a reference. Surveys of weight changes with age reveal that the young-old are more likely to be overweight, whereas the old-old tend to be underweight (Andres et al, 1985). With age there is a loss of lean body mass and an increase of body fat; therefore body weight alone can be misleading. Older adults should be cautioned against extreme leanness. Andres et al (1985) report an increased mortality risk in lean older adults compared with older adults who have 10% to 15% more body weight. With this information, Andres created a table of heights and weights (Table 10-1).

Recently, measuring body surface area has been recommended to detect those overweight and underweight for their height. Other types of anthropometric measurements include triceps skinfold and midarm muscle circumference. These measurements are of limited value when measured only one time and are also of limited use in their applicability to older adults. The standards for "normal" anthropometric ranges are based on a healthy middle-aged population; however, methods of comparing anthropometric measurements over time for older adults have been published (*Nutritional assessment of the elderly through anthropometry*, 1988). Measurements such as triceps skinfold and midarm muscle circumference may be of value when the initial reading is used as its own standard for a given individual. Measurements over time may reveal changes in fat stores and muscle mass. Standardization in measurement of both these parameters is of importance to ensure accuracy. The midarm muscle circumference should be measured at the midpoint of the distance between the tip of the acromial process of the scapula and the olecranon process of the ulna. Triceps skinfold should be measured with calipers that have a known degree of accuracy. An in-depth discussion of how to perform anthropometric measurements is presented in most nutrition texts (Williams and Schlenker, 2003).

Another fast, noninvasive, and highly accurate method for assessing lean tissue and bone mass is dual-energy x-ray absorptiometry (DXA). These relatively new scanning devices allow the practitioner to evaluate bone density at several sites and to evaluate body fat in a minimum amount of time (generally less than 20 minutes) with minimum radiation exposure (less than 5 mrem) (DXA: Hologic, Inc., Bedford, MA). The disadvantage of DXA scanning is the client must be mobile and able to get to a clinic site to take advantage of the most efficient and advanced equipment.

Laboratory Values. No single laboratory test is diagnostic of malnutrition. Several tests that reflect protein synthesis can also reflect nutritional status. Serum albumin is the serum protein most frequently cited in reference to malnutrition; it reflects the liver's ability to synthesize plasma protein. Albumin has a half-life of about 21 days, so it is not always reflective of current nutritional status. Albumin values can also be affected by immune status and hydration. Given these limitations, albumin levels below 3.5 g/dl may indicate some degree of malnutrition.

Transferrin is a carrier protein for iron and has a shorter half-life of 8 to 10 days. It is a more rapid predictor of protein depletion. Levels below 200 mg/dl may indicate mild-to-moderate depletion. Levels below 100 mg/dl may indicate severe depletion.

Prealbumin is a carrier protein for retinol-binding protein and has a half-life of 2 to 3 days. It is sensitive to sudden demands on protein synthesis and is often used in the acute care setting. Prealbumin levels that range from 15 to 5 mg/dl reflect mild to moderate protein depletion. Levels below 5 mg/dl are considered reflective of severe protein depletion.

Total lymphocyte count (TLC) is sometime used as a nutritional marker. In severe or prolonged malnutrition, immune proteins are depleted and the TLC is decreased.

NUTRITIONAL GUIDELINES FOR ALL AGES

Healthy eating is important for all Americans, regardless of age. Nutritional guidelines have been published by a number of organizations. The Food Guide Pyramid is a well-recognized

TABLE 10-1 A New Weight Table for Older Adults

This age-adjusted weight chart, devised by Johns Hopkins University gerontologist Dr. Reubin Andres, indicates medically sound weight ranges for people in their 50s and 60s. The ideal weight for most people is around the midpoint for each person's age and height. Those in the lower ranges are probably heavy enough to maintain good health, as long as there is no sudden or unexplained weight loss. Weights in the upper ranges may also be acceptable, but if a client finds himself or herself on the high side, he or she should talk with a physician about the possibility of losing weight. A physician makes recommendations based on where the client tends to store fat and his or her general health.

HEIGHT	WEIGHT (lb) AGES 50 TO 59	WEIGHT (lb) AGES 60 TO 69*
4′10″	107-135	115-142
4′11″	111-139	119-147
5′0″	114-142	123-152
5′1″	118-148	127-157
5′2″	122-153	131-163
5′3″	126-158	135-168
5′4″	130-163	140-173
5′5″	134-168	144-179
5′6″	138-174	148-184
5′7″	143-179	153-190
5′8″	147-184	158-196
5′9″	151-190	162-201
5′10″	156-195	167-207
5′11″	160-201	172-213
6′0″	165-207	177-219
6′1″	169-213	182-225
6′2″	174-219	187-232
6′3″	179-225	192-238
6′4″	184-231	197-244

Reprinted with permission from Health after 50, *Johns Hopkins Medical Letter* 7(1):5, 1999.
*Those over age 69 should use the ranges for individuals in their 60s.

tool for assisting Americans to eat a more nutritious and balanced diet (Fig. 10-3). This pyramid has undergone revision and boasts a new design in 2005. The new Food Guide Pyramid points the reader to an interactive website that can be tailored to individual needs (www.MyPyramid.gov). A typical meal plan for 2000 kilocalories based on the Food Guide Pyramid is shown in Fig. 10-3. The U.S. Department of Agriculture (USDA) and the Department of Health and Human Services (HHS) created a list of dietary guidelines for Americans (Box 10-2). They provided recommendations that are consistent with those of other organizations such as the American Heart Association and the American Cancer Society, whose guidelines are intended to reduce the incidence of heart disease and cancer.

Studies have suggested that the typical American diet is deficient in fruit and vegetable intake (USDA/US Department of Health and Human Services [DHHS], 1995). Adequate intake of fruits and vegetables rich in fiber, antioxidants, beta-carotene, and other vitamins is associated with a reduction in the risk of cancer, cardiovascular disease, macular degeneration of the eye, and other diseases (Alpha-Tocopherol, Beta Carotene Cancer Prevention Study Group, 1994; Omenn et al, 1996), yet only 28% of the American population consume the recommended number of fruits per day, and 45% consume the recommended number of vegetables (Consumer Nutrition Research, 2000). Despite growing awareness and early research reports of undernutrition among middle-aged and older adults in the 1980s, a survey from May to August 1992 still found inadequate energy and nutrient intake among a sizable percentage of the 474 surveyed individuals ages 65 to 98 (Ryan, Craig, and Finn, 1992). In 1997 the American Dietetic Association (ADA) published a position statement endorsing liberalized diets for older adults in long-term care settings (ADA, 2002). Noting physical problems that are common for institutionalized older adults, such as poor appetite, infections, weight loss, pressure ulcers, and polypharmacy, the ADA called for a careful evaluation of the risks versus benefits of restrictive diets for adults in long-term care settings. As a result of several pieces of legislation, HCFA defined adequate care for residents of long-term care, which includes writing a standardized assessment tool and delineating a process for incorporating assessments into a care plan for each resident. The document can be used to develop, review, evaluate, and revise care plans for residents (*Minimum Data Set Reference Manual,* 1993). Nutrition interventions may play an important role in addressing the health care problems identified in the minimum data set (MDS) and resident assessment protocols (RAPs) established by HCFA (*Nutrition interventions based on OBRA resident assessment protocols,* 1995). The triggers established in the MDS and RAPs may have a nutritional basis and should be considered as part of the assessment process.

Recommended Dietary Allowances and Dietary Intakes

In 1989 the Food and Nutrition Board of the U.S. National Research Council published the tenth edition of the RDAs for nutrients (Table 10-2). The RDAs list protein, vitamins, minerals, and selected trace elements with their recommended daily intake for infants and children, women and men, and for pregnant and lactating women. Although grouped by age ranges, the U.S. RDAs end at age 51 and over. Because of this limitation, the Canadian RDAs may provide more useful information for the aging (Table 10-3). The Canadian RDAs address fewer nutrients but include recommendations for ages 19 to 24, 25 to 49, 50 to 74, and 75 and older. Some of today's older adults are at risk for malnutrition as a function of a number of factors noted earlier. The Food and Nutrition Board attempts to address the differential in energy requirements and estimated minimum requirements of additional vitamins and minerals for men and women over the age of 50.

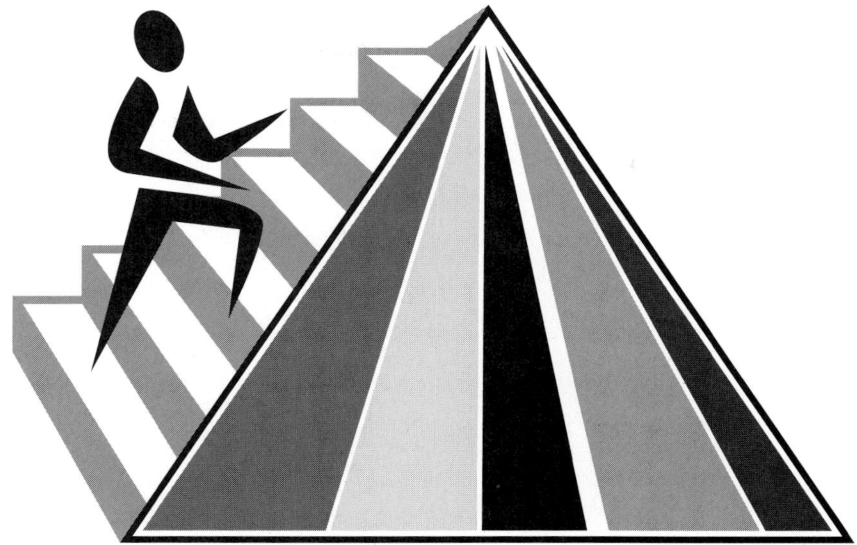

Grains	**Vegetables**	**Fruits**	**Oils, fats**	**Milk products**	**High-protein foods**
At least half should be whole-grain	Fresh, frozen, canned, dried, juices	Fresh, frozen, canned, dried, juices	Liquid, not solid	Low- or no-fat, calcium-rich types	Lean meat, poultry, fish; eggs; beans, nuts, seeds; tofu; peanut butter

MyPyramid.gov

STEPS TO A HEALTHIER YOU

GRAINS Make half your grains whole	VEGETABLES Vary your veggies	FRUITS Focus on fruits	MILK Get your calcium-rich foods	MEAT & BEANS Go lean with protein
Eat at least 3 oz. of whole-grain cereals, breads, crackers, rice, or pasta every day 1 oz. is about 1 slice of bread, about 1 cup of breakfast cereal, or 1/2 cup of cooked rice, cereal, or pasta	Eat more dark-green veggies like broccoli, spinach, and other dark leafy greens Eat more orange vegetables like carrots and sweet potatoes Eat more dry beans and peas like pinto beans, kidney beans, and lentils	Eat a variety of fruit Choose fresh, frozen, canned, or dried fruit Go easy on fruit juices	Go low-fat or fat-free when you choose milk, yogurt, and other milk products If you don't or can't consume milk, choose lactose-free products or other calcium sources such as fortified foods and beverages	Choose low-fat or lean meats and poultry Bake it, broil it, or grill it Vary your protein routine – choose more fish, beans, peas, nuts, and seeds
For a 2,000-calorie diet, you need the amounts below from each food group. To find the amounts that are right for you, go to MyPyramid.gov.				
Eat 6 oz. every day	Eat 2 1/2 cups every day	Eat 2 cups every day	Get 3 cups every day; for kids aged 2 to 8, it's 2	Eat 5 1/2 oz. every day

Find your balance between food and physical activity

- Be sure to stay within your daily calorie needs
- Be physically active for at least 30 minutes most days of the week.
- About 60 minutes a day of physical activity may be needed to prevent weight gain.
- For sustaining weight loss, at least 60 to 90 minutes a day of physical activity may be required.
- Children and teenagers should be physically active for 60 minutes every day, or most days.

Know the limits on fats, sugars, and salt (sodium)

- Make most of your fat sources from fish, nuts, and vegetable oils.
- Limit solid fats like butter, margarine, shortening, and lard, as well as foods that contain these.
- Check the Nutrition Facts label to keep saturated fats, *trans* fats, and sodium low.
- Choose food and beverages low in added sugars. Added sugars contribute calories with few, if any, nutrients.

Fig. 10-3 The Food Guide Pyramid. (Courtesy the US Department of Agriculture, 2005.)

BOX 10-2 Health Promotion

The Dietary Guidelines for Americans were designed to advise how to make food choices that promote health and prevent disease.

- Eat a variety of foods.
- Maintain healthy weight.
- Choose a diet low in fat, saturated fat, and cholesterol.
- Choose a diet with plenty of vegetables, fruits, and grain products.
- Use sugars only in moderation.
- Use salt and sodium only in moderation.
- If you drink alcoholic beverages, do so in moderation.

From US Department of Agriculture, US Department of Health and Human Services: Nutrition and your health: dietary guidelines for Americans, *USDA, DHHS Home and Garden Bulletin* 232, Washington, DC, 1995, US Government Printing Office.

However, these modifications still do not adequately consider the diversity of the older adult population. A major problem in developing guidelines that more specifically address the aging population is simply a lack of data.

RDAs are being replaced by RDIs, or recommended dietary intakes. RDIs are divided into four levels of intake: estimated requirements, RDAs, adequate intake, and tolerable upper intake limitation RDI. In addition, the RDIs include reference takes for older adults in categories 51 to 70 years and beyond 70 years, adjusting for a major limitation of the RDAs. However, not all nutrients have been evaluated with data available for the RDIs. Those available include calcium, phosphorus, magnesium, fluoride, vitamin D, thiamin, riboflavin, niacin, vitamin B_6, folate, and vitamin B_{12} (*Nutrition, aging and the continuum of care,* 2000).

It is important to keep in mind that recommended guidelines are simply that—guidelines. The RDAs have a built-in standard deviation, plus or minus the peak of the bell curve for outliers in a population category. Therefore each RDA is set to allow plenty of room for each age category given individual variations in need. In the elderly population, individuals are in complex situations, including consuming many types of medications, having a variety of underlying medical conditions, and perhaps taking vitamins and other supplements. It is always advisable to consult a dietitian when considering special dietary needs.

Food Labeling

In 1990 the Nutrition Labeling and Nutrition Act enabled the Food and Drug Administration (FDA) to develop and enforce labeling for the food industry. The label law requires a label to include the amount of protein in grams, the energy as calories, the fat-soluble vitamin content (A, D, E, and K), the water-soluble vitamin content (vitamin C, thiamine, riboflavin, niacin, B_6, folate, and B_{12}), calcium, phosphorus, magnesium, iron, zinc, iodine, and selenium. The label must also specify calories

TABLE 10-2 Recommended Dietary Allowances for Persons Ages 51 and Over (Revised in 1989)

	MEN	WOMEN
Weight*		
kg	77	65
lb	170	143
Height*		
cm	173	160
in	68	63
Protein (g)	63	50
Vitamin A (mg RE)†	1000	800
Vitamin D (mg)‡	5	5
Vitamin E (mg α-TE)§	10	8
Vitamin K (mg)	80	65
Vitamin C (mg)	60	60
Thiamine (mg)	1.2	1.0
Riboflavin (mg)	1.4	1.2
Niacin (mg NE)¶	15	13
Vitamin B_6 (mg)	2.0	1.6
Folate (mg)	200	180
Vitamin B_{12} (mg)	2.0	2.0
Calcium (mg)	800	800
Phosphorus (mg)	800	800
Magnesium (mg)	350	280
Iron (mg)	10	10
Zinc (mg)	15	12
Iodine (mg)	150	150
Selenium (mg)	70	55

*Weights and heights given are actual median values for the U.S. population ages 51 and over as reported by National Health and Nutrition Examination Survey II. These height-to-weight ratios may not be ideal.
†*RE*, retinol equivalents: 1 RE = 1 mcg retinol or 6 mcg beta-carotene.
‡As cholecalciferol: 10 mcg cholecalciferol = 400 IU of vitamin D.
§*α-TE*, α-tocopherol equivalents: 1 mg d-α-tocopherol = 1 α-TE.
¶*NE*, niacin equivalent: 1 NE = 1 mg niacin or 60 mg dietary tryptophan.

based on a serving size and indicate the number of servings. In addition, the label specifies the percentage of a Recommended Dietary Intake that the product provides, which is typically based on 2000 kcal a day.

Although the label law did much to standardize labeling of foods and provided a clearer means of comparing the nutrient content of foods, label claims, such as "low-fat," "lite," or "free" continued to confound consumers. In September 1993 the FDA provided a dictionary that included common labeling claims and standardized the meaning of these terms (Table 10-4).

DRUG-NUTRIENT INTERACTIONS

Medication use is common in older adults. A medication history should include prescription and over-the-counter drugs, herbal therapies, and alternative medicines. The interactions between nutrients and medicines may affect metabolism, absorption, digestion, or excretion of drugs. Table 10-5 lists the

TABLE 10-3 Recommended Nutrient Intakes for Canadians

AGE	GENDER	ENERGY (kcal)	THIAMIN (mg)	RIBOFLAVIN (mg)	NIACIN NE*	N-3 PUFA* (G)	N-6 PUFA* (G)
0-4 months	Both	600	0.3	0.3	4	0.5	3
5-12 months	Both	900	0.4	0.5	7	0.5	3
1 year	Both	1100	0.5	0.6	8	0.6	4
2-3 years	Both	1300	0.6	0.7	9	0.7	4
4-6 years	Both	1800	0.7	0.9	13	1.0	6
7-9 years	M	2200	0.9	1.1	16	1.2	7
	F	1900	0.8	1.0	14	1.0	6
10-12 years	M	2500	1.0	1.3	18	1.4	8
	F	2200	0.9	1.1	16	1.2	7
13-15 years	M	2800	1.1	1.4	20	1.5	9
	F	2200	0.9	1.1	16	1.2	7
16-18 years	M	3200	1.3	1.6	23	1.8	11
	F	2100	0.8	1.1	15	1.2	7
19-24 years	M	3000	1.2	1.5	22	1.6	10
	F	2100	0.8	1.1	15	1.2	7
25-49 years	M	2700	1.1	1.4	19	1.5	9
	F	1900	0.8	1.0	14	1.1	7
50-74 years	M	2300	0.9	1.2	16	1.3	8
	F	1800	0.8†	1.0†	14†	1.1†	7†
75+ years	M	2000	0.8	1.0	14	1.1	7
	F‡	1700	0.8†	1.0†	14†	1.1†	7†

From Scientific Review Committee: *Nutrition recommendations,* Ottawa, 1990, Health and Welfare.
**NE,* niacin equivalents; *PUFA,* polyunsaturated fatty acids.
†Level below which intake should not fall.
‡Assumes moderate physical activity.

interactions between nutrients and drugs that are commonly taken by older adults. As the client's drug profile changes, the nurse must continue to screen for drug-drug or drug-nutrient interactions and consult with a pharmacist as needed.

NURSING DIAGNOSES ASSOCIATED WITH NUTRITIONAL PROBLEMS

Nursing diagnoses are derived from an assessment of the client during a comprehensive health history and physical examination, during a client interview, or while carrying out nursing interventions. The nursing diagnoses subsequently become the basis for the nursing care plan and goals for nursing care. Box 10-3 lists nursing diagnoses associated with a primary nutrition problem and diagnoses that commonly have a nutritional component.

Alterations in nutrition require a care plan that specifically addresses the nutritional problem. Nursing interventions related to nutrition include instruction and counseling regarding a diet that is adequate in a specific nutrient or nutrients, calories, and fluids. Therapeutic diets have been modified to include more or less than the RDA and RDI for a specific nutrient or nutrients and are usually prescribed to manage or treat a chronic disease or illness. Examples of therapeutic diets include those which are restricted in sodium, protein, cholesterol, total calories, or fat. Therapeutic diets may also include modifications in the texture of foods, such as a low-fiber or high-fiber diet, liquid diet, semiliquid diet, or clear liquid diet. Finally, therapeutic diets may include specialized nutrition such as parenteral nutrition, enteral tube feeding, or oral supplements.

Oral supplements are often prescribed for clients who are unable to ingest adequate protein or calories because of early satiety or fatigue during eating. By adding a concentrated liquid oral supplement to the meal plan, the client may improve protein or overall caloric intake. Supplements should be timed so that they do not become a "meal substitute." Most often, supplements are given between meals and at bedtime, but the nurse must carefully assess the impact of the supplement on overall intake. Commercial oral supplements, such as Ensure, Nutren, Osmolite, and Complete Modified, are available at most pharmacies and grocery stores without a prescription. In addition, supplements are available as soups, nutrient bars, and slushes. Commercial products are convenient, but are often more costly than using regular food or dry powder products, such as Carnation Instant Breakfast mixed with whole milk, cream soups, puddings, regular candy bars, ice cream, and powdered fortified milk.

TABLE 10-4 FDA-Approved Definitions of Label Claims

	TERMINOLOGY	DEFINITION
Sugar	Sugar free	Less than 0.5 g per serving (1) No sugars added during processing or packing, including ingredients that contain sugars. (2) Processing does not increase sugar content above the amount naturally present in the ingredients. (3) Compared foods normally contain added sugars.
	No added sugar; without added sugar; no sugar added	
	Reduced sugar	At least 23% less sugar than in compared food
Calories	Calorie free	Fewer than 5 calories per serving
	Low calorie	40 calories or less per serving, if the serving is 30 g or less or 2 tbsp or less; 40 calories or less per 50 g of food
	Reduced or fewer calories	At least 25% fewer calories than in compared food
Fat	Fat free	Less than 0.5 g of fat per serving
	Saturated fat free	Less than 0.5 g of saturated fat per serving, and the level of trans fatty acids does not exceed 1% of total fat
	Low fat	3 g or less per serving and, if the serving is 30 g or less or 2 tbsp or less, per 50 g of the food
	Low saturated fat	1 g or less per serving and not more than 15% of calories from saturated fatty acids
	Reduced or less fat	At least 25% less per serving than compared food
Cholesterol	Cholesterol free	Less than 2 mg of cholesterol and 2 g or less of saturated fat per serving
	Low cholesterol	20 mg or less and 2 g or less of saturated fat per serving and, if the serving is 30 g or less or 2 tbsp or less, per 50 g of the food
	Reduced or less cholesterol	At least 25% less than compared food
Sodium	Sodium free	Less than 5 mg per serving 140 mg or less per serving and, if the serving is 30 g or less or 2 tbsp or less, per 50 g of the food
	Very low sodium	35 mg or less per serving and, if the serving is 30 g or less or 2 tbsp or less, per 50 g of the food
	Reduced or less sodium	At least 25% less per serving than compared food
Fiber	High fiber	5 g or more per serving
	Good source of fiber	2.5 to 4.9 g per serving
	More or added fiber	At least 2.5 g more per serving than compared food

Adapted from Food Labeling Education Information Center, Beltville, Md; and Robert Famighetti, editor: *The world almanac book of facts.* Copyright World Almanac Education Group, New York, 1985.

Dysphagia is a problem that often affects nutritional status and can occur because of a cerebrovascular accident, oral or neck cancer treatment, or neuromuscular and neurologic disorder. Dsyphagia after stroke can be successfully treated with swallowing exercises and retraining. Referral to a speech therapist is indicated for clients who display dysphagia. The nurse can help the client who is not totally dysphagic to ingest thickened liquids and solids; thin liquids are most difficult for clients with dysphagia to swallow. Thickeners can be added to liquids to achieve a consistency that clients can ingest, usually about the consistency of mashed potatoes. Clients with dysphagia must be assisted during meals, and the nurse or caregiver should carefully observe that foods are successfully swallowed instead of being trapped in the mouth. Aspiration of liquids or solids can occur and may lead to aspiration pneumonia. Clients with severe dysphagia require enteral tube feeding.

SPECIALIZED NUTRITIONAL SUPPORT

Specialized nutrition is used when a client is unable to ingest, digest, or absorb nutrients. Common indications for enteral tube feeding include conditions in which a client is unable to swallow foods, such as cerebrovascular accident, myasthenia gravis, amyotrophic lateral sclerosis, and multiple sclerosis. Enteral nutrition is also used when there is obstruction of the upper gastrointestinal tract, as in cancer or severe esophageal stenosis. A feeding tube is placed below the area of obstruction. Feeding tubes can be placed into the stomach or the intestine. The tubes are placed through the nose (nasogastric or nasointestinal), directly into the stomach (gastrostomy, percutaneous endoscopic gastrostomy [PEG], or radiology assisted gastrostomy), or directly into the jejunum (jejunostomy or percutaneous endoscopic jejunostomy). For decompression of the stomach and simultaneous feeding into the intestine, a PEG tube is placed into the stomach and a smaller feeding tube is threaded through the PEG and guided, using endoscopy, into the small intestine. The PEG tube is used for decompression, and the intestinal tube is used for feeding.

Enteral formulas include standard (whole proteins and complex carbohydrates), modified protein (peptides), and elemental (amino acids) formulas. Some enteral formulas have added soluble or insoluble fiber. Disease-specific formulas

TABLE 10-5 Common Drug Interactions That May Affect Older Adults

DRUG CATEGORY AND DRUGS	NUTRIENT INTERACTION OR NUTRITIONAL SIDE EFFECTS
ANTACIDS	
Sodium bicarbonate	Decreased absorption of folate, phosphate, copper, and calcium
Aluminum hydroxide	Decreased absorption of folate, phosphate, copper, and calcium
ANTICOAGULANTS	
Warfarin	Vitamin K antagonist
ANTIBIOTICS/ANTIBACTERIALS	
Amoxicillin	Food reduces absorption
Ampicillin	Food reduces absorption
Amphotericin G	Can affect taste and smell
Gentamicin	Decreased potassium and magnesium
Metronidazole	Antabuse-type reaction can occur with alcohol
Neomycin	Malabsorption of fat, nitrogen, lactose, sucrose, sodium, potassium, and calcium
Penicillin G	Food reduces absorption
Sulfa drugs	Food delays absorption
Tetracycline	Food reduces absorption
ANTICANCER DRUGS	
Methotrexate	Antagonist of folate
Prednisone	Decreased calcium levels
Cisplatin	Decreased magnesium levels
ANTIGOUT AGENTS	
Colchicine	Malabsorption of fat, vitamin B_{12}, lactose, sodium, and potassium
CARDIAC AGENTS (ANTIHYPERTENSIVES, CHOLESTEROL-LOWERING AGENTS, DIURETICS, POTASSIUM REPLACEMENTS)	
Cholestyramine	Malabsorption of fat; fat-soluble vitamins A, D, E, and K; vitamin B_{12}; and iron
Digoxin	Absorption delayed by food
Methyldopa	Malabsorption of vitamin B_{12}, folic acid, and iron
Potassium chloride	Malabsorption of vitamin B_{12}; gastrointestinal distress
Thiazide diuretics	Depletes potassium
H_2-RECEPTOR ANTAGONISTS	
Cimetidine, ranitidine	Decreased vitamin B_{12}
LAXATIVES	
Mineral oil	Fat and fat-soluble vitamin malabsorption
Phenolphthalein	Potassium depletion
Senna	Fat malabsorption; decreased calcium
STEROIDS	
Glucocorticoids	Decreased calcium transport

Adapted from Morrison SG: Feeding the elderly population, *Nurs Clin North Am* 32:791, 1997; Williams SR: *Nutrition and diet therapy,* ed 7, St Louis, 1993, Mosby; Hennessy KA, Orr ME, editors: *Nutrition support nursing core curriculum,* ed 3, Silver Spring, Md, 1996, American Society of Parenteral and Enteral Nutrition.

are also available for use with the dietary treatment of diseases, such as reduced protein for clients receiving renal dialysis, an increased lipid percentage of total calories for clients with diabetes and pulmonary disease, and an increased percentage of branched-chain amino acids for clients with hepatic disease. Specialized enteral formulas are considerably more expensive than standard formulas and should be used only when clearly indicated. Short-term enteral feeding is often used after surgery, traumatic injury, and burns. Transition to an oral diet occurs as soon as is feasible, generally when the client is able to consume about 50% to 75% of nutrient and fluid needs (ASPEN, 1998).

Parenteral nutrition consists of intravenous solution that includes dextrose, amino acids, vitamins, minerals, elec-

BOX 10-3 Nursing Diagnoses Associated With Nutritional Problems

PRIMARY NUTRITIONAL PROBLEM

Altered nutrition: less than body requirements
Altered nutrition: more than body requirements
Altered nutrition: risk for more than body requirements

NUTRITIONAL COMPONENT

Risk for aspiration
Diarrhea
Altered family processes: alcoholism
Fluid volume deficit
Self-care deficit: feeding
Sensory/perceptual alterations: gustatory
Impaired swallowing
Altered tissue perfusion: gastrointestinal

From Kim MJ, McFarland GK, McLane AM: *Pocket guide to nursing diagnoses*, ed 7, St Louis, 1997, Mosby.

trolytes, trace elements, and water. A lipid emulsion is commonly added to produce a total nutrient admixture, but it can be given by separate infusion. The dextrose and lipids provide calories to support metabolic needs, while amino acids are administered to meet daily protein requirements.

Parenteral nutrition is indicated when the gastrointestinal tract cannot be used for enteral feeding or cannot absorb adequate nutrients to maintain health. Diseases and conditions typically associated with the need for parenteral nutrition include severe inflammatory bowel disease, fistula, acute pancreatitis, and massive bowel resection. Research has shown that feeding into the bowel is protective of bowel mucosa and maintains immunity (Kudsk et al, 1996); thus critically ill older adults may receive both parenteral and enteral nutrition.

Parenteral nutrition is administered through a vascular access device, such as a central venous catheter, tunneled catheter, peripherally inserted central catheter, or implanted port. Most parenteral nutrition solutions are hypertonic and must be administered into a large central vein.

Clients receive enteral and parenteral nutrition in various health care settings or at home. Nurses educate home care clients about the use and care of their access devices, administration of the enteral formula or parenteral solution, use of an enteral or intravenous pump, management of common problems associated with specialized feeding, and signs and symptoms of complications. Although specialized nutrition is prescribed to clients of all ages, a large percentage of the clients who receive enteral tube feeding and parenteral nutrition are older adults.

FAILURE TO THRIVE

Failure to thrive is a label originally applied to infants who did not gain weight and grow despite the apparent absence of a physiologic or psychologic pathologic condition. In fact, failure to thrive in infants often does have disease as its source, and failure to perform a comprehensive diagnostic workup on these infants can delay appropriate treatment. Failure to thrive in older adults is similar. It is characterized by refusal to eat, loss of weight and lean body mass, and subsequent malnutrition.

Sarkisian and Lachs (1996) have described commonly impaired domains associated with failure to thrive in older adults, including impaired physical functioning, malnutrition, depression, and cognitive impairment. Each of the domains has contributors; for example, contributors for the malnutrition domain are changes in food preference, dentition problems, and speech or swallowing problems. These investigators suggest that failure to thrive is a complex process involving interactions among the various domains and contributors; it should be approached from a broad perspective.

Physiologic changes associated with aging; mental disorders such as dementia and depression; and medical, social, and economic factors have been cited as causes of failure to thrive in older adults (Marcus and Berry, 1998). Although initial treatment is directed toward correcting the malnutrition through the use of diet, oral supplements, or specialized nutrition as necessary, a thorough diagnostic evaluation is warranted.

SUMMARY

Food has had strong cultural, spiritual, religious, and social connotations, which were recognized by physicians, statesmen, and scholars throughout history. Interest in homeopathic remedies and the pharmaceutical and disease prevention properties of food and nutrients has resurfaced as a major area of research in the past decade.

The older adult population is increasing as a percentage of the total population, and the percentage of older adults will peak around 2030 with the aging of the "baby boom" generation. General perceptions of older adults do not correlate with reality, and differentiation should be made between healthy older adults and older adults with chronic disease.

Malnutrition is detected through nutritional screening and nutritional assessment. Anthropometrics, diet history, and laboratory studies are components of a nutritional assessment. Organizations that provide accreditation of hospitals and home care agencies and the CMS require nutritional screening of all patients receiving clinical services, with referral for a comprehensive assessment if the client is found to be at risk of malnutrition.

Although a number of organizations have published nutrient requirements and ideal weight tables, none of these resources is well researched for the aged. Surveys of eating patterns of older adults have found inadequate energy and nutrient intake. In comparison to recommendations in the Food Guide Pyramid and *Healthy People 2010*, many older

Americans do not consume enough fruits, vegetables, and whole grains.

Specialized nutrition therapies, such as parenteral nutrition and enteral tube feeding, can provide nourishment to clients who are unable to ingest, digest, or absorb nutrients. Although parenteral nutrition is lifesaving, research has shown that nutrients provided via the gastrointestinal tract enhance recovery and improve immune response.

The nurse plays an important role, along with the dietitian, in identifying alterations in nutrition and in developing nursing interventions that restore nutritional adequacy. The nurse collaborates with the physician, dietitian, pharmacist, and other members of the health care team to promote nutritional health of clients.

Key Points

- Appropriate food intake for health maintenance was recognized by Hippocrates (460-377 BC) and other early scholars.
- Explosion of the older population to more than 32 million people calls for the control of lifestyle factors such as adequate nutrition.
- Among middle-aged and older adults, age alone is the poorest predictor of capacities, interests, performance, and health status. Exercise with maintenance of muscle mass is a good predictor of vitality.
- Wellness, as contrasted to health, is an ongoing dynamic process in the state of becoming; it is the prime objective of health promotion and disease prevention.
- Recent literature has determined a correlation between nutrients and chronic disease.
- A balanced dietary intake, using the Food Guide Pyramid and the *Healthy People 2010* guidelines, can promote nutritional health.
- Nurses have the opportunity and responsibility to assess nutritional status and can collaborate with other members of the health care team to formulate a comprehensive and coordinated nutritional care plan.

Critical Thinking Exercises

1. A 67-year-old man with chronic obstructive pulmonary disease has been referred for home health nursing services for medication instruction and respiratory assessment. During the nurse's first visit, the following information is obtained during the nursing history: overweight for height by about 30 pounds, weight loss of 10 pounds over past 2 months, complaints of shortness of breath while eating, and unable to get to the grocery store (relies on a neighbor for assistance). How would this information relate to the development of a nursing care plan?
2. An 81-year-old woman who is 5 foot, 4 inches tall, weighs 152 pounds, and is in generally good health records the following 24-hour intake:

   Breakfast: 1 glass orange juice, 2 slices whole wheat toast, 1 tablespoon butter

   Lunch: ½ cup cottage cheese, 1 bag cheese curls, ½ peanut butter and jelly sandwich, 1 cup tea

   Dinner: 1 cup wheat flakes cereal, ½ cup skim milk

   Snack: 1 candy bar, 1 cup ice cream

   Analyze this client's diet. What conclusions, if any, can be made about her dietary status based on this 24-hour recall?
3. A 71-year-old man is a Seventh Day Adventist and practices vegetarianism. He does not eat fish, but he does eat eggs. His physician has recommended that he ingest more protein. What recommendations can the nurse offer?

Home Care

1. Instruct caregivers and homebound older adults to keep a nutritional log for a defined period to enable the home care nurse to compare it with the Food Guide Pyramid.
2. Instruct caregivers and homebound older adults on nutrients and selected food sources that supply required vitamins and minerals.
3. Be aware that geographic location, culture, and religion play a part in food patterns, preferences, and the meaning of food for homebound older adults.
4. Assess physiologic conditions and psychosocial issues that may place homebound older adults at risk for nutritional deficiencies.
5. Assess homebound older adults' medications for any that may predispose them to nutritional deficiencies.
6. Instruct caregivers and homebound older adults on assistive devices that promote independence in eating (e.g., strong plastic plates and bowls with suction cups or padded utensils). An occupational therapist can evaluate the client and provide assistive devices.
7. Instruct caregivers and homebound older adults on any treatments that provide nutritional support (e.g., enteral nutrition).
8. Ensure that appliances (such as the stove and microwave) are functioning safely. Assess older adults' functional ability to use appliances safely.

REFERENCES

AARP, Administration on Aging: *A profile of older Americans*, Washington, DC, 1994, US Department of Health and Human Services.

Alpha-Tocopherol, Beta Carotene Cancer Prevention Study Group: The effect of vitamin E and beta carotene on the incidence of lung cancer and other cancers in male smokers, *N Engl J Med* 330:1029, 1994.

American Dietetic Association: *Position of the American Dietetic Association: liberalized diets for older adults in long-term care*, Chicago, 2002, The Association.

American Dietetic Association: Position of the American Dietetic Association: cost-effectiveness of medical nutrition therapy, *J Am Diet Assoc* 958891, 1995a.

American Dietetic Association: *Position of the American Dietetic Association: nutrition, aging, and the continuum of care,* Chicago, 1995b, The Association.

American Society for Parenteral and Enteral Nutrition, Board of Directors: *Clinical pathways and algorithms for delivery of parenteral and enteral nutrition support in adults,* Silver Spring, Md, 1998, The Society.

American Society for Parenteral and Enteral Nutrition, Board of Directors: Standards for nutrition support: hospitalized patients, *NCP* 10:208, 1995.

Andres R et al: Impact of age on weight and goals, *Ann Int Med* 103:1030, 1985.

Balon R: Dine-out customers in post-9/11 world value affordable comfort food in family setting, *Nations Restaurant News,* p 26, Sept 16, 2002.

Bower RH: Early enteral administration of a formula (impact supplemented with arginine, nucleotides, and fish oil) in intensive care unit patients: results of a multicenter, prospective, randomized clinical trial, *Crit Care Med* 23:436, 1995.

Comforted but unfattened, *Adweek Western Ed* 52(38):34, 2002.

Cress ME et al: Exercise: effects on physical functional performance in independent older adults, *Gerontol A Biol Sci Med Sci* 54A:M242, 1999.

Dwyer JT: *Screening older Americans' nutritional health: current practices and future responsibilities,* Washington, DC, 1991, Nutrition Screening Initiative.

Health Care Financing Administration: *Outcome and assessment information set: implementation manual,* Washington, DC, 1998, US Department of Health and Human Services.

Joint Commission on Accreditation of Healthcare Organizations: *Comprehensive accreditation manual for home care,* Oakbrook Terrace, Ill, 1998, The Association.

Keithley JK: Geriatrics. In Hennessy KA, Orr ME, editors: *Nutrition support nursing,* ed 3, Silver Spring, Md, 1996, American Society for Parenteral and Enteral Nutrition.

Kudsk KA et al: Randomized trial of isonitrogenous enteral diets following severe trauma: an immune-enhancing diet (IED) reduces septic complications, *Ann Surg* 224:531, 1996.

Marcus EL, Berry EM: Refusal to eat in the older adults, *Nutr Rev* 56:163, 1998.

Mendez C et al: Effects of an immune-enhancing diet in critically ill patients, *J Trauma* 42:933, 1997.

Minimum data set for nursing home resident assessment and care screening form in the minimum data set reference manual, Natick, Mass, 1993, Elliot Press.

Moore MC: *Pocket guide to nutrition and diet therapy,* ed 2, St Louis, Mosby, 1993.

Nutrition, aging and the continuum of care, *J Am Dietetic Assoc* 100:580, 2000.

Nutrition interventions based on OBRA resident assessment protocols, Columbus, Ohio, 1995, Ross Laboratories.

Nutritional assessment of the elderly through anthropometry, Columbus, Ohio, 1988, Ross Laboratories.

Omenn GS et al: Effects of a combination of beta carotene and vitamin A on lung cancer and cardiovascular disease, *N Engl J Med* 334:1150, 1996.

Ponza M, Ohls JC, Millen BE: *Serving elders at risk: the older Americans nutrition programs, national evaluation of the elderly nutrition program,* Washington, DC, 1996, Mathematica Policy Research.

Robinson G, Goldstein M, Levine GM: Impact of nutritional status on DRG length of stay, *JPEN* 11:49, 1987.

Ryan AS, Craig D, Finn SC: Nutrient intakes and dietary patterns of older Americans: a national study, *J Gerontol Med Sci* 47(5):M145, 1992.

Sarkisian CA, Lachs MS: "Failure to thrive" in older adults, *Ann Intern Med* 124:1072, 1996.

Schilling J et al: Clinical outcome of postoperative arginine, omega-3 fatty acids, and nucleotide-enriched enteral feeding: a randomized prospective comparison with standard enteral and low calorie/low fat IV solutions, *J Nutr* 12:423, 1996.

Stadler KM, Teaster PB: As you age ... basics about an aging population, Pub. No. 348-190, Virginia Cooperative Extension, Jan 2002.

Tannahill R: *Food in history,* New York, 1988, Crown Publishers.

US Census Bureau, March 2003. Accessed at website: *www.census.gov/population/* projections/mation/nas/npas.*

US Department of Agriculture, US Department of Health and Human Services: Nutrition and your health: dietary guidelines for Americans, *USDA, DHHS Home and Garden Bulletin* 232, Washington, DC, 1995, US Government Printing Office.

Weinberg AD, Minaker KL: Dehydration: evaluation and management in older adults, *JAMA* 274:1552, 1995.

Williams SR, Schlenker E: *Essentials of nutrition and diet therapy,* ed 8, St. Louis, 2003, Mosby.

Zulkowski K, Albrecht D: How nutrition and aging affect wound healing, *Nursing 2003* 33(8):70, 2003.

11 Sleep and Activity

LYNN FEREBEE, MSN, RN, FNP

Learning Objectives

On completion of this chapter, the reader will be able to:

1. Identify three age-related changes in sleep.
2. Describe the features of insomnia.
3. Discuss four factors influencing sleep in older adults.
4. Discuss two sleep disorders.
5. List four components of a sleep history.
6. Describe three sleep hygiene measures.
7. Describe the effects of lifestyle changes in older adults on sleep and activity.
8. Define basic and instrumental activities of daily living.
9. Discuss the benefits of physical activity for older adults.
10. Identify three characteristics of meaningful activities for older adults with dementia.

Sleep and activity are two universal, dichotomous functions of all human beings. Sleep is a natural, periodically recurring, physiologic state of rest for the body and mind; sleep is a state of inactivity or repose that is required to remain active. Activity includes the things we do while awake, such as personal care, daily tasks, exercise, and recreation. The kind, amount, and intensity of the activities pursued vary widely among individuals according to personal choices, lifestyle, and health status. This chapter considers age-related changes in sleep and activity and the role of the nurse in assisting older individuals to adapt to those changes.

SLEEP AND OLDER ADULTS

Biologic Brain Functions Responsible for Sleep

Regulation of sleep and wakefulness occurs primarily in the hypothalamus, which contains both a sleep center and a wakefulness center. The thalamus, limbic system, and reticular activating system are controlled by the hypothalamus and also influence sleep and wakefulness. The hypothalamus consists of several masses of nuclei, interconnected with other parts of the nervous system, and is located below the thalamus, where it forms the floor and part of the lateral walls of the third ventricle. Sleep is a state of consciousness characterized by the physiologic changes of reduced blood pressure, pulse rate, and respiratory rate along with a decreased response to external stimuli.

Stages of Sleep

Normal sleep is divided into rapid eye movement (REM) sleep and four stages of non-REM sleep (Table 11-1). Approximately 75% to 80% of sleep is non-REM sleep (Foreman and Wykle, 1995). The remaining 20% to 25% of sleep is REM sleep. A night's sleep begins with the four stages of non-REM sleep, continues with a period of REM sleep, and then cycles through non-REM and REM stages of sleep for the rest of the night. Sleep cycles range from 70 to 120 minutes in length, with four to six cycles occurring in a night.

Stage 1 of non-REM sleep is the lightest level of sleep. During stage 1 an individual can be easily awakened. Sleep progressively deepens during stages 2 and 3 until stage 4, the deepest level, is reached. Muscle tone, pulse, blood pressure, and respiratory rate are reduced in stage 4 (Abrams, Beers, and Berkow, 1995). In REM sleep, pulse, blood pressure, and respiratory rate increase. However, there is muscle atonia (Foreman and Wykle, 1995). The REMs of this stage are associated with dreaming. When the amount of REM sleep is reduced, an individual may experience difficulty concentrating, irritability, or anxiety the next day.

Variations in the REM and non-REM sleep stages occur with advancing age. REM sleep is interrupted by more frequent nocturnal awakenings, and the total amount of REM sleep is reduced. The amount of stage 1 sleep is increased. Stage 3 sleep and stage 4 sleep are less deep. In the very old, especially men, the amount of slow wave sleep on electroencephalogram (EEG) is greatly reduced (Kryger et al, 2004).

Sleep and Circadian Rhythm

The sleep-wake cycle follows a circadian rhythm, which is roughly a 24-hour period. The hypothalamus controls many circadian rhythms, which include the release of certain hormones during sleep. Numerous factors can gradually strengthen or weaken the sleep and wake aspect of circadian rhythm, including the perception of time, travel across time zones, light exposure, seasonal changes, living habits, stress,

TABLE 11-1 Normal Stages of Sleep

STAGES	TYPE OF SLEEP	SELECTED CHARACTERISTICS
NON-REM SLEEP (4 STAGES)		
Stage 1	Light sleep	Easily awakened
Stage 2	Medium deep sleep	More relaxed than in stage 1 Slow eye movements Fragmentary dreams Easily awakened
Stage 3	Medium deep sleep	Relaxed muscles Slowed pulse Decreased body temperature Awakened with moderate stimuli
Stage 4	Deep sleep	Restorative sleep Body movement rare Awakened with vigorous stimuli
REM SLEEP		
	Active sleep	Rapid eye movement Increased or fluctuating pulse, blood pressure, and respirations Dreaming occurs

Modified from Ebersole P, Hess P, Luggen, AS: *Toward healthy aging*, ed 6, St Louis, 2004, Mosby.

illness, and medication (Allen, 1994). The decrease in nighttime sleep and the increase in daytime napping that accompanies normal aging may result from changes in the circadian aspect of sleep regulation (Bundlie, 1998).

Insomnia

Insomnia, the inability to sleep, is a complex phenomenon. Reports of insomnia include difficulty falling asleep, difficulty staying asleep, frequent nocturnal awakenings, early morning awakening, and daytime somnolence. Insomnia may be transient, short term, or chronic (Abrams, Beers, and Berkow, 1995). Transient insomnia lasts only a few nights and is related to situational stresses. Short-term insomnia usually lasts less than a month and is related to acute medical or psychologic conditions such as postoperative pain or grief. Chronic insomnia lasts more than a month and is related to age-related changes in sleep, medical or psychologic conditions, or environmental factors. Insomnia may affect the older adult's quality of life with excessive daytime sleepiness, attention and memory problems, depressed mood, nighttime falls, and possible overuse of hypnotic or over-the-counter medications (Kryger et al, 2004).

Age-Related Changes in Sleep

Many older adults experience changes in sleep, which are considered "normal" age-related changes (Box 11-1). However, while some older adults either do not experience these common changes or do not consider them sources of distress, other older adults find these changes problematic (Fichten et al, 1995). The sleep changes experienced by many older adults include increased sleep latency, reduced sleep efficiency, more awakenings in the night, increased early morning awakenings, and increased daytime sleepiness (Bundlie, 1998).

BOX 11-1 Age-Related Changes in Sleep

- Increased sleep latency
- Reduced sleep efficiency
- Increased nocturnal awakenings
- Increased early morning awakenings
- Increased daytime sleepiness

Sleep latency, a delay in the onset of sleep, increases with age. Older adults report that it takes longer to fall asleep at the start of the night and after being awakened during the night. Because the time spent awake in bed trying to fall asleep increases, sleep efficiency decreases. Sleep efficiency is the relative percentage of time in bed spent asleep. For young adults sleep efficiency is approximately 90%. However, this percentage drops to 75% for older adults (Bundlie, 1998).

Nocturnal awakenings contribute to an overall decrease in the average number of hours of sleep. The frequency of nocturnal awakenings increases with age. The interruptions of sleep contribute to the perception that the amount of sleep is inadequate or of poor quality. If the person has little difficulty falling back to sleep, the decrease in the number of hours of sleep may be slight. However, some older adults report increased periods of wakefulness following nocturnal awakening. The reasons for nocturnal awakening include trips to the bathroom, dyspnea, chest pain, arthritis pain, coughing, snoring, leg cramps, and noise (Whitney et al, 1998). Early morning awakening and inability to fall back to sleep may be related to changes in circadian rhythm or to any of the reasons for nocturnal awakening.

Daytime sleepiness is often reported by older adults and may be due to frequent nocturnal awakening or other sleep disturbances. However, in some older adults, daytime sleepiness suggests underlying disease, contributes to the risk of motor vehicle accidents, and, when cognitive dysfunction is present, is a predictor of mortality (Whitney et al, 1998). Daytime sleepiness may also be due to medication side effects.

Daytime napping is common in older adults and does not necessarily indicate problems with nighttime sleep. Naps, voluntary and involuntary episodes of daytime sleep, occur throughout the day. Floyd (1995) found that there was no difference in the length of nighttime sleep between individuals who took naps and individuals who did not take naps, and that the amount of nighttime sleep and the duration of naps were not correlated. Floyd concluded that the time spent napping supplemented the total daily amount of sleep.

Although some of the sleep changes experienced by older adults are related to aging, other sleep changes are associated with chronic disease and other health problems (Foley et al, 1995). When older adults describe the ways their sleep has changed as they have aged, they offer nurses valuable clues. Their descriptions indicate health problems (actual or potential), safety concerns, and possible interventions to improve sleep quality.

Factors Affecting Sleep

Proper sleep is essential for a person's sense of well-being and health. Sleep is often defined subjectively and linked to an individual's feelings on awakening. A good night's sleep is described as one that refreshes, restores, and leaves a person ready for the coming day's activities. Feeling tired and less alert after a poor night's sleep may lead to a less active and productive day. Factors that influence sleep quality in older adults include the following, alone or in combination: environment, pain, lifestyle, dietary influences, medication use, medical conditions, depression, and dementia. Nursing interventions can modify these factors and promote a good night's sleep.

Environment. The environment can positively or negatively influence the quality and amount of sleep persons receive. For older adults, environments conducive to relaxation are likely to be soporific. Such environments include low levels of stimuli, dimmed lights, silence, and comfortable furniture.

Home Environments. The home environment supports a good night's sleep by its very familiarity. The bed and bedding, the people, and the noises are all familiar. The routines leading up to bedtime are natural and individualized.

Hospitals and Long-Term Care Facilities. The environment of a health care institution can detract from the quality of sleep. Not only are these environments unfamiliar, but they typically feature bright lights, noisy people and machines, limited privacy and space, and uncomfortable mattresses. There may be physical discomfort or pain from invasive procedures such as Foley catheterization, intravenous line placement, venipuncture, or mechanical ventilation, or from equipment such as oxygen masks, casts or traction devices, and monitors. The hospital patient or long-term care facility resident is often awakened to receive medications or treatments or to be assessed for changes in vital signs and condition. Nocturnal awakenings for incontinence care or for other care procedures such as repositioning and skin care interrupt the normal sequence of sleep stages (Nagel et al, 2003). Fear of the unexpected or unknown may also keep older adults awake in health care institutions. The quality of sleep in institutional settings improves as nursing interventions address the scheduling of procedures and care activities to avoid unnecessary awakenings; modification of environmental factors to promote a quiet, warm, relaxed sleep setting; and orientation of older adults to the institutional setting.

Noise. Environmental noise potentially interferes with sleep in all health care settings. The consequences of environmental noise can include (1) sleep deprivation, (2) alteration in comfort, (3) pain, and (4) stress or difficulty concentrating, which can interfere with the enjoyment of activities. Sources of noise include personnel, roommates, visitors, equipment, and routine activities on the nursing unit (Box 11-2). Interventions to reduce environmental noise include closing the doors of client and resident rooms when possible, adjusting the volume control on telephones, rescheduling nighttime cleaning routines, and reminding staff and visitors to speak quietly. Some older adults may appreciate headphones to provide relaxing music and block background noise. Headphones will also reduce noise from late evening television watching. Noise reduction may include asking the facility's maintenance staff to clean and lubricate the wheels on all of the unit's utility carts. Reducing environmental noise in institutions involves employees from other departments and visitors as well as nurses.

Lighting. Most individuals are accustomed to sleeping in darkened rooms. The lights in hallways and nurses' stations in some health care institutions interfere with the sleep of clients and residents. The nurse should assess environmental lighting in the institutional setting for glare, brightness, and uneven levels of illumination. Selectively dimming the institution's lights at night may promote better sleep. However, safety concerns must be considered. Nightlights in rooms, bathrooms, and hallways may be a safe compromise—promoting sleep by reducing the glare of bright lights while allowing enough light to see.

Temperature. Falling asleep and staying asleep are difficult when a person is cold. Older adults may wake during the night because of a nighttime reduction in core body temperature related to reduced metabolic rate and reduced muscle activity. Being too warm will also disrupt sleep, but some older adults sleep better if simple measures are used to keep them warm. The ambient temperature of the bedroom should be no lower than 65° F (Worfolk, 1997). Several light

BOX 11-2 Sources of Nighttime Noise in Nursing Facilities

- Talking and calling out by residents
- Talking by staff
- Television
- Intercoms, bells, alarms
- Equipment (e.g., linen carts, floor cleaning equipment)

Modified from Schnelle JF et al: Sleep hygiene in physically dependent nursing home residents: behavioral and environmental intervention implications, *Sleep* 21:515, 1998.

thermal blankets and flannel sheets (both fitted and flat) make for a warmer bed. Flannel pajamas or nightgowns, bed socks, and nightcaps help sleepers stay warm. If bed socks are worn, slippers should be used when out of bed to prevent slipping on uncarpeted floors. To avoid thermal injury to the fragile skin on the feet and lower legs, heating devices such as heating pads or hot water bottles should be avoided.

Pain and Discomfort. Body pain, acute or chronic, interferes with falling asleep and with staying asleep. Nursing interventions to relieve pain begin with assessment of the location, severity, and type of pain, and any aggravating or alleviating factors (see Chapter 15). The effect of the pain on older adults' lifestyles, including sleep quality, should also be assessed. Both nonpharmacologic and pharmacologic measures may be used to relieve pain. When body pain interferes with sleep, analgesics are more effective for sleep promotion than sedative or hypnotic medications. However, the alterations in pharmacokinetics that are common in older adults make the careful selection of analgesics important. Drugs with long half-lives linger longer in many older adults. Small initial doses that may be titrated upward to achieve analgesia may be better tolerated than generous initial doses. Attention must be paid to common side effects such as constipation.

Even when there is no report of body pain, some older adults find just being in bed uncomfortable. For the older individual whose discomfort prevents sleeping in a standard bed, comfortable chairs may be a solution. Reclining chairs with soft cushions may be more comfortable for individuals with chronic congestive heart failure or severe chronic obstructive pulmonary disease (COPD). The rhythmic motion of a rocking chair may comfort some individuals and thus promote sleep. If being out of bed is not feasible, modifying the bed with extra pillows to support painful limbs and promote comfortable body positioning, or using special mattresses (such as air or water mattresses), can be effective. Elbow and heel protectors cushion sensitive joints. Nighttime garments should be made of a soft material such as cotton and should not be restrictive to allow freedom of movement. Blankets should be light to avoid adding weight to sensitive body areas.

Lifestyle Changes

Loss of Spouse. Widowhood is a common life event in the older adult population. For older women, widowhood is much more common than it is for older men. Almost half (47%) of women over the age of 65 are widows, while only 14% of men are widowers (AARP, 1997). Widowhood leaves older adults without "touch partners." Loss of a bed partner can make sleep psychologically less comforting. Older widows and widowers describe the strangeness of going to bed alone after many years of marriage. This change in bedtime routine may interfere with the onset of sleep. If the widow or widower experiences depression, the depression should be treated.

Retirement. Retirement brings about changes in schedule and activities. For decades the older adults' times for going to bed and awakening were influenced by the work schedule; retirement removes that variable. The structure of a day in retirement is not imposed by the demands of a job. The work activities that caused fatigue have ceased. It is no longer necessary to get a good night's sleep to be restored from the day's work and prepared for the next day's efforts. The activities that remain are personal care activities, activities around the house, recreational activities, and any new activities adopted with the coming of retirement. These changes create the potential for alterations in sleep. Some retired older adults may follow the same schedule they observed while working. It is familiar; it feels comfortable. But other retired older adults find their days and nights without structure. In the absence of old routines, sleep is disturbed. Unless other activities replace work activities, retired older adults may not feel fatigued at the end of the day or sleepy at bedtime. Sleep may also be disturbed by the uncertainties that come with retirement. Questions about family relationships, finances, and future activities may lead to sleep-disturbing stress.

Relocation. Some older adults experience relocation as a change of residence from house or apartment to the home of children or siblings, a retirement community, assisted living facility, or nursing facility. Sleep is adversely affected by the transition to these unfamiliar surroundings. Deciding to move from the familiar place of residence to another residence, even if that other residence is desirable and the relocation voluntary, engenders stress during the time of decision making, during the actual move, and during the time of adjustment to the new residence. The unfamiliar environment of the new residence also contributes to disturbed sleep. As older adults become accustomed to a new residence, sleep should improve.

Having a Roommate. Having a roommate (or a bed partner in the case of a spouse) may interfere with sleep. Some sleep-related problems occur in long-term care facilities when roommates do not get along with one another because of different interests or lifestyles. For example, one older adult may watch television to fall asleep, and the other may find this disruptive to sleep. The nursing staff must make every effort to review significant psychosocial interests with residents and to match roommates accordingly. Ideally residents should be allowed to select roommates with whom they share common interests. The roommate or bed partner who snores loudly, sleepwalks, talks in his or her sleep, or has restless leg syndrome is also a cause of sleeplessness. Treatment must be directed toward the cause of the roommate's problem; if treatment is impossible or ineffective, separate bedrooms may be needed.

Dietary Influences. Sleep is influenced by what we eat and drink. Popular caffeine-containing beverages (coffee, tea, cola drinks) make falling asleep more difficult for some older adults. The effects of caffeine include restlessness, nervousness, insomnia, tremors, reduced peripheral vascular resistance, increased heart rate, and relaxation of bronchial smooth muscle.

The standard advice is to avoid caffeine-containing beverages for several hours before going to bed. This diminishes the likelihood that the stimulant effect of caffeine will interfere with falling asleep and staying asleep. Other sources of caffeine include hot chocolate, chocolate candy, some over-the-counter pain analgesics and cold remedies, and some brands of decaffeinated tea and coffee (Cochran, 2003). Some herbal products also contain caffeine (Miller, 1998). Alternative choices for late evening beverages are fruit juices, milk, and water.

Alcohol occupies an equivocal position among beverages that influence sleep. Many adults include alcohol as part of their normal lifestyle and continue to do so in advancing age. They enjoy a glass of wine or sherry with an evening meal or an occasional beer or mixed drink. Small amounts of alcoholic beverages may cause a slight drowsiness or a relaxation that promotes falling asleep. However, larger amounts of alcohol reduce the amount of both REM sleep and deep sleep and impair the overall quality of a night's sleep (Gambert, 1997). The diuresis caused by alcohol-induced inhibition of antidiuretic hormone secretion leads to nocturnal awakenings for urination. When discussing the use of alcohol with older adults, the nurse must determine how they define a "small" or "large" amount of alcohol and the circumstances of alcohol use. These details of alcohol use vary from group to group and from culture to culture (see Chapter 18).

Fluid intake in the evening and immediately before going to bed is associated with nocturia. Although nocturia may have other causes, such as urinary retention related to benign prostatic hypertrophy or diuretic therapy for congestive heart failure, many older adults reduce the kind and volume of fluid intake in the evening. However, it is important that older adults, who as a group are at risk for inadequate fluid intake and dehydration, not reduce the total amount of liquids drunk in 24 hours.

Hunger and thirst can be causes of sleeplessness. Bedtime snacks and small amounts of liquids may provide the touch of comfort that promotes sleep. Warm snacks containing protein are better at bedtime than cold snacks (Cochran, 2003). Milk, eggnog, creamed soup, or flavored gelatin may all be served hot to provide warmth and calories. Pudding, custard, or tapioca may be more palatable than crackers or graham crackers. For older adults with diabetes, bedtime snacks should be included in their diabetic diets. Falling back to sleep after awakening during the night with a dry mouth is facilitated when there is a cup of water close to the bed.

Drugs Influencing Sleep. Both prescription and over-the-counter drugs can contribute to sleep and to sleep disturbance. Drugs affect sleep in three ways: (1) causing sleep by intent, (2) causing drowsiness by side effect, and (3) causing insomnia or other sleep disturbances by side effect.

Drugs Used to Promote Sleep. Medications are often used to treat insomnia, although there are also nonpharmacologic interventions for insomnia. Tranquilizers and sedatives decrease activity and calm the recipient. Sleep may follow the calming effect. Hypnotics produce drowsiness and facilitate the onset and maintenance of sleep by causing central nervous system depression. Hypnotics should be used only for a short course of therapy (3 weeks or less) or for intermittent use in chronic insomnia (once every two or three nights) (Cochran, 2003). Long-term use of hypnotics may lead to tolerance of the drug and rebound insomnia (Marchello, Boczko, and Shelkey, 1995). When selecting a medication to promote sleep, nurses should avoid barbiturates, chloral hydrate, antihistamines, and over-the-counter preparations because of their side effects (Abrams, Beers, and Berkow, 1995).

Benzodiazepines are the most commonly prescribed hypnotics for the older adult because of the safety profile and efficacy of the medications (Cochran, 2003). Benzodiazepines alter both non-REM and REM sleep and increase the total sleep time. When benzodiazepines are used with older adults, the risk of side effects is increased because some benzodiazepines have long half-lives and active metabolites that prolong the sedating effect of the drug (Abrams, Beers, and Berkow, 1995). Age-related changes in the clearance of benzodiazepines increase the risk of prolonged sedation. Complications of benzodiazepine use include daytime drowsiness, increased risk of falls during the night or in the early morning, confusion, and disorientation.

Drugs with Drowsiness as a Side Effect. Many medications, prescription and over-the-counter, have drowsiness as a side effect. While this side effect may be welcomed as a benefit beyond the intended therapeutic purpose of the medication, the use of these medications to induce sleep is problematic. Some of these medications have other side effects that negate the sleep-beneficial effect. Two types of medications will serve as examples: antihistamines and tricyclic antidepressants (Tatro, 1996). While drowsiness is one side effect of antihistamines, the other side effects include increased intraocular pressure; dry mouth; constipation; urinary retention; and, paradoxically, confusion, agitation, restlessness, and insomnia. As another example, tricyclic antidepressants may be slightly sedating but may also cause insomnia and nightmares (see Chapter 22).

Drugs Causing Insomnia or Sleep Disturbances. Several types of medications have insomnia as a side effect or have side effects that lead to disturbed sleep or nocturnal awakening (Table 11-2). Over-the-counter medications that interfere with sleep include nasal decongestants containing amphetamine-like substances, and analgesics containing caffeine. Many prescription medications have side effects that affect sleep.

Natural or Herbal Remedies. Various natural or herbal remedies have been recommended as aids for securing a good night's sleep. Unlike prescription drugs, the composition of

TABLE 11-2 Examples of Medications That Disturb Sleep

TYPE OF SLEEP DISTURBANCE	EXAMPLES OF MEDICATIONS
Alteration of REM sleep	Alcohol, barbiturates, benzodiazepines
Insomnia	Haloperidol, risperidone, phenytoin, sertraline, theophylline, amitriptyline
Delayed onset of sleep	Caffeine, amphetamines, theophylline, nasal decongestants containing stimulants
Nocturnal awakening	Diuretics
Nightmares, vivid dreams	Atenolol, nifedipine, carbidopa-levodopa, propranolol, amitriptyline
Daytime sleepiness	Antipsychotics (haloperidol, risperidone), long-acting benzodiazepines, cold remedies containing antihistamines, atenolol, diltiazem, nifedipine, ranitidine, cimetidine

Compiled from Abrams WB, Beers MH, Berkow R: *The Merck manual of geriatrics,* ed 2, Whitehouse Station, NH, 1995, Merck Research Laboratories; Foreman MD, Wykle M: Nursing standard-of-practice protocol: sleep disturbances in elderly patients, *Geriatr Nurs* 16:238, 1995; and Tatro DS, editor: *Nurses drug facts,* St Louis, 1996, Facts & Comparisons.

BOX 11-3 Tips for Older Adults Using Herbal and Homeopathic Remedies

1. Before treating any symptom with a nonprescription product, make sure there are no conditions that require medical attention.
2. Discuss the use of any nonprescription product with your physician and other health care providers.
3. Be cautious about viewing herbal or homeopathic products as a substitute for prescribed medications.
4. Use single-ingredient products rather than combinations.
5. Observe for beneficial and harmful effects.
6. Report any possible side effects to your physician for evaluation.
7. Seek information from objective sources, rather than relying on promotional materials and package information.
8. Check any warnings on the label or package, and check for information from additional sources.
9. Consider the fact that herbal and homeopathic products are not required to meet standards for safety and efficacy.
10. Be skeptical about exaggerated claims—if it sounds too good to be true, it probably is!

From Miller CA et al: Alternative healing products, *Geriatr Nurs* 17(3):145, 1996.

these compounds is not readily available, and their side effects and interactions with prescription or over-the-counter drugs have not been fully explored (Box 11-3). However, because some herbal remedies contain active ingredients that resemble prescription and over-the counter drugs, some risk for drug-drug interaction exists (Cochran, 2003).

Depression. Depression among older adults is a treatable condition that is frequently accompanied by insomnia. Clients awaken in the early morning and are unable to return to sleep. Clients may also report excessive daytime somnolence. Evaluation and treatment are essential once depression is suspected (see Chapter 14).

Dementia and Disturbed Sleep. Older adults with Alzheimer's disease or other dementias may experience disturbed sleep. Increased confusion at night, nocturnal wandering, and agitation have been reported.

The causes of the sleep disruption may be no different from causes that disturb sleep in any older adult. However, the cognitive impairment complicates assessment, intervention, and evaluation. The nurse may not receive a clear response when asking about sleep or any conditions that contribute to insomnia. Instead nurses must anticipate the needs of older adults with dementia. Interventions include reducing confusion with an explanation of what is expected of the older adult ("Now it's time to sleep"), identification of the place for sleeping ("This is your bed"), and reassurance that going to bed is the right thing to do ("Your bed is ready for you"). Assisting older adults with dementia to perform bedtime routines redirects their behavior. Nocturnal wandering behaviors may signal a need that cannot be expressed verbally, such as hunger or a need for toileting (Coltharp, Richie, and Kaas, 1996). Wandering may also be an expression of pain or of a need for exercise. Once the meaning of the wandering is discerned, appropriate interventions follow naturally. Medications such as sedatives or antipsychotics should be avoided as much as possible because of their side effects, which may worsen confusion, interfere with safe ambulation, and alter the sleep-wake cycle.

Sleep Disorders and Conditions

The two most common sleep disorders experienced by older adults are sleep apnea and periodic limb movements in sleep (PLMS). Both disorders are seen with excessive daytime sleepiness and reports of insomnia. However, PLMS is essentially a benign condition, while the hypoxia related to sleep apnea may lead to serious consequences.

Sleep Apnea. During sleep, individuals with sleep apnea experience recurrent episodes of cessation of respiration. These apneic episodes may last from 10 seconds to 2 minutes. The number of apneic episodes may range from 10 to more than 100 per hour of sleep (Ancoli-Israel, 1997). The incidence of sleep apnea increases with age, and it is more common in men than in women. Conditions linked to sleep apnea include sudden death during the night, cardiac arrhythmias, angina, myocardial infarction, hypertension, stroke, renal dysfunction, impotence, depression, and cognitive impairment.

There are two major types of sleep apnea: central and obstructive. In central sleep apnea there is a cessation of respiratory efforts, both diaphragmatic and intercostal. Central sleep apnea usually is seen with insomnia, mild or intermittent snoring, and depression. The causative mechanisms underlying central sleep apnea include decreased responsiveness to central chemoreceptors (as in COPD or pickwickian syndrome), increased responsiveness of chemoreceptors (as at a high altitude), and delayed transit of information (as in stroke or heart failure) (Ancoli-Israel, 1997). The usual treatment for central sleep apnea is medication.

Obstructive sleep apnea is more common in older adults than central sleep apnea (Abrams, Beers, and Berkow, 1995). In obstructive sleep apnea, air flow ceases because of airway obstruction, while respiratory efforts continue. Factors associated with obstructive sleep apnea include obesity, short neck or neck circumference of less than 43 cm, jaw deformities, large tonsils, large tongue or uvula, narrow airway, and deviated septum (Olson et al, 2003). Older adults with obstructive sleep apnea report excessive daytime sleepiness, awakening with a headache, and awakening confused. The families of older adults with obstructive sleep apnea describe loud snoring and choking or gasping sounds during the person's sleep. Treatment includes weight loss, body positioning during sleep to prevent lying supine, and continuous positive airway pressure (CPAP) (see Research box and Nursing Care Plan).

Periodic Limb Movement in Sleep. Approximately 45% of older adults experience PLMS (Kryger et al, 2004). In PLMS there are repetitive kicking leg movements throughout the night. The kicking movements may occur every 20 to 40 seconds, and each kick causes a brief disruption of sleep. Some older adults are unaware of their leg movements; others wake up and have difficulty falling back asleep. Older adults with PLMS report insomnia and excessive daytime sleepiness. Their bed partners report being kicked during the night. Medications such as carbidopa-levadopa (Sinemet), pramipexole hydrochloride (Mirapex), pergolide mesylate (Permax), ropinirole hydrochloride (Requip), and gabapentin (Neurontin) are commonly prescribed. If the movements are frequent, the nurse may suggest that older adults sleep alone to allow their bed partners less disturbed nights' sleep (Ancoli-Israel, 2004).

Getting a Good Night's Sleep

Whether sleep is disturbed by the environment, diet, medications, lifestyle changes, or sleep disorders, the first step in developing interventions to improve the amount and quality of sleep is a thorough sleep history. Supplementing the sleep history are measurement tools to assess sleep quality and quantity, direct observation of the older adult during sleep, a sleep diary, and diagnostic studies such as EEG monitoring and sleep study evaluation. After assessment, interventions to improve sleep usually begin with basic sleep hygiene measures.

Research

PURPOSE

The purpose of this literature review was to obtain information about heart failure patients with sleep-disordered breathing. The target population of the literature review was primary care providers.

METHODS

A literature review was conducted of scientific literature, classic studies, and Internet sources over the past 10 years.

FINDINGS

Obstructive sleep apnea and central sleep apnea are prevalent and harmful to heart failure patients and may affect prognosis if not treated. The severity of apnea ranged from mild to severe hypoxia. Sleep apnea is not typically screened in heart failure patients.

IMPLICATIONS

Heart failure patients should be screened and treated for sleep apnea to improve their quality of life and prognosis.

Spieker ED, Motzer SA: Sleep-disorder in patients with heart failure: pathophysiology, assessment and management, *J Am Acad Nurse Pract* 15(11):487, 2003.

Components of the Sleep History. A complete sleep history begins with the client's self-report of his or her sleep pattern and sleep-related problems (Box 11-4). The quality of sleep is usually described along a continuum of poor, fair, good, or excellent. The quantity of sleep refers to the amount of sleep in a 24-hour period, including daytime naps. Quantity may be difficult to calculate, especially in the client with frequent nocturnal awakenings who cannot recall if sleep occurred after the awakening. The nurse should determine when the client retires for bed, falls asleep, and usually awakens. The number of nocturnal awakenings and length of time awake at night are important to review with the client. If a client retires at 9 PM, does not fall asleep until 11 PM, arises at 4 AM, and takes a daytime nap from 4 to 5 PM daily, then this individual has slept a total of 6 hours. Information about a person's typical bedtime rituals or practices should also be obtained.

The older adult is likely to seek additional help in achieving satisfaction with sleeping habits. If the older adult is too tired or fatigued to perform normal activities, then the sleep

Nursing Care Plan
Sleep Pattern Disturbance

Clinical Situation: Mr. B is a 78-year-old single white man who is admitted to the nursing facility for convalescence following a tracheotomy for obstructive sleep apnea. Before hospitalization, he was living alone on the third floor of an apartment complex for older adults. He describes himself as limited in activities such as driving, traveling, and cooking because of respiratory distress. He reports daytime fatigue associated with grooming, dressing, feeding, and toileting. He admits to sleeping poorly, with several nighttime awakenings and general fatigue all day long, which prompts him to take a daytime nap.

Medical history includes hypertension, obesity, COPD, severe peripheral vascular disease with a stage II venous stasis ulcer of the lower leg, and recent tracheotomy for obstructive sleep apnea.

While at the nursing facility, Mr. B tells you that he plans on discharging himself home in 1 to 2 weeks. He is observed to need assistance in mobility and uses a wheelchair to wheel himself around his room. He refuses to go to the dining room but requests to have a refrigerator in his room. He eats all his meals in his room and rarely socializes with any resident or staff member. His pastimes include playing solitaire in his room and watching television. He is a retired salesman, having worked in the business for more than 40 years.

Nursing Diagnosis

Sleep pattern disturbance related to obesity and reduced activity level

Outcomes

Client will identify personal lifestyle habits contributing to sleep pattern disturbance.
Client will achieve weight loss of 1 lb per week.
Client will eat a well-balanced diet, as evidenced by food diary.
Client will participate in one group activity a day.
Client will walk 100 feet twice daily, increasing distance to tolerance.
Client will report increased length of uninterrupted periods of sleep.

Interventions

Teach relationship between weight and sleep pattern, and importance of losing weight to improve sleep pattern.
Explore motivators with client to lose weight; reinforce as needed.
Teach about the Food Guide Pyramid, and assist him in identifying nutritious foods.
Teach use of food diary for self-monitoring.
Offer nutritious foods as snacks.
Encourage client to increase level of activity on the unit by increasing mobility and engaging in nonsedentary activities; review list of available activities with client. Offer to accompany client on a walk on the unit to his tolerance at least twice a day to help with wound healing and weight reduction.
Introduce client to fellow residents on the unit who share common interests.
Encourage client to join other residents in activities to tolerance.
Explore with client his likes or dislikes, previous hobbies, and level of activity during middle adulthood.
Schedule an activity with the client that will be part of his daily routine.
Discourage daytime napping; instead, replace it with a stimulating activity.
Teach client to monitor pulse, to watch for symptoms of respiratory distress when engaging in activities on the unit, and to stop if respiratory distress occurs or increase in heart rate causes adverse symptoms.
Offer praise and positive reinforcement when he performs a nonsedentary activity and when weight loss is achieved.
Observe client during sleep for signs of obstructive apnea such as loud snoring or periods of apnea. Observe for daytime fatigue and somnolence.
Encourage client to assume a side-lying position for sleep.
Discuss with client plans for discharge, and explore alternative living arrangements, which can include residence on a first-floor apartment, especially if mobility is impaired.

problem may be viewed as disruptive to the daily routine and may require further evaluation. The nurse should ascertain if the older adult experiences daytime sleepiness or has a strong desire to nap.

A client's activities before bedtime and his or her exercise and activity pattern provide additional information about sleep habits. In general, strenuous activity should be avoided at least 2 hours before bedtime. The nurse should identify what the client does to relax before bedtime, such as reading or drinking a warm beverage. The nurse should question the client having difficulty with sleep about the consumption of alcohol, caffeinated beverages, sedative-hypnotics, over-the-counter medications, and other practices before bedtime.

Questions about the type of bed in which the person sleeps are also important. Does the client sleep in the same bed every night? Is it comfortable? Is the mattress soft or unsupportive? Some individuals who are unable to sleep in a recumbent position because of medical problems may be able to sleep in a semirecumbent position in a lounge chair or recliner. Clients who are unable to fall asleep supine and who need several pillows or cushions in bed require further medical evaluation for heart failure, pulmonary disease, or

BOX 11-4 Sleep History Components

- Sleep quality
  —The self-report of the older adult, described as poor, fair, good, or excellent
- Sleep quantity
  —The number of hours asleep per 24 hours, including daytime naps
- Bedtime routines
- Place of sleep
- Characteristics of the bed, bedding, and bedroom environment
- Food and fluid intake in the evening and at bedtime
- Use of alcohol and caffeine-containing beverages
- Medications (prescription and nonprescription)
- Characteristics of the sleep disturbance
  – Difficulty falling asleep
  – Difficulty staying asleep
  – Frequent nocturnal awakenings
  – Early morning awakening
  – Daytime sleepiness
- The older adult's account of the reasons for the disturbed sleep

musculoskeletal problems. Common problems that cause pain and discomfort in bed include COPD; rheumatologic problems such as osteoporosis; degenerative joint disease of the spine, hips, or neck; and rheumatoid arthritis. Nocturia occurring several times in the course of one night must be further evaluated. Older men with prostatic enlargement need to urinate several times during the night. Older adults with congestive heart failure or urinary tract infections may also have nocturia.

Further Assessment of Sleep. A sleep diary kept by the older adult is helpful in recalling the amount of sleep, bedtime routines, and possible symptoms of disturbed sleep over a 24-hour period. The type and quantity of activities are also noted in the diary for the same 24-hour period. To complete the sleep diary, the older adult may need the assistance of a family member or the nurse. The nurse can suggest measures such as tape recording entries to help clients with visual impairment or difficulty writing to enter information in the diary.

Sleep laboratories specialize in treating clients with primary sleep disorders. Clients are asked to spend the night so that a sleep study can be administered. This often includes a polysomnogram, which provides data about the stages of sleep and ventilation, and an EEG for graphic tracing of the variations in the brain's electric force. Physicians specially trained in sleep disorders evaluate the history and objective findings, including a review of basic sleep hygienic measures, to arrive at a diagnosis and treatment plan.

Additional information about sleep may be collected using questionnaires for research purposes, as well as for clinical evaluation. Two examples of instruments are the Stanford Sleepiness Scale (SSS) and the Epworth Sleepiness Scale (ESS). The SSS measures feelings of sleepiness or tiredness at specific times. The ESS also measures sleepiness, but it measures in terms of sleep propensity, the likelihood of falling asleep at a particular time. The person completing the ESS considers certain situations and indicates the likelihood (low to high) that he or she would fall asleep in those situations (Cochran, 2003). A third instrument is the Pittsburgh Sleep Quality Index, which subjectively measures sleep quality and includes five additional questions for the bed partner. In addition to instruments that only address sleep, questions about sleep may be included in other instruments (Cohen, 1997).

Sleep Hygiene. Basic sleep hygiene includes those activities that foster normal sleep and that can be practiced by individuals on a routine basis. The goal of sleep hygiene measures is to achieve normal sleep. The various measures reinforce habits, routines, and attitudes that promote sleep and advocate changes in habits and routines that do not contribute to a good night's sleep (Hohagen, 1996). Sleep hygiene measures emphasize stable schedules and bedtime routines, a sleep-friendly environment, avoidance of any substances that would interfere with sleep, regular exercise (but not immediately before trying to sleep), and stress reduction.

Retiring at the same time every night and awakening at the same time every morning help establish a routine. A client can condition himself or herself to such a routine over time. Likewise, limiting the amount of time spent in bed to only the time spent sleeping establishes a routine for sleep. Retiring in the same location, such as the bedroom and not a couch or chair on some nights, also helps solidify the routine. If unable to fall asleep, the person should get up and move to another area to perform other activities until sleepy. Eliminating noise and creating a darkened environment promotes sleep. Limit day time napping. Have warm beverages and light nutritious snacks at bedtime.

Avoiding caffeinated beverages, sleeping pills, and alcohol can reduce the chances of sleep-related breathing disorders. The basic measures to help reduce episodes of sleep apnea include losing weight, sleeping on one's side or stomach, avoiding central nervous system depressants such as sedative-hypnotics and alcohol, and treating any obvious nasal or upper airway diseases.

Fostering Normal Sleep among Homebound Older Adults. It is important for the nurse to assess risk factors (e.g., environment, pain, or equipment such as a Foley catheter) that would predispose homebound older adults to sleep disturbances. Review all medications to identify those which may interfere with homebound older adults' sleep patterns. Instruct caregivers and homebound older adults on activities that would foster normal sleep, such as the avoidance of caffeinated beverages and alcohol. Assist caregivers and homebound older adults with environmental changes that would foster normal sleep, such as using a rocking chair or taking a warm bath. Remember that worry and anxiety concerning safety and welfare can be an obstacle to sleep. A system of notification and monitoring to link older adults living alone with the outside world is important to a sense of security.

Other Therapies to Promote Sleep. In addition to sleep hygiene measures, other nonpharmacologic interventions may be used to promote sleep. Among these measures are relaxation therapies, stimulus control therapy, and sleep restriction therapy. Relaxation therapies reduce either somatic arousal or cognitive arousal. Progressive muscle relaxation is one example of a therapy to reduce somatic arousal. Cognitive arousal is reduced by attention-focusing therapies such as guided imagery or meditation. Stimulus control therapy attempts to reestablish the bedroom environment as the stimulus for sleep by banning activities not related to a good night's sleep from the bedroom. Examples of such activities include eating and watching television. Stimulus control therapy is helpful for individuals with sleep-onset insomnia (Cochran, 2003). Sleep restriction therapy limits the amount of time spent in bed. Individuals stay in bed only for the number of hours they estimate as their average time asleep, plus 15 minutes (Ancoli-Israel, 1997). These measures may be combined with basic sleep hygiene to improve sleep.

The assessment of sleep for older adults should include questions about sleep habits, bedtime routines and rituals, medications, diet, and the sleep environment. Physiologic factors such as pain, sleep disorders, and other health problems that might affect sleep should be included in the assessment (Foreman and Wykle, 1995). The nursing interventions that follow the assessment include educating clients about normal age-related changes in sleep; basic sleep hygiene measures; and strategies to improve sleep that are specific to the client's health status, lifestyle, and environment. Evaluation of the effectiveness of the intervention depends on the older adult's report of sleep quantity and quality (Table 11-3).

ACTIVITY AND OLDER ADULTS

Activity, as discussed in this chapter, includes routine daily activities, diversional activities, and physical exercise. Changes occur in the activities pursued by older adults as they age or experience acute or chronic illness. Other changes in activities occur in response to major lifestyle changes such as retirement, relocation, or loss of a spouse. There is also the case of specialized activities to meet the needs of older adults with Alzheimer's disease or a related dementia. Whether cared for at home or in a long-term care facility, the older

TABLE 11-3 Nursing Standard of Practice Protocol: Sleep Disturbance in Older Adult Clients

ASSESSMENT	INTERVENTION	EVALUATION
SLEEP-WAKE PATTERNS Inquire about usual times for retiring, falling asleep, and rising; frequency and duration of nighttime awakenings; frequency and duration of daytime naps; daytime physical and social activity. Have person provide a subjective evaluation of the quality of sleep.	**MAINTAIN NORMAL SLEEP PATTERN** Maintain usual bedtime. Schedule nighttime activities to provide uninterrupted periods of sleep of at least 2-3 hours. Balance daytime activity and rest. Discourage daytime naps. Promote social interaction.	**OBJECTIVE EVIDENCE** Time required to fall asleep: should fall asleep within 30-45 minutes Time for awakening: at usual reported time Behavior, alertness, attention, ability to concentrate, reaction time Observe duration of sleep: should remain asleep for at least 4-hour intervals
BEDTIME ROUTINES/RITUALS Inquire about activities performed before bedtime (e.g., personal hygiene, prayer, reading, watching TV, listening to music, snacks). **MEDICATIONS** Obtain information relative to all prescribed and self-selected over-the-counter medications used by person, especially sleep-aids, diuretics, laxatives. Determine types of medications and length of time used by person.	**SUPPORT BEDTIME RITUALS/ROUTINES** Offer a bedtime snack or beverage. Enable bedtime reading or listening to music. Assist with aspects of personal hygiene at bedtime (e.g., a bath). Encourage prayer or meditation. **AVOID OR MINIMIZE DRUGS THAT NEGATIVELY INFLUENCE SLEEP** Pharmacologic treatment of sleep disturbances is treatment of last resort. Discontinue or adjust dose or dosing schedule of any offending medications. Consider drug-drug potentiation. Administer medications to promote sleep; give diuretics at least 4 hours before bedtime.	**SUBJECTIVE EVIDENCE** Verbalizations about the quality and quantity of sleep (e.g., statements of difficulty falling asleep, frequent awakenings; having slept well, feeling well-rested/refreshed; or an increased sense of well-being)

TABLE 11-3 Nursing Standard of Practice Protocol: Sleep Disturbance in Older Adult Clients—cont'd

ASSESSMENT	INTERVENTION	EVALUATION
DIET EFFECTS Obtain information about consumption of caffeinated and alcoholic beverages.	**MINIMIZE OR AVOID FOODS THAT NEGATIVELY INFLUENCE SLEEP** Discourage use of beverages containing stimulants (e.g., coffee, tea, sodas) in afternoon and evening. Encourage use of warm milk. Provide snacks according to client preference. Generally discourage use of alcoholic beverages. Decrease fluid intake 2-4 hours before bedtime.	
ENVIRONMENTAL FACTORS Evaluate noise, light, temperature, ventilation, bedding.	**CREATE OPTIMAL ENVIRONMENT FOR SLEEP** Keep noise to absolute minimum. Set room temperature according to client preference. Provide blankets as requested. Use nightlight as desired. Provide soft music or white noise to mask noise of hospital activity.	
PHYSIOLOGIC FACTORS Evaluate breathing pattern during sleep, with attention to pauses. Observe for periodic movement or jerking during sleep. Inquire about usual position and number of pillows used during sleep. Note diagnoses of sleep disorders (e.g., sleep apnea, narcolepsy). Note diagnoses of specific health problems that adversely affect sleep (e.g., congestive heart failure).	**PROMOTE PHYSIOLOGIC STABILITY** Elevate head of bed as required. Provide extra pillows per client preference. Administer bronchodilators, if prescribed, before bedtime. Use medical therapeutics (e.g., CPAP machine) as prescribed.	
ILLNESS FACTORS Inquire about pain, affective disturbances (e.g., depression, anxiety, worry), fatigue, and discomfort.	**PROMOTE COMFORT** Provide analgesia as needed 30 minutes before bedtime. Massage back or feet to help client relax. Use warm and cool compresses on painful areas as indicated. Assist with progressive relaxation or guided imagery. Encourage client to urinate before going to bed. Keep path to bathroom clear, or provide bedside commode.	

Bibliography for the development of protocol from Jenike MA: *Geriatric psychiatry and psychopharmacology: a clinical approach*, St Louis, 1989, Mosby; Johnson JE: Bedtime routines: do they influence the sleep of elderly women? *J Appl Gerontol* 7:97, 1988; National Institutes of Health: Treatment of sleep disorders of older people, *Consensus Statement* 8(3):1, 1990.
From Foreman MD, Wykle M: Nursing standard-of-practice protocol: sleep disturbances in elderly patients, *Geriatr Nurs* 16:238, 1995.

adult with dementia benefits from an activity program that includes both diversional activities and activities to promote independence in activities of daily living (ADLs). Physical exercise deserves special attention because of its health-promoting benefits for all older adults. Although the activities pursued by a particular older adult are influenced by his or her preferences, situation, and health, there are some general considerations for activity and older adults. In some settings nurses participate in planning activities, adapting activities to the older adult's current situation, and evaluating the effects of activities on health.

Activities of Daily Living

ADLs include the things that most adults do every day, often without special attention or effort (see Chapter 1 for more discussion on ADLs and IADLS). Until something happens to interfere with normal daily routines, little thought may be given to bathing, dressing, eating, or attending to elimination needs. But with advancing years, and with changes in health and circumstances, activities that once were accomplished with ease may require modified approaches or the assistance of others. In addition to providing direct assistance with

ADLs, nurses assist older adults in the modification of routines and the use of assistive devices that help maintain independence. Nurses also support and advise family members and friends who assist the older adult with ADLs.

Instrumental activities of daily living (IADLs) include activities such as driving, shopping, cooking, housekeeping, and using a telephone. Older adults modify their approaches to IADLs because of commonly experienced changes in aging, such as reduced strength, impaired vision, or impaired hearing. Assistive devices make the tasks of cooking or housekeeping easier and safer. Driving may be restricted to familiar areas and daylight hours. Family members, friends, or paid caregivers may help with shopping and other tasks. During episodes of acute illness or recovery from hospitalization, additional help may be needed. However, if sufficient assistance with IADLs is available in the home, relocation to a long-term care facility is not required.

Basic ADLs include the everyday personal care tasks related to hygiene, nutrition, and elimination. Remaining independent in these activities is highly prized by older adults. Dependency in basic ADLs increases the risk of relocation to a long-term care facility or to the home of a family member. To remain independent in basic ADLs, older adults use assistive devices and modify their care routines. Handheld shower sprays, raised toilet seats, sturdy grab bars in bathrooms, plate guards, and built-up handles on toothbrushes and eating utensils are examples of assistive devices. Clothing with Velcro instead of buttons, ties that clip on rather than tie, and shoes that slip on rather than lace are examples of modifications to help with dressing. However, for some older adults the amount of assistance needed with personal care exceeds their ability to modify routines and the capacity of family members and friends to help. Home care nurses may supplement the care provided by family members and friends, or relocation to a long-term care facility may be necessary.

Physical Exercise

Physical activity is important for older adults to maintain health, preserve the ability to perform ADLs, and improve the general quality of life. The benefits of physical activity include prevention of heart disease, reduction of elevated blood pressure, reduced risk of osteoporosis, promotion of appropriate weight, and promotion of more restful sleep (Jones and Jones, 1997). Exercise may also improve hyperlipidemia and glucose tolerance (Gunnarsson and Judge, 1997). Exercise preserves mobility by promoting muscle strength and joint flexibility, and it reduces the risk of falling by increasing agility.

Older adults exercise for a variety of reasons (Jones and Jones, 1997). They exercise to have fun, to socialize with friends and neighbors, and to simply feel better. Exercise is used to reduce stress, to promote relaxation, and, together with a good nutritional program, to control weight. Jones and Jones (1997) recommend walking and suggest 30 minutes or more of moderate-intensity physical activity every day. The 30 minutes may be divided into smaller segments. To measure the appropriate intensity while walking for exercise, they describe the "talk test": the person exercising should be able to carry on a conversation while walking. Breathing may be slightly labored, but a conversation should still be possible. The walker should not be out of breath.

If the older adult has not been exercising every day, starting with only 5 minutes of exercise each day and gradually working up to 20 or 30 minutes a day is appropriate (Butler et al, 1998). Gunnarsson and Judge (1997) also recommend a gradual progression in an exercise program for older adults who have been sedentary. A sedentary lifestyle is not unusual for older adults. In a study of physical activity and the risk of osteoporosis, 40% of the older women in the sample reported 6 to 8 hours of sitting per day (Gregg et al, 1998). Another 27% reported sitting more than 8 hours per day.

In addition to recommending gradual increases in the amount of exercise time for older adults who have not been exercising regularly, the nurse may pass along other safety tips. Drinking water before and after exercise is important because water will be lost during exercise. Clothing worn for exercise should allow for easy movement and perspiration. Athletic shoes provide both support and protection. Outdoor exercise should be avoided in extremely hot or extremely cold weather. Enclosed shopping malls are sheltered places for walking during the extremes of weather or when there are concerns about neighborhood safety. Exercising with a partner provides both encouragement to continue exercising and safety. Nurses should advise older adults to stop exercising and seek help if they experience chest pain or tightness, shortness of breath, dizziness or lightheadedness, or palpitations during exercise (Gunnarsson and Judge, 1997).

Activity As Affected by Lifestyle Changes

Retirement, relocation, and the loss of a spouse influence older adults' activity levels and the types of activities they pursue. These lifestyle changes are directly experienced by many older adults; others experience them indirectly when a spouse retires or is admitted to a long-term care facility.

Retirement. Retirement represents a major lifestyle change for older adults. During most of their adult lives, older adults have gone to work or watched a spouse go to work each day. With retirement the daily schedule changes. The hours spent on the job and in transit to and from the job are no longer committed. For couples where only the husband has worked, the wife's daily routine is affected by her husband being home. If the wife is still working outside the home when the husband retires, the husband finds himself at home alone. For the unmarried retired person, retirement may be a transition from a companionable work setting to a lonely, empty house. Key issues for the retired older adult are the replacement of work with meaningful activities, and the replacement of work-related friends with new acquaintances.

Activities in retirement may be chosen to be meaningful and to meet socialization needs. Choices about activities are influenced by past interests. If past interests have focused only on work-related topics, retirement choices may be restricted unless the retired older adult develops new areas of interest. Finances may also impose practical restrictions on the types of activities chosen. Health status issues such as limited mobility, limited endurance, or sensory deficits may also restrict activity choices. But for many older adults, retirement is a time to become involved in activities that could not be pursued while still working because of time and energy constraints. Many older adults volunteer in community organizations, return to school for the joy of learning, or even start second careers. For older adults, nurses are empathetic listeners to accounts of the changes retirement brings and sources of information about different activities available.

Relocation. Relocation is movement from one place of residence to another. Relocation may be from the long-time home in a cold climate to a house or apartment in a warmer part of the country. Older adults may also move from their home to the home of their children or grandchildren. Still other older adults may move to a retirement community or an assisted living or skilled nursing facility. Regardless of the destination, relocation is always an uprooting, a disordering of usual routines. Even when the move is from an unpleasant or unsafe situation, there is still a risk that relocation may adversely affect well-being.

Relocation disrupts the usual patterns of activity. Adaptations that maintained independence in ADLs may no longer function. The walk through a familiar neighborhood for exercise may no longer be possible. The new community or long-term care facility will have different options for activities. There will be new social networks to establish. The nurse's role during relocation is to support efforts to become accustomed to new situations and opportunities, and to monitor the effect of the stress of relocation on health.

Activity programming in long-term care facilities is the responsibility of recreational therapists. A sufficient variety of activities is provided to allow residents to have choices. Although residents are encouraged to participate in a variety of activities, they always have the right to determine the degree of their participation. The activity preferences of each resident are assessed on admission. The individualized care plan includes activities that are appropriate for the resident. Individual (one-on-one activities), small group, and large group activities are typically provided (Fig. 11-1). Some facilities provide mechanisms for residents to participate in planning future activities and for families and friends of the residents to be part of the activity program (Box 11-5).

Loss of Spouse. The loss of a spouse disrupts both joint activities and those activities where one spouse supported the other. If death is preceded by an illness, activities are altered in advance of death. During the period of grief, activities may be reduced. For example, the older adult may not feel up to participating in an exercise class. But part of the process of grief and recovery from grief is the adoption of a new pattern of life. That new pattern includes new activities, but also includes the resumption of former activities, although these may be altered by the absence of the spouse.

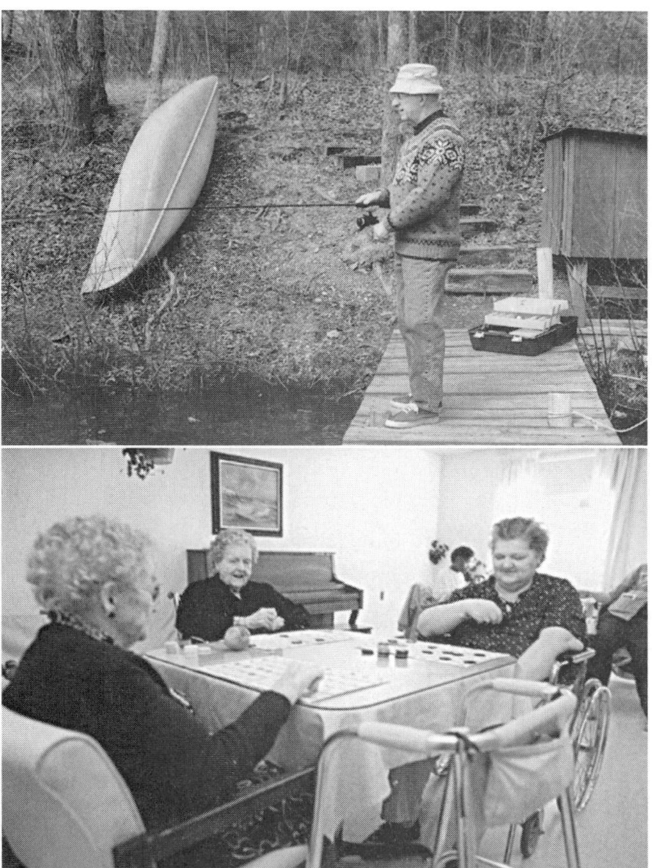

Fig. 11-1 Recreational activities, performed individually or in a group, are important for older adults. (*Top photo* courtesy Loy Ledbetter, St Louis; *bottom photo* from Sorrentino SA: *Mosby's textbook for nursing assistants*, ed 3, St Louis, 1992, Mosby.)

Nurses assist the older adult who has experienced the loss of a spouse by listening attentively and supporting the development of new activities. Some of these new activities may require learning new skills such as handling finances, cooking, doing the laundry, or maintaining the car. Other activities may involve making new friends. Information from nurses about available programs and services may help with the acquisition of new skills and the reestablishment of social connections. During the period of adjustment after the loss of a spouse, nurses also monitor the client's physical and mental health, remembering that stress may lead to alterations in health.

Activity As Affected by Alzheimer's Disease and Other Dementia

Alzheimer's disease and other dementias, conditions causing cognitive failure, affect an estimated 4 million to 5 million

BOX 11-5 Examples of Activities in Long-Term Care Facilities

EXERCISE

Walking programs (indoor, outdoor)
Dancing (balloon, square, line)
T'ai Chi (or similar disciplines)

SPECTATOR ACTIVITIES

Television (selected programming, including telecourses)
Videotaped movies
Live performances at the facility

PARTICIPATIVE ACTIVITIES

Games
Cards, bingo, and board games
Adapted versions of bowling and volleyball
Adaptations of TV game shows (*Jeopardy, Wheel of Fortune)*
Yard games, such as croquet, miniature golf, bocci ball, and horseshoes
Field trips to museums, sports events, restaurants, shopping malls, and parks
Picnics and barbecues
Fishing

CREATIVE ACTIVITIES

Art projects (painting)
Crafts (woodworking, stitchery)
Gardening (indoor or outdoor)
Cooking or planning menus for special meals at the facility
Music (vocal or instrumental performances by residents)
Writing a newsletter for the facility

INTERGENERATIONAL ACTIVITIES

Visits from children's groups
Adopting (and being adopted by) a schoolroom or scout troop

PETS AND OTHER ANIMALS

Domestic animals kept at the facility (dogs, cats, rabbits, songbirds, parrots, fish, sheep, goats, llamas, chickens, ducks, and geese)
Other animals brought to the facility by zoos or conservation groups (owls, hawks, chimpanzees, nonvenomous snakes)

people in the United States (Abrams, Beers, and Berkow, 1995). As the disease progresses, cognitive impairment increases, adversely affecting the ability to initiate and participate in routine daily activities. The older adult with advancing dementia also loses the ability to initiate diversional activities and to participate in activities that were once enjoyed. Caregivers gradually assume more and more responsibility for supervising behavior; performing basic personal care tasks; and providing opportunities for physical exercise, cognitive stimulation, and entertainment.

At the heart of planning activities for an older adult with dementia is the desire to preserve the remaining physical and cognitive abilities and to promote independence. Activities should draw on assets rather than deficits and should maximize the remaining abilities (Maddox and Burns, 1997). When planning activities, nurses or other caregivers must consider the extent of cognitive impairment, any concomitant physical constraints caused by aging or other diseases, and safety concerns.

Activities for older adults with dementia should be meaningful (Zogla, 1995). A meaningful activity has a purpose. The purpose may be to exercise arthritic joints or simply to have fun, but the activity should not be aimless. Meaningful activities are also voluntary. No one is compelled to participate. Instead individuals are invited to participate and given encouragement and explanations of the activity. Meaningful activities foster a sense of well-being for the participants. If an older adult with dementia is stressed by the activity or indicates discomfort, that person should be allowed, or assisted, to stop or leave the activity. Activities should also be consistent with the older adult's social status and support his or her dignity. Older adults may choose to participate in an activity that appears childish, but they must also have the option to refuse to participate. Activities should promote good feelings, not feelings of embarrassment, distress, or failure. To successfully plan and implement activities for older adults with dementia, nurses and other caregivers must be flexible, patient, and sensitive to the environment (Chavin, 1995). Communication is enhanced when the nurse or other caregiver speaks to the older adult as one adult to another and assumes the older adult will understand. If the older adult does not understand, repetition or rephrasing may be necessary, but it is best to begin with the positive expectation that the older adult will understand. Scolding, addressing the older adult as a child, or issuing negative instructions ("don't . . .") should be avoided.

As cognitive impairment increases, the older adult with dementia requires more supervision and assistance with personal care activities such as bathing, dressing, grooming, toileting, oral hygiene, and eating. Personal care activities are best accomplished in regular routines that involve simple, single-step instructions and visual cues. The environment should be quiet, soothing, uncluttered, and unhurried. To promote independence and preserve functional ability, nurses should encourage older adults with dementia to do the personal care tasks, or parts of tasks, that are within their abilities.

While physical exercise for the older adult with dementia is important for general physical well-being, exercise may also reduce agitation or wandering. The rhythmic movement of a rocking chair may reduce agitation. Going for a walk may redirect the impulse to wander. Whether the benefit is due to the change of setting, the removal of the older adult from a provocative stimulus, or the physical effects of walking, the end result is often an older adult who appears more comfortable. Exercise is also important to preserve muscle strength, flexibility, and ambulation. Other activities providing physical exercise include dancing, marching in place or swinging the arms to music, and gardening.

Older adults with dementia gradually lose the ability to select diversional activities. Yet when diversional activities are provided, they appear to enjoy themselves and participate to the extent of their abilities. Activities for older adults with dementia range from playing simple games to dancing to watching birds at a bird feeder. Activities may include simple housekeeping tasks such as dusting or folding towels. Activities may be one-on-one activities, such as taking a walk with a caregiver, or group activities, such as attending a church service.

Activities that tap into the older adult's past life experiences and interests may stimulate memory. Older adults with dementia may enjoy reminiscence, in groups or individually, because long-term memory may be preserved in the early stages of dementia. Activities that involve making or growing things evoke pride in the self and in accomplishments. Even in later stages of dementia, an object or a song may evoke a memory. Song lyrics or the familiar motions of cooking or painting may be remembered when many other things have been forgotten.

The benefits of activity for older adults include the promotion of health and the preservation of independence. Nurses help older adults adapt their activities to the situations that arise in the later years. Nurses also work with older adults to identify new activities. Whether the activities involve daily activities, physical exercise, or diversion, older adults and nurses should work together to design and select activities that improve the quality of life.

SUMMARY

Sleep and activity are two halves that combine to make the wholeness of our days. Without sleep we are not restored from the previous day's efforts, and today's activities are slowed by fatigue. Without activities we face going to bed without feeling the necessity of rest. Without the appropriate balance of rest and activity we are at risk of alterations in health. Nurses, by recognizing the changes that come with age and with alterations in health status, are able to assist older adults with their sleep and activity needs.

Home Care

1. Assess risk factors (e.g., environment, pain, or equipment such as a Foley catheter) that would predispose homebound older adults to sleep disturbances.
2. Review all medications to identify those which may interfere with homebound older adults' sleep patterns.
3. Instruct caregivers and homebound older adults on activities that would foster normal sleep, such as the avoidance of caffeinated beverages and alcohol.
4. Assist caregivers and homebound older adults with environmental changes that would foster normal sleep, such as using a rocking chair or taking a warm bath.
5. Remember that anxiety concerning safety and welfare can be an obstacle to sleep. A system of notification and monitoring to link older adults living alone with the outside world is important to a sense of security.

Key Points

- The sleep changes experienced by many older adults include increased sleep latency, decreased sleep efficiency, increased awakening in the night, increased early morning awakening, and increased daytime sleepiness.
- Some of the sleep changes experienced by older adults are associated with chronic disease and other health problems.
- Factors influencing sleep quality include environmental factors, pain, lifestyle changes, diet, medication use, medical conditions, depression, and dementia.
- Sleep apnea and PLMS are two common sleep disorders that may result in excessive daytime sleepiness and reports of insomnia.
- The first step in developing interventions to improve the amount and quality of sleep is a thorough sleep history.
- The sleep history includes questions about sleep amount and quality, bedtime routines, the sleep environment, activities, diet, and medications.
- Direct observation of the older adult during sleep, reports from a roommate or bed partner, a sleep diary, measurement instruments to assess sleep quality and quantity, and diagnostic studies in a sleep laboratory may be used to supplement the sleep history.
- Sleep hygiene measures include activities that promote sleep, emphasis on stable schedules, bedtime routines, a sleep-friendly environment, avoidance of substances that interfere with sleep, exercise, and stress reduction.
- Activities pursued by a particular older adult are influenced by that individual's preferences, lifestyle, and health.
- With advancing years and changes in health and lifestyle circumstances, performance of ADLs may require modified approaches or the assistance of others.
- Physical exercise is important for older adults to maintain health, preserve the ability to perform ADLs, and improve the general quality of life.
- Safe exercise requires gradual increases in the amount of exercise for older adults who have not been exercising regularly, adequate hydration before and after exercise, and suitable clothing and footwear.
- Retirement, relocation, and the loss of a spouse influence the ways older adults are active and the types of activities that they pursue.
- The goals of activities for older adults with Alzheimer's disease and other dementias include preservation of physical and cognitive abilities and promotion of independence.

Critical Thinking Exercises

1. A nursing facility resident tells you she has not been sleeping well and asks you to have the doctor order a sleeping pill. What questions do you ask to assess her sleep quality and quantity? Because you are aware of the drawbacks to the use of sedatives and hypnotics, what other interventions do you suggest to improve her sleep?
2. In the clinic you meet with an older gentleman who is accompanied by his wife. She reports that he is snoring loudly every night and is always falling asleep during the day. He denies snoring but admits that he is often very sleepy during the day. What sleep disorder do you suspect? What reports and symptoms would strengthen your suspicion? What recommendations do you make to the client?
3. You are checking blood pressures at a senior citizen health fair. After you check the blood pressure of an older woman, she asks you about starting an exercise program. She has not been exercising, but some of her friends have told her that she should start to exercise regularly. What recommendations do you give her? What precautions do you include in your recommendations?

References

Abrams WB, Beers MH, Berkow R: *The Merck manual of geriatrics*, ed 2, Whitehouse Station, NH, 1995, Merck Research Laboratories.

Allen T: Sleepless in Seattle . . . and San Francisco . . ., *Adv Nurse Pract* 2(4):26, 1994.

American Association of Retired Persons: *A profile of older Americans*, Washington, DC, 1997, The Association.

Ancoli-Israel S: Sleep disorders in older adults: a primary care guide to assessing 4 common sleep problems in geriatric patients, *Geriatrics* 59(1):37, 2004.

Ancoli-Israel S: Sleep problems in older adults: putting myths to bed, *Geriatrics* 52(1):20, 1997.

Bundlie SR: Sleep in aging, *Geriatrics* 53:S41, 1998.

Butler RN et al: Physical fitness: exercise prescription for older adults, *Geriatrics* 53(11):45, 1998.

Chavin M: The do's and don'ts of working with persons with dementia. In *Activity programming for persons with dementia: a sourcebook*, Chicago, 1995, Alzheimer's Association.

Cochran, H: Diagnosis and treatment of primary insomnia, *Nurse Pract* 28(9):13, 2003.

Cohen FL: Measuring sleep. In M Frank-Stromborg, SJ Olsen, editors: *Instruments for clinical health-care research*, ed 2, Sudbury, Mass, 1997, Jones & Bartlett.

Coltharp W, Richie MF, Kaas MJ: Wandering, *J Gerontol Nurs* 22(11):5, 1996.

Fichten CS et al: Poor sleepers who do not complain of insomnia and lifestyle characteristics of older good and poor sleepers, *J Behavioral Med* 18:189, 1995.

Floyd JA: Another look at napping in older adults, *Geriatr Nurs* 16:136, 1995.

Foley DJ et al: Sleep complaints among elderly persons: an epidemiologic study of three communities, *Sleep* 18:425, 1995.

Foreman MD, Wykle M: Nursing standard-of-practice protocol: sleep disturbances in elderly patients, *Geriatr Nurs* 16:238, 1995.

Gambert SR: Alcohol abuse: medical effects of heavy drinking in late life, *Geriatrics* 52(6):30, 1997.

Gregg EW et al, for the Study of Osteoporotic Fractures Research Group: Physical activity and osteoporotic fracture risk in older women, *Ann Intern Med* 129:81, July 15, 1998.

Gunnarsson OT, Judge JO: Exercise at midlife: how and why to prescribe it for sedentary patients, *Geriatrics* 52(5):71, 1997.

Hohagen F: Nonpharmacological treatment of insomnia, *Sleep* 19:S50, 1996.

Jones J, Jones KD: Promoting physical activity in the senior years, *J Gerontol Nurs* 23(7):40, 1997.

Kryger M et al: Sleep, health, and aging: bridging the gap between science and clinical practice, *Geriatrics* 59(1):24, 2004.

Maddox MK, Burns T: Positive approaches to dementia care in the home, *Geriatrics* 52(suppl 2):S54, 1997.

Marchello V, Boczko F, Shelkey M: Progressive dementia: strategies to manage new problem behaviors, *Geriatrics* 50(3):40, 1995.

Miller CA: How safe are herbs? *Geriatr Nurs* 19:163, 1998.

Miller CA et al: Alternative healing products: herbal and homeopathic remedies, *Geriatr Nurs* 17:145, 1996.

Nagel C et al: Sleep promotion in hospitalized elders, *Med Surg Nurs* 12(5):279, 2003.

Olson EJ et al: Obstructive sleep apnea-hypopnea syndrome, *Mayo Clin Pro* 78:1545, 2003.

Schnelle JF et al: Individualizing nighttime incontinence care in nursing home residents, *Nurs Res* 47:197, 1998.

Spieker ED, Motzer SA: Sleep-disorder in patients with heart failure: pathophysiology, assessment and management, *J Am Acad Nurse Pract* 15(11):487, 2003.

Tatro DS, editor: *Nurses drug facts*, St Louis, 1996, Facts & Comparisons.

Whitney CW et al: Correlates of daytime sleepiness in 4578 elderly persons: the cardiovascular health study, *Sleep* 21:27, 1998.

Worfolk JB: Keep frail elders warm! *Geriatr Nurs* 18:7, 1997.

Zogla J: Activities: an overview. In *Activity programming for persons with dementia: a sourcebook*, Chicago, 1995, Alzheimer's Association.

12 Safety

SUE E. MEINER, EdD, APRN, BC, GNP

Learning Objectives

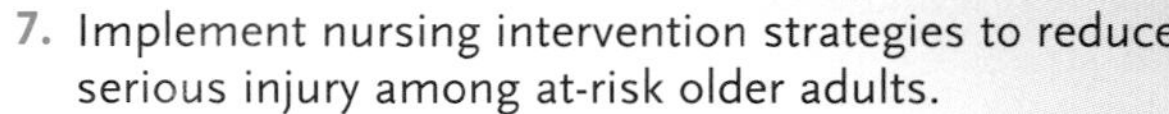

On completion of this chapter, the reader will be able to:

1. Identify the nurse's role in the promotion of safety for older adults.
2. Name various community, state, and federal safety-related resources for older individuals.
3. Identify safety hazards in the health care setting that can lead to litigation.
4. Differentiate between intrinsic and extrinsic causes of falling in older adults.
5. Identify common treatable causes of falling in older adults.
6. Implement the nursing standard of practice for clients experiencing falls.
7. Implement nursing intervention strategies to reduce serious injury among at-risk older adults.
8. Use home safety tips to prevent burns, accidental poisoning, smoke inhalation, and foodborne illnesses among community-dwelling older adults.
9. Differentiate among the various types of elder abuse.
10. List clinical syndromes and conditions that could impair older individuals and lead to safety hazards on the roadway.
11. Describe the pros and cons of having firearms in the homes of older adults.

Safety is a broad concept that refers to security and the prevention of accidents or injuries. When working with older clients, the gerontologic nurse must provide a standard of care that promotes safety and prevents foreseeable accidents or injuries, while also respecting individuals' autonomy to make decisions. This standard of care should pervade all aspects of the nurse's health care relationships with older adult clients.

Part of the nurse's role in ensuring safety is educating older adults so they can make informed choices. Education allows one to weigh benefits versus risks and to choose the best option in the presenting situation. In situations where clients are unable to make informed choices, family members or significant others are sought as advocates for the clients. If clients are unable to make informed choices and no family members are available, the nurse must use nursing judgment and follow an acceptable standard of care to promote safety and security.

This chapter presents common problems that can jeopardize client safety and lead to accidents, injuries, and death. These include falls, restraint use, accidental injuries, crime and victimization, elder abuse, and safety in the home environment. Attention will be given to safety tips and interventions for injury prevention.

*Deanna Gray Miceli, MSN, RN, CS, contributed much of the content to the "Falls" section of the second edition.

FALLS

Overview and Magnitude of the Problem

Falls are a common clinical problem affecting nearly one third of community-dwelling older adults and over half of institutionalized older persons in the United States. Falling is a major health problem for those over age 65 (Hausdorff, Rios, and Edelber, 2001). In 2001 more than 1.6 million seniors were treated in emergency departments for fall-related injuries, and nearly 388,000 were hospitalized (Centers for Disease Control and Prevention [CDC], 2003). Falling occurs among people of all ages, but falling results in higher rates of morbidity and mortality among those over the age of 75 because of the higher incidence of frailty and a limited physiologic reserve among the aging population (CDC, 2003; Murphy, 2000). In terms of serious injury, falls are the leading cause of hip fractures, accounting for over 270,000 occurrences annually. Older individuals who fall are also more likely to be hospitalized or institutionalized as a result of falling or concomitant serious injury than other age-groups. Fall-related injuries account for 5.3% of all hospitalizations for those 65 years and older (Bell, Talbot-Stern, and Hennessy, 2000; Jager et al, 2000). Women sustain about 80% of all hip fractures (Stevens and Olson, 2000). In a research study by Tideiksaar (2005), falls accounted for nursing facility placement in 40% of the population seeking institutionalization.

BOX 12-1 Client Statements Indicating Falling as a Normal Age Expectation

- "You know, I'm getting older."
- "I can't get around like I used to."
- "What's the use? I'll just fall again."
- "I'm doing okay the way I am now."

BOX 12-2 General Fall Prevention Guidelines

GENERAL CARE

- Wear low-heeled shoes with small wedge platforms.
- Wear leather- or rubber-soled shoes.
- Leave nightlights on at night.
- Keep items within reach to avoid overreaching.
- Check the tips of canes and walkers for evenness.
- Paint the last step a different color, indoors and outdoors.
- Dangle the legs between positional changes and rise slowly.
- Avoid the use of alcohol.
- Avoid rushing.
- Avoid risky behavior, such as standing on ladders unaided.

STEPS AND FLOOR SURFACES

- Be careful to avoid slippery floors and frayed carpets.
- Watch for the last step when descending the stairs.
- Count the number of steps as a cue while ascending and descending the stairs.
- Install and use sturdy banisters on both sides of staircases.
- Tack down throw rugs or remove them entirely.
- Remove obstacles in the path of traffic.
- Use carpeting on landing surfaces that has color contrast.

BATHROOM

- Install grab bars in the tub and shower and near the toilet.
- Avoid throw rugs; install carpeting.
- Avoid bar soaps; use liquid soap from a dispenser mounted in the shower.

Falling has numerous antecedents and consequences that can be identified and managed. Most clinical research demonstrates a reduction in fall frequency as a result of intervention strategies to modify risk factors. Clinical programs targeting high-risk older adults have incorporated intervention strategies aimed at medication modification, environmental improvements, and behavioral modification. Clinical research findings demonstrate variability in the effectiveness of these interventions. It has been estimated that about 30% of falls can be prevented through a combination of multitargeted interventions (Tinetti, McAvay, and Claus, 1996). Not all falls are preventable; therefore goals for individuals who fall frequently are fall reduction, prevention of serious injury, and modification of significant risk factors.

It is also important to note that because falls are multifactorial, not all individuals fall as a result of the same antecedents. For instance, an older woman may lose her balance and fall when hurrying to answer the telephone, and then experience a second fall the next morning when getting up from bed too quickly. In this example there are two distinct causes of falling, both of which can be modified through education and behavioral modification. Thus, because falls tend to be multifactorial in this age-group, care must be taken to perform a comprehensive assessment of falling individuals; this includes a detailed history and physical examination.

Client education is the cornerstone of fall prevention and management. The gerontologic nurse must explore client beliefs and misconceptions about falling. Older individuals may consider falling to be a normal part of the aging process. For some, it is an expectation of growing old. Client statements that may indicate this belief are presented in Box 12-1. Individuals who hold these stereotypes must be educated about the normal aging process, which is distinct from diseases and the adverse effects of medications. It is important to tell older adults that the etiology of falling can most often be determined by a health care professional who has expertise in fall assessment, and that falls can be reduced and even prevented through some simple interventions (Box 12-2). The treatable causes of falling must also be emphasized in continuing education and staff development programs in all health care settings. Once the clients' and staff's knowledge of falling improves, the reporting of falls in an effort to seek treatment may improve.

Falling Defined

It is crucial for the gerontologic nurse to recognize that how older individuals define falling is variable and influenced by perceptions of aging and disease and the context of the situation. For instance, older individuals may not perceive a slip that results in a fall to the floor to be an actual "fall." Rather it may be termed a *slip*, *trip*, or *accident*, but not a *fall*. Box 12-3 illustrates some common reasons given by older adults to explain the fall. The falling event needs to be reviewed in detail to determine if the person fell to the lowest level or ground. Moreover, how individuals define falling is likely to influence the reporting of falls.

History taking should be detailed enough for the examiner to envision the details leading to the fall. Refer to the later section "Evaluation of Clients Who Fall" for specific questions to ask during history taking (Tideiksaar, 2005).

BOX 12-3 Common Explanations for Falling Given by Older Adults

- "I think I slipped."
- "I don't remember what happened."
- "I was in a hurry."
- "I tripped."
- "I lost my balance."

Meaning of Falling to Older Adults

Falling in a broad sense is a concept that holds negative connotations, since it is associated with a decline, drop, or descent to a lower level. As it relates specifically to client falling, the same negative connotation appears to hold true, as evidenced by the plethora of research that presents the significant negative consequences of falling. However, to clients falling may mean something entirely different. It may not be associated with an actual dropping to a lower level, such as the ground; falling might mean a perceived loss in status. In a research investigation of community-dwelling older adults' statements about falls, the extent to which the fall was attributed to a person's own limitations instead of the environment depended on self-rated health, among other variables (Arfken et al, 1994). Thus the meaning of falling involves several related variables and most likely is determined according to an individual perception of how serious the fall is in terms of daily living.

The health care professional may equate a fall with a decline in client health or function or a worsening of a client's condition. Falling may be viewed as a marker of future decline. In fact, the concept of *prodromal falling* refers to a series of falls that occurs before the onset of illness or disease, as a prelude (or *prodrome*). Events such as infections are classic examples of medical conditions associated with falling.

Normal Age-Related Changes Contributing To Falling

Numerous age-related changes can predispose older adults to falling, especially when these changes affect functional ability and give rise to sensory impairment or gait and balance instability. This section highlights the salient age-related changes related to falling, along with nursing interventions directed at modifying the impact of these changes to prevent falling. Normal age-related changes in organ function can contribute to an intrinsic risk for falling (Tideiksaar, 2005).

Vision. Accompanying the aging of the eye are structural changes in eye shape and crystalline lens flexibility. It is the latter change—inflexibility of the lens—that causes presbyopia, a reduction in the eye's accommodation for changes in depth, such as when ascending or descending the stairs. If older individuals are experiencing presbyopia, instruction must be given for them to carefully watch door edges, curbs, and landing steps, which signal a change in height. Additionally, because of the tendency for the crystalline lens to become cloudy and form a cataract with advancing years, eye glare can occur and cause temporary visual disturbances. This effect is particularly evident outdoors on sunny days or indoors as bright light reflects off shiny floors. Instruction must be given to older individuals with this problem to wear wide-brimmed hats or sunglasses to shield the glare effect and to shade indoor windows with drapes or blinds to minimize the effects of sun glare.

Hearing. An age-related change affecting the inner ear is atrophy of the ossicle in the inner ear, which causes changes in sound conduction, including a loss of high-tone frequencies, called presbycusis. Other age-related changes include an amplification of background noise and a decrease in directional hearing. The vestibular system is an integral part of maintaining balance and to a large degree is dependent on intact hearing. Therefore older individuals with hearing impairments are more susceptible to falling when feedback to the brain is altered.

Assessment of hearing difficulties begins during the initial interview. In some individuals with significant hearing loss it becomes necessary to use alternative forms of visual cues to signal where their feet and bodies are in space so they can maintain stability. For instance, when hearing loss cannot be corrected, one aim of the management of hearing problems is to introduce vibratory or visual cues to compensate for hearing loss. The use of bells on shoelaces causes a vibratory sense that can be felt by older adults when a foot is placed on the ground. Nursing interventions include instructing older clients to observe foot placement on the floor by literally "watching their step" and to be especially cognizant of environmental conditions such as floor surfaces.

Cardiovascular. One of the most common problems facing older adults is the loss of tissue elasticity, which affects the arteries. This lack of elasticity leads to a decrease in tissue recoil, resulting in changes in blood pressure with position changes. Older adults who lie supine and then get up quickly are likely to experience the effects of lack of tissue elasticity when the blood pressure drops and a feeling of lightheadedness develops. It is important to educate older individuals to change position slowly and to dangle the legs a few minutes when arising from a supine position. Older adults should be encouraged to wait between position changes and to hold onto the side of the bed or other furniture should an episode of lightheadedness occur. The use of a single bed rail specially manufactured for transferring can aid older adults with getting in and out of bed.

Musculoskeletal. The bones of aging individuals, particularly the weight-bearing joints, undergo "wear and tear," which causes a loss of supportive cartilage. As a result, joints can become unstable and "give way," leading to a fall. In many instances osteoarthritis occurs in the weight-bearing joints, causing pain with weight bearing and further eroding joint stability. Interventions are directed at identifying such problems and correcting them through the use of antiinflammatory agents, prescribed activity and exercise, braces, and/or joint replacement. If joint pain develops and remains untreated, it can cause older adults to become sedentary or immobile. This phenomenon of disuse and muscle atrophy contributes to muscle weakness. This cycle of pain, reduced mobility, disuse, and atrophy can become a vicious one unless interrupted by regular mobility and pain control through topical or systemic medication use. Nursing interventions are directed at encouraging, supervising, or assisting with regular ambulation; appropriate use of ambulation aids; joint range of motion; and the modalities such as ice, hot packs, and physical therapy.

Another normal age-related musculoskeletal change is the reduction in steppage height, which can place older adults at risk for tripping, especially when door edges are not visible or carpeting is frayed. The gerontologic nurse's role is to identify these changes and offer suggestions for improvement, depending on the etiology. In some cases an assistive device can be employed to aid mobility and avoid further joint damage.

Neurologic. One of the most universal age-related changes affecting the neurologic system is a slowing in reaction time. It takes older individuals a longer time to respond both verbally and physically to changes in position. Older adults who lose their balance are able to right themselves to an upright position, provided the musculoskeletal strength of hips, ankles, and shoulders is adequate. However, those with functional impairments and diseases, muscle weakness, or adverse effects from medications might lose their postural stability and fall. For these individuals, uneven surfaces in the environment such as steps, sidewalks, and curbs can lead to a loss of footing and subsequent falls. Nursing interventions for those with impaired righting reflex include monitoring mobility for signs of unsteadiness and offering supervision and assistance when needed. In an effort to promote autonomy, it is important to allow older clients to continue to perform their usual activities independently and safely.

When independent activity is no longer possible, older adults require a physiatry evaluation or physical therapy evaluation for the use of a walking aid, such as a straight cane, stationary walker, or posterior walker. Nursing interventions also include the use of chair or bed alarms or call buttons worn around the neck to signal that assistance is needed. Shoes should be inspected for sturdy heels that are low and preferably wedge-type. Observation of an older adult client's ability to walk is crucial. For instance, is the walking path straight, or does the client deviate from it? Does the client trip when walking because of inappropriate shoes? For some older adults with gait disorders, rubber soles, like those on sneakers, worn on high-pile carpeting can actually be a hindrance and result in shuffling or stumbling while walking. Leather soles are preferable, as are those which are low heeled and have laces, providing extra ankle and foot support.

Fall Risk

Overall, most published research on falls and falling pertains to determining fall risk. There are clearly identified antecedents (e.g., diseases such as stroke, delirium, dementia, or urinary incontinence) that can lead to falls (Box 12-4), but many individuals with these disease-related risk factors do not fall. Thus fall risk is not determined solely on the basis of the number and kind of diseases, but also on how these risk factors influence an older adult's functional ability, specifically in the areas of mobility, transferring, and negotiating within the environment.

Fall risk is best determined by observation of mobility. Fall risk can be categorized according to intrinsic (illness or disease-related) or extrinsic (environmental) risk. A risk for falling according to these categories is different from the intrinsic or extrinsic causes of falling. *Risk* is determined by the clinician and is a term that reflects a judgment, based on a thorough evaluation of a client, known hazards for falling, and foreseeable events. Older clients at "risk" for falling may not experience a fall at all. There are numerous extrinsic risks for falling, such as lack of color contrast on curbs, poor lighting, frayed carpeting, and unsteady furniture. Intrinsic risks for falling include conditions such as orthostatic hypotension, blindness, or advanced dementia. The presence of these

BOX 12-4 Treatable Causes of Falling in Older Adults

- Orthostatic hypotension
- Dehydration
- Profound anemia
- Cardiac arrhythmia (e.g., bradyarrhythmia, tachyarrhythmia, sick sinus syndrome)
- Overdosing with medication or alcohol
- Urinary tract infection
- Vitamin B_{12} deficiency
- Osteoporosis
- Hypoglycemia
- Seizures
- Carotid hypersensitivity
- Carotid stenosis
- Delirium*

*Mental status is an important determinant of fall risk because changes in mental status, such as those incurred with delirium, can cause older individuals to have difficulty negotiating within the environment. Delirium causes individuals to misperceive sensory input, as well as stimuli and objects in the environment.

risk factors, however, does not mean that an older client will actually fall—just that he or she is *likely* to fall given certain circumstances. In fact, some individuals who are at risk for falling, as evidenced by the presence of these risk factors, do not fall. Some of the circumstances that can lead to falling in older adults include unsteady gait or balance instability, delirium or side effects of medications causing unsteadiness, and an inability to right themselves when footing is lost or balance is unstable.

As mentioned, risk for falling is different from actual intrinsic or extrinsic causes of falling. In the latter case, a fall has actually occurred and is the result of either intrinsic disease, extrinsic causes in the environment, or a combination of the two. These falls are likely to occur among those deemed at "risk for falling." The workup seeks to identify the underlying etiology so it can be treated to ultimately prevent or reduce recurrent falling. One aim of fall management is the reduction of risk factors to promote safety while still respecting client autonomy. Because falling is individually determined and not always preventable or predictable, it is important to avoid classifying clients according to the clinician's perception of their risk for falling (i.e., high risk versus low risk). As previously discussed, falling does not necessarily occur among individuals who are deemed at greatest risk. The effect of functional ability has significance as it relates to falling older individuals. Research has shown that the individual with frailty and physical functional limitations is at greatest risk for falling (Tideiksaar, 2005).

Intrinsic Risk. Intrinsic risk for falling refers to the combined effect of normal age-related changes and concurrent disease. The most salient observations for intrinsic risk relate to gait, balance, stability, and cognition. This requires the gerontologic nurse to observe and analyze older individuals' gait and balance and determine if impairment exists. Measurement tools have been developed to rate both gait and balance. These tools identify key components of gait such as step length and height, step symmetry, and path. Important areas of balance assessment include sitting and standing balance, turning, and the ability to sit without loss of balance. The Tinetti Gait and Tinetti Balance instruments are measurement tools that quantitatively score gait and balance. These tools have been tested through clinical research and hold acceptable validity and reliability ratings (Tinetti, 1986). Before managing gait or balance impairments with assistive aids or physical therapy, older individuals require medical workups for treatable causes of gait and balance abnormalities (Table 12-1).

Extrinsic Risk. Numerous environmental hazards, both indoors and outdoors, can predispose individuals to falling. Research has found that older persons continue to perform the same types of risk-taking behaviors in their later years of life as before. Modification of risky behaviors in the face of functional impairment can prevent accidental falls in and around the home. Instruction in home safety tips should be incorporated into health encounters with older individuals who experience falling.

TABLE 12-1 Treatable Causes of Gait and Balance Abnormalities

PHYSICAL EXAMINATION FINDING	POSSIBLE ASSOCIATED GAIT OR BALANCE IMPAIRMENT
Peripheral neuropathy	Inability to feel feet on the floor
Charcot's joint	Foot instability and/or foot pain
Loss of proprioception	Foot placement on floor altered
Hemiparesis	Leaning to one side; gait instability
Hammer toe	Foot pain during weight bearing
Decreased steppage height	Shuffling gait; tripping

The modification of environmental risk factors is also critical for fall prevention. Environmental hazards are those which contribute to accidental falls. Research has found that about 30% of falls can be prevented through environmental modification (Warde, 1997). The key areas that require evaluation for safety are steps, floor surfaces, edges and curbs, lighting, and grab rails; nursing interventions are directed at environmental assessment of the indoor living space in these key areas. Whenever possible, steps that are uneven should be repaired or at least have a sturdy handrail to hold onto for support. Floor surfaces should have low-pile carpeting in good repair. Tears should be sewn to prevent shoe heels from becoming caught. Throw rugs should be eliminated to avoid tripping. Curbs and cement landing surfaces should be painted with a contrasting color to outline edges. Lighting should be adequate in high-traffic and dimly lit areas. On a more global scale, a community effort to notify the local Housing Commission of areas needing improvement is an important step in the design of future homes that are safe for older adults.

Steps. The most commonly cited place where falls occur in the home is the last step of a staircase. The last step is a problem area primarily because of visual changes or functional impairment. Handrails should be present on both sides of a staircase or series of steps. The handrail typically ends at the second to last step; if a person descending the stairs is using the handrail as a guide for the landing surface, it will place the individual at the second to last step. Interventions to correct this include educating clients about this situation, teaching individuals to count the steps (i.e., keeping a mental tally of the number of steps ascending or descending), and reinstalling handrails that meet individuals' needs. Another problematic area on the staircase is an unevenness of steps (Fig. 12-1). Observation and correction of this phenomenon may be the first step toward fall prevention in the home.

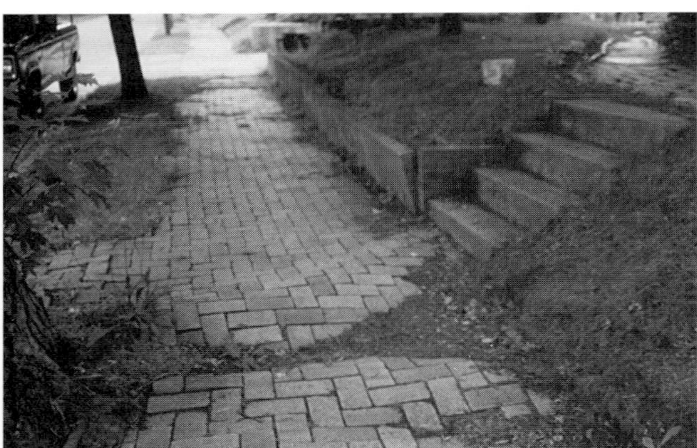

Fig. 12-1 Steep stairs with handrail missing on the right. (Created by Deanna Gray Miceli.)

Floor Surfaces. Floors that have been waxed or polished are common slippery surfaces that are a safety risk for older adults, especially persons with visual impairments. Carpeting that is frayed or torn can also catch heels. Throw rugs can lead to tripping or sliding (if on a hardwood or tile surface). In general, it is advisable to tack down throw rugs or remove them altogether. Floor surfaces should also be clutter free, as clutter can lead to tripping and accidental falls.

Edges and Curbs. Edging that lacks a contrasting color can lead to falls as surfaces tend to blend together. In the interior of the home, carpeting on the staircase and landing surface that are the same color can lead to falling. In the exterior of the home, concrete steps that are homogeneous in color can lead to misperceptions and subsequent falling. Uneven pavement outdoors can cause falling (Fig. 12-2). Curbs that are not clearly marked with a bold contrast in color can also cause falling. Simple modifications include painting the outdoor steps at the landing surface a contrasting color and using carpet borders in a contrasting color (or adhesive tape) to distinguish changing indoor surfaces.

Lighting. Dimly lit rooms cause difficulty for aging eyes and also for those with low levels of vision or impaired vision. Bright lights can lead to glare and temporary visual impairment. Lighting should ideally be evenly distributed and have consistent brightness. Diffuse overhead lighting is often preferable to one bright light source.

Grab Bars or Rails. Grab bars and rails can aid those with functional impairments and serve those who accidentally slip in the tub or shower. Grab bars to steady balance can be placed around the toilet, in the shower, or on the tub. Grab bars should be strategically placed to be most beneficial for the person with the impairment (Fig. 12-3). Misplaced grab bars, which cause older persons to reach, can actually lead to falls. Tubs and showers should have adhesive mats, be well lit, and be free of bar soap that can lead to accidental falls during showering.

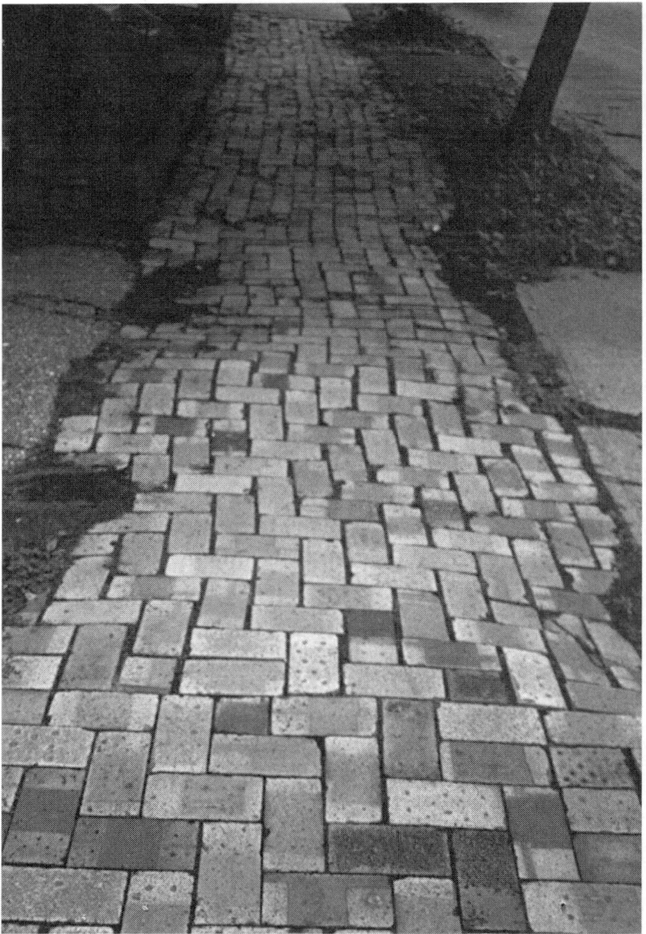

Fig. 12-2 Uneven sidewalk in the community. (Created by Deanna Gray Miceli.)

Risk for Serious Injury. A small percentage of older individuals who fall are at the greatest risk for serious physical injury (Box 12-5). It is vital for the gerontologic nurse to identify these individuals because they possess intrinsic risk factors that can be identified and often modified to prevent serious injury. Additionally, recognition and treatment of these individuals are part of the gerontologic nurse's role in preventing foreseeable events. Serious injuries such as hip fractures, head trauma, and internal bleeding affect only a relatively small percentage of older individuals who fall. Although falls are the leading cause of hip fractures, only about 5% to 6% of older individuals who fall sustain them (CDC, 2004). There is a high mortality associated with hip fracture, and their treatment costs place great economic strain on society for rehabilitation and other ancillary services (Liporace et al, 2005).

In addition, the use of physical restraints can increase the risk for serious injury. Individuals who are physically restrained can injure themselves attempting to remove the restraints. Incidents of strangulation and asphyxiation have

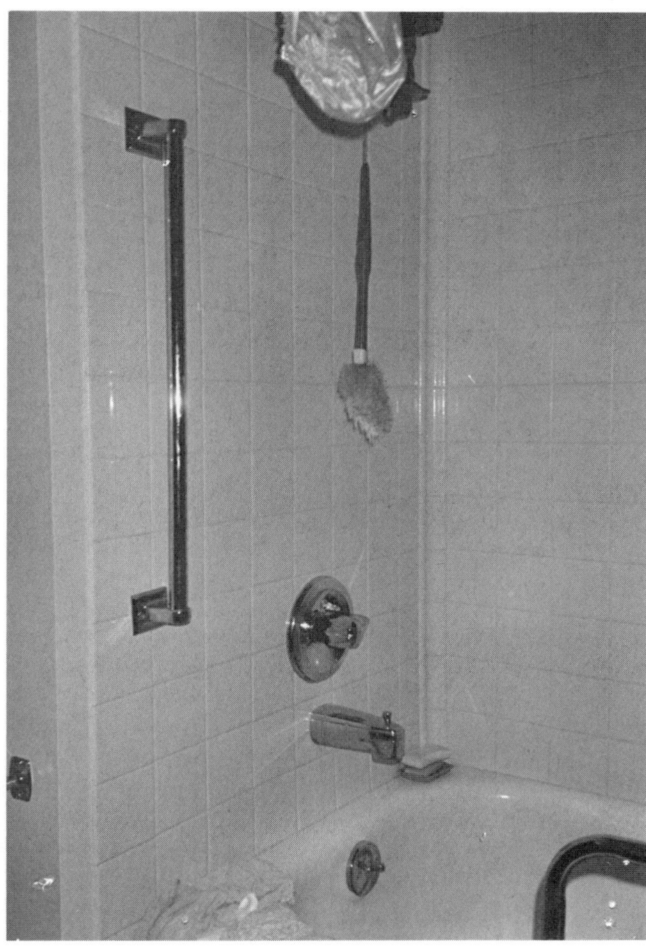

Fig. 12-3 Grab rails in the shower and bathtub. (Created by Deanna Gray Miceli.)

been reported secondary to restraint use. The elevation of both side rails can lead demented or delirious older adults to fall in attempting to climb over the side rails. These individuals are at risk for serious injury because of the height of the fall, and thus the impact is greater than if the side rails had not been elevated. Physical restraint use does not prevent falls and therefore should never be employed for "safety precautions."

BOX 12-5 Conditions Associated With Greatest Risk for Serious Injury

- Mental status changes (e.g., those related to delirium and dementia)
- Osteoporosis
- Gait or balance instability
- Concurrent fractures (e.g., of the hip, pelvis, humerus, ulna)
- Restraint use

Reducing the Risk of Serious Injury. *Behavioral modification* is a broad term applied to interventions that alter behavior to effect positive outcomes. The gerontologic nurse is in a pivotal position to educate older individuals, especially those at risk for serious injury from falling, about fall prevention measures. Older individuals' knowledge base and receptivity to changing behavior are important aspects for the gerontologic nurse to assess before initiating a teaching program. Specific teaching points will vary individually, but general guidelines for fall prevention and home safety can be illustrated through a pictorial display of high-risk environmental hazards or by issuing a handout with teaching points. As they relate to those conditions most likely to result in serious injury, specific interventions can be reinforced (Table 12-2).

Behavioral modification and instruction, such as teaching an older client who has orthostatic hypotension to rise slowly or an individual with dizziness who moves too quickly to slow down, may not be as easy as it seems. Behavior modification first requires older clients to recognize behaviors that

TABLE 12-2 Behavioral Interventions to Prevent Serious Injury

CONDITION	CLIENT INTERVENTIONS
Osteoporosis	Take medications prescribed for increasing bone mineral density. Take vitamin D and calcium supplements. Eat well-balanced, nutritious meals high in calcium. Perform moderate weight-bearing exercises on a routine basis. Avoid smoking. Avoid excessive alcohol ingestion. Avoid strain on the spine (e.g., heavy lifting, bending).
Gait instability	Wear footwear with nonskid soles. Use mobility aids and assistive devices as prescribed. Make deliberate attempts to scan the environment while walking to look for possible hazards. Participate in an exercise program that includes muscle strengthening and gait training. Make environmental modifications as needed.
Balance instability	Change positions slowly and carefully. Stabilize position before moving. Use mobility aids and assistive devices as prescribed. Assume a seated position during high-risk activities, such as bathing and dressing.

are contributing to problems. Often, the causes and effects of these behaviors need to be pointed out to clients in a clear and concise manner. However, this is not a foolproof method, because while clients are modifying behaviors, falls might not occur. The client's behavior may thus be negatively reinforced, and he or she may feel justified in continuing to perform the same behaviors. Behavioral modification requires older clients to make conscious attempts, whenever a behavior is performed, to change or alter it. Much of what the nurse teaches must be remembered for later action; the use of notes and tape recorders as daily reminders can help (see Table 12-2).

Disease or condition modification to reduce the risk of serious injury from falls includes appropriate treatment of the actual disease. In the case of osteoporosis, agents to prevent bone demineralization and build bone mass are prescribed and used with calcium and vitamin D supplements. The nurse plays a key role in teaching clients with osteoporosis about the importance of calcium-rich foods and ways to incorporate these foods into the diet on a daily basis. Teaching about the risk factors associated with the development of osteoporosis is also important.

In cases of delirium, condition modification includes a determination of the underlying etiology; unless the cause is identified and treated, the condition will not resolve and clients will remain at increased risk of serious injury from a fall. It is imperative for the nurse to recognize that the etiology is often multifactorial, thus requiring a variety of interventions based on the identified causes. While the delirium is resolving, injury can be prevented through additional nursing interventions, including padding of side rails, increased surveillance, assistance with activities of daily living (ADLs), and measures to promote a calm and reassuring environment.

Fall Antecedents and Fall Classification

Falling occurs when persons are upright and ambulatory, termed *bipedal* or *ambulatory*, or when they are sitting or lying down, termed *nonbipedal*. Falls may also be considered serious or nonserious, depending on the consequences for clients. Individuals who fall but not to the lowest level (the ground) and those who catch themselves are considered to be experiencing "near falls"; those who actually fall to the ground are experiencing true falls. Falling can be classified according to the cause of the fall (intrinsic, extrinsic, or multifactorial), frequency of falling, and the timing of falling in relation to other diseases. Most falls in the older adult are *multifactorial* in etiology, a combination of both intrinsic and extrinsic factors. Because so many different circumstances lead to falls in older adults, it is important to determine the type of fall according to a classification system (Box 12-6).

BOX 12-6 Fall Classification

- Multifactorial
- Extrinsic (environmental)
- Intrinsic (illness or disease related)
- Intentional
- Isolated
- Cluster
- Premonitory
- Prodromal

Isolated falling refers to a one-time event that was most likely purely accidental. The term *accidental* fall has been avoided in the literature during the last decade because most falls are not accidental, but rather indicate specific disease processes or conditions.

Cluster falls can be observed among individuals with specific diseases who decompensate. The classic example is an older individual with congestive heart failure who falls with the onset of oxygen desaturation or cerebral hypoperfusion associated with overexertion. Usually several falls occur over a short period and are markers for a decline in health.

Premonitory falls are those produced by specific medical illnesses. These types of falls have key symptoms that can be elicited on history taking; physical examination findings and diagnostic tests may also confirm this type of falling. Classic examples of premonitory falls are the new onset of stroke, seizure activity, hypoglycemia, and positional vertigo.

Prodromal falling refers to the onset of frequent falling heralding an acute medical problem; thus falling is a prodrome to later disease onset. An infectious disease typically causes this type of fall. Falls have also been associated with a clinical syndrome called *drop attack*. A drop attack has been defined as sudden leg weakness without loss of consciousness. Drop attacks are diagnosed when all other medical illness and environmental conditions have been excluded and clients continue to fall.

Intentional falls refer to falls by individuals who fall on purpose, possibly with a desire to do harm. Older clients with significant depression or suicidal ideation may throw themselves down to cause bodily harm. Other types of intentional falls include when one resident pushes another resident to the ground. This is frequently observed among demented residents in long-term care institutions.

Thus classifications of falls will often aid in determining the underlying causes of the falls. Box 12-7 illustrates the underlying medical diseases associated with the various types of falls. It is important to note that individuals can experience any one of these types of falls singularly or in combination. If an older resident experiences a premonitory fall on one occasion, the next fall may be from a different cause altogether. Since falls are often unpredictable and therefore not always preventable, it behooves the clinician to start the evaluation with the goal of identifying and managing those falls which are treatable.

BOX 12-7 Fall Typology with Common Causes of Falls

MULTIFACTORIAL FALLS

- Visual loss from macular degeneration, cataracts, hemianopia, retinal artery or vein occlusion, or temporal arteritis
- Hearing loss from sensorineural factors, conductive problems, or neuromas
- Orthostatic hypotension from age, volume depletion, medications, or diseases (e.g., diabetes mellitus, Parkinson's disease)
- Peripheral neuropathies of the lower extremities from vitamin B_{12} deficiency, diabetes mellitus, spinal lesions or tumors, or cervical arthritis
- Lower extremity weakness from degenerative joint disease, hypothyroidism, hyperthyroidism, electrolyte imbalances, cerebrovascular accidents, or polymyalgia rheumatica
- Poor balance from cerebrovascular accidents, Parkinson's disease, and parkinsonism (related to medications and cerebrovascular dementia)
- Gait abnormalities from dementia (e.g., apraxic gait), Parkinson's disease, normal pressure hydrocephalus, vitamin B_{12} deficiency, and posterior column diseases

PREMONITORY FALLS

- Seizure associated with postictal state, stroke, de novo Alzheimer's disease, or loss of urine control from previous head trauma
- Cerebrovascular accident associated with palpitations or shortness of breath from sick sinus syndrome, sinus bradycardia or tachycardia, junctional rhythms or blocks, or uncontrolled atrial fibrillation
- Orthostatic hypotension associated with lightheadedness with positional changes, caused by diuretics or other factors
- Vertigo associated with dizziness with room or person seeming to move, caused by labyrinthitis or vertebrobasilar insufficiency
- Syncope from sudden blood loss, vasovagal maneuvers, postmicturation, hypersensitive carotids or carotid stenosis, or a neurologic etiology

PRODROMAL FALLS

- Congestive heart failure
- Infections
- Functional decline with impairment in mobility and performance of ADLs

EXTRINSIC FALLS

- Improper footwear (e.g., poor soles, poor fit)
- Loose or frayed carpeting
- Poor lighting
- Cluttered environment with obstacles
- Difficult-to-see edging on sidewalks
- Tripping over cords or walkers (among those with dementia)
- Slips on the floor from spills or slippery substances
- Sitting or leaning on a movable object (e.g., unlocked bed or wheelchair)
- Glare on the floor (causing temporary loss of vision)
- Poorly repaired steps
- Lack of grab rails or devices to lean on
- Missing step(whitedescending orascending the stairs)

From Gray Miceli D: Evaluation and treatment of falls—ideas for protocols and practice, *Adv Nurs Pract,* November, pp 29-32, 50, 1995. Reprinted with permission from ADVANCE News magazines.

Fall Consequences

Physical Injury. The incidence of fall-related injuries spans from trivial trauma, such as skin tears and sprains, to serious injury, such as hip fractures, internal bleeding, or subdural hematomas. Each year thousands of older Americans fall at home. Many of them are seriously injured, and some are disabled. In 2001 more than 11,500 people over age 65 died because of falls (CDC, 2004). Overall the rate of serious injury is low, ranging from 5% to 6% of falls resulting in hip fracture (Nevitt and Cummings, 1994). Research investigations have found that cognitive impairment, gait and balance impairment, low body mass index, and at least two chronic conditions were factors independently associated with serious injury during a fall (Tinetti, McAvay, and Claus, 1996). The majority of injuries to older adults caused by falling are considered minor. Perhaps because of the low incidence of serious injury, older individuals often do not perceive falling to be a problem that warrants reporting or a medical evaluation.

Serious injury from falling is more likely to occur among those with osteoporosis. Bones weakened by osteoporosis, particularly weight-bearing bones like the femur, are more susceptible to breakage. Injury prevention measures to reduce the impact of falling, such as lowering the distance an older client falls to the ground and even using padding over the bony prominences of the hips, are required. Undergarments such as girdles with extra padding over the high-risk bony prominences have been designed for women. Individuals with osteoporosis should also be placed on medications to increase bone mineral density and strength over time. Exercise can aid in increasing bone mass.

Psychologic Trauma. Older individuals who fall may or may not experience psychologic trauma after the fall. Many factors influence the development of postfall trauma, including personality, depression, anxiety, and stress-related syndromes. Overall, little research has been done to elucidate the incidence, prevalence, and occurrence of postfall psychologic trauma. One significant consequence of falling may be fear of falling again or fear of being able to get up independently after a fall. Both these conditions have been researched more extensively than other psychologic trauma associated with the postfall period. But the fear is not limited to those who fall; it has also been reported among nonfallers (Howland et al, 1998).

Fear of falling appears to occur variably in the older adult population. One study found the majority of a sample of community-dwelling older adults expressed no fear of falling (Arfken et al, 1994). Still in other community-based research of older adults, fear of falling existed among falling and nonfalling individuals and was evenly distributed between the groups (Gray Miceli, 1997). Some research has shown that if older persons express a fear of falling, they may avoid activities (Vellas et al, 1997; Tideiksaar, 2005) and become physically dependent (Burker et al, 1995). One researcher found that chronic dizziness is strongly associated with fear of falling (Franzoni et al, 1994).

The gerontologic nurse's role is to determine if fear of falling or other psychologic trauma has occurred after the fall. The best time to elicit this information is during history taking with older individuals who fall. The nurse focuses attention on how confident the older adults are in performing activities that might predispose them to falling. One exception to consider, however, is an older individual who falls when nonambulatory, as in the case of a fall from bed. In this case, confidence may be unaffected during mobility. Possible indicators of fear of falling are presented in Box 12-8.

Defining and Measuring Fear of Falling. There are several ways to assess an older adult's fear of falling. A simple method is to simply ask the older individual an open-ended question such as, "How do you define fear of falling and what does it mean to you?" Responses will provide insight into the client's perception about falling and then give direction for intervention.

While interviewing an individual who falls, the nurse can also assess his or her fear of falling by simply asking the respondent to quantify fear using a visual analog scale that measures (on a 100 mm line) perception of how fearful the client is during ambulation. Yet another measure is the Fear of Falling Questionnaire, which evaluates self-perceived fear and potential harm based on answers to 21 items (Dayhoff et al, 1998).

Fear of falling has been operationally defined by some researchers as low perceived self-efficacy at avoiding falls during nonhazardous ADLs (Tinetti, 1986). The Tinetti Falls Efficacy Tool lists a series of questions, on a Likert scale, related to how confident the person is during activities such as walking, reaching into cabinets, or hurrying to answer the telephone. This tool is based on Bandura's self-efficacy theory and is reported as a measure of fear of falling self-efficacy or confidence. The validity and reliability of the tool have been established in limited studies (Howland et al, 1998).

BOX 12-8 Possible Indicators of Fear of Falling (as Observed by the Clinician)

- Apprehension or anxiety during ambulation (observed in facial expressions)
- Sweating, trembling, or difficulty breathing while ambulating (not present before ambulation)
- Clutching person or objects while ambulating or transferring
- Watching own footsteps during ambulation
- New onset of wobbly, reduced mobility after a fall
- Reluctance to change position
- Reluctance to ambulate

From Gray Miceli D: Falling among older individuals: exploring psychological issues, *Adv Nurs Pract* 5(7):41, 1997.

Evaluation of Clients Who Fall

History. Most often the underlying cause of falling will be identified during the health history. Because there is a tendency to underreport symptoms, the gerontologic nurse must be sure to ask about key symptoms that could be related to a treatable cause or causes of falling. At the onset of the interview an older individual should be informed that falling is not a result of normal aging and therefore information about the fall onset, location, activity associated with the fall, and other details is essential to the evaluation. It is important to elicit the client's own words about the circumstances surrounding the fall. Inquiries should be made about fall frequency and what usually happens immediately before a fall. The acronym SPLATT can help in further evaluation (Tideiksaar, 2005):

- **S**ymptoms at the time of the fall
- **P**revious fall
- **L**ocation of the fall
- **A**ctivity at the time of the fall
- **T**ime of the fall
- **T**rauma postfall

A fall history depends on fall recall and intact memory. If the client who falls suffers from dementia or delirium, it is advisable to seek additional information from witnesses or significant others. Often a fall diary can be useful in retrieving detailed information about the fall that the individual may have forgotten. Key symptoms to inquire about are related to diseases that are known to cause falls. Every older adult needs to be asked about a series of key symptoms that will help to further identify the underlying cause of the fall. If these symptoms occurred at the time of the fall or precipitated the fall, it is likely that a treatable cause does exist (Box 12-9).

BOX 12-9 Key Symptoms to Elicit during History of Falling Clients

SYMPTOM	ASSOCIATED MEDICAL CONDITION
Sudden onset of visual or hearing loss	Stroke
Sudden leg weakness (unilateral)	Stroke
Lower extremity weakness (bilateral)	Arthritis
Dizziness	Vertigo, labyrinthitis
Lightheadedness with standing	Orthostatic hypotension
Tremors or confusion	Hypoglycemia, hypoxia
Loss of consciousness	Syncope
Involuntary loss of urinary or bowel function immediately after the fall	Seizure
Difficulty breathing or shortness of breath	Arrhythmia
Palpitations	Arrhythmia

Physical Examination. The physical examination of an individual who falls includes a focused examination based on the client's presenting complaints in addition to the sensory, cardiovascular, musculoskeletal, and neurologic systems. Many treatable causes of falling can be identified on physical examination. Sensory input originates from visual, auditory, tactile, cardiovascular, and motor response systems. Sensory inputs from vision and hearing, proprioception of the distal lower extremities, and the peripheral sensory system all provide stimuli for the brain to process in regard to the maintenance of balance. The cardiovascular system is also critical because blood pressure regulation aids in homeostasis. Changes in apical heart rate such as bradycardia, tachyarrhythmias, or irregular rhythms can alter cerebral perfusion and thus affect balance. In particular, a drop in blood pressure when a client goes from supine to standing can lead to falling because of cerebral hypoperfusion as blood pools in the lower extremities.

Assessment of the motor response system includes muscle strength testing, with particular attention to hip and knee extension and ankle dorsiflexion. Several research investigations have found that poor ankle dorsiflexion affects the ability to right oneself during the phases of a fall (Tideiksaar, 2005). Manual muscle strength testing can show weakness in particular muscle groups, which can then be targeted for exercise. Gait analysis includes evaluation of footwear, base of support, limb stability, and clearance. The neurologic examination focuses on position sense, vibratory sense, Romberg"s test, and cranial nerve assessment. Refer to an assessment textbook for details regarding the examination of older adults.

The physical examination should identify any findings that might explain a client's symptoms. For instance, if a client complains of dizziness while getting up in the morning, the nurse should check orthostatic blood pressures. Other causes of dizziness for older adults include carotid artery hypersensitivity, cervical arthritis, carotid stenosis, and positional vertigo, all of which can cause dizziness with head movement and can often be reproduced during a physical examination.

Special Testing. A few tests will aid the nurse in further evaluating gait and balance. One helpful test for static balance is the sternal nudge. This is a test of the righting reflex and can be done with two persons and the client. One examiner stands in front of the client and one behind; the examiner in front pushes on the client's sternum to displace the client. If the test is positive, the client will begin to fall. A negative test results when the client is able to maintain standing balance despite the nudge. Tests of dynamic balance include observance of the client walking and changing position. Additional tests of balance include administration of the Tinetti assessment tool for balance (Box 12-10). The timed "get up and go test" is a measure of the client's quickness in getting up from a seated position, walking, and sitting down. The test is timed, and results are correlated with the prognosis of risk for falling . Results of less than 20 seconds have a good prognosis compared with those individuals who finish the test in greater than 30 seconds (Tinetti, 1993).

NURSING MANAGEMENT OF FALLS

The management of falls is challenging to the nurse, especially when older individuals experience multiple or recurrent falls. In these cases it is helpful to identify a pattern, if any, to the falling. Similarities in antecedents that lead to falling or specific symptoms might help identify the underlying cause. The goals of management are to identify the underlying cause, to reduce the incidence of recurrent falling, and to prevent serious injury.

Several aids for monitoring and preventing falls are available. The fall diary helps to monitor fall occurrences, injury, and patterns. Community-dwelling older clients can use the fall diary to jot down all the important information that led to the fall, occurred during the fall, or followed the fall. This information is extremely useful in determining antecedents and consequences of falling. Fall diaries are inexpensive or can be created by the nurse using a pen, paper, and ruler (Box 12-11).

For institutionalized older individuals at risk for serious injury from bed or chair falls, the use of bed or chair alarms can alert the nurse when movement is initiated. A sensor is attached to a client and to the chair or bed via a long thin wire. When the client attempts to get up, the wire falls off the sensor and signals an alarm. These alarms are noninvasive and do not restrict voluntary movement in any way. The alarm is fairly loud and may startle an older adult, so it is important to alert the client and family about the noise to be expected when the alarm is triggered. In the corridors of hospitals and nursing facilities, video surveillance cameras can help staff view ambulatory clients around the corner or in

BOX 12-10 Tinetti Balance and Gait Evaluation

INSTRUCTIONS: CLIENT IS SEATED IN A HARD, ARMLESS CHAIR. THE FOLLOWING MANEUVERS ARE TESTED:

1. Sitting balance
   0 = Leans or slides in chair
   1 = Steady and safe
2. Arise
   0 = Unable without help
   1 = Able, but uses arm to help
   2 = Able without use of arms
3. Attempts to arise
   0 = Unable without help
   1 = Able, but requires more than one attempt
   2 = Able to arise in one attempt
4. Immediate standing balance (first 5 seconds)
   0 = Unsteady (e.g., staggers, moves feet, marked trunk sway)
   1 = Steady, but uses walker or cane or grabs another object for support
   2 = Steady without walker, cane, or other support
5. Standing balance
   0 = Unsteady
   1 = Steady, but has a wide stance (i.e., medial heels >4 inches apart) or uses a cane, walker, or other support
   2 = Narrow stance without support
6. Nudge (with subject at maximum position with feet as close together as possible. Examiner pushes lightly on client's sternum three times with palm of the hand).
   0 = Begins to fall
   1 = Staggers, grabs, but catches self
   2 = Steady
7. Eyes closed (with subject at maximum position as in #6)
   0 = Unsteady
   1 = Steady
8. Turn 360°
   0 = Discontinuous steps
   1 = Continuous steps
   0 = Unsteady (e.g., grabs, staggers)
   1 = Steady
9. Sit down
   0 = Unsafe (e.g., misjudges distance, falls into chair)
   1 = Uses arms or does not use a smooth motion
   2 = Safe, smooth motion

   ________/ 16 BALANCE SCORE

From Brady R et al: Geriatric falls: prevention strategies for the staff, *J Gerontol Nurs* 19(9):26, 1993.

BOX 12-11 Designing a Fall Diary

1. Gather several pieces of 8 1/2 × 11 inch paper.
2. Across the longest margin write or type the headings "Date," "Time of Fall," "Activity at the Time of Fall," "Symptoms," and "Injury."
3. Instruct clients to write, in the space underneath each heading, the information pertaining to each fall soon after the fall occurs.
4. At the bottom of the fall diary include an "Emergency Contact Number" for clients to call in case a fall results in serious injury.
5. Instruct clients who have experienced a fall to keep a record of the fall events and to bring it to the health care provider's office at the next scheduled appointment.

distant areas. These cameras are prohibited, however, in private areas such as client rooms because of privacy laws. Other safety aids include safety belts in wheelchairs and the "lap buddy," which is a soft foam cushion that fits on the client's lap and wraps underneath the armrests of a wheel chair. However, if a client is unable to remove these devices voluntarily, they are considered restraining devices. If the use of these aids fits the criteria for "restraint" for a particular client, then the clinical guidelines for restraint use must be instituted. Health care providers must ensure that the use of these aids is the least restrictive alternative available for the client and that the aids do not replace observation or inhibit purposeful activity.

Injury epidemiology is the study of the interaction of effects of injury on the host, the environment, and the agent. The process of aging, along with the effects of disease, results in changes that affect the host. One aim of injury prevention is to alter factors that impinge on the host by maximizing client health and functional status, reducing unnecessary medications, and altering risk-taking behaviors. These combined efforts will reduce the risk of unintentional injuries. Alterations in environment through the elimination of environmental hazards will reduce accidental injuries that occur in older clients' homes. Improved technology through research seeks to alter the transfer of energy and thus modify those agent-related factors contributing to injuries in older adults. One such example is the alteration in the transfer of energy by use of super-soft mats and floor surfaces designed to absorb the impact of a falling body and redistribute its mass. Thus when an older client falls on a special floor surface, the rate of injury is likely to be lower than on a conventional surface.

For all older clients at risk for falls, and those at risk for serious injury from a fall, it is advisable to discuss with them the possibility that falling will result in serious injury, and how to reduce the potential for such injury. Clients should be given the choice of reducing mobility to prevent serious injury or continuing ambulation, knowing that the risk of serious injury is present. Client autonomy should be promoted and respected; it is the client's choice. In instances in which clients are demented or unable to make informed choices, discussion with the families or guardians is required. In any event the goal of the gerontologic nurse is to promote safety.

Fall and injury prevention modalities have received much attention in recent years. There is evidence that certain activities that improve flexibility and balance will prevent injury (Agostini, Han, and Tinetti, 2004). It is advisable to follow the recommendations presented in Box 12-12 and the Nursing Care Plan in an effort to reduce falling. The Emergency Treatment box gives recommendations for treating a client who has fallen.

SAFETY AND THE HOME ENVIRONMENT

Environmental hazards in the homes of older adults are common. These hazards are found in all living areas and entrances to homes of community-living older adults. Hazards have been observed less frequently in housing that is age-restricted to older adults (Gill et al, 1999) or has been remodeled or designed with older adults in mind. Hazards especially injurious are those associated with temperature-regulating equipment and household chemicals. The equipment includes fire, heat-related, and ventilation sources, while the chemicals include household cleaners, herbicides, and pesticides (Warde, 1997).

BOX 12-12 Fall and Injury Prevention Strategies

PHYSICAL MODIFICATIONS

- Cushion the landing surface.
- Use specialized tile that absorbs the impact of falls.
- Pad the floor.
- Cushion bony prominences.
- Use padding around high-risk bony prominences.
- Gain weight (if appropriate).
- Lower the distance to the floor surface.
- Use low-rise beds.
- Use futon beds or a mattress on the floor.
- Sit during dressing and shaving whenever possible.
- Sit in a shower chair instead of standing in a tub.
- Avoid high heels; use wedge heels or flat shoes.

BEHAVIORAL MODIFICATION

- Slow the pace of activities.
- Avoid risk-taking behaviors such as climbing on ladders if unsteady.
- Rise slowly and dangle the legs before changing position.
- Pay attention to the environment, terrain, and uneven or slippery surfaces.

ENVIRONMENTAL SAFETY

- Paint curbs and edges.
- Remove intravenous tubing in the hospital setting.
- Remove urinary catheter and drainage bag.
- Install grab bars or rails.
- Use the "Lifeline" for fall detection.
- Set a predetermined schedule for "checking in" with neighbors or friends.

Burn Injuries in the Home

Burns. Residential fires are directly related to the increase in deaths of older adults as the result of burns to the body. Although hot food or beverages often cause scald burns, they do not account for the large percentage of deaths from burns. The major cause of scald burns is the temperature of the hot water coming from the faucets (Harper and Dickson, 1995). Warde (1997) stated that scalds resulting from bathing or showering were caused by hot water tank temperatures in excess of 140° F (60° C). Scalds can be prevented by turning down the thermostat on the household water heater to 120° F. At temperatures of 140° F, only 3 seconds of exposure are needed to produce third-degree burns on sensitive skin (Warde, 1997).

The nurse should instruct older adults to use a meat thermometer and a container with a padded or safety handle to check the hot water temperature in the kitchen and bathroom: Let the water run until steam is noted; fill the container and wait until the thermometer registers a stable temperature; then adjust the hot water tank controls accordingly. The temperature should not be above 120° F.

Cigarette Smoking. Smoking in the home has been associated with the dangers of secondhand smoke for many years (Ashley et al, 1998). Smoking in bed or in a chair has also resulted in the deaths of numerous older adults from unintentional home fires. The environmental hazards of cigarette smoking include the careless disposal of cigarette butts and cigarettes dropped onto cloth surfaces (e.g., stuffed furniture, curtains, carpets, clothing). Multiple injuries and deaths have been attributed to older persons falling asleep while smoking (Carleton et al, 1979; Leistikow and Shipley, 1999; Warde, 1997).

The nurse should obtain information from the National Safety Council regarding smoking in the home, prepare an instructional plan to offer to older adults who smoke, and review the materials with them on a quarterly basis to refresh the safety steps associated with smoking at home. These include (1) never smoke in bed, (2) do not smoke in a chair when there is a possibility of falling asleep, (3) do not smoke after taking any mind-altering medications (e.g., sleeping pills, tranquilizers, narcotic pain medicine), and (4) place all smoking debris in a container away from all combustible items (e.g., curtains, furniture, clothing, trash). Have fire extinguishers available for use. Several types of fire extinguishers are available, but the best type for home use is a multipurpose "ABC" type extinguisher. ABC extinguishers generally use ammonium phosphate as the active chemical and are capable of putting out most common fires (National Agricultural Safety Database [NASD], 2002a).

Nursing Care Plan
Risk for Injury: Fall

Clinical Situation: Ms. S is an 85-year-old woman admitted to the hospital from home with acute congestive heart failure secondary to aortic stenosis and new onset pneumonia. Her medical history includes osteoporosis and a hip fracture 3 years ago. She is short of breath with minimum exertion despite a recent diuresis and the loss of 10 pounds. She is receiving intravenous diuretics and antibiotics. Vital signs include a temperature of 98° F, a pulse of 100 beats/min at rest, respirations of 26 breaths/min at rest, and a blood pressure of 90/60 mm Hg; her pulse oximetry on 2 L of oxygen is 90%. She insists on walking by herself to the bathroom to "stay independent." As a result of the diuretic, the client has to rush to the bathroom to prevent urinary incontinence. On examination, the client complains of dizziness when first getting up.

Nursing Diagnosis

Risk for injury: fall related to altered mobility, urinary urgency, and treatment modalities secondary to osteoporosis and respiratory compromise

Outcome

Client will maintain autonomy and independence while avoiding falls during the hospital stay.

Interventions

Observe client during basic ADLs, instructing her regarding ways to conserve energy while still encouraging independence.
Check blood pressure and pulse, supine and standing, to determine if orthostatic hypotension exists.
Keep immediate environment free of obstacles.
Instruct client to dangle legs before standing up from a supine position.
Place call light within reach to encourage client to call for assistance.
Provide temporary use of bedside commode to limit exertional activities while still encouraging independence; instruct in the use of safe transfer procedures.
Monitor electrolytes, blood urea nitrogen, and serum creatinine for evidence of drug-induced dehydration.
Weigh client daily to monitor fluid status.
Monitor intake and output.
Provide nonskid slippers.
Eliminate intravenous tubing and use Heplock to avoid tripping over clear tubing.

EMERGENCY TREATMENT

Mr. T is an 80-year-old man who was found lying on the floor in his bedroom, located in a residential care facility. He says, "I just fell down, but I feel okay." Closer examination reveals a large hematoma over the right temporal area and swelling of the right ankle and lower extremity. The distal dorsalis pedis pulse on the right is obscured by the edema. A right lower extremity fracture is suspected. To stabilize the client, the following interventions are carried out:

1. Immobilize the suspected fractured extremity with a splint or board and Ace wrap.
2. Apply ice to right lower extremity and to right temporal area.
3. Check apical pulse immediately to ascertain if an arrhythmia occurred, resulting in the fall; monitor vital signs, especially blood pressure and apical pulse.
4. Perform neurologic assessment and inquire about postfall headache.
5. Check environment for any spills or hazards that could have led to the fall.
6. Elicit a health history for symptoms of medical conditions that could have led to the fall, such as syncope, seizures, or vertigo.
7. Contact emergency transportation to move client to local emergency department for x-ray and evaluation.

Fireplace Hazards. The risk of starting a residential fire exists when using a wood or gas fireplace. Wood fireplaces need to be cleaned of ash and soot buildup regularly when used during winter and in geographic areas where cold weather persists for many months. When ash and other wood debris accumulate over time, the flue may become blocked, causing the smoke or flames to enter the living area instead of exiting through the chimney or vent. All chimneys, vents, and flues need to be checked annually for patency. The ash and wood debris must be removed to prevent blocking the exit of fire and smoke. If proper cleaning is not done regularly, the resulting inhalation of smoke can lead to substantial airway damage and pulmonary complications (Carrougher, 1993; Warde, 1997).

During the past 20 years, natural gas fireplaces have replaced many wood-burning fireplaces. Although the danger of ash and wood debris is eliminated, the draft element of the fireplace must be checked regularly to ensure a patent opening for the gas fumes to escape. In many municipalities a regulation on the use of gas fireplaces includes installation of safety valves and permanent vents to prevent the introduction of natural gas into the home (Lee-Chiong, 1999; Tearle, 1998).

The nurse should discuss fireplace safety and maintenance with older adults who acknowledge using fireplaces, and suggest having the flues checked for blockages on a routine basis.

Kitchen Hazards. Kitchen fires are frequently the result of a "dry fire" from an unattended stove with water boiling in a pan or kettle. Older adults in homes or congregate residences frequently put water on a stove to heat for instant soup, coffee, or tea. Forgetfulness concerning the boiling water is the major reason for dry fires in the homes of older adults (CDC, 1998; Warde, 1997).

The nurse should instruct older adults living alone about the possibility of dry fires. Clients with mild dementia need to be evaluated for cooking safety because of their forgetfulness. Three basic rules to instruct older adults are:

1. Be on the lookout for potential hazards.
2. Accidents can be prevented by doing things the right way and not taking short cuts.
3. Use protective equipment when needed.

Space Heaters. A space heater can be overturned by accident, causing a fire that may not be noticed until it is fully engulfing the home. All space heaters should have a safety mechanism that will turn the unit off as soon as it changes position (e.g., falls forward or backward). This safety device can shut off the heater and prevent the ignition of a fire in carpeting, curtains, or upholstery (CDC, 1998; Warde, 1997).

The nurse should recommend that older adults have home inspections; programs are often available through the local fire departments. When space heaters are used, an emergency shutoff must be operable. The equipment housing and the electrical cords must be intact. The cords must be appropriate for the electrical outlets being used (i.e., a three-prong plug cannot be placed in a two-prong adapter, which negates a grounded outlet).

Fire Safety Tips. Local fire districts across the country are encouraging families to keep fire extinguishers, smoke detectors, and carbon monoxide detectors in their homes. Home fire drills are recommended for all families, but especially for households with older adults. Box 12-13 lists safety tips to protect the home from the hazards of fire. Identification of exits and a plan for meeting outside the building are necessities for independent older persons or couples living alone in a private residence (Harvey et al, 1998; Warde, 1997). The nurse should instruct older adults and families with older adult members regarding prevention measures.

Nonburn Injuries in the Home

Knife Injuries. The use of knives, particularly in the kitchen, provides the potential for injury. The nurse should instruct older adults in six basic rules (NASD, 2002b):

1. When using knives, always cut away from the body on a proper cutting surface.
2. Keep the blades sharp and clean.
3. Keep the knife grips clean.
4. Never leave knives lying in water, since this can injure an unsuspecting dishwasher.
5. When wiping blades, always point the cutting edge away from the hand.
6. If a knife should fall, do not try to catch it; pick it up after it has fallen.

BOX 12-13 Safety Tips to Protect the Home from Fire

- Never spend more than 30 seconds fighting a home fire. Warn all others in the home and then leave. Call 911 from a neighbor's home.
- Conduct household fire drills on a monthly basis.
- Establish a meeting place outside the home for all members of the household.
- Keep a fire extinguisher in the kitchen, basement, and garage. Check the expiration date on the days that daylight saving time begins and ends each year.
- Install smoke and carbon monoxide detectors in areas near sleeping quarters, at the top of stairwells, and near the furnace. Check the expiration date of the batteries on the days that daylight saving time begins and ends each year.

Adapted from Warde J: *The healthy home handbook: all you need to know to rid your home of health and safety hazards,* New York, 1997, Random House.

Carbon Monoxide Poisoning. Carbon monoxide toxicity from use of heating oil or natural gas can occur during the winter months. Furnaces that do not have flues checked for patency can be the cause of this silent killer (Drescher et al, 1999). The condition of furnace venting should be checked annually just before the furnace is turned on for the home heating season (Warde, 1997).

Power interruptions during cold weather increase the risk of unintentional carbon monoxide poisoning. Often the electricity is interrupted during severe winter storms. This can create a need for alternative heating methods. Methods associated with carbon monoxide exposure are gasoline generators, propane or kerosene heaters, and charcoal grills (Houck and Hampson, 1997; Wrenn and Conners, 1997; Yoon, Macdonald, and Parrish, 1998). Warnings regarding the use of alternative heating methods during electrical outages should become part of all home safety instructions.

The nurse should include a recommendation for installation of a carbon monoxide detector in all home safety programs. Box 12-14 lists ways to prevent carbon monoxide in the home.

Chemical Injuries. Inadvertent skin exposure or ingestion of household chemicals, herbicides, or pesticides has been linked to deaths or injuries requiring long-term medical care (Lee, Chen, and Wu, 1999). Reading labels and properly storing chemicals used in and around the home are essential for the protection of health and safety. Many chemicals available

BOX 12-14 **Prevention of Carbon Monoxide in the Home**

- Check exhaust connection.
- Check ventilation.
- Service furnace regularly.
- Arrange for chimney inspections and cleaning as needed.
- Do not use a gas stove to heat a room.
- Use barbecue grills outdoors only.
- Do not start automobile engines in a closed garage.
- Vent space heaters (except electric models) to the outside.

Adapted from Warde J: *The healthy home handbook: all you need to know to rid your home of health and safety hazards,* New York, 1997, Random House.

for household and yard or garden use require mixing before administration. Proper ventilation during mixing and storage is mandatory for most chemicals approved for home use.

Misinterpretation of the label, or visual difficulties in older persons, may lead to improper mixing and storage. All home safety programs should include information related to the correct reading of labels and storage of herbicides and pesticides (Warde, 1997). When labels are written in small print, older adults with visual deficits should be instructed to ask for a large print version of the label. These can usually be obtained from the manufacturer (Lanson, 1997).

To prevent accidental poisoning, all hazardous household cleaning substances should be kept in a locked cabinet. This cabinet should be difficult for an older adult with cognitive impairment to access. Some household cleaning agents (e.g., disinfectants, oven or drain cleaners) are caustic or corrosive to human skin or mucous membranes and can cause critical injuries or death if swallowed. These agents are labeled with cautions and require gloves and eye protection during use. Immediate action is required if an agent is ingested or comes into contact with the eyes or mucous membranes. Where poison centers are available, one should be contacted immediately and given the name and contents of the product that caused the injury. The emergency system (911 in most areas) should be contacted for any accidental poisoning when antidotes are not immediately available in the home (Lanson, 1997; Warde, 1997).

Cooling Fans. Ceiling, floor, and table fan injuries occur over the summer months when air conditioning is unavailable, not used, or ineffective. Floor and table fans need to have screening surrounding the entire mechanism of the fan blade. The electric cords should be placed in no-traffic or low-traffic areas and checked monthly during use for any defect or fraying of the wires. During seasonal use of fans, cleaning should be done with floor and table fans unplugged and ceiling fans completely turned off (Potts, 1999). To avoid falls while climbing ladders to clean ceiling fans, extension poles with dusting attachments made for fan blades should be used (Warde, 1997).

Foodborne Illnesses

Food handling, preparation, and consumption behaviors associated with foodborne diseases are common in the homes of older adults. Fruits and vegetables are available all year in most of the United States because of the long-distance trucking industry. These foods are shipped from unknown locations, where pesticides and other sprays may have been used. Therefore washing fruits, vegetables, and hands before beginning food preparation is a must to prevent foodborne illnesses. Ground meat and ground poultry are more perishable than most foods. In the danger zone between 40° and 140° F, bacteria can multiply rapidly. Since bacteria can't be seen, smelled, or tasted, ground meats should be kept cold to keep them safe. Safe handling and safe storage are a must when preparing ground meat and poultry (NASD, 2002b).

Cleaning all surfaces before and after food preparation is essential to prevent the spread of bacteria and fungus that are common on raw foods. Common household bleach diluted with tap water can be sprayed and wiped off preparation surfaces following cleaning with soap and water. Cleaning procedures should be done after each different type of food is prepared (Parashar et al, 1998; Yang et al, 1998) (see Research box).

SEASONAL SAFETY ISSUES

Older adults are at particular risk for environmental temperature–induced illnesses. Predisposing medical conditions and side effects from a variety of medications can render older persons vulnerable to heat- or cold-related symptoms ranging from weakness, dizziness, and fatigue to exhaustion, coma, and death (Ballester and Harchelroad, 1999; Barrow and Clark, 1998).

The nurse should prepare seasonal information materials that deal with the dangers of hyperthermia or hypothermia for all older adults living independently. Additionally, the nurse should identify those clients at risk for illnesses associated with temperature extremes and promote ways of initiating a neighborhood watch program for dangerous climatic changes.

Hyperthermia

Environmental heat–related deaths and illnesses are preventable. Prevention strategies include recognizing which persons are at risk for heat-related illnesses and initiating a client-teaching program to aid in recognition of the signs and symptoms of potential heat stroke. Preventive care should include drinking plenty of fluids before, during, and after any activities that can increase the effect of the ambient tempera-

> **Research**
>
> **SAMPLE/SETTING**
>
> A sample of 19,356 completed questionnaires (2461 in Colorado, 3335 in Florida, 2212 in Indiana, 1572 in Missouri, 3149 in New Jersey, 2477 in New York, 2110 in South Dakota, and 2040 in Tennessee) on food safety practices, including food handling, preparation, and consumption behaviors, were collected over a 12-month period.
>
> **METHODS**
>
> The 1995 Behavioral Risk Factor Surveillance Systems (BRFSS) Questionnaire was administered by the CDC, the Food and Drug Administration (FDA), and several state health departments.
>
> **FINDINGS**
>
> Questionnaire analysis revealed that 50.2% reported eating undercooked eggs, 23.8% ate home-canned vegetables, 19.7% ate pink (undercooked) hamburgers, 8% ate raw oysters, and 1.4% drank raw (unpasteurized) milk. The prevalence of not washing the hands with soap after handling raw meat or chicken and not washing a cutting board with soap or bleach after using it for cutting raw meat or chicken was 18.6%.
>
> **IMPLICATIONS**
>
> Health care professionals should develop and present teaching programs to the public that discuss the dangers inherent in questionable food preparation and handling practices to prevent foodborne illnesses.
>
> Yang et al: Multistate surveillance for food handling, preparation, and consumption behaviors associated with food-borne diseases: 1995 and 1996 BRFSS food-safety questions, *Morbid Mortal Weekly Rep: CDC Surveillance* 47(4):33, 1998.

ture and the production of excess body heat (Ballester and Harchelroad, 1999; Barrow and Clark, 1998; Davis, 1997).

Heat stroke is a life-threatening problem that must be treated immediately for maximum recovery. Fast and effective cooling of the body is the cornerstone of treatment for heat stroke. The community response to heat emergencies can greatly decrease morbidity and mortality of older adults through neighborhood contact programs. These programs can identify older adults who are living without air conditioning or who do not have funds to pay high utility bills to keep their homes cooled to a safe temperature zone (i.e., 72° to 78° F) (Hett and Brechtelsbauer, 1998).

Hypothermia

Ambient household temperatures below 65° F are associated with hypothermia in older adults. When the air temperature remains below optimum levels for even short periods, older adults often fail to sense the cold. This failure can lead to other thermoregulatory impairments that include (Worfolk, 1997):

- Failure of the body to perform adequate vasoconstriction in response to the cold
- Failure of or reduced shivering response to the cold
- Failure of a person's metabolic rate to increase in response to the cold

Further complicating the thermoregulatory failures are reactions to specific medications or substances that interfere with the body's ability to increase heat production. These medications or substances include phenothiazines, barbiturates, benzodiazepines, tricyclics, vasodilators, alcohol, and narcotics. When a client is taking one or more of these medications or has known alcohol consumption, instruction should contain warnings for potential problems with hypothermia recognition (Worfolk, 1997).

STORAGE OF MEDICATIONS AND HEALTH CARE SUPPLIES IN THE HOME

The majority of older adults take medications on a regular basis. The storage of medications at home can become a safety and drug-effectiveness issue. Some storage areas in the home are not safe for keeping medications. The windowsill in the bathroom or kitchen is frequently used to shelve medication bottles. Most drugs degrade when left in direct sunlight, with or without excessive heat. Heat can change the chemical makeup of specific compounds in the medication, and moisture is considered an undesirable element for solid-based drugs, such as medications in tablet form.

The nurse should review the home conditions and instruct clients to identify those places which are undesirable areas for medication storage (e.g., kitchens, bathrooms, laundry rooms, basements, windowsills) (Skidmore-Roth and McKenry, 2005). Clients should be instructed to appropriately dispose of all outdated prescriptions when new ones are written. The most common method for disposing of outdated or unused medications is to flush them down the toilet. Instructions for older adults to throw away old medications must have explicit directions to not dispose of them in trash or garbage containers.

If health care has been delivered in the home setting, dressings and other medical supplies may remain after the treatment ends. Clients should be instructed on how to dispose of used wound dressings and needles or syringes according to local health department regulations. Dressings and bandages touched by infectious disease drainage require special disposal instructions by home care nurses. The nurse should provide and collect biohazard containers for contaminated dressings and sharp objects (e.g., needles, syringes) when home care is being provided. The nurse should also prepare instructional material related to safety and the use of sharp objects that can be left with clients after home care is discontinued. These materials must not be disposed of among regular paper trash in home trash collection.

Arrangements for disposal should be made through the local health department or hospital.

LIVING ALONE

Fear of crime reduces the subjective well-being of older adults, while also curtailing neighborhood mobility (Bazargan, 1994). The fear of crime differs somewhat between crimes at home versus outside of the home. In one study a gender variable was identified: women were significantly more fearful of crime outside the home and much less fearful of crime inside the home. Among factors that affected the perception of personal fear was previous victimization, media exposure, trust of neighbors, and length of residence in the neighborhood (Bazargan, 1994).

Community action groups have developed neighborhood strategies to protect older adults living alone. Among those strategies are (Chu, 1998):

- Daily telephone calls to specific persons on a call list
- Raising and lowering window shades or curtains at specific times of the day and evening, which will be monitored by a specific person
- Mail carrier alerts when mail is not picked up daily from mailboxes of enrolled older persons

AUTOMOBILE SAFETY

Maintaining independence after retirement includes the ability to travel to shopping centers and health care providers' offices, to visit family and friends, and to participate in recreational activities. A decline in an older adult's ability to drive safely may result in the loss of driving privileges. This decline may be a result of presbyopia, decreased dark adaptation, decreased depth perception, susceptibility to glare, and the general slowing of reflexes and cognitive processing (Ebersole, Hess, and Luggen, 2004).

The U.S. Department of Health and Human Services (1995) estimated that 20% of American drivers are ages 65 and older. Persons over age 70 have been associated with greater than 23% fatalities per 100,000 drivers. Because driving is a complex skill that involves rapid cognitive and psychomotor coordination, and many older adults have age-related changes, have illnesses, or are taking medications that slow down their responses to road conditions, automobile safety eventually becomes an issue. For post-stroke drivers, vision and attention essential for safe driving are often impaired. The severity of these deficits could influence driving behaviors (Fisk, Owsley, and Mennemeier, 2002)

Operating a motor vehicle can often require quick reflexes and reaction time, especially in the event of road hazards. As response time diminishes with advancing age, health care professionals and their clients must address driving safety issues. Driving evaluations are essential for older adults with suspected dementia.

Carr et al (1998) established a traffic sign identification test that can differentiate drivers with mild or moderate senile dementia of the Alzheimer's type from cognitively normal older adults. This test was devised to protect the driving rights of older adults while identifying those persons at risk for automobile accidents because of dementia.

Alzheimer's disease causes impaired visual-spatial ability and misperception of the environment. Because of damage to neurons and a lack of neurotransmitter substances, thinking and reflexes are slowed, impulse control and judgment are impaired, short-term memory loss occurs, and attention span is reduced. When dementia affects language function, road signs and signals may be misinterpreted or ignored. Persons suspected of having early (mild) dementia should have a driving evaluation that can determine their continued ability for safe driving (Carr et al, 1998).

Guerrier, Manivannan, and Nair (1999) found that older drivers have difficulty at intersections, especially when making left turns. Their work indicates that a deficit in information-processing abilities of older persons was responsible for accidents at intersections. The three deficits identified were in visual field dependence, visual search skills, and working memory of decision making to complete a left turn maneuver. Box 12-15 lists common reasons for pedestrian accidents.

When Finelli and Lee (1996) studied the effects of stroke and automobile accidents among older adults, visual field defect, impaired consciousness, and loss of motor control were major contributing factors to accidents. Data analysis revealed that few strokes were caused by accidents, and accidents caused by stroke were not common. When stroke survivors were questioned about driving practices, 50% reported they did not receive advice about driving, and 87% reported they did not receive any type of driving evaluation. These

BOX 12-15 Most Commonly Cited Reasons for Pedestrian Accidents

- Vehicles turning left are more dangerous than vehicles turning right. Pedestrians step off the curb before being sighted by vehicles turning left.
- Pedestrians are most vulnerable when first stepping off the curb because there is less time for driver or pedestrian to react or respond.
- Vehicles leaving an intersection are more dangerous because they are picking up speed.
- Pedestrians or vehicles may initially be hidden from each other's view by visual screens.
- Immediate action by pedestrians often occurs as the signal turns green or changes to "Walk," often while a vehicle is still in the intersection.
- "Walk" or green signal does not give sufficient time to allow older persons to cross safely.

From Automobile Association of America: Pedestrian safety for the older (65+) adult, *Motorist* 14, May-June 1993.

individuals were driving 6 or 7 days a week or 100 to 200 miles a week (Fisk, Owsley, and Pulley, 1997).

Older adults with mild to moderate Parkinson's disease have been found to have diminished driving performance (Heikkila et al, 1998). When medical treatment is effective, driving performance may improve during remission of symptoms.

Other disorders that can adversely affect driving ability are (Heikkila et al, 1998):

- Vertigo
- Seizure disorders
- Stroke sequelae
- Macular degeneration or retinal hemorrhage
- Unstable cardiac arrhythmias

Nursing assessment and instruction of older clients must include inquiry about driving as a separate and independent component of functional assessment (Gallo, Rebok, and Lesikar, 1999). When a functional assessment strongly indicates that a driving safety issue exists, discussion regarding cessation of driving may become necessary. Since an older adult's lack of driving may place a burden on other members of the family, this discussion is best done in the presence of significant others viewed as trustworthy by the client. States laws and policies differ as to mandatory reporting of high-risk individuals and to licensing provisions. The nurse must be aware of the significance that driving has for older adults. If driving is an important quality-of-life issue for an older person and he or she wants to continue to drive, the nurse should provide the following guidelines for safe travel (Ebersole, Hess, and Luggen, 2004):

- Preplan the route of travel.
- Bring someone else to assist in navigation.
- Maintain space between oneself and the vehicle in front.
- Avoid night driving.
- Continue to wear appropriate hearing aids and glasses while driving.
- Avoid driving in poor weather conditions (e.g., ice, snow, rain, fog).
- Keep the automobile's maintenance records up to date.
- Avoid driving if medications warn against using mechanical devices while under the influence of the drug.

The issues of quality of life, personal autonomy, and safety dictate that older adults need to be supported in their desire to continue to drive automobiles. As the number of drivers over the age of 70 continues to grow, new ways of evaluating driving safety while supporting personal autonomy are needed (Ebersole, Hess, and Luggen, 2004).

ABUSE AND NEGLECT

With the estimated number of older adults suffering mistreatment by neglect or actual physical abuse reaching 2 million by the year 2020, the nurse needs to assess clients for risk factors to identify those who are most vulnerable (Bird et al, 1998). When signs of injury are evident, the nurse should screen for risk factors of substance abuse; familial violence; dependency needs; or stresses in the spouses, roommates, or guardians of older persons. A suggested scale for determining levels of abuse and neglect was studied by Bird et al (1998). The four-level scale placed clients in one of the following categories:

- Low risk for abuse
- Self-neglect
- Neglect
- Abuse

By using a scale to rate the potential for abuse or neglect, nursing personnel can become aware of the incidence and prevalence of this tragedy. Once aware, they can initiate action to remove a client from an abusive environment.

Older persons with physical or mental frailties are more vulnerable to abuse and neglect than are independent older adults. When they need assistance to perform basic ADLs such as bathing, dressing, toileting, walking around the immediate living area, and eating meals, stress may overtake the caregivers (Cromwell, 1999). For older spouses or adult children with heavy financial and family responsibilities, the stress and strain of caregiving tasks is often the cause for the initial abuse or neglect (Butler, 1999; Jones, Holstege, and Holstege, 1997; Phillips, 1988). Some abusive family members report the reasons that led to abuse as irritable feelings or constant illnesses and fatigue that were never relieved. Often they lacked knowledge about caregiving skills and community resources available to provide relief to caregivers before they become abusive or neglectful (Cromwell, 1999).

Elder abuse or neglect reached such magnitude that the U.S. Congress passed the Family Violence Prevention and Services Act of 1992. The act mandated a national study, which reported that 450,000 older persons living in the community were abused or neglected in 1996 (Administration on Aging [AOA], 1998). The identified cases were broken down into five areas of abuse or neglect:

- Neglect (reported by 49% of persons)
- Emotional abuse (35%)
- Exploitation or financial abuse (30%)
- Physical abuse (26%)
- Abandonment (3%)

In nearly 90% of abuse and neglect cases, a family member was identified as the perpetrator. The spouse or adult child of the abused or neglected older person was identified as being responsible for nearly 68% of the poor care. When ethnic and cultural diversity is used to identify cases of abuse or neglect, the following breakdown results (AOA, 1998):

- Whites, 84% of reported cases
- Blacks, 8.3%
- Hispanics (of any color), 5.1%
- Asian/Pacific Islanders, 2.1%
- Native Americans/Alaskan Natives, 0.4%

Each state has an adult protective service (APS) agency. When geriatric assessment teams work with APS agencies, the chances of identifying the perpetrator and taking corrective action are greatly increased (Dyer et al, 1999).

A newly developing nursing specialty is forensic nursing. These nurses care for the injuries and emotional distress of the victims, while collecting and preserving evidence of the crimes for the legal system. Through continued support, these nurses can aid the healing process and provide information to prevent further victimization. This focus is added to that of psychiatric nursing specialists, who intervene with perpetrators of violent or sexual acts (Barton, 1995).

FIREARMS

A firearm in the home can potentially offer both benefits and risks. "Having a gun in the home might affect the risk of homicide, suicide, or unintentional firearm injury," stated Cummings and Koepsell (1998). Community training programs for the care and safe use of legal firearms have addressed gun safety issues for several decades. However, firearms are associated with high rates of suicide among older men and women (Adamek and Kaplan, 1996; Kaplan et al, 1997). When mortality records of three age-groups of white and black men ages 65 and older were examined, firearms accounted for 80% of all suicides (Adamek and Kaplan, 1996).

Contrary to myths about methods of suicide among women, firearms have become the most common suicide method among women ages 65 and older. A study found that the risk of suicide by firearms varied significantly across culturally diverse groups of older women (Kaplan et al, 1997). Suicide rates among older adults continue to be the highest of any age-group. The age-group with the highest rate of successful suicide attempt with firearms is persons ages 80 and over. In one retrospective study a large percentage of suicide victims saw a health care provider within 6 months before their death (Purcell, Thrush, and Blanchette, 1999). Suicide is often associated with alcohol or drug dependence. In fact, in addition to advancing age in men, alcohol and drug dependence are among the greatest risk factors (see Chapter 18).

Other dangers of firearms in the home of older adults include the potential for accidental injury during weapon cleaning and handling. Another concern is the risk of a criminal entering a home and taking the weapon away from an older person, which often has fatal consequences.

Home Care

1. Assess the home environment for the presence of hazards and risk factors that predispose homebound older adults to falls.
2. Carefully assess the physical status of homebound older adults for risk factors that predispose them to falls (i.e., examine feet, gait, vision, posture, muscle control, and memory).
3. Instruct caregivers and homebound older adults on tools and techniques to maximize independent functioning.
4. Assist caregivers and homebound older adults in planning a safe environment for the older adults based on the identified risks and hazards.
5. Emphasize the value of physical therapy in assessing the home setting; determine what environmental adaptations should be made to make it safer and easier for homebound older adults.
6. Teach older adults the effects of prescribed medications, focusing on the potential risks associated with falling. Instructions to decrease the effects of orthostatic hypotension, such as rising slowly and waiting 1 to 2 minutes before standing, are important in preventing falls.
7. For frail older adults, ascertain that emergency phone numbers are located in accessible locations throughout the home; identify emergency call buttons or boxes and alarms.
8. Assess community-dwelling older adults' homes for hazards associated with fire and heat, chemicals, food handling, storage of medications and health care supplies, and firearms, and instruct or make recommendations to promote a safe, hazard-free environment.
9. Assess the temperature of the home environment during seasons of extremely high or low temperatures. Refer homebound older adults to area energy-assistance programs if indicated, or to other community agencies that provide heating and cooling assistance.
10. Be alert to signs of abuse and neglect of homebound older adults by caregivers. If abuse or neglect is suspected, follow the reporting laws of the given state.

SUMMARY

The concept of safety encompasses many aspects of an older person's internal and external environment. The challenge for the nurse caring for older clients is to conduct individualized safety assessments, to identify age-related risk factors that affect safety, and to develop interventions aimed at the prevention of harm and injury.

Fall-related injuries are common among older adults. It is essential to identify some of the more common risk factors before planning nursing interventions or preventive measures. Risk factors include environmental issues and existing health conditions.

Nurses must also consider nonfall-related injuries such as burns; poisoning with carbon monoxide or pesticides; seasonal safety issues with hyperthermia and hypothermia; motor vehicle accidents; crimes and abuse; and suicide. Gerontologic nurses can be on the cutting edge for developing nursing interventions and seeking research opportunities that highlight safety issues among independent older adults. Client assessment and education concerning safety matters must be incorporated into every discharge plan and, in the case of primary care, into each clinic or office visit. The most challenging step to promoting safety in the homes of older adults is the prevention of injuries and illnesses from environmental hazards.

Key Points

- Safety and freedom from harm are essential to an older adult's sense of well-being.
- A direct correlation exists between an older person's sense of autonomy and his or her sense of personal safety.
- Risk factors contributing to falls in older adults include sensory impairment, cognitive impairment, unsafe living environments (e.g., poor lighting, staircases and walkways in poor repair or without hand rails, lack of grab bars in bathrooms, unsecured or worn rugs, and unstable furniture), and a history of falls.
- Thorough and accurate assessment of the risk factors related to falls is essential.
- Methods for preventing falls in older adults may include exercise programs, alarms, and safer environmental conditions.
- As a leading cause of injury in older adults, burns can occur from scalds associated with bathing, cooking, fireplace hazards, use of space heaters, and careless smoking in the home. Chemical burns or injuries can occur when mixing or storing household chemicals, including pesticides and herbicides.
- Carbon monoxide poisoning is preventable through maintenance and repair of heating sources in the home and detection with properly placed carbon monoxide detectors.
- Fan injuries can occur when proper guards are not in place over the fan blade housing on floor and table fan models, or during the cleaning of overhead fans. Maintenance is essential to the safe use of fans and all other electrical equipment in the home.
- Foodborne illnesses can be prevented through careful cleaning of all foods before cooking and cleaning of the food preparation area before, during, and after meal preparation.
- Seasonal safety issues include hyperthermia during hot weather and hypothermia during cold weather. Extra precautions are needed when older adults experience decreased sensation to extremes in weather conditions.
- Neighborhood safety programs for older adults, especially homebound persons or those living alone, should become a component of all neighborhood watch organizations.
- Operating a motor vehicle is often a basic ingredient in an older adult's independence. Yet with this independence comes increased risk for accidents, mainly as a result of decreased visual acuity and peripheral vision.
- Many older adults are victims of abuse, usually from a relative. Risk factors include poor health, physical or mental dependency, advanced age, and alcohol abuse.
- The maintenance of firearms in the homes of older adults can present special problems. The safety of the equipment, need for its use, ability to manage firearms, and safety of others in the home must be considered.
- Suicide is a leading cause of death in older adults. It is often associated with poor physical or psychologic health, alcohol or drug abuse, a history of suicide attempts, and social isolation.
- Nurses must be aware of the risk factors associated with safety and injury in older adults, and they must implement the necessary methods to prevent injuries.

Critical Thinking Exercises

1. A 72-year-old woman is hospitalized for management of her diabetes. She has a history of functional urinary incontinence and poor vision from the diabetes. The nursing staff observes her climbing over the side rails on numerous occasions at night en route to the bathroom. She is quite agitated during this time. The nursing assistant requests that you obtain an order for a body restraint at night to prevent her from falling out of bed. Should this client be restrained to prevent injury? Would you request the order for a body restraint? Why or why not? What other information is relevant to this case? What nursing interventions could be tried before considering a restraint?
2. A 75-year-old woman, hospitalized on a medical/surgical unit, shares a room with another older adult. You see her sitting on the edge of her bed with her feet dangling about 2 feet from the floor. She has two intravenous lines and a Foley catheter. The Foley catheter is hanging on the floor beneath her feet as she sits on the edge of her bed. Her bed is next to a window, which is usually left open. In the middle of the night she climbs over the side rails to get out of bed and walks barefoot to the bathroom, which is about 30 feet away. She tells you she hangs onto her intravenous pole to steady her balance and drags her Foley catheter bag alongside. What environmental hazards can you identify, and what environmental modifications could you make to improve her safety?
3. You are a home care nurse visiting a 72-year-old man in his small second-story apartment, following his discharge from the hospital after having two toes amputated due to frostbite injuries. During your initial visit you note that he lives in a two-room, dimly lit, musty-smelling apartment. Stacks of newspapers and old mail are scattered in both rooms. The temperature is noted to be 68° F on the wall thermostat. Cold drafts can be felt around the large window in the bedroom. List the safety hazards in this apartment and identify nursing interventions that will improve the client's living conditions.

References

Adamek ME, Kaplan MS: Firearm suicide among older men, *Psychiatr Serv* 47(3):304, 1996.

Administration on Aging: The national elder abuse incidence study: final report, Washington, DC, 1998, National Aging Information Center, US Department of Health and Human Services.

Agostini JV, Han L, Tinetti ME: The relationship between number of medications and weight loss or impaired balance in older adults, *J Am Geriatr Soc* 52(10):1719-1723, 2004.

Arfken CL et al: The prevalence and correlates of fear of falling in elderly persons living in the community, *Am J Pub Health* 84(4):565, 1994.

Ashley MJ et al: Smoking in the home: changing attitudes and current practices, *Am J Pub Health* 88(5):797, 1998.

Ballester JM, Harchelroad FP: Hypothermia: an easy-to-miss, dangerous disorder in winter weather, *Geriatrics* 54(2):51, 1999.

Barrow MW, Clark KA: Heat-related illnesses, *Am Fam Phys* 58(3):749, 1998.

Barton S: Investigating forensic nursing, *Kansas Nurse* 70(6):3, 1995.

Bazargan M: The effects of health, environmental, and socio-psychological variables on fear of crime and its consequences among urban black elderly individuals, *Int J Aging Human Development* 38(2):99, 1994.

Bell AF, Talbot-Stern JK, Hennessy A: Characteristics and outcomes of older patients presenting to the emergency department after a fall: a retrospective analysis, *Med J Australia* 173(4):176, 2000.

Bird PE et al: Elder abuse: a call to action, *J Burn Care Rehabil* 19(6):522, 1998.

Burker EJ et al: Predictors of fear of falling in dizzy and nondizzy elderly, *Psychol Aging* 10(1):104, 1995.

Butler RN: Warning signs of elder abuse, *Geriatrics* 54(3):3, 1999.

Carleton RA et al: Fire deaths from smoking, *N Engl J Med* 301(7):389, 1979.

Carr D et al: Differentiating drivers with dementia of the Alzheimer type from healthy older persons with a traffic sign naming test, *J Gerontol A Biol Sci Med Sci* 53(2):135, 1998.

Carrougher GJ: Inhalation injury, *AACN Clin Issues Crit Care Nurs* 4(2):367, 1993.

Centers for Disease Control and Prevention: *Check for safety: a home fall prevention checklist for older adults*, Atlanta, 2004, The Centers.

Centers for Disease Control and Prevention: Web-based injury statistics query and reporting system (WISQARS), 2003, National Center for Injury Prevention and Control, Centers for Disease Control and Prevention. Accessed Nov 28, 1999, from website: www.cdc.gov/ncipc/wisqars.

Centers for Disease Control and Prevention: *National summary of injury mortality data, 1988-1994*, Atlanta, 1996, The Centers.

Centers for Disease Control and Prevention: Deaths resulting from residential fires and the prevalence of smoke alarms—United States, 1991-1995. *JAMA* 280(16):1395, 1998.

Chu NL: Environment/home. In Luggen AS, Travis SS, Meiner S, editors: *NGNA core curriculum for gerontological advanced practice nurses*, Thousand Oaks, Calif, 1998, Sage.

Cromwell S: Social issues: abuse and violence. In Robinson DL, editor: *Core concepts for advance practice nursing*, St Louis, 1999, Mosby.

Cummings P, Koepsell TD: Does owning a firearm increase or decrease the risk of death? *JAMA* 280(5):471, 1998.

Davis LL: Environmental heat-related illnesses, *Med Surg Nurs* 6(3):153, 1997.

Dayhoff NE et al: Balance and muscle strength as predictors of frailty among older adults, *J Gerontol Nurs* 24(7):18, 1998.

Drescher MJ et al: Heating oil company responses to inquiries concerning carbon monoxide toxicity, *Ann Emerg Med* 33(4):406, 1999.

Dyer CB et al: Treating elder neglect: collaboration between a geriatrics assessment team and adult protective services, *Southern Med J* 92(2): 242, 1999.

Ebersole P, Hess P, Luggen AS: *Toward healthy aging: human needs and nursing response*, ed 6, St Louis, 2004, Mosby.

Finelli P, Lee N: Stroke and automobile accidents, *Conn Med* 60(3):145, 1996.

Fisk GD, Owsley C, Mennemeier M: Vision, attention, and self-reported driving behaviors in community-dwelling stroke survivors, *Arch Phys Med Rehab* 83(4):469-477, 2002.

Fisk GD, Owsley C, Pulley LV: Driving after stroke: driving exposure, advice, and evaluations, *Arch Phys Med Rehabil* 78(12):1338, 1997.

Franzoni S et al: Fear of falling in nursing home patients, *Gerontology* 40(1):38, 1994.

Gallo JJ, Rebok BW, Lesikar SE: The driving habits of adults aged 60 years and older, *J Am Geriatr Soc* 47(3):335, 1999.

Gill TM et al: A population-based study of environmental hazards in the homes of older persons, *Am J Pub Health* 89(4):553, 1999.

Gray-Miceli D: Falling among older individuals: exploring psychological issues, *Adv Nurse Pract* 5:7, 1997.

Guerrier JH, Manivannan P, Nair SN: The role of working memory, field dependence, visual search, and reaction time in the left turn performance of older female drivers, *Applied Ergonomics* 30(2):109, 1999.

Harper RD, Dickson WA: Reducing the burn risk to elderly persons living in residential care, *Burns* 21(3):205, 1995.

Harvey PA et al: Residential smoke alarms and fire escape plans, *Pub Health Rep* 113(5):459, 1998.

Hausdorff JM, Rios DA, Edelber HK: Gait variability and fall risk in community-living older adults: a 1-year prospective study, *Arch Phys Med Rehab* 82(8):10050, 2001.

Heikkila HV et al: Decreased driving ability in people with Parkinson's disease, *J Neurol Neurosurg Psychiatr* 64(3):325, 1998.

Hett HA, Brechtelsbauer DA: Heat-related illness: plan ahead to protect your patients, *Postgrad Med* 103(6):107, 1998.

Houck PM, Hampson NB: Epidemic carbon monoxide poisoning following a winter storm *J Emerg Med* 15(4):469, 1997.

Howland J et al: Covariates of fear of falling and associated activity curtailment, *Gerontologist* 38(5):549, 1998.

Jager TE et al: Traumatic brain injuries evaluated in U.S. emergency departments, 1992-1994, *Acad Emerg Med* 7(2):134, 2000.

Jones JS, Holstege C, Holstege H: Elder abuse and neglect: understanding the causes and potential risk factors, *Am J Emerg Med* 15(6):579, 1997.

Kaplan MS et al: Firearm suicide among older women in the U.S., *Soc Sci Med* 44(9):1427, 1997.

Lanson S: Pesticide poisoning: an environmental emergency, *J Emerg Nurs* 23(6):516, 1997.

Lee HL, Chen KW, Wu MH: Acute poisoning with a herbicide containing imazapyr (arsenal): a report of six cases, *J Toxicol Clin Toxicol* 37(1): 83-89, 1999.

Lee-Chiong TL: Smoke inhalation injury, *Postgrad Med* 105(2):55, 1999.

Leistikow BN, Shipley MJ: Might stopping smoking reduce injury death risks? A meta-analysis of randomized, controlled trials, *Prevent Med* 28(3):255, 1999.

Lindsay R: The burden of osteoporosis: cost, *Am J Med* 98:9S, 1995.

Liporace FA et al: What's new in hip fractures? Current concepts, *Am J Orthop* 34(2):66-74, 2005.

Murphy SL: Deaths: final data for 1998, *National Vital Statistics Reports*, 48(11), Hyattsville, Md, 2000, National Center for Health Statistics.

National Agricultural Safety Database: A consumer guide to safe handling and preparation of ground meat and ground poultry, 1996, Accessed from website: www.cdc.gov/nasd/docs/d001201-d001300/d001229/d001229.html.

National Agricultural Safety Database: Fire extinguishers, 2002a. Accessed from website: www.cdc.gov/nasd/docs/d0001101-d001200/d001102/d001102.html.

National Agricultural Safety Database: Kitchen safety, 2002b. Accessed from website: www.cdc.gov/nasd/docs/d000801-d000900/d000825/d000825.html.

Nevitt MC, Cummings SR: Type of fall and risk of hip and wrist fractures: the study of osteoporotic fractures, *J Am Geriatr Soc* 42(8):909, 1994.

Parashar UD et al: An outbreak of viral gastroenteritis associated with consumption of sandwiches: implications for the control of transmission by food handlers, *Epidemiol Infect* 121(3):615, 1998.

Phillips LR: The fit of elder abuse with the family violence paradigm, and implications of a paradigm shift for clinical practice, *Pub Health Nurs* 5:222, 1988.

Potts JR: Ceiling fan injuries: the Townsville experience, *Med J Australia* 170(3):119, 1999.

Purcell D, Thrush CR, Blanchette PL: Suicide among the elderly in Honolulu County: a multiethnic comparative study (1987-1992), *Int Psychogeriatr* 11(1):57, 1999.

Skidmore-Roth L, McKenry L: *Mosby's drug guide for nurses 2005*, ed 6, St Louis, 2005, Mosby.

Stevens JA, Olson S: Reducing falls and resulting hip fractures among older women. In Centers for Disease Control and Prevention: Recommendations regarding selected conditions affecting women's health, *Morbid Mortal Weekly Rep* 49(RR-2):3, 2000.

Tearle P: Fire awareness in the office and laboratory, *Commun Dis Pub Health* 1(4):290, 1998.

Tideiksaar R: *Falls in older persons: prevention and management*, ed 3, Baltimore, 2005, Health Professions Press.

Tinetti ME: Tinetti balance and gait evaluation. In Brady R, Chester F, Pierce L, editors: Geriatric falls: prevention strategies for the staff, *J Gerontol Nurs* 19(9):26, 1993.

Tinetti ME: Performance oriented assessment of mobility problems in elderly patients, *J Am Geriatr Soc* 34:199, 1986.

Tinetti ME, McAvay G, Claus E: Does multiple risk factor reduction explain the reduction in fall rate in the Yale FICSIT Trial? Frailty and injuries cooperative studies of intervention techniques, *Am J Epidemiol* 144(4):389, 1996.

US Department of Health and Human Services: *Healthy people 2000: midcourse review and 1995 objectives*, Washington, DC, 1995, National Institutes of Health.

Vellas BJ et al: Fear of falling and restriction of mobility in elderly fallers, *Age Aging* 26(3):189, 1997.

Warde J: *The healthy home handbook: all you need to know to rid your home of health and safety hazards*, New York, 1997, Random House.

Worfolk JB: Keep frail elders warm, *Geriatr Nurs* 18(1):7, 1997.

Wrenn K, Conners GP: Carbon monoxide poisoning during ice storms: a tale of two cities, *J Emerg Med* 15(4):465, 1997.

Yang S et al: Multistate surveillance for food handling, preparation, and consumption behaviors associated with foodborne diseases: 1995 and 1996 BRFSS food-safety questions, *Morbid Mortal Weekly Rep: CDC Surveillance* 47(4):33, 1998.

Yoon SS, Macdonald SC, Parrish RG: Deaths from unintentional carbon monoxide poisoning and potential for prevention with carbon monoxide detectors, *JAMA* 279(9):685, 1998.

13 Intimacy and Sexuality

PHYLLIS J. ATKINSON, MS, RN, APRN, BC

Learning Objectives

On completion of this chapter, the reader will be able to:

1. Identify the myths surrounding sexual practice in older adults.
2. Explore the possible reasons for a nurse's hesitancy in assisting older adults with fulfilling their sexual desires.
3. Describe the normal changes of the aging male and female sexual systems.
4. Describe the pathologic problems of the aging male and female sexual systems.
5. Explain the influence of dementia on older adults' sexual desires and practices.
6. Discuss the environmental barriers to older adults' sexual practices and the ways to manipulate these barriers.
7. Conduct an assessment interview related to an older adult's sexuality and intimacy.
8. State two nursing diagnoses applicable to older adults' sexual practices.
9. Plan nursing interventions for assisting older adults in fulfilling their sexual desires.
10. State one alternative to an older adult's sexual practice other than sexual intercourse.

OLDER ADULTS' SEXUAL NEEDS

Sexuality is an important part of health, general well-being, and quality of life (Nusbaum, Singh, and Pyles, 2004). Human sexuality includes various types of intimate activity, as well as the sexual knowledge, beliefs, attitudes, and values of individuals. Not only does sexual activity provide pleasure for older adults, it may also help maintain a sense of usefulness and self-esteem, aspects of life often diminished following retirement. Sexual activity can help each partner express love, affection, and loyalty. It can also enhance personal growth, creativity, and communication. Older persons, especially older women, who feel desirable and attractive often feel younger as well (Messinger-Rapport, Sandhu, and Hujer, 2003).

In the 1999 AARP/*Modern Maturity* sexuality study, older adults reported that a satisfying sexual relationship is an important part of life. Although the need to express sexuality continues among older adults, they face several barriers to sexual expression, including problems arising from aging, disease, and medications; societal beliefs; and changes in social circumstances (AARP, 1999; Messinger-Rapport, Sandhu, and Hujer, 2003). Nurses are in a pivotal position to assess normal aging changes, along with those caused by disabling medical conditions and medications, and to intervene at an early point to enhance sexuality in older adults. This chapter explores both normal and pathologic aspects of sexuality for older adults. The obstacles in assessing and managing sexuality in the various care settings in which older adults reside are discussed. Finally, it proposes the application of the nursing process to older adults' intimacy and sexuality needs.

THE IMPORTANCE OF INTIMACY AMONG OLDER ADULTS

Despite the fact that the literature supports the existence of sexual interest and practice in older adults, health care professionals carry out few interventions to facilitate older adults' expression of sexuality. One reason for this is that society continually equates sexuality with sexual intercourse. However, sexuality extends beyond sexual intercourse. In fact, if sexuality among older adults is viewed as a need for intimacy, society and health care professionals may be more comfortable in helping older adults meet those needs.

The absence of male partners for older women propagates the stereotype that older adults should not participate in sexual relationships. The life span of men in the United States is shorter than that of women. For every man over the age of 85 there are 2.5 women (*Older Americans 2000,* 2004). This often leaves older women without sexual partners. The loss of a partner does not necessarily mean that the woman does not have continuing sexual needs. In a recent study Nusbaum, Singh, and Pyles (2004) found that older women had a similar number of sexual concerns as younger women, but were less likely to have the topic of sexual health raised during health care visits. It is imperative that health care professionals value the continuing sexual needs of older women as much as those of younger individuals and provide interventions for fulfilling sexuality.

At times such interventions might include increasing socialization for older women to assist them with finding new partners. Older adults may be reluctant to begin dating, feeling unfamiliar with dating practices. How to date and make new relationships can be challenging (Butler and Lewis, 2000). Alternatively, masturbation is a method in which both men and women can be sexually fulfilled in the absence of partners. Negative generational attitudes about masturbation and homosexuality can interfere with sexual expression (Butler and Lewis, 2000). Assisting older adults with masturbation may appear beyond a nurse's ability; however, there are excellent references available within commercial bookstores to help older adults use this method to become sexually fulfilled.

The literature has established that in addition to older adults' ongoing need to express their sexuality through traditional sexual methods, older adults also must fulfill the human need to touch and to be touched. A person's need for intimacy and closeness to another does not end at any age (Kaiser, 2000a, 2000b). There is little information about the role of touch as a substitute or addition to the sexual practices of older adults. It is known that touch is an overt expression of closeness, intimacy, and sexuality and is an integral part of sexuality.

The importance of touch is often undervalued by society. In fact, touch is often thought of as the invasion of a person's space. For legal as well as privacy reasons, many people have shied away from touching. To older adults experiencing touch deprivation, the social rules that govern touch may be devastating. It is important to remember that touch is a way in which older adults may fulfill their sexuality with each other. Touch may be both a welcome addition to traditional sexual methods and an alternative means of sexual expression when intercourse is not desired or possible.

When older adults are not able to participate in sexual relationships with others, the nurse's use of touch is fundamental in preventing touch deprivation. Therapeutic touch is an alternative nursing intervention developed by Kreiger and Kunz. Based on Martha Roger's Science of Unitary Human Beings, therapeutic touch has been widely used to diminish anxiety, accelerate healing, and decrease pain. The use of therapeutic touch in fulfilling the sexuality of older adults is an exciting, yet understudied, area of nursing.

Despite the continuing need for sexuality, older adults may have difficulty accepting and understanding their sexuality. Sexuality and sexual expression were not formally or informally taught during the developmental years of today's cohort of older adults. In fact, sexuality was hidden behind closed doors for most of these older adults' lives. Therefore the sexuality assessment of an older adult may be the first opportunity he or she has to openly discuss sexuality. Embarrassment, shyness, and apprehension in this area are common. In addition, the client may view the normal changes of aging as embarrassing or indicative of illness and may be reluctant to discuss these matters with a nurse. Some are misinformed about sexuality and may refuse to discuss sexual issues about which they harbor feelings of guilt and shame (Butler and Lewis, 2000; National Council on Aging, 2004). Understanding older adults' attitudes and myths about aging will help the nurse assess and intervene to sensitively promote the expression of sexuality.

NURSING'S RELUCTANCE TO MANAGE THE SEXUALITY OF OLDER ADULTS

Over the past few years the literature exploring the sexuality of older adults has expanded greatly. However, this information is not always applied clinically. Several reasons account for this lack of implementation. The most obvious continues to be society's distaste for and lack of insight into the sexual behavior of older adults. The thought of older, often disabled, people engaging in sexual intercourse is not appealing to society. Nurses often share society's ageist beliefs about the asexuality of older adults, which can lead to nurses discouraging sexual activity (Messinger-Rapport, Sandhu, and Hujer, 2003).

In long-term care facilities, there is an increased need to address the sexual needs of older adults because of the prevalence of disabilities. Long-term care residents face many barriers to sexual expression. Absence of a suitable partner and lack of privacy have been cited as the two most common impediments. Family members of nursing home residents often believe that older adults are or should be asexual and encourage staff not to allow sexual activity (Messinger-Rapport, Sandhu, and Hujer, 2003).

Acute care nurses are in a key position to address newly developed or potential sexual dysfunctions before discharge to a community setting or long-term care environment. However, because of discomfort, myths, and lack of training in the area of sexuality, these problems are often ignored. The end result is that older adults are discharged home or to another setting with a newly developed or chronic sexual dysfunction that prevents them from functioning sexually.

In the community setting, nurses have access to the client's entire family unit in his or her natural surroundings. The information needed to make a sexual assessment is therefore readily accessible. Yet nurses may feel intimidated or uncomfortable questioning older adults about their sexual desires and needs. Consequently, the information needed for proper intervention is not obtained.

As a result of these factors, nurses have recoiled from venturing into such uncharted territory. The end result is that sexually interested older adults are in a situation in which they may have multiple disabilities, no privacy, no support, and no appropriate way in which to express their sexual feelings (Wallace, 2004).

NORMAL CHANGES OF THE AGING SEXUAL RESPONSE

To assist older adults in fulfilling their sexual desires most effectively, it is critical nurses understand the normal changes of the aging sexual system. Knowledge about these normal changes enables the nurse to work more confidently with the client to compensate for these changes, to assist the client in understanding these changes, and to become aware of possible pathologic problems within the aging sexual system.

The four sequential responses to sexual stimulation (excitement, plateau, orgasm, resolution) are affected in a similar manner by the aging process in both men and women (Messinger-Rapport, Sandhu, and Hujer, 2003):

- The excitement phase prolongs with age in both men and women.
- A longer period of stimulation is typically required for both men and women to reach orgasm.
- The refractory period following orgasm is also longer for both men and women.

In both genders the reduced availability of sex hormones in older adults results in less rapid and less extreme vascular responses to sexual arousal (Butler and Lewis, 2000). Although some older adults view this gradual slowing as a decline in function, others do not consider it an impairment, since it merely results in them taking more time to achieve orgasm (Butler and Lewis, 2000).

Common physiologic changes associated with aging men are an erection that is less firm and shorter acting, less preejaculatory fluid, and semen that is less forceful at ejaculation (Butler and Lewis, 2000; Messinger-Rapport, Sandhu, and Hujer, 2003). The refractory period between ejaculations is long. Andropause (male menopause) has several physical, sexual, and emotional symptoms. A decline in concentration of testosterone is believed to be the cause of andropause (Matsumoto, 2002). Testosterone levels diminish with age from a reduction in both testosterone production and metabolic clearance. These hormonal changes lead to a loss of libido, decreased muscle mass and strength, alterations in memory, diminished energy and well-being, increase in sleep disturbance, and possibly osteoporosis secondary to a decrease in bone mass. Testosterone appears to influence the frequency of nocturnal erections; however, low testosterone levels do not affect erections produced by erotic stimuli (Kaiser, 2000a; Messinger-Rapport, Sandhu, and Hujer, 2003). Despite these physiologic changes, aging men can still experience orgasmic pleasure (Messinger-Rapport, Sandhu, and Hujer, 2003).

Erectile dysfunction (impotence), the inability to develop and sustain an erection for satisfactory sexual intercourse in 50% or more attempts at intercourse, can occur at any age but does increase with age (Kaiser, 2000a). Causes of erectile dysfunction include structural abnormalities of the penis; the adverse effects of drugs; psychologic disorders; and vascular, neurologic, and endocrine disorders. It is most common to have more than one cause of erectile dysfunction (Kaiser, 2000a).

Women usually do not have difficulty maintaining sexual function in older age unless a medical condition intervenes. The infrequency of sexual activity for older women is usually not a result of their own sexual capacity and desire but a result of the age, health, and sexual function of their partner, as well as the availability of a partner (Butler and Lewis, 2000). Most sexual changes occur with menopause, including atrophic vaginitis, with dryness of the vaginal mucosa leading to irritation or pain and bleeding during intercourse (Butler and Lewis, 2000; Messinger-Rapport, Sandhu, and Hujer, 2003). Urinary incontinence from detrusor insufficiency or stress can cause embarrassment during intercourse (Messinger-Rapport, Sandhu, and Hujer, 2003). The age-related shortening and narrowing of the vagina may further compromise pleasurable intercourse (Butler and Lewis, 2000). Women may also have increased facial hair from decreased estrogen levels, causing them to feel less attractive (Butler and Lewis, 2000).

Libido appears to be testosterone dependent in both men and women. Women experience a decline in both ovarian hormones and adrenal androgens in the years preceding menopause. This can cause a diminished sense of well-being, loss of energy, loss of bone mass, and decrease or loss of libido (Kaiser, 2000b). Some of the causes of decreased libido include low bioavailable testosterone, elevated prolactin, and, indirectly, decreased estrogen. Incontinence can also decrease libido and inhibit arousal (Kaiser, 2000b). Dyspareunia, painful intercourse or pain with attempted intercourse, is a condition older women often experience, resulting in a decreased desire to participate in sexual activity. About one third of sexually active women over the age of 65 experience dyspareunia. Causes of dyspareunia include inadequate vaginal lubrication, irritation and dryness of the external genitalia, urethritis, improper entry of penis, anorectal disease, altered anatomy of the female genital tract, vulvovaginitis, local trauma (e.g., episiotomy scars), and even arthritis (Kaiser, 2000b). Vaginismus, involuntary painful contraction (spasm) of the lower vaginal muscles, is also often experienced by older women, again decreasing their desire to participate in sexual activity. Causes may be related to dyspareunia, vaginal infections, or vaginal mucosal irritation. It may be triggered by fear of losing control or of being hurt during intercourse (Kaiser, 2000b).

Changes associated with the aging sexual system may have important consequences. It is common for older adults to be uncomfortable with the changes in their internal and external sexual systems.

PATHOLOGIC CONDITIONS AFFECTING OLDER ADULTS' SEXUAL RESPONSES

Illness, Surgery, and Medication. Sexual function is a process that depends on the neurologic, endocrine, and vascular systems. It is also influenced by several psychosocial factors, including family and religious beliefs, the sexual partner, and the individual's self-esteem (Nusbaum, Hamilton, and Lenahan, 2003). Several medical disorders common to older adults can affect sexual function (Box 13-1).

BOX 13-1 Medical Conditions That Affect Sexual Function

CARDIAC CONDITIONS
Congestive heart failure
Myocardial infarction
Angina
Arrhythmias
Hypertension

ENDOCRINE CONDITIONS
Diabetes mellitus
Hypothyroidism

GENITOURINARY CONDITIONS
Prostatitis
Cystitis and urethritis
Chronic renal failure

IMMUNE CONDITIONS
HIV/AIDS
Cancer

MUSCULOSKELETAL CONDITIONS
Arthritis
Pain syndromes

NEUROLOGIC CONDITIONS
Parkinson's disease
Dementia
Stroke

RESPIRATORY CONDITIONS
Chronic emphysema
Bronchitis
Sleep apnea

Modified from Messinger-Rapport B, Sandhu S, Hujer M: Sex and sexuality: is it over after 60? *Clin Geriatr* 11(10):45, 2003; Nusbaum M, Hamilton C, Lenahan P: Chronic illness and sexual functioning, *Am Fam Phys* 67:347, 2003; American Association for Geriatric Psychiatry: Annual meeting—axis III and beyond: social function and sexuality in late life, 2003. Accessed May 15, 2004, from website: www.cmecorner.com/macmcm/AAGP/aagp2003_06.htm; Butler R, Lewis M: Sexuality. In Beers M, Berkow R, editors: *The Merck manual of geriatrics*, Rahway, NJ, 2000, Merck.

Surgeries can also affect an older adult's sexual responses. Some of theses surgeries include coronary artery bypass surgery; hysterectomy; mastectomy; prostatectomy; orchiectomy; and removal of anus and rectum. In addition, many drugs adversely affect sexuality (Table 13-1).

Human Immunodeficiency Virus

Older adults continue to be a considerable proportion of population infected by human immunodeficiency virus (HIV) (Linsk, 2000). According to the National Center for HIV, STD and TB Prevention's 2002 statistics, those over the age of 50 with acquired immunodeficiency syndrome (AIDS) represent between 11% and 15% of all AIDS cases (National Association on HIV over Fifty, 2004). Statistics indicate older adults are more likely than younger persons to develop AIDS less than 12 months after diagnosis of HIV infection. The estimated number of new diagnoses of HIV/AIDS has also increased among older adults over 65 years of age, from 382 in 1999 to 432 in 2002 (Centers for Disease Control and Prevention, 2004).

Older adults may be at risk for HIV infections if they engage in sex (Linsk, 2000). Despite the fact that older adults do engage in behavior that puts them at risk for HIV infection, they are less likely than younger persons to adopt safer sexual practices, since they do not perceive themselves as being at risk. Some of the reasons older adults do not practice safer sexual behaviors include:

- They see sexually transmitted diseases (STDs) as something that happens to somebody else, since they were settled in marriages when the safe sex battles of the 1980s were raging.
- Older women do not fear pregnancy, since they are postmenopausal, so wearing a condom is not a concern.
- Women outnumber men, giving men many partners to choose from; therefore women try to please their male partners by agreeing to unprotected sex
- Older adults grew up when men made most of the decisions in a relationship, and if a man does not want to use a condom, then it is not used.

Age-related changes also increase the risk of HIV infection. For example, age-related thinning of the vaginal mucosa and the subsequent vaginal tissue disruption, as well as age-related reductions in immune function, place older adults at increased risk for HIV infection. Older adults who do contract HIV are more likely to be diagnosed late in disease and experience progression more quickly, with death from AIDS coming sooner after diagnosis than their younger counterparts (Resnick, 2003).

Malignancies. Breast cancer, one of the leading cancers affecting older women, has clear implications for self-esteem and sexual functioning. The presence of medical illnesses, as well as myths about sexuality and the benefit of treatment to older adults, often prevents clinicians from aggressively treating older women with breast cancer.

Prostate cancer is the most common cancer in men and the second leading cause of death from cancer in men in the United States. The risk of developing prostate cancer increases with age. Radical prostatectomy, a curative treatment, involves massive disturbance of hormone-producing glands, surrounding nerves, and urinary structures. This often results in temporary urinary incontinence and impotence, both affecting a male's sexuality.

Dementia. Clients with dementia should be given special attention to ensure their safety when they decide to engage in sexual relationships. Health care professionals working with

TABLE 13-1 Drugs Adversely Affecting Sexuality

DRUG CLASS	EXAMPLE	EFFECT ON SEXUALITY
Dopamine agonists	Levodopa Ropinirole hydrochloride (Requip) Pramiprexole dihydrochloride (Mirapex) Pergolide mesylate (Permax)	Increased desire
Diuretics	Furosemide (Lasix) Bumetanide (Bumex) Spironolactone (Aldactone)	Incontinence
Anticholinergics	Tolterodine tartrate (Detrol) Metoclopramide (Reglan) Benadryl Lasix NOTE: Many drugs have anticholingeric properties.	Impaired ejaculation
Antipsychotics	Risperidone (Risperdal) Olanzapene (Zyprexa)	Inhibited erection Inhibited ability to ejaculate, even when the capacity for erection remains
Sedatives-hypnotics	Zolpidem tartrate (Ambien) Temazepam (Restoril)	Depressed sexual arousal
Antidepressants	Peroxetine hydrochloride (Paxil) Fluoxetine hydrochloride (Prozac)	Inhibited sexual desire Lack of orgasm
Antihypertensives	Hydrochlorothiazide (HCTZ) Aldactone Atenolol Clonidine Lisinopril Diltiazem hydrochloride (Cardizem)	Erectile dysfunction Incontinence Inhibition of orgasm
Alcohol		Erectile dysfunction Women's sexual function
Antianxieties/benzodiazepines	Lorazepan (Ativan) Alprazolam (Xanax)	Decreased sexual desire Inhibition of orgasm
Anticonvulsants	Phenytoin (Dilantin) Carbamazepine (Tegretol)	Decreased desire Erectile dysfunction

Data from Messinger-Rapport B, Sandhu S, Hujer, M: Sex and sexuality: is it over after 60? *Clin Geriatr* 11(10):45, 2003; Nusbaum M, Hamilton C, Lenahan P: Chronic illness and sexual functioning, *Am Fam Phys* 67:347, 2003; Butler R, Lewis M: Sexuality. In Beers M, Berkow R, editors: *The Merck manual of geriatrics,* Rahway, NJ, 2000, Merck.

cognitively impaired older adults need to determine if the individual is actually consenting to a sexual activity. If the person is unable to consent to participation in a sexual activity and has a surrogate decision maker, that person should be involved with judgments regarding the benefits or potential harm associated with that person's sexual expression (Messinger-Rapport, Sandhu, and Hujer, 2003).

One behavior common among clients with dementia is sexual deviance. Older adults with dementia may masturbate in public, strip themselves of clothing, expose themselves, or make overt gestures to other clients or staff. These behaviors are disturbing to others and often difficult to address. Although there may be no apparent explanation for such behavior, family and staff should consider the possibility that these behaviors are triggered by unmet intimacy needs (Messinger-Rapport, Sandhu, and Hujer, 2003).

The research division of the Hebrew Home for the Aged, under a state-sponsored grant, completed a training video titled, "Freedom of Sexual Expression: Dementia and Resident Rights in Long-Term Care Facilities." More information on the video can be found at www.terranova.org.

ENVIRONMENTAL AND PSYCHOSOCIAL BARRIERS TO SEXUAL PRACTICE

One of the most difficult problems encountered when intervening to assist older adults with meeting sexual needs is overcoming environmental barriers. In the community setting, older couples may be hindered by a lack of assistive equipment needed to safely fulfill their sexual desires. In long-term and acute care facilities, lack of privacy often prevents older clients from pursuing sexual relationships.

Interventions used to overcome these environmental barriers are discussed later in this chapter.

Sexual dysfunction may signal other psychosocial disorders, such as depression, delirium, and dementia. Sexuality can also be affected by anxiety concerning partner availability and lifestyle issues. Substance abuse, including smoking, alcohol, and street drugs, is often associated with sexual dysfunction (American Association for Geriatric Psychiatry, 2003).

ALTERNATIVE SEXUAL PRACTICE AMONG OLDER ADULTS

In addition to the burden caused by society's lack of understanding of the sexuality of older adults, aging homosexuals have the additional burden of society's lack of understanding of homosexuality. Brotman, Ryan, and Cormier (2003) looked at the health and social service needs of older gays and lesbians in Canada. They found much discrimination regarding health and access to health services. Older gays and lesbians who have "come out" to others often need to go into hiding when they need health care services. Aging networks' attitudes and practices toward gays and lesbian older adults have gone unchallenged, resulting in a senior health care system that is even more homophobic than other health care systems (Brotman, Ryan, and Cormier, 2003). Despite prevailing stereotypes, it is important for nurses to recognize that same-sex companionship is an acceptable expression of sexuality for both men and women.

Although change in providing health care to gays and lesbians has been slow, some progress has been made. In Broward County, Florida, for example, Edith Lederberg has been working on opening an adult day care center for frail gay and lesbian elders, which will be the first of its kind (Kanapaux, 2003).

Nurses need to be sure that their own personal beliefs about alternative sexual practices do not prevent older homosexual clients from fulfilling their sexual desires. Examination of his or her own feelings toward this alternative sexual practice may allow the nurse to recognize the meaning of the homosexual lifestyle to the client. This allows the nurse to enter into a therapeutic relationship with these older adults without the interference of personal feelings. Homosexual clients' partners should be encouraged to participate in the sexual assessment and planning when appropriate. Nurses should also remember that no information about the sexual orientation of clients should be shared with a client's family unless permission has been given. See Box 13-2 for questions that can be added to an assessment.

NURSING MANAGEMENT

Assessment

Sexual health may have a direct impact on the well-being of an individual with chronic illnesses (Nusbaum, Hamilton, and Lenahan, 2003). Therefore it is essential to obtain a sexual history, but one of the greatest obstacles in assessing the sexuality of older adults occurs at the beginning of the assessment.

BOX 13-2 Questions on Sexuality

- Are you currently sexually active? If so, with one or more than one partner?
- Male or female partner?
- Are your sexual desires being met?
- Do you have any questions or concerns about your sexual function? About your partner's sexual function?
- What kind of information would you like?

Getting started with the sexual history becomes easier with experience. One challenge nurses face is to help older adults develop and sustain the intimate relationship they desire. This involves active assessment, including actively reviewing health concerns and conditions that affect sexual functioning (Szwabo, 2003). Although discomfort in this area is understandable, increased proficiency comes with experience. According to the Association of Reproductive Health Professionals (ARHP) (2002), healthy sexuality depends on good communication between the health professional and the patient. Nurses are in a pivotal position to begin this communication. A simple sexual history can be performed by nurses and can include questions such as those found in Box 13-2.

Some nurses are more comfortable than others in completing a sexual assessment; however, most can develop skills to (ARHP, 2002):

- Be a sympathetic listener.
- Reassure the patient who has sexual concerns that strategies exist for addressing those concerns.
- Make an appropriate referral if needed.

A detailed sexual history should be completed by the primary care practitioner (nurse practitioner or physician). The PLISSIT model continues to be used to assess and to manage the sexuality of adults (Annon, 1976). The model involves obtaining *p*ermission from clients to initiate sexual discussion, providing the *l*imited *i*nformation they need to function sexually, giving *s*pecific *s*uggestions for individuals to proceed with sexual relations, and providing *i*ntensive *t*herapy regarding the issues of sexuality for clients. The goal of the assessment, regardless of the model used, is to gather information that allows clients to express sexuality safely and to feel uninhibited by normal or pathologic problems.

It is common for nurses and nursing students to feel uncomfortable and embarrassed when assessing the sexual desires and functions of older clients. Regardless, a sexual assessment should be performed as a routine part of the nursing assessment. Knowledge, skill, and a sense of comfort are necessary for the nurse to assess the sexuality of older adults. Nusbaum, Singh, and Pyles (2004) found that although the sexual health care needs of older woman varied, the greatest need was the desire for their health care provider to talk to them about their sexuality (see Research box).

According to ARHP (2002), nurses can take a number of steps to create a nonthreatening environment conducive to communication. They should provide a quiet, private meeting place, and avoid interruptions during the discussion. Nurses should sit at eye level with the patient and ask questions in a manner that is not threatening. Nurses need to avoid using terms that may suggest they are making assumptions about sexual behavior or orientation. For example, when asking about an older adult's sexual orientation, they should avoid using the term *husband* or *wife*, instead using the term *partner*. They also need to avoid medical terminology and the use of slang words (Nusbaum and Hamilton, 2002).

Other components of the sexual history taking include reviewing medications and medical conditions that may contribute to a sexual dysfunction, as discussed earlier. In addition, the nurse should review the older adult's early experiences, if he or she is willing to share. Earlier experiences can have a direct effect on the individual's ability to respond positively to sexuality later in life (Kallejian, 2000). A physical assessment of the breasts and genital tissue is an essential part of the assessment of sexuality. Laboratory tests may be useful in determining reductions in hormone levels that may contribute to decreased libido or erectile dysfunction. Box 13-3 lists laboratory tests relevant to a sexual assessment for older adults.

The nurse should also obtain information on sexual preferences. An assessment of the environments in which clients live should follow. The nurse should determine where clients plan to participate in sexual activity. In acute and long-term care settings the environment should be assessed for privacy and safety. This enables older adults to proceed with sexual activity safely and comfortably. In the community setting the environment should be assessed for safety and the availability of adaptive equipment such as side rails, trapezes, and specialized beds, which may be needed to allow older adults to practice sexual activity safely within the home.

BOX 13-3 Laboratory Tests to Guide Sexual Assessment

- Total serum testosterone
- Dihydrotestosterone
- Estradiol
- Mean gonadotropin-releasing hormone
- Serum luteinizing hormone
- Serum prolactin
- Prostate-specific antigen
- Complete blood count
- Complete metabolic panel
- Thyroid-stimulating hormone

The nursing staff should be cognizant of indications of sexual interest in older adults. Overt gestures of sexuality in public areas or hints of sexual interest during conversations with clients should not be ignored or punished; they should be viewed as an indication of sexual interest between two older adults.

Older adults should not thoughtlessly enter into sexual relationships. Among older adults, there is the added risk factor of potential cognitive impairments, which may hinder clients' decision-making ability. Before a sexual relationship commences, it may be appropriate for the nurse to meet with both clients individually and together to discuss their intentions and expectations regarding the sexual relationship. In so doing, the clients' fears and apprehensions may be expressed and their questions answered. In addition, such a discussion may reveal whether one client is being coerced into the relationship or is not mentally competent to decide to enter into such a relationship.

A cognitive assessment such as a MiniMental State Examination (MMSE) should be performed as part of the assessment of older adults. The information gained from this assessment is useful if the nurse suspects clients are cognitively impaired and unable to make decisions to participate in sexual relationships. If the MMSE does not provide sufficiently clear information regarding clients' decision-making abilities, a more thorough assessment by a psychologic team may be necessary to prevent anyone from taking advantage of these clients.

Research

SAMPLE/SETTING

Departments of Family Practice and Obstetrics and Gynecology at Madigan Army Medical Center, Tacoma, Washington

METHODS

Self-reported sexual concerns and interests in and experience with discussing these concerns with their physicians

FINDINGS

Older women had similar number of sexual concerns as younger women and were more likely to be concerned about their partner's sexual difficulties. Older women are less likely to have the topic of sexual health raised during health care visits. Most women said they would have discussed their concerns had their physician raised the topic.

IMPLICATIONS

Older women want to discuss their sexuality with their health care provider if the topic is raised. All health care providers should have the responsibility of discussing sexuality with the older adults they care for.

Nusbaum M, Singh A, Pyles A: Sexual healthcare needs of women aged 65 and older, *J Am Geriatr Soc* 52:117, 2004.

Diagnosis

After the assessment of older adults' sexuality, the nurse is prepared to make a nursing diagnosis. Several nursing diagnoses are appropriate for older adults experiencing actual or potential sexual problems. The first, "ineffective sexuality patterns," is defined as the expression of concern regarding one's own sexuality (Gulanick et al, 2003). The expected outcome would be that the patient or couple verbalizes satisfaction with the way they express physical intimacy. Both members of the couple exhibit behaviors that are acceptable to the partner (Gulanick et al, 2003). This diagnosis is appropriate when the older adult has experienced a life change that causes a new impediment to sexual functioning. Related factors for this diagnosis in older adults are knowledge or skill deficits about alternative responses to health-related transitions, altered body function or structure, illness or medical treatment, lack of privacy, lack of significant other, conflicts with sexual orientation or variant preferences, fear of acquiring STDs, or impaired relationship with significant other (see Nursing Care Plan on Altered Sexuality Patterns).

Another diagnosis that may be appropriate for older adults experiencing a sexual problem is "sexual dysfunction." The expected outcome would be for the patient to adapt sexual techniques and engage in sexual activity with assistive devices as needed (Gulanick et al, 2003). This diagnosis is appropriate if an older client is exhibiting unacceptable sexual activity, such as exposure. This diagnosis might also be applicable if an aging woman is experiencing dyspareunia or decreased or absent sexual desire (see Nursing Care Plan on Sexual Dysfunction).

Nursing Care Plan
Altered Sexuality Patterns

Clinical Situation: Mr. B, a 76-year-old retired brick layer, comes to the clinic complaining of headaches that have been increasing in severity over the past several months. His initial assessment shows severe hypertension. During the nursing assessment, it is revealed that Mr. B is a widower who lives alone. However, he has a female friend who visits him often, and they have sexual intercourse every 1 to 2 weeks. To date, he has not experienced any problems with his sexual performance. He was placed on a beta-blocker to control his hypertension.

Nursing Diagnosis

Potential altered sexuality patterns related to potential side effects from antihypertensive medication

Outcome

Client will not experience a disruption in his sexual patterns.

Interventions

Instruct client on the normal aging changes of the male and female sexual systems.

Instruct client that impotence is not a normal aging change and may be a side effect of his antihypertensive medication.

Instruct client to notify his physician or advanced practice nurse if impotence or any other sexual problem is noticed.

Suggest that client's partner meet with the nurse and client to discuss current medical condition, normal changes of aging, and the precautions outlined by the CDC.

Nursing Care Plan
Sexual Dysfunction

Clinical Situation: Mr. J is a 74-year-old retired boxer who has resided at a nursing facility for 3 years. He has Parkinson's disease and uses a walker. He is generally happy and pleasant. Mrs. H is an alert 75-year-old widow who was admitted to the facility 1 month ago after a stroke left her wheelchair bound and unable to perform her activities of daily living independently. She was upset when she arrived at the nursing facility and had some difficulty adjusting to her new home.

Over the past 2 weeks a close relationship has developed between the two residents. Mrs. H has been happier than she was on admission, and both residents appear to have a new sense of energy and enthusiasm for life. Recently, the nursing staff has noticed that they display sexual expression and signs of intimacy to each other in public areas.

Nursing Diagnosis

Sexual dysfunction related to lack of privacy

Outcome

Clients will be free to pursue their sexual relationship in private.

Interventions

Perform sexual assessment of both clients.

Provide climate in which both can openly discuss the situation and respond with trust and confidence.

Pay close attention to verbal and nonverbal cues while listening.

Provide reassurance as needed.

Meet with both clients individually to assess each one's desire regarding sexual activity and each one's degree of competence.

Assess level of comfort in discussing topic and issues alone or with each other present; provide opportunity for both.

Provide teaching on normal changes of the aging sexual system (see Box 13-1 and the Client/Family Teaching boxes on p. 276).

Compensate for any physical disabilities assessed.

Implement precautions against the spread of STDs.

Find a safe, private location for the couple to pursue their sexual interests.

Other potential appropriate nursing diagnoses include knowledge deficit, risk for ineffective coping or ineffective coping, self-esteem or body imagine disturbance, social isolation, anxiety, and fear (Gulanick et al, 2003; Swearingen, 2004).

Planning and Expected Outcomes

The nurse should develop an individualized care plan, which includes the information elicited during clients' histories, physical assessments, and discussion about specific sexual relationships. This plan should (1) compensate for the physical disabilities of older adults, (2) prevent the spread of infection, (3) provide for the emotional well-being of older adults, (4) satisfy the needs of family members when possible, and (5) ensure client safety. Expected outcomes of the care plan should result from specific, time-limited goals aimed at restoring or promoting the client's sexual satisfaction.

Expected outcomes include, but are not limited to:

1. Client attains satisfactory level of sexual activity as evidenced by resumption of sexual activity at a level acceptable to the client.
2. Client verbalizes his or her sexual concerns and discusses them with his or her significant other.
3. Client explores alternative sexual activities and practices to attain sexual satisfaction.
4. Client verbalizes his or her feelings about sexual performance.

Intervention

Older adults should be given information, education, and concrete direction to assist them in creating and sustaining intimate relationships (Szwabo, 2003). This needs to start by educating older adults about changes associated with aging. Teaching and reassurance by the nurse that some changes are a normal part of aging helps clients understand their bodies and feel comfortable learning how to compensate for these changes (see Client/Family Teaching boxes). Teaching regarding coital positioning for couples with physically disabling conditions is often a necessary intervention (Fig. 13-1).

As discussed previously, cognitively impaired clients often display inappropriate sexual behavior, such as exposure or advances toward other clients and staff. It is important for the nurse to manage these difficult behaviors while maintaining the dignity of these older adults. Ignoring the behavior or punishing the older adults does not curtail the behavior. A thorough assessment of mental status and sexuality is necessary to isolate the cause of the behavior. Inappropriate behaviors may best be managed by redirecting cognitively impaired older adults' sexual interest toward socially acceptable behaviors, such as providing a quiet place for masturbation and provision of sexually explicit materials (magazines or videos) (Messinger-Rapport, Sandhu, and Hujer, 2003).

When sexual intercourse is not the preferred method of intimacy or is not possible for an older couple, the couple may be taught alternative methods of intimacy in the form of touch. The physical and psychosocial changes of aging affect the ability of older adults to be intimate with one another. Touch is a means of expressing intimacy and closeness that may fulfill older clients' sexual needs and desires. Touch can best be fulfilled by finding a comfortable environment in which an older adult couple can expose parts of their bodies to each other as they feel comfortable. A shower or bath may be enjoyable. The couple should be taught to move their fingertips slowly or lightly over each other's skin while enjoying

Client/Family Teaching

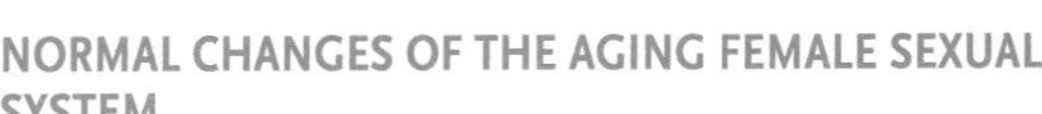

NORMAL CHANGES OF THE AGING FEMALE SEXUAL SYSTEM

Instruct female clients that, with aging:

- Vaginal secretions diminish; the use of an artificial water-based lubricant helps decrease discomfort.
- The vagina becomes shorter and does not expand as well to accommodate the penis. Some discomfort may be experienced, so alternative positions for intercourse (see Fig. 13-1) may help decrease discomfort.
- Orgasmic contractions are fewer and may be accompanied by painful uterine contractions. However, these generally do not indicate pathologic problems.
- Vaginal irritation and clitoral pain are common and do not signify illness.
- The breasts lose tone, and the areolar area does not enlarge as considerably.
- Infrequent rectal sphincter contractions that do not interfere with orgasm and the postcoital need to void may be experienced.

Client/Family Teaching

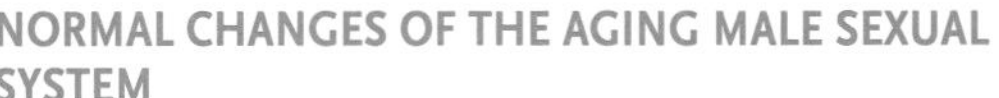

NORMAL CHANGES OF THE AGING MALE SEXUAL SYSTEM

Instruct male clients that, with aging:

- The penis may take longer to become firm and may not be as firm as at a younger age; therefore a longer period of foreplay should be planned.
- Ejaculation may take longer to achieve, may be less expulsive, and may be shorter in duration. The client should conserve strength and not work hard at the beginning of intercourse, which could result in tiring before climax.
- The erection diminishes more quickly after climax, so if condoms are being used, the client should plan to withdraw immediately after climax.
- It takes longer to achieve a second orgasm, so the client should plan to resume foreplay or use this time to touch or talk.
- Rectal sphincter contractions may be experienced, but these do not interfere with orgasm.

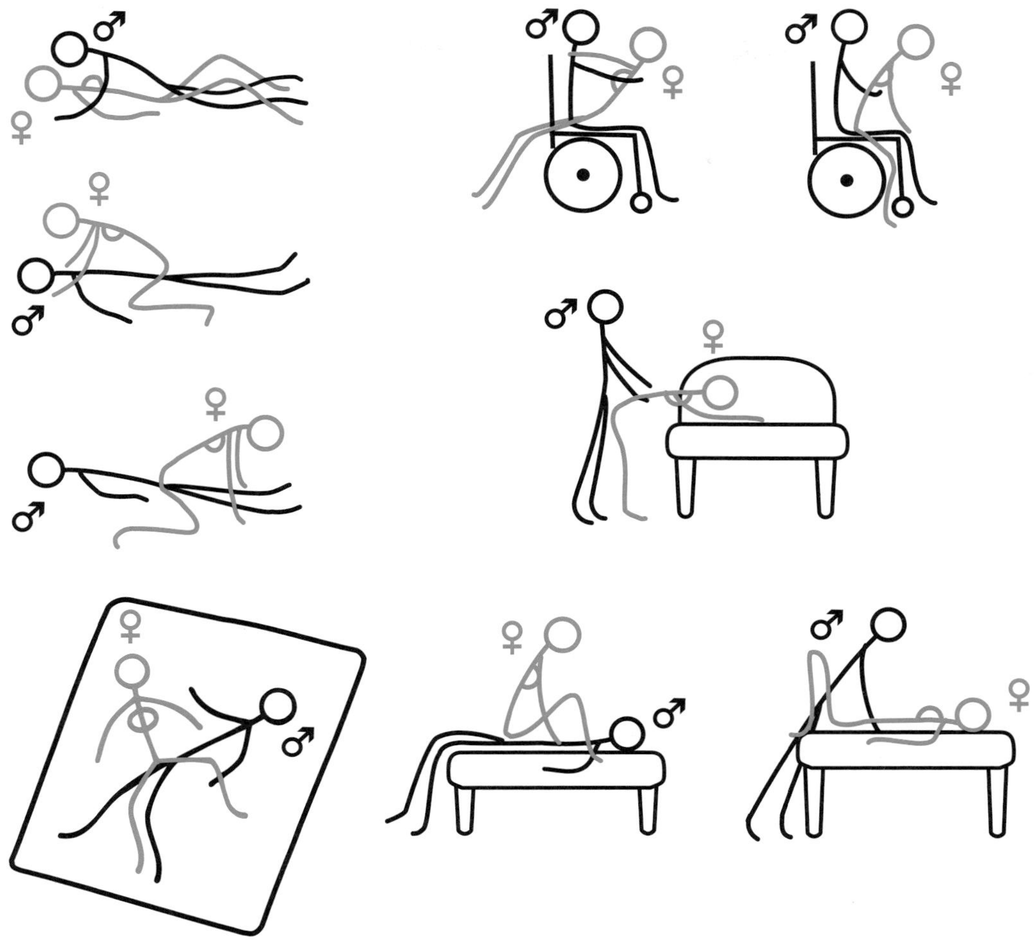

Fig. 13-1 Coital positioning for couples.

the closeness of the other person. Massage therapy, books, and videos may provide older adults a way to touch that results in the fulfillment of sexual desires. Soft music may add to the conducive environment for older couples.

Proper precautions need to be implemented to prevent the spread of disease from one client to another. Older adults are rarely the focus of existing HIV prevention and care services. Low-risk behaviors should be encouraged, such as practicing monogamous relationships, partner reduction, and aggressive use of condoms (male and female versions) (Resnick, 2003). According to the National Association on HIV over Fifty (2004) and AIDS Action (2001), several actions need to occur to prevent the spread of HIV among older adults (Box 13-4).

If an older adult is concerned about his or her family's feelings regarding a sexual relationship, further counseling should be provided and should include the family when possible. At this time family members may bring forth their concerns regarding the relationships, and the older adult may answer them with a nurse present. It is important for the older adult's family to understand and accept his or her decisions about

BOX 13-4 Actions to Prevent Spread of HIV among Older Adults

- Implement specific education programs for older adults on the transmission and prevention of HIV infection.
- Hold workshops and training sessions devoted to basic HIV/AIDS information—including safe sexual practices—all in relationship to aging.
- Fund and support more research pertaining to older adults' sexual behaviors.
- Educate health care professionals on HIV risk behaviors, symptoms of HIV infection, misdiagnoses, testing technologies, treatments, support groups, case management, and the importance of being actively involved in the health and well-being of their older clients.
- Increase media and social marketing campaigns, which can raise awareness of HIV/AIDS in older people and reinforce the need for educational programs, while promoting respect and validation for older adults as a group.

From National Association on HIV over Fifty and AIDS Action, 2004.

relationships. However, if no agreement can be reached that is amenable to both the older adult and family, the older adult's needs must be the nurse's primary consideration.

Becoming more prevalent are policies that incorporate the sexual needs of older adults in care plans (Messinger-Rapport, Sandhu, and Hujer, 2003). Acute and long-term care facilities should make proper arrangements for privacy during older adults' sexual experiences. The physical facilities within each setting vary. The ideal situation is to set up a pleasant room that can be used for a variety of activities but may also be reserved by older adults for private visits with a spouse or partner. In most settings this may not be possible, and client rooms may be used while the nursing staff gains permission from and plans alternate activities for clients' roommates.

In any setting, client safety should be maintained. The call lights should be easily accessible. Side rails on the bed should be used if necessary, and the room should be situated so that the nursing staff is aware of when it is in use. Although the clients' privacy is important, they should not be alone in any situation in which they may injure themselves.

In the community setting, adaptive equipment such as hospital beds, side rails, or trapezes may be needed to allow clients to function safely. Based on the information gathered from assessments, the nurse may assist clients in ordering the necessary devices. The nurse may also need to demonstrate the transfer process to ensure that clients are able to transfer and to function independently, or with the help of the partner. See Box 13-5 for strategies that can enhance sexual function.

Education of nursing staff in issues related to sexuality in older adults has been shown in the past to improve the attitudes toward sexual issues in nursing homes; however, no current studies exist to support this (Kamel, 2001). Open discussion of attitudes and sexual issues among staff can increase comfort with sexual issues. Case studies can be an effective means of education. Education should also be available to the family. The training should begin by discussing and dispelling the myths surrounding older adults' sexual desires and activity. The training should include normal changes associated with older men and women, and how to compensate for specific physical disabilities. A more positive attitude toward the sexual expression of older adults may develop with increased knowledge and may allow such expression to become a natural part of the aging process.

Training should conclude with discussion groups to allow staff and family to discuss their own feelings about sexuality and its role in the life of older adults. Role-playing may be an effective technique to gain understanding of the effect of the staff and family's personal values on older adults.

The use of medications such as sildenafil citrate (Viagra), tadalafil (Cialis), and vardenafil hydrochloride (Levitra) has increased public awareness of the prevalence of impotence among men in the United States. These medications, classified as erectile enhancers, have been thought to be overprescribed and misused among men who are seeking erectile enhancement to increase sexual potency. It has also been suggested that these drugs contributed to the transmission of HIV and other sexual diseases among older adults (Paniagua, 1999). These medications may be effective in treating erectile impotence in older men when appropriately prescribed and therefore may enhance the quality of life for older adults.

BOX 13-5 Strategies To Enhance Sexual Function in Older Adults

DIETARY STRATEGIES

Avoid alcohol or tobacco.
Discuss well-balanced meals with a registered dietitian.

MEDICATION STRATEGIES

Take pain medications before sexual activity if needed.
Discuss with primary care provider (medical doctor or nurse practitioner) discontinuing medications that may impair sexual function.

ENVIRONMENTAL ADAPTATIONS

Plan for sexual activity when most rested.
Allow conjugal visits or home visits.
Live pets provide sensory stimulation.
Offer objects to touch, fondle, and hold such as dolls or stuffed animals for demented older adult.

PSYCHOLOGIC STRATEGIES

Communicate desires to partner.
Discuss fears and concerns with primary care provider.
Encourage routine visits to hairdresser to promote self-esteem and well-being.
Join a support group.
Use relaxation techniques.

PHYSICAL STRATEGIES

Improve exercise tolerance by participating in supervised exercise program.
Use touch, kissing, and hugging.
Use pillows under painful joints.
Take a warm shower before activity.
Get regular check-ups.

Modified from Nusbaum M, Hamilton C, Lenahan P: Chronic illness and sexual functioning, *Am Fam Phys* 67:347, 2003; Kallejian V: It never ends: aging and sexuality, part I: health and age, 2000. Accessed May 15, 2004, from website: www.healthandage.com/Home/?gid2=599&fa=1&path=null&x=43&y=8; National Council on the Aging: Sex after 60: a natural part of life. Accessed May 16, 2004, from website: www.ncoa.org/content.cfm?sectionID=109&detail=134; Kamel H: Sexuality in aging: focus on institutionalized elderly, *Ann Long-Term Care* 9(5):64, 2001.

Evaluation

Evaluation of older adults with sexual health–related concerns is based on client achievement of the established expected outcomes. Older adults can attain a satisfying level of sexual activity that is compatible with functional capacity with the help of sound, sensitive nursing interventions. When total sexual functioning cannot be restored, alternative sexual practices should be explored. The use of touch and massage may be an alternative to sexual intercourse and may help older adults achieve sexual satisfaction. Although many stereotypes hinder the ability of professionals to promote sexuality among older adults, older adults can and should be allowed to achieve their sexual outcomes with the full assistance of the staff. It is important to continue to assess and intervene until the goals have been met. Documentation within the care plan of the sexual diagnosis is an essential method of communicating the interventions and progress toward meeting the expected outcomes. Interventions that have been attempted, including the procurement of artificial aids and teaching, should be documented.

SUMMARY

The need and desire to function sexually continues throughout the life span. It is the nurse's role to disregard the myths of society toward the sexual practices of homosexual, heterosexual, and bisexual older adults, and to assist older adults in reaching their sexual potential. Many normal and pathologic changes are common in older men and women. However, most of these changes can be compensated for so that older adults can continue to practice sexually.

With a thorough nursing assessment and management of the normal and pathologic changes of the aging sexual system, older adults are free to pursue sexuality as desired. The end result can be older adults who are able to pursue the highest quality of life attainable.

Home Care

1. Assess sexual patterns in homebound older adults who have chronic conditions.
2. Provide information regarding sexual positions or sexual function to accommodate environmental barriers (e.g., a Foley catheter) to both homebound older adults and their significant others.
3. Foster a supportive environment for homebound older adults and their partners to discuss sex-related fears, concerns, and feelings.
4. Explain pathologic conditions that may affect older adults' sexual responses, such as types of medications and chronic illnesses.
5. Teach safer sex practices to homebound older adults and their partners.
6. Teach alternate methods of intimacy to both homebound older adults and their significant others, based on identified sexual dysfunctions or alterations.

Key Points

- Sexual desire and interest persist throughout the life span of older adults.
- Nurses are often subject to myths surrounding the sexual practices of older adults and often lack the knowledge and training on how to assist older adults in fulfilling their sexual desires.
- Older adults may experience normal, age-related changes in their sexual systems, which may hinder their sexual response.
- Pathologic problems with the aging sexual response are often related to illnesses and medication.
- Older adults with dementia may display inappropriate sexual behavior and may not be competent to participate in sexual relationships.
- Environmental barriers in the home, as well as in acute and long-term care settings, may prevent older adults from fulfilling their sexual desires.
- It is imperative that all older adults receive a sexual assessment so that normal and pathologic changes can be identified.
- Normal changes of aging can be compensated for by teaching older adults about the changes.
- Interventions used to assist older adults in adapting to age-related changes include manipulation of the environment and procurement of assistive equipment and devices needed to continue to function sexually.
- Touch can be an alternative to sexual intercourse and can provide the intimacy needed by some older adults.

Critical Thinking Exercises

1. A 73-year-old female client confides that she is embarrassed because her 75-year-old male friend wants to know why he is having difficulty getting an erection. She confesses she is very uncomfortable and does not know how to help her friend. What suggestions can you offer in dealing with this sensitive but important matter?
2. A married couple resides in the long-term care facility where you are employed. The husband is ambulatory, but his wife needs a great deal of assistance with her daily care. One afternoon as you enter their room with medication, you find the couple in bed together, and it is obvious they are attempting to have sex. How should you respond? Discuss your feelings about this situation.

REFERENCES

AARP/*Modern Maturity*: Sexuality survey: summary of findings, Aug 1999. Accessed May 15, 2004, from website: http://research.aarp.org/health/mmsexsurvey_1.html.

AIDS Action: Older Americans and HIV/AIDS, 2001. Accessed April 28, 2004, from website: www.aidsaction.org.

American Association for Geriatric Psychiatry: Annual meeting—axis III and beyond: social function and sexuality in late life, 2003. Accessed

May 15, 2004, from website: www.cmecorner.com/macmcm/AAGP/aagp2003_06.htm.

Annon J: The PLISSIT model: a proposed conceptual scheme for behavioral treatment of sexual problems, *J Sex Ed Therapy* 2:1-15, 1976.

Association of Reproductive Health Professionals: Mature sexuality, clinical proceedings, April 8, 2002. Accessed May 15, 2004, from website: www.arhp.org.

Brotman S, Ryan B, and Cormier R: The health and social service needs of gay and lesbian elders and their families in Canada, *Gerontologist* 43(2):192, 2003.

Butler R, Lewis M: Sexuality. In Beers M, Berkow R, editors: *The Merck manual of geriatrics,* Rahway, NJ, 2000, Merck.

Centers for Disease Control and Prevention, Division of HIV/AIDS Prevention, National Center for HIV, STD and TB Prevention: Statistics. Accessed May 11, 2004, from website: www.cdc.gov/hiv/stats.htm.

Gulanick M et al, editors: *Nursing care plans: nursing diagnosis and interventions,* ed 5, St Louis, 2003, Mosby.

Kaiser F: Sexual dysfunction in men. In Beers M, Berkow R, editors: *The Merck manual of geriatrics,* Rahway, NJ, 2000a, Merck.

Kaiser F: Sexual dysfunction in women. In Beers M, Berkow R, editors: *The Merck manual of geriatrics,* Rahway, NJ, 2000b, Merck.

Kallejian V: It never ends: aging and sexuality, part I: health and age, 2000. Accessed May 15, 2004, from website: www.healthandage.com/Home/?gid2=599&fa=1&path=null&x=43&y=8.

Kamel H: Sexuality in aging: focus on institutionalized elderly, *Ann Long-Term Care* 9(5):64, 2001.

Kanapaux W: Homosexual seniors face stigma, *Geriatric Times* p 3, Nov/Dec 2003.

Linsk N: HIV among older adults: age-specific issues in prevention and treatment, *AIDS Reader* 10(7):430, 2000.

Matsumoto A: Andropause: clinical implications of the decline in serum testosterone levels with aging in men, *J Geront: Med Sci* 57(2):M76, 2002.

Messinger-Rapport B, Sandhu S, Hujer M: Sex and sexuality: is it over after 60? *Clin Geriatr* 11(10):45, 2003.

National Association on HIV over Fifty: Educational tip sheet: HIV/AIDS and older adults. Accessed May 15, 2004, from website: www.hivoverfifty.org/tip.html.

National Council on Aging: Sex after 60: a natural part of life. Accessed May 16, 2004, from website: www.ncoa.org/content.cfm?sectionID=109&detail=134.

Nusbaum M, Hamilton C: The proactive sexual health history, *Am Fam Phys* 66(9):1705, 2002.

Nusbaum M, Hamilton C, Lenahan, P: Chronic illness and sexual functioning, *Am Fam Phys* 67:347, 2003.

Nusbaum M, Singh A, Pyles A: Sexual healthcare needs of women aged 65 and older, *J Am Geriatr Soc* 52:117, 2004.

Older Americans 2000: Key indicators of well-being. Accessed April 28, 2004, from website: www.agingstats.gov/chartbook2000/.

Paniagua F: Commentary on the possibility that Viagra may contribute to transmission of HIV and other sexual diseases among older adults, *Psychol Rep* 85:942, 1999.

Resnick B: Risky behaviors in older adults, 2003. Accessed April 28, 2004, from website: www.medscape.com/viewarticle/464727? src=search.

Swearingen P: *All-in-one: care planning resource,* St Louis, 2004, Mosby.

Szwabo P: Counseling about sexuality in the older person, *Clin Geriatr Med* 19(3):595, 2003.

Wallace M: Best practices in nursing care to older adults: sexuality, Jan 2004. Accessed April 28, 2004, from website: www.medscape.com/viewarticle/466153?src=search.

14 Mental Health

MARY J. REED, PhD, APN, CS, BC

Learning Objectives

On completion of this chapter, the reader will be able to:

1. Discuss why many older persons with mental and behavioral symptoms are often not diagnosed and treated.
2. Relate the concept of ageism to the psychiatric diagnosis of older adults.
3. State the prevalence of mental morbidity among nursing facility residents.
4. Explore major factors that contribute to mental health wellness.
5. Recognize the prevalence and significance of mental illness or disorders in older adults.
6. Describe the range of mental illness or disorders experienced by older adults.
7. Distinguish between the identified mental illnesses or disorders.
8. Apply the nursing process to older adult clients experiencing mental illnesses or disorders.
9. Identify appropriate nursing interventions when caring for older adults using psychotropic medications.
10. Evaluate the extent of mental health resources available in the care of older adults.
11. Describe trends in the mental health treatment and care of older clients.
12. Identify needs for research in geropsychiatric nursing.

Mental illnesses or disorders can occur throughout the life span, affecting older adults as well as other age-groups. Of the nearly 35 million Americans ages 65 and older, an estimated 2 million have a depressive illness (major depressive disorder, dysthymic disorder, or bipolar disorder), and another 5 million may have *subsyndromal depression,* or depressive symptoms that fall short of meeting full diagnostic criteria for a disorder (National Institute of Mental Health, 2003). Screening instruments are available to primary care providers for detecting mental disorders, but the actual diagnoses are based on criteria detailed in the *Diagnostic and Statistical Manual for Mental Disorders, Fourth Edition, Text Revised* (DSM-IV-TR) (American Psychiatric Association [APA], 2000). The content of the DSM-IV-TR reflects the breadth of mental disorders, providing diagnostic criteria for several hundred of them (Novosel, 2004). A multiaxial system involves an assessment on several axes, each of which refers to a different domain of information that may help the clinician plan treatment and predict outcome. The DSM-IV-TR multiaxial classification includes five axes:

- **Axis I:** Clinical Disorders
  —Other Conditions That May Be a Focus of Clinical Attention
- **Axis II:** Personality Disorders
  —Mental Retardation
- **Axis III:** General Medical Conditions
- **Axis IV:** Psychosocial and Environmental Problems
- **Axis V:** Global Assessment of Functioning

This chapter focuses on depressive disorders, suicide, anxiety, schizophrenia, delusional disorders, mental retardation (an increasing problem as persons reach older adulthood), and disorders caused by medical conditions. Delirium is briefly discussed; dementia and the other cognitive disorders are discussed in greater detail in Chapter 29. Substance abuse disorders are discussed in Chapter 18.

DIFFICULTY IN DIAGNOSIS

One of the major problems in the care of older persons with mental disorders is the difficulty with diagnosis. Some of the problems are "under diagnosis, [client] reluctance to undergo treatment, and the safety and tolerability of various therapies" (Waite, 2004). Several chronic physical health problems often take precedence in the minds of older persons, family members, and primary care physicians. However, multiple physical health problems may be the cause of depression or an anxiety disorder. Paranoid beliefs may be caused by a decreasing ability to perceive the environment correctly because of declining vision or hearing. Both physical and mental illnesses or disorders may be caused by polypharmacy—taking multiple prescription and over-the-counter medications that together cause adverse side effects and complications. Two of the most common side effects of many medications taken by older adults are mental confusion and disorientation, since some medications cross the blood-brain barrier more easily in this age-group than in younger persons. Therefore the question becomes: Are early signs of memory loss and confusion caused by a reversible physical condition such as an infection, an adverse effect of a medication taken for a chronic physical condition, or the beginning symptoms of depression or irreversible dementia?

Older adults are often reluctant to seek care from a mental health professional, especially a psychiatrist, because they grew up during a period when a strong stigma was attached to mental illness, mental hospitals, and mental treatment (Morris, 2001). Many older persons are independent and self-reliant and still believe that a mental or emotional problem is a sign of weak character. They do not want family or friends to know they have a mental disorder of some kind and are seeking treatment for it, since they think that it might reflect negatively on other family members. A geriatric care manager, geriatric mental health specialist, home health care nurse, or social worker can perform a screening mental health assessment in the home and, if a mental disorder is suspected, can convince the older person to see a mental health specialist such as a psychiatrist or psychologist for further evaluation and treatment.

Depression often co-occurs with other serious illnesses such as heart disease, stroke, diabetes, cancer, and Parkinson's disease. Because many older adults face these illnesses as well as various social and economic difficulties, health care professionals may mistakenly conclude that depression is a normal consequence of these problems—an attitude often shared by patients themselves. These factors together contribute to the underdiagnosis and undertreatment of depressive disorders in older people. Depression can and should be treated when it occurs with other illnesses, since untreated depression can delay recovery from or worsen the outcome of the other illnesses. The relationship between depression and other illness processes in older adults is a focus of ongoing research (National Institute of Mental Health, 2003).

Effect of Ageism on Diagnosis and Treatment

Older individuals usually seek care from their primary care physician for a physical problem, even though the underlying cause could be a mental or emotional problem. When the older person visits a primary care physician in family practice or internal medicine, the physician may not see that the real cause is mental or emotional because he or she may lack specialized education or experience in the needs of older clients. The physician may not order the appropriate number and type of diagnostic tests needed to make an accurate diagnosis because of the additional expense or a false belief that the observed behavior is "part of the normal aging process" or that mental health treatment is "not effective in older clients." These are examples of ageism, a negative, prejudiced view of aging and older persons (see Chapter 1). In addition, the physician may note vague symptoms of a cognitive disorder and give the client an outdated diagnosis such as senile dementia, or a meaningless diagnosis such as organic brain syndrome, without the benefit of specific diagnosis or treatment.

Prescription medications may be ordered for anxiety or depression without determining the cause. Medications may be ordered for aggressive, disruptive, paranoid-type behavior without assessing the reasons for the behavior. Thus symptoms may be suppressed without determining the cause and possible cure. This type of action is similar to giving medication for pain without knowing what causes the pain, which may result in severe complications later, such as a ruptured appendix or gallbladder.

Preventing Premature Institutionalization

Adequate, accurate diagnosis is essential. Some conditions (e.g., Alzheimer's disease) have no specific cure, but it is essential to know if the symptoms and behavior are reversible. Even those irreversible disorders can and should be treated with appropriate medications, if useful, and with effective communication techniques and environmental strategies as needed.

Approximately 5% of people in this country live in extended care facilities, and the lifetime risk of admission to an extended care facility in the United States is 25% to 50%. By 2040 as many as 4 million Americans will live in long-term care settings. The incidence of dementia and other psychiatric disorders in this growing population will range from 51% to 94% (Antai-Otong, 2003). The changing demographics of our society and the anticipated growth of the elderly population during the next few decades have created a need for nurse practitioners and other health care providers to develop age-related interventions that address the mental health needs of an aging population.

MENTAL HEALTH WELLNESS

Mental health wellness is one of the major components of successful aging, together with physical health, adequate income, and a strong support system (e.g., family, friends, church, and neighbors). Koenig (1994), a geriatric psychiatrist, has defined successful aging as "how an older person feels, thinks, and acts in whatever circumstances he or she finds them self." This definition is broader than the traditional concepts of physical health, financial security, a strong support system, and family or occupational successes.

Many aspects of aging are difficult. The well-known phrase "old age is not for sissies" is probably true. Examples of losses in old age abound in the literature on gerontology and depression. Much of the depression in older adults is caused by situational factors in the environment (e.g., the loss of family, the stresses of physical illness, or the loneliness of a nursing facility). Therefore, "where symptoms are mild or antidepressants are contraindicated or unsafe (the majority of cases), then treatment should be directed at relieving the situation" (Koenig, 1994). However, medications are all too often considered the first part of treatment rather than the last.

The loss of physical health, employment and income, family and friends, and house and comfortable environment are difficult to accept, especially if they all occur within a relatively short period. Retirement can be difficult and depressing for many, especially those who were involved in interesting, rewarding work. Comorbidity, or the presence of multiple chronic health problems, may prevent older adults from enjoying life and may lead to depression.

One of the keys to successful aging is adjusting to—or, perhaps more accurately, adapting to while not necessarily accepting—changes that occur in one's life. Some people adapt to change better than others, depending on their self-concept and feelings of self-worth. For example, a man who has always been independent in decisions about personal matters may find it difficult to accept suggestions if his physical condition prevents him from performing all the activities he has in the past. Alternatives and substitutions should be evaluated carefully and used slowly. A woman whose self-concept and feelings of self-worth have primarily been based on her perception of personal beauty may develop insecure feelings or self-hatred and may consider self-destruction when age-related changes occur. She may seek all kinds of artificial beauty aids such as breast implants, eye tucks, and face lifts. These substitutions may be essential to her feelings of self-worth. Another woman who was never beautiful in her younger years may not even be aware of, or at least concerned about, physical changes in appearance. A French woman whose age in 1995 was documented to be 120 stated, "I was never very pretty, or ugly either, and aging actually suits me rather well." She also said, "I see badly, I hear badly, I can't feel anything, but everything's fine" (Whitney, 1995). She evidently adapted well to many losses and years of aging (Box 14-1).

Prevention of Mental Illness

The focus on prevention of physical illnesses among older adults has increased in recent years. However, there has been less focus on the prevention of mental illness, especially among older adults. As previously mentioned, part of this problem may be a result of ageism. Another reason may be the lack of specific, well-considered, planned programs and activities for older persons, the primary focus of which is the prevention of mental and emotional problems.

Retirement planning seminars and workshops have been provided by some employers for many years. However, these sessions often focus on financial planning, with some time spent on living arrangements, physical health, and leisure activities. Perhaps it can be concluded that all these factors are related to mental health wellness. However, specific discussion of mental health wellness, issues, and prevention of mental disorders during retirement is not usually stressed. With the many losses that may accompany retirement, such as the loss of challenging and stimulating work, the loss of relationships with colleagues, and the reduction of income, these issues should be considered and plans should be made.

BOX 14-1 Mental Health Promotion and Prevention of Problems

PROMOTION OF MENTAL HEALTH

- Continued physical and mental activity, including exercise and mental stimulation
- Optimum nutrition, including supplements
- Strong support system, including family, friends, and health care providers (when needed)
- Regularly scheduled activities based on personal preferences and interests

PREVENTION OF MENTAL ILLNESSES OR DISORDERS

- Avoidance of social isolation
- Seeking help when symptoms occur
- Use of essential prescribed medications; questioning use of multiple medications
- Choosing physicians and other health care providers who know how to treat mental illnesses or disorders in older adults

Physical Wellness

Physical wellness is obviously important to mental health wellness. The young-old, those ages 65 to 74, are increasingly interested in health promotion activities such as good nutrition, mild aerobic exercise, and routine health assessments by a qualified health care professional. They attend health education classes at wellness centers, senior centers, AARP chapter meetings, and church meetings, where they learn about good health practices and the dangers of polypharmacy, thus contributing to their mental health wellness. They learn that continued physical and mental activities are essential to good health.

Activities that contribute to mental health wellness may be volunteer activities based on experience and expertise; part-time employment; continuing education to seek a degree (an increasing number of people in their 70s and 80s are completing baccalaureate, master's, and doctoral degrees); attendance at local or regional workshops or seminars; and participation in political organizations, activities, and hostel programs on university campuses.

Older adults who experience acute physical illnesses and recover quickly are probably not as at risk for mental illnesses or disorders as those who develop chronic, long-lasting, incurable diseases that cause them to become frustrated, depressed, and sometimes suicidal.

Support Systems

Another factor essential in maintaining mental health wellness in old age is a strong support system. Support may be provided by family members, the church, friends, neighbors, and others. A person needs someone to turn to, confide in, and have available during times of wellness *and* illness. This type of support is especially important when people reach the older ages, especially the late 80s, 90s, and 100s, because they are more likely to develop physical and dependency needs.

The family continues to be the first source of support for older adults. This support may be regular contact through visiting or telephoning; participation in recreational activities with them; social and psychologic support; assistance with transportation, shopping, and financial matters such as paying bills; or direct physical caregiving.

The church is the second source of support for many older adults. For some it may be the first place they turn. They may have lost their spouses, siblings, and adult children to death. Or, in today's mobile society, adult children may live thousands of miles away and not be readily available in times of need.

Social contact is an essential human element that has direct effects on health and emotional well-being. Relationships also act as potential buffers against stress (Calandra, 2003a). Both informal and formal fulfilling human connections can be healthful. Formal supports may include a member of the clergy, housekeeper, visiting nurse, or psychotherapist. Informal relations are family members and casual contacts, perhaps the grocery store clerk. For some elderly persons, close neighbors are a crucial source of informal support. Studies indicate that pets are a source of relational support. Elderly pet owners have been shown to be less depressed, better able to tolerate social isolation, and more active than those without pets (Ebersole and Hess, 2001).

Role of the Nurse in Mental Health Wellness

Nurses need to be aware of their personal attitudes and opinions about aging and the care of older persons. Ageism is usually the result of inaccurate information and inadequate knowledge. "Age also influences how health care professionals respond to [clients]. Adverse incidents in older [clients] often lead to interventions such as administering psychotropic medications, applying physical restraints, and inserting urinary catheters—interventions that carry their own intrinsic risks" (*Geriatric models of care: which one's right for your institution?* 1994). The nurse who understands the aging process and the conditions that may accompany the aging process does not label an acutely ill hospitalized older adult as demented when the client's behavior is most likely a symptom of delirium, a reversible, temporary condition brought on by a change in environment, anesthesia, medication, or another physical factor, such as pain or infection (see Chapter 29). The nurse should communicate with and attentively listen to the older person, taking into consideration any sensory deficits identified during the admission history and physical examination. The nurse should involve the older client and his or her family in the care plan. The nurse should do everything possible to maintain or to enhance the older client's feelings of self-worth by providing privacy, seeking his or her opinion in matters of care, treating the older client with respect, and, if needed, seeking referrals for specific diagnosis and treatment of possible mental illnesses or disorders.

A nurse often functions as a coordinator of the care provided to older adult clients. As a coordinator attempting to provide a holistic approach, the nurse assesses the client's mental health needs and provides intervention based on the assessment. Older adult clients benefit from nurses who have a comprehensive knowledge of the community's mental health resources available to older adults. The ability to anticipate client needs and respond in a proactive manner to mental health issues by referral to a community resource (e.g., a support group) can significantly enhance a nurse's effectiveness.

Nurses with specialty training and experience in geropsychiatric issues may take an expanded role in the provision of services designed to enhance mental health wellness in the older adult population. For example, a specialty nurse could meet with individuals preparing to retire to discuss emotional experiences common to new retirees. Another nurse might moderate a support group for older adults who have recently moved to the homes of adult children. By acknowledging their shared issue of decreased independence, the older persons can explore available coping skills and improve their adjustment techniques.

MAJOR MENTAL HEALTH PROBLEMS

The older population—persons 65 years or older—numbered 35.9 million in 2003 (the latest year for which data are available). They represent 12.3% of the U.S. population, about one in every eight Americans. Census 2000 Data on the Aging identified "Persons with Mental Disability" at 3,592,912, with the United States (50 states and Washington, DC) equaling 10.8% of the population (Administration on Aging, 2004). These statistics indicate a significant impact on American society and a challenge for nurses as the role of nursing in interdisciplinary care of older adults and their family members increases.

To adequately perform the nursing role, nurses require a comprehensive body of knowledge that includes theories of aging, health and illness, mental health, biopsychosocial interplay, and clinical skills. Nurses must also understand the relevant neurobehavioral theories, the use of psychotherapeutic medications, and the potential adverse reactions or drug interactions that can be seen when these drugs are used (Calandra, 2003a). The goals for which nurses strive when working with older adults experiencing major mental health problems include optimizing individual functioning, independence, and quality of life; providing support for clients and their families; adapting interventions to multiple settings, such as home, community, and long-term care institutions; lowering morbidity; decreasing suffering; improving older adults' self-esteem and integrity; enhancing clients' daily life experiences; and ensuring continuity of care with smooth transitions between the various levels of care.

Depression

In primary care settings, depression has been identified in 17% to 37% of elderly patients, 30% of whom had major depression. In medically hospitalized patients 11% have major depression; 25% have less severe, yet clinically significant, depressive symptoms. In long-term care settings 12% and 30% of elderly patients are affected with major and less severe depression, respectively (Serby and Yu, 2003). Unfortunately depression in older adults is often overlooked and therefore left untreated. When left untreated, depression can lead to an increase in both morbidity and mortality among older adults. Equally problematic is the fact that depressive disorders are often misdiagnosed as a result of the unique symptoms manifested by depressed older adults. Symptoms that may appear to be representative of a cognitive disorder are often really symptoms of depression (Box 14-2 and Nursing Care Plan).

A number of theories attempt to explain the cause of depression. Each theory presents a different viewpoint or causative factor, but the depression that clinicians see in older adults seems to represent an interplay of biologic, psychologic, and social factors. Older adults at the highest risk for depressive symptoms are women over age 85 who are unmarried, living in an urban area, living in a long-term care setting, experiencing physical illness or disability, lacking adequate social support, of a low socioeconomic status, or experiencing a significant loss; a combination of these factors may also exist. Factors that seem to protect older adults from depression include hardiness (defined as a personal characteristic of

BOX 14-2 Common Symptoms of Depression in Older Adults

- Apathy
- Lack of interest in pleasurable activities
- Withdrawal from friends
- Anorexia resulting in weight loss
- No pleasures in life
- Not sleeping well
- Feelings of uselessness, hopelessness, or helplessness
- Increased dependency
- Multiple vague somatic (physical) complaints
- Other behavioral changes

Nursing Care Plan
Major Depression

Clinical Situation: Mrs. S is an 81-year-old widow whose husband died suddenly 4 years ago after a massive myocardial infarction. She has one daughter who lives 800 miles away and visits once a year. Her major source of support and friendship since her husband's death had been a neighbor, Mrs. J, who died 1 month ago after suffering a stroke. Mrs. S tells the nurse practitioner at a recent office visit, "I just don't know how to deal with this. I handled things well after my husband died, but when my neighbor died last month, I just fell apart. I don't feel like eating. I can't fall asleep at night. And my daughter tells me I sound like I'm going to pieces." On assessment, the nurse practitioner finds Mrs. S has symptoms that include slow motor movements and thought processes. Her grooming is poor, and she appears to be sleep deprived. She has lost 12 pounds since her last visit 5 weeks ago. She is tearful with frequent sobbing.

Nursing Diagnosis

Ineffective individual coping related to death of husband 4 years ago and recent death of neighbor

Outcomes

Short term: Client will verbalize two coping strategies that have been effective for her in the past at the time of the next appointment (3 days).

Long term: Client will develop a prioritized list of issues that she plans to address with the identified coping strategies within 1 month of the initial assessment.

Interventions

Assess client's risk for injury as a result of self-directed violence by completing an assessment of suicidal risk.

If client is suicidal, arrange for a higher level of care, such as partial hospitalization or inpatient care.

Develop a therapeutic relationship with client based on trust and empathy.

Assist client in identifying coping strategies that she has successfully used in the past.

Help client develop a list of individuals (with phone numbers) who have been or could be supportive.

Help client outline a daily schedule that can guide her completion of ADLs.

Assist client in developing a list of problems from most to least urgent.

Assess need for initiation of antidepressant medication.

Educate client and family of need for ongoing support.

Refer client to local grief support group.

commitment, control, and ability to handle challenges) and the development of healthy attitudes toward death.

Depression in older adults may be divided into the two broad categories of depressive disorder and bipolar disorder. Depressive disorders can range from an acute major depression to dysthymia, which is a chronic (2 years or more) range of depressive symptoms. In bipolar disorders the depressive symptoms alternate with manic symptoms, which are seen as an abnormal elevation of mood. The swings between depression and mania can be drastic, as seen in bipolar I disorder; can alternate between major depression and less severe manic behavior (hypomania), as seen in bipolar II disorder; or may alternate between signs of dysthymia and other hypomanic symptoms; these latter clients are referred to as cyclothymic (APA, 2000).

Although the course of depressive symptoms varies from individual to individual, some common elements can be found in the development of depression in older adults. The change in self-concept, combined with a sense of loneliness and isolation, often leads to a feeling of increased dependence on family members or other caregivers. This sense of dependency can lead to a progressive decline as the depression begins. Also contributing to the development of depression are factors such as preexisting mental illness and the loss of loved ones, especially if multiple losses occur in a short period. A number of physical disorders are associated with the development of depression in older adults. These include congestive heart failure, diabetes mellitus, infectious diseases, changes in gastrointestinal function, cancer, seizure disorders, anemia, and sleep disorders. A number of medications used by older adults are associated with depressive symptoms; in particular, cardiovascular agents, antianxiety drugs, amphetamines, narcotics, and hormone medications may all play a role in the development of depression. Substance abuse of alcohol, illegal drugs, prescription medications, or over-the-counter medications can pose a significant risk for depression (Morris, 2001) (Box 14-3).

Symptoms of depression in older adults can include distressful feelings, cognitive changes, behavioral changes, and physical symptoms. Feelings that older adults may experience when they are depressed include malaise, fatigue, lack of interest, inability to experience pleasure, sense of uselessness, hopelessness, helplessness, decreased sexual interest, increased dependency, and anxiety. Cognitive changes include a slowing or unreliability of memory, paranoia, agitation, a focus on the past, thoughts of death, and thoughts of suicide. Older adults with depression may show behavioral changes such as difficulty completing activities of daily living (ADLs), change in appetite (most commonly, a decrease), changes in sleeping patterns (usually insomnia), lowered energy level, poor grooming, and withdrawal from people and interests they have enjoyed in the past. Physical symptoms commonly seen in older adults experiencing depression include muscle aches, abdominal pain or tightness, flatulence, nausea and vomiting, dry mouth, and headaches (Baldessarini, 2003; Calandra, 2003b).

BOX 14-3 Medications That Can Cause Depression

- Amphetamines
- Antineoplastic agents
- Antiparkinsonian agents
- Barbiturates
- Benzodiazepines
- Digoxin
- Estrogen
- Phenothiazines
- Sulfonamides

Compiled from Semia TP, Beizer JL, Higbee JD: *Geriatric dosage handbook*, ed 3, Hudson, Ohio, 1997-1998, American Pharmaceutical Association; Shannon MT, Wilson BA, Stang CL: *1998 drug guide*, Stanford, Conn, 1998, Appleton & Lange.

NURSING MANAGEMENT

Assessment

Depression in older adults can be assessed with standardized rating scales or with a comprehensive nursing assessment that includes an evaluation of several key components of depression. A number of instruments have been developed to screen older adults for depression, and other instruments provide a standardized approach to rating its severity. One of the most commonly used scales in assessing the presence or absence of depression in older adults is the Geriatric Depression Scale (see Chapter 4). The simplicity and versatility it provides the clinician make it particularly useful (Stevens, Friedman, and Baldwin, 1998).

When the nursing assessment indicates the possibility of depression, the nurse can further assess the symptoms of depression previously mentioned. The comprehensive assessment includes a health history, physical examination, medication history, mental status examination, nutritional history, family assessment, and performance of ADLs. Diagnostic tests that may be useful in ascertaining the presence of depression instead of another illness include certain laboratory tests (complete blood count [CBC], thyroid function studies, urinalysis, dexamethasone suppression test), electrocardiogram (ECG), electroencephalogram, magnetic resonance imaging, and computed tomography scans.

Diagnosis

After a comprehensive assessment of depression has been completed, nursing diagnoses may be used to delineate identified human responses. The following is a list of sample nursing diagnoses commonly identified in older adults experiencing depression, with examples of possible causes:

- Altered family processes related to death of spouse
- Anxiety related to recent retirement
- Body image disturbance related to decreased mobility
- Dysfunctional grieving related to denial of death of loved one
- Fear related to sensory alteration
- High risk for self-directed violence related to depressed mood
- Hopelessness related to change in living environment
- Impaired social interaction related to activity intolerance
- Ineffective individual coping related to numerous recent losses
- Powerlessness related to impaired decision making
- Risk for loneliness related to social isolation
- Risk for self-directed violence related to hopelessness
- Risk for self-mutilation related to body image disturbance
- Self-care deficit related to depressed mood
- Self-esteem disturbance related to retirement
- Social isolation related to recent move
- Spiritual distress related to frequent thoughts of death

Planning and Expected Outcomes

In planning care for older adults with depression, the nurse should set both short- and long-term goals appropriate for the nursing diagnoses identified for a given client. Expected outcomes for clients with depression include the following:

1. Client demonstrates improved coping strategies as evidenced by establishment of a support system and use of two additional coping skills that have proved successful in the past.
2. Client demonstrates acceptance of the aging process as evidenced by verbal acknowledgment of limitations and fears.
3. Client demonstrates a decrease in social isolation as evidenced by participation in a weekly therapeutic group session and one outing outside the home per week.
4. Client demonstrates resolution of grief as evidenced by verbalization of loss, adequate sleep, improved concentration, appropriate energy level, and the ability to accomplish ADLs.

Intervention

Nurses have a unique role in the interdisciplinary team approach that is most often used in the treatment of depression. The focus of nursing care is to assist with the human responses that occur as a result of the depression. Nursing intervention can occur at numerous points along the continuum of care in settings ranging from clients' homes to outpatient clinics to partial hospitalization programs or inpatient units.

Regardless of the setting in which nursing care is provided, safety is the primary goal. Depressed older adults are often at risk because of their inability to care for themselves; they may also be at risk as a result of self-destructive behavior or suicidal plans. The nurse must constantly assess the level of risk for clients with whom they work and must take appropriate steps to ensure their clients' safety.

Physical needs are also a priority for frequent intervention in depressed older adults. They may be unable to perform their own ADLs and need assistance or motivation to do so. They may also have numerous somatic concerns such as insomnia, decreased appetite, pain, gastrointestinal distress, and headaches.

The nurse's ability to positively effect change in older adults' responses to depression lies in the development of therapeutic relationships. The nurse must show unconditional positive regard and empathy in a professional manner so that trust can be developed. Once trust has been established, clients become far more open to the nurse's intervention.

In an inpatient setting a professional nurse is most often considered the milieu manager and, as such, must provide an optimum environment for client treatment. Nursing has considered the role that the environment plays in client recovery as far back as the experiences of Florence Nightingale. Environmental factors include color, light, art, movement, level of activity, and interpersonal environment.

A number of psychotherapeutic modalities are used to respond to depression in older adults. These include milieu, individual, family, and group therapy. Group therapy is particularly effective with older adults because it allows them to express and to receive support. A specific type of group therapy that seems to be useful with older adults is reminiscence therapy, in which they are encouraged to discuss past events to identify problem-solving skills that have worked for them in the past. Reminiscence groups involve a caring facilitator (who does not have to be a health care professional) who encourages and listens to group members share experiences from the past. The facilitator may initiate a topic of interest to the group, such as childhood and early school experiences, certain family holiday rituals, marriage and the time when their children were young, or popular movies and music from the past. Most reminiscing is about happy or pleasant events from the past. If sad, unhappy, or unresolved problems begin to emerge, the group facilitator should obtain the assistance of a trained mental health professional. Older adults who display unhealthy behavioral changes in response to their depression may also benefit from behavior therapy. The key to behavior therapy in older adults is to use a direct, structured approach that maintains the clients' integrity and autonomy. Offering clients options with clearly delineated consequences for their choices enables them to maintain a sense of control. Some older people do not feel comfortable sharing emotions and feelings in a group, so individual therapy or medication may be the best choice.

Nurses also play a significant role in the biologic interventions that are used to treat depression. A thorough understanding of the appropriate use of psychotherapeutic medications, drug-drug interactions, drug-food interactions, potential adverse reactions, and legal and ethical implications of these medications is necessary for the nurse to intervene appropriately with depressed older adults. Electroconvulsive therapy (ECT) is sometimes used for depression in older adults. The nurse who intervenes with clients receiving ECT must have a comprehensive understanding of the indications, benefits, and risks inherent in this therapeutic intervention.

Nursing intervention for older adults who are depressed occurs on three levels: primary, secondary, and tertiary. Primary intervention involves actions that promote health and decrease the likelihood of depression. Secondary intervention includes the nurse's response when clients are experiencing the acute symptoms of depression. Tertiary intervention is the restorative or rehabilitative functions that the nurse performs to assist clients in their recovery process. An important aspect of tertiary intervention involving clients with depression is teaching new coping skills to lessen the likelihood of recurring depression (see Client/Family Teaching box).

Evaluation

In evaluating the care provided to older adults experiencing depression, the nurse should initially compare client outcomes with the short- and long-term goals outlined in the planning phase of the nursing process and document client progress toward achievement of the goals. Appropriate alterations should then be made to the continuing treatment plan to ensure optimum client response. It is helpful to assess the level of satisfaction that clients and their families feel with the nursing care that has been provided. It is also important for nurses to assess their own reactions to clients and the care that has been provided to ascertain the effect (positive or negative) that the clients have had on the nurse.

Suicide

Older Americans are disproportionately likely to die by suicide. Making up only 13% of the U.S. population, individuals ages 65 and older accounted for 18% of all suicide deaths in 2000. Among the highest rates (when categorized by gender and race) were white men ages 85 and older: 59 deaths per 100,000 persons in 2000, more than five times the national rate of 10.6 per 100,000 (National Institute of Mental Health, 2003). Affective illness has been referred to as the predominant psychopathology associated with suicide in later life. Among older persons who commit suicide, three fourths (76%) have diagnosable mood disorders and nearly two thirds (63%) have depression. Contributing risk factors include alcoholism and substance abuse, axis II disorders, and dementia. In later life, bereavement, loss of independence, or financial reversals may lead to depression. Older persons who take their own lives also tend to have greater physical health burdens and more functional disabilities than those who do not commit suicide (Montross et al, 2003).

Client/Family Teaching 

Older adults and their family members need to be taught the following:

- Depression is not a normal part of aging.
- Symptoms of depression may be vague (e.g., decreased appetite).
- A key indicator may be a change in the level of functioning without any physiologic cause.
- Depression in older adults can be treated.
- Older adults have a potential for suicide when they are depressed.

Despite these sobering statistics, American society continues to ignore suicide in older adults. Older adults are less likely to communicate their intent to commit suicide; as a result, many health care professionals have assumed erroneously that suicide is not a significant issue among older adults. Some older adult suicides are attempts to remain in control by deciding the appropriate time to die. Such attempts are sometimes called *benign suicides* or *rational suicides*. These terms refer to suicides planned by individuals because they perceive their life to have no value. These types of suicide pose an ethical dilemma for nurses regarding client autonomy versus the value of life, and often also pose a legal issue, as evidenced by the recent publicity resulting from reexamination of laws in several states. Despite the inherent uncertainty in these cases, nursing scholars have supported a nursing perspective that affirms life by enhancing the individual's quality of life rather than ensuring them of their right to die (Baldessarini, 2003; Fontaine, 2003).

Another issue that nurses deal with in caring for older adults is passive suicide, or subintentioned suicide. It is a passive attempt to hasten one's death. This type of self-destructive behavior often goes unrecognized and can range from noncompliance with the health care regimen (e.g., refusing safe and appropriate use of needed medication), to behaviors that harm the individual in a more active manner (e.g., continued smoking, alcohol abuse, or an eating disorder), to participating in dangerous situations (e.g., reckless driving).

Risk Factors. The risk factors for suicide in older adults are presented in Box 14-4. At highest risk for suicide are Protestant white men living alone in their homes. They often have a neat appearance and calm behavior and take either antianxiety or antipsychotic medications. Many of the steps outlined in the nursing process of older adults with depression are also appropriate for older adults at risk for suicide. The following steps are more specific to suicidal clients.

NURSING MANAGEMENT

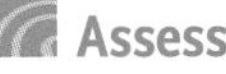

Assessment

In assessing clients for the potential for suicide, it is helpful to have a series of interview questions (Box 14-5). Although

BOX 14-4 Risk Factors for Suicide in Older Adults

- Age (especially those between 75 and 85)
- Low socioeconomic status
- Male gender
- White race
- Living alone
- Chronic illness
- Chronic pain
- Alcoholism
- Recent personal loss (especially spouse's death within past year)
- Other losses (such as economic, social, or prestige) or cumulative losses
- Substance abuse (e.g., alcohol, prescription medication, over-the-counter medication, or illegal substances)
- Family history of suicide
- Prior suicide attempts or threats
- Fear of institutionalization or increasing dependence
- Recent retirement
- Social isolation
- Chronic sleep problems
- Symptoms of depression (related to 50% to 70% of suicides by older adults)
- Impulsivity
- Unemployment
- Widowed or never married

Compiled from Browning MA: Depression, suicide and bereavement. In Hogstel MO, editor: *Geropsychiatric nursing*, ed 2, St Louis, 1995, Mosby; Courage M et al: Suicide in the elderly: staying in control, *J Psychosoc Nurs* 31(7):25, 1993; Holzapfel SK: The elderly. In Varcarolis EM, editor: *Foundations of psychiatric mental health nursing*, ed 2, Philadelphia, 1994, WB Saunders; Varcarolis EM: People who contemplate suicide: aggression toward self. In Varcarolis EM, editor: *Foundations of psychiatric mental health nursing*, ed 2, Philadelphia, 1994, WB Saunders; Kelsey JE: The use of antidepressants in long-term care and the geriatric patient: primary care issues, *Geriatrics* 53(suppl 4):512, 1998.

not all questions are needed or appropriate for all clients, it is helpful to have a progressive series of assessment items in mind that can be adapted to the situation. The basic components of suicide assessment include evaluating suicidal ideation (thoughts), any prior attempts, a client's suicide plan, the plan's lethality, the availability of the implements of the plan, coexisting substance abuse, and the pervasiveness of the despair a client is experiencing.

Diagnosis

Nursing diagnoses for older adults at risk for suicide include:

- Ineffective individual coping related to multiple perceived losses
- Dysfunctional grieving related to multiple perceived losses
- Hopelessness related to deteriorating health
- High risk for violence related to perceived loss of control
- Spiritual distress related to hopelessness

BOX 14-5 Questions for Assessing the Potential for Suicide

- What has been the most difficult moment for you in the recent past?
- Have things been so bad that you have thought about escaping? If so, how?
- Are there times when death seems like an attractive option to you?
- Have you thought of harming yourself?
- Have you thought about killing yourself?
- If you were to harm yourself, how would you do it?
- Do you have access to the items you would need to carry out your plan (e.g., gun, quantities of medication, rope, enclosed garage)?
- Have you thought about harming yourself or attempted to harm yourself in the past?
- What has kept you from harming yourself thus far?
- What might keep you from harming yourself in the future?

Planning and Expected Outcomes

Planning care for a suicidal older adult client requires a strong interpersonal connection with the client. Expected outcomes include:

1. Client identifies and verbalizes thoughts and feelings related to emotional state.
2. Client reports absence of suicidal ideation.
3. Client demonstrates effective coping skills for managing stress and frustration, as evidenced by reported use of two coping strategies.
4. Client experiences behavior control with assistance of others, as evidenced by absence of suicidal ideation.
5. Client expresses satisfaction with spiritual well-being, as evidenced by verbalization of positive statements about self and life, including a sense of purpose in life.

Intervention

When a risk of suicide is identified in an older adult client, appropriate safety measures must be taken. These safety measures can be tailored to the client's suicide plans, the setting in which the nurse is intervening (e.g., the client's home, an inpatient setting), and the extent of human connection the client has. It may be necessary for the nurse to arrange with the local mental health authorities for inpatient hospitalization (voluntary or involuntary) if client safety cannot be ensured in an outpatient setting. The client's significant other can often be helpful in helping develop a plan of safety. It is essential for nurses to remember that no extent of environmental precautions can take the place of a strong interpersonal connection with a client. Clients who are suicidal may be creative and adaptive in finding alternative methods of suicide. Without a strong therapeutic relationship to assist a client, the nurse's best efforts to keep him or her safe may prove fruitless.

Asking clients about potential suicidal thoughts does not plant the idea in their minds. If the nurse has reason to believe a client may be suicidal, it is quite likely that he or she already considered this option. A useful tool with suicidal individuals is a "no-suicide contract." This is an agreement (ideally written and signed) between a client and a health care provider that the client will not harm himself or herself. The specific wording of the agreement may differ based on the client's risk factors and the setting in which the care is occurring. For example, on an inpatient unit an agreement might state, "I commit that I will not harm myself while in the hospital, and if I have thoughts of harming myself, I will immediately inform a staff member."

Once a client is past the immediate danger of suicidal behavior, it is helpful to help him or her develop suicide prevention plans. Such plans can include alternatives to consider other than suicide and may also include specific steps that a client can take if he or she again experiences suicidal thoughts. These plans encourage clients to take a problem-solving (active) approach to the potential for self-harm and therefore increase their sense of control. Nurses can play a significant role in suicide prevention for older adults. Essential components in such preventive intervention include assessing all older adults for potential self-harm issues, proactively identifying and treating depression in older adults, developing community programs focused on prevention of older adult suicide, and teaching health care professionals who work with older adults in different settings about the risk for suicide.

Evaluation

Unfortunately, despite excellent nursing assessment and intervention, older adults do continue to commit suicide at a distressingly high rate. When an older adult has committed suicide, the nurse's focus may be to assist the survivors of the suicide in coping with the resulting grief and trauma. A psychologic autopsy, or the processing of events and behaviors surrounding the client's suicide, may be useful to both the health care professionals and the surviving family and friends. It is also helpful to encourage the survivors to obtain assistance from a support group for survivors of suicide.

Delirium

Many individuals accept a decline in intellectual functioning as a normal part of aging. But, although there may be changes in older adults' intellectual functioning, a recognizable impairment such as confusion, hallucination, or delusion is not a normal aspect of aging and may represent an active disease process. Accurate diagnosis of these impairments becomes essential to successfully treat or cure some processes or to provide optimum intervention in those which cannot be cured (Richardson, 2003).

The APA's DSM-IV-TR divides the cognitive disorders into four categories: delirium, dementia, amnestic disorders, and other cognitive disorders. Dementia and delirium are discussed in greater detail in Chapter 29. The delirium disorders may be related to a general medical condition or substance withdrawal, be substance induced, have multiple causes, or fit into a broad category labeled "not otherwise specified" (APA, 2000).

Delirium disorders are brain disorders evidenced by a change in the individual's level of consciousness and cognition. Delirium develops rapidly over a short period. Dementia is a disorder of multiple cognitive deficits and memory impairment. It is important to differentiate between delirium and dementia. Symptoms from both include memory impairment, but delirium disorders also show a change in a client's level of consciousness. In delirium disorders the symptoms may fluctuate over time, whereas in dementia the symptoms are more stable. Delirium may occur in older adults who have previously experienced symptoms or a diagnosis of dementia (APA, 2000). When delirium symptoms are superimposed on dementia symptoms, it becomes vital to sort out the difference and the illness process that the delirium symptoms may represent. Essentially, delirium is a disorder with an acute onset and a reversible cause, whereas dementia is a disorder with a chronic onset and an often irreversible cause (Byrd, 2003).

Systematic tools for assessing a client's cognitive function such as the MiniMental State Examination (MMSE) or the Short Portable Mental Status Questionnaire (SPMSQ) (see Chapter 4) are useful in differentiating delirium from other disorders (Richardson, 2003).

Anxiety

Anxiety is one of the most common symptoms seen in older adults; the most common anxiety disorder seen in older persons is obsessive-compulsive disorder (OCD) (Morris, 2001). OCD comprises obsessive symptoms (e.g., persistent intrusive thoughts) and compulsive symptoms (e.g., repetitive behavior performed in an attempt to reduce anxiety). For example, older adults may manifest OCD in morning routines so ritualistic that they miss both their breakfast and their lunch. Other anxiety disorders seen in older adults may be generalized anxiety disorder (GAD) and phobic disorders. GAD is excessive worry that is beyond the individual's control (APA, 2000) and may be evidenced by symptoms such as restlessness, fatigue, decreased concentration, irritability, muscle tension, or disturbed sleep. A phobic disorder is manifested by a persistent, irrational fear provoked by the feared object or situation.

Anxiety disorders in older adults may develop as a result of a specific event or a general pattern of change seen by clients as threatening. Such changes can include declines in health, illness, financial strain, an actual or potential change in living situation, the death of a significant other, or a loss of independence. Retirement is a change that often is associated with the development of an anxiety disorder in older adults.

NURSING MANAGEMENT

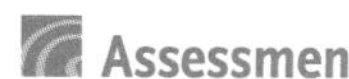

Assessment

Older adult clients with anxiety disorders are usually able to describe their anxiety without the nurse needing to probe extensively. They may also exhibit behavioral clues such as pacing, irritability, and fidgeting. When clients lack insight into their anxiety, the nurse may find it helpful to describe the symptoms observed as indicating anxiety. The nurse should also assess associated changes that may accompany the anxiety, such as sleeping habits and appetite, the presence or absence of depression, and any complaints of physical pain. Box 14-6 lists factors that should be assessed in older adults with an anxiety disorder.

Somatic complaints are often seen in older adult clients experiencing anxiety. This may be due to the physical toll that anxiety places on the physical systems or to a client being more comfortable reporting a physical health concern rather than a mental health one. If the nurse believes the somatic concerns may be related to anxiety, a thorough anxiety assessment should be conducted.

Diagnosis

The nursing diagnoses for older adults with an anxiety disorder usually include:

- Anxiety related to situational crisis
- Ineffective individual coping related to perceived vulnerability

Planning and Expected Outcomes

Expected outcomes include:

1. Client identifies his or her own anxiety and coping patterns.
2. Client reports an increase in psychologic and physiologic comfort.
3. Client demonstrates effective coping skills as evidenced by ability to solve problems and meet self-care needs.
4. Client demonstrates use of appropriate relaxation techniques.

BOX 14-6 Factors to Assess in Older Adults With Anxiety Disorder

- Recent changes in a client's life
- Degree of anxiety
- Interference of the anxiety with performance of ADLs
- Physical symptoms (e.g., vital signs, gastrointestinal function, headaches, tremor)

Intervention

The nurse can intervene with older adults experiencing anxiety in a number of ways. It may be helpful to assist clients in examining their own "worst case scenario." By developing strategies that could be used to cope with the worst possible situation, clients may feel an increased ability to cope with their current situation. Relaxation strategies such as progressive muscle relaxation, breathing techniques, therapeutic use of music, and exercise are useful in helping clients alleviate the acute anxiety states that are most distressing to them. The nurse should help clients learn to identify increasing anxiety early in the anxiety cycle so they can take steps to reduce it to a lower level. Family education may also be beneficial to obtain support systems for clients. Clients experiencing moderate to panic-level anxiety may need a referral for antianxiety medications. Clients who continue to experience distress as a result of anxiety may benefit from psychotherapy. Behavior modification techniques are especially effective with phobic disorders.

Evaluation

The nurse can evaluate the care that has been provided to clients experiencing anxiety by monitoring their progress toward achievement of the expected outcomes and documenting the results. Effectiveness of any health teaching is evident in a client's ability to use relaxation techniques and constructive problem solving.

Schizophrenia

Schizophrenia is a thought disorder characterized by altered perceptions of reality, alterations in thought processes (both form and content), and declines in clients' ADLs and occupational and social functioning. The onset of schizophrenia usually occurs between the late teens and the mid-30s. However, in rare cases schizophrenia has an onset after the age of 45 (APA, 2000).

Typically older adult clients with schizophrenia have been dealing with the disorder for a long time but may experience exacerbations of the schizophrenic symptoms with the stress of the aging process. Presentation is more likely to include delusions and hallucinations and less likely to include disorganized and negative symptoms (Calandra, 2003b).

Schizophrenia is divided into five types: paranoid, disorganized, catatonic, undifferentiated, and residual (APA, 2000) (Table 14-1).

NURSING MANAGEMENT

Assessment

The reader is referred to a general psychiatric nursing textbook for a complete review of the assessment process in individuals with a diagnosis of schizophrenia.

TABLE 14-1 Types of Schizophrenia

TYPE SYMPTOMS	CHARACTERISTICS	MOST COMMON
Paranoid	Preoccupied with delusions and/or hallucinations	Mistrustful of others May be hostile at times
Disorganized	Disorganized speech and behavior	Flat or inappropriate affect (feeling state)
Catatonic	Motor dysfunction ranging from near stuporous to excessive activity	Resistance to interaction Peculiar movements or speech patterns
Undifferentiated	Schizophrenia that does not meet the criteria for paranoid, disorganized, or catatonic type	Vague
Residual	Continued evidence of schizophrenia	No prominent symptoms (such as hallucinations or delusions)

Diagnosis

Nursing diagnoses appropriate to the older adult with schizophrenia include:

- Social isolation related to altered mental status
- Altered thought processes related to feelings of distress over altered perception of reality
- Sensory or perceptual alterations related to poor symptom management
- Sleep pattern disturbance related to psychologic status

Planning and Expected Outcomes

Schizophrenia is an illness that shows periods of exacerbation and remission. The goal of nursing intervention in individuals with schizophrenia is safe, effective treatment, rather than a cure. A reduction in symptoms and an improved quality of life are goals that a nurse should work toward. Other goals include reducing client anxiety (anxiety usually exacerbates the schizophrenic symptoms), building a therapeutic relationship with a client, providing continuity of care, and eliciting the support of family and friends to enhance a client's function and experience. Expected outcomes include:

1. Client develops a trusting relationship, as evidenced by the presence of supportive significant others.
2. Client maintains contact with mental health caregivers as evidenced by weekly meetings with a counselor.
3. Client experiences a decrease in hallucinations and distress as evidenced by verbalized reports of fewer hallucinations and feelings of distress, as well as demonstration of methods to handle hallucinations.
4. Client gets adequate sleep as evidenced by reports of sleeping through the night or verbalization of feeling rested after a night's sleep.

Intervention

Nursing interventions for older adults with schizophrenia should provide a comprehensive approach to the maintenance of ADLs, nutrition, hygiene, health promotion, and reality orientation. The reader is referred to a general psychiatric nursing text for a thorough review of nursing interventions for clients with schizophrenia. Interventions that may be most essential in dealing with older adults with schizophrenia include providing adequate family or social support, responding to client symptoms, using touch appropriately, and dealing with aggressive behavior.

If clients give evidence (verbal or nonverbal) of hallucinations or delusions, the nurse should focus on responding to the feelings without arguing about the reality of their perceptual experiences. For example, if a client states that the television is broadcasting his or her thoughts, the nurse could respond by saying, "That must be frightening," rather than saying, "Now Mr. D, you know that the television can't do that!" Attempting to argue perception with clients only escalates their anxiety. It may, however, be helpful to reorient clients without being confrontational.

Clients with schizophrenia may easily misinterpret touch by the nurse as being harmful or threatening to them. Therefore the nurse should only touch clients when there is a purpose and then only after asking permission.

Older adults with schizophrenia may at times present a danger to themselves or others. The nurse should assess the level of danger with each client. If the assessment shows that a client has a potential for aggression, the nurse should take steps to deescalate the client's anger and to provide safety for the client and others.

Evaluation

Evaluation is based on achievement of the identified expected outcomes. The nature of the disorder may make it difficult for the nurse to establish a relationship with a client; thus the nurse may feel hopeless, frustrated, and inadequate while attempting to provide care. It is often helpful to establish short-term goals for clients with schizophrenia that are easily achievable and specific. The nurse is responsible for documenting progress toward achievement of the objectives, as well as the level of safety achieved.

Delusional Disorders

Delusional disorders involves nonbizarre delusions. (An example of a "nonbizarre" delusion would be a person with the false belief that he or she is under surveillance by the police. An example of a "bizarre" delusion would be that one's bodily organs have been removed and replaced by someone else's organs.) Aside from the delusion, thinking is normal. Hallucinations rarely occur. These patients usually do not respond well to antipsychotic medications (Calandra, 2003b).

The following types are assigned based on the predominant delusional theme (APA, 2000):

- **Erotomanic type:** delusions that another person, usually of higher status, is in love with the individual
- **Grandiose type:** delusions of inflated worth, power, knowledge, identity, or special relationship to a deity or famous person
- **Jealous type:** delusions that the individual's sexual partner is unfaithful
- **Persecutory type:** delusions that the person (or someone to whom the person is close) is being malevolently treated in some way
- **Somatic type:** delusions that the person has some physical defect or general medical condition
- **Mixed type:** delusions characteristic of more than one of the above but with no one theme predominant
- **Unspecified type**

Mental Retardation

Mental retardation is characterized by below-average intellectual functioning. The onset occurs before age 18 and is accompanied by an alteration in an individual's ability to cope with life's demands and to function independently (APA, 2000). The individual's functioning, including such things as communication, self-care ability, performance of ADLs, interpersonal relationships, occupational functioning, and health and safety behaviors, may all be affected by the mental retardation. There are multiple causes related to mental retardation. The functioning of clients with mental retardation is affected throughout the life span, including the later years. These individuals are also more susceptible to alterations in emotional states.

NURSING MANAGEMENT

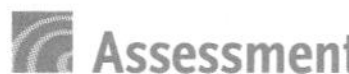

Assessment

Variables that may determine a client's level of functioning should be assessed to determine the extent to which they enhance or detract from client well-being (Box 14-7).

BOX 14-7 Factors to Assess in Older Adults With Mental Retardation

- Sociocultural factors (e.g., financial resources)
- Community setting (e.g., availability of needed services)
- Family support (e.g., their level of acceptance)
- Functional status (e.g., living independently)
- Education (e.g., highest grade level completed)
- Personal characteristics (e.g., level of happiness)
- Occupational opportunities (e.g., employment status)
- Social setting (e.g., peer group)

Diagnosis

The most common nursing diagnosis seen in older adults with mental retardation is altered thought processes. This may be evidenced by delusions, a decreased attention span, or impaired problem solving. This diagnosis represents the ongoing challenge with which older adults with mental retardation are living. Other common nursing diagnoses for older adults with mental retardation include self-care deficit and a potential for violence directed at self or others.

Planning and Expected Outcomes

In planning short- and long-term goals, the nurse should customize the care plan to a client's intellectual abilities. Adaptations to routine interventions may be needed to assist clients in comprehending their care, thereby allowing them to participate in the care. It may be useful to know a client's intellectual functioning in terms of age level, so interventions can be adapted accordingly. Expected outcomes include:

1. Client demonstrates ability to maintain personal safety as evidenced by ability to communicate anger and frustration, appropriately use methods for coping with feelings, and exhibit appropriate self-control.
2. Client demonstrates ability to care for self independently within limitations, as evidenced by demonstration of appropriate self-care activities on regular, consistent basis with minimum supervision.

Intervention

Nursing interventions that are specifically useful in dealing with older adults with mental retardation primarily involve customizing the care routines to their level of intellectual functioning. When communicating with a client, the nurse should use clear, simple instructions. Caregivers may be assigned a parental role by clients with mental retardation. This role may represent a challenge for these clients because of their continued dependence throughout their life span; this is especially true if parents or other family members who have cared for clients throughout their life have become disabled or are now deceased. Therefore many mentally retarded older adults with physical problems are admitted to nursing facilities for care.

Evaluation

In evaluating the care provided to older adult clients with mental retardation, the nurse should also be aware of the need for an expanded nursing focus in this population. The opportunities for nursing research and service, especially in community settings, are varied and abundant. Documentation focuses on achievement of the expected outcomes and on the adaptations that are required as a result of age-related changes superimposed on the mental retardation.

Conditions Associated With Physical Problems

This category includes mental illness symptoms that result from a physiologic process or a general medical condition, as well as the somatoform disorders. An example of a mental illness symptom that may be a result of a physiologic process would be a cognitive disorder resulting from head trauma. An example of a mental illness symptom that may be a result of a general medical condition can be personality changes that are a result of hypothyroidism (APA, 2000). Somatoform disorders are seen in a higher incidence among older adults. They are described as complaints of physical symptoms without the medical conditions that would explain the existence of the symptom. Box 14-8 outlines the various types of somatoform disorders.

NURSING MANAGEMENT

Assessment

The initial priority when assessing these clients is their physical status, which determines the interplay between their physical and mental status. Therefore a thorough health history, medication history, physical assessment, and mental status examination should be completed. Physical symptoms should not be ignored. Their presence should be explained by a physical illness, or their possible causes should be ruled out.

BOX 14-8 Types of Somatoform Disorders

TYPE	CHARACTERISTICS
Somatization	Multiple symptoms, usually a combination of symptoms and/or pain, often including gastrointestinal or sexual symptoms
Conversion	Unexplained neurologic motor disorders or sensory deficits
Pain disorder	Pain with unexplained onset, severity, or duration
Hypochondriasis	Preoccupation with or fear of serious disease that leads to an inordinate focus on body functions or symptoms; the most common somatoform disorder seen in older adults
Body dysmorphic	Preoccupation with an exaggerated or imagined physical appearance deficit

Health care professionals often minimize the physical complaints exhibited by older adults with somatoform disorders, but this can be a fatal mistake. Diagnoses can be missed, and clients who have true somatoform disorders may develop physical illnesses unrelated to their disorder. Failure to diagnose and appropriately treat such illnesses can be disastrous. In addition to assessing the physical and mental status of clients, the nurse should attempt to understand the secondary gain that clients may receive from the somatoform disorder. Often this information is best elicited by assessing the impact of the somatoform disorder on a client's family members and friends.

Diagnosis, Planning, and Expected Outcomes

The care of older adults with somatoform disorders is often planned around the nursing diagnosis of ineffective individual coping. The short- and long-term goals are then centered around enhancing client coping skills.

Intervention

The nurse should reinforce positive, healthy well-role behaviors and attitudes that clients may demonstrate. At the same time the nurse can encourage and reward client discussion of non–symptom-related topics. When clients attempt to focus on their physical symptoms, the nurse can respond with a caring but neutral attitude that does not encourage this focus. The nurse should not try to convince clients they are not ill or are not really experiencing the physical symptoms. Such efforts can be futile and frustrating for the clients and the nurse. The nurse should respond to clients' emotional feelings rather than focusing on the symptom. The nurse should be alert to the possibility of clients using multiple physicians who are unaware of one another, as well as the possibility of clients overusing both prescription and over-the-counter medications.

Evaluation

The nurse may become easily frustrated if all evaluation criteria center around a client's somatoform symptoms. These symptoms are not easily treated or readily relinquished. It may be helpful to use markers such as the consistency of the care a client received, any decrease seen in the client's levels of anxiety, or the client's improved awareness of his or her emotions, and then document based on these markers.

MEDICATION MANAGEMENT

Psychotropic Medications

The second most common type of medication used by older adults is psychotropic agents. These drugs affect client brain function, behavior, or experience (Antai-Otong, 2003). Older adults exhibit changes in the absorption, distribution, metabolism, and excretion of medications, as well as in the central nervous system neurotransmitters and receptor sites that these drugs affect. Therefore there is a corresponding change in the indications and contraindications for appropriate use of these medications (see Chapter 22).

In the past, psychotropics have been commonly used among long-term care residents. This use was often inappropriate or excessive. In 1987 federal regulations were developed (the Omnibus Budget Reconciliation Act) to decrease the inappropriate use of antipsychotic medications. There has been a corresponding decline in the frequency of use of antipsychotic agents in long-term care residents. Psychotropic medications are appropriate when used in long-term care settings for what Drinka (1993) terms the *three Ds*: "Danger, to the resident or others; distress for the resident; dysfunction of the resident including interference with basic nursing care."

A primary goal in medication management with older adult clients is to find the lowest effective dose with the least adverse effects. When psychotropic medications are used in older adults, it is also essential to remain aware of drug-drug interactions, drug-food interactions, nonadherence issues, and substance abuse and dependency issues. The nursing implications of antianxiety medications, antidepressants, antimanic agents, antipsychotics, and other psychoactive medications used in older adults are discussed in this section (Mohundro and Ramsey, 2003).

Antianxiety Agents. Antianxiety medications are also called anxiolytics. In the past, barbiturates were the main types of drugs used for anxiety; however, benzodiazepines are now used because of their improved safety compared with barbiturates. Long-term use (usually defined as longer than 1 to 2 months) of benzodiazepines does put clients at risk for the development of dependence, and they do have potential adverse interactions, especially with sedative agents and alcohol. There are two broad categories of benzodiazepines: short-acting (e.g., alprazolam [Xanax], lorazepam [Ativan], and oxazepam [Serax]) and long-acting (e.g., diazepam [Valium], chlordiazepoxide [Librium], and clonazepam [Klonopin]). The short-acting agents are preferred for older adults because of their lower potential for buildup leading to sedation and depression.

When used for anxiety, benzodiazepines should be given in the lowest possible dose for the shortest possible time. Therefore the precipitating cause of the anxiety needs to be evaluated and addressed while the benzodiazepine is being used. Although alprazolam may be used on a long-term basis for panic in older adults, most benzodiazepines should be used for less than 30 days. When used for longer periods, clients may experience withdrawal symptoms that can be as severe as seizures. When a drug is discontinued, it should be tapered slowly to prevent withdrawal symptoms or rebound anxiety symptoms. Of particular concern in older adults is the potential for benzodiazepines to exacerbate sleep apnea. Therefore older adults should be assessed for alterations in sleep patterns (especially snoring) before using a benzodiazepine.

There are other options besides benzodiazepines for older adults who need an anxiolytic. Buspirone (BuSpar) is a chemically unique antianxiety agent that does not produce dependence or interaction with benzodiazepines or alcohol. Its drawback lies in its slow onset of action (often up to 2 weeks), which tends to limit client compliance. Nurses can play an important role in educating clients about the slow onset of buspirone, thereby improving the clients' adherence to their medication regimens and giving older adults a safer option for reducing anxiety. Other medications used to manage anxiety in older adults include antidepressants and beta-blockers such as propranolol (Inderal).

Antidepressants. Antidepressant medications include monoamine oxidase inhibitors (MAOIs), tricyclics, and selective serotonin reuptake inhibitors (SSRIs). The MAOIs (e.g., phenelzine [Nardil] and tranylcypromine [Parnate]) affect the monoamine neurotransmitter system but are rarely used because of their potential drug-food interaction with tyramine, which can precipitate a hypertensive crisis. They are used for older adults with refractory depression or cardiac arrhythmias, since they do not produce the cardiovascular side effects of other antidepressants. Clients taking MAOIs must adhere to a tyramine-free diet and must be warned of the potential for a hypertensive crisis from drug-drug interactions with a number of other medications. Their physicians and pharmacists should monitor any new prescription or over-the-counter medications.

Tricyclic antidepressants such as amitriptyline (Elavil), imipramine (Tofranil), desipramine (Norpramin), and nortriptyline (Pamelor) block the reuptake of norepinephrine and serotonin. The side effects include anticholinergic effects, sedation, hypotension, dry mouth, tachycardia, blurred vision, constipation, and urinary retention. These medications are contraindicated in clients with recent myocardial infarction or cardiac arrhythmias. They are rarely used since the development of the new SSRIs.

The most recent additions to the antidepressant category are SSRIs such as fluoxetine (Prozac), sertraline (Zoloft), paroxetine (Paxil), fluvoxamine (Luvox), citalopram (Celexa), and escitalopram (Lexapro). All are selective and potent inhibitors of serotonin reuptake, but each differs slightly in its effect on other neurotransmitter receptors and enzymes, which may make the difference in tolerability and efficacy to individual agents. When using SSRIs with the older population, start with a low dose and go slowly. When withdrawing the antidepressants, do so over 2 to 6 weeks to avoid withdrawal symptoms. The SSRIs are considered safe in the elderly because of a low risk of central nervous system, anticholinergic, and cardiovascular effects. However, the older population is at increased risk for impaired balance and falls with any antidepressant, especially at a higher dose. Older patients may need up to 12 weeks on these medications for evaluation of a full response. It is important to monitor for drug-drug interactions and for excessive weight loss, especially in those who are debilitated. Improved cognitive function has been noted in the elderly patient with depression when treated with antidepressants (Bezchilibnyk-Butler and Jeffries, 2001; de la Fuente, 2001).

Bupropion (Wellbutrin, Wellbutrin SR, and Wellbutrin XL) is the one norepinephrine dopamine reuptake inhibitor. The main consideration is screening out patients with a history of seizures, organic brain disorder, or alcohol withdrawal. The elderly are at risk for increased accumulation of bupropion because of decreased clearance of the drug and its metabolites.

Venlafaxine (Effexor, Effexor SR), a selective serotonin norepinephrine reuptake inhibitor, is considered three drugs in one. At the lower dose it is a potent inhibitor of serotonin; at moderate doses both serotonin and norepinephrine reuptake occurs; and at the higher doses neuronal uptake pumps for serotonin, norepinephrine, and dopamine are inhibited. This is an excellent choice for anxiety with comorbid depression and for GAD.

Mirtazapine (Remeron) is a nonadrenergic-specific serotonergic antidepressant and is very sedating at 15 mg and below and less sedating at doses greater than 15 mg. It can increase appetite and weight gain because of its strong antihistaminic properties, but the side effects sometimes diminish over time. Monitor for sedation, hypotension, and anticholinergic effects, and taper this medication gradually, like all antidepressants, to avoid withdrawal symptoms. Clearance of the medication is reduced in elderly men by up to 40% and in elderly women by up to 10% (de la Fuente, 2001). A new drug, duloxetine hydrochloride (Cymbalta), is being launched for the treatment of major depressive disorder.

Additional helpful information about antidepressants includes the course of treatment. Antidepressants are commonly used until clients have been free of the symptoms of depression for 6 months to 2 years. Clients are then gradually taken off the medication to prevent the development of rebound depression. Some clients with recurrent major depression may continue to use antidepressants indefinitely. Compliance problems may be more common in older adults because of side effects of the medication. However, because of the concern about side effects, drug prescribing in this age group has been to start low, go slow, and never go high, often resulting in doses that do not achieve "a full response." Careful monitoring of drug dosage and drug interactions will aid in client adherence, safety, and recovery (de la Fuente, 2001). ECT may be used in clients with life-threatening depression if antidepressants have not been effective. The usual course of ECT would be 10 to 14 treatments every other day. ECT is now considered a humane and effective treatment for depression because of the use of anesthesia and muscle relaxants during the procedure.

Mood Stabilizers. In the older population with bipolar disorder, lithium and anticonvulsants are used as mood stabilizers. The older adult is more sensitive to lithium and is at a higher risk for neurotoxicity and cognitive impairment, even at therapeutic plasma levels. Before beginning lithium use, clients should have baseline ECG; CBC; and renal, thyroid, and liver function studies. In the older adult lithium begins at a low dosage (e.g., 300 mg/day), and a blood level is obtained in 3 or 4 days. This level should be drawn 12 hours after the last dose of lithium. The dose is then titrated until a therapeutic blood level is reached (usually 0.4 to 1.5 mEq/L). Blood levels are drawn every 3 or 4 days until the therapeutic level is attained. The frequency of obtaining blood levels can then be decreased to once a month for the first 6 months, then every 2 to 3 months indefinitely. Renal, liver, and thyroid studies should be evaluated every 6 months because of potential toxicity (de la Fuente, 2001).

Side effects seen in older adults who are taking lithium include gastrointestinal distress, hand tremors, ataxia, and weight gain. Cardiovascular side effects may also occur; therefore periodic ECGs may be obtained as needed. Lithium toxicity can be evident in blood levels greater than 1.5 mEq/L; moderate to severe toxicity can be seen in levels greater than 2 mEq/L; and death may occur with blood levels greater than 2.5 mEq/L. Clients should inform all physicians and pharmacists involved in their care of any lithium use because of the potential for drug-drug interactions.

Anticonvulsants are also considered a good option for use in bipolar mood disorders, but again, dosing should be gradual in the older population and those with liver impairment. These drugs may cause confusion, cognitive impairments, or ataxia that can lead to falls. There is an additive caution in combining them with other drugs that affect the central nervous system or have anticholinergic properties. Valproate, one of the anticonvulsants, causes an increased risk for thrombocytopenia in the older population (de la Fuente, 2001). Symbyax (fluoxetine and olanzapine) is a new combination drug for bipolar disorder, depressive episode.

Antipsychotic Medications. Antipsychotic medications are also called neuroleptics. They work by blocking the action of dopamine. Neuroleptics are used in schizophrenia, acute psychosis, and delirium; they may be used to treat the agitation and aggression sometimes seen in dementia. The specific choice of a neuroleptic agent is made both by considering clients' clinical symptoms and examining the side-effect profiles of the various neuroleptic agents. Older adults are usually started on lower doses (one half to one third of the normal dose) of the high-potency neuroleptics such as haloperidol (Haldol), thiothixene (Navane), or trifluoperazine (Stelazine). The high-potency neuroleptics have a lower frequency of anticholinergic, cardiovascular, and sedative side effects than do the low-potency neuroleptics such as chlorpromazine (Thorazine) and thioridazine (Mellaril). However, the high-potency neuroleptics have an increased rate of extrapyramidal symptoms (EPSs) in comparison with the low-potency neuroleptics. Therefore it is essential to monitor all clients on neuroleptics for EPSs, which are discussed later in this chapter. Haloperidol and fluphenazine (Prolixin) are neuroleptics that are available in long-acting deaconate forms for nonadhering clients, and may be administered weekly to monthly. However, the deaconates are rarely used in older adults because of their long half-life of 1 to 4 weeks. This treatment could be dangerous should side effects become problematic.

Clozapine (Clozaril), risperidone (Risperdal), quetiapine (Seroquel), ziprasidone (Geodon), and aripiprazole (Abilify) are newer, atypical antipsychotics with a decreased incidence of side effects and EPSs. Unfortunately, clozapine carries with it the potentially dangerous side effect of agranulocytosis; therefore weekly CBCs must be obtained for all clients receiving clozapine. The safety of the newer, atypical antipsychotics for older adult clients is uncertain because of limited data, but unpublished trials seem to indicate promising results (American Medical Directors Association, 1998).

Side Effects

Extrapyramidal Symptoms. Nurses play a vital role in the monitoring, education, and evaluation of EPSs in clients who are receiving neuroleptic medications. EPSs are described in Box 14-9.

EPSs are treated with anticholinergic or antiparkinsonian agents such as diphenhydramine (Benadryl), benztropine (Cogentin), or trihexyphenidyl (Artane). Amantadine (Symmetrel), a dopamine agonist, may be used, especially in older clients and those with cardiovascular dysfunction, because of its reduced anticholinergic effects.

Tardive Dyskinesia. Tardive dyskinesia (TD) is a potentially permanent neurologic side effect of neuroleptic medications. Clients and their families must be informed of the risk of TD before initiating neuroleptic therapy. TD is characterized by involuntary movements, especially in the face, lips, and tongue. The trunk and extremities may also be involved. TD is most likely to develop in clients who have used neuroleptics longer than 2 years. Clients should be evaluated for TD at each appointment. Unfortunately, no effective treatment for TD exists. The best prevention is using the lowest possible dose of a neuroleptic for the shortest time necessary.

BOX 14-9 Extrapyramidal Symptoms

SYMPTOM	CHARACTERISTICS
Acute dystonic reaction	Muscle rigidity; eyes fixed in deviated position; arched posture; should be treated with an anticholinergic agent such as diphenhydramine
Akathisia	Inability to sit still
Akinesia	Decreased psychomotor movements; shuffling gait
Pseudoparkinsonism	Tremor in the extremities that resembles Parkinson's disease
Perioral tremor (rabbit syndrome)	Fine, rapid lip movements

Neuroleptic Malignant Syndrome. Neuroleptic malignant syndrome (NMS) is a rare but serious side effect that may lead to death. Its frequency increases with the use of high-potency antipsychotics. The initial symptoms include a decreased temperature, the development of EPSs, and delirium. If untreated, it then progresses to hyperthermia, stupor, severe EPSs, and coma. It is treated by immediately discontinuing any neuroleptic medication. Dantrolene sodium, which can cause liver toxicity, or bromocriptine may also be used. Because of the potential for death from NMS, all clients receiving neuroleptic medications in an inpatient or long-term care setting should have their vital signs measured daily. Clients who take neuroleptics on an outpatient basis should be educated on the signs of NMS, particularly the cardinal sign of a temperature change.

EPSs, TD, and NMS all present significant risks for clients taking neuroleptic medications. It is therefore essential that nurses educate clients and their caregivers of the need for routine monitoring for the development of these side effects.

Other Psychoactive Medications Used With Older Adults

Anafranil. Clomipramine (Anafranil) is a tricyclic antidepressant that is specifically helpful for OCD. Its side-effect profile is consistent with that of other tricyclics.

Antiparkinsonian Agents. As discussed earlier, antiparkinsonian agents such as benztropine and trihexyphenidyl are used to treat side effects elicited by antipsychotic medications.

Sedative-Hypnotic Agents. Sleep patterns change with age, and older adults may experience a decrease both in the quantity and quality of sleep. Delayed onset of sleep and nighttime awakenings are not uncommon in older adults. Sedative-hypnotic agents can be dangerous when used in older adults; therefore they are used only if clients are unable to function on a daily basis as a result of insomnia. Long-term use of sedative-hypnotics can produce a disturbed sleep-wake cycle and can lead to dependence and a decrease in the sense of being rested, even after an adequate amount of sleep. In older adults whose symptoms include insomnia, other causes should first be ruled out. Early-night insomnia may be indicative of anxiety or pain (e.g., arthritis), and middle-of-the-night to late-night insomnia may be seen with depression. Additional information on the nursing management of sleep disorders in older adults is found in Chapter 11.

MENTAL HEALTH RESOURCES

The number and quality of resources for the care of mental illness in older adults are minimum because geropsychiatric care is a relatively new specialty within gerontology. These resources include human resources (e.g., mental health professionals [physicians and nurses], physical resources (e.g., hospitals, clinics, nursing facilities, and dementia units), and financial resources needed to pay for mental health care (e.g., Medicare, Medicaid, and health insurance coverage).

Human Resources

Geriatric psychiatrists are physicians trained as psychiatrists with special preparation in the care of older adults with mental and behavioral problems. They may be nationally certified in general psychiatry with additional qualifications in geriatric psychiatry. They work with older individuals and their families in private practice, group practice, clinics, and hospitals, using a wide variety of treatment modalities. Psychiatrists trained in geriatrics are more likely to meet the needs and satisfaction of older clients.

However, according to Koenig (1994), "Few health professionals . . . choose geriatrics as their primary specialty," especially when psychiatrists receive such low reimbursement from Medicare and managed care organizations. Therefore few young physicians are motivated to choose a career in geriatric psychiatry.

Geropsychiatric nurses and geriatric mental health nurses are trained at the master's level, usually in programs that offer some combination of psychiatric or mental health nursing and gerontologic nursing course work (Hoeffer, 1994). The primary major is usually psychiatric or mental health nursing with some courses in gerontologic nursing. These nurses may be certified by the American Nurses Credentialing Center as clinical nurse specialists in adult psychiatric and mental health nursing, as gerontologic nurses, or as both, if they have master's degree preparation in one or both specialties. These specialists should be prepared to assess and care for individuals who often have multiple, complex, physical *and* mental or emotional problems. There is no national certification in geropsychiatric nursing.

More geropsychiatric nurses are needed to work as staff or consultants in hospitals, nursing facilities, outpatient clinics, day treatment centers, adult day services programs, and home health agencies. Geropsychiatric advanced practice nurses, often working with geriatric psychiatrists, provide much needed care in nursing facilities. They do assessments, manage medications, participate in individual and group therapy on a regular schedule, and provide in-service education for the nursing staff. As previously mentioned, many older adults are never adequately diagnosed or treated for underlying psychopathologic problems. Nurses in these settings can help prevent this occurrence. These nurses are also greatly needed to teach technical nursing staff members, who have close contact with clients, in how to communicate with and relate to older adults with mental and emotional disturbances. Client abuse may occur when nonprofessional staff does not know how to respond to aggressive, hostile, and combative behavior.

Because an interdisciplinary approach is important in the health care of older adults, psychiatrists, social workers, dietitians, clergy, speech pathologists, and physical and occupational therapists with some formal preparation in geriatrics and gerontology are also essential to provide high-quality care for geropsychiatric clients.

Physical Resources

Older clients with mental and emotional problems are increasingly being treated on an outpatient basis, primarily because of available methods of payment. Some of these outpatient choices are:

- Community mental health centers (which may include emergency psychiatric services during the evening or night)
- The clinic or offices of a geriatric psychiatrist, geriatric mental health nurse, or advanced practice nurse specializing in geriatric mental health
- Senior partial hospitalization programs where clients receive assessment, diagnosis, and treatment (including various types of medications and other therapy), then return home in the late afternoon
- In-home assessments, diagnosis, treatment, care, and follow-up in clients' own residences

These types of programs may be more effective for older clients than residential treatment in hospitals, which can cause relocation confusion, loss of familiar environmental and sensory stimulation, and functional decline associated with the hospitalization. On the other hand, individuals without family members or an adequate support system may have problems managing difficult medication regimens alone at home. Those with major depression are at greater risk for potential suicide.

Some general hospitals have geropsychiatric units staffed and equipped to care for the mental *and* physical needs of older clients. These units provide thorough assessments and an interdisciplinary approach to total care and rehabilitation on a relatively short-term basis for older clients with primarily mental and emotional problems. Unless the general psychiatric hospital has a specific unit planned for older clients, such a facility may have difficulty meeting their needs. In fact, many general psychiatric hospitals do not even admit clients who also have physical problems and needs. Most geropsychiatric units are located in psychiatric facilities associated with medical schools, where fellowships are available to psychiatrists specializing in this area. Some psychiatric hospitals have well-developed day hospitalization programs that provide treatment, care, and supervision on a daily basis. However, adequate transportation to and from the hospital each day can be a problem for older persons. Some hospitals and community agencies provide this type of medical transportation when individuals or their families cannot provide it. However, escort services from the van to the area of treatment may not be available, so that the older person cannot make the trip alone for safety reasons.

The large majority of older persons who have some type of chronic mental illness or disorder are found in long-term care nursing facilities with some type of dementia or depression related to physical or environmental factors. In fact, Brower (1993) has stated that nursing facilities "are in reality mini-geropsychiatric facilities but without the trained psychiatric staff." Many of the residents in these facilities have not had the benefit of a thorough mental status assessment and diagnosis and therefore lack proper treatment and care. In addition to ageism, another reason for this problem is the lack of adequate financial resources for the necessary assessment and treatment.

Few nursing facilities have special units or programs exclusively for the treatment and care of residents with mental illness, excluding those with dementia. In an attempt to determine to what extent mental health services and personnel were available in nursing facilities in one metropolitan area, the Mental Health and Aging Coalition mailed a survey to 67 facilities. Thirty-two (48%) of the surveys were returned. Most of them were completed by the facility social worker. Only six (19%) used a mental health screening test on admission. The most common mental diagnoses *documented* on the medical record were major depression, anxiety disorder, schizophrenia, and bipolar disorder. The most common types of interventions used were psychotropic medications (97%), referral to an outside mental health professional (94%), and behavioral therapy (75%) (Hogstel and Weeks, 1998).

Financial Resources

One of the greatest issues in the care of mental illnesses or disorders in older adults is the lack of adequate financial resources to provide for needed care. For adults ages 65 and older, Medicare coverage is limited (Box 14-10).

Inequality in the provision of health insurance coverage exposes a person with mental or emotional distress to disproportionately high copayments and out-of-pocket expenses. Many health plans provide fewer "covered days" for psychiatric hospitalization and limited visits to mental health specialists when compared with general medical coverage. This practice is especially hurtful to Medicare beneficiaries, who are required to pay a 20% copayment for medical and surgical services but are held responsible for 50% of the cost of mental health services. The General Accounting Office (GAO) reported that approximately 90% of all insurance plans impose some restrictions on mental health benefits that are not placed on general medical care (Novosel, 2004).

Medicaid is a federal-state program that differs somewhat from state to state. Services for mental health care for both inpatient and outpatient care are limited for Medicaid recipients (Hogstel and Weeks, 1998). A current trend in many states is to place people on Medicaid in coordinated (managed) care plans to save money. States must receive a waiver from the federal government for this plan because partial federal funds are used. How this proposal works will be of interest, especially as if affects those with dementia who reside in nursing facilities. If nursing facilities bid on Medicaid-coordinated (managed) care contracts for their residents on Medicaid, there is concern that less money will be available for total care and even less for mental health care. Managed care plans have generally not "established systemic policies for how mental health is to be delivered" (Colenda, Banazak, and Mickus, 1998).

BOX 14-10 Medicare Coverage for Mental Health Care

MEDICARE	COVERAGE
Part A (hospital)	Lifetime limit of 190 days of inpatient care in a participating psychiatric hospital Inpatient psychiatric care in a general hospital the same as any other Medicare inpatient hospital care
Part B (outpatient after initial $100 deductible)	Partial hospitalization (day treatment) for approved care in a Medicare-participating facility Pays 50% of approved amount of mental health care by physicians, clinical psychologists, clinical social workers, and other nonphysician practitioners in a mental health care center, skilled nursing facility, or physician's office 20% copayment for psychotropic prescription drugs

From US Department of Health and Human Services: *Your Medicare 1997 handbook*, Baltimore, 1997, Pub. No HCFA 10050, Social Security Administration; Colenda CC, Banzak D, Mickus M: Mental health services in managed care: quality questions remain, *Geriatrics* 53(8):60, 1998.

TRENDS AND NEEDS

The need to focus more on the mental and emotional health care needs of older adults will continue to increase (Box 14-11). Nurses and family members must advocate for older persons who have mental illnesses or disorders and who are not being adequately diagnosed and treated. State and local ombudsmen programs are expanding, with plans to have at least one or two certified trained volunteer ombudsmen in all long-term care facilities, including nursing facilities, hospital skilled nursing

BOX 14-11 Trends and Needs in Mental Health Care of Older Adults

- Strong advocacy
- Increased outpatient care
- Expanded community resources
- Improved quality of long-term care
- Additional legislation and regulations related to psychosocial training for staff in long-term care facilities
- More emphasis on gerontologic, geriatric, and geropsychiatric education for health care providers
- More educational programs for family members
- Short-term respite care for family members

units, and assisted living facilities (sometimes called personal care homes).

Long periods of hospitalization in a psychiatric hospital are rare. More people are treated in the home setting and in partial hospitalization and outpatient settings. Other community organizations such as churches and congregations, senior citizens' groups, and other social organizations are developing programs to help older persons maintain their mental health by preventing loneliness and depression. There will be increased emphasis on improving the quality of care in long-term care facilities. The primary need is to focus more on mental illnesses or disorders, psychosocial issues, and communication skills (e.g., in-service training for all personnel). Perhaps this goal will be accomplished through state legislation or regulatory agencies. Emphasis will also be placed on increasing gerontologic, geriatric, and geropsychiatric content in the curricula of medical, nursing, and social work educational programs. Advocacy groups should work toward including more of such content in state licensing examinations.

Family members also need to learn more about the aging process, especially the normal, common, and abnormal changes in behavior as one ages, so that they will be better able to relate to and care for their older family members in the home if needed. Although respite care (e.g., adult day programs and nursing facilities) is available to some extent for those family members who care for older persons with mental and behavioral problems, additional short-term respite care is greatly needed. Family members caring for older persons in the home need a couple of hours of relief now and then, perhaps by a volunteer from a church, so that they can take a walk, go to a movie, or go shopping. Trained volunteers can easily provide this kind of short-term respite care to assist the caregiver and, ultimately, the older family member.

More emphasis needs to be placed on the cultural and ethnic influences on mental health, especially since minority populations are increasing every year. Not only must nurses learn more about the special needs and customs of various ethnic groups, but nursing also needs to recruit students from these groups into the profession. Some older adults who are immigrants from other countries retain more of their cultural beliefs and practices than younger adults. Health practices they have used successfully in the past should not be devalued or discouraged as long as they do not interfere with current essential treatment modalities (see Cultural Awareness boxes).

Cultural Awareness

SELECT CULTURE-BOUND SYNDROMES

GROUP	DISORDER	REMARKS
Black/Haitian	Blackout	Collapse, dizziness, inability to move
	Low blood	Not enough blood or weakness of the blood; often treated with diet
	High blood	Blood that is too rich; a result of ingestion of too much red meat or rich foods
	Thin blood	Occurs in women, children, and older persons; renders the individual more susceptible to illness in general
	Diseases of hex, witchcraft, or conjuring	Sense of being doomed by spell; gastrointestinal symptoms such as vomiting; hallucinations; part of voodoo beliefs
Chinese/ Southeast Asian	Koro	Intense anxiety that penis is retracting into the body
Eskimo	Pibloktoq	Traumatic anxiety state; bizarre, overdramatized behavior such as running naked through the snow
Greek	Hysteria	Bizarre complaints and behavior; belief that the uterus leaves the pelvis for another part of the body
Hispanic	Empacho	Food forms into a ball and clings to the stomach or intestines, causing pain and cramping
	Fatigue	Asthma-like symptoms
	Pasmo	Paralysis-like symptoms of the face or limbs; often prevented or relieved by massage
	Susto	Anxiety, trembling, phobias from sudden fright

Cultural Awareness—cont'd

SELECT CULTURE-BOUND SYNDROMES—cont'd

GROUP	DISORDER	REMARKS
Native American	Ghost	Terror, hallucinations, sense of danger
	Trance disassociation Soul loss	Caused by the loss of one's soul or the invasion of a benign or evil spirit; viewed as a mystical state; some vision quests result in altered states of consciousness
Japanese	Wagamama	Apathetic childish behavior with emotional outbursts
Korean	Hwa-Byung	Multiple somatic and psychologic symptoms, including "pushing up" sensation of chest, palpitations, flushing, headache, epigastric mass, dysphoria, anxiety, irritability, and difficulty concentrating; mostly affects married women

Cultural Awareness

CULTURAL INFLUENCES ON MENTAL HEALTH AND MENTAL ILLNESS

- Regardless of whether they are understood, people of all cultures have reasons for their behavior.
- Normal and abnormal behaviors are cultural phenomena.
- Culture influences the expression, presentation, recognition, labeling, explanations, acceptance, and distribution of mental illness, as well as its treatments and healers.
- Mental health and mental illness are more difficult to delineate than physical disorders. For example, visions and dream states, hallucinations, trances, delusions, belief in spirits, speaking in "tongues," drug or alcohol intoxication, and suicide may be judged normal or abnormal according to the cultural context.
- At times, cultural groups encourage altered states of consciousness that may be viewed as mental disturbances to outsiders.
- Although mental disorders occur in every society, cultural tolerance for variations in human behavior varies markedly from one cultural group to the next.

Needs for Research

There is much need for research in the nursing care of older persons with mental, emotional, and behavioral problems. Some questions and needs to consider include:

- Should some type of mental status screening tool be used in the assessment of all older adults admitted to general hospitals and nursing facilities to detect possible problems for earlier treatment? If so, which tool or tools?
- To what extent are licensed nurses in nursing facilities knowledgeable about the diagnosis, treatment, and nursing care of residents with mental health disorders?
- What can nurses do to decrease loneliness and depression in older persons, especially in home health care and nursing facilities?
- Is group psychotherapy effective in decreasing depression in nursing facility residents? Who should lead these groups?
- To what extent do home health care nurses assess mental status in their clients?
- What will be the effect of decreasing Medicare, Medicaid, and managed care funding for mental health treatment and care of older persons?
- To what extent do coordinated (managed) care plans (e.g., Medicare, health maintenance organizations, and Medicaid) provide mental health care for older adults? What is the quality of that care? Is there a focus on prevention of mental illnesses or disorders?
- Which psychotropic medications and doses are the most effective and have the fewest side effects in older adults?

Home Care

1. Assess for any changes in behavior.
2. Insist on a specific diagnosis by the physician.
3. Assess situational factors in the environment that may predispose older clients to depression.
4. Chronic, long-lasting incurable diseases predispose clients in the home to feelings of frustration and depression; they may even lead to suicide.
5. In assessing older adults, look for signs of depression, including behavioral changes such as difficulty completing ADLs, decrease in appetite, changes in sleep patterns, lowered energy levels, poor grooming, and withdrawal from people and interests.
6. Physiologic symptoms that may be seen in clients at home who are experiencing depression include muscle aches, abdominal pain or tightness, flatulence, nausea and vomiting, dry mouth, and headaches.

Home Care—cont'd

7. The Geriatric Depression Scale is an effective screening tool that can be used to assess depression in older clients.
8. Assess the perception of the future in all clients in the home, since this population has an increased incidence of suicide.
9. Use psychiatric and mental health specialists to provide counseling to clients and caregivers.
10. Early recognition of delirium can be helpful in obtaining diagnosis, treatment, and care for clients.

SUMMARY

Many older persons experience mental, emotional, and behavioral disorders. One of the major problems is that they are often not diagnosed or treated. Some of the reasons for this problem are a false belief that mental symptoms are a part of the normal aging process, a belief that these symptoms are not treatable or curable (which is a reflection of ageism), or a reluctance on the part of older persons to admit a need and seek treatment and care from mental health professionals because of a stigma about mental illness.

Important factors in maintaining mental health wellness among older adults are physical wellness, especially good nutrition, exercise, and limited prescription medications; physical and mental activity and stimulation; and a strong support system comprising family, church, friends, and neighbors.

Nurses play important and varied roles in the management of mental illnesses or disorders experienced by older adults. The nurse has the opportunity to enhance the quality of life in older adult clients by maintaining an awareness of the illnesses or disorders that may be seen in this population and appropriately intervening when they are recognized. The establishment of effective communication, a therapeutic relationship, and health promotion activities are functions that are integral in the treatment of mental illnesses or disorders. These are also functions that nurses have the education, skills, and experience to implement in an expert manner. The nursing focus on promoting a biopsychosocial approach, encouraging family involvement, and developing an effective continuity of care also allows nurses to play a unique and vital role in the treatment of mental illnesses or disorders in older adults.

The major mental illnesses or disorders experienced by older adults include depression, suicide, delirium, dementia, anxiety, schizophrenia, delusional disorders, mental retardation, and somatoform disorders. The major psychotropic medication groups were summarized with a focus on their nursing implications.

Resources for the treatment and care of mental illness in older adults are limited. These resources include geriatric psychiatrists, geropsychiatric nurses, and other mental health professionals prepared in geropsychiatry; geropsychiatric units and psychiatric hospitals; dementia special care units in nursing facilities; and special stand-alone dementia care facilities. Medicare, Medicaid, and private health insurance companies provide only limited coverage and care for mental illnesses or disorders, in part because these often are chronic long-term conditions and the benefits of diagnosis, treatment, and care are less predictable than for physical illness.

More geropsychiatric diagnoses and treatments are being carried out on a partial hospitalization or outpatient basis for older adults. However, there continues to be a great need to provide more mental health care and support to older residents in the 23,000 nursing facilities in the United States. Nurses need to be strong advocates for their older clients by helping them maintain their independence, self-respect, and self-worth; by referring them for specific diagnosis and treatment when mental or emotional problems are noted; and by improving the quality of psychosocial communication and care of older persons in all health care settings.

Key Points

- Health care providers and older persons themselves often blame mental and emotional problems on the aging process.
- Many older persons with mental illnesses or disorders are never diagnosed and treated.
- Physical wellness, mental and physical activity, adaptation to the changes of aging, and a strong support system contribute to mental health wellness.
- To positively affect older adult clients who are experiencing alterations in mental health, the nurse must first develop therapeutic relationships based on trust.
- Nurses who care for older adult clients must be aware of the clients' significant risk for suicide.
- The reduction of anxiety is a central focus of nursing interventions in caring for older adults experiencing delusions.
- A central goal in psychotropic medication use in older adults is finding the lowest effective dose with the least adverse effects.
- There are few geropsychiatrists and geropsychiatric nurses in the United States.
- Most acute mental illnesses or disorders in older persons are treated in a partial hospitalization program or on an outpatient basis.
- There is a disparity in the insurance coverage for mental and physical disorders.
- Nurses need to be strong advocates for their older clients in obtaining accurate diagnosis and treatment of mental illnesses or disorders.

Critical Thinking Exercises

1. The wife of a 68-year-old man died 1 year ago. During a routine blood pressure screening, he admits to the nurse that he is depressed. What additional data should the nurse obtain?
2. On admission to the hospital of an older woman with longstanding chronic emphysema, the nurse performs a thorough physical assessment but overlooks the psychologic assessment. Should this oversight be called to the nurse's attention? Why is a psychologic assessment of particular importance in this older adult?
3. Analyze sociocultural, economic, and technologic trends into the early twenty-first century. How might future trends affect the mental and emotional health care needs of older persons? What role will the nurse play in meeting the mental health needs of this population?

References

American Medical Directors Association: Symposium coverage: psychopharmacology update, *Ann Long-Term Care* 5(A):1, 1998.

American Psychiatric Association: *Diagnostic and statistical manual of mental disorders: DSM-IV-TR*, ed 4, Washington, DC, 2000, The Association.

Antai-Otong D: Optimizing psychotropic use in older adults: strategies for nurse practitioners, *Adv Nurse Pract* 11(8):32, 2003.

Baldessarini R: Reducing suicide risk in psychiatric disorders, *Current Psychiatry* 2(9):15, 2003.

Bezchilibnyk-Butler KJ, Jeffries JJ. In de la Fuente E: Pharmacologic and nonpharmacologic options for anxiety and depression in late life, *J Am Psych Nurses Assoc* 7(6):S8, 2001.

Brower HT: Special care units for dementia, *J Gerontol Nurs* 19(2):3, 1993.

Byrd L: Terminal dementia in the elderly, *Adv Nurse Pract* 11(9):65, 2003.

Calandra J: Mental health and older adults: mental illness in later life, part 1, *NurseWeek* 4(23):21, 2003a.

Calandra J: Mental health and older adults: mental illness in later life, part 2, *NurseWeek* 4(24):25, 2003b.

Colenda CC, Banazak D, Mickus M: Mental health services in managed care: quality questions remain, *Geriatrics* 53(8):49, 1998.

de la Fuente E: Pharmacologic and nonpharmacologic options for anxiety and depression in late life, *J Am Psych Nurses Assoc* 7(6):S8, 2001.

Drinka D: OBRA-1987 nursing home regulations, *J Am Geriatr Soc* 41(4):466, 1993.

Ebersole P, Hess P: *Geriatric nursing and healthy aging*, St Louis, 2001, Mosby.

Fontaine K: *Mental health nursing*, ed 5, NJ, 2003, Prentice Hall.

Hoeffer B: Essential curriculum content, *J Psychosoc Nurs* 32(4):33, 1994.

Hogstel MO, Weeks S: Mental health issues in long-term care, *Issues Mental Health Nurs* 1998.

Koenig HG: *Aging and God*, Binghamton, NY, 1994, Haworth Press.

Mohundro M, Ramsey L: Pharmacologic considerations in geriatric patients, *Adv Nurse Pract* 11(9):21, 2003.

Montross L et al: Preventing late-life suicide: 6 steps to detect the warning signs, *Current Psychiatry* 2(8):15, 2003.

Morris PL: Geriatric mental health: an overview, *J Am Psych Nurses Assoc* 7(6):82, 2001.

National Institute of Mental Health: Older adults: depression and suicide facts, 2003. Accessed on website: http://www.nimh.nih.gov/publicat/elderlydepsuicide.cfm.

Novosel L: Securing mental health parity: the struggle to become law, *Am J Nurse Pract* 8(6):9, 2004.

Richardson S: Delirium: assessment and treatment of the elderly patient, *Am J Nurse Pract* 7(1):9, 2003.

Salzman C in de la Fuente E: Pharmacologic and nonpharmacologic options for anxiety and depression in late life, *J Am Psych Nurses Assoc* 7(6):S8, 2001.

Serby M, Yu M: There's good news about depression in the elderly, *Clinical Advisor* Sept 2003, p 64.

Stevens GL, Friedman SD, Baldwin BA: Geriatric psychiatric nursing. In Stuart GN, Laraia, MT, editors: *Principles and practice of psychiatric nursing*, ed 6, St Louis, 1998, Mosby.

Waite R: Successful aging: mental health, *National Black Nurses Assoc News* Spring 2004, p 33.

Whitney CR: Oldest person in the world turns 120, *Fort Worth Star Telegram* Sec A:1, Feb 22, 1995.

15 Pain

MARGARET LOUIS, PhD, RN, BC, and SUE E. MEINER, EdD, APRN, BC, GNP

Learning Objectives

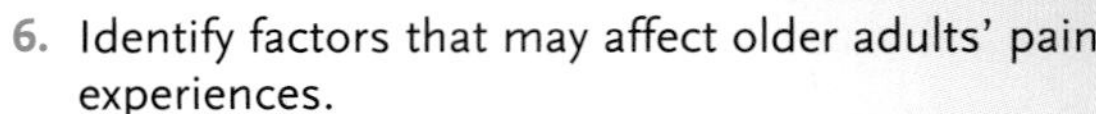

On completion of this chapter, the reader will be able to:

1. Define the concept of pain, including types and sources.
2. Identify the potential effects of pain on an older adult.
3. Discuss the goals of pain management in older adults.
4. Identify barriers that affect pain assessment or its management in older adult clients.
5. Describe the effect of pain on quality of life for older adult clients.
6. Identify factors that may affect older adults' pain experiences.
7. Use a pain assessment tool to rate clients' pain intensity.
8. Describe the use of pharmacologic and nonpharmacologic therapies for older adults with pain.

Pain is not part of growing old (Kedziera, 2001). There are many misconceptions about pain and age; predominant among the ones held by health care professionals is the myth that pain is a normal aspect of growing old (Pasero, Reed, and McCaffery, 1999). Many health care practitioners have only encountered older adults in an emergency room or hospitals where they are in need of unusually intense medical or nursing treatment; this is not a good way to understand that these patients are not representative of normal aging.

UNDERSTANDING PAIN

Definition

Understanding pain and how to efficaciously treat it calls for a look at how pain is defined. There are multiple definitions of pain; most include the mind-body relationship. According to some, pain is an unpleasant sensory and emotional experience associated with actual or potential tissue damage (McCaffery, Frock, and Garguilo, 2003; McCaffery and Pasero, 1999). McCaffery (2000) further states that pain is "whatever the experiencing person says it is, existing whenever he or she says it does." Aronoff's (2002) definition is more specific: "a subjective, personal, unpleasant experience involving sensations and perceptions that may or may not relate to bodily or tissue damage." Pain is also defined as an unpleasant sensory and emotional experience (Merskey and Bogduk, 1994). The literature on pain is in agreement that pain is a complex phenomenon derived from sensory stimuli or neurologic injury and modified by individual memory, expectations, and emotions (Sternbach, 1978) and that it is usually associated with injury or a pathophysiologic process that causes an uncomfortable experience. These authors clearly note pain is individual and can be very different for different persons with the same disease or injury.

Pain Classification

Pain can be defined as acute or chronic. Acute pain is defined by rapid onset and relatively short duration and a sign of a new health problem requiring diagnosis and analgesia. Treatment usually involves treating the underlying disease or injury and short-term use of analgesics. In contrast, chronic or persistent pain continues after healing or is not amenable to cure. This pain usually has no autonomic signs and is associated with longstanding functional and psychologic impairment. It is likely to require a multidimensional approach to relief (Kedziera, 2001). The American Geriatrics Society (2002) advocates the use of the term *persistent* rather than *chronic* pain, which may be associated with negative images and stereotypes.

The AGS Panel on Persistent Pain identified four categories of pain that encompass most syndromes (Box 15-1) (AGS, 2002):

1. Nociceptive pain may be visceral or somatic and is usually a result of stimulation of pain receptors. It may arise from tissue inflammation, mechanical deformation, ongoing injury, or destruction of tissue. This type pain usually responds well to common analgesic medication and nonpharmacologic strategies.
2. Neuropathic pain results from pathophysiologic process involving the peripheral or central nervous system. These types of pain do not respond as predictably as do nociceptives to analgesic therapy. They do respond to unconventional analgesic drugs, such as tricyclic antidepressants, anticonvulsants, or antiarrhythmic drugs.

BOX 15-1 Pathophysiologic Classification of Chronic Pain

NOCICEPTIVE PAIN

Arthropathies (e.g., rheumatoid arthritis, osteoarthritis, gout, posttraumatic arthropathies, mechanical neck and back syndromes)
Myalgia (e.g., myofascial pain syndromes)
Skin and mucosal ulcerations
Nonarticular inflammatory disorders (e.g., polymyalgia rheumatica)
Ischemic disorders
Visceral pain (pain of internal organs and viscera)

NEUROPATHIC PAIN

Postherpetic neuralgia
Trigeminal neuralgia
Painful diabetic polyneuropathy
Poststroke pain (central pain)
Postamputation pain
Myelopathic or radiculopathic pain (e.g., spinal stenosis, arachnoiditis, root sleeve fibrosis)
Atypical facial pain
Causalgia-like syndromes (complex regional pain syndromes)

MIXED OR UNDETERMINED PATHOPHYSIOLOGY

Chronic recurrent headaches (e.g., tension headaches, migraine headaches, mixed headaches)
Vasculopathic pain syndromes (e.g., painful vasculitis)

PSYCHOLOGICALLY BASED PAIN SYNDROMES

Somatization disorders
Hysterical reactions

From American Geriatrics Society Panel on Chronic Pain in Older Persons: Clinical practice guidelines, *J Am Geriatr Soc* 46:635, 1998.

3. Mixed or unspecified pain has mixed or unknown mechanisms. Treatment is unpredictable and may require more trials of different or combined approaches.
4. Other types of pain may be rare conditions such as conversion reaction or psychologic disorders. Persons with these disorders may benefit from specific psychiatric treatments, but traditional medical interventions for analgesia are not indicated.

Age-associated changes in pain perception have been observed in some older persons with unusual manifestations of common illnesses. Neuroanatomic and neurochemical findings have shown that the perception of pain and its treatment in the central nervous system are elaborate and complex (Gibson and Helme, 2001). Alteration of transmission along A-delta and C-nerve fibers may be associated with aging, but it is not clear how it affects the individual experience of pain (Chakour et al, 1996). An AGS panel concluded age-related changes in pain perception are probably not clinically significant (AGS, 2002).

Scope of Problem of Pain

Even though pain is *not* part of normal, healthy aging, pain is a common problem among older adults, with persistent physical pain being widespread in the older population (AGS, 2002). It is estimated that 50% of community-dwelling older adults experience significant pain problems (Herr, 2002; Mosby et al, 1994). A Louis Harris telephone survey found that nearly 20% of older Americans are taking analgesic medications regularly (several times a week or more) and 63% had taken prescription pain medications for more than six months (Cooner and Amorosi, 1997). Pain is even greater in nursing homes, where it has been shown that 70% to 80% of residents have substantial pain that is undertreated (AGS, 2002; Ferrell, 1995; Weiner, Peterson, and Keefe, 1999; Werner et al, 1998).

Stereotyping older persons as having less pain because of their age contributes to less frequent pain assessment and consequently less appropriate and effective treatment for the pain. Older adults commonly report less pain because they do not want to be complainers, fear more tests and medicines, and fear losing their independence (AGS, 2002). In addition, "Many elderly have become resigned to pain. They are ambivalent about benefit of any action for their pain. Older adults are often reluctant to express their pain" (Yates, Dewar, and Fentiman, 1995). Some of these responses by older persons may be due to health practitioners saying such things as, "What do you expect at *your* age?" supporting the belief nothing can be done to control or stop their pain.

Adding to this problem is the fact that older patients have been systematically excluded from clinical trials of analgesic drugs despite the fact that they are more likely to experience the side effects of analgesic medications.

Consequences of Unrelieved Pain

Consequences of persistent pain are numerous. Depression, anxiety, decreased socialization, sleep disturbance, decreased or impaired ambulation, prolonged recovery periods, increased use of health care resources, premature death, and increased health care use and costs have been documented with the presence of pain in older patients (Agency for Health Care Policy and Research [AHCPR], 1994; Ferrell, Ferrell, and Osterweil, 1990). Unrelieved pain has been shown to result in decreased ambulation, impaired posture, sleep disturbance, anxiety, and impaired appetite in nursing home residents. Pain can make getting to the bathroom so difficult that incontinence occurs. Constipation can also be related to unrelieved pain when the person changes diet plans, decreases activity, and has difficulty getting to a toilet before the urge passes (Ferrell, Ferrell, and Osterweil, 1990). Weiner and Rudy (2002) found that nursing home residents who were functionally disabled believed that the staff labeled them as less deserving of pain treatment than more independent residents.

Pain research and literature on pain management have increased dramatically over the past four decades. Despite these advances, pain remains underrecognized and undertreated in older adults, especially those 75 and older. This situation has developed because the study of pain has generally been limited to the young and to those with cancer-related pain in acute care settings. More recently, though, studies have focused on the special needs of older adults in other care settings such as the nursing facility (Loeb, 1999; Morley et al, 1995; Stein and Ferrell, 1996; Wagner et al, 1997), the home, and the community (Cooner and Amorosi, 1997; Huber and Spirig, 2004; Keef et al, 2004; Mosby et al, 1994). Pain in cognitively impaired older adults is a relatively new field of inquiry (Farrell, Katz, and Helme, 1996; Ferrell, Ferrell, and Rivera, 1995; Kovach et al, 2001) along with gender differences in pain response (Bradbury, 2003; Giles and Walker, 2000; Luggen, 1996; Roberto, 1994; Vallerand, 1995). Accountability for undertreatment of pain is also gaining attention, given the results of court cases against professionals who undertreat pain in older adults (Pasero and McCaffery, 2001).

Older adults offer unique challenges to health care professionals in the diagnosis and treatment of pain. The nurse caring for older adults in pain needs to understand the special needs of this diverse population. Although older adults are at risk for chronic disease and the often painful conditions that accompany those ailments, their pain is often underrecognized. Therefore accurate and ongoing assessment is essential for effective pain management in older adults. Goals for pain management in older adults include:

- Relief from the pain
- Control of chronic disease conditions causing pain
- Maintenance of mobility and functional status
- Promotion of self-care and maximum independence
- Improved quality of life

These goals can be achieved through education of clients, families, and health care professionals, and through good nursing care.

Epidemiology of Pain

The causes of pain in older adults are both chronic and acute. Chronic diseases that cause pain are especially prevalent in this age-group. Some of the major chronic illnesses causing pain in older adults are arthritis, polymyalgia rheumatica, temporal arteritis, peripheral vascular disease, diabetic neuropathy, postherpetic neuralgia, and cancer. It is suggested that sex hormones influence the neural circuitry that detects and controls pain, although their role has not been clearly identified (Giles and Walker, 2000). Animal study findings also support gender differences in pain and response to pain (Proceedings of the National Academy of Science, 2003).

PATHOPHYSIOLOGY OF PAIN IN OLDER ADULTS

Pain has multiple components that affect one's physical and psychosocial functioning. Although older adults develop more chronic diseases as they age, pain does not need to be an expectation of normal aging. An understanding of pain physiology and pain theories is essential to effective pain management in older adults.

The three major components of the nervous system that cause the sensation and perception of pain are the afferent pathways (reception), central nervous system (perception), and efferent pathways (reaction). Afferent pathways have nociceptors and are found on the skin. Pacinian corpuscles that mediate sensation—including pain, pressure, and itch—are the nerve endings that are distributed in the skin. Stimulation of these nerve endings by vibrations such as massage or sound wave vibrations can reduce perception of pain such as chronic rheumatoid arthritis. The free nerve endings of nociceptors are sensitive to mechanical, thermal, electrical, or chemical stimuli and are responsible for transmitting sensory pain information. This stimulation flows through peripheral sensory nerves (afferent pathways) to the spinal cord. A painful stimulus (e.g., pinprick) sends an impulse to a nociceptor (a receptor for painful stimuli) along a peripheral nerve fiber, which enters the gray matter of the spinal cord. Nociceptors terminate in the spinal cord (McCaffery and Pasero, 1999). Here the nociceptor stimulation flows to the brain through a series of relay neurons.

When the pain stimulus or signal reaches the central nervous system, it is evaluated and interpreted in the limbic system, reticular formation, thalamus, hypothalamus, medulla, and cerebral cortex. The brain's interpretation is based on both physical and psychologic aspects. Modulation of the pain stimulus can occur in the gray matter, the dorsal horn of the cord. Here, transmission occurs from the nociceptor to the spinothalamic tract neuron. Substance P, a neurotransmitter, facilitates transmission of the stimulus from the afferent (peripheral) neuron across the synapse to the spinothalamic tract neuron. Uninhibited by medications or other modalities, the pain impulse travels to the cerebral cortex of the brain, where the brain interprets the quality of pain, processing past experiences with pain, knowledge of pain, and cultural associations related to pain perception. The interpretation is relayed back through the peripheral nervous system (efferent) pathways that are made up of fibers connecting the reticular formation, midbrain, and substantia gelantinosa. Pain modulation takes place in the efferent neural pathways and may involve chemical factors of neuropeptides, which can increase the sensitivity of the afferent pain receptors to noxious stimuli. These pathways result in the sensation and perception of pain (McCance and Huether, 2002.)

The mind-body connection of pain can be affected by mind-body therapies that are useful in reducing symptoms of pain, especially persistent (chronic) pain. Some mind-body therapies are meditation, relaxation, guided imagery, and cognitive behavioral counseling. Study findings also reveal that factors such as emotion, attitudes, and stress can directly influence physiologic functions and health outcomes (Astin et al, 2003). A more detailed explanation may be obtained in any extensive book or chapter on pain physiology.

Atypical Acute Pain in Older Adults

Atypical silent myocardial infarction occurs more commonly in older adults. The acute pain of appendicitis in young adults is often not experienced by older adults (McCaffery and Pasero, 1999). The reason for this difference is unknown. Nevertheless, studies demonstrate that older adults have the same intensity of pain as younger adults and are as sensitive to it (Harkins and Scott, 1996). Older persons may have decreased pain tolerance (Leo and Huether, 1998).

BARRIERS TO EFFECTIVE PAIN MANAGEMENT IN OLDER ADULTS

Many barriers impede the assessment and management of pain in older adults. Although reports on age-associated changes in pain perception are controversial, many health care professionals, as well as older clients and their family members, believe that pain is a natural occurrence of aging and chronic disease. This belief can lead to underreporting of pain and can prevent accurate pain assessment and appropriate use of pain relief measures. This lack of interventions for pain relief has many negative outcomes, including decreased function and exacerbation of the cause of the pain.

Laboratory study findings that suggest an age-related decline in pain sensitivity and perception are questionable (Ferrell, Rhiner, and Ferrell, 1993; Harkins and Scott, 1996). One review concluded that age has no significant effect on the perception of acute pain (Harkins and Scott, 1996). Furthermore, the intensity and frequency of pain increase with increasing age. Pain sensitivity and perception should be examined in relation to analgesic use, coexisting disease, and comorbid conditions.

Accurate assessment and pain management is also inhibited when older clients underreport their pain. Older clients may underreport pain because they believe that stoicism and refusal to "give in" to the pain are appropriate behaviors or attitudes. Pain assessment may also be hindered by older clients who do not report pain because they "don't want to bother anyone" or they believe their report of pain will not be believed.

Older adults with cancer may fear the meaning of pain and its implications of worsening disease and possible death. Clients experiencing cancer-related pain may believe this is a natural outcome of cancer and cannot be relieved. These clients and their family members needlessly suffer from the clients' experiences of pain.

Inadequate access to diagnostic services is another barrier to appropriate pain assessment for older residents of nursing facilities and frail older adults in the community. Often it is difficult to schedule appointments and arrange transportation so that a family member or health care professional can accompany the client to a diagnostic testing facility. Furthermore, many older adults do not have children who live near them and have lost their social networks (Luggen and Rini, 1995).

Pain assessment tools such as visual analog scales, word descriptor scales, and numeric scales have not been validated in the older adult population. Cognitive, visual, hearing, and motor impairments may prevent accurate use of these pain assessment methods. When using any pain assessment tool, the nurse must evaluate each client's ability to use that tool. The use of a second tool may help confirm the value obtained with the first tool used. The AGS panel (1998) found the most accurate and reliable indicator of pain intensity and experience is the patient's self-report.

An additional barrier to effective pain management may be the nurse's extensive use of pain-related behavior assessment to identify and to validate the presence of pain in older adults with dementia. Confused older adult clients have difficulty interpreting painful stimuli. They may be unable to identify its location or communicate the nature of their distress to caregivers (Wold, 1999). They do not respond to pain typically. They may demonstrate changes in body language, vital signs, and level of confusion as indicators of pain. Pain may result in agitation, as well as increased pulse, respiration, blood pressure, and confusion (Wold, 1999). Researchers have tried to verify pain behaviors such as facial grimacing, agitation, restlessness, groaning, and attempting to leave or escape as valid signs indicating pain. However, the assessment of pain through behavior indicators should be done with caution because clients in pain may not portray any visible signs of pain or distress, or may be unable to communicate their pain.

The compromised ability of people with moderate to severe dementia to clearly or consistently report on their internal states provides both challenges and opportunities to nurses who want to improve care and comfort. The Serial Trial Care Protocol (STCP), developed to assess and treat physical pain and affective discomfort in people with dementia who are no longer able to clearly and consistently verbalize needs, addresses critical steps in the breakdown and disconnection between nurses' understanding of the person's need and the provision of care for that unmet need (Fig. 15-1). The STCP is an innovative approach that has concrete specifications but allows discretion in individualizing assessments and interventions to the situation.

The STCP is based on the assumption that behaviors associated with dementia (e.g., fidgeting, exiting, pacing, decreased appetite, combative behavior) signal an unmet need. When the sources of these behaviors are not easily identified, the nurse begins the STCP protocol by doing a physical assessment. If the physical assessment reveals a problem, the nurse institutes an intervention to target the problem. If the physical assessment is negative or the intervention provided is ineffective in returning behaviors to baseline, the nurse assesses for common psychosocial and

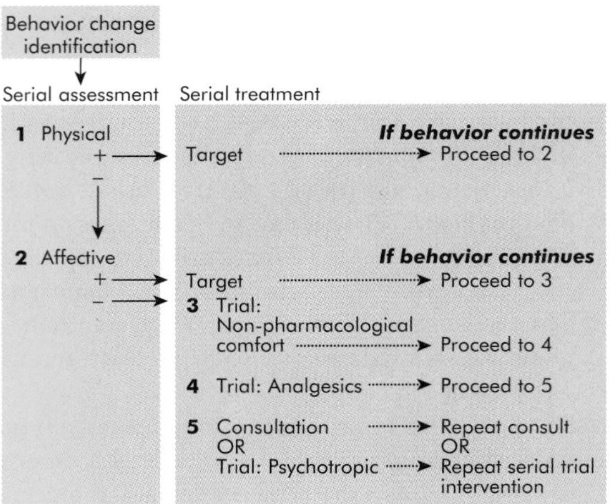

Fig. 15-1 Serial Trial Intervention to assess and treat physical pain and affective discomfort in people with dementia unable to clearly and consistently verbalize needs. (Courtesy Christina Kovach, Milwaukee, Wisc)

environmental needs. Intervention trials are pharmacologic or nonpharmacologic treatments provided when specific domains of assessment or intervention have failed to uncover the source of the problem or failed to ameliorate behaviors. The STCP is a systematic process for using intervention trials that proceeds from nonpharmacologic comfort interventions, to a trial of analgesics, and then perhaps to a trial of psychotropics (Kovach, 2004).

Studies have documented that physicians and nurses tend to underestimate their clients' pain. This seems to be based on limited education and on the belief that older adults have less sensitivity to pain, which has not been demonstrated in fact. Older adult clients actually underreport pain and are therefore at risk for undertreatment of pain, which may cause unnecessary suffering, exacerbation of the underlying disease, and reduction in activities of daily living (ADLs) and quality of life. Nurses must always be aware of the negative influence ageism has on pain management for older adults (Keefe et al, 2004).

For health care professionals, clients, and their families, fear of addiction is a barrier to effective pain management. However, the risk of addiction is not an issue for those older adults who require opioids for pain relief. In fact, because of side effects, especially constipation, older adults have a high rate of discontinuation of opiates (Reuben, Yoshikawa, and Besdine, 1996). Nonetheless, clinicians are reluctant to provide opioids to those with chronic painful conditions in a community setting (American Academy of Pain Medicine [AAPM] and American Pain Society [APS], 1997). Unwarranted fear of addiction should not inhibit the appropriate use of pain-relieving medications.

Tolerance to opioids may occur a few days after treatment (McCaffery and Pasero, 1999), supporting a need for monitoring for a period. Tolerance is defined as the diminished effect of a drug while maintaining the same dosage over time. With opiates, higher and higher doses of a drug are required to maintain its effect. This should not be confused with addiction; it is a characteristic of these drugs when given over time. The drug dosage must be increased to avoid causing needless pain to clients. There is no ceiling (level for effectiveness of the drug) for the amount of drug that can be given, in contrast to drugs that have a level at which additional drug does not offer increased relief. Tolerance to the nonanalgesic effects (i.e., the side effects) of opioids also develops (McCaffery and Pasero, 1999). Tolerance to nausea and mental clouding, which commonly occur when the drug is first given, will develop. These symptoms diminish in days or weeks. However, tolerance to constipation does not occur, so no program of pain relief with opiates should be started without an accompanying bowel regimen, including diet, fluids, activity, and stool softeners.

Inadequacy of the pain education provided to medical and nursing students is also a barrier to effective pain management (Gloth, 2000; Zalon, 1995). Changes in demographics and health care delivery, as well as increasing research, have increased the awareness of the prevalence of pain (Davis, 1998). Furthermore, gerontology is still not a priority in nursing school curricula despite the age of the clients in need of nursing care (Luggen, 1997). As Gloth (2000) notes, "It is difficult to find space for additional instruction in a busy medical school curriculum but here remains a disproportionate allotment to subjects such as obstetrics (which many physician use very little), compared with pain management and care of the dying (which most physicians will encounter, regardless of specialty)."

Lack of education does not fully account for undertreatment of pain. It is a multifaceted problem (McCaffery and Pasero, 1999). Institutional rituals of practice and care are persistent barriers to effective pain management. An interdisciplinary team approach can provide the impetus for blending continuous quality improvement with other strategies for changing systems and practices, such as those described in the Client/Family Teaching box.

The pharmacodynamics and the pharmacokinetics of commonly prescribed medications are different in older adults than in individuals in other age-groups (see Chapter 22). Older adults are especially vulnerable to the effects of drugs because of age-related physiologic changes and altered pharmacodynamics. The limited research in this area supports the importance to start with low doses and slowly titrates upward until the desired effect is achieved (Nagle and Erwin, 1996).

Although opioids have been accepted as a treatment for acute pain and cancer-related pain, they have not been widely accepted as a treatment modality for chronic, nonmalignant pain. Physicians' reluctance to prescribe opioids for chronic, nonmalignant pain may have a negative effect on pain management for older adults experiencing this type of pain. Pain

Client/Family Teaching

CONTROLLING PAIN THROUGH A TEAM APPROACH

The best way to control pain is through a team approach involving the client, the family, and the nurse and physician. In addition to a client telling the others the extent of his or her pain, he or she should be asked the following:

- Where is your pain located?
- When did the pain start?
- Describe the pain. Is it sharp? Dull? Throbbing? Burning?
- Does the pain come and go, or is it constant?
- What makes the pain worse?
- What makes the pain better?
- What medications are you taking for the pain?
- Are you using any other methods to relieve your pain, such as relaxation, a heating pad, or a cold pack? Do they seem to help?

management specialists are prepared to diagnose and treat pain without the prejudice that often accompanies treatment by general practitioners.

Undertreating Pain: Abuse

Inadequate treatment of pain in older people may ultimately lead to legal action. In 2001 a California court found a doctor guilty of recklessness and abuse under California's Elder Abuse and Dependent Adult Care Protection Act (Pasero and McCaffery, 2001). The charge was one of not providing adequate pain medication for an 85-year-old man with cancer pain. An increased number of cases of this type are expected in the future. To reduce the risk of such legal action, institutional guidelines and education for individual nurses and physicians are suggested (Pasero and McCaffery, 2001). Guidelines for pain treatment, as suggested by Yonan and Wegener (2003), include using a baseline report of activity or pain level of the individual to set the initial goals for pain treatment outcomes at about 75% of the established baseline for the individual. This is believed to be a reasonable initial goal for pain control.

PAIN ASSESSMENT

Pain assessment begins when the nurse accepts the client's self-report of pain and takes that report seriously. Assessment is essential in differentiating acute, life-threatening pain from longstanding, chronic pain. Otherwise, disease progression and acute injury may go unrecognized and be attributed to preexisting disease or illness. Table 15-1 identifies components of the clinical assessment of pain in older adults.

Pain assessment should include a thorough history and a physical examination. These assessments are especially important for older clients because effective pain management often depends on the appropriate treatment of underlying disease or illness. When the underlying disease is unknown, multidisciplinary consultation is indicated (AGS, 2002).

Some of the following are general principles on pain assessment from the AGS Panel on Persistent Pain in Older Persons (2002):

- There are no biologic markers for the presence of pain.
- The client's report is the most accurate and reliable evidence of pain and its intensity.
- Clients with mild to moderate cognitive impairment can be assessed with simple questions and screening tools.
- Older clients may be reluctant to report pain despite substantial impairments.
- Older persons expect pain with aging.
- Older adults may use words like "discomfort," "aching," and "hurting," rather than "pain."
- They may see pain as a metaphor for serious disease or death.
- Pain may represent "God's will" or atonement for "bad" deeds.
- Assess clients for evidence of chronic pain.
- Recognize pain that significantly affects functional ability or quality of life as a significant problem.
- For clients with cognitive or language impairments, observe nonverbal pain behaviors, recent functional changes, and vocalizations (e.g., groans, cries).
- For clients with cognitive or language impairments, seek caregiver reports and input.
- Seek specialist consultation for clients with debilitating psychiatric problems, substance abuse problems, or intractable pain.
- Monitor clients with chronic pain by recording pain intensity, medication use, response, and associated activities in a pain log or diary.
- Reassess all clients with chronic pain regularly for improvement, deterioration, positive or negative effects of medications, and complications of treatment. Use the same pain instruments at each client visit.

Cultural Pain Assessment

Pain is an individual experience. Clients' pain intensity and pain distress are related to factors such as culture, past pain experiences, individual attributes, and pain threshold. Nurses need to take an individual approach with each client.

Little research has been conducted on pain in clients of any age from different cultures. Because of increasing racial and ethnic diversity in the United States, nurses must work closely with culturally diverse clients to identify mutual goals, including clients' preferences about specific remedies and practices from their culture (McCaffery and Pasero, 1999; Sakauye, 2005) (see Cultural Awareness box). In a notable study of hospital nurses caring for Arabic clients, nurses who spoke Arabic rated their clients' pain similarly to the way

TABLE 15-1 Assessment of Pain in Older Adults

HISTORY	PHYSICAL EXAMINATION	ASSESSMENT OF OTHER VARIABLES
MEDICAL HISTORY Acute illnesses Chronic illnesses Previous surgeries Timed events leading to present pain complaint	ROUTINE EXAMINATION	PERTINENT LABORATORY DATA AND TESTS DEPRESSION SCALES Beck Depression Inventory Zung Self-Rating Scale Geriatric Depression Scale
	MUSCULOSKELETAL EXAMINATION Neuromuscular: Weakness Hyperalgesia Numbness	COGNITIVE ASSESSMENT MiniMental State Examination Short Portable Mental Status Questionnaire Philadelphia Geriatric Center MSQ
PAIN HISTORY Intensity Character Frequency Pattern Location Precipitating factors Relieving factors Alleviating factors	**SIGNS OF TRAUMA** Bruises Inflammation Tenderness Guarding Swelling	**FUNCTIONAL ASSESSMENT** Katz Activities of Daily Living Lawton Instrumental Activities of Daily Living Stanford Health Assessment Questionnaire Barthel Index
HISTORY OF TRAUMA Recent falls Other injuries	**FUNCTIONAL PERFORMANCE** Range of motion Up-and-Go test Tinetti Gait and Balance Test	**PSYCHOSOCIAL ASSESSMENT** Finances Social networks Dysfunctional relationships
MEDICATION HISTORY Prescription Over-the-counter Herbal or natural Side effects		**PAIN ASSESSMENT SCALES:** Visual analog scale Word descriptor scale Numeric scale Faces scale
PAIN MEDICATIONS Drugs that worked Drugs that did not work Prescription or over-the-counter Natural remedies Side effects		**QUALITY OF LIFE MEASURES** Dartmouth COOP Project Profile of Mood States Pain/Quality of Life Scale
PREVIOUS PAIN EXPERIENCES		

From American Geriatrics Society Panel on Chronic Pain in Older Persons: Clinical practice guidelines, *J Am Geriatr Soc* 46:635, 1998.

clients' rated their own pain. This was not true of non-Arabic–speaking nurses, whose pain ratings were notably dissimilar to the ratings of their Arabic clients (Harrison, Busebar, and Al-Kaabi, 1996).

Pain Assessment Tools

Pain assessment tools assist health care professionals in objectively and accurately measuring a client's report of pain and any relief or change in that pain. Pain assessment tools include numeric pain rating scales, such as a 0 to 10 scale where 0 means no pain and 10 means the worst pain; visual analog scales; descriptive pain intensity scales, using descriptions such as "no pain," "a little pain," "a lot of pain," and "too much pain"; pain diaries; and pain logs. Examples of pain assessment tools are illustrated in Fig. 15-2.

A client's report of pain should also be evaluated for pain intensity and pain distress. Pain intensity is a measure of the amount of pain that the client is experiencing and is measured by a numeric pain rating scale, such as the 0 to 10 scale. The numeric pain rating scale translates the client's report of pain into a number that provides the health care pro-

Cultural Awareness

ALTERNATIVE PRACTICES IN PAIN MANAGEMENT

Culture often influences older adults' choices of interventions for dealing with pain. The following is an illustrative, though not exhaustive, list of alternative or complementary practices sometimes used by clients from culturally diverse backgrounds:

- Herbal remedies
- Meditation
- Progressive relaxation
- Hypnosis
- Yoga
- Imagery
- Therapeutic touch
- Acupuncture or acupressure
- Application of heat or cold
- Music
- Humor

Modified from Supportive Care Services Committee: *City of Hope patient handbook for cancer pain management*, Duarte, Calif, 1994, City of Hope National Medical Center.

fessional with an objective description of the client's pain. This measure of pain can then be used to gauge relief, assuming that the number is lower after treatment for the pain. These measures should be recorded in the client's pain log or chart.

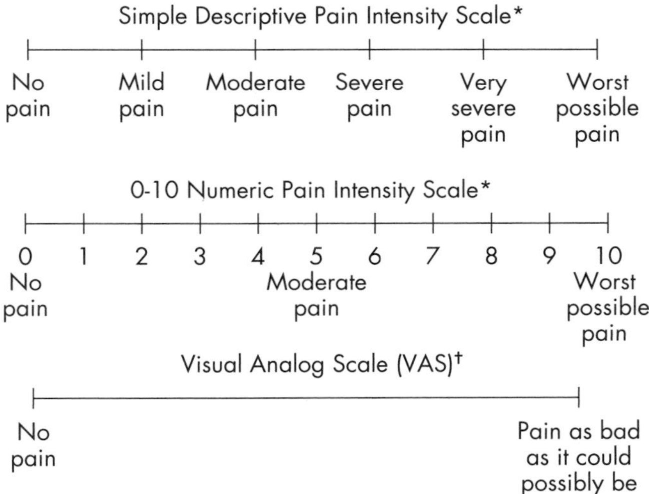

Fig. 15-2 Examples of pain assessment tools. (From Acute Pain Management Guideline Panel: *Acute pain management: operative or medical procedures and trauma*, AHCPR Pub No 92-0032, Rockville, Md, 1992, Agency for Health Care Policy and Research, US Public Health Services, US Department of Health and Human Services.)

A self-care pain management log (Fig. 15-3) is a useful tool. Older adult clients and family members can record pain intensity, pain distress, actions (pharmacologic or nonpharmacologic) taken to relieve the pain, and the outcome of the actions (McCaffery and Pasero, 1999). The self-care pain management log furnishes clients, family members, and clinicians with the information needed to provide effective pain assessment and management. (For another method of recording, see the daily pain diary in Fig. 15-4.) Researchers have found that the use of self-care pain management log and diaries may involve an excessive focus on pain, resulting in a negative client response (Kerns and Habib, 2004).

Gloth (2000) suggests the following three-pronged assessment guide:

1. Pain history: Focus on concurrent medications, prior adverse drug reactions, concomitant illnesses, duration, type, onset, and relieving factors of pain.
2. Physical examination: Recognize that pain in the older patient may present differently than in younger patients (e.g., less pain may indicate more serious problems).
3. Prescribing: Resist prescribing analgesics without a diagnosis; begin with low doses (often less than the minimum recommended doses, especially with oldest old) and increase while frequently monitoring pain status; continually review medications (including over-the-counter drugs) and decrease or remove medications when indicated; monitor for adverse effects and changes in mental status.

A pain scale that relies on level of activity rather than a subjective rating on pain alone can provide more specific data that are helpful in assessing level of pain and effectiveness of pain interventions when it is used in the posttreatment period (Table 15-2). Using other terms in addition to the word *pain* is shown to more accurately reflect how many older persons view their discomfort or pain.

History. The nurse should carefully question and thoroughly assess a client's report of pain. This is especially important in older adults because of their tendency for multiple sources of pain from multiple chronic problems occurring simultaneously. Acute pain is often attributed to chronic illness, but it should be evaluated with the knowledge that older adults often demonstrate an altered presentation of common acute illnesses, including "silent" myocardial infarctions and "painless" intraabdominal emergencies. In addition, chronic pain is characterized by variable intensity and character, and thus is often overlooked.

Physical Examination. Pain assessment for older adults includes a comprehensive physical examination of the musculoskeletal and nervous systems. This is an important aspect of pain assessment in this population because many older adults experience painful traumatic and degenerative

Please use this pain assessment scale to fill out your self care log:

0 1 2 3 4 5 6 7 8 9 10

No pain Worst pain

Date	Time	How severe is the pain?	How distressing is the pain to you?	Describe action or medicine taken	How severe is the pain after 1 hour?

Fig. 15-3 Self-care pain management log. (From Ferrell BR, Ferrell BA: Pain in the elderly. In McGuire DB, Yarbro CH, Ferrell BR, editors: *Cancer pain management*, Boston, 1995, Bartlett & Jones.)

musculoskeletal problems. A thorough neurologic assessment includes an evaluation for autonomic, sensory, or motor deficits, which may indicate neuropathic conditions or nerve injuries.

Evaluation for Functional Impairment. Impaired functional status is a major problem for older adults. An evaluation of an older adult's level of function is important so that mobility and independence can be maximized. Evaluation of functional status includes the assessment of ADLs, ambulation, psychosocial well-being, and overall quality of life. Functional activities may be restricted by the presence and intensity of pain. Functional evaluation includes an assessment of factors that contribute to or help alleviate pain. Functional status can be significantly improved through aggressive pain management. It is important to assess for new or different causes for pain, not just to assume increased pain represents an exacerbation of a previous diagnosis. It is also imperative to assess the older person for the cause of a complaint of pain, not to simply attribute it to age. Age does not cause pain; disease and injury do.

Evaluation of Quality of Life. Pain is not an isolated phenomenon; it is an experience that influences all dimensions of an individual's quality of life. Pain assessment should include an evaluation of the impact of pain on a client's quality of life. According to Albert (2000), most available quality-of-life tools have been developed for research purposes, are long and detailed instruments, and require time and energy that may not he available to chronically ill older adults. Albert recommends using a tool that has been tested in older adults and found to be reliable and valid—such as the Dartmouth COOP Project Functional Assessment Charts. This nine-chart system measures health and quality-of-life issues and can be administered by nurses (Luggen and Meiner, 2000).

It is imperative to remember that quality of life can mean different things to different people. Some want freedom from pain and clear cognition; others will trade one for another if given sufficient information concerning alternative treatment regimens. Albert (2000) suggests that elements of quality of life include social relationships; a spiritual element; energy; sexual health; daily activity functions; independence; freedom from pain and depression; positive coping patterns; personal strength; and freedom from symptoms such as fatigue, constipation, chronic pain, loss of appetite, and nausea. Nurses can focus on interventions in any or all of these areas to help older adult clients maintain or improve their quality of life (Albert, 2000).

Practitioners can get a "quick and dirty" assessment of their patient's quality of life by asking "How is life for you?" "Are you doing and enjoying what you want to do and enjoy?" and "Has there been a recent change in your life activities?" Such questions may be as effective and accurate as more scientific tools that are not practical for use in daily practice.

Evaluation for Depression. Pain assessment of older adults also includes an evaluation for depression. A high incidence of depression is associated with chronic pain. Persistent depression affects a person's ability to cope with the pain, so it must be treated. Anxiety may also affect the

FORM 3.5B Pain Control Record: Patient Example

This is a record of how your pain medicines are working. Please keep this record until you and your nurse/doctor find the dose and frequency of medicine that provides satisfactory pain relief for you most of the time. After that, you only need to keep this record when you have problems related to your pain medicines.

Name: *Martin* Date: *Friday*

GOALS Satisfactory pain rating: *3* Activities: *Sleep through the night; walk around the house*

My pain rating scale:

0 1 2 3 4 5 6 7 8 9 10

No pain — Moderate pain — Worst possible pain

Directions: Rate your pain before you take pain medicine and 1 to 2 hours later.

Time:	Pain rating:	Medicine I took:	Side effects (drowsy? upset stomach?)	Other:
12:15 am	*6*	*30 MS IR*	*No*	
3	*6*	*30*		*can't sleep*
5:15	*5*	*30*		
8:30	*6*	*30* *+ ibuprofen* *+ MS Contin*		*staying in bed*
10:30	*4*			*MS IR 45* *8 p.m. MS Contin* *150 mg*
11	*6*	*45*		
12	*3*			

If pain is greater than *5*, or if you have other problems with your pain medicine, call:

Nurse: Name/phone *C. Adams 555-1234*

Doctor: Name/phone *Jones 555-4321*

FORM 3.5B Patient example. This patient has been receiving the following analgesics ATC every day: ibuprofen, 400 mg qid; amitriptyline, 100 mg HS; MS Contin, 100 mg q12h (8 AM and 8 PM). His supplemental (breakthrough, rescue) dose is morphine immediate release (MS IR), 30 mg PO q2h. He usually takes two supplemental doses a day. This has relieved his pain to a 3 or less, and he has been able to sleep through the night uninterrupted by pain and walk around his home. The record reveals that his pain ratings now are greater than 3 and that he is taking supplemental doses every 3 to 4 hours. Pain keeps him awake and he stays in bed. The patient talks with the nurse at 10:30 AM. The nurse contacts the physician and the decision is to increase his morphine doses by 50% to 45 mg MS IR q2h and to MS Contin 150 mg q12h. (This dose of MS Contin requires five 30-mg tablets. However, depending on the tablet strength the patient has on hand, the MS Contin dose may be slightly more or less than 150 mg.) When an opioid dose is safe but ineffective, a 50% increase will usually produce a moderate increase in pain relief. When the patient takes more than two supplemental doses during a 12-hour period, the controlled-release should be increased.

Fig. 15-4 Daily pain diary. (From McCaffery M, Pasero C: *Pain: clinical manual*, ed 2, St Louis, 1999, Mosby.)

TABLE 15-2 Functional Pain Scale

SCORE	DESCRIPTION OF PAIN BY PATIENT FUNCTION
0	No pain
1	Tolerable (and does not prevent any activities)
2	Tolerable (but does prevent some activities)
3	Intolerable (but can use telephone, watch TV, or read)
4	Intolerable (cannot use telephone, watch TV, or read)
5	Intolerable (and unable to verbally communicate because of pain)

From Gloth FM et al: The Functional Pain Scale (FPS): Reliability, validity, and responsiveness in a senior population, *J Am Med Dir Assoc* 2(3):110-114, 2001.

management of chronic pain, especially if the outcome of the chronic problem is uncertain. An observer-rated scale used to diagnose depression in older persons with dementia is the National Institute of Mental Health (NIMH) Dementia Mood Assessment Scale (Sunderland, Alterman, and Young, 1988). The reader is also referred to Chapter 4 for additional tools for effective assessment.

End of Life. Singer, Martin, and Kelner (1999) studied client perspectives on quality of life at the end of life. The authors found that clients valued:

- Receiving adequate pain and symptom management
- Avoiding inappropriate prolongation of dying
- Achieving a sense of control
- Relieving burden
- Strengthening relationships

These clients' main concern was pain, which reinforces the need to assess and provide adequate interventions for pain. Other symptoms of concern, which commonly occur with painful problems and made pain distress worse, were vomiting, breathlessness, and diarrhea. One client said, "If I'm in pain, severe pain, and the doctors can do nothing, the pain persists and there's nothing to take the pain away, I don't think it's fair to let me suffer like that, or anybody" (Singer, Martin, and Kelner, 1999). Pain continues to be an end-of-life problem that clearly severely impairs quality of life. Lynn, Teno, and Phillips (1997) found that 4 out of every 10 clients who were dying had severe pain most of the time. Nurses are in a key position to assess clients in pain and then recommend appropriate pain management to improve their quality of life.

PRINCIPLES OF PAIN MANAGEMENT

Ferrell (1991) suggested 10 principles of pain management for elderly people. These offer an excellent base for a practitioner working with older persons to provide care that meets needs of the individual in relation to pain:

1. Always ask elderly persons about pain or whether their activity is limited by discomfort or pain.
2. Accept the patient's word about pain and its intensity.
3. Never underestimate the potential effects of chronic pain on a patient's overall condition and quality of life.
4. Be compulsive in the assessment of pain. An accurate diagnosis will lead to the most effective treatment.
5. Treat pain to facilitate diagnostic procedures. Don't wait for a diagnosis to relieve suffering.
6. Use a combined approach of drug and nondrug strategies when possible.
7. Mobilize patients physically, and involve patient in their therapy psychosocially.
8. Use analgesic drugs correctly. Start doses low and increase slowly. Achieve adequate doses and anticipate side effects.
9. Anticipate and attend to anxiety and depression.
10. Reassess responses to treatment. Alter therapy to maximize functional status and quality of life.

NURSING CARE OF OLDER ADULT CLIENTS WITH PAIN

Pharmacologic Treatment

Older adults often respond with unpredictable sensitivity and frequent side effects to many classes of drugs, including analgesics (Nagle and Erwin, 1996). Aging probably affects drug absorption: distribution, metabolism, and excretion (see Chapter 22). Changes that require ongoing assessment of a client's response to a medication, with subsequent adjustments in dose and dosing intervals or prescribed drug, are:

- Changes in physiologic factors such as decreased gastric acid production and gastrointestinal motility
- Changes in body composition such as decreased total body water, lean body mass, and serum protein, and increased body fat
- Changes in organ function such as decreased hepatic blood flow and reduced glomerular filtration rate

These changes, especially in liver and renal function, can increase the risk of accumulation of lipid-soluble drugs such a fentanyl and may slightly delay the onset of action and increase the risk for accumulating agents used to control pain (Lee, 1996). Age-related changes in absorption, distribution, metabolism, and elimination demand that prescribers be conservative, especially since recommendations for age-adjusted doses are not available for most analgesics (Kedziera, 2001). Continued follow-up is critical for the older adult to monitor for effects and side effects. Baseline blood work should include a complete blood cell count, stool for occult blood, blood urea nitrogen, creatinine, and potassium, with levels being monitored about every 3 months (Forman and Stratton, 1991). Nonsteroidal antiinflammatory drugs (NSAIDs) can interact with beta-blockers, angiotensin-converting enzyme inhibitors, diuretics, phenytoin, sulfonylureas, warfarin, and digoxin

(Kedziera, 2001). Monitoring should include an up-to-date review of all medications being taken by the patient. Having patients bring *all* medications in their medicine chest to the office visit can be helpful, since many forget something they take only as needed. Patients should be reminded to include any over-the-counter or "natural" items, since they may not consider these "real medicine" because they do not require a prescription. Nurses are especially good at making this review.

It is important to remember that drug selection depends on the type of pain and its intensity. For example, a client who reports mild to moderate pain that is poorly tolerated and not responsive to a nonopioid analgesic may require a weak opioid analgesic such as oxycodone (OxyContin). Oxycodone is the only opioid analgesic besides morphine currently available in the United States in an oral, 12-hour controlled-release form allowing for twice-daily dosing. It is described as an "ideal opioid": it has a short half-life (4 1/2 hours), it provides analgesia of long duration, it has no clinically significant active metabolites, onset of action is rapid, and titration is easy (Levy, 2001). It does have the same adverse effects of other opioids, including constipation, nausea, sedation, and respiratory depression. The controlled-relapses oxycodone should always be taken whole and never broken, chewed, or crushed, since this would cause a rapid release of the entire dose, which could be fatal (Pasero and McCaffery, 2004).

Pain therapy must always be individualized for the client, especially those in their eighth decade or older. Effective pain management requires ongoing assessment of the medication used in relation to its analgesic effect and side effects.

Analgesic drugs can be classified into three broad categories: (1) mild analgesics, including nonopioid analgesics and some weak opioid analgesics such as codeine and oxycodone; (2) strong opioid analgesics, including morphine; and (3) adjuvant drugs, including those agents which enhance the analgesic effects of opioids and those which have intrinsic analgesic activity.

Mild Analgesics. Mild analgesics are used as a first-line approach to pain management. Acetaminophen (Tylenol), ibuprofen (Motrin, Advil), and naproxen (Naprosyn, Aleve) are examples of mild analgesics. These drugs block pain by inhibiting pain reception at the local level. As with all medications, usage by older adults must be continuously monitored. Acetaminophen seems to be well tolerated by older adults and does not affect platelet function. It is the drug of choice for relieving mild to moderate musculoskeletal pain (AGS, 2002). The maximum dosage of acetaminophen is between 3200 and 4000 mg/day. Long-term use should be discouraged in those with compromised renal function because the drug is excreted by the kidneys and may accumulate to toxic levels. Acetaminophen is as effective as aspirin in its analgesic and antipyretic properties but less effective than aspirin in its antiinflammatory properties. Although acetaminophen has not been associated with renal or gastric problems, it can result in hepatic toxicity in clients with a history of alcohol abuse or after the ingestion of very high doses (Table 15-3).

NSAIDs are especially effective for treating mild to moderate arthritic pain and bone pain caused by malignant metastases. NSAIDs have been associated with a variety of adverse side effects in older adults, including stomach ulcers, renal insufficiency, and a tendency to bleed. The most common complaint associated with NSAIDs is indigestion. Indigestion may be reduced with antacid use or food consumption timed to coincide with analgesic intake. However, the health care professional must remember that gastrointestinal irritation may occur without symptoms. Severe ulceration can result in perforation and extensive bleeding. An older adult's response to the medication must be evaluated closely. NSAIDs should be avoided in high doses, for long periods, in clients with abnormal renal function, and in clients with a history of ulcer disease or bleeding (AGS, 1998). NSAIDs most likely to cause gastrointestinal irritation are aspirin, indomethacin (Indocin), sulindac (Clinoril), tolmetin (Tolectin), and naproxen (McCaffery and Pasero, 1999). The COX-2 inhibitors are said to provide similar relief from pain as NSAIDs, but without the side effects of gastric damage and renal insufficiency. The COX-2 inhibitors, celecoxib and valdecoxib, are as effective as NSAIDs for relief of mild to moderate pain and are associated with lower risk of gastrointestinal bleeding, but have similar risk for other side effects. Celecoxib should not be used with persons who have sulfa sensitivities (Gorman, 1998; Horgas, 2003).

Ketorolac (Toradol) is an NSAID that has similar side effects to other NSAIDs. It carries a high risk of gastric problems with continued use beyond 5 to 7 days parenterally or 10 to 14 days orally. Ketorolac is intended for short-term use, generally in the postoperative period. Acetaminophen is considered the drug of choice for relief of musculoskeletal pain because it has few side effects and is probably the safest nonopioid for most people. However, it should be used with caution in people with underlying hepatic or renal disease (Horgas, 2003).

The analgesic effect of NSAIDs and acetaminophen is also limited by a ceiling effect. In other words, raising the drug's dose beyond a given level does not result in added analgesia.

Opioid Analgesics. For clients with mild to moderate pain that is poorly tolerated or cannot be adequately managed with a mild analgesic, the clinician should consider using an opioid analgesic. Clinical experience suggests that older adults are particularly sensitive to the effects of opioid analgesics because they experience a higher peak and longer duration of pain relief (Vanegas, 1998) (Table 15-4).

Older adults may be more sensitive to opioids, supporting the advice to "start low and go slow" and monitor until titrated for adequate pain relief. Problems with opioids usually involve those with long half-lives, such as methadone (Dolophine) or levorphanol (Levo-Dromoran). The half-life

TABLE 15-3 Acetaminophen and NSAIDs: Dosing Information*

CHEMICAL CLASS	GENERIC NAME	HALF-LIFE (HR)	DOSING SCHEDULE	RECOMMENDED STARTING ORAL DOSE (mg)	RECOMMENDED MAXIMUM ORAL DOSE (mg/day)	COMMENTS
P-Aminophenol derivatives	Acetaminophen	2	q4-6h	650	3200-4000	Overdosage produces hepatic toxicity. No GI or platelet toxicity. Available as liquid and for rectal administration.
Salicylates	Aspirin	3-12	q4-6h	650	6000	Standard for comparison. May not be as well tolerated as some of newer NSAIDs. Available for rectal administration.
	Diflunisal	8-12	q12h	500	1500	Less GI toxicity than aspirin.
	Choline magnesium trisalicylate	9-17	q12h	500-1000	4000	Minimal GI toxicity. No effect on platelet aggregation. Available as liquid.
	Choline salicylate	2-3	q3-6h	870	5352	Liquid. Minimal effect on platelet function.
	Magnesium salicylate		q4-6h	1000	4000	
	Salsalate	16	q12h	500-1000	4000	
Proprionic acids	Ibuprofen	2	q6h	400	3200	Available as a suspension.
	Naproxen	13	q12h	250	1025-1375	
	Fenoprofen	2-3	q6-8h	200	3200	
	Ketoprofen	2-3	q6-8h	25	300	Available for rectal administration and as a topical gel.
	Flurbiprofen	5-6	q12h	100	300	
	Oxaprozin	40	q24h	600	1800	
Acetic acids	Indomethacin	4-5	q8h	25	150	Higher incidence of GI and central nervous system side effects than proprionic acids. Available in slow-release preparations and for rectal administration.

May be duplicated for use in clinical practice. As appears in McCaffery M, Pasero C: *Pain: clinical manual,* ed 2, St Louis, 1999, Mosby. (Modified from Coyle N, Cherny NL, Portenay RK: Pharmacologic management of cancer pain. In McGuire DB, Yarbro CH, Ferrell BR, editors: *Cancer pain management,* ed 2, Boston, 1995, Jones & Bartlett.)
GI, Gastrointestinal; *h,* hour; *q,* every.

TABLE 15-4 Equianalgesic Chart: Nonopioids and Opioids for Mild to Moderate Pain

NONOPIOIDS	ORAL DOSE (mg)	OPIOIDS	ORAL DOSE (mg)
Acetaminophen	650	Codeine	32-60
Aspirin	650	Hydrocodone	5
Choline salicylate	1000	Oxycodone	3-5
Magnesium salicylate	1000		
Sodium salicylate	1000		

From McCaffery M, Pasero C: *Pain: clinical manual,* ed 2, St Louis, 1999, Mosby.

of an opioid is defined as the time it takes for the drug to decrease to half its initial plasma concentration. Plasma levels of drugs that have long half-lives rise slowly over several days after the initiation of a dosing schedule. Thus the risk of delayed toxicity is much greater with these drugs than with drugs having shorter half-lives. Codeine, hydromorphone (Dilaudid), and morphine, in appropriate doses, can safely be used for older adults with pain (see Nursing Care Plan).

Moderate-to-severe pain can commonly be relieved with opioids such as codeine and morphine. However, in spite of their effectiveness and relative safety, most providers are reluctant to use these in older adults (Horgas, 2003).

TABLE 15-3 Acetaminophen and NSAIDs: Dosing Information*—cont'd

CHEMICAL CLASS	GENERIC NAME	HALF-LIFE (hr)	DOSING SCHEDULE	RECOMMENDED STARTING ORAL DOSE (mg)	RECOMMENDED MAXIMUM ORAL DOSE (mg/day)	COMMENTS
	Tolmetin	2-5	q8h	200	2000	
	Sulindac	14	q12h	150	400	Not recommended for prolonged use because of increased risk for GI toxicity.
	Diclofenac	2	q9h	25	150	
	Ketorolac	4-7	q6h	10	40	Use limited to 5 days. Recommended parenteral dose ≤30 mg; total daily dose ≤120 mg.
Oxicams	Piroxicam	50	q24h	20	40	
Fenamates	Mefenamic acid	2	q6h	250	1000	Use limited to 7 days.
	Meclofenamate	2	—	—	400	Not recommended for analgesia.
Pyranocarboxylic acids	Etodolac	7	q8h	200	1200	
Other	Nabumetone	24	q24h	1000	2000	Minimal effect on platelet aggregation.

CLINICAL RELEVANCE OF INFORMATION PRESENTED

- *Half-life.* Half-life is the time required for 50% of the dose to be eliminated from the body. A short half-life (approximately 2 to 7 hours) is recommended for some clients, such as older adults. Drugs with a short half-life are usually preferred for occasional or unexpected pain because they tend to have a quicker onset of analgesia than drugs with a long half-life.
- *Dosing schedule.* Dosing intervals may range from every 4 hours to once a day. Drugs with short half-lives have shorter dosing intervals than those with long half-lives. If clients can tolerate a drug with a long half-life, dosing once or twice a day is usually preferred. The fewer the doses, the more likely it is the client will remember to take the drug.
- *Recommended starting dose.* This dose should be reduced by one half to two thirds in older adults, those taking multiple drugs, or those with renal insufficiency.
- *Recommended maximum dose.* Data are lacking, but the dose listed is thought to be the maximum needed by most clients for analgesia and the dose beyond which side effects are more likely. However, in some clients, careful dose titration may identify clients who need and tolerate 50% to 100% more than the maximum dose recommended. Others may require or tolerate less. For some clients at risk for side effects, the maximum daily dose may be one half or less than recommended.

*Table based on the clinical experience of the authors and a variety of published sources, including: Agency for Health Care Policy and Research: *Management of cancer pain: adults. Quick reference guide for clinicians,* AHCPR Pub No 94-0593, 1994; American Pain Society: *Principles of analgesic use in the treatment of acute pain and cancer pain,* ed 3, Skokie, Ill, 1992, The Society; Insel PA; Analgesic-antipyretic and antiinflammatory agents and drugs employed in the treatment of gout. In Hardman JL, Limbird LE: *Goodman and Gilman's the pharmacological base of therapeutics,* ed 9, New York, 1996, McGraw-Hill; Portenoy RK, Kanner RM: Nonopioid and adjuvant analgesics. In Portenoy RK, Kanner RM, editors: *Pain management: theory and practice,* Philadelphia, 1996, FA Davis; and Sunshine A, Olson NZ: Nonnarcotic analgesics. In Wall PD, Melzack R, editors: *Textbook of pain,* ed 3, New York, 1994, Churchill Livingstone.

Transdermal fentanyl is an opioid alternative that may be appealing to older adults. Fentanyl is given subcutaneously as a patch. It is delivered over a 72-hour period but may be active longer in older adult clients (AGS, 2002). Consequently, transdermal fentanyl should be used with caution in older adults. It is useful in clients who have stable pain. It can also be very useful for those older adult clients who need a more simplified pain medication regimen, have compliance problems, or cannot take medications by mouth (Maxwell, 2000). Older adult clients seem to prefer transdermal fentanyl over sustained-relief morphine, probably because of a superior side-effect profile, including less constipation and sedation (Maxwell, 2000). Also, it is likely that the transdermal route is less "stigmatizing" than morphine to older adults.

Side Effects. Common side effects of opioids include nausea, vomiting, constipation, and urinary retention, especially in individuals with prostatic hypertrophy. Older adults are more sensitive to sedation and respiratory depression, probably as a result of altered distribution and excretion of medications. This is especially true in opioid-naive clients, that is, those who have not had earlier exposure to opioids.

Constipation as a side effect of opioid use is of particular concern in older clients, since many of them have preexisting bowel problems. It is a good practice to start a client on a bowel program when starting an opioid (see Client/Family

Nursing Care Plan
Prostate Cancer with Bone Metastases

Clinical Situation: Mr. V is a 79-year-old retired telephone company executive who has been admitted to the local hospital-based home care program. Mr. V had always been in good health until diagnosed with prostate cancer 2 years ago. He and his wife have enjoyed an active social life. Her four adult children live in cities throughout the United States. The couple does not have any church affiliation. Mr. and Mrs. V have been married for 10 years and live in a mobile home park in the desert. They also own a condominium in the city but do not have any resources for support in that neighborhood. Three years ago, they acquired a puppy named Max. Up until the last 2 to $2\frac{1}{2}$ months, Mr. V had taken morning and evening walks with Max throughout the neighborhood and local park.

In the last 2 months Mr. V has complained about a great deal of pain in his legs and back. He has lost 35 pounds in the past month. He tires easily and is unable to walk outside his home or for distances longer than 25 feet without resting. Mr. V's first wife died 20 years ago from breast cancer. Mr. V relates how she suffered intensely from the effects of chemotherapy and severe pain. He had refused all treatment for his cancer until 6 months ago, when he started receiving hormone therapy. He has refused to take the long-acting opioid prescribed by his physician because he does not "want to get hooked." Mr. V rates his pain as a 9 on a scale of 0 to 10, with 0 meaning no pain and 10 meaning the worst pain. Mrs. V is having difficulty caring for him and dealing with his impending death.

Nursing Diagnosis

Chronic pain related to inadequate knowledge of pain management

Potential for alteration in bowel elimination related to analgesic use

Impaired physical mobility related to pain@B list flush:

Outcomes

Client will report decreased pain (between 0 and 3) at rest and with activity as evidenced by self report.

Client will continue his usual bowel elimination pattern—a soft, formed stool every day.

Client will maintain ADLs and other physical activities as he is able.

Interventions

Discuss general pain content information with client and his wife.

Elicit client's description of his pain, including the quality of the pain, its location, and its precipitating and relieving factors.

Identify the intensity of client's pain using a pain assessment tool.

Identify the distress client experiences in relation to his pain.

Evaluate client's current use of pharmacologic and nonpharmacologic pain relief methods.

Discuss with client his fear of addiction and his need to maintain control of his life and remain alert and functional.

Implement use of a self-care pain management log, including the use of a pain rating scale.

Instruct client and his wife about around-the-clock scheduling for analgesics.

Discuss the current pain management regimen and plans for further treatment with client's physician.

Identify client's current bowel elimination pattern.

Explain the physician's prescription for a stool softener.

Discuss the use of a mild laxative if there is no bowel movement after 2 days.

Encourage a fluid intake of at least eight glasses of water each day.

Modify client's diet to increase his intake of high-fiber foods.

Discuss the effect of analgesics on bowel elimination with client.

Reinforce the fact that although constipation is an expected side effect of opioids, it can be prevented.

Instruct client to take analgesic medications on a regular basis.

Identify activities that are important to client and that he would like to maintain.

Encourage him to take short walks with his dog and sit in the dining room for his meals.

Encourage use of the self-care log.

Instruct client about energy conservation and about the need to space activities with periods of rest.

Evaluate the environment to determine the need for equipment for ambulation or other activities.

Teaching box). Careful assessment of bowel habits, including the use of stool softeners and laxatives and the dietary intake of high-fiber foods, is essential when using opioids. The health care professional must emphasize to the client and his or her family the importance of being proactive, that is, preventing the occurrence of constipation rather than waiting for it to occur. To deal with the side effect of constipation, the Oncology Nursing Society recommends the following (Kuck and Ricciardi, 1998):

- Increase fluid intake.
- Modify diet; add high-fiber foods (see Nutritional Considerations box).
- Maintain or increase activity levels.
- Adapt a daily evacuation schedule that takes into account when gastrocolic reflexes are most active.
- Take medications such as stool softeners, expanders, or natural laxative mixtures, avoiding pharmaceutical laxatives when possible.

Client/Family Teaching

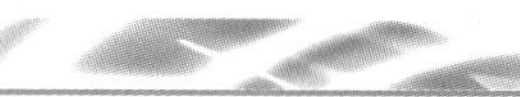

WHAT CAN YOU DO FOR CONSTIPATION?

Opioid analgesics cause constipation in most people. The following suggestions help prevent constipation from becoming a problem and causing discomfort:

- Eat foods high in fiber, such as uncooked fruits and vegetables and whole-grain breads and cereals.
- Add 1 or 2 tbsp of unprocessed bran to foods.
- Drink plenty of liquids—eight to ten glasses per day.
- Eat foods that have helped relieve constipation in the past.
- Plan your bowel movement for the same time each day if possible.
- Try to use the toilet or bedside commode to have a bowel movement.
- Have a hot drink about 30 minutes before the planned time for a bowel movement.
- Consult with a physician about using a bulk laxative, such as Metamucil, or any other laxative or stool softener.

Modified from American Cancer Society and National Cancer Institute: *Questions and answers about pain control: a guide for people with cancer and their families*, Atlanta, 1992, The Society.

Although nausea and vomiting caused by opioid use usually disappear after a few days of taking the medication, it is critical that clinicians take a preventive approach in treating these side effects. As with all medications, antiemetics must be evaluated for their effectiveness in controlling nausea and vomiting in older adults, as well as for side effects such as sedation. The nurse should advise clients and family members that sedation may occur as a result of the antiemetic. If nausea persists beyond a few days of starting the opioid, a new opioid should be tried (AGS, 1998) (Table 15-5).

Sedation and impaired cognitive performance should be anticipated when starting opioids (AGS, 1998). The sedation usually decreases in 1 to 3 days. In case it does not, the patient needs to be informed orally and in written form that the health care provider should be notified. Sedation may also be related to sleep deprivation resulting from unrelieved pain. A fact that must be stressed is that sedation can occur without adequate pain relief. This type of sleep does not result in the expected rejuvenation offered by sleep. Nurses should monitor for respiratory depression (less than 8 breaths/min or oxygen saturation of less than 90% [AGS, 1998]), especially during rapid, high-dose escalations. Table 15-6 identifies analgesics that should be avoided in older adults.

Nutritional Considerations

High-Fiber Foods to Relieve Constipation

Oatmeal, bran, whole wheat, rye

Apples, pears, strawberries, peaches, plums

Citrus

Beans, dry beans

Peas, cabbage, root vegetables, fresh tomatoes, green beans, carrots

Opioids for Chronic Pain. Three situations in which opioids are appropriate for the treatment of nonmalignant pain are to (1) provide pain relief during procedures and those times when other treatment regimens are being incorporated into a client's care, (2) provide pain control during times of exacerbation, and (3) control the discomfort and suffering associated with severe chronic pain. Nurses and other health care professionals must remember that the majority of individuals using opioids for pain relief stop taking opioids when the pain stops. The literature reveals that the risk of addiction to opioids is very low in clients without a prior history of addiction (AAPM and APS, 1997). There is no national consensus on the management of chronic pain that is not caused by cancer (AAPM and APS, 1997).

Adjuvant Medications. Adjuvant medications—defined as medications without intrinsic analgesic properties—are helpful in treating certain types of chronic pain. Adjuvant medications include anticonvulsants, antidepressants, and some sedatives. The treatment of underlying depression or mood disorders may enhance other pain management strategies.

Anticonvulsants, drugs usually used to treat seizures, are often helpful in controlling painful conditions such as postherpetic neuralgia, diabetic neuropathy, and phantom limb pain. An anticonvulsant that is useful in the treatment of older adult clients and has few side effects is gabapentin (Neurontin) (McCaffery and Pasero, 1999). Anticonvulsants may cause blood dyscrasia, however, and laboratory data must be assessed on a regular basis. For older adults, some sedatives or tranquilizers may cause side effects such as increased confusion and constipation. Thus the use of these medications in older adults must be continuously monitored. Short-acting benzodiazepines, such as alprazolam or low-dose haloperidol, and phenothiazines are suggested (Stein, 1997). Tricyclic antidepressants (TCAs) are found to be useful in neuropathic pain (Kelly and Payne, 1993). TCAs do not seem to help musculoskeletal pain; higher doses are needed for therapy superimposed on cancer pain. Desipramine hydrochloride (Norpramin) seems to be better tolerated by older adults, with fewer anticholinergic side effects than certain other medications such as amitriptyline. However, TCAs can cause constipation, blurred vision, dry mouth, urinary retention, and sedation; they should be avoided by those with glaucoma and benign prostatic hypertrophy. They can cause arrhythmias, cognitive changes, orthostatic hypotension, and falls (Gloth, 1996). Selective serotonin reuptake inhibitors (SSRIs) seem to have relatively low side-effect profiles (McDonald, 1999). These include sertraline (Zoloft), paroxetine (Paxil), and fluoxetine (Prozac). These drugs appear to block pain-transmission pathways.

TABLE 15-5 Equianalgesic Dose Chart

A GUIDE TO USING EQUIANALGESIC DOSE CHARTS

Equianalgesic means approximately the same pain relief.
The equianalgesic chart is a guideline. Doses and intervals between doses are titrated according to an individual's response.
The equianalgesic chart is helpful when switching from one drug to another or switching from one route of administration to another.
Doses in this equianalgesic chart are not necessarily starting doses. They suggest a ratio for comparing the analgesia of one drug to another.
The longer the client has been receiving opioids, the more conservative the starting doses of a new opioid.

OPIOID	PARENTERAL (IM/SC/IV) (OVER ≈4 HR)	ORAL (PO) (OVER≈4 HR)	ONSET (min)	PEAK (min)	DURATION[1] (HR)	HALF-LIFE (HR)
MU AGONISTS						
Morphine	10 mg	30 mg	30-60 (PO) 30-60 (CR)[2] 30-60 (R) 5-10 (IV) 10-20 (SC) 10-20 (IM)	60-90 (PO) 90-180 (CR)[2] 60-90 (R) 15-30 (IV) 30-60 (SC) 30-60 (IM)	3-6 (PO) 8-12 (CR)[2] 4-5 (R) 3-4 (IV)[1,3] 3-4 (SC) 3-4 (IM)	2-4
Codeine	130 mg	200 mg NR	30-60 (PO) 10-20 (SC) 10-20 (IM)	60-90 (PO) UK (SC) 30-60 (IM)	3-4 (PO) 3-4 (SC) 3-4 (IM)	2-4
Fentanyl	100 mcg/h parenterally and transdermally ≅ mg/h morphine parenterally; 1 mcg/h transdermally ≅ morphine 2 mg/24 h orally	—	5 (OT) 1-5 (IV) 7-15 (IM) 12-16 h (TD)	15 (OT) 3-5 (IV) 10-20 (IM) 24 h (TD)	2-5 (OT) 0.5-4 (IV)[1,3] 0.5-4 (IM) 48-72 (TD)	3-4[4] 13-24 (TD)
Hydrocodone (as in Vicodin, Lortab)	—	30 mg[5] NR	30-60 (PO)	60-90 (PO)	4-6 (PO)	4
Hydromorphone (Dilaudid)	1.5 mg[6]	7.5 mg	15-30 (PO) 15-30 (R) 5 (IV) 10-20 (SC) 10-20 (IM)	30-90 (PO) 30-90 (R) 10-20 (IV) 30-90 (SC) 30-90 (IM)	3-4 (PO) 3-4 (R) 3-4 (IV)[1,3] 3-4 (SC) 3-4 (IM)	2-3
Levorphanol (Levo-Dromoran)	2 mg	4 mg	30-60 (PO) 10 (IV) 10-20 (SC) 10-20 (IM)	60-90 (PO) 15-30 (IV) 60-90 (SC) 60-90 (IM)	4-6 (PO) 4-6 (IV)[1,3] 4-6 (SC) 4-6 (IM)	12-15
Oxycodone (as in Percocet, Tylox)	—	20 mg	30-60 (PO) 30-60 (CR) 30-60 (R)	60-90 (PO) 90-180 (CR) 30-60 (R)	3-4 (PO) 8-12 (CR) 3-6 (R)	2-3 4.5 (CR)
Oxymorphone (Numorphan)	1 mg	(10 mg R)	15-30 (R) 5-10 (IV) 10-20 (SC) 10-20 (IM)	120 (R) 15-30 (IV) UK (SC) 30-90 (IM)	3-6 (R) 3-4 (IV)[1,3] 3-6 (SC) 3-6 (IM)	2-3
AGONIST-ANTAGONISTS						
Buprenorphine (Buprenex)	0.4 mg	—	5 (SL) 5 (IV) 10-20 (IM)	30-60 (SL) 10-20 (IV) 30-60 (IM)	UK (SL) 3-4 (IV)[1,3] 3-6 (IM)	2-3

May be duplicated for use in clinical practice. From McCaffery M, Pasero C: *Pain: clinical manual,* ed 2, St Louis, 1999, Mosby.
CR, Oral controlled release; *hr,* hour; *IM,* intramuscular; *IV,* intravenous; *mcg,* microgram; *mg,* milligram; *min,* minute; *NR,* not recommended; *NS,* nasal spray; *OT,* oral transmucosal; *PO,* oral; *R,* rectal; *SC,* subcutaneous; *SL,* sublingual; *TD,* transdermal; *UK,* unknown.

TABLE 15-5 Equianalgesic Dose Chart—cont'd

OPIOID	PARENTERAL (IM/SC/IV) (OVER ≈4 HR)	ORAL (PO) (OVER≈4 HR)	ONSET (min)	PEAK (min)	DURATION[1] (hr)	HALF-LIFE (hr)
AGONIST-ANTAGONISTS—cont'd						
Butorphanol (Stadol)	2 mg	—	5-15 (NS) 5 (IV) 10-20 (IM)	60-90 (NS) 10-20 (IV) 30-60 (IM)	3-4 (NS) 3-4 (IV) 3-4 (IM)	3-4
Dezocine (Dalgan)	10 mg	—	5 (IV) 10-20 (IM)	UK (IV) 30-60 (IM)	3-4 (IV)[1, 3] 3-4 (IM)	2-3
Nalbuphine (Nubain)	10 mg	—	5 (IV) <15 (SC) <15 (IM)	10-20 (IV) UK (SC) 30-60 (IM)	3-4 (IV)[1, 3] 3-4 (SC) 3-4 (IM)	5

[1]Duration of analgesia is dose dependent; the higher the dose, usually the longer the duration.
[2]As in, for example, MS Contin.
[3]IV boluses may be used to produce analgesia that lasts approximately as long as IM or SC doses. However, of all routes of administration, IV produces the highest peak concentration of the drug, and the peak concentration is associated with the highest level of toxicity (e.g., sedation). To decrease the peak effect and lower the level of toxicity, IV boluses may be administered more slowly (e.g., 10 mg of morphine over a 15-minute period) or smaller doses may be administered more often (e.g., 5 mg of morphine every 1 to 1½ hours).
[4]At steady state, slow release of fentanyl from storage in tissue can result in a prolonged half-life of up to 12 hours.
[5]Equianalgesic data not available.
[6]The recommendation that 1.5 mg of parenteral hydromorphone is approximately equal to 10 mg of parenteral morphine is based on single dose studies. With repeated dosing of hydromorphone, it is more likely that 2-3 mg of parenteral hydromorphone is equal to 10 mg of parenteral morphine.

Other adjuvant medications that may be tried include antihistamines such as hydroxyzine (Atarax, Vistaril), stimulants such as caffeine (Luggen, 2000), and corticosteroids, which should only be used for short-term therapy (AGS, 1998). Baclofen (Lioresal) may be used for neuropathic pain and muscle spasm (AGS, 1998), and an antiarrhythmic, mexiletine (Mexitil), is also used for neuropathic pain.

It is important that the nurse notify clients and their family members when these adjuvant medications are being used to treat the client's pain. Clinical experience has shown

TABLE 15-6 Drugs to Avoid in Pain Management of Older Adults

DRUG	PRECAUTIONS	POTENTIAL SOLUTIONS
Meperidine (Demerol)	Extremely low oral potency; metabolite normeperidine; may accumulate and cause confusion, agitation, and seizure activity, especially among clients with renal impairment.	Choose a drug with higher oral potency; there are no advantages of either oral or parenteral meperidine over other opioid drugs.
Pentazocine (Talwin)	Mixed opioid agonist/antagonist activity often leads to central nervous system excitement, confusion, and agitation.	Avoid all use in frail older adults.
Propoxyphene (Darvon)	Potency no better than aspirin; significant potential for abuse and renal injury.	Choose an NSAID or weak opioid.
Methadone (Dolophine)	Plasma half-life may be extremely prolonged in older adults; analgesic half-life relatively short.	Short-acting or long-acting morphine is a better alternative.
Levorphanol (Levo-Dromoran	The optimal analgesic dose varies widely among patients. Doses should be titrated to pain/prevention. Use with caution in patients with hypersensitivity reactions to morphine, hydrocodone, hydromorphone, oxycodone, or oxymorphone.	For use in relief of moderate-to-sever pain.

Modified from Ferrell BR, Ferrell BA: Pain in the elderly. In McGuire DB, Yarbro CH, Ferrell BR, editors: *Cancer pain management*, Boston, 1995, Jones & Bartlett.

that a client may discontinue the analgesic when an adjuvant medication is added, especially if he or she thinks it is for a psychologic problem. The client may also take an adjuvant medication such as an antidepressant without realizing that it is being used in conjunction with the analgesic to treat pain. As with all analgesics, the nurse must continue to assess the client's reports of pain and the effectiveness and side effects of the adjuvant medication.

Routes of Administration. The majority of clients can be effectively treated with oral analgesics. The use of "high-tech" routes such as intravenous or epidural analgesic administration must be evaluated from the perspectives of cost, comfort, risk for complications, and caregiver burden. A conservative approach to high-tech pain management is advised. The transdermal patch and the oral transmucosal lozenge forms of fentanyl are recent new routes of pain medication administration that may be useful in older adults (Rhiner and Kedziera, 1999).

Breakthrough Pain. As many as 67% of older adult clients report breakthrough pain (Rhiner and Kedziera, 1999). Breakthrough pain can be incident pain, meaning it is triggered by certain activities and can be predicted; spontaneous pain, which is common with neuropathic pain, fleeting, and difficult to predict; or end-of-dose failure, when analgesic levels have decreased to the point of allowing breakthrough pain before the next scheduled dose of medication (AGS, 1998). Nurses used to increase the around-the-clock dose with breakthrough pain, but this could cause sedation or higher analgesia than needed. The goal is to treat the breakthrough pain with a fast-acting opioid such as morphine, hydromorphone, or oxycodone. However, unless given intravenously, this could take 30 minutes or more to take effect. A newer therapy is oral transmucosal fentanyl citrate, a lozenge with a handle, which can begin to act as quickly as intravenous medications (Rhiner and Kedziera, 1999). This medication is only for use by clients who are already opioid tolerant to around-the-clock doses.

Placebos. Numerous organizations have endorsed the Oncology Nursing Society position statement against placebo use in pain control (Pasero, 1998). An example of a placebo is a saline injection or sugar pill given to elicit a therapeutic effect in a client. The use of placebos "represents flagrant disregard for ethical tenets relative to patient rights and professional conduct" (Pasero, 1998).

Alternative Therapies

The combined use of pharmacologic and nonpharmacologic pain management therapies works well in older adults. Individually, most of the nondrug therapies work well only with mild pain. With moderate pain, drug therapy must complement the other therapies. Clinical experience suggests that many of these techniques are effective in individual cases. As with all treatment modalities, individual response must be evaluated. In one study 96% of older adults reported using at least one complementary or alternative therapy modality (Dunn and Horgas, 2000). Individuals differ greatly in their preferences for and use of nonpharmacologic interventions to manage their pain. Some find spiritual or religious coping strategies effective, whereas others may use imagery or relaxation techniques. However, cognitively impaired persons may not be able to use these techniques. Family and individual input is essential in use of these types of therapies (Horgas, 2003).

Alternative therapies can be categorized as physical or cognitive and behavioral. Some major alternative therapies are highlighted in the following sections.

Physical Therapies. Physical therapies include cutaneous stimulation with heat and cold, as well as counterstimulation methods such as massage, acupuncture, and nerve stimulation.

Heat and Cold. Heat is useful in decreasing pain and discomfort. It increases blood flow to skin and superficial tissues, increases oxygen and nutrient delivery, and decreases joint stiffness by increasing the elasticity of muscles (AHCPR, 1994). Heat is delivered by hot water bottle, heating pad, compresses, tub baths, soaks, and heat lamps. Clients and caregivers must be cautioned to avoid thermal burns, which can occur in older adult clients during prolonged use of these methods.

Cold reduces inflammation and edema and reduces pain, especially after an acute injury such as a fall. It may reduce muscle spasms not relieved by heat therapy (AHCPR, 1994). Cold can be given via ice bags and cold packs (with caution), compresses, cool soaks, and baths. Often, older adults have preferences for either heat or cold for pain relief (Luggen, 2000).

Massage. Most forms of touch are pleasurable to older adults (Ebersole, Hess, and Luggen, 2004). Massage can be deep pressure, such as rubbing and kneading, or it can be light stroking and smoothing. It should be used with caution in clients with bone metastases or very osteoporotic bones. Older adult clients may have preferences for certain odors in massage oils and creams.

Exercise. Exercise and physical therapy prevent stiffness, maintain function, relieve muscle spasm, and increase one's sense of well-being (Luggen, 2000). Medical consultation should be obtained for clients before instituting physical therapy. Many clients need pretreatment analgesic medication shortly before starting the regimen.

Acupressure and Acupuncture. Acupuncture is the insertion of needles at specific body sites, followed by manual or electrical stimulation. The stimulation competes for placement on pain receptor sites, which stops the progression of pain messages to the higher brain centers. Acupressure is manual pressure at the acupuncture sites. This is not a therapy that nurses can perform without extensive training; rather, it should be done by a health professional certified by a national program.

Transcutaneous Electrical Nerve Stimulation. Transcutaneous electrical nerve stimulation (TENS) has been found to be useful in the management of pain in older adults (Eiman et al, 1996). The client controls the electrical stimulation through electrodes on his or her skin and can increase or decrease the stimulation as needed. TENS is useful for neuropathic pain in diabetes, spinal pain, and neuralgias.

Percutaneous Electrical Nerve Stimulation. Percutaneous electrical nerve stimulation (PENS) utilizes stainless steel acupuncture-like needle probes that deliver stimulation that counters pain (Ghoname et al, 1999). It has been compared with TENS and exercise therapy and found to be superior to both in clients with low back pain. Pain scores were significantly decreased after therapy. Although it is said to be useful in osteoarthritis, there has been no extensive testing in older adult clients at this time. Percutaneous neuromodulation therapy (PNT) is used to desensitize continuous sensory pain (Shah, Ericksen, and Lacerte, 2003).

Cognitive and Behavioral Therapies. Cognitive and behavioral pain management strategies are meant to change the perception of pain, to alter pain behaviors, and increase a client's sense of control over pain (AHCPR, 1994). They can help change negative thoughts and attitudes (McCaffery and Pasero, 1999). Nurses can teach new skills that can influence a client to practice positive behaviors and emotions. Those clients with maladaptive behaviors, ongoing depression, or poor coping skills can be referred to mental health practitioners or pain clinics (McCaffery and Pasero, 1999). The following are some of the cognitive and behavioral therapies that nurses can use with their clients.

Meditation. Meditation is focusing on an object or word to achieve a calm, receptive mental state in a quiet environment. The client breathes slowly, adopts a passive attitude, and exhales while focusing on a word such as "peace."

Visualization or Imagery. This is a state of pleasure and peace achieved by creating a vivid picture in one's mind. This picture might be a setting sun, a serene forest, or rolling waves at sunrise. It might be recalled from the past or simply imagined. It is a concentrated focus on an image formed in the mind, involves all five senses. It transports the person to another place—a real, imaginary, or ideal place (Hoffart and Keene, 1998). It is described as altering the relationship between endorphins and the immune system, thereby reducing pain.

Progressive Relaxation. This is an alternating contraction and relaxation of the various muscle groups. One may move head to toe, or toe to head, or hand to head to toe. It is usually done lying down on a mat or bed, with a quiet, often darkened, environment. It can be accompanied by soft music or relaxation tapes, which are readily available at bookstores.

Jaw Relaxation. This cyclical method can be used anywhere and anytime and is useful for managing tension. First, the jaw is dropped and the tongue comes to the back of the front teeth. The lips relax. Then deep, rhythmic inhalation is followed by a slow exhale. This cycle is repeated 8 to 10 times (Clair, 1996). This is usually accompanied by music, though not the "toe tapping" type.

Distractions. Distractions can be almost anything that takes one's mind off the pain. They can include radio, television, videos, music, memories, pet therapy, projects such as games or puzzles, a story or newspaper read aloud, or spectator events. This is useful only for mild pain unless it is accompanied by pain medication.

Music Therapy. This therapy can be incorporated into many other therapies presented here. Furthermore, it is one therapy that has been used extensively in clinical practice with older adults (Clair, 1996). The music should be of a category appreciated by the client and at a volume that the client can control. Clair's book, *Therapeutic Use of Music with Older Adults* (1996), is worth reviewing by practitioners interested in this pain management modality.

Aroma Therapy. Aroma therapy involves using essential oils in a medium such as a vapor pot. Louis and Kowalski (2002) found increased relaxation and sense of well-being in a controlled repeated measures study of hospice patients. The calming effect was observed in the family members present during the procedure as well as in the patients. However, this therapy did not replace any pharmacologic interventions being used. It was seen as an agent to facilitate the action of the regularly prescribed treatments.

Hypnosis. Hypnosis includes some of the other cognitive modalities such as deep concentration, imagery, and breathing exercises. Self-hypnosis and imagery begin with developing a relaxed state; closing the eyes; focusing on the pain; and visualizing its color, shape, and size. Then the pain is projected out into space. It is made bigger, then smaller, and then allowed to be any size. Its color is changed, and then put back as it was. Finally, the eyes are reopened.

Therapeutic and Healing Touch. Therapeutic touch is a five-phase process in which a nurse combines "compassionate intent" with hand movements that "rebalance" a client's energy (Hutchison, 1999). It is associated with the Chinese qi, or "life energy." The therapy directs energy to the client to provide pain relief and promote healing. The therapist centers, reaching a meditative state that is sensitive to the client's needs. The energy flow is assessed by detecting differences in energy, temperature, and rhythm. The achievement of balance or harmony is the goal of therapy. There is considerable interest in this alternative therapy (Tyson, 1999). The reader is advised to pursue the Hutchison reference or the many new books and articles in the literature.

Healing touch is "hands-on healing" (Hutchison, 1999), using touch to balance the energy system. It is useful for controlling pain, decreasing anxiety, increasing relaxation, decreasing depression, and increasing the sense of well-being. There has been a tremendous growth in the practice of healing touch in recent years, and a three-level training program for certification has been developed for its practitioners. It is being used in hospitals, nursing facilities, and independent practices with considerable anecdotal evidence of its success.

Education. Education is a cognitive therapy that involves teaching a client about pain and the role of cognition in pain perception. The client learns to track the pain and record episodes of pain and distress. The nurse helps the client interpret the thoughts that accompany pain. Relaxation is incorporated to divert attention from the pain of the body. The goal is to help a client develop some mastery over his or her pain.

Financial Cost of Pain Management

For older adult clients and their caregivers, who may have already assumed the high costs of surgery, other treatments can be financially overwhelming. Financial considerations are particularly problematic for older persons because of fixed, limited incomes and third-party reimbursement schedules that may be restrictive. The cost/benefit ratio in pain treatment can best be achieved by using the least invasive, least costly treatment method. All pharmacologic and nonpharmacologic interventions should be carefully evaluated for cost and benefit. When selecting or implementing analgesic treatments, nurses should do the following (also see Research box):

- Use the ladder approach of the World Health Organization (1990); that is, a stepwise progression of pain drugs for increasing levels of pain.
- Provide adequate analgesia consistent with the intensity of a client's pain.
- Aggressively treat side effects such as constipation and nausea.
- Continuously reevaluate a client's status to determine the optimum treatment approach.
- Develop expertise in the use of high-dose morphine; read current pain literature.
- Assist with the development of hospital-wide guidelines on treatment modalities and procedures.
- Consider the impact of psychosocial influences on the effectiveness of a pain relief method.
- Use a multidisciplinary approach to pain management, including nursing, medicine, pharmacy, social services, physical therapy, and pastoral care.

Research

SAMPLE/SETTING

Subjects included 126 participants from three client groups: dialysis clients (48 participants), clients with HIV infection (40 participants), and residents of a long-term care facility in Toronto (38 participants).

METHODS

This qualitative study used data to conduct a content analysis.

FINDINGS

The subjects identified five domains of high-quality end-of-life care: (1) receiving adequate pain and symptom management, (2) avoiding inappropriate prolongation of dying, (3) achieving a sense of control, (4) relieving burden, and (5) strengthening relationships with loved ones.

IMPLICATIONS

Clients who are dying are often in pain. Having control of that pain is very important to any client. As client advocates, nurses need to expect such pain in their clients, assess and treat for pain, and then assess for adequate pain control. Implications for educators include increased gerontologic content in the basic curriculum, including content on pain assessment, measurement, treatment, and management.

Singer PA, Martin DK, Kelner M: Quality end-of-life care: client perspectives, *JAMA* 281(2):163, 1999.

Planning Pain Relief

The primary consideration in selecting pain relief methods is individual planning. Clients vary greatly in their medication requirements, choices of nonpharmacologic interventions, and prior pain experiences. Clients should be involved in choosing pain management methods and should share responsibility for implementing pain relief measures. Active involvement of clients and family caregivers is essential to the successful implementation of pain management regimens. This applies to both pharmacologic and nonpharmacologic pain relief measures.

Home Care

1. The nurse caring for homebound older adults should know the effects pain has on functional status and quality of life.
2. The home care nurse should evaluate a client's pain at each home visit.
3. The nurse should assess factors that may influence effective pain control in homebound older adults (e.g., motor, cognitive, and functional impairments).
4. When using a pain assessment tool, a home care nurse must evaluate a homebound older adult's ability to use the tool.
5. Caregivers are an important source of information when assessing homebound older adults with pain.
6. The nurse should instruct homebound older adults and their caregivers on adjunctive therapies that can be used with analgesics to enhance pain management.
7. The nurse should assess and identify barriers for homebound older adults and caregivers related to pain and its management.
8. The nurse should encourage around-the-clock pain management to provide optimum pain control.

SUMMARY

Pain continues to be underrecognized and undertreated in older adults despite dramatic increases in the knowledge of pain and pain management. Pain in clients in nursing facilities is a large problem. Older adults suffer many painful chronic illnesses such as arthritis and cancer. When conducting client assessments, the practicing nurse must look for pain in older adult clients and be alert to chronic diseases that may cause pain. There are many excellent pharmacologic treatments for pain today and many routes of administration; thus it is possible to individualize care for each client. Though pharmacology is the main therapy for most chronic illnesses, many alternative and complementary therapies are available that will benefit the nurse's older adult clients.

Key Points

- Pain often remains underrecognized and undertreated in older adults, mainly because of limited gerontologic pain research. Therefore nurses must have a special understanding and conduct an accurate and ongoing assessment of the pain needs of this population.
- Goals for pain management in older adults include control of chronic disease conditions that cause pain, maintenance of mobility and functional status, promotion of maximum independence, and improvement of quality of life.
- Barriers to effective pain management in older adults include the misconception that intolerance to pain is age related, underreporting of pain, lack of access to diagnostic services, cognitive and functional impairment, the inability to communicate pain effectively through pain behavior scales, fear of addiction, and inadequacies in pain education.
- Accurate and ongoing assessment, as well as a thorough understanding of pain physiology, is essential to effective pain management for older adults.
- The nurse's clinical assessment of older adults' pain includes a number of important components: medical history; pain history; history of trauma, medications, and previous pain experiences; physical examination, focusing on signs of trauma; musculoskeletal examination; assessment of range of motion; and functional impairments. A variety of tools and scales are available for these assessments.
- The quality-of-life assessment is a vital part of pain assessment in older adults. This assessment may include sleeping, ADL function, pain, social relationships, and a number of other areas. Different areas will have different values based on an individual's preferences.
- Pharmacologic pain management includes the use of analgesics, opioid analgesics, and adjuvant medications. Nonpharmacologic therapies include physical methods using cold, heat, and massage; relaxation or distraction; imagery; TENS; hypnosis; and therapeutic and healing touch. For the pain management to be effective, the nurse must continually assess a client's response to pain when employing any of these methods.
- A standard assessment scale that differentiates between pain intensity and pain distress in older adult clients is a useful tool for nurses when planning successful pain interventions. Consistent use of this tool, coupled with accurate record keeping, helps promote effective pain management.
- Family members often play an integral role in the pain management of older adults. Family members can provide insight into older adult clients' pain experiences by offering the nurse information that the clients may not be willing or able to accurately share.

Critical Thinking Exercises

1. A 90-year-old woman with a small bowel obstruction is admitted to the hospital from a long-term care facility. She also has a history of dementia and is incoherent. Discuss how you would revise your assessment and evaluation techniques in managing her pain.
2. What criteria should you use to determine if an older adult client requires an adjustment in dose or dosing interval, or which drug is prescribed for pain management?
3. In caring for a 77-year-old man who has had a prostatectomy, a nurse practitioner (APN) might have an option of administering meperidine (Demerol) (50 mg intramuscular), morphine sulfate (10 mg intravenous), Toradol (30 mg intramuscular), or pentazocine (Talwin) (50 mg intramuscular). If you are an APN, are there any additional data that you would need to know before making your choice?

REFERENCES

Agency for Health Care Policy and Research, US Department of Health and Human Services: *Clinical practice guideline no. 9, Management of cancer pain,* Rockville, Md, 1994, US Public Health Service.

Albert E: Quality of life assessment for older adults. In Luggen A, Meiner S, editors: *Care of the older adult with cancer,* Pittsburgh, 2000, Oncology Nursing Society Press.

American Academy of Pain Medicine, American Pain Society: A consensus statement regarding the use of opioids for the treatment of chronic pain, *ASPMN Pathways* 6(2):9, 1997.

American Geriatrics Society Panel on Chronic Pain in Older Persons: Clinical practice guidelines, *J Am Geriatr Soc* 46:635, 1998.

American Geriatrics Society Panel on Persistent Pain in Older Persons: The management of persistent pain in older persons, *J Am Geriatr Soc* 50:S205, 2002.

Aronoff G: Drawing the line between pain management and addiction, *Psychopharmacol Update* 12(9):1, 2002.

Astin J et al: Mind-body medicine: state of the science, implications for practice, *J Am Board Fam Practice* 16(20):131, 2003.

Bradbury J: Why do men and women feel and react to pain differently? *Lancet* 361(9374):2052, 2003.

Chakour MC et al: The effect of age on A-delta and C-fiber thermal r perceptions, *Pain* 64:143, 1996.

Clair AA: *Therapeutic use of music with older adults,* Baltimore Health Professional Press.

Cooner E, Amorosi S: *The study of pain and older Americans,* 1997, Louis Harris.

Davis GC: Nursing's role in pain management across the health care continuum, *Nurs Outlook* 46(1):19, Jan-Feb 1998.

Dunn K, Horgas AL: The prevalence of prayer as a spiritual self-care modality in elders, *J Holistic Nurs* 18:337, 2000.

Ebersole P, Hess P, Luggen A: *Toward healthy aging: human needs and nursing response,* ed 6, St Louis, 2004, Mosby.

Eiman M et al: Geriatric pain management. In Salerno E, Willens J, editors: *Pain management handbook,* St Louis, 1996, Mosby.

Farrell M, Katz B, Helme RD: The impact of dementia on the pain experience (review article), *Pain* 67:7, 1996.

Ferrell BA: Pain evaluation and management in nursing homes, *Ann Intern Med* 123:681, 1995.

Ferrell BA: Pain management in elderly people, *J Am Geriatr Soc* 39:64, 1991.

Ferrell BA, Ferrell BR, Osterweil D: Pain in the nursing home, *J Am Geriatr Soc* 38:409, 1990.

Ferrell BA, Ferrell BR, Rivera R: Pain in cognitively impaired nursing home patients, *J Pain Symptom Manage* 10(8):591, 1995.

Ferrell BR, Rhiner M, Ferrell BA: Development and implementation of a pain education program, *Cancer* 72:3426, 1993.

Forman WB, Stratton M: Current approaches to chronic pain in older patients, *Geriatrics* 46:47, 1991.

Ghoname EA et al: Percutaneous nerve stimulation for low back pain, *JAMA* 281(9):818, 1999.

Gibson SJ, Helme RD: Age-related differences in pain perception and report, *Clin Geriatric Med* 17:433, 2001.

Giles BE, Walker JS: Sex differences in pain and analgesia, *Pain Rev* 7(3/4):181, 2000.

Gloth FM: Factors that limit pain relief and increase complications, *Geriatrics* 55(10):46, 2000.

Gloth FM: Concerns with chronic analgesia therapy in elderly patients, *Am J Med* 101(suppl 1A):195, 1996.

Gorman C: Aspirin without ulcers, *Time* July 7, 1998.

Harkans SW, Kwentus J, Price DD: Pain and suffering in the elderly. In Bonica JJ, editor: *The management of pain,* ed 2, Philadelphia, 1990, Lea & Febiger, p 522.

Harkins SW, Scott RB: Pain and presbyalgos. In Birren JE, editor: *Encyclopedia of gerontology: age, aging and the aged,* vol 2, San Diego, 1996, Academic Press.

Harrison A, Busebar A, Al-Kaabi A: Does sharing a mother tongue affect how closely patients and nurses agree when rating the patient's pain, worry and knowledge? *J Adv Nurs* 24:229, 1996.

Herr K: Chronic pain: challenges and assessment strategies, *J Gerontol Nurs* 2:20, 2002.

Hoffart MB, Keene EP: The benefits of visualization, *Am J Nurs* 98(12):44, 1998.

Horgas AL: Pain management in elderly adults, *J Infusion Nurs* 26(3):161, 2003.

Huber E, Spirig R: Living with pain—elderly women as experts in the management on their chronic musculoskeletal pain, *Pflege* 17(5):296-305, 2004.

Hutchison CP: Healing touch—an energetic approach, *Am J Nurs* 99(4):43, 1999.

Kedziera PL: Easing elders' pain, *Holistic Nurs Pract* 15(2):4, 2001.

Keefe FJ et al: Psychological aspects of persistent pain: current state of the science, *J Pain* 5(4):195-211. 2004.

Kelly J, Payne R: Pain management in the elderly. In Barclay L, editor: *Clinical geriatric neurology,* Philadelphia, 1993, Lea & Febiger.

Kerns RD, Habib S: A critical review of the pain readiness to change model, *J Pain* 5(7):357-367, 2004

Kovach CR: Personal communication, July 29, 2004.

Kovach CR et al: Use of the assessment of discomfort in dementia protocol, *Applied Nurs Res* 14(4):193, 2001.

Kuck AW, Ricciardi E: Alterations in elimination. In Itano JD, Taoka KN, editors: *Core curriculum for oncology nursing,* ed 3, Philadelphia, 1998, WB Saunders.

Lee M: Drugs in the elderly: do you know the risks? *Am J Nurs* 96:24, 1996.

Leo J, Huether SE: Pain, temperature regulation, sleep, and sensory function. In McCance K, Huether S, editors: *Pathophysiology,* ed 3, St Louis, 1998, Mosby.

Levy MH: Advancement of opioid analgesia with controlled-release oxycodone, *Eur J Pain* 5(suppl A):113, 2001.

Loeb JL: Pain management in long term care, *Am J Nurs* 99(2):48, 1999.

Louis M, Kowalski S: Use of aromatherapy with hospice patients to decrease pain, anxiety and depression and to promote an increased sense of well being, *Am J Hospice Palliative Care* 19(6):381-386, 2002.

Luggen A: Cancer pain management in older adults. In Luggen A, Meiner SE, editors: *Care of the older adult with cancer,* Pittsburgh, 2000, Oncology Nursing Society Press.

Luggen A: NGNAs strategic plan: report of a delphi survey, *Geriatr Nurs* 18(1):33, 1997.

Luggen A: Review: older women and chronic pain, *Contemp Gerontol* Winter 1996.

Luggen AS, Meiner SE: Handbook for the care of the older adult with cancer, Pittsburgh, *2000, Oncology Nursing Press.*

Luggen A, Rini A: Assessment of social networks and isolation in community-based elderly men and women, *Geriatr Nurs* July-Aug 1995.

Lynn J, Teno JM, Phillips RS: Perceptions by family members of the dying experience of older and seriously ill patients, *Ann Intern Med* 126:97, 1997.

Maxwell T: Cancer pain management in the elderly, *Geriatr Nurs* 21(3):158-163, 2000.

McCaffery M: *Pain: nursing management of the patient with pain,* ed 3, Philadelphia, 2000, Lippincott.

McCaffery R, Frock T, Garguilo H: Understanding chronic pain and the mind-body connection, *Holistic Nurs Pract* 20(3):281, 2003.

McCaffery M, Pasero C: *Pain: clinical manual,* ed 2, St Louis, 1999, Mosby.

McCance KL, Huether SE: *Pathophysiology: the biologic basis for disease in adults and children,* ed 4, St Louis, 2002, Mosby.

McDonald M: Assessment and management of cancer pain in cognitively impaired elderly patients, *Geriatr Nurs* 20(5), Sept-Oct 1999.

Merskey H, Bogduk N, editors: *Classification of chronic pain,* ed 2, Seattle, 1994, IASP Press, p xi.

Mogil JS et al: The melanocortin-1 receptor gene mediates female-specific mechanisms of analgesia in mice and humans, *Proc Natl Acad Sci* 100:4867-4872, 2003.

Morley JE et al: Perception of quality of life by nursing home residents, *Nurs Home Med* 3(8):191, 1995.

Mosby PR et al: An epidemiologic analysis of pain in the elderly: the Iowa 65+ Rural Health Study, *J Aging Health* 6:138, 1994.

Nagle B, Erwin WG: Geriatrics. In DePiro JT et al, editors: *Pharmacotherapy: a pathophysiological approach,* ed 3, Norwalk, Conn, 1996, Appleton & Lange.

Pasero C: Pain control, *Am J Nurs* 98(1):52, 1998.

Pasero C, McCaffery M: Controlled-release oxycodone: it's worth considering when treating around the clock pain, *Am J Nurs* 104(1):30, 2004.

Pasero C, McCaffery M: The under-treatment of pain: are providers accountable for it? *Am J Nurs* 101(11):62, 2001.

Pasero C, Reed B, McCaffery M: Pain in the elderly. In McCaffery M, Pasero C, editors. *Pain: a clinical manual,* ed 2, St Louis, 1999, Mosby, p 674.

Reuben D, Yoshikawa T, Besdine R: *Geriatrics review syllabus: a core curriculum in geriatric medicine,* ed 3, Dubuque, Iowa, 1996, Kendall/Hunt.

Rhiner ME, Kedziera P: Managing breakthrough pain: a new approach, *Am J Nurs* (suppl):99(3):S3-S14, March 1999.

Roberto KA: *Older women with chronic pain,* New York, 1994, Haworth.

Sakauye K: Cultural influences on pain management in the elderly, *Comp Ther* 31(1):78-82, 2005.

Shah RV, Ericksen JJ, Lacerte M: Interventions in chronic pain management. 2. Frontiers: invasive nonsurgical interventions, *Arch Physical Med Rehab* 84(3 suppl):S39-S44, 2003.

Singer PA, Martin DK, Kelner M: Quality end-of-life care, *JAMA* 281(2):163, 1999.

Stein W: Pain management in long term care facilities, *Clin Geriatr* 5(3):24, 1997.
Stein W, Ferrell BA: Pain in the nursing home, *Clin Geriatr Med* 12(3):601, 1996.
Sternbach RA: Clinical aspects of pain. In Sternbach RA, editor: *The psychology of pain,* New York, 1978, Raven Press, p 223.
Sunderland T, Alterman I, Young D: A new scale for the assessment of depressed mood in demented patients, *Am J Psychiatry* 145(8):955-959, 1988.
Tyson ST: *Gerontological nursing care,* Philadelphia, 1999, WB Saunders.
Vallerand AH: Gender differences in pain, *Image* 27(3):235, 1995.
Vanegas G: Side effects of morphine administration in cancer patients, *Cancer Nurs* 21(4):289-297, 1998.
Wagner A et al: Pain prevention and pain therapies for residents in Oregon nursing homes, *Geriatr Nurs* 18(6):268, 1997.
Weiner D, Peterson B, Keefe F: Chronic pain-associated behaviors in the nursing home: resident versus caregiver perceptions, *Pain* 15:92, 1999.
Weiner DK, Rudy TE: Attitudinal barriers to effective treatment of persistent pain in nursing home residents, *J Am Geriatr Soc* 50(12):2035-2040, 2002.
Werner P et al: Pain in participants of adult day care centers: assessment by different raters, *J Pain Symptom Manage* 15:8, 1998.
Wold GH: *Basic geriatric nursing,* ed 2, St Louis, 1999, Mosby.
World Health Organization: *Cancer pain relief and palliative care,* Geneva, 1990, The Organization.
Yates P, Dewar A, Fentiman B: Pain: the views of elderly people living in long-term residential care settings, *J Adv Nurs* 21:667, 1995.
Yonan CA, Wegener ST: Assessment and management of pain in the older adult, *Rehab Psychol* 48(1): 4, 2003.
Zalon ML: Pain management instruction in nursing curricula, *J Nurs Educ* 95(34):262, 1995.

Internet Addresses

American Academy of Hospice and Palliative Medicine (www.aahpm.org)
American Academy of Pain Medicine (www.painmed.org)
American Geriatrics Society (www.americangeriatrics.org)
American Pain Society (www.ampainsoc.org)
International Hospice Institute and College (www.hospicecare.com)
National Hospice and Palliative Care Organization (www.nho.org)
Pain.com (www.pain.com)
SeniorHealthCare.org (www.seniorhealthcare.org)
Worldwide Congress on Pain (www.pain.com)

16 Infection

DIANNE THAMES, DNS, RN, and SUE E. MEINER, EdD, APRN, BC, GNP

Learning Objectives

On completion of this chapter, the reader will be able to:

1. Describe alterations in the immune system related to aging.
2. Describe nutritional factors that influence immune status.
3. Describe psychosocial factors that influence immune status.
4. Describe the effect of exercise on immune status.
5. Describe the effect of lifestyle factors on immune status.
6. Describe the effect of medications and drugs on immune status.
7. Identify strategies to prevent nosocomial and/or community-acquired infections.
8. Incorporate nutritional, psychosocial, and lifestyle factors into a nursing care plan.

The importance of investigating infections in the elderly cannot be overstated. Moran (2003) states that "infectious diseases account for 1 of 5 leading causes of death and 1 of the top 10 indications for hospitalization in persons 65 or older." Infections in the elderly are often masked in their presentation, which can lead to delayed treatment. The immune system, which enables the body's to defend itself against outside infections and altered cells such as neoplasms within the body, is vital to human survival. Yet with aging this system exhibits a diminished ability to provide such protection (Sunderkötter et al, 1997). Considering this system's fundamental importance to maintaining health, a clear understanding of the age-related changes in the immune system is crucial.

The immune system has two primary functions: (1) to discriminate between that which is self and that which is nonself and (2) to remove from the body that which is recognized as nonself. The system accomplishing this comprises several organs, cells, and proteins (Porth, 2004). Furthermore this system interacts with the neurologic and endocrine systems in a highly complex manner to modulate function of the human immune response. Thus immunologic functioning can be mediated by psychologic and behavioral factors. There is an increasing awareness of the impact of mood, activity level, stress, and nutrition on the capacity of this system to provide optimum protection.

This chapter examines the age-related changes in the immune system. The influence of other factors, such as psychosocial influences and nutrition, on the immune status of older adults is also discussed. Cancer, autoimmune diseases, human immunodeficiency virus (HIV), and significant nosocomial pathogens are presented.

THE CHAIN OF INFECTION

For an infection to occur, there must be a reservoir of an infectious disease, a portal of entry, and a susceptible host. The source of an infectious disease is the reservoir or substance from which the infectious agent was acquired. The source may be a person's own microbial flora (endogenous) or something in the environment (exogenous), such as water, air, food, soil, or another person. Infectious diseases passed from other animal species to humans are *zoonoses*; these include cat-scratch disease and rabies. Infections acquired in the hospital are called *nosocomial*; those acquired outside the health care facility are called *community acquired*. The source of transmission may also be a body substance, such as feces, blood, and body fluids. Infections can be transmitted from person to person through shared inanimate objects (fomites) contaminated with infected body fluids. Examples of this mechanism of transmission would include *Clostridium difficile* infection from a contaminated rectal probe or an electronic thermometer, and HIV infection from the use of shared syringes by intravenous drug users.

The portal of entry is the way a pathogen enters the body and gains access to susceptible tissues to cause disease. A portal of entry may be gained through penetration, direct contact, ingestion, or inhalation. Any disruption or penetration in the integrity of the skin and mucous membranes is a potential portal of entry. The break may be accidental (e.g., abrasion, burn), the result of a medical procedure (e.g., surgery, catheterization), or the result of direct inoculation from animal or arthropod bite (e.g., Lyme disease, malaria). In direct contact, pathogens are transmitted directly from infected tissue or secretions to exposed intact mucous membranes.

Sexually transmitted diseases such as gonorrhea and chlamydia are examples of direct contact transmission. A more efficient portal of entry is through the oral cavity and gastrointestinal tract. The pathogens are ingested and successfully compete with the normal bacterial flora to cause infection. Cholera, food poisoning, and hepatitis A are examples of diseases that occur through ingestion. Pathogens must be able to survive low pH and the enzymes of the gastric acid secretions to establish infection. People with reduced gastric acidity (because of disease or medications) are more susceptible to this route of infection because more types of pathogens survive the gastric environment in larger numbers.

A number of pathogens can invade the body through inhalation into the respiratory tract and cause disease. These diseases include influenza, common cold, and bacterial pneumonia. The portal of entry does not limit the site of infection. Ingested pathogens may penetrate the mucosa, disseminate through the circulatory system, and cause disease in other organs (Porth, 2004). Hepatitis A and vancomycin-resistant *enterococci* are examples of ingested pathogens causing infection in the liver and bloodstream, respectively.

The host is an important factor in determining whether a pathogen will succeed in causing infection and clinical disease (Soule, Larson, and Preston, 1995). Fig. 16-1 illustrates

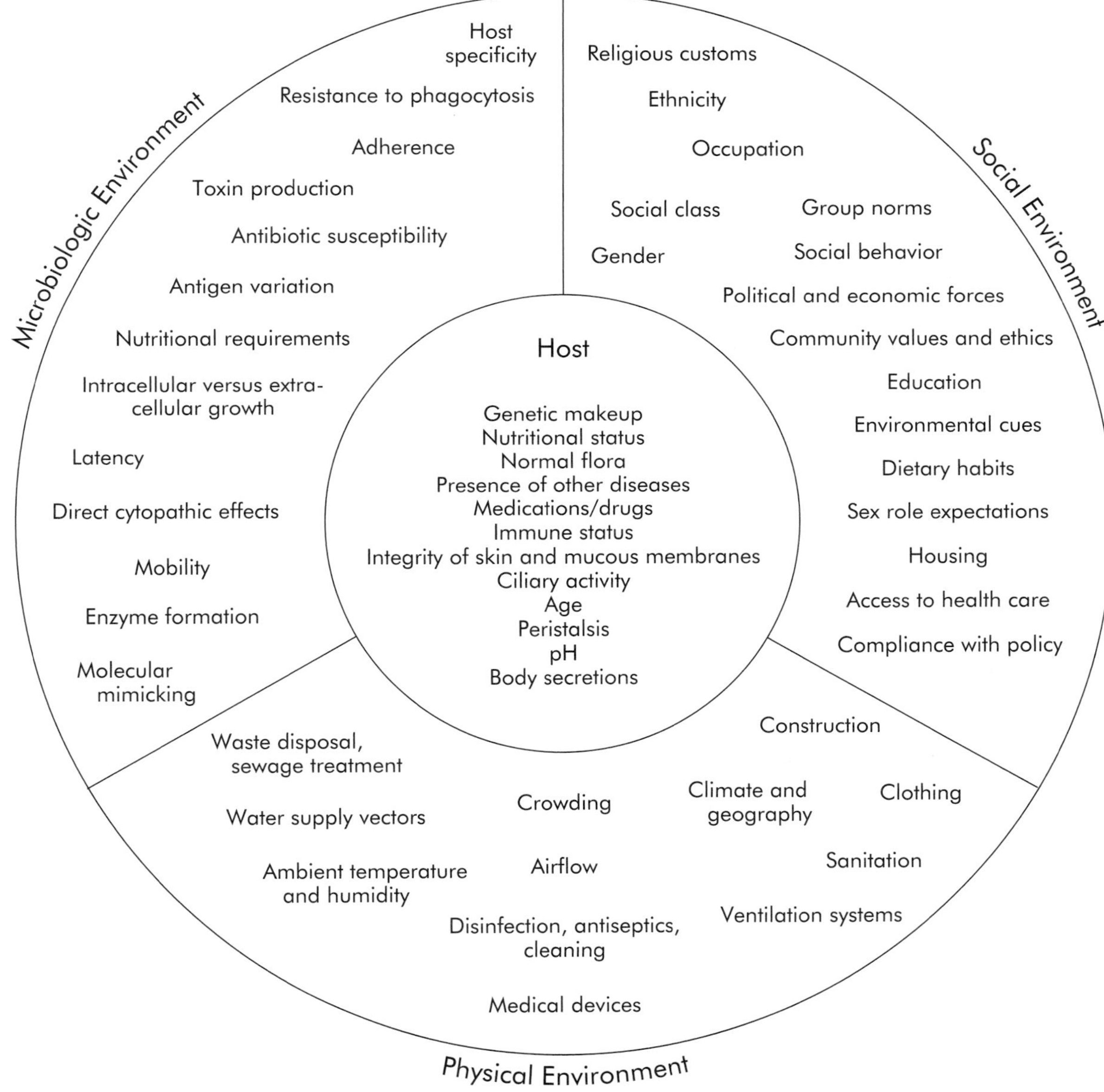

Fig. 16-1 Host-environment interaction. (From Soule B, Larson E, Preston G: *Infections and nursing practice*, St Louis, 1995, Mosby.)

host factors that influence the outcome of a pathogen's interaction with the human host. These host factors are unique for each individual and influence whether an individual becomes ill or remains well.

AGE-RELATED CHANGES IN THE IMMUNE SYSTEM

Some researchers believe that much of the illness seen in older adults may be the direct consequence of declining immunocompetence (Soule, Larson, and Preston, 1995; Sunderkötter et al, 1997). Alterations in immune status can be responsible for infections, cancer, and autoimmune processes, all of which can be life threatening (Porth, 2004). Scientists have tried to determine whether the diminished immunocompetence noted with age is a result of decreased numbers of immune cells or merely decreased functioning of the cells. However, since immunocompetence is affected by numerous other factors, it has been difficult to isolate changes that are related to age alone. Thymic atrophy, which occurs naturally with aging, affects T lymphocyte function (Porth, 1994). Diminished cellular (T cell–mediated) and humoral (B lymphocyte) immunity have both been associated with aging. Box 16-1 summarizes age-related changes in the immune system.

BOX 16-1 Age-Related Changes in the Immune System

LYMPHOCYTES

No change in total number of lymphocytes
No change in number of B cells
No change or increase in T_h-cells
Decrease in suppressor T cells
Decreased T cell responsiveness
Decreased CD_4 and CD_8 cells

POLYMORPHONUCLEAR LEUKOCYTES

Reduced migration ability

ANTIBODY

Decrease of T cell–dependent antibody responsiveness
Decreased primary response to new antigens
Maintenance of secondary response to antigens
Increased globulins associated with secondary response and autoimmunity
Increased incidence of antibodies to self-antigens

LYMPHOID TISSUE

Involution of thymus
Atrophy of thymic cortex
Atrophy or hypertrophy of some lymph nodes

MECHANICAL BARRIERS

Changes in skin and mucous membranes, resulting in reduced effectiveness of physical barriers

From Porth CM: *Pathophysiology: concepts of altered health status*, ed 4, Philadelphia, 1994, JB Lippincott; Sunderkötter C et al: Aging and the skin immune system, *Arch Dermatol* 133(10):1256, 1997.

Changes in Cell-Mediated Immunity

Cell-mediated immunity is the ability of the host to differentiate between self and nonself. Diminished cell-mediated immunity in older adults is generally associated with declining T cell function. Some researchers also report a decrease in the number of T cells, but this finding has not been consistently demonstrated. T cells in older adults seem to have a decreased ability to produce the cytokines needed to facilitate growth and maturation of B cells. Furthermore, T cells exhibit a diminished ability to proliferate when exposed to an antigen (Sunderkötter et al, 1997).

Changes in Humoral Immunity

Two components of humoral immunity are *complement* and *antibody*. Complement attracts more phagocytes to the site of microbial invasion, enhances phagocytosis, and causes lysis of bacteria by puncturing their cell walls (Soule, Larson, and Preston, 1995). Antibodies in the form of immunoglobulin are produced by B cells. Some antibody functions are to (1) assist phagocytosis by clumping the bacteria, (2) enhance phagocytosis, (3) activate complement, (4) recruit killer cells, (5) inhibit microbial motility, and (6) neutralize toxins (Soule, Larson, and Preston, 1995). The effect of aging on B cells is less clear. With aging, B cells exhibit a decreased production of immunoglobulin (Sunderkötter et al, 1997). B cells do retain their normal numbers with aging. However, with the decreased immunoglobulin production there is a concurrent decrease in hypersensitivity or allergic reactions. Primary immunity (natural immunity), which is composed of phagocytosis, killer cells, and complement, is not generally thought to be affected by age. Because prior exposure to the pathogen is not a prerequisite to this type of immunity, secondary immunity (acquired immunity) has exposure to the causative agent as a prerequisite. This initial exposure will activate T cells and antigen-presenting macrophages. These T cells are negatively affected by aging and thus negatively affect secondary immunity (Cantrell and Norman, 1998).

Changes in Natural Killer Cell Activity

Natural killer (NK) cells support host resistance to infection through immune surveillance (Porth, 2004). Although some researchers have documented a decrease in NK cell activity in the older adult population, most research on humans has failed to confirm an age-related loss of NK function (Porth, 2004).

Changes in Barrier Protection

The skin is the largest immunologically active system of the body and its first line of defense. The skin contains cells of the immune system, such as macrophages; B lymphocytes and T lymphocytes; and skin-specific immunocompetent cells, such as Langerhans' cells, keratinocytes, and endothelial cells (Sunderkötter et al, 1997). With aging, the skin becomes more fragile and prone to breakdown or abrasion (Cantrell and Norman, 1998).

FACTORS AFFECTING IMMUNOCOMPETENCE

Nutritional Factors

Nutritional and dietary status is of critical importance to immune function. This is especially true in the older adult population. Older adults are at high risk for nutritional deficits, with at least one third of individuals over age 65 having nutritional deficiencies (see Chapter 10). Risks associated with the development of a nosocomial infection include poor nutrition, unintentional weight loss, and low serum albumin levels (Soule, Larson, and Preston, 1995). Numerous factors that may contribute to this tendency toward inadequate nutrition include altered taste, social isolation, physical inability to prepare food, altered absorption, and poverty. Individuals with nutritional deficiencies have been shown to have significant reductions in delayed cutaneous hypersensitivity (Eliopoulos, 2001).

Protein-Energy (Caloric) Malnutrition. Significant deprivation of protein and energy (caloric) nutrients has been shown to result in major alterations in immune function (Porth, 2004; Soule, Larson, and Preston, 1995). Maturation of T cells is impaired, and serum immunoglobulin G and immunoglobulin M levels are decreased. Microbicidal activity is reduced because phagocytic cells are decreased in number and function abnormally; complement is also decreased (Soule, Larson, and Preston, 1995). These changes result in increased susceptibility to infectious disease. Restoring nutritional balance, especially protein balance, can improve older adults' immune status (Porth, 2004; Soule, Larson, and Preston, 1995).

Iron and Trace Element Deficiency. Although the effects of iron deficiency on immunocompetence and susceptibility to infection have not yet been fully determined, it has been established that lymphocyte and granulocyte function is compromised in the presence of iron deficiency (Soule, Larson, and Preston, 1995). Low levels of iron also decrease the number of circulating T cells. Iron deficiency contributes to decreased functioning of neutrophils, macrophages, and B cells and T cells. In addition, iron deficiency contributes to a delayed responsiveness to antigens.

Three trace metals—zinc, selenium, and copper—are thought to be associated with immune function. A prolonged zinc deficiency leads to impaired cell-mediated immunity, wound healing, and protein synthesis (Keegan, 1996). Improved immune function following the administration of moderate amounts of zinc to older adults has been reported. These improvements include increases in circulating T cells and appropriate delayed cutaneous hypersensitivity to a variety of antigens (Soule, Larson, and Preston, 1995).

Evidence suggests that other trace metals such as selenium and copper enhance humoral immunity (Keegan, 1996). Trace metals, especially selenium, are thought to be particularly important in maintaining resistance to malignancy. These trace metals are readily available in the diet, provided foods rich in these minerals are normally eaten. Selenium is present in fish and grain, depending on the selenium content of the soil in which the grain was grown. Good dietary sources of copper include organ meats, nuts, seeds, and legumes. The best sources of zinc are meats (especially beef), seafood (especially oysters), eggs, and poultry. Although zinc is also present in legumes and whole grain foods, with these sources it is less readily available for use by the body. Thus people on vegetarian diets may be at increased risk for zinc deficiency (Keegan, 1996).

Vitamin Deficiencies. Numerous vitamins have been shown to affect immune function. These include vitamins A, B_6 (pyridoxine), B_{12}, C, D, and E. Vitamins influencing cell-mediated immunity include vitamins A, C, D, E, and B_6 (Keegan, 1996; Soule, Larson, and Preston, 1995). Vitamin C (ascorbic acid) supplements (500 mg/day) have been shown to enhance lymphocyte responsiveness and skin reactivity to purified protein derivative (PPD) (Kennes et al, 1983). Dietary supplements of vitamins A, C, and E have also been shown to enhance cellular immunity in institutionalized older adults (Keegan, 1996).

Fat Intake. Both the amount and type of fat consumed may affect immune function. Unsaturated fat, especially in excessive amounts, may depress immune function and increase the likelihood of autoimmune disease (Calder, 1998; Griffini et al, 1998). Polyunsaturated fats have been associated with diminished T cell function. Animal studies have found that polyunsaturated fat enhances the proliferation and aggressiveness of cancer cells (Griffini et al, 1998). In humans receiving kidney transplants, supplementation of the diet with fish oil results in a decreased transplant rejection rate because of the immunosuppressive effect of fat (Calder, 1998). However, saturated fats have been associated with increased responsiveness of T cells.

Psychosocial Factors

Awareness is growing of the potential impact of psychosocial factors on immune status. These factors include chronic and acute stress, depression, bereavement, and social relationships. Recognition that such factors influence immune status is relatively recent, and our understanding of the nature of these relationships is constantly changing. Therefore the clinical relevance of these changes remains a source of investigation and controversy.

In the late 1980s into the 1990s, psychoneuroimmunology emerged as a discipline for examining the reciprocal influences between the immune and nervous systems (Soule, Larson, and Preston, 1995). Findings from this field will have important nursing implications because of the holistic (mind-body) approach to care. Older adults endure so many psychosocial assaults, the potential impact on immune status must be considered. Older adults often have to deal with bereavement as they lose family and friends. They also often endure a shrinking sphere of social relationships and exhibit a high incidence of depression. These factors are also particularly relevant for older individuals' immune status.

Stress. There is a growing awareness of the impact of stress on the immune system (Soule, Larson, and Preston, 1995). The exact influence that stress has on the immune system is unknown. The stress response induces changes in several hormonal factors that affect the immune response. The hallmark of the stress response is increased cortisol production, which suppresses the inflammatory and immune response (Porth, 2004). Research has found a variety of links between psychologic stress and the development of infectious diseases, especially colds (McNeil, 1998).

Stress depresses the immune system, causing diminished numbers and activity of NK cells, inhibition of lymphocyte proliferation, and decreased production of interferon (Soule, Larson, and Preston, 1995). Chronic stressors such as depression, bereavement, and caregiving affect the ability of NK cells to lyse a target cell or tumor cell. Clients with low NK cell activity are at higher risk for infection than those with normal activity (Anderson, 1998).

Depression. Depression has also been associated with decreased immune capacity. This is significant because approximately 15% of community-dwelling older adults have symptoms of depression (see Chapter 14). Furthermore, suicide is more common in older adults than in any other age-group (Cohen and Rabin, 1998). Individuals suffering from depression generally have fewer T-helper (T_h) cells and fewer suppressor T cells. Stress may increase the autoimmune response and the development of autoimmune diseases (Porth, 2004; Soule, Larson, and Preston, 1995). There is some evidence that the negative impact of depression on the immune system increases with age. Thus older adults who are depressed may be at risk for greater immune deficiencies than younger depressed individuals.

Bereavement. It has long been noted that bereaved spouses are at higher risk for illness or death than the general population (Anderson, 1998). Diminished immune function may account for this higher risk. Studies have consistently shown that the lymphocytes of bereaved spouses are less responsive, thus weakening both cellular and humoral immunity. Admittedly, bereavement and depression may go hand in hand. Yet in the population of older adults, where so many individuals are surviving the death of a spouse, the effect this event may have on immune status must be noted. In addition, the compacting effect of depression along with bereavement must be considered.

Social Relationships. Social relationships, either by their presence or absence, can have a substantial effect on immune status. Loneliness and divorce have been strongly associated with a diminished immune response (Anderson, 1998). On the other hand, the presence of interpersonal relationships may have a positive effect on immune status. There is evidence that the provision of social support may be associated with increased NK cell cytotoxicity and may influence the progression of disease (Cohen, 1998). Social relationships are important in quality as much as, or more so, than in quantity. It is the closeness of a relationship that contributes positively to immune status.

Lifestyle Factors

Activity Level. Activity level has been shown to affect immune status (Evans et al, 1998). Physical exercise has been shown to induce increased cell-mediated tumor cytotoxicity and NK cell activity in older adult women. Improvements in NK cell activity have been shown with as little as 5 minutes of moderate physical activity in healthy adults. Exercise also increases blood monocytes and neutrophils needed for phagocytosis (Evans et al, 1998).

Smoking. Smoking may have a detrimental effect on the immune system. Research has linked smoking with changes in lymphocyte populations, decreased IgA secretion, and increased immunoglobulin E secretion (Fischer and Konig, 1994). Smoking also inhibits respiratory ciliary action and enhances attachment of certain pathogens to pharyngeal epithelium (Soule, Larson, and Preston, 1995). Research indicates that individuals who smoke and who are seropositive for HIV progress to acquired immunodeficiency syndrome (AIDS) more quickly than their nonsmoking counterparts. Specifically, the smokers developed *Pneumocystis carinii* pneumonia sooner than nonsmokers (Nieman et al, 1993). Thus smoking, in addition to its carcinogenic effects, may also suppress immune function.

Medications

A variety of medications can affect the immune system; these include immunosuppressants and immunoenhancers. Many drugs given for therapeutic purposes have an immunosuppressant effect. Some of these drugs include corticosteroids, cyclosporine, and chemotherapeutics for cancer. Corticosteroids such as prednisone are given for a variety of reasons, including treatment of autoimmune processes such as rheumatoid arthritis. Individuals receiving corticosteroids have a diminished inflammatory process and decreased immunity. People taking these drugs in high doses or over prolonged periods probably have greater levels of immunosuppression than those individuals taking lower doses for shorter periods. Similarly, individuals taking cyclosporine after a transplant to diminish the chance of organ rejection, or individuals taking certain anticancer drugs, are at higher risk for infection.

Other drugs potentially affecting the immune system are usually taken for less therapeutic reasons. These include alcohol and marijuana. Chronic alcohol use has long been associated with a higher incidence of diseases such as tuberculosis and cancer (Soule, Larson, and Preston, 1995). Alcohol is thought to inhibit cell-mediated immunity (Porth, 2004). This effect is both direct in its suppression of immune function and indirect through alcohol-associated nutritional deficits that also compromise immune status.

Herbs

Because herbs are thought to be products of common plants, many believe that they can do no harm. Actually, individually or in concert with other herbs or medications, selected herbs can be harmful and negatively affect the immune system. Some believe that Echinacea and garlic prevent infection and may even enhance the immune system. Others believe that ginseng protects the body from negative stress (Eliopoulos, 2001)

COMMON PROBLEMS AND CONDITIONS

The immune deficits seen so often in older adults make this population more vulnerable to both infection and cancer, thus contributing to increased rates of infections such as pneumonia and influenza, as well as a wide variety of malignancies. As people age, the likelihood increases that autoimmune antibodies will be found in serum, suggesting an increased likelihood of autoimmune processes. However, there is controversy on whether such autoimmune processes are actually age related (Sunderkötter et al, 1997).

Numerous infections are possible for individuals with diminished immune capacity. Some of the more common infections in older adults include influenza, pneumonia, tuberculosis, urinary tract infections (especially in women), and shingles (herpes zoster) (Davies, 1996; Monto and Terpenning, 1996). (See Chapter 24 for additional information about specific respiratory diseases.) With diminished IgA production, the barriers of skin and mucous membranes are less effective. Furthermore, as these barriers become more fragile with aging, the entry of pathogens is more easily achieved. Weakening of respiratory muscles and decreased clearance of bacteria by the mucociliary system make older adults susceptible to respiratory infections (Soule, Larson, and Preston, 1995). Medical management of infections consists primarily of determining the source of the infection and prescribing the appropriate antibiotic or antiviral medication.

Influenza and Pneumonia

Pneumonia and influenza are tied as the fourth leading cause of death in the elderly (Eliopoulos, 2001). Nosocomeal pneumonia is documented to be the second most common nosocomial infection (Brooks, 2001). As with the United States, data from other developed countries show influenza and pneumonia are among the 10 leading causes of death (Monto and Terpenning, 1996). The cost of treating these clients has been estimated to be more than $550 million a year (Ely, 1998).

Host factors associated with influenza include age and underlying cardiovascular, pulmonary, metabolic, or renal disease (Soule, Larson, and Preston, 1995). Influenza attack rates of 60%, with 30% mortality, have been reported in nursing facilities (Soule, Larson, and Preston, 1995). The predominant portal of entry is inhalation of small droplets transmitted through sneezing, coughing, or talking. The virus can also survive on environmental surfaces for 1 or 2 days, providing an opportunity for contamination and transmission via health care workers' hands. Closed populations such as those in long-term care facilities provide an ideal setting for the spread of influenza. The social environment in these institutions also facilitates transmission of influenza through group activities, communal dining rooms, and rehabilitation activities.

The most effective measure to control influenza is the vaccination of persons at high risk. Influenza vaccination is a Medicare-covered benefit for older adults (Monto and Terpenning, 1996). Cost analysis of the flu vaccine revealed that a 40% vaccination rate and a vaccination effectiveness of 42% in a "severe" year or 21% in a "mild" year had a zero net cost to the system. At higher vaccination levels the benefit would actually save money for Medicare (Monto and Terpenning, 1996). Other strategies to control nosocomial spread of influenza include the early identification and grouping of infected clients; careful hand washing; and the use of barrier precautions when handling bodily substances, especially respiratory secretions.

Pneumonia may follow influenza or develop independently. The organisms involved depend on the setting in which pneumonia appeared (Ely, 1998). Community-acquired pneumonia is most frequently due to *Streptococcus pneumoniae*; in nursing facilities, *Haemophilus influenzae* is often the cause; and in hospital-acquired pneumonia, the most frequent pathogens are *Pseudomonas aeruginosa, Klebsiella pneumoniae,* and *Staphylococcus aureus.* Pneumonia represents approximately 20% of nosocomial infections among older adults, second only to urinary tract infections (Ely, 1998). The pneumonia-causing pathogens may migrate from the lungs to the bloodstream, causing a bacteremia. Pneumonia coupled with a bloodstream infection is very serious and has up to a 90% mortality rate in older adults (Ely, 1998).

The major host factor associated with community-acquired pneumonia is advanced age (Soule, Larson, and Preston, 1995). Smoking, alcohol abuse, chronic lung disease, recent history of viral upper respiratory tract infection, and neurologic disease (which may contribute to microaspiration of secretions from the oropharynx) are other contributing factors. Pneumonia follows aspiration of the organism into the lungs. The aging lung has impaired elasticity and mucociliary clearance, which allows the organisms to survive and multiply. Social environments such as congregate housing, communal dining rooms, churches, crowded shopping centers, day care centers, or nursing facilities place older adults at risk for exposure and infection (Soule, Larson, and Preston, 1995). However, social isolation is not recommended because of its negative psychologic consequences. Older adults should be encouraged to select activities that may reduce the infection risk during the colder months.

Vaccination against pneumococcal infection is the primary prevention strategy, although it is underused (Ely, 1998). The pneumococcal vaccine has been a Medicare-covered benefit since 1981. Cost analysis shows a net savings of $141 to third-party payers for each person vaccinated (Monto and Terpenning, 1996). Vaccines are currently being developed for bacilli such as *P. aeruginosa, K. pneumoniae,* and *Escherichia coli* (Ely, 1998). Other infection control measures include hand washing, meticulous suctioning technique, careful attention to nutritional and fluid intake, and prompt disposal of items contaminated with respiratory secretions (Ely, 1998; Soule, Larson, and Preston, 1995). Older persons and their families should be instructed to seek early medical attention for subtle changes that may signal the onset of infection. For example, pneumonia may be seen in patients with confusion or tachypnea but no other findings (Ely, 1998) (see Chapter 24).

Precautions recommended to individuals throughout their lives take on added importance with aging. For example, older adults need to maintain tetanus immunization every 10 years because their immune response may be diminished. Older adults also become more vulnerable to tuberculosis, which has increased in prevalence in recent years. The age-related changes in the immune system contribute to the emergence of tuberculosis in previously infected individuals (Davies, 1996). The great majority of cases in persons ages 65 and older are likely to be due to reactivation of endogenous infection. Older adults are also more likely to contract the bacillus in environments where tuberculosis is prevalent. Older adults who live in congregate housing, eat communally, or are impoverished have increased rates of infection and disease (Davies, 1996).

Cancer

Neoplasms occur with greater frequency in older adults. The weakened immune system evidently loses some of its ability to maintain surveillance for aberrant cell growth (Sunderkötter et al, 1997). Thus cells within the body that would normally be eliminated by the immune system are able to grow uncontrolled. A wide variety of types of cancer are possible in older adults (see Chapter 19).

Common types of cancer in older adults include lung cancer, breast cancer, and prostate cancer. However, the potential for numerous other forms of cancer should not be overlooked. The presence of the cancer itself reveals the presence of an immune deficiency. Cancer cells are normally detected by the immune system and eliminated after being recognized as abnormal cells. It is only when the immune system fails to carry out this function that cancer occurs. However, the cancer and the cancer treatment can induce additional immune deficits. For example, cancer is often accompanied by a decrease in appetite, which increases the possibility of malnutrition. Furthermore, anticancer drugs often deplete immune cells, causing further debilitation of the immune system. Since many of these drugs have their greatest effect on rapidly dividing cells, the rapidly dividing immune system cells are attacked concurrently with the cancer cells. Neutropenic individuals (such as cancer clients undergoing immunosuppressive therapy) are at risk for developing invasive disease from aspergilli. The duration of neutropenia appears to be the strongest predictor of subsequent development of invasive aspergillosis (Soule, Larson, and Preston, 1995). *Aspergillus* is a genus of common mold, easily suspended in the air and inhaled. The illness first is seen as an acute pneumonia, which leads to tissue invasion (invasive aspergillosis) and disseminates into systemic disease. The prognosis for cancer is highly variable depending on the time of diagnosis, the client's general health, and the type of cancer.

Autoimmunity

Autoimmune antibodies increase with aging, while suppressor T cells decrease. But there is no firm evidence that these changes result in an increase in autoimmune diseases (Sunderkötter et al, 1997). Therefore, although older adults may have autoimmune diseases such as rheumatoid arthritis, these cannot necessarily be considered age associated. Older adults with autoimmune diseases are more likely to take immunosuppressant drugs as treatment for their disease processes, and they still risk the immune deficits that accompany aging. Therefore these older adults carry higher risks for infection than other older adults without autoimmune disease.

The event or events that trigger the development of an autoimmune disease are not known. The body may form antibodies against itself or fail to recognize native antigens as self (Porth, 1994). Criteria for identifying autoimmune disease are based on (1) evidence of autoimmune reaction, (2) determination that immunologic findings are not secondary to another condition, and (3) lack of other identified causes for the disorder.

There is a striking prevalence of autoimmune disease in women. Estrogen alone is not responsible for the female connection to autoimmune diseases. Systemic lupus erythematosus (SLE) is seen predominantly in women in their childbearing years, yet most clients with temporal arteritis are older women, and rheumatoid arthritis peaks in postmenopausal women (Merrill et al, 1998). Box 16-2 lists autoimmune diseases more prevalent in women. Box 16-3 provides a fuller list of autoimmune diseases.

Systemic Lupus Erythematosus. SLE can affect many parts of the body, including the joints, skin, kidneys, heart, lungs, blood vessels, and brain. The most common symptoms are extreme fatigue, painful or swollen joints, unexplained fever, skin rashes, and kidney problems. The antinuclear antibody (ANA) is one of the more specific tests for lupus; clients with lupus have a positive ANA. There is no cure for lupus at this time. The management objectives are controlling severity of symptoms and preventing a flare. The warning signs of a flare are increased fatigue, pain, rash, fever, stomach discomfort, headache, and dizziness. Clients must monitor their health and learn to recognize symptoms of disease activity. Avoiding the sun, exercising, complying with medications, limiting stress, and having regular health care visits are important.

BOX 16-2 Autoimmune Diseases More Prevalent in Women

DISEASE	FEMALE/MALE RATIO
Scleroderma	15:1
SLE	10:1
Takayasu's arteritis	10:1
Giant cell arteritis	4:1
Rheumatoid arthritis	3:1

From Merrill J et al: *Autoimmunity: the female connection.* Accessed July 1998 from website: http://www.medscape.com.

BOX 16-3 Examples of Autoimmune Diseases

SYSTEMIC DISEASES

Polymyositis-dermatomyositis
Rheumatoid arthritis
Scleroderma
SLE

BLOOD DISEASES

Autoimmune hemolytic anemia
Idiopathic thrombocytopenic purpura

DISEASES OF OTHER ORGANS

Autoimmune hepatitis
Goodpasture's syndrome
Hashimoto's disease
Insulin-dependent diabetes mellitus
Myasthenia gravis
Temporal arteritis
Thyrotoxicosis
Ulcerative colitis

From Lawrence R et al: Estimates of the prevalence of arthritis and selected musculoskeletal disorders in the United States, *Arthritis & Rheumatism* 441(5):778, 1998; Newton J et al: Autoimmune hepatitis in older patients, *Age & Aging* 26:441, 1997; Porth CM: *Pathophysiology: concepts of altered health status,* ed 4, Philadelphia, 1994, JB Lippincott.

Rheumatoid Arthritis. Rheumatoid arthritis is characterized by an inflammatory polyarthritis of unknown cause. Symptoms include morning stiffness, tenderness, pain on motion, limited range of motion, and joint deformity in the small joints of the hands and feet. Extraarticular signs are pulmonary (e.g., pleuritis, pneumonitis), cardiac (e.g., pericarditis, myocarditis), renal (e.g., amyloidosis), and ocular (e.g., scleritis); rheumatoid (subcutaneous) nodules also develop. The course of rheumatoid arthritis is highly variable; most people develop progressive functional limitation and physical disability. The prevalence of rheumatoid arthritis among adults in the United States is approximately 10 per 1000. Clients with rheumatoid arthritis have a higher mortality rate than the general population. Traditional management for rheumatoid arthritis follows the pyramid model of rest, exercise, and physical therapy with applications of heat and cold. The treatment protocol builds over time by increasing the strength of various prescriptions, ending with disease-modifying drugs. Researchers now advise starting disease-modifying drugs at the time of diagnosis, since the cytotoxic agents and corticosteroids are not as toxic to individuals as previously thought.

Autoimmune Hepatitis. Autoimmune hepatitis has an unknown etiology and is characterized by progressive destruction of the liver parenchyma, leading to hepatic fibrosis and cirrhosis (Newton et al, 1997). Although it was once thought to be rare in older adults, autoimmune hepatitis is now thought to be underrecognized in this population. Liver biopsy is essential to confirm the diagnosis and assess for disease activity and the presence of cirrhosis. Clients usually respond to immunosuppressive treatment with steroids (Newton et al, 1997).

HIV IN OLDER ADULTS

Americans generally do not believe HIV infection is a problem among the older adult population. Many erroneously believe the incidence of AIDS in older adults is rare and can be attributed to blood transfusions. But the spread of HIV and AIDS is a multigenerational crisis. The low clinical suspicion of HIV infection and delayed recognition of AIDS-defining infections contributes to the poor prognosis of HIV infection in older adults. In older adults there is only a short interval from HIV infection to the development of AIDS and death. The aging immune system is not able to eliminate the HIV residing in macrophages, lymphoid tissue, or the brain. Since the immune system's regenerative capacity is diminished and not all replacement cells are fully functional, the disease progresses more rapidly (Adler et al, 1997). The proportion of older adult AIDS cases attributed to heterosexual transmission and intravenous drug use has continued to rise since 1988. Only a small proportion of older adults exhibiting an AIDS risk behavior reported the use of condoms during sex.

These findings hold major implications for nursing practice. In assessing older adults, nurses must complete a sexual history. Nurses need to discuss HIV and risk behaviors for acquiring HIV. Sex education, the use of condoms, and how and when to take an HIV test should be taught to older adults. The primary prevention strategies of HIV transmission among older adults needs to focus on sexual transmission (National Association of Social Workers, 2003).

SIGNIFICANT NOSOCOMIAL PATHOGENS

Older adults are more likely to be affected by different microorganisms that those that affect younger adults (Cantrell, 1998). Richards et al (2000) found that 72% of reported nosocomial infections occurred in patients over the age of 55; 13% of those occurred in patients 85 years of age or older.

Clostridium difficile

At one time, antibiotic-associated diarrhea was considered noninfectious. Now it is recognized that it is caused by *C. difficile,* a significant nosocomial pathogen. *C. difficile* is an anaerobic, spore-forming bacillus. The presence of *C. difficile* alone does not indicate infection. Disease occurs when the organism is present and the normal flora of the bowel are disturbed. During antibiotic administration, *C. difficile* produces spores to enable its survival. When antibiotic levels in the colon are low, *C. difficile* reverts to vegetative form. *C. difficile* produces toxins A and B, which cause hemorrhage and cellular damage, resulting in fluid accumulation in the intestines. The hallmark diarrhea is caused by a motility-altering factor that stimulates muscle contractions.

C. difficile is transmitted person to person, primarily from health care worker hands. *C. difficile* has also been transmitted indirectly through contaminated equipment such as rectal probes and electronic thermometers. Consistent hand washing between contacts with clients and the use of gloves when handling body substances such as feces are imperative. Clients with *C. difficile* should be placed in a private room with their own bathroom or commode. Antibiotic restriction is a useful adjunct for decreasing the frequency of symptomatic disease.

Vancomycin-Resistant Enterococcus

From 1989, when VRE was first identified in the United States, through 1993, the proportion of enterococcal isolates resistant to vancomycin increased 35-fold (Weber and Rutala, 1997). Multiple factors predispose a person to infection with VRE, but colonization precedes most infections. No effective antimicrobial therapy is available for VRE, and attributable mortality is approximately 40% (Weber and Rutala, 1997). Vancomycin use has increased dramatically in the past 20 years as a result of various factors, including increases in the incidence of methicillin-resistant *S. aureus* (MRSA), prosthetic device–related infection, *C. difficile* infection, and inappropriate drug use (McDonald, 1997). Risk factors for VRE acquisition include an age of more than 65 years, antimicrobial therapy, chronic renal failure, malignancies, organ transplants, and prolonged hospitalization.

VRE is transmitted person to person via the hands of health care workers. VRE is also transmitted by contaminated medical devices, including electronic thermometers, fluidized beds, and environmental surfaces. VRE can survive on environmental surfaces up to 7 days (Weber and Rutala, 1997). To control transmission of VRE, health care workers must perform a meticulous 15-second hand washing with an antimicrobial soap. Dedicated equipment such as stethoscopes are required for infected clients. Colonized and infected clients should be isolated in private rooms or grouped with other infected clients in the acute care setting. Barrier precautions, gloves, and gowns should be implemented for client care. However, the use of gowns remains controversial because VRE has been shown to survive on fabric in laboratory experiments. Restrictions on vancomycin use are also recommended; however, this control measure has not been subject to rigorous scientific tests of efficacy (Weber and Rutala, 1997).

Methicillin-Resistant *Staphylococcus aureus*

S. aureus is a gram-positive cocci. In the early 1940s, when penicillin first became available, *S. aureus* was highly susceptible to antibiotic treatment. By the early 1950s, 80% of nosocomial *S. aureus* was resistant to penicillin. Today, more than 90% of community- and hospital-acquired *S. aureus* is resistant to penicillin. Methicillin became available in the 1960s, and by the mid-1970s MRSA became a significant problem.

The antibiotic of choice for MRSA infection is vancomycin. However, exposure to vancomycin is a risk factor for the acquisition of VRE.

MRSA is transmitted client to client via the hands of health care workers. MRSA may also be transmitted via contaminated equipment, especially in burn units. Risk factors for acquiring MRSA are insulin-dependent diabetes mellitus, chronic hemodialysis, illicit intravenous drug use, prolonged hospitalization, prolonged antibiotic therapy, stays in intensive care or burn units, and rooming next to a client colonized or infected with MRSA. Control of MRSA focuses on health care worker hand washing to reduce transmission. Health care workers should wear gloves for all contact with clients who are either colonized or infected. MRSA-positive clients should be placed in private rooms or grouped together in the acute care setting (Olmstead, 1996).

NURSING MANAGEMENT

Assessment

Obviously, with such a spectrum of possible infections, the clinical assessment varies widely. However, there are some crucial aspects to assessing older adults for the presence of infection (Box 16-4). Older adults with possible immune deficits may not exhibit classic symptoms of infection. Diminished inflammatory responses may lead to false negatives for skin tests used in the diagnosis of disease; for example, the PPD skin test for tuberculosis (Sunderkötter et al, 1997). Similarly, redness, swelling, or inflammation may be reduced with infections. These reduced responses are even more likely to occur in people who have diseases or drug treatments that further suppress the immune system, such as people with cancer or those taking immunosuppressants.

Another classic example of a reduced response to infection is the absence of fever. With an infection, local or systemic fever is provoked by the immune response. In healthy adults an elevated temperature provides an indicator of the presence of infection. However, certain individuals, such as older adults who have immune deficits, may experience only a limited temperature increase or no increase at all (Riquelme et al, 1997). Symptoms of pain may also be reduced or absent. Thus infection in these older adults can progress to life-threatening stages before it is detected.

Because of this reduced immune response, mild symptoms such as a low-grade fever must be taken seriously. Close observation is needed to detect subtle symptoms. Changes in the behavior of clients (such as increased malaise or fatigue, especially combined with other symptoms) may indicate the onset of infection. Fever and inflammation may be reduced, whereas the white blood cell (WBC) count can still reflect an increased value (Soule, Larson, and Preston, 1995). Yet if immunosuppression is present from drug treatment for diseases such as cancer or AIDS, elevations in WBC counts may not be seen, even with severe infection.

In addition to observed data, subjective and historical data are valuable when evaluating older adults with infection. A history of previous episodes of infection, including the timing, nature, and severity of the infection, is important. Infections in older adults can often recur. Although individuals normally develop immunity following the first infection, older adults may be unable to develop an adequate immune response and are therefore more likely to be susceptible to the same infection again. Information regarding exposure to others with infections may also be helpful. Older adults are more susceptible to infection, especially if they are living in environments conducive to the spread of pathogens. Such environments include nursing facilities, hospitals, and crowded environments, where hygiene standards are difficult to maintain. Immunization records also provide important information that needs to be kept on file.

It is also important to determine other disease processes for which clients may currently be receiving treatment. Persons with cancer may be experiencing assaults on their immune systems from the disease and from cancer treatments. Older adults with autoimmune diseases may be receiving antiinflammatory immunosuppressant drugs. Individuals with HIV infection are obviously experiencing an extreme assault on their immune system. All of these make older adults more prone to a variety of infections. In such situations the most likely infections are often those resulting from an individual's own normal flora, such as *Candida* organisms. Respiratory infections are also very likely (Ely, 1998).

A thorough record of medications is necessary to detect the potential for drug-related immunosuppression. This record should include both prescription and over-the-counter drugs. Clients receiving drugs with immunosuppressant qualities are obviously more prone to infections. In addition, information on the use of alcohol, tobacco, and other drugs, as well as exposure to toxic substances, should be obtained.

Information about a client's lifestyle can provide invaluable information in developing a care plan. This should include a thorough nutritional history and an indication of activity and exercise. An understanding of an individual's social support system should be acquired, and indicators of life stressors should be elicited. A classic life stressor is bereavement, especially for a spouse. However, the loss of friends and other family members should not be overlooked. Even the loss of a home or relocation to another place can yield a sense of bereavement.

BOX 16-4 Assessment of Individuals at High Risk for Infection

SUBJECTIVE

Take history.

- Previous infections
- Predisposing illnesses
- Medications
- Vaccinations
- Living environment
- Lifestyle factors (e.g., smoking, activity level, chemical exposures)
- Social support system

OBJECTIVE

Assess for signs and symptoms of infection.

- Fever—high grade or low grade
- Inflammation—pronounced or slight
- Pain—slight or severe
- Malaise, fatigue
- Turbidity, odor, and amount of body fluids
- CBC with differential

Diagnosis

Several nursing diagnoses may be applicable to older clients who either have infections or are at high risk for developing infections (Box 16-5). The risk factors determined during the assessment indicate some potential nursing diagnoses. For example, many older adults are either inadequately or inappropriately nourished. Thus a diagnosis of "altered nutrition: less than body requirements" is likely. People with cancer may be malnourished because of lack of appetite or side effects resulting from medications. Poor nutrition may also be attributed to a self-care deficit in preparing and eating food; older adults sometimes have difficulty preparing their own meals. These difficulties may be related to a variety of problems such as visual deficits, arthritis, or depression. Regardless of the cause, if these self-care deficits result in poor nutrition, the older adults are then at higher risk for infection.

The diagnosis "high risk for infection" is applicable to those at high risk for getting an infection and those with existing infections. The presence of an infection indicates that the immune system is already challenged. This increases the likelihood of a secondary infection. For instance, it is not unusual for an individual with viral influenza to later develop a secondary bacterial infection of pneumococcal pneumonia.

A diagnosis of "knowledge deficit" is also a possibility. Knowledge deficits may involve (1) immunizations, (2) nutrition, or (3) protection against infection from oneself or others. Clients may be unaware of their nutritional needs or the relationship between nutritional and immune status. If they have this knowledge, older adults may be more likely to consume appropriate foods. Similarly, older adults may be unaware of available vaccinations or the benefit such vaccinations may hold for them. Older individuals need information on ways to protect themselves from contracting infections to reduce their risk.

Finally, "social isolation" may be a relevant diagnosis associated with the individual at risk for infection, since social support has also been associated with immune status.

Planning and Expected Outcomes

In planning care for older clients, the health care team and clients must set goals together. Goals must be congruent with realistic expectations and with clients' desired outcomes. For individuals at increased risk for infection, goals include (1) avoiding primary or secondary infection and (2) maintaining or improving immune status. A careful assessment of client knowledge in areas related to infection prevention, maintenance of immune status, and health practices determines the goals for client teaching.

In setting nutritional goals, the nurse might find a consultation with a registered dietitian appropriate. They must consider clients' dietary preferences and financial ability to buy food (if not in an institutional setting). An outcome might be that a client consumes a well-balanced, high-caloric diet on a daily basis. Clients with cancer may have even more extreme nutritional needs. An outcome for these individuals might be that they stabilize body weight, and then gradually increase it at a rate of 1 pound every 3 weeks. Another outcome may be that a client performs self-care activities with minimum energy expenditure and risk of injury. For clients with activity deficits, an appropriate goal might be to participate in 15 minutes of moderate exercise 3 times a week. The exact target goal for exercise should be established in consultation with the primary care provider, and possibly achieved through physical therapy.

BOX 16-5 NANDA Nursing Diagnoses Appropriate for Older Adults with Autoimmune Diseases

Risk for infection
Altered nutrition: less than body requirements
Self-care deficit: feeding
Knowledge deficit: immunizations, nutrition, protection from infection
Social isolation

Intervention

Nursing management of older adults with alterations in immunity focuses on the prevention of infections. Interventions addressing this goal are targeted at (1) preventing exposure to infections and (2) enhancing the immune system to enable clients to better resist infections. Totally preventing exposure to pathogens is impossible, especially since one source of pathogens is the body's own natural flora. However, exposure can be minimized for individuals with diminished immune capacity (see Research box). During times of epidemic, such as influenza season, the client can avoid crowds of people. In an institutional or home setting, visitors can be screened for respiratory infections. If contact is unavoidable, infected visitors can be given a mask to wear to minimize potential contamination of the clients. Any catheters, intravenous fluids, or similar therapeutic devices should be carefully assessed for pathogen growth. Teaching clients to drink at least 2000 ml of fluid a day, unless contraindicated, will aid in preventing urinary tract infection and constipation. In addition, teaching stress management techniques to promote immune system function may be indicated. Finally, hygiene standards should be rigorously maintained, especially for clients experiencing treatment-induced immune suppression, as is seen with some anticancer drugs. In addition to normal bathing, careful attention should be paid to oral and perineal care. Both clients and caregivers should be alert for changes in the color, consistency, and odor of body fluids to detect the onset of infections.

Nutrition Interventions. Other measures can be taken to strengthen the immune system to better enable clients to resist infection. As previously mentioned, optimum nutrition status is important. To achieve this status, clients must receive adequate energy and protein, as well as sufficient vitamins, iron, and trace minerals, with a special emphasis on zinc, sele-

Research

SAMPLE/SETTING

The subjects were staff members and older adult participants of two senior day care sites.

METHODS

Surveillance for acute respiratory tract illness (ARTI). Staff members reported to the project nurse any such possible illness among the day care participants or staff. ARTI is defined as nasal congestion, sore throat, new or increased cough, wheezing, sputum production, or respiratory difficulty, with or without fever. ARTI cases were evaluated through physical examination and nasopharyngeal swabs obtained for culture.

FINDINGS

The overall rate was 10.8 cases of ARTI per 100 persons a month, which was higher than in previous studies of respiratory illness in older adults. Explanations for the higher rates include (1) adults in day care setting had increased exposure to infectious agents, and (2) older adults who attend day care are more debilitated and susceptible to infection than independently living older adults. More older adults experienced cough, dyspnea, and sputum production than did the staff. Older adults had a high hospitalization and death rate, suggesting ARTI in older adults has a significant impact on this population.

IMPLICATIONS

Because of the small sample size, it is difficult to generalize these findings to include all older adult day care participants. However, well-documented alterations in the immune system of older adults suggest the need for nursing interventions aimed at the prevention of infection in this specific population.

Falsey A et al: Acute respiratory tract infection in day care centers for older persons, *J Am Geriatr Soc* 43(1):30, 1995.

nium, and copper. Although all nutritional needs for healthy older adults can be met through normal dietary intake, many older adults have dietary deficiencies. For clients with cancer the nutritional deficits can be extreme. After assessment, efforts should be made to resolve detected deficiencies. In institutional settings dietary supplements and frequent meals can be supplied. Food can be prepared specifically to suit the clients' tastes and needs. For older adults in the community it is helpful to have services such as Meals on Wheels, assistance with food preparation, or the ability to visit a senior center nutrition site. Liquid food supplements or over-the-counter vitamins are other alternatives. However, these may be beyond the financial resources of some clients.

The inability to feed oneself is another barrier to proper nutrition. Individuals feeding clients, either in the home or institutional setting, must ensure that the clients receive a balanced, nutritional diet. Family members or nonprofessional care providers may need special instruction on how best to accomplish this with clients (see Nutritional Considerations box).

Psychosocial Interventions. Based on the relationships between psychosocial factors and immunity, a variety of modalities are available that may enhance immunocompetence. These include (1) relaxation and visualization, (2) social support, and (3) exercise.

Relaxation training, either alone or in conjunction with imagery, has been associated with increased levels of NK cell activity and T cell responsiveness (McNeil, 1998). Since social support has been associated with immune status, facilitating the maintenance or development of a system of social support may have immunity benefits. This may be accomplished by mobilizing a group of existing friends and relatives or introducing the client to support groups (McNeil, 1998). One possibility might be to establish a network of people who check on each other, either by phone or letters or in person. Another possibility is to get people with similar interests together for activities or discussion groups. For example, one group might get together to discuss politics, another to discuss literature, and a third to do quilting or woodcarving. Many of these groups may already be active in senior centers or churches.

Nutritional Considerations

Alterations in nutrition: less than body requirements related to:

TASTE/OLFACTORY CHANGES

Use tart food to stimulate taste buds.
Use extra seasoning.
Try sauces.
Substitute fish and chicken for red meat.

DYSPHAGIA

Eat soft foods.
Try sauces and gravies.
Eat small meals frequently.

DYSPEPSIA

Avoid fatty, spicy, or gas-producing foods.
Use antacids.
Avoid lying down after meals.

ANOREXIA

Vary surroundings.
Eat with family and friends.
Try new foods and recipes.
Use smaller plates.
Eat high-calorie snacks.
Drink high-protein shakes.

From Otto S: *Pocket guide to oncology nursing*, St Louis, 1997, Mosby.

Nursing Care Plan
Pneumococcal Pneumonia

Clinical Situation: Mrs. T is a 78-year-old woman, admitted to the hospital for treatment of pneumococcal pneumonia, which she developed while she had influenza. She lives alone in a low-rent housing development in a large city, having moved there 2 years ago after the death of her husband. Without his income, she was unable to afford the rent on her previous home. Her nearest family member, a niece, lives 75 miles away and rarely visits. Her former neighbors, who live across town, are unable to visit because of the distance and because of their own debilities. Mrs. T is 20% underweight for her height and is anemic. Her WBC count is high. Her blood values are as follows: red blood cell count of 3.7/ml, hematocrit of 34%, hemoglobin of 10.8, WBC count of 18,200/ml, and serum albumin of 2.6 g/dl.

Nursing Diagnosis

High risk for infection related to compromised immune status

Altered nutrition: less than body requirements related to low income, transportation difficulties, and social isolation

Social isolation related to loss of friends and limited contact with family

Knowledge deficit: influenza and pneumococcal vaccine related to new experience

Outcome

Client will not experience additional infections as evidenced by (1) WBC count returning to normal limits, (2) afebrile state, and (3) other vital signs being within normal limits.

Client will verbalize a knowledge of infection prevention strategies.

Client will have adequate nutrition as demonstrated by (1) weight gain of 1/2 pound per week, (2) increased hemoglobin, and (3) increased serum protein.

Client will consume a well-balanced, sufficient caloric diet, as evidenced by (1) calorie counts showing an intake of at least 1800 calories per day and (2) consumption of food from all food groups, including protein sources, breads, fruits and vegetables, and dairy products.

Client will acquire social contacts desirable to her as evidenced by (1) spending time each week with others and (2) voicing satisfaction with social contacts.

Client will identify the advantages of the influenza and pneumococcal vaccine.

Interventions

Screen all visitors with infection who may come into direct contact with client.

Provide family and visitors with information on transmission of infection.

Teach client that she is at high risk for additional infections because of her depressed immune status and should limit her exposure to additional pathogens.

Observe for slight increases in temperature every 4 hours or more often as needed.

Be aware that client may develop subtle or undetected signs and symptoms of infection, and that slight changes in temperature may be highly significant.

Observe for increased respiratory difficulty.

Auscultate the client's lungs every shift.

Have the client report any sore throat.

Monitor dietary intake using calorie counts.

Teach what constitutes a well-balanced diet, high in protein.

Ensure adequate intake of vitamin and trace minerals through diet or through supplements.

Encourage client to eat foods that include vitamins and minerals, as well as trace minerals such as zinc and magnesium.

Provide vitamin and mineral supplements in addition to the high-protein diet, as needed.

Arrange for Meals on Wheels on discharge, or facilitate attendance at a nutrition site to provide better nutrition after discharge.

Contact churches or other organizations to include client in their social gatherings to reestablish a social support system.

Assess client's level of stress to determine if an easily accessible, low-exertion relaxation program is indicated. (A relaxation program may provide an easily accessible, low-exertion intervention with immune benefit.)

Plan a program of graduated exercise designed to fit client's tolerance.

Contact social services or a local senior citizen center to identify center activities and transportation.

Contact area organizations or churches for information about activities.

Provide information to client and develop a plan of action with her.

Provide information for client regarding the influenza vaccine: (1) influenza can be a serious, life-threatening condition in older people; (2) yearly immunization (in early fall) is important to protect her from getting influenza; (3) the signs and symptoms of influenza are weakness, cough, headache, sudden increase in temperature, aches, chills, and occasional vomiting; and (4) pneumonia is a common complication of influenza.

Refer client to the primary care provider for specific advice regarding recuperation time before taking the vaccine.

Provide information for client on pneumococcal vaccine—primarily that she should be immunized once in her lifetime.

Inform her that the vaccine should not be administered soon after having pneumonia.

Refer client to the primary care provider for the specific timing of administration following her illness.

As previously discussed, exercise, even in moderate amounts, may have an immunoenhancing effect. Therefore implementation of an exercise program may be beneficial. Exercise programs should be tailored to individual abilities. For clients with physical debilities, exercise programs can be tailored to meet their specific needs and interests. Possible exercises include walking, dancing or dancelike movement, water exercises, or swimming. It is important to develop exercise programs that are moderately difficult rather than strenuous for older individuals.

As the relationships between immune status and numerous variables are explored, new modalities are developed. Modalities currently being explored include biofeedback, therapeutic touch, and hypnosis.

Evaluation

Monitoring the success of interventions is based on clients' responses in meeting their goals and outcomes. One standard for evaluation is whether a client contracts an infection, either through contact with others or from his or her own flora. Improving or at least maintaining immune status may be more difficult for some clients, since the understanding of the immune system and the concomitant changes that occur with aging is incomplete. Furthermore, many individuals are enduring severe assaults on their immune systems. Persons with cancer receive anticancer drugs that can literally destroy the immune response. In persons with AIDS, the immune system is directly targeted by viral attack. Interventions such as diet, exercise, and psychosocial enhancement are rarely sufficient in overcoming such odds, although unexplained recoveries have been known to occur. For the majority of situations, it may be unreasonable to expect a return to normal status for immunocompromised individuals. However, any improvement in immune status, or even maintenance, may allow older clients to live better lives (see Nursing Care Plans).

SUMMARY

This chapter explored the age-related changes of the immune system. The influences of other factors on the immune status of older adults, such as psychosocial influences and nutrition, were also discussed. Cancer, autoimmune diseases, HIV, and significant nosocomial pathogens were presented.

A key role of the nurse in caring for older adults in all settings is to recognize the potential for infection in this population and develop care plans to prevent, as well as promote early detection of, infection. Because of the increased risk of morbidity and mortality associated with infection in this age-group, immunizations and interventions specific to various body systems should be implemented for those identified as susceptible to infection.

Nursing Care Plan
Effects of Chemotherapy

Clinical Situation: Ms. A is a 69-year-old woman who is receiving chemotherapy following a modified radical mastectomy for breast cancer. Although she was previously well nourished, chemotherapy has diminished her appetite and stomatitis has made eating painful. In addition, the chemotherapy has decreased her WBC count to 2000. Ms. A lives with her husband in their home. She receives her chemotherapy on an outpatient basis but is visited daily by a home health nurse to maintain her Hickman catheter.

Nursing Diagnosis

High risk for infection related to suppressed immune system

Altered nutrition: less than body requirements related to inability to eat secondary to side effects of chemotherapy

Outcome

Client will not develop an infection, as evidenced by (1) no temperature elevation; (2) no elevation in WBC count; (3) no sore throat or mouth; and (4) no redness or irritation around wounds, intravenous tubes, or catheters.

Client will have adequate intake of proteins, vitamins, and minerals, as evidenced by (1) calorie counts of at least 2000 calories per day and (2) maintenance of body weight.

Interventions

Teach client to minimize exposure to pathogens and to screen visitors with contagious infections.

Explain the need to maintain careful hygiene (e.g., daily shower; proper oral, foot, and perineal care).

Use sterile technique when working with Hickman catheter.

Monitor mouth and throat for signs of infection such as white patches or redness; teach Ms. A to report the same to the nurse.

Auscultate lungs at each visit.

Teach client to monitor body fluids for alterations in color, odor, or consistency.

Encourage fluid intake of at least 2000 ml a day unless otherwise indicated.

Teach client to eat small, frequent meals, rich in protein, vitamins, and minerals.

Teach client food sources high in calories, protein, vitamins, and minerals.

Use food supplements to increase intake if needed.

Teach the importance of eating nutrient-dense foods (e.g., those with high nutritional content in small volumes).

Acquire oral anesthetic for stomatitis.

Teach client how to prepare bland foods of moderate temperature.

Home Care

1. Assess nutritional and dietary status to ensure proper immune function in homebound older adults.
2. Instruct older adults and caregivers about the need to receive a balanced nutritional diet and the role of vitamin supplements in promoting proper immune function.
3. An altered emotional state may lead to a decreased immune function in homebound older adults.
4. Vaccinations are imperative for homebound older adults (e.g., annual influenza vaccine, Pneumovax).
5. Assess and report any signs of impaired immunity (e.g., fever, changes in WBCs).
6. Bedridden older adults and immunocompromised older adults are at high risk for infections. Instruct older adults and caregivers about ways to protect the older adults from infection from themselves and others.
7. Tailor an exercise program that can be done by homebound or bedridden older adults to enhance their immune system and to prevent infection.
8. Assess how homebound older adults manage personal hygiene, and teach them the importance of hand washing.
9. Practice appropriate cleaning and maintenance of humidifiers, catheters, respiratory equipment, and other devices used in home care–related treatment.
10. Develop a plan for alternative care in case a caregiver develops an infection.

Key Points

- With aging, the immune response diminishes.
- The diminished immune response reduces the normal responses to infection, such as fever, which makes infection in older adults more difficult to detect.
- Nutrition, especially in regards to protein, energy, vitamins, and trace minerals, has a substantial effect on immune status.
- Activity has a substantial effect on immune status. Even moderate amounts of daily exercise can enhance immune status.
- Mood can influence immune status. Depression is associated with a decreased immune response.
- Stress, both chronic and acute, is associated with decreased immune responses.
- Interventions dealing with infection and decreased immune response must address nutrition, exercise, mood, stress, and physical protection.

Critical Thinking Exercises

1. Your neighbor is a 68-year-old woman whose husband died last year. Since his death, she has become sedentary and withdrawn. Concerned, you decide to stop by to see her. She explains that she has been ill off and on for the past few weeks and does not understand why she keeps getting sick. She says she is losing faith in her doctor. Recognizing that her depression and sedentary lifestyle can alter her immune response, how might you intervene to help her?

References

Adler W et al: HIV infection and aging: mechanisms to explain the accelerated rate of progression in the older patient, *Mech Aging Devel* 97:137, 1997.

Anderson B: Stress and immune response after surgical treatment for regional breast cancer, *J Natl Cancer Inst* 90(1):30, 1998.

Anderson R et al: Report of final mortality statistics 1995, *Monthly Vital Statistics Rep* 45(11; suppl 2), 1997, National Center for Health Statistics.

Brooks JA: Postoperative nosocomial pneumonia: nurse-sensitive interventions, *AACN Clin Iss* 12(2)304-323, 2001.

Calder P: Fat chance of immunomodulation, *Immunology Today* 19(6):244, 1998.

Cantrell M, Norman D: *Infections, practice of geriatrics*, ed 3, Philadelphia, 1998, Saunders.

Cohen S, Rabin B: Psychologic stress, immunity and cancer, *J Natl Cancer Inst* 90(1):3, 1998.

Davies P: Tuberculosis in the elderly, *Drugs & Aging* 8(6):436, 1996.

Eliopoulos C: Acute conditions. In Eliopoulos C: *Gerontological nursing*, Philadelphia, 2001, Lippincott.

Ely W: Pneumonia in the elderly: diagnostic and therapeutic challenges, *Infection in the elderly*. Accessed July 1998 from website: http://www.medscape.com.

Evans W et al: Exercise and treatment of wasting: aging and human immunodeficiency virus infection, *Sem Oncol* 25(92; suppl 6):112, 1998.

Fischer A, Konig W: Modulation of in-vitro immunoglobulin-synthesis of human peripheral-blood mononuclear-cells by nicotine and cotinine, *Clin Invest* 72(3):225, 1994.

Gordon S, Thompson S: The changing epidemiology of human immunodeficiency virus infection in older persons, *J Am Geriatr Soc* 43(1):7, 1995.

Griffini P et al: Dietary Ω-3 polyunsaturated fatty acids promote colon carcinoma metastasis in rat liver, *Cancer Res* 58(15):3312, 1998.

Gueldner S: The elderly: the silent population, *J Assoc Nurses AIDS Care* 6(5):9-10, 1995.

Keegan L: *Healing nutrition*, Albany, NY, 1996, Delmar.

Kennes B et al: Effect of vitamin B supplements on cell-mediated immunity in old people, *Gerontology* 29:305, 1983.

McDonald C: Vancomycin-resistant enterococci outside the health care setting: prevalence, sources and public health considerations, *Emerg Infect Dis* 3(3):311, 1997.

McNeil C: Stress reduction: three trials test impact on cancer progression, *J Natl Cancer Inst* 90(1):12, 1998.

Monto A, Terpenning M: The value of influenza and pneumococcal vaccines in the elderly, *Drugs & Aging* 8(6):445, 1996.

Moran D: Infections in the elderly, *Topics Emerg Med* 25(2):174-181, 2003.

National Association of Social Workers: The aging of HIV, 2003. Accessed April 2005 from website at www.naswdc.org.

National Institutes of Health: *Systemic lupus erythematosus*, Bethesda, Md, 1998, The Institutes.

Newton J et al: Autoimmune hepatitis in older patients, *Age & Aging* 26:441, 1997.

Nieman RB et al: The effect of cigarette-smoking on the development of AIDS in HIV-1 seropositive individuals, *AIDS* 7(5):705, 1993.

Olmstead R: *APIC infection control and applied epidemiology: principles and practice*, St Louis, 1996, Mosby.

Pagano M, Swift L: *Rheumatoid arthritis: an update*. Accessed July 1998 from website: http://www.medscape.com.

Porth CM: *Pathophysiology: concepts of altered health state*, ed 7, Philadelphia, 2004, JB Lippincott Williams & Wilkins.

Riquelme R et al: Community acquired pneumonia in the elderly: clinical and nutritional aspects, *Am J Respir Crit Care Med* 156(6):1908, 1997.

Soule B, Larson E, Preston G: *Infections and nursing practice*, St Louis, 1995, Mosby.

Sunderkötter C et al: Aging and the skin immune system, *Arch Dermatol* 133(10):1256, 1997.

Weber D, Rutala W: Role of environmental contamination in the transmission of vancomycin-resistant enterococci, *Infect Control Hosp Epidemiol* 18(5):306, 1997.

17 Chronic Illness and Rehabilitation

PAMALA D. LARSEN, PhD, RN, CRRN

Learning Objectives

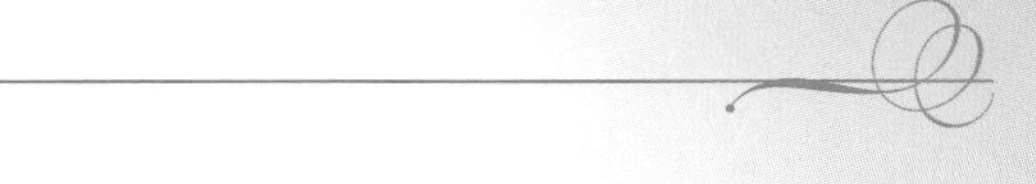

On completion of this chapter, the reader will be able to:

1. Define chronic illness and rehabilitation.
2. Apply the trajectory concept to a client with a chronic condition.
3. Identify potential goals for older adults with chronic illness.
4. Plan interventions that support an older adult's adaptation to a chronic illness or disability.
5. Analyze the nurse's role in assisting older adults in managing chronic conditions.
6. Identify opportunities for change in the health care system to improve care for older adults with disabilities.

CHRONICITY

Chronic disease affects the physical, psychologic, and social aspects of the lives of individuals and families. It is important to distinguish between the terms *chronic disease* and *chronic illness*. Chronic disease is the problem viewed from a biomedical model, whereas chronic illness reflects the human experience of the symptoms and suffering and how the disease is perceived, lived with, and managed (Lubkin and Larsen, 2002).

The impact of chronic illness is great. Living with a chronic disease affects a person's lifestyle and interactions with others. Many adults with chronic illness become homebound, and this decreased contact with the community leads to social isolation and affects interpersonal relationships. Individuals with chronic illness may perceive themselves as a burden, and families often experience caregiver stress. By nature, chronic illnesses are long term and expensive. Funding the chronic care, whether it is curative, restorative, maintenance, or palliative in nature, is another challenge for older adults and their families or caregivers. Because funding of chronic care is complex, the nurse must understand the payment systems that are regulated by state and federal governments so that they can address reimbursement issues when planning care.

Over 125 million Americans had one or more chronic conditions in 2000, and it is predicted that 157 million individuals will have chronic conditions by 2020 (Partnership for Solutions, 2002). Medical costs associated with individuals with chronic conditions amount to over $1.5 trillion each year (Groessl and Cronan, 2000). Seventy-six cents out of every dollar being spent on direct medical costs is associated with chronic disease (Siebens, 2002). More than 33 million Americans are over the age of 65, and that number is expected to double over the next 30 years. The aging population, with the first "baby boomers" born in 1946 becoming 65 in 2011, will significantly affect a health care delivery system that is far behind in addressing the needs of the *current* population of older adults with chronic illness.

The prevalence of chronic conditions is increasing due to lifesaving technologies, an expanding population of older adults, and increasing life expectancy. Individuals who in the past would have succumbed to an acute illness now recover, age, and develop and live with chronic conditions. The occurrence of two or more chronic conditions, often called comorbidities, is particularly common in older adults. Currently 62% of the population 65 and older has two or more chronic conditions (National Center for Health Statistics, 2003). One in five Americans (of all ages) has multiple chronic conditions.

Even though the prevalence of chronic conditions has created additional complex issues for the health care system, most health care services remain oriented to acute, episodic illness. The result is often a conflict between the expectations of the individual with the chronic illness and those of the health care providers. The conflict may result in dissatisfaction on the part of the client and a diminished level of care from the system.

The acute care model of care is based on diagnosis, treatment, and interventions designed to cure illness. In contrast, the care of a client with a chronic condition is based on the assumption that cure is not possible. Consequently, nursing care focuses on increasing functional ability; preventing complications; promoting the highest quality of life; and, when the end-stage of life occurs, providing comfort and dignity in dying. A key role for the nurse caring for an older adult with a chronic condition is to help the client achieve optimum physical and emotional health. Health care providers typically view an ill older person within a disease framework, whereas individuals with chronic conditions, of any age, see the disease process as only one part of themselves. More important to the client may be the economic, work-related, and role changes within the family that occur because of the illness. Older adults may face problems accessing community resources and may confront legislative barriers or the stigma of having a chronic illness.

Defining Chronic Illness

The Commission on Chronic Illness (1957) defined *chronic illness* as:

> All impairments or deviations from normal that have one or more of the following characteristics: (a) are permanent, (b) leave residual disability, (c) are caused by nonreversible pathological alteration, (d) require special training of the client for rehabilitation, and (e) may be expected to require a long period of supervision, observation, or care.

The Centers for Disease Control and Prevention (CDC) (1998) defines chronic disease as illnesses that are prolonged, do not resolve spontaneously, and are rarely cured completely. However, another definition is:

> Chronic illness is the irreversible presence, accumulation, or latency of disease states or impairments that involve the total human environment for supportive care and self-care, maintenance of function, and prevention of further disability (Curtin and Lubkin, 1995).

Prevalence of Chronic Illness

Hypertension is the most common chronic condition in non-institutionalized people in the United States. Box 17-1 lists the most common chronic conditions in the population over age 65. Individuals with chronic conditions typically have repeated hospitalizations to treat exacerbations of their illness. For both men and women ages 65 to 74, the most common reasons for hospitalization are heart disease, cancer, pneumonia, and stroke (Table 17-1). However, as both men and women reach 75 and older, the reasons for hospitalization don't vary, but the rank order of the cause of hospitalizations does (Table 17-2). Hospitalizations resulting from injuries, particularly in women (e.g., hip fractures), jump significantly, as does heart disease in this age category. Using these statistics, elderly women have significantly more hospitalizations than do men of the same age.

BOX 17-1 Prevalence of Selected Chronic Conditions in Individuals 65 and Older (in Order of Prevalence): United States, 1997-2001

Hypertension
Arthritis
Heart disease
Cancer
Sinusitis
Ulcer
Diabetes

From Centers for Disease Control and Prevention, National Center for Health Statistics, National Hospital Discharge Survey: *Health, United States, 2003.*

TABLE 17-1 Hospital Discharges and Average Lengths of Stays by Diagnosis (Ages 65-74): 2001

DIAGNOSIS	NO. OF DISCHARGES (IN THOUSANDS)	AVERAGE LENGTH OF STAY (DAYS)
WOMEN 65-74		
Heart disease	489	4.9
Cancer	147	7.3
Pneumonia	115	6.5
Stroke	118	5.3
Diabetes	59	6.1
Osteoarthritis	100	4.7
Injuries	189	6.2
MEN 65-74		
Heart disease	566	4.6
Cancer	149	7.6
Pneumonia	111	5.6
Stroke	109	4.7
Diabetes	41	5.1
Hyperplasia/prostate	35	2.4
Osteoarthritis	65	4.5
Injuries	143	7.4

From Centers for Disease Control and Prevention, National Center for Health Statistics, National Hospital Discharge Survey: *Health, United States, 2003.*

TABLE 17-2 Hospital Discharges and Average Lengths of Stay by Diagnosis (Ages 75 and Older): 2001

DIAGNOSIS	NO. OF DISCHARGES (IN THOUSANDS)	AVERAGE LENGTH OF STAY (DAYS)
WOMEN 75 AND OLDER		
Heart disease	1010	5.0
Cancer	192	7.6
Pneumonia	286	6.8
Stroke	301	5.2
Diabetes	67	5.2
Osteoarthritis	107	4.4
Injuries	503	6.1
MEN 75 AND OLDER		
Heart disease	727	5.1
Cancer	156	6.9
Pneumonia	248	6.4
Stroke	157	5.2
Diabetes	38	6.5
Hyperplasia/prostate	45	3.5
Osteoarthritis	52	4.4
Injuries	199	6.5

From Centers for Disease Control and Prevention, National Center for Health Statistics, National Hospital Discharge Survey: *Health, United States, 2003.*

The picture of chronic conditions broadens when leading causes of death for people over age 65 are added. Chronic conditions are not only the leading cause of disability and activity restriction but also the leading cause of death. Each of the causes of death noted in Table 17-3 (with the exception of "other causes") is a chronic condition or results from one. The first atlas to map the leading causes of death by race and gender for small geographic areas throughout the United States has identified high-risk areas for heart disease, cancer, and stroke, and reveals important geographic patterns (Pickle et al, 1997). Death rates for heart disease are higher in the Southeast than in the Northeast, previously the region with the highest rates. Cancer, the second leading cause of death, has two areas of concentration: the highest rates for black men are in urban centers, and the highest rates for white men are along the Mississippi River and southern Atlantic coast. The stroke belt, a band of southeastern states excluding Florida, has now dispersed, with rates dropping in this area and increasing to the north and west.

TABLE 17-3 Percentage of Deaths from Leading Causes among Persons Ages 65 and Over: United States, 2000

CAUSE OF DEATH	NUMBER	PERCENT
All causes	1,799,825	100
Heart disease	593,707	32.9
Cancer	392,366	21.8
Stroke	148,045	8.2
Chronic lower respiratory disease	106,375	5.9
Influenza and pneumonia	58,557	3.3
Diabetes	52,414	2.9
Other causes	448,361	24.9

From National Center for Health Statistics: *Health, United States, Chartbook on trends in the health of Americans,* Hyattsville, Md, 2003,The Center.

Chronic Illness Trajectory

The term *illness trajectory* was first used by Anselm Strauss, Barney Glaser, and Jeanne Quint Benoliel in the early 1960s as they studied the care of dying patients. Their insight into this care was that dying took time, and many strategies shape the course of the dying patient (Corbin and Strauss, 1992). They coined the phrase *trajectory* from the physical sciences. A trajectory is defined as the course of an illness over time, plus the actions that patients, families, and health care providers take to manage that course (Corbin, 1998). The trajectory model of chronic illness provides a framework for caring for the client in a comprehensive, holistic manner with a focus on nursing care.

There are nine phases in the trajectory model, and although it could be conceived as a continuum, it is not linear. Clients may move through these phases in any direction or may plateau. Additionally, having one or more other chronic diseases will affect movement on the trajectory. The trajectory model begins with the *pretrajectory phase,* or preventive phase, in which the course of illness has not yet begun; however, genetic factors or lifestyle behaviors place an individual at risk for a chronic condition. During the *trajectory* phase, signs and symptoms of the disease appear and a diagnostic workup may begin. In the *stable* phase the illness symptoms are under control and management of the disease occurs primarily at home. A period of inability to keep symptoms under control occurs in the *unstable* phase. The *acute* phase brings severe and unrelieved symptoms or disease complications. Critical or life-threatening situations requiring emergency treatment occur in the *crisis* phase. The *comeback* phase signals a return to an acceptable way of life with the symptoms that the disease imposes. The *downward phase* is characterized by progressive deterioration and an increase in disability or symptoms. The trajectory model ends with the *dying phase,* characterized by gradual or rapid shutting down of body processes (Corbin, 1998).

The illness trajectory of a disease is not the same as the disease course. A disease course is the physical progression of a disease. The illness trajectory is not only the physiologic changes and symptoms that occur, but the "work" (both physical and psychosocial) of the patient, family, and health care provider during the illness. As we talk about "shaping" the illness, this may or may not mean altering the direction or course of the disease. The trajectory of chronic illness varies with the individual, family, and illness. Additionally, patients and families make treatment choices that influence the illness trajectory, whether it is aggressive treatment, minimum treatment, palliative care, or withdrawal of treatment. The illness trajectory may progress slowly or quickly, predictably or unpredictably, with exacerbations and remissions, or it may be influenced by other acute and chronic conditions. Box 17-2 depicts a potential trajectory of a client with diabetes mellitus.

Maslow's model of the five levels of need that affect function and self-perception complements the trajectory model. An older adult's perception of needs and biologic and functional limitations can predict movement within the illness trajectory. For example, an older adult with chronic obstructive pulmonary disease may be malnourished because of increased energy expenditure for breathing. Malnutrition and inadequate oxygen exchange threaten this older person's biologic integrity. Weakened by malnutrition and unable to breathe sufficiently, the older adult will not be interested in exploring productive, sedentary activities to increase self-esteem until treatment meets these basic survival needs. If such survival needs are not met, the trajectory of the illness proceeds downward. Wellness in chronic illness is a continuum, from treatment to maximizing life satisfaction (Lindsey, 1997). The nurse's approach to wellness with an older adult who has a chronic condition should include interventions to assist the older adult in meeting as many levels of Maslow's defined needs as possible.

The concept of health within chronic illness is beginning to gain recognition in nursing (Lindsey, 1996). The prolonged nature of chronic illness creates expertise in these people that is rarely recognized or respected by health care professionals (Lindsey, 1997). Lindsey (1995, 1996, 1997) identified themes in a chronically ill person's journey to a state of wellness: (1) in the beginning, taking control; (2) hitting the wall, seeking knowledge; (3) letting go, connecting with others; (4) creating opportunities, accessing alternate healing modalities; (5) letting in, celebrating life; (6) the gift, transcending self, acquiring a state of grace; and (7) an altered relationship with health care providers. These themes can result in a reconceptualization of health and illness, and a transformation in nursing care from a focus on problems and deficits to a focus on personal capacity and promotion of health and well-being (Lindsey, 1996).

Thorne and Patterson (1998) collaborated on a meta-study of 158 studies from 1980 to 1996 that analyzed client roles in the chronic illness experience. Results demonstrated a shift from a focus on loss and burden toward health within illness, transformation, and normality. Awareness of these themes provides nurses an opportunity to respond to the experiences of clients with chronic illness with interventions that enhance their autonomy.

For example, to achieve optimum health and wellness, clients with diabetes must modify their lifestyle. Initial priorities include (1) restoring fluid and electrolyte balance, which may be associated with osmotic diuresis from hyperglycemia; and (2) correcting metabolic abnormalities related to insulin deficiency. This deficiency causes decreased uptake and use of glucose by the tissues, which results in increased protein and fat metabolism. After homeostasis is achieved, the nurse can teach older adult diabetics about the disease process, disease management, self-care needs, and the therapeutic regimen. The nurse and older adults can work together to identify food preferences, incorporating these, along with other ethnic and cultural choices, into the meal plan. The nurse can teach older adults how to perform fingerstick glucose testing and how to administer insulin (Fig. 17-1). By incorporating older adults' preferences into their therapeutic regimens, the nurse promotes their feelings of involvement. As older adults learn how to control diabetes, they can make the necessary adaptations to achieve wellness and control over the chronic illness. These adaptations include dietary modifications, glucose monitoring, use of medications, steps to prevent or reduce the risk of infection, establishment of an exercise regimen, and smoking cessation.

Continued support is usually necessary to sustain lifestyle changes and to promote well-being. The nurse can provide older adults with information on community resources such as the American Diabetes Association, home health nursing, and weight loss or smoking cessation clinics. Without lifestyle adaptation, an older adult's diabetes may enter the unstable phase of the illness trajectory model.

BOX 17-2 Trajectory of Diabetes Mellitus

Pretrajectory—Risk factors for diabetes: hypertension, atherosclerosis, smoking, obesity, hyperlipidemia, and family history of diabetes

Trajectory—Disruption of metabolism (glucose), increased appetite, increased thirst, increased urine volume, pruritus vulvae, weight loss, weakness, and fatigue

Stable—Blood glucose levels stable; free from infection; adapting to lifestyle changes

Unstable—Disruption of metabolism that may be a result of infection; poor compliance with methods to control or monitor; illness

Acute—Severe and unrelieved symptoms caused by uncontrollable blood glucose levels

Crisis—Cardiovascular, renal, and neurologic sensory problems; uncontrollable blood glucose levels; possible ketoacidosis

Comeback—Systemic problems of uncontrollable blood glucose under control; may involve physical healing and rehabilitation

Downward—Cardiovascular, renal, and neurologic complications; blindness, dementia, or amputations as a result of vascular changes

Dying—Multisystem organ failure resulting from degenerative changes, diabetic ketoacidosis, myocardial infarction, gastroparesis, end-stage renal failure, and stroke

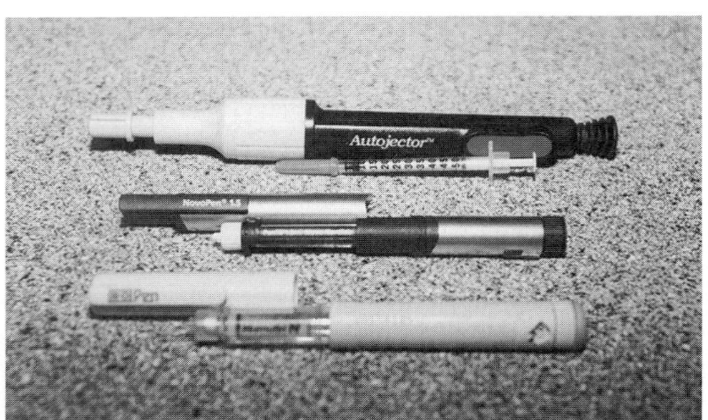

Fig. 17-1 Insulin injection devices. (From Phipps WJ, Sands JK, Marek JF: *Medical-surgical nursing: concepts and clinical practice,* ed 6, St Louis, 1999, Mosby.)

The following case study demonstrates how these features of chronic illness and the trajectory of one illness are influenced by the superimposition of other disorders (see Research box).

Case Study

Mr. A, a 67-year-old black man, is hospitalized for a unilateral below-knee amputation. He also has end-stage renal disease (ESRD), for which he has been receiving hemodialysis 3 times a week for 2 years. The length of his hospital stay and rehabilitation is 54 days, compared with the average person's stay of 36 days. On discharge he is walking independently with his prosthesis. The factors that affect the trajectory of his illness are ESRD, anemia, deconditioning, and depression. These factors imposed exercise and endurance limitations, which lengthened his stay, recovery, and rehabilitation.

Depression in older adults also contributes to a lack of physical energy that can further impede recovery. The amputation further interfered with Mr. A's level of function because of the high-energy cost of using a prosthetic limb. Energy requirements increase at least 25% in unilateral below-knee amputees (Sioson, Kerfoot, and Ziat, 1993).

In addition to nursing care, Mr. A requires a variety of ancillary services, including physical and occupational therapy, hemodialysis, a prosthetist, a psychiatrist, and social services. His stay was more expensive because of the comorbidity of ESRD; medical and nursing efforts were also directed at maintaining his ESRD in the stable phase of its trajectory.

Research

SAMPLE/SETTING

57 men and women with arthritis, ages 66 to 95, living in their own homes or in congregate retirement settings

RESEARCH QUESTION

To explore barriers to pain management, identify common barriers, and develop a theoretic model of these relationships

METHOD

Focus groups

FINDINGS

Themes were identified, including relationships with health care providers, knowledge deficits, personal decision making, age-related expectations, lack of access to health care, pain-movement cycle, use of diversional activities, and use of adaptive resources.

IMPLICATIONS

Better understanding of the barriers to pain management will assist the health care provider in enhancing the older adult's ability to manage pain.

Davis G et al: Barriers to managing chronic pain of older adults with arthritis, *J Nurs Scholarship* 34(2):121, 2002.

As we care for older adults with chronic illness, a paradigm shift is needed when deciding what constitutes wellness. As previously mentioned, health care providers may see older adults within a disease framework. After learning and mastering the physical care requirements imposed by the condition, older adults may view themselves as "well." The greatest factor in achieving wellness is adaptation (Ebersole, Hess, and Luggen, 2004). The physical traits of chronic illness should not determine an older adult's state of wellness. Many older adults are now more involved in their health care and accept responsibility for their wellness. They seek education about health promotion and management of their illness. The nurse can support older adults by working with them to identify areas that may hinder progress along the wellness continuum and by teaching self-care management in these areas.

Little is known about how members of ethnic minority and cultural groups view chronic illness or how they manage it in daily life. Ethnic minorities do not necessarily subscribe to the values or tenets associated with this country's medical system. The unique ways in which different cultural groups interpret illness affect their response to symptoms, treatment, and modifications of daily life. In the study by Becker et al (1998), blacks understood their condition to be chronic and were able to explain their illness, regardless of their level of education. Reports of self-care practices such as diet, exercise, and attempts to be realistic about physical limitations were common. Hispanics did not express understanding of chronicity. Symptom remissions were seen as a cure, and each exacerbation was seen as a separate illness unrelated to previous episodes. They knew they must take their medications, yet they did not perceive themselves as responsible for changing any aspect of their lifestyle. Hispanics believed medications alone would control their illness. Filipino Americans were knowledgeable about their illness, yet they minimized its seriousness. They consistently used prescribed medications and recognized the value of sound health practices. However, Filipino Americans did not link responsibility for following good health practices to their chronic illness. Instead, the concept of maintaining good health was the responsibility of the family and social group. An emphasis on cultural diversity in educating nurses, especially on the differential effect of culture on illness management, could positively affect nurse-client relationships.

Case Study

Ms. B, a 70-year-old insulin-dependent woman who has had diabetes for 10 years, is able to self-monitor her blood glucose and administer her insulin. She confides in her nurse that when she cheats on her diet, she "ups the insulin a little and that fixes it." The nurse also discovers that Mrs. B trims her corns with a razor blade. Ms. B expresses great pride in taking care of herself and being independent.

How can the nurse in this case channel Ms. B's desire for independence into safer actions that promote health? The goal is to assist and to support Ms. B in making attitude and lifestyle changes to maintain the stable phase of her diabetes and prevent complications. To achieve these goals, the nurse emphasizes Ms. B's abilities rather than limitations. For example, the nurse reviews the relationship between insulin and diet, as well as proper foot care. The nurse and Ms. B review her dietary program, usual eating pattern, and recent intake to identify deficits and deviations from her therapeutic needs. The nurse reinforces that, with correct insulin dosage, glucose can enter the cells and be used for energy. Complex carbohydrates such as corn, peas, carrots, and broccoli can decrease glucose levels and insulin needs and promote satiation.

The nurse also reminds Ms. B that her peripheral circulation may be impaired, which places her at risk for skin breakdown and infection. The nurse teaches Ms. B to inspect her feet daily for signs of infection and inflammation, including redness, flushed appearance, and open sores or drainage. Ms. B learns to dry her feet thoroughly after bathing and to keep her skin dry. She is instructed to keep her feet warm but avoid hot water or the use of a heating pad. The sudden development of cold hands or feet may reflect hypoglycemia; in this case, her blood glucose level should be tested. Ms. B comes to the understanding that receiving foot care from the podiatrist is not being dependent; it is a responsible decision. Ms. B also accepts the referral to the dietitian; together they create a diet plan that includes more of her favorite foods but remains within her caloric limitations.

Quality of Life and Health-Related Quality of Life

Advancements in medical and rehabilitative care have increased interest in the quality of life of persons with chronic illness. There are multiple definitions of quality of life, but most include physical, psychologic, and social components; disease and treatment-related symptoms; and spirituality. There is no consensus on the definition, however (Haas, 1999). The following definition can be applied to the older adult with a chronic illness:

> Quality of Life: An individual's perceptions of well-being that stem from satisfaction or dissatisfaction with dimensions of life that are important to the individual (Ferrans and Powers, 1985)

To further confuse the issue, most researchers draw a distinction between quality of life (QOL) and health-related quality of life (HRQOL). Most suggest that HRQOL is a subset of QOL. Brown, Renwick, and Nagler (1996) believe that HRQOL should be used in a narrow sense within the medical-nursing environment for those who are interested in the outcomes and quality of changes resulting from medical and nursing interventions. Patrick and Erickson (1993) conceptualize HRQOL in terms of opportunity, health perceptions, functional status, impairment, and death and duration of life.

How QOL and HRQOL intersect is salient to the client with chronic illness and those providing care. For example, a person who has adjusted to a wheelchair for mobility might perceive his HRQOL and his QOL as excellent, whereas the health care provider may not rate the person's HRQOL high because a wheelchair may not be his optimum state of function and wellness. The subjective and objective components of both of these concepts are important.

Compliance in Chronic Illness

Compliance is an encompassing term for all behaviors consistent with health care recommendations (Holroyd and Creer, 1986). However, compliance with those medical recommendations is poor across all chronic disease regimens (Berg, Evangelista, and Dunbar-Jacob, 2002). Fawcett (1995) suggests that compliance can be improved through a stronger therapeutic relationship between the health care provider and the client. The therapeutic relationship is the foundation for teaching and supporting a client's behavioral changes. Therapeutic regimens require adherence to certain behaviors, and perseverance in these behaviors is necessary for success.

Many complex issues surround noncompliance. Factors affecting compliance include (1) client characteristics, (2) psychologic factors, (3) regimen characteristics, (4) somatic factors, (5) social support, (6) prior health behavior, (7) economic and sociocultural factors, (8) motivation, and (9) client-provider interactions (Berg, Evangelista, and Dunbar-Jacob, 2002).

Another issue related to compliance is self-destructive behavior. An older adult may have engaged in a lifetime habit of self-destructive behaviors. What does the individual gain from these behaviors? Does an older adult with congestive heart failure receive more attention from his family if he does not comply with his sodium restriction? Does he equate scolding from his family with love? What is his definition of quality of life? Is quality of life related to a long life that depends on a program of lifestyle changes or to a shortened life of doing exactly as he wants? If his chronic illness becomes stable, does his role in the family change? How do members of society contribute to noncompliance through regulations and policies? These are just a few of the issues of noncompliance for older adults.

The degree of an individual's physical and social disability increases with the number of chronic conditions he or she experiences. But in spite of highly technical and advanced acute care, many individuals with chronic illness are readmitted to hospitals with the same problem. This self-defeating process may be offset by the present-day emphasis on rehabilitation. However, the success of any therapeutic regimen depends on compliance, and the nurse plays an important role in facilitating the older adults' adherence to the prescribed treatment regimen. The nurse must first assess an older adult's belief in the mutually established outcomes and the amount of energy required for compliance (Ebersole, Hess, and Luggen, 2004). The assessment should include identification of strengths such as self-motivation. Studies suggest that self-motivation does not change with age; therefore an older adult is as likely to comply as any other age-group (Rhodes, Morrissey, and Ward, 1992).

The cost of today's health care requires that nurses be aware of specific needs of older adults when structuring their therapeutic regimens. Regimens should emphasize activities that build endurance and self-reliance and that facilitate self-care and quality of life. Older adults must believe that a therapeutic regimen aids in the recovery or maintenance of their functional level (see Research box).

Research

SAMPLE/SETTING

Subjects were 147 women and 62 men, ages 78 to 95, living in the community.

RESEARCH QUESTION

To describe the incentives and disincentives for participating in an exercise program

METHOD

Phone interviews

FINDINGS

The three main incentives focused on health benefits, psychologic benefits, and positive program features. Disincentives included competing commitments, doubts about exercise, and negative program features.

IMPLICATIONS

Exercise programs need to be tailored to the older adult, keeping in mind lifestyle, age-specific obligations, and values that may affect their participation.

Schneider J et al: Exercise training program for older adults: incentives and disincentives for participation, *J Gerontol Nurs* 29(9):21, 2003.

Positive Coping

Adaptation is largely determined by how individuals cope with stress. Living with a chronic illness on a daily basis is a stressor and hampers an individual's ability to realize aspirations, satisfy needs, and respond positively to the challenges of the environment (McWilliam et al, 1996). Personal perception and coping strategies can be the most important aspects of dealing with a chronic illness (Kart, 1997). Kart (1997) identified three broad categories of coping response: (1) responses that modify the situation, (2) responses that are used to reappraise the meaning of problems, and (3) responses that help individuals manage tension. The way older persons view their situations and their personality strengths is often more crucial than how a situation is handled. Older adults may perceive chronic illness in terms of loss (e.g., loss of income, personal relationships, or independence), or they may view their situation as requiring one more adaptation in a changing life. An older adult's decreased interest in life may undermine his or her ability to deal with a chronic illness. Personal coping strategies include the ability to solve problems in managing care, including environmental changes and adaptation to untoward events in the illness. An older adult must also maintain his or her self-image, including social relationships.

Case Study

Mrs. D is a 65-year-old woman who has been married for 40 years. She is receiving home health services following a cerebrovascular accident (CVA) with left hemiparesis. On the nurse's first visit to Mrs. D's home, she notices that Mrs. D appears depressed and withdrawn. Mrs. D establishes eye contact only when discussing her role as a wife and homemaker. Mrs. D feels significant loss regarding these roles, which were crucial to her self-image. But her husband does not understand her feelings; he thinks she should appreciate everything he is doing for her. The nurse assists Mr. and Mrs. D in confronting both Mrs. D's loss of identity and Mr. D's response to his wife's disability. The nurse also focuses on homemaking tasks that Mrs. D can perform from her wheelchair, such as meal preparation and laundry. The nurse refers Mr. and Mrs. D to a community agency that provides homemaker assistance. Mrs. D now plans the meals, and the homemaker does the grocery shopping. Mrs. D makes decisions about how her house should be run, and she has regained her sense of purpose. The nurse successfully identified the stresses Mr. and Mrs. D were experiencing as a result of their role reversals and helped them cope with Mrs. D's disability.

Changes in positions within the family affect family duties and responsibilities. Successful coping requires a positive attitude toward new roles and the ability to obtain a feeling of independence and security. Traditional roles are often masked in the hospital, and clients may think that everything will be fine on returning home. However, the transition from hospital to home is often difficult for clients and their families. They discover how much has changed and begin to face their losses. Roles may need to be renegotiated, and those which are no longer applicable must be acknowledged and mourned (Hibbard et al, 1996).

The nurse can guide, educate, and support older adults and their families in developing positive coping strategies. Understanding the illness and what to expect is directly related to the ability to cope. In providing support to older adults and their families, the nurse assists them in identifying their feelings. A reduction in the distress that accompanies chronic illness or disability may be achieved with nursing interventions that encourage an active problem solving and coping orientation and interrupt avoidant, passive coping patterns (Aikens et al, 1997). Direct questions such as, "How are you dealing with this illness? What helps you deal with this change in your family? What interferes with your ability to deal with this illness?" will provide an indication of a client's coping strategies and their effectiveness (Twibell, 1998). The nurse can also observe older adults and family members for signs of stress that may result from ineffective coping.

One of the most difficult tasks in adjustment is balancing hope and realism (Miller, 1992). A client and his or her family may need to express frustration and anger with the course of the illness and rehabilitation. By setting mutually agreed on goals, divided into small increments, the nurse and older adult can succeed. Sharing goals with family members may elicit their support or assist them in accepting the need to avoid active involvement (Twibell, 1998). Personal coping also involves problem solving. The nurse serves as a resource for older adults and their families in solving care management problems.

A supportive social network also has been found to have significant impact on stress (Tremethick, 1997). The roles of home, neighborhood, friends, and family need to be considered in assessing the adequacy of social support. Referrals for day care, home health nursing, temporary long-term care, or respite care may be needed.

Another obstacle is understanding and coping with role reversals. The nurse can guide older adults in finding tasks and responsibilities within their new roles and assist in conflict resolution as old roles are redefined. Chronic illness requires long-term adaptation on the part of older adults and their families. Ongoing support by health care professionals is crucial for them to find enough strength to continue coping.

Orem's Self-Care Model

Orem (1995) identified three basic variations in nursing systems based on the belief that the client can perform self-care, that the nurse can provide care, or that the care can be provided in combination. The basic nursing systems are (1) wholly compensatory, (2) partly compensatory, and (3) supportive-educative.

The client's condition determines which nursing system applies. Clients move from system to system as their care needs change. A wholly compensatory system is required when the client is entirely dependent on others for sustenance and well-being. A partly compensatory system is used when the client can and should perform some self-care. A supportive-educative system is needed when the client is able to perform or learn to perform self-care, but requires professional assistance. In this system the areas for help are confined to making decisions, controlling behavior, and gaining new knowledge or skills.

Orem's conceptual framework of self-care is useful in planning care because older adults are concerned about maintaining independence and adapting to aging. Orem's framework allows older adults to retain control and physical functioning, both of which are usually lost when the nurse does not involve the older adult in the caregiving process. The framework provides a method to assess clients for variables that could affect their ability to care for themselves. The framework also directs the nurse in developing an individual and realistic care plan. Nurses can assist older adults in exercising self-care agency and successfully meeting therapeutic self-care demands by focusing on psychosocial needs and physical interventions.

Case Study

Ms. F, age 75, is admitted to the emergency department after her son found her on the floor of her home. An x-ray study confirms an intertrochanteric fracture; a prosthetic device is used to repair the fracture. After the operation, using Orem's self-care model, the nurse assesses Ms. F's universal self-care requisites: air, water, food, elimination, activity, rest, solitude, social balance, safety, and promotion of normalcy. The nurse plans the appropriate level of care for Ms. F based on her capacity to care for herself. For the first few days after the operation, Ms. F requires a wholly compensatory nursing system because of her immobility. The nurse plans interventions that assist Ms. F in progressing to a partially compensatory system before discharge. After discharge, a supportive-educative system can be provided through home health care. The goals for Ms. F focus on her retaining her control and dignity and gradually assuming self-care as her condition progresses. By moving Ms. F toward the supportive-educative system, the nurse is preparing her for independence. Orem's theory also allows the nurse to act in roles such as teacher, change agent, and referral agent (Metha, 1993).

Case Study

Mr. G is 80 years old and has been referred to a home health agency because of his poorly controlled insulin-dependent diabetes and noncompliance with diet and medications. On initial assessment, the nurse finds that although he can see the numbers on the syringe, Mr. G lacks the fine motor control needed to withdraw the insulin and inject himself. His 70-year-old wife suffers from dementia and is dependent on Mr. G for care. They rely on neighbors and their son for grocery shopping. They have no reliable transportation and often miss medical appointments.

The nurse identifies several factors contributing to Mr. G's noncompliance: Mr. G's inability to administer his insulin, difficulty obtaining groceries, lack of transportation, and abundance of caregiving demands. Had the nurse not personally observed his home setting, important information needed for a realistic care plan would have been missed.

Psychosocial Needs of Older Adults With Chronic Illness

The nurse needs to understand the relationship between social, psychologic, and biologic factors of aging to assist older adults in preserving independence. Although many studies on aging have emphasized losses, other researchers contend that the beneficial effects of diet, exercise, personal habits, and psychosocial factors on aging have been underestimated. "It is not merely a matter of what aging does to people but also of what people do with aging" (Smits and Kee, 1992). Understanding the interplay of these factors can help the nurse assist older adults in adapting to aging and maintaining independence.

An older adult's self-concept plays an important role in adaptation to aging and chronic illness. Morris (1985) defined *self-concept* as a person's appraisal of appearance, background, origins, abilities, resources, attitudes, and feelings that culminates in a force that directs behavior. Past research has found that physical alterations, whether from illness or normal aging, can be integrated into self-concept with both positive and negative results. The way an older adult reminisces can help indicate his or her success in integrating negative events (Tremethick, 1997). The capacity for self-concept to change in response to new demands is consistent with Holtzclaw's (1985) statement that self-concept is "permanent yet permeable."

Powerlessness. An older adult's self-concept can also be affected if he or she feels unable to control an illness or disability or feels that self-care patterns have contributed to the present disorder. Feelings of powerlessness can be a result of normal aging changes, an altered body image, or numerous losses. Older people grieve the loss of function or the loss of their former self. How they grieve is individual, and the significance of the loss also influences the grieving process. The result of powerlessness is a loss of hope. In addition, older adults who feel powerless may lose their independence to family members or health care professionals who take over and make decisions for them. This cycle of powerlessness, loss of control, and dependence may be perpetuated by well-meaning caregivers.

Case Study

Mr. J is a 62-year-old man, a small store owner who recently had a mild cardiovascular accident. He told his wife and the nurse that he would never return to work and that he would have to give up everything. His wife cannot understand his sudden decision to abandon his store. She tells the nurse that his store was his life. Mr. J worked two jobs as a young man to save money to start his business. At last, with considerable embarrassment, he reveals to the nurse that he experienced episodes of fecal incontinence. "Losing this control means losing everything. I can't work like this. I'll never be independent again." A long history of constipation led him to frequent laxative use, and the cardiovascular accident has damaged his rectal enervation. Mr. J is not always aware of the sensations of a full bowel.

After an assessment, the nurse develops a short-term plan with Mr. J to use incontinence pads and take a change of clothes to work. The nurse develops a mid-range plan with Mr. J to increase his daily exercise and intake of water and other noncaffeinated fluids. He gradually adds high-fiber foods, establishes a consistent daily toileting time, and avoids using laxatives. Several weeks later Mr. J reports a more regular bowel pattern with decreased incontinent episodes. His morale has improved, and he feels in control of his life. The nurse's assistance with Mr. J's fecal incontinence returned his feeling of control and enabled him to focus on other rehabilitation goals.

Meaning of Life in Adjustment. Adaptation and adjustment to chronic illness or disability are also affected by the meaning an older adult attaches to life. According to Frankl (1962), a person's search for meaning in life is the primary source of motivation. An older adult with a disability or illness faces a variety of losses, including loss of his or her former self, changes in body image, loss of control over a disease process, and possibly loss of work and changes in residence. The older adult may experience other losses associated with age-related changes, such as deaths of significant others, retirement, and declining health status.

Research has suggested that loss of the meaning of life is a serious threat to older adults because of the multiple changes and losses they encounter. Researchers have found a significant correlation between purpose in life and physical health status. A study by Kivinen et al (1998) found that age was the most important factor for physicians' estimates of the health of older adults. However, from the older adults' perspective, capacity to perform activities of daily living (ADL) and depression were the strongest determinants of self-perceived health. Clients feeling a loss of meaning need to be identified and interventions planned to increase their feelings of fulfillment. To ascertain an older adult's meaning of life in the psychosocial assessment, the nurse may ask, "Is there any one thing or things so important to you as to give your life meaning?" By asking clients to describe things that are meaningful, the nurse can gain insight into their needs and behaviors.

As the nurse learns what is meaningful, interventions can be planned to support or strengthen these areas, such as supporting an existing relationship, finding ways for clients to continue an enjoyable hobby, or arranging transportation to church. Through the interaction of the assessment, the nurse assists older adults in redefining their situation and rediscovering meaning. These discussions lead to descriptions of situations that are important, and as these situations are defined, the meaning emerges. Through interactions with others, older adults can discover and define meaning in all aspects of life.

Nursing Interventions to Assist Psychosocial Adjustment. The ability of older adults to cope with the issues and problems encountered in the course of living with and managing a chronic illness determines the nurse's role and the type of interventions needed. A collaborative relationship may be most effective in facilitating psychosocial adjustment (Strauss and Corbin, 1988). This type of relationship allows older adults to participate in their care planning and retain control and dignity; independence is a major concern, especially for older persons in the American culture, where it is highly valued. In addition, the nurse often uses the supportive-educative nursing system. Teaching older adult clients the trajectory model may actually help them cope with acute exacerbations (Strauss and Corbin, 1988).

Adjustment is an individual process and depends on the circumstances of the disability. Developmental changes, life transitions, and meaning placed on the disability or illness influence this ongoing process. Interventions may include supporting existing relationships or referring older adults who have lost significant relationships to a senior center where they can establish new relationships. The nurse may also explore interventions that meet spiritual needs. The nurse can refer and encourage older adults to participate in formal or informal learning opportunities available in the community.

The group process is one way to assist clients in their psychosocial adjustment. Self-help groups provide a support system in which older adults redefine themselves, focus on issues, adjust to new roles, or learn about their disease processes and how others manage (Ebersole, Hess, and Luggen, 2004). The group may encourage greater self-understanding and responsibility and provide older adults the opportunity to reshape for the family how to live with life's imperfections, with love and compassion for the self and others (Holkup, 1998).

Physiologic Needs of Chronically Ill Older Adults

A thorough nursing health history includes a comprehensive review of body systems, as well as medication and treatment review (see Chapter 4). The medication review should include both prescription drugs and over-the-counter medications (see Chapter 22). An older adult may have more than one physician prescribing drugs and additionally may be using nonprescription remedies.

Pain. A major issue with chronic disorders is the management of pain. In evaluating pain, the nurse should note its characteristics, location, and intensity (on a scale of 1 to 10). The nurse should make an assessment of causes of possible discomfort other than the chronic illness. In addition to analgesia, the nurse can teach the client relaxation techniques, deep breathing exercises, guided imagery, and visualization. These techniques can relieve muscular and emotional tension, enhance the sense of control, and possibly improve coping abilities (see Chapter 15 for a more detailed discussion of pain management and treatment strategies).

Fatigue. Older adults living with a chronic disorder often experience fatigue. Fatigue can be unpredictable, making it difficult to manage or alleviate. The nurse can help older adults identify causes and patterns of fatigue. Older persons may need to be taught how to conserve energy to enjoy meaningful activities. Emphasizing the benefits of periodic rest, a slower pace of activity, and more time to complete tasks may help older clients cope and feel in control. The nurse should encourage older adults to choose where to expend energy and should respect the priorities established.

Immobility and Activity Intolerance. Activity may be the most important factor in maintaining or recovering health and wellness in the older adult (Easton, 1999). Older adults commonly perceive health in relation to their level of activity (Kivinen et al, 1998). Physical activity and psychosocial interaction are important in maintaining chronically ill older adults on the continuum of wellness. Inactivity may result from functional loss, and as activity levels decline, even more function may be lost. Problems as a result of inactivity are compounded when clients, families, and health care professionals display reduced expectations of debilitated older adults. In the United States, people ages 65 and older can expect to live an additional 17.5 years, and therefore care based on preserving or restoring functional ability is essential (National Center for Health Statistics, 2003). One possible nursing goal may be to prevent complications of prolonged inactivity during an acute exacerbation of illness.

Sexual Activity. Aging, alone, causes changes to the reproductive system in both men and women. Chronic disease may further affect the sexual activity and functioning of the older adult. These changes in a client's sexual life may cause psychologic distress. Effects of the condition, medications, treatments, fatigue, changes in body image, and the feeling that one is no longer attractive may present difficult emotional barriers. Open communication between partners, including frank discussion of needs and feelings, may result in helpful adjustments in sexual practices and deeper commitments to the relationships. Counseling partners or individual clients may smooth over these transitions. In addition to a medication review, a sexual history provides the nurse with insight into a client's needs. The nurse should create an open, accepting atmosphere to facilitate discussion of sexuality and provide information in a nonjudgmental manner. Only when concerns are identified and discussed can problem solving occur (see Chapter 13).

Effect of Chronic Illness on Family and Caregivers

More and more families are faced with providing care for older family members with chronic illness because of the rapidly aging population and the present ability to manage chronic illness. Family caregivers constitute the overwhelming majority of unpaid caregivers and provide the equivalent of billions of dollars of care annually (Shirey and Summer, 2000). Studies have enhanced our awareness of family caregiver stress and the difficulty of balancing caregiving with activities such as personal time or social activities (Fig. 17-2). The primary family caregiver often receives little help from siblings or children and considers institutionalization only when he or she is physically or emotionally exhausted.

Situational factors related to caring for chronically ill older adults contribute to caregiver stress. As noted previously, chronic illnesses are both long term and uncertain. Periods of improvement, stability, and exacerbations in the trajectory of the illness cause uncertainty. Anticipation of these phases can also produce stress. Some chronic conditions develop slowly, and planning for crisis periods is possible. Advance notice of impending stress can allow the caregiver to activate coping strategies and reduce the stress experienced. However, anticipation can also be related to fear of the worst possible outcome.

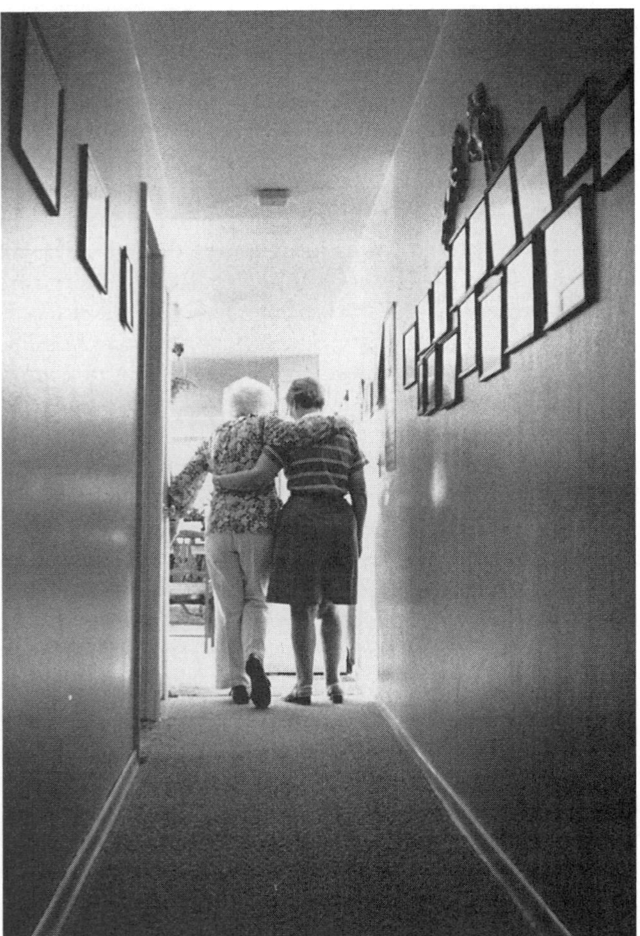

Fig. 17-2 Daughter caregiver assisting her mother down the hallway of her home. (Courtesy Rod Schmall, West Linn, Ore.)

The characteristics of a chronic illness can contribute to caregivers' stress. Caregivers report stress when the client does not recognize family members or does not remember previous relationships because of cognitive changes. Behavioral problems resulting from illness also contribute to stress. The client's functional ability and the type and amount of care needed affect caregiver stress. Ongoing care or the perception that ongoing care is needed can be physically and psychologically draining. When a caregiver is faced with a spouse's illness, the marital relationship may be affected (Knop et al, 1998). The quality of the past and present relationship contributes to how a spousal caregiver copes. In questioning a spousal caregiver, the nurse should determine if unresolved marital problems exist, because these problems may affect the caregiver's reactions to the caregiving experience. Interventions that focus on resolution of issues in relationships and identification of negative coping skills may improve relationships and decrease the possibility of depression in spousal caregivers (Knop et al, 1998).

Role strain is a problematic feature inherent in balancing the role as primary caregiver with other roles within the family network. Most caregivers feel a strong sense of responsibility to caregiving, and although most have a family system in place, it is rarely used as a source of support. Maintaining a healthy sense of self and successfully coping with role strain requires a balance of caregiving and caring for one's self. Personal activities may include work outside the home. As many as 67% of caregivers experience work conflicts that result in changes in work schedules or performance. Many caregivers have to quit their employment completely.

Caregivers may feel powerless when they seem to have no control over events and perceive the stressors in their life as irreversible. Fewer than 15% of all "helper days of care" for people needing help with ADLs are provided by paid caregivers or sources outside the family. Factors that influence coping with caregiver stress and powerlessness are personal characteristics (e.g., age, sex, marital status, health, social roles), knowledge of the illness, knowledge of available resources, and personal perceptions and coping strategies. Female caregivers experience a greater sense of burden and stress than male ones. Burden and feelings of being overwhelmed are related to a subsequent decline in mental and physical health (Hibbard et al, 1996). Assumption of a role previously assigned to an older adult with chronic illness can significantly affect stress levels.

Nursing Implications of Caregiver Stress

Effective nursing care of a client with chronic illness requires providing care not only to the identified client but also to the caregiver. The caregiver's personal characteristics, social and emotional support, financial resources, and perception of the caregiving situation should be assessed in relation to feelings of powerlessness. Personal coping strategies, including the ability to solve problems in managing care, need to be explored by the nurse. Questions such as, "Many family member caregivers have trouble with [such and such]. Have you found that to be true for you?" can help the nurse determine stressors and problem-solving abilities in a nonthreatening manner.

Support can be sought from other resources such as community social service agencies, local church members, visiting nurse organizations, and other family members. Support groups for caregivers also are becoming more prevalent. Group participation decreases the sense of isolation and may help a caregiver cope with new situations. The nurse can provide information about the illness and reassurance that feelings of frustration or helplessness are not unusual reactions. Referral to a social worker may be necessary to provide detailed information regarding Medicare coverage and Medicaid eligibility, as well as other means of obtaining assistance in the health care system. Stress may be reduced by the use of adult day care or home health nursing. Temporary placement in a nursing facility provides the caregiver much-needed respite.

Caring for older adults with chronic disorders requires long-term adaptation on the part of family members. To continue in a caregiving role, a family member caregiver needs ongoing support by all involved health care professionals (see Chapter 6).

REHABILITATION

Rehabilitation refers to services and programs designed to assist individuals who have experienced a trauma or illness that results in an impairment which creates a loss of function—physical, psychologic, social, or vocational (Remsburg and Carson, 2002). Rehabilitation may also be referred to as a philosophic approach of care to promote recovery from acute illness or promote an optimum quality of life in those with chronic illness.

Gerontologic rehabilitation nursing is a specialty practice that focuses on the unique requirements of elderly rehabilitation clients (Association of Rehabilitation Nurses, 1995). Interestingly, the specialty did not arise from gerontologic nursing but from rehabilitation nursing as a subspecialty. It was seen as a need because of the large number of older clients with more disease-related conditions, rather than injury or trauma conditions. Clearly these older clients needed a different approach to their care. The main goal of the gerontologic rehabilitation nurse is to assist elderly clients in achieving their personal optimum level of health and well-being by providing holistic care in a therapeutic environment (Easton, 1999). What is unique about the role is that these nurses consider the special needs, roles, social relationships, and potential comorbidities that occur in the aging process.

The 85-plus age-group, the oldest-old, is the fastest growing segment of the population (Resnick, 2002). The highest percentage of people with disabilities is in the oldest-old age-group (Hobbs, 1997). More strokes occur after age 65, and the incidence of stroke doubles with every decade after age 55 (Reddy and Reddy, 1997). Hip fractures peak in the eighth decade of life and are expected to double by the year 2040 (Ethans and MacKnight, 1998). Older drivers have more crashes per mile driven than do middle-age drivers (Foley and Mitchell, 1997). These data suggest an increasing need for rehabilitation with a gerontologic focus. Rehabilitation planning should begin at the time an older adult is first seen or hospitalized.

The growth of the older population has specific implications for disability, and it affects the nurses who provide preventive, restorative, and rehabilitation services to this population. Age-related physiologic changes can slow recovery and increase residual debilitation from an acute illness or injury. Age-related changes also increase the likelihood of physical limitations from a chronic illness (Lohr, 1997). Studies agree that older adults are more likely to be functionally impaired in ADLs and mobility.

Treatment Environments

Rehabilitation services are offered in a variety of settings. Bedside therapy on acute medical-surgical units can assist a client in maintaining strength when confined to bed. However, the acute medical environment offers little opportunity to apply skills learned in therapy and often emphasizes bedrest and inactivity. Rehabilitation services lasting 1 to 2 hours a day are available in intermediate rehabilitation facilities and skilled care facilities (Fig. 17-3). This environment is suitable for an older adult who has the goal of returning home, who is unable to tolerate more therapy, or who only requires one therapy discipline. Intensive rehabilitation—3 hours of therapy or more—is available in the rehabilitation units of acute care hospitals, freestanding rehabilitation hospitals, and some geriatric assessment/rehabilitation units. Outpatient rehabilitation therapy services may be available to older adults in their homes.

Reimbursement Issues

Medicare becomes available to older adults at age 65 whether they remain working or not. Part A, or basic coverage (inpatient hospital coverage), is without cost to those who qualify. Part B (more comprehensive coverage) is available for a monthly premium with deductibles. A variety of private insurance plans are available to cover the "Medigap," or the 20% of service cost not reimbursed under Medicare guidelines. Medicare is a fee-for-service delivery system. Medicare also contracts with health maintenance organizations

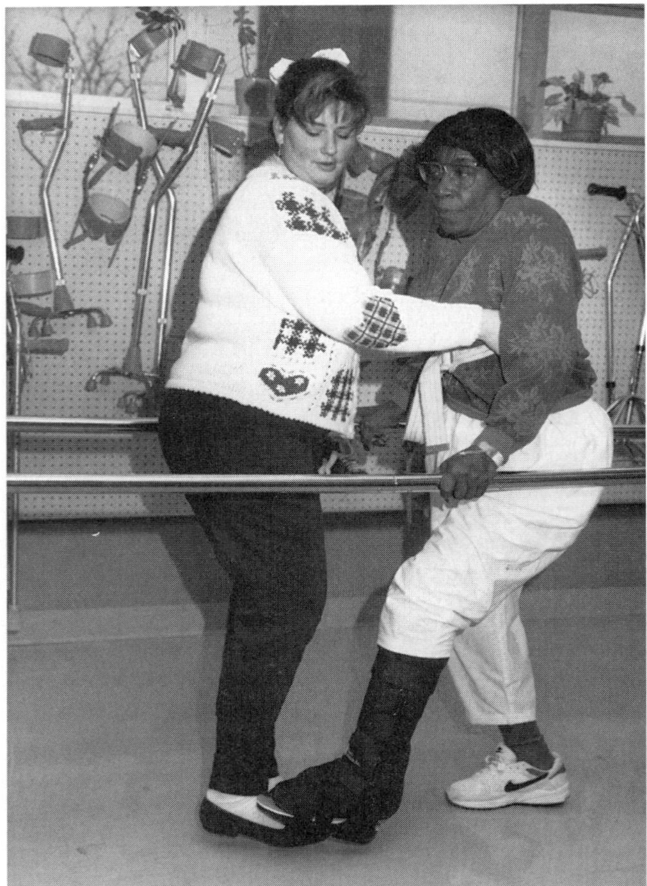

Fig. 17-3 Client receiving therapy in a rehabilitation setting. (Courtesy Loy Ledbetter, St Louis, Mo.)

BOX 17-3 Managing Chronic Illness through Managed Care

The expansion of managed care can be the catalyst to reform chronic disease management. Needed reforms include:

1. A chronic care information system (IS).
2. Use of a chronic care IS to develop a system of parameters (a glidepath) for each chronic condition; at each client encounter, data on these parameters are obtained and the client's deviations from the glidepath are displayed graphically.
3. Management of deviations in the treatment plan by the clinician.

The glidepath facilitates consistent collection of information about client outcomes. Chronic care should include:

1. Annual screening to identify those who have potentially treatable conditions or those who have a generalized risk score, indicating likelihood of hospitalization in the near future.
2. An assessment program to establish the cause of the risk condition and to guide development of the plan of care.
3. A tracking system to ensure the plan of care is implemented and evaluated for its effectiveness throughout the glidepath.

Aging of the population has resulted in calls for better research to prevent and treat age-related conditions; an equally important strategy is to improve the efficiency of care delivery.

From Kane R: Managed care as a vehicle for delivering more effective chronic care for older persons, *Am Geriatr Soc* 46(8):1034, 1998.

(HMOs). HMOs provide the full range of Medicare benefits and may offer additional benefits at little or no additional charge. Box 17-3 outlines how managed care could enhance chronic care for older adults.

Medicaid is a state-specific medical care source of funding for people with low incomes. It varies from state to state, but generally the costs of inpatient, outpatient, home health, and nursing facility rehabilitation services are partially reimbursed. Increasing fiscal constraints in local, state, and federal agencies will affect rehabilitation reimbursement and may further decrease resources available to older adults (Lohr, 1997).

Public Policy and Legislation

Nurses have the power to influence public policy and legislation by advocating for the needs of older adults with disabilities and supporting and conducting relevant nursing research. The process of national public policy making started in 1951 when the first White House Conference on Aging was held. This conference made the problems of older adults visible and since then has been held each decade. The Older Americans Act of 1965 introduced the concept of a focal point of services for older adults. Also in 1965, Medicare and Medicaid were established, having been revised in the subsequent years. In 1982 the Tax Equity and Fiscal Responsibility Act introduced prospective reimbursement for hospitals under Medicare diagnosis-related groups.

The Americans with Disabilities Act (ADA) of 1990 outlawed discrimination on the basis of disability in employment, programs and services provided by state and local governments, the provision of goods and services provided by private companies, and commercial facilities (ADA, 1998). However, the ADA did not eliminate the discrimination inherent in the current system of risk-based health insurance. Insurers may continue to discriminate on the basis of risk, provided that risk classifications are based on sound actuarial data.

The National Council on Disability (NCD), founded in 1978, champions the disability movement. The NCD strives to ensure full participation, equal opportunity, independent living, and economic self-sufficiency for all Americans with disabilities. A 1998 survey by the NCD found that Americans with disabilities still face difficulties in securing employment, education, and accessible public transportation. The most notable finding was the significant difference in employment rates of people with disabilities versus people without them. Approximately 29% of people with disabilities (ages 18 to 64) work full or part time, compared with 79% of people without disabilities (NCD, 1998). Of the unemployed persons with disabilities, 72% say they want to work. This survey also found that only 54% of adults with disabilities have heard of the ADA.

Enhancement of Fitness and Function

The goal in caring for disabled older adults is to maintain or improve function. Maintaining mobility, even when hospitalized, can prevent or decrease the effects of deconditioning. Referral to physical therapy assists the nurse in developing and implementing an exercise plan. Many activities that older adults enjoy such as walking, swimming, cycling, rowing, and dancing can be incorporated into exercise and endurance training. In teaching older adults that deconditioning can be reversed, the nurse should stress that activity and exercise not only increase muscle strength and endurance but also help reduce diastolic blood pressure, body fat, and the risk of coronary artery disease. Other benefits include increased bone mineral density, improved joint flexibility, and improved mental health.

Many of the nation's chronic health problems could be reduced by increases in physical activity. Finding ways to increase fitness levels, in all ages, is a national public health priority. As an example, women over 65 are among the least physically active groups in the nation. Increases in their physical activity would likely reduce or prevent osteoporosis and heart disease. A recent longitudinal study examined environmental factors that affect the physical activity of older women. The investigators followed up a walking intervention from 1982 to 1985 among 229 white women in Pittsburgh. Long-time outcomes of this study suggest that creating environments that encourage exercise (e.g., stores within walking distance; biking or walking trail close) may increase their physical activity levels (King et al, 2003).

Functional Assessment

Regular, comprehensive assessment of older adults is a central principle of gerontologic care. As early as 1959, a World Health Organization advisory group stated, "Health in the elderly is best measured in terms of function; improved function rather than cure is a therapeutic goal for the chronically ill person" (McWilliam et al, 1996). Function is a useful measure in the diagnosis of illness and self-care deficits. Functional assessment can help older adults, their families, and health care providers identify problem areas and plan appropriate interventions that assist in treatment or provision of support measures.

In rehabilitation, assessment tools measure functional status of clients. These tools can provide baseline data, progress data, and outcomes of therapy. A commonly used tool is the Functional Independence Measure (FIM). This tool measures physical abilities (such as ability to eat, bathe, dress, and toilet), communication, and social cognition. It includes 18 items, all measured on an ordinal scale from 1 (dependent) to 7 (independent). Functional assessment is incorporated into the initial nursing assessment and provides information about a client's level of functioning before illness. Establishing a client's baseline level of functioning helps the nurse identify the client's strengths and rehabilitation potential. In long-term care and rehabilitation settings, functional assessment data are used in a resident's care plan.

Keys for Completing a Functional Assessment

To successfully complete a functional assessment:

- The nurse should understand a client's mental status before assessment. For example, some people with cognitive impairment deny any and all problems, whereas people with depression may just respond, "I don't know."
- The assessment approach should be adapted to the degree of potential or actual disability. Healthy older adults may only need to be assessed in areas of social function, ADLs, and independent activities of daily living. Older adults with complex problems need specific assessments of their abilities and disabilities.
- Both self-report and observation may be used along with a functional assessment tool. Some older adults may deny any functional difficulty or may minimize the amount of assistance needed. The nurse should ask older adults what they have done rather than what they can do.
- The nurse should screen for factors that limit older adults in their self-care or in their ability to remain in their home: (1) confusion, (2) safety awareness, (3) toileting, (4) continence, (5) depression or poor motivation, (6) falls, and (7) transfer ability. The most important physical task for an older adult is the ability to transfer in and out of a bed or chair. A person who cannot transfer from bed to chair or chair to toilet cannot be left alone for long periods.
- Geriatric assessment and interventions must consider older adults' values and beliefs. An older client's cultural and spiritual beliefs, feelings regarding health practices, and beliefs about quality-of-life issues should be incorporated into the care plan.

Deconditioning

The effects of deconditioning can be reversible to the extent of the age-related decline in physiologic systems (Lavie and Milani, 1997). Cardiac changes include a decrease in maximum aerobic capacity, cardiac output, left ventricular function, and stroke volume. Associated changes in other body systems include lower extremity venous stasis; decreased vital capacity; negative nitrogen balance; and progressive loss of strength, endurance, and coordination. Deconditioning in older adults appears earlier, is more severe, and takes longer to reverse than it does in younger people.

Exercise training and endurance training can be used to reverse the effects of disuse and maintain the health status of older adults. Strength training improves muscle strength, and muscle building can be achieved through the tenth decade (Lavie and Milani, 1997). Endurance training is beneficial, and circuit training is a safe method to improve strength and endurance for older adults (Means, Currie, and Gershkoff, 1993).

Health Promotion

Health promotion is defined as a combination of health education and related organizational, political, and economic changes aimed at improving health (Hooyman and Kiyak, 1999). Research over the years has demonstrated that pursuing a healthy lifestyle and making lifestyle changes prevents disease; however, health care providers and clients continue to have difficulty implementing needed changes in lifestyle. If health promotion activities enhance function, what motivates older adults to pursue health promotion? Skinner (1951) stated that all activity is motivated behavior. *Motives* are desires, intentions, and goal sets, whereas *incentives* are praise, rewards, and punishments. Although chronic disease and disability cannot be eliminated, health promotion in rehabilitation allows older adults to achieve a maximum level of functioning and increase longevity. Determining reasons why an older adult participates in rehabilitation may provide the nurse with insight to further promote health in the client. Some authors have promoted self-efficacy as a major determinant of behavior (Resnick, 2002). Others suggest that the rehabilitation environment continues to focus on disease process versus a health promotion model (Gunderson and Tomkowiak, 2004) and thus is not an appropriate environment for clients. Studies have found that fitness, health, independence, and socialization are important incentives to older adults (Lavie and Milani, 1997; McWilliam et al, 1996) (Fig. 17-4). Perhaps motivational assessment tools can be used in rehabilitation programs to facilitate planning of interventions that enhance participation and compliance.

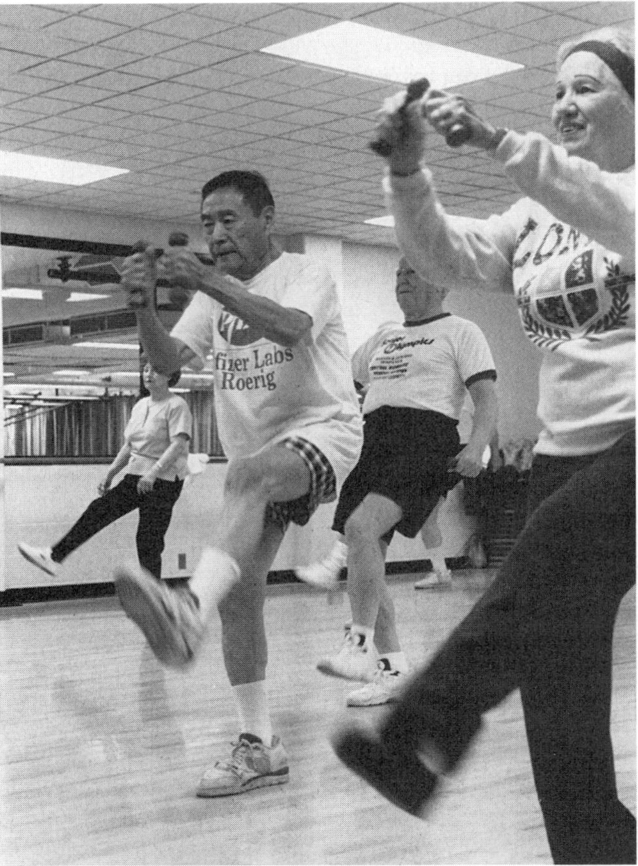

Fig. 17-4 Older adults in exercise class, practicing health promotion. (Courtesy Ursula Ruhl, St Louis, Mo.)

Nursing theories illuminate how health is created and promoted (McWilliam et al, 1996). The nurse can use King's theory of goal attainment in an older adult's rehabilitation. King (1981) states that the goal of nursing is to "help individuals maintain their health so they can function in their roles." Nurses assist clients through purposeful interaction to set goals and agree on actions that achieve those goals. As a result of interactions, transactions occur. Transactions involve bargaining, negotiating, and social exchange. Role performance and role expectations of the nurse and client influence these transactions. Therefore any misunderstanding of roles or distortions in perception may influence the outcome of care. Newman (1986) views health as an evolving process, and discovering the meaning of life and health assists health care providers in determining health promotion interventions. Nurses applying Newman's theory focus on promoting awareness of personal strategies and resources (McWilliam et al, 1996).

Case Study

Mr. P is a 76-year-old man who has been married for 50 years and has three children. Mr. P has been diagnosed and treated for prostate cancer. He developed bladder incontinence, which he has had difficulty accepting. Mrs. P calls his home health nurse for assistance. Using King's theory, the nurse suggests to Mr. P that they talk about the situation. Mr. P agrees only because he wants to enjoy the company of his grandchildren with minimum embarrassment and disruption. The nurse agrees with this goal, and they plan a course of action. The nurse shows Mr. P how to use a Texas catheter and incontinence pads. Mr. P practices application and develops a comfortable means of wearing the protection. Bargaining allows the nurse to function in her role as a facilitator and educator and Mr. P to function in his role as a client. By assisting Mr. P in maintaining his roles of man and grandfather, the nurse protects his self-esteem and ability to function with comfort.

Had Mr. P's incontinence not been managed to his satisfaction, his embarrassment would have hindered continued role performances and impeded further interaction and consequent goal attainment. By supporting Mr. P in roles that satisfied him, the nurse facilitated continued interaction between herself and Mr. P. This led to the plan of action and short-term goal. King's theory provided the nurse with a means of coping with the potentially debilitating effect of conflict between two roles or two perceptions of a role.

Management of Disabling Disorders

Progressive disablement is a process influenced by advancing age, comorbid conditions, and frailty (Ferrucci et al, 1997). It is important for the nurse to understand the normal physiologic effects of aging and their effect on rehabilitation. For example, a cardiac rehabilitation program should focus on exercise training, education, secondary prevention, and vocational counseling. Modifications in exercise training may be needed for older adults with other physical impairments.

Peripheral vascular disease frequently limits activities of endurance. A graded reconditioning program to increase endurance is most successful. If amputation is required, rehabilitation goals and prosthetic candidacy should be determined by premorbid function, condition of the residual limb, and goals of the amputee.

An older adult who is incapacitated with pulmonary disease can improve the quality of life and ease functional tasks through pulmonary rehabilitation. Success depends on the client's motivation, since there may be improvement in symptom management but a lack of improvement in pulmonary function testing.

Acute presentation of neurologic disorders in older clients is confounded by comorbid conditions. About 50% of all strokes occur in persons over age 75 (Reddy and Reddy, 1997). With pharmacologic reduction of blood pressure, an older adult stroke client is at greater risk for compromised cerebral perfusion. Functionally an older adult who survives a brain injury needs more personal assistance and is more likely to require institutional care for some time. Only 30% of stroke survivors over age 75 return home, compared with 73% of those less than 65 years old (Reddy and Reddy, 1997).

Older adults with Parkinson's disease experience postural problems and contracture of the hips and shoulders. As many as half of them experience depression. Essential elements of rehabilitation are stretching, coordination, and gait training. Depression also needs to be assessed as part of the overall management (see Chapter 14).

Late-Life Effects of Early-Life Disabilities

A small body of literature, most of it descriptive, focuses on late-life complications of congenital or early-onset acquired disabilities. Little research is directed toward how to prevent or treat late-life complications. As more becomes known about aging with disabilities, it may be possible to prevent some causes of functional loss (Gulick, 1998).

Aging with cerebral palsy is a prototype for aging with a neuromuscular disorder because it has been studied extensively. Nutritional problems of older adults with early-life disabilities range from obesity (from overeating and inactivity) to malnutrition (from dysphagia). The musculoskeletal system displays changes in young adulthood that are usually seen much later in life, such as degenerative joint disease and osteoporosis with pathologic fractures. Therefore aggressive range-of-motion exercises should be avoided. Destructive behavioral factors in young adulthood, such as restricting or withholding fluids and voluntary retention of urine and feces, leads to urinary tract dysfunction, constipation, diverticula, and hemorrhoids in older adults.

Postpolio syndrome (PPS) is new weakness, fatigue, joint and muscle pain, and loss of function occurring decades after acquisition of the original disability of poliomyelitis. Longitudinal studies of older adults with PPS show a loss of strength of about 1% per year until a functional loss occurs. Other problems contributing to weakness include arthritis, deconditioning, obesity, and coronary artery disease. Rehabilitation programs include the use of lightweight splints and braces to reduce muscular overuse, and adaptive equipment and techniques for energy conservation, weight reduction, postural training, and stress reduction. Introduction of assistive devices is often difficult for older adults with PPS to accept in light of the efforts expended over many years to avoid such devices.

Multiple sclerosis (MS) is generally diagnosed between 20 and 40 years of age, and most individuals have a normal life expectancy despite their disabilities. An important aspect of self-care is the ability of the person to monitor his or her own health status (Orem, 1991). Through client self-reporting data, nurses can obtain information about a client's health status and illness trajectory (Gulick, 1998). Gulick's (1998) 10-year longitudinal study found slow but significant decreases in three system components: motor, brainstem, and elimination. There is also a downward trajectory in all ADL functions, including fine and gross motor control, socialization and recreation, sensation and communication, and intimacy. Reduction in the ability to perform fine and gross motor functions indicates the need for adaptive devices and a modified environment to aid in control of symptoms, enhance ADL performance, and foster independence. The MS pattern of exacerbations and remissions makes providing appropriate care for these clients challenging.

Currie, Gershkoff, and Cifu (1993) give the following generalizations about older adults with childhood onset disabilities:

- Many have a limited social life.
- Few live independently.
- Few are or were competitively employed.
- Intellectual potential has more influence on vocational outcome than does physical ability or disability.
- Many lose access to the health care system after age 21.

These generalizations have not changed over time. The NCD (1998) found that approximately 95% of federal funds spent on persons with disabilities are targeted to support dependency. The younger a disabled individual is when Supplemental Security Income (SSI) begins, the longer that individual is likely to stay on the rolls. The percentage of beneficiaries under age 30 increased by 43% between 1989 and 1993. Acceptance for SSI benefits automatically confers Medicaid coverage in most states. The average SSI federal payment in 1995 was $334 a month, at or below poverty level. The current Social Security system does not encourage persons with disabilities to develop their capabilities toward independent living. The NCD recommends the unlinking of benefits to eliminate the "cliff effect" that people experience when they leave the Social Security rolls and simultaneously lose health insurance and long-term services such as personal assistance, housing subsidies, and food stamps. The government's economic security policy should support maximum employment and independence. The NCD envisions a system that "serves as a trampoline, rather than a safety net, supporting people as they maximize their potential, catching them when they fall, and supporting their efforts toward independence again, always moving toward the goal of maximal employment." The system would include access to health insurance, tax credits to ensure that the transition from benefits to employment does not produce financial disincentive, and flexibility to accommodate disabilities that intermittently limit the ability to work.

Life Issues

Complications and continued deterioration of function may go unrecognized as a result of inadequate transition from pediatric to adult health services. People with disabilities treated by rehabilitation are usually not "sick," but have a narrower margin of health. Many persons with disabilities state that they must constantly educate health professionals about the idiosyncrasies of their condition and how it needs to be considered when prescribing treatment.

There is a wide range of response to disability. An individual who has had arthritis for many years may attach little significance to the condition. An individual faced with a long rehabilitation after a stroke may respond with shock, fear, and disbelief. The human spirit is remarkably resilient, adjusting to seemingly unbearable circumstances. In time most people (in their own way) accept the reality of their condition.

A person with a chronic illness or disability finds that taking health or ability for granted is no longer possible. Symptoms may spoil plans for the day, week, or month. Side effects from medication may present a variety of problems from dry mouth to ataxia. A short trip to the store may be impossible if the day is windy or the sidewalks are wet or icy. As discussed previously, fatigue is a constant companion for many older adults with chronic disabilities.

Older adults must also reorganize their lives to enhance their functional ability and rehabilitation. The nurse can assist older adults in their organization. For example, calendars, schedules, and lists can assist with organizing self-care activities. Home blood glucose and blood pressure monitoring, weight measurement, self-assessments of physical condition based on the specific illness, and records of findings are examples. Organizing medication and treatments might include establishing a schedule for medications or treatments such as catheterization, toileting, or home dialysis. Organizing for working with professionals might include establishing a means to make and keep appointments, preparing for a visit, and obtaining the information needed to improve self-care.

The nurse can help older adult clients maximize financial resources by interpreting insurance coverage and making referrals to community agencies. For example, more than 250,000 adults ages 75 and older need assistive devices but cannot afford them (Ebersole, and Hess, and Luggen, 2004). Most assistive devices, hand rails, canes, walkers, and hearing aids are paid for out of pocket. The nurse should encourage clients to shop around, ask questions, try the equipment, and inquire about service and cost of repairs. Used equipment may be purchased at medical supply stores or privately from individuals. Nurses need to influence legislators regarding the insurance industry's coverage of monitoring equipment, adaptive equipment, and supplies needed to maintain health. The NCD (1998) has proposed that Congress periodically review the Medicare and Medicaid benefits packages to ensure inclusion of assistive technologies that accurately reflect contemporary health and medical practices. The NCD also recommends the insurance term *medical necessity* be clarified to include the concept of maintaining and improving the functional capacity of individuals.

Nursing Strategies

In addition to helping older adults with rehabilitation, the nurse can assist in setting and achieving goals that facilitate reintegration to former environments. Goals that older adults need to achieve in rehabilitation include:

- Improving range of motion
- Improving endurance and tolerance for activity
- Restoring functional ability to an acceptable level
- Improving ambulation (if appropriate)
- Maintaining safety

An important tenet of rehabilitation is setting goals; however, the goals must be the client's goals, not the health care provider's goals of care. Often health care providers make assumptions as to what is most important to clients (often what is most important to them) as opposed to listening to the client and identifying his or her priorities. Drawing up a contract with a client may clarify expectations. The strategy of providing homelike routines is consistent with teaching clients how to live with their illnesses and disabilities.

Incorporating a client's normal routine into teaching content can provide a sense of security that facilitates learning. Showing interest by listening to older adult clients and involving them in all decision making increases their confidence in their ability to achieve care outcomes. Studies suggest that clients who believe in their internal locus of control progress further in rehabilitation than those who believe in powerful others or an external locus of control (Lindsey, 1997; McWilliam et al, 1996; Tate et al, 1997). Rehabilitation is a process, not an end unto itself, in which the greatest steps are usually small ones.

Case Study

Mrs. W is a 73-year-old woman, admitted to a skilled nursing facility for rehabilitation following a CVA with right hemiparesis. She has a history of hypertension. In addition to the hemiparesis, she displays fatigue and emotional lability. She receives physical and occupational therapy twice a day. Her goal is to return home to be with her husband. The priorities in her care are to (1) prevent complications and permanent disabilities; (2) achieve independence in ADLs; (3) support the coping process and integration of changes into her self-concept; and (4) provide information about the CVA, prognosis, and treatment.

The nursing staff assists Mrs. W in turning and repositioning until she masters bed mobility in physical therapy. Mrs. W becomes tearful and frustrated with her attempts at self-care. She is upset with the length of time and effort needed to complete tasks. The nurse supports Mrs. W by anticipating the time required for the self-care and getting her started. The nurse provides assistance only as necessary, maintaining a supportive but firm attitude. The nurse praises Mrs. W's efforts, and slowly Mrs. W gains a sense of self-worth that encourages her continued endeavors. She loudly expresses her feelings about her body. She refers to the affected side as "it." The nurse acknowledges Mrs. W's feeling about the betrayal of her body but retains a matter-of-fact attitude that Mrs. W can still use the unaffected side and learn to control the affected side. The staff uses words such as "weak," "affected," "right," and "left" to treat that side as a part of her body. Small gains in function are celebrated. Mrs. W is also referred to social services for additional support.

After 60 days Mrs. W is independent in ambulation with a quad cane and independent in self-care. She can assist in meal preparation while sitting. She is discharged home with her husband. Follow-up home care includes an assessment of the home environment by the occupational therapist and additional physical therapy in the home. Homemaker assistance is not necessary because of family support.

Rehabilitation and the Future

At present there is no system of primary care after rehabilitation, and once a person is discharged, they have an "orphaned condition" that is not the province of any one medical discipline (NCD, 1998). Preparing people with disabilities to live independently or productively is undermined when they face recurring health problems that limit their ability to participate fully in life. The following five health care service issues dominate the lives of most people after rehabilitation: (1) a high rate of unscheduled rehospitalization, (2) a lack of access to primary care, (3) development of new health problems as a person with a disability ages, (4) a lack of access to long-term services such as home care and personal assistance services, and (5) a lack of access to appropriate health insurance coverage and its subsequent effects on a person's willingness to accept gainful work (NCD, 1998).

These five health care service issues have many implications for nursing. Nursing can help reduce rehospitalization of older adults with disabilities through assessment, early detection, and treatment of changes in their medical conditions. Acting as an advocate for older adults with disabilities, the nurse can arrange a continuum of health care services before discharge from a rehabilitation program to ensure a plan for primary care. In interactions with chronically ill older adults or older adults with disabilities, the nurse should focus on maintenance and restoration of function. Rehabilitation health care professionals must take leadership roles in addressing the ongoing needs of clients with disabilities through education, advocacy, and direct provision of primary care.

Five factors affecting the future of rehabilitation are (1) multidisciplinary and multiagency collaboration and cooperation, (2) awareness of the efficacy of rehabilitation, (3) better

Home Care

1. Arthritis, the number two chronic illness, is commonly found in homebound older adults.
2. Homebound older adults with chronic conditions most likely have functional limitations that can affect their independence.
3. Use caregivers as sources for data about homebound older adults' abilities to cope with chronic conditions.
4. Refer caregivers and homebound older adults to equipment vendors for assistive devices (e.g., canes, walkers, shower chairs, grab bars, glucose monitoring machines) that promote independence at home.
5. Use social workers as sources for identifying community resources for financial assistance for homebound older adults.
6. Assist caregivers and homebound older adults in adjusting to the necessary lifestyle changes to promote coping with chronic illnesses.
7. Encourage caregivers to attend support groups to help ease the burden of caring for homebound older adults with chronic illnesses.
8. Physical or occupational therapists can assess older adults and provide assistive devices that help maintain functional ability.

research of rehabilitation outcomes, (4) adequate community and caregiver support, and (5) access to rehabilitation in a variety of settings (Lohr, 1997; NCD, 1998).

SUMMARY

Our health care system is based on acute and episodic care and does not fit with long-term chronic disease and disability. The aging of the population and increasing prevalence of chronic disease will continue to challenge the health care system. Currently 75 cents of every dollar spent on direct medical costs is associated with chronic disease (Siebens, 2002). One major shortcoming in the health care system is the manner in which it pays for health care. The current system offers little incentive for providers and payers to make investments up front to avert medical problems later, that is, health promotion and disease prevention.

However, the health care system is changing in the face of competition, rapid cost growth, and health care reform. These changes offer a window of opportunity to address the health care needs of older adults with chronic disease and disability.

Key Points

- The trajectory of chronic illness varies with each individual and each illness.
- Orem's model of self-care provides the nurse with a framework to assess variables that affect older adults' abilities to care for themselves.
- Regular, comprehensive assessment is a central principle of the care of older adults.
- Assessing what is meaningful to older adults helps the nurse plan interventions to support psychosocial adjustment to a chronic condition or illness.
- Rehabilitation of older adults focuses on improving functional ability.
- Health promotion incentives that are important to older adults are fitness, health, independence, and socialization.

Critical Thinking Exercise

1. A 75-year-old woman, independent and in relatively good health, has had a nagging cough for the past several months. She is concerned that the cough may indicate a serious illness. She is reluctant to seek help because she does not want to prolong her life if it means a loss of quality. Make a judgment about where she fits within the illness trajectory and explain how a nurse can be of assistance.

REFERENCES

Aikens J et al: A replicated prospective investigation of life stress, coping and depressive symptoms in multiple sclerosis, *J Behav Med* 20(5):433, 1997.

Americans with Disabilities Act: Accessed from website: http://www.usdoj.gov/crt/ada/.

Association of Rehabilitation Nurses: *The gerontological rehabilitation nurse: role description,* Skokie, Ill, 1995, The Association.

Becker G et al: Knowledge and care of chronic illness in three ethnic minority groups, *Fam Med* 30(3):173, 1998.

Berg J, Evangelista L, Dunbar-Jacob J: Compliance. In Lubkin I, Larsen P, editors: *Chronic illness: impact and interventions,* ed 5, Sudbury, Mass, 2002, Jones & Bartlett.

Brown I, Renwick R, Nagler M: The centrality of quality of life in health promotion and rehabilitation. In Renwick R, Brown I, Nagler M, editors: *Quality of life in health promotion and rehabilitation,* Thousand Oaks, Calif, 1996, Sage, pp 3-13.

Centers for Disease Control and Prevention: *Prevent chronic diseases,* Atlanta, 1998, The Centers.

Commission on Chronic Illness: *Chronic illness in the United States, prevention of chronic illness,* Cambridge, Mass, 1957, Harvard University Press.

Corbin J: The Corbin and Strauss chronic illness trajectory model: an update, *Scholarly Inquiry Nurs Pract* 12(1):33, 1998.

Corbin J, Strauss A: A nursing model for chronic illness management based upon the trajectory framework. In Woog P, editor: *The chronic illness trajectory framework: the Corbin and Strauss Nursing Model,* New York, 1992, Springer.

Currie D, Gershkoff A, Cifu D: Geriatric rehabilitation: mid- and late-life effects of early life disabilities, *Arch Phys Med Rehab* 74(5):413, 1993.

Curtin M, Lubkin I: What is chronicity? In Lubkin I, editor: *Chronic illness: impact and interventions,* ed 3, Sudbury, Mass, 1995, Jones & Bartlett, p 6.

Easton K: *Gerontological rehabilitation nursing,* Philadelphia, 1999, WB Saunders.

Ebersole P, Hess P, Luggen A: *Toward healthy aging: human needs and nursing response,* ed 6, St Louis, 2004, Mosby.

Ethans K, MacKnight C: Hip fracture in the elderly, *Post Grad Med* 103(1):157, 1998.

Fawcett J: Compliance: definition and key issues, *J Clin Psychiatr* 56(suppl 1):4, 1995.

Ferrans C, Powers M: Quality of life index: development and psychometric properties, *Adv Nurs Sci* 8: 15, 1985.

Ferrucci L et al: Hospital diagnoses, Medicare charges and nursing home admissions in the year when older persons become severely disabled, *JAMA* 227(9):728, 1997.

Foley K, Mitchell S: The elderly driver: what physicians need to know, *Cleveland Clin J Med* 64(8):423, 1997.

Frankl V: *Man's search for meaning,* New York, 1962, Simon & Schuster.

Groessl E, Cronan T: A cost analysis of self-management programs for people with chronic illness, *Am J Community Psychol* 28(4):455, 2000.

Gulick E: Symptom and activities of daily living trajectory in multiple sclerosis: a 10 year study, *Nurs Res* 47(3):137, 1998.

Gunderson A, Tomkowiak J: Dynamic health promotion for the geriatric population, *Rehab Nurs* 29(2):45, 2004.

Haas B: Clarification and integration of similar quality of life concepts, *Image: J Nurs Scholarship* 31(3):215, 1999.

Hibbard J et al: Gender differences in the support networks of caregivers, *J Gerontol Nurs* 22(9):15, 1996.

Hobbs F: Sixty-five plus in the US, *Current population reports series,* Washington, DC, 1997, US Census Bureau.

Holkup P: A therapy group to facilitate understanding of intergenerational behavior patterns and to promote family healing, *J Psychosocial Nurs* 36(2):20-26, 1998.

Holroyd K, Creer T: *Self-management of chronic disease,* New York, 1986, Academic Press.

Holtzclaw LR: The importance of self-concept for the older adult, *J Religion Aging* 1(3):23, 1985.

Hooyman N, Kiyak H: *Social gerontology: a multidisciplinary perspective,* Needham Heights, Mass, 1999, Allyn & Bacon.

Kane R: Managed care as a vehicle for delivering more effective chronic care for older persons, *Am Geriatr Soc* 46(8):1034, 1998.

Kart C: *The realities of aging*, ed 5, Boston, 1997, Allyn & Bacon.

King I: *A theory of nursing*, New York, 1981, Wiley & Sons.

King WC et al: The relationship between convenience of destinations and walking levels in older women, *Am J Health Promotion* 18(1):74, 2003.

Kivinen P et al: Self-rated health, physician-rated health and associated factors among elderly men: the Finnish cohorts of the seven countries study, *Age & Ageing* 27:41, 1998.

Knop D et al: In sickness and in health: an exploration of the perceived quality of the marital relationship, coping and depression in caregivers of spouses with Alzheimer's disease, *J Psychosoc Nurs* 36(1):16, 1998.

Lavie C, Milani R: Benefits of cardiac rehabilitation and exercise training in elderly women, *Am J Cardiol* 79(5):664, 1997.

Lindsey E: Experiences of the chronically ill: a covert caring for the self, *J Holist Nurs* 15(3):227, 1997.

Lindsey E: Health within chronic illness: experiences of chronically ill/disabled people, *J Adv Nurs* 24(3):465, 1996.

Lindsey E: The gift of healing in chronic illness/disability, *J Holist Nurs* 13(4):287, 1995.

Lohr K: Improving health care outcomes through geriatric rehabilitation, *Med Care* 35(6):121, 1997.

Lubkin I, Larsen P: What is chronicity? In Lubkin I, Larsen P, editors: *Chronic illness: impact and interventions*, ed 5, Sudbury, Mass, 2002, Jones & Bartlett.

McWilliam C et al: Creating health with chronic illness, *Adv Nurs Sci* 18(3):1, 1996.

Means K, Currie D, Gershkoff A: Geriatric rehabilitation: assessment, preservation and enhancement of fitness and function, *Arch Phys Med Rehab* 74(5):417, 1993.

Metha S: Applying Orem's self-care framework, *Geriatr Nurs* 14(4):182, 1993.

Miller J: The psychosocial aspects of rehabilitation, *Caring* 4:20, Aug 1992.

Morris CA: Self-concept as altered by the diagnosis of cancer, *Nurs Clin North Am* 20:611, 1985.

National Center for Health Statistics: *Health, United States, 2003 with Chartbook on trends in the health of Americans*, Hyattsville, Md, 2003, The Center.

National Council on Disability: *Bulletin*, July 1998.

Newman M: *Health as expanding consciousness*, St Louis, 1986, Mosby.

Orem D: *Nursing: concepts of practice*, ed 5, St Louis, 1995, Mosby.

Orem D: *Nursing: concepts of practice*, ed 4, St Louis, 1991, Mosby.

Partnership for Solutions: *Chronic conditions: making the case for ongoing care*, Baltimore, 2002, Johns Hopkins University.

Patrick D, Erickson P: *Health status and health policy: quality of life in healthcare evaluation and resource allocation*, New York, 1993, Oxford.

Pickle L et al: *Atlas of United States mortality*, Hyattsville, Md, 1997, National Center for Health Statistics.

Reddy M, Reddy V: After a stroke: strategies to restore function and prevent complications, *Geriatrics* 52(9):59, 1997.

Remsburg R, Carson B: Rehabilitation. In Lubkin I, Larsen P, editors: *Chronic illness: impact and interventions*, Sudbury, Mass, 2002, Jones & Bartlett.

Resnick B: Geriatric rehabilitation: the influence of efficacy beliefs and motivation, *Rehab Nurs* 27(4):152, 2002.

Rhodes R, Morrissey M, Ward A: Self-motivation: a driving force for elders in cardiac rehabilitation, *Geriatr Nurs* 13(2):94, 1992.

Schneider J et al: Exercise training program for older adults: incentives and disincentives for participation, *J Gerontol Nurs* 29(9):21, 2003.

Shirey L, Summer L: *Caregiving: helping the elderly with activity limitations*, Washington, DC, 2000, National Academy on an Aging Society.

Siebens H: The domain management model: organizing care for stroke survivors and other persons with chronic disease, *Topics Stroke Rehab* 9(3):1, 2002.

Sioson ER, Kerfoot S, Ziat LM: Rehabilitation outcome of older patients with end-stage renal disease and lower extremity amputation, *J Am Geriatr* 41(6):667, June 1993.

Skinner BF: How to teach animals, *Sci Am* 185:26-29, 1951.

Smits M, Kee C: Correlates of self-care among the independent elderly, *J Gerontol Nurs* 18(9):13, 1992.

Strauss A, Corbin J: *Shaping a new health care system*, San Francisco, 1988, Jossey-Bass.

Tate D et al: Quality of life issues among women with physical disabilities or breast cancer, *Arch Phys Med Rehab* 78:518, 1997.

Thorne S, Patterson B: Shifting images of chronic illness, *Image: J Nurs Scholarship* 30(2):173, 1998.

Tremethick M: Thriving, not just surviving the importance of social support among the elderly, *J Psychosoc Nurs* 35(9):27, 1997.

Twibell R: Family coping during critical illness, *Dimensions Crit Care Nurs* 17(2):100, 1998.

APPENDIX 17A

Resources

AARP
601 E Street NW
Washington, DC 20049
(888) 687-2277
http://www.aarp.org/

ADA Information Line
(800) 514-0301
(800) 514-0383 TDD
http://www.usdoj.gov/crt/ada/adahom1.htm

Alzheimer's Disease Education and Referral Center
PO Box 8250
Silver Springs, MD 20907-8250
(800) 438-4380
Fax: (301) 495-3334
E-mail: adear@alzheimers.org
http://www.alzheimers.org/

American Academy of Physical Medicine and Rehabilitation
One IBM Plaza, Suite 2500
Chicago, IL 60611-3604
(312) 464-9700
Fax: (312) 464-0227
E-mail: info@aapmr.org
http://www.aapmr.org/

American Parkinson Disease Association
1250 Hylan Blvd., Suite 4B
Staten Island, NY 10305
(800) 223-2732
Fax: (718) 981-4399
E-mail: apda@apdaparkinson.org
http://www.apdaparkinson.org/

Arthritis Foundation
PO Box 7669
Atlanta, GA 30357-0669
(404) 872-7100 or (800) 568-4045
www.arthritis.org

National Caucus and Center on Black Aged
1220 L Street NW, Suite 800
Washington, DC 20005
(202) 637-8400
http://www.ncba-aged.org/

National Council on Disability
1331 F Street NW, Suite 850
Washington, DC 20004
(202) 272-2004
(202) 272-2074 TTY
Fax: (202) 272-2022
www.ncd.gov

National Institute on Aging
Building 31, Room 5C27
31 Center Drive, MCS 2292
Bethesda, MD 20892
(800) 222-2225
(800) 222-4225 TTY
www.nia.nih.gov

National Rehabilitation Information Center
4200 Forbes Blvd., Suite 202
Lanham, MD 20706
(800) 346-2742
(301) 459-5984 TTY
E-mail: naricinfo@heitechservices.com
http://www.naric.com/

National Stroke Association
9707 E. Easter Lane
Englewood, CO 80112
(303) 649-9299
(800) 787-6537
Fax: (303) 649-1328
www.stroke.org

U.S. Senate Special Committee on Aging
G31 Dirksen Senate Office Building
Washington, DC 20510
(202) 224-5364
Fax: 202-224-8660
E-mail: mailbox@aging.senate.gov
http://aging.senate.gov/

18 Substance Abuse

MARY J. REED, PhD, APN, CS, BC

Learning Objectives

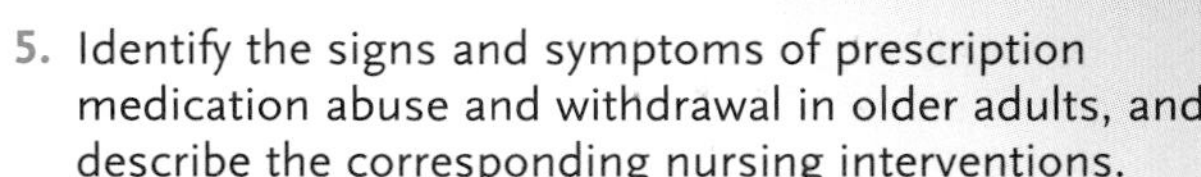

On completion of this chapter, the reader will be able to:

1. Identify key physiologic, psychologic, and sociologic changes associated with aging that make it difficult to identify and treat substance abuse in older adults.
2. List the key components of assessing older adults for substance abuse.
3. Identify the key multidisciplinary and nursing interventions for older adults who abuse substances.
4. Identify the signs and symptoms of alcohol abuse and withdrawal in older adults, and describe the corresponding nursing interventions.
5. Identify the signs and symptoms of prescription medication abuse and withdrawal in older adults, and describe the corresponding nursing interventions.
6. Identify the signs and symptoms of nonprescription medication abuse and withdrawal in older adults, and describe the corresponding nursing interventions.
7. Identify the signs and symptoms of nicotine abuse and withdrawal in older adults, and describe the corresponding nursing interventions.
8. Identify the signs and symptoms of caffeine abuse and withdrawal in older adults, and describe the corresponding nursing interventions.

Many older adults enjoy leisure activities as a result of decreased work schedules and retirement. However, some are unable to enjoy leisure activities because of the emotional, physical, social, and economic effects of growing older. Illicit drugs, such as cocaine, opiates, and marijuana, are more commonly used by younger adults than older adults. Among older persons, commonly abused substances are alcohol, prescription drugs, nonprescription drugs, nicotine, and caffeine. Alcohol abuse is prevalent in 10% to 15% percent of older adults. Frequently, the symptoms are subtle or atypical, or they mimic symptoms of other age-related illnesses and remain undiagnosed. Clients' presenting symptoms may be erratic changes in affect, mood, or behavior; malnutrition; bladder and bowel incontinence; gait disturbances; and recurring falls, burns, and head trauma (Morris, 2001; Videbeck, 2004). Approximately one third of older adults began to abuse alcohol late in life because of bereavement, retirement, loneliness, and physical and emotional illnesses. Denial is more intense in older adults because of cognitive and memory problems and shame that substance abuse is immoral. Prescription drug abuse in older adults is two or three times higher than in the general population. Benzodiazepine abuse and dependence are more common than in the general population, and the drugs are usually prescribed over longer periods, resulting in excessive daytime sedation, ataxia, falls and accidents, and cognitive impairments such as attention and memory problems (Fontaine, 2003).

DEFINITIONS AND COMMON USAGE

Nurses must understand definitions associated with substance abuse to correctly assess substance abuse and plan appropriate interventions for older adults. The fourth edition of the *Diagnostic and Statistical Manual of Mental Disorders* (DSM-IV-TR) is used by physicians to aid in diagnosing clients. The DSM-IV-TR distinguishes between substance abuse and substance dependence. *Substance abuse* is defined as "a maladaptive pattern of substance use manifested by recurrent and significant adverse consequences related to the repeated use of substances." *Substance dependence* is defined as "a cluster of cognitive, behavioral, and physiologic symptoms indicating that the individual continues use of the substance despite significant substance-related problems" (American Psychiatric Association [APA], 2000). Substance dependence also comprises the distinct phases of tolerance, withdrawal, and compulsive drug-taking and drug-seeking behaviors. Box 18-1 lists the DSM-IV-TR diagnostic criteria for substance abuse and substance dependence. *Substance misuse* is a problem for many independent living older adults. It includes not following instructions on a prescription by either taking too much or not enough medication or taking someone else's prescribed drugs. Misuse also means self-medicating with old prescriptions kept long after the reason for the prescription has passed (Meiner, 1997; Meiner, 2004).

BOX 18-1 DSM-IV-TR Diagnostic Criteria

SUBSTANCE ABUSE

A. A maladaptive pattern of substance use leading to clinically significant impairment or distress, as manifested by one (or more) of the following, occurring within a 12-month period:
   1. Recurrent substance use resulting in a failure to fulfill major role obligations at work, school, or home (e.g., repeated absences or poor work performance associated with substance use; substance-related absences, suspensions, or expulsions from school; or neglect of children or household)
   2. Recurrent substance use in situations in which it is physically hazardous (e.g., driving an automobile or operating a machine when impaired by substance use)
   3. Recurrent substance-related legal problems (e.g., arrests for substance-related disorderly conduct)
   4. Continued substance use despite having persistent or recurrent social or interpersonal problems caused or exacerbated by the effects of the substance (e.g., arguments with spouse about consequences of intoxication, physical fights)

B. The symptoms have never met the criteria for substance dependence for this class of substance.

SUBSTANCE DEPENDENCE

A. A maladaptive pattern of substance use, leading to clinically significant impairment or distress, as manifested by three (or more) of the following, occurring at any time in the same 12-month period:
   1. Tolerance, as defined by either of the following:
      a. A need for markedly increased amounts of the substance to achieve intoxication or desired effect
      b. Markedly diminished effect with continued use of the same amount of the substance
   2. Withdrawal, as manifested by either of the following:
      a. The characteristic withdrawal syndrome for the substance
      b. The same (or a closely related) substance is taken to relieve or avoid withdrawal symptoms
   3. The substance is often taken in larger amounts or over a longer period than was intended
   4. There is a persistent desire or unsuccessful efforts to cut down or control substance use
   5. A great deal of time is spent in activities necessary to obtain the substance (e.g., visiting multiple doctors or driving long distances), use the substance (e.g., chain-smoking), or recover from its effects
   6. Important social, occupational, or recreational activities are given up or reduced because of substance use
   7. The substance use is continued despite knowledge of having a persistent or recurrent physical or psychologic problem that is likely to have been caused or exacerbated by the substance (e.g., current cocaine use despite recognition of cocaine-induced depression or continued drinking despite recognition that an ulcer was made worse by alcohol consumption)

Difficulty in Identification of Abuse

The physiologic, psychologic, and sociologic changes associated with aging make the identification and treatment of substance abuse in older adult clients difficult. Most studies report that the average older person is not taking the prescribed medication at all or is taking unnecessary drugs with dosages that are too high, even though a safer alternative to the drug prescribed is available. Age-related psychologic and sociologic changes and symptoms can be subtle or atypical and can mimic symptoms of substance abuse (Mohundro and Ramsey, 2003; Videbeck, 2004).

Physiologic Changes

The pharmacokinetics, or the activity or fate of a drug within the body, includes absorption, distribution, plasma protein binding, hepatic metabolism, and elimination or clearance of a drug. These processes can be affected by age, nutritional status, altered physiology, and pathologic conditions. Absorption in the elderly can be influenced by a decreased ability to swallow, increased gastric pH, delayed gastric emptying, and decreased intestinal motility. The absorption issues may reduce the bioavailability of a drug or reduce its clinical efficacy or onset. Distribution of a drug in the elderly is affected by decreased muscle mass, decreased total body water, and increased total body fat. Because many drugs are lipophilic, an increase in body fat can lead to an increase in a drug's half-life without changing the plasma steady state. Plasma protein binding can be affected by changes in albumin and alpha-1-acid glycoprotein levels, and both levels can be somewhat altered by age, malnutrition, and increased medical burden. The clinical significance of protein binding on drugs is highly variable and is affected by age, gender, health, and specific medication. However, one important aspect is that only an unbound drug can cross the blood-brain barrier and reach its intended receptor site. An unbound drug may also interact with peripheral sites of action and cause unintended and unwanted side effects.

Nurses should be aware of these age-related physiologic changes of absorption, distribution, plasma protein binding, hepatic metabolism, and elimination or clearance of a drug.

The assessment of these changes in relation to substance use is essential in planning interventions to prevent or halt substance abuse and misuse in the older adult population.

Psychologic Changes

Psychologic changes in older adults result primarily from the numerous losses this age-group may experience in a relatively short period. Separation from family and friends, retirement, decline in physical health, and decreased ability to participate in previous social activities can contribute to feelings of loss. Two thirds of this age-group have longstanding problems with alcohol and multiple medical complications. One third develop the drinking problem late in life, often in response to bereavement, retirement, loneliness, relationship stress, and physical illness (Eliopoulos, 2001) (Fig. 18-1).

In addition, nurses should be aware of the misconception that select prescribed or over-the-counter substances can help the client deal with unmet psychologic needs. For example, an older adult may become anxious if sleep has decreased to less than 8 hours and may seek sedatives. In addition, some older adults tend to use certain substances to mask negative feelings about themselves; they may eventually attribute some of their positive personality characteristics to substances. Examples of such substances include alcohol and benzodiazepines (e.g., diazepam [Valium]). Clients who are given a benzodiazepine by a physician for a limited period may become dependent on the medication. An older adult client who is dependent may find another physician to prescribe the medication when the original physician discontinues it.

The nurse must also assess older adult clients for suicidal ideations. Clients should be asked whether they have had thoughts of harming themselves and if they have a plan to carry out these thoughts. Advancing age and substance abuse are among the greatest risk factors for suicide. Suicide rates tend to increase with age in white men, and it should be noted that suicide is a leading cause of death in older adults.

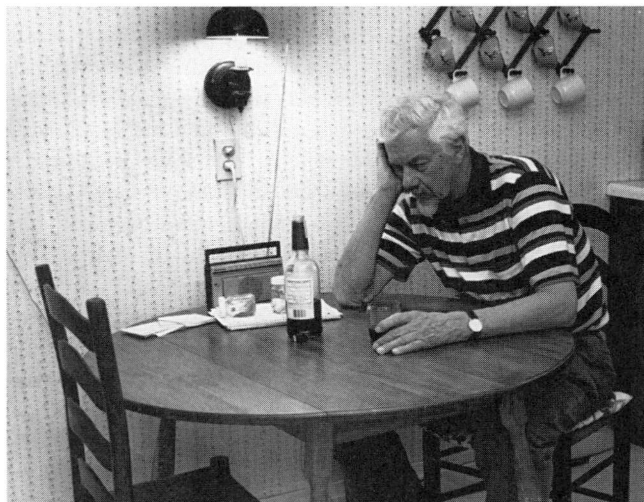

Fig. 18-1 Loneliness and hopelessness may be manifestations of alcohol abuse. (Courtesy Ursula Ruhl, St Louis, M.)

Sociologic Changes

Sociologic changes—such as decreases in finances, transportation, and social support—tend to place older adults at risk for substance abuse and misuse. As a result of decreased finances and transportation, many older adults fill prescriptions through mail-order pharmacies. Mail-order pharmacies tend to increase the potential for drug abuse and misuse as a result of prescription errors, late arrivals, and large quantities of drugs. Social conditions such as low income, difficulty shopping, and lack of socialization tend to affect the nutrition of older adult clients. The nurse should educate older adults about the dual effects of poor nutritional status and drug metabolism.

Sociologic changes are based on the cultural values and attitudes about substance abuse behaviors that are passed from one generation to another. There is a lower incidence of substance abuse in cultures whose religious and moral values prohibit or limit their use. Older adults are targeted by advertisements for prescription and nonprescription drugs because they experience minor aches, pains, and major health problems. Substance abuse is symptomatic of the larger social problems among minority groups (e.g., poverty, substandard housing, inadequate health care, and lack of power). The lack of culturally competent care is an additional barrier to substance abuse care for the older adult.

ASSESSMENT

The following section is a general overview of the key concepts in assessing and planning nursing interventions for substance abuse in the older adult population. Nurses should be aware of the specific assessment and nursing intervention strategies for abuse of alcohol, prescription medications, nonprescription medications, nicotine, and caffeine. Substance abuse in older adults is challenging in that it requires expertise in gerontology, geriatrics, psychiatric mental heath, and the specific presentation and management of disorders in this population.

Substance Abuse History

The DSM-IV-TR criteria for substance abuse are developed for the general population, not specifically for the older adult population (see Box 18-1). Therefore it is essential for the nurse to assess clients' medical and psychologic histories. After a history is complete, the nurse should identify whether the key medical and psychologic manifestations of substance abuse are present (Boxes 18-2 and 18-3).

BOX 18-2 Medical Manifestations of Substance Abuse in Older Adults

Peripheral neuropathy
Diminished proprioception
Alcoholic liver disease (hepatitis or cirrhosis)
Alcoholic pancreatitis
Gastrointestinal bleeding
Esophageal varices
Peptic ulcer or gastritis
Malignancies
Cardiomyopathy
Protein-calorie malnutrition
Hypovitaminosis (particularly B vitamins)
Anemia
Osteopenia
Susceptibility to infections
Electrolyte disturbances
Hypercortisolemia
Delirium tremens (occurs after recent cessation of or reduction in alcohol intake; is marked by signs of delirium with autonomic hyperactivity—tachycardia, sweating, hallucinations, delusions, agitation, tremor, fever, and seizures)
Seizures
Hypertension
Acquired immunodeficiency syndrome (AIDS)
Peripheral muscle weakness
Falls
Orthostatic hypotension

From Solomon K et al: Alcoholism and prescription drug abuse in the elderly: St Louis University Grand Rounds, *J Am Geriatr Soc* 41:57, 1993.

BOX 18-3 Psychologic Manifestations of Substance Abuse in Older Adults

Manic (expansively elevated) mood or behavior
Depressed mood
Social withdrawal
Vegetative symptoms of depression
Apathy or poor motivation
Suicidal ideation, plans, or behavior
Violent threats or behavior
Paranoid or nonparanoid delusions
Auditory, visual, olfactory, or gustatory hallucinations
Anxiety
Panic attacks
Phobias
Poor personal hygiene
Poor activities of daily living (ADLs) skills
Personality change
Irritability
Sleep disturbances
Memory loss (immediate, recent, or remote)
Delirium (intoxication or withdrawal)
Flashbacks
Marital, social, or legal difficulties
Noncompliance with medical care
Hallucinations
Alcoholic dementia (Wernicke-Korsakoff syndrome)

From Solomon K et al: Alcoholism and prescription drug abuse in the elderly: St Louis University Grand Rounds, *J Am Geriatr Soc* 41:57-69, 1993.

Screening Tools

A number of screening tools are available to assess alcohol use (Boxes 18-4 to 18-6). The two most commonly used tools are the CAGE (Mayfield, McLeod, and Hall, 1974) and the Michigan Alcoholism Screening Test (MAST) (Selzer, 1971).

BOX 18-4 CAGE

1. Have you ever felt the need to **C**ut down on drinking?
2. Have you ever felt **A**nnoyed by the criticism of drinking?
3. Have you ever had **G**uilty feelings about drinking?
4. Have you ever taken a morning **E**ye opener?

NOTE: If the client answers "yes" to any of the above questions, further assessment for alcohol abuse is warranted.

From Mayfield D, McLeod G, Hall P: The CAGE questionnaire: validation of a new alcoholism screening instrument, *Am J Psychiatr* 131:1121-1123, 1974. Reprinted with permission from the Aamerican Journal of Psychiatry, Copyright 1994. American Psychiatric Association.

The Brief Michigan Alcoholism Screening Test (BMAST) is a modified form of the MAST (Pokorny, Miller, and Kaplan, 1972). Frederick Blow developed the Michigan Alcoholism Screening Test—Geriatric Version (MAST-G) (Morton, Jones, and Manganaro, 1996). Results indicate that the MAST-G is an instrument that is more reliable and valid in the older adult population than the MAST (Knight and Mjelde-Mossey, 1995). Even though further research is required to validate the use of these tools for the assessment of abused substances besides alcohol, positive clinical results have been demonstrated with the use of these tools, substituting the words "substance" or "prescription medication" for "drink."

Clients undergoing detoxification from alcohol abuse should be assessed on an ongoing basis using the Clinical Institute Withdrawal Assessment tool. The tool measures the severity of alcohol withdrawal based on 10 common signs and symptoms: nausea and vomiting; tremor; paroxysmal sweats; anxiety; agitation; tactile, auditory, and visual disturbances; headache; and orientation. The maximum score is

BOX 18-5 MAST*

		YES	NO
1.	Do you enjoy having a drink now and then?	0	
2.	Do you feel you are a normal drinker? (By normal, we mean do you drink less than or as much as most other people, and you have not gotten into any recurring trouble while drinking?)		2
3.	Have you ever awakened the morning after some drinking the night before and found that you could not remember a part of the evening?	2	
4.	Do either of your parents, or any other near relative, or your spouse, or any girlfriend or boyfriend ever worry or complain about your drinking?	1	
5.	Can you stop drinking without a struggle after one or two drinks?		2
6.	Do you feel guilty about your drinking?	1	
7.	Do friends or relatives think you are a normal drinker?		2
8.	Are you able to stop drinking when you want to?		2
9.	Have you ever attended a meeting of Alcoholics Anonymous (AA)?	5	
10.	Have you gotten into physical fights when you have been drinking?	1	
11.	Has your drinking ever created problems between you and either of your parents, another relative, your spouse, or girlfriend or boyfriend?	2	
12.	Have any of your family members ever gone to anyone for help about your drinking?	2	
13.	Have you ever lost friends because of your drinking?	2	
14.	Have you ever gotten into trouble at work or at school because of drinking?	2	
15.	Have you ever lost a job because of drinking?	2	
16.	Have you ever neglected your obligations, school work, your family, or your job for 2 or more days in a row because you were drinking?	2	
17.	Do you drink before noon fairly often?	1	
18.	Have you ever been told you have liver trouble? Cirrhosis?	2	
19.	After heavy drinking have you ever had severe shaking, heard voices, or seen things that really weren't there (e.g., delirium tremens [DTs])?	2 (DTs: 5)	
20.	Have you ever gone to anyone for help about your drinking?	5	
21.	Have you ever been a patient in a psychiatric hospital or on a psychiatric ward of a general hospital where drinking was part of the problem that resulted in hospitalization?	2	
22.	Have you ever been seen at a psychiatric or mental health clinic, or gone to any doctor, social worker, or clergy for help with any emotional problem, where drinking was part of the problem?	2	
23.	Have you ever been arrested for drunk driving, driving while intoxicated, or driving under the influence of alcoholic beverages or any other drug? (If YES, how many times?)	2 each	
24.	Have you ever been arrested, or taken into custody, even for a few hours, because of other drunk behavior as a result of either alcohol or another drug? (If YES, how many times?)	2 each	

Modified and reprinted with permission from Selzer ML: The Michigan Alcoholism Screening Test: the quest for a new diagnostic instrument, *Am J Psychiatr* 127:1653, 1971. Reprinted with permission from the American Journal of Psychiatry, Copyright 1994. American Psychiatric Association.
*Interpretation: Standard MAST—0 to 3 points probable normal drinker; 4 points borderline score; 5 to 9 points 80% associated with alcoholism/chemical dependence; 10 or more points 100% associated with alcoholism.

67, and clients who score higher than 20 should be admitted to a hospital (Fontaine, 2003).

Nursing Caveats

In assessing older adults for substance abuse, the nurse must be aware of his or her own perceptions and attitudes regarding substance abuse in the older adult population. Many health care providers overlook the possibility that the presenting symptoms in an older adult may be related to substance abuse. It is important to have a healthy collaborative relationship with patients, showing respect for their values and choices.

Inherent changes in tissue and organ function are highly variable and individual. Hence the response to medication is just as variable and as unpredictable in this population. Guiding principles are to start low and go slowly when prescribing medications; change or add only one medication at a time; review each medication to see whether the patient is still taking it; and determine the dose, frequency, and time (see Research box).

BOX 18-6 BMAST*

		YES	NO
1.	Do you feel that you are a normal drinker?		2
2.	Do friends think that you are a normal drinker?		2
3.	Have you ever attended an AA meeting?	5	
4.	Have you ever lost friends, girlfriend or boyfriend because of drinking?	2	
5.	Have you ever gotten into trouble at work because of drinking?	2	
6.	Have you neglected your obligations, family, or work for 2 or more days in a row because you were drinking?	2	
7.	Have you ever had DTs, heard voices, or seen things that were not there after heavy drinking?	2	
8.	Have you ever gone to anyone to help stop your drinking?	5	
9.	Have you ever been in a hospital because of drinking?	5	
10.	Have you ever been arrested for drunk driving or driving after drinking?	2	

Modified from Pokorny AD, Miller BA, Kaplan HB: The brief MAST: a shortened version of the Michigan Alcoholism Screening Test, *Am J Psychiatr* 129:342-345, 1972. Reprinted with permission from the American Journal of Psychiatry, Copyright 1994. American Psychiatric Association.
*Alcoholism is indicated by a score of greater than 5. Test scores are determined by tallying values for answers that are on a progressive scale of 0, 2, and 5.

Research

SAMPLE/SETTING

The subjects included 826 older adults living in a small Eastern Ontario community. The participants were interviewed in their homes by nurses.

METHODS

This was a survey design of older adults living in a small community. Participants were interviewed for 30 to 210 minutes about self-reports of alcohol use, medication use, and health status. The study was part of a larger health promotion study.

FINDINGS

The study explored the relationship between drinking practices and self-reported health as identified through such indicators as overall rating of health and hospital admissions. Even when the variables of sex, age, education, and antidepressant medication use were controlled, the results indicated that the quantity and volume of alcoholic beverage intake significantly contributed to perceived health.

IMPLICATIONS

The findings assist in improving the assessment skills of nurses in identifying the risk level for alcohol use and abuse in older adults. Early identification will assist with early intervention for this population.

Graham K, Schmidt G: The effects of drinking on the health of older adults, *Am J Drug Alcohol Abuse* 24(3):465, 1998.

NURSING DIAGNOSES

The following list identifies nursing diagnoses that can be used for older adult clients who abuse substances:

- Impaired adjustment
- Anxiety
- Risk for altered body temperature
- Acute confusion
- Ineffective individual coping
- Altered family processes: alcoholism
- Altered nutrition: less than body requirements
- Self-care deficit
- Self-esteem disturbance
- Sleep pattern disturbance
- Impaired social interaction
- Risk for violence

Interventions

Multidisciplinary interventions are appropriate for all individuals overcoming substance abuse, since no single intervention is appropriate. Effective interventions attend to the multiple needs of individuals, not just their drug or substance use. Interventions must address medical, nursing, psychologic, social, vocational, and legal problems.

Interventions and treatment options include brief therapy, intensive outpatient or inpatient treatment, and residential treatment. Brief therapy is usually provided by a trained professional in a community drug treatment center. Goal setting, self-monitoring, and identifying high-risk situations are specific behaviors clients learn for stopping or reducing their substance abuse. Intensive outpatient programs allow clients to remain at home and continue working while they participate in treatment in an unrestricted setting for four to five hours every day. Intensive inpatient treatment occurs in the emergency department or acute care inpatient units for clients at risk for severe withdrawal symptoms, those who are psychiatrically disabled, and those who have not responded to less intensive treatment efforts. Residential treatment programs are downsizing and closing because third-party reimbursement is rapidly decreasing. Traditionally treatment lasted 7 to 21 days and offered a safe and structured environment for those who lacked social and vocational skills and drug-free social supports to be abstinent in a less restricted setting (Fontaine, 2003).

Older adults resist referrals to substance abuse programs and are more comfortable in senior-oriented programs. Some are unable or unwilling to leave their homes; thus programs should be specific for older adults and use special approaches such as slow-paced and emotionally supportive therapy instead of the confrontive style used with younger adults.

Complementary or alternative therapies (herbs and nutrients) and a nutritional supplement called SAMe (pronounced "sammy") may be effective in substance use disorders. SAMe (*S*-adenosylmethionine), a compound made by every cell in the body, helps produce dephenylchlorarsine, 5-hydroxytryptamine, and norepinephrine. SAMe may be used for depression that accompanies withdrawal from psychoactive substances. It may also reverse some of the effects of alcoholic hepatitis and cirrhosis (Brown and Gerbarg, 2000). Acupuncture is another effective treatment for substance use disorders. It eases the symptoms of withdrawal, decreases the intensity of cravings, and decreases the number of relapses. Acupuncture is a safe and relatively low-cost form of treatment.

Evaluation

The evaluation of the treatment of older adults who abuse substances consist of the assessment of safe detoxification, adherence to the sobriety treatment plan, and outpatient support. Detoxification is safe if a client has been weaned from the abused substance without seizures, delirium tremens (DTs), changes in vital signs, or other complications of withdrawal. Adherence is measured by noting if the client is abstaining from substance use and attending meetings (e.g., Alcoholics Anonymous [AA] or Narcotics Anonymous [NA]) and individual or family group sessions. Finally, outpatient support is assessed to determine if the client is maintaining the relationship with a sponsor. A *sponsor* is someone who can be a mentor and support the client during abstinence.

COMMONLY ABUSED SUBSTANCES IN OLDER ADULTS

Alcohol

Prevalence. Alcohol abuse can be difficult to assess as a result of the drug's legal status and socialization as a recreational activity in the United States. The difficulty in identifying alcohol abuse notwithstanding, the incidence of older adults identified as abusing alcohol is from 10% to 15% of the older adult population. The number of older adults who abuse alcohol may appear low, but the current cohort of older adults grew up during Prohibition and the Great Depression, when alcohol was illegal, was considered immoral, or was too expensive. The prevalence rate of alcohol abuse is projected to increase as younger generations move into old age. The pattern of illicit drug use may change and become a major concern (Colyar, 2003; Morris, 2001).

Some heavy drinkers with an early-onset addiction survive into old age; others are late-onset drinkers who may have started drinking in late middle age and began to exhibit health problems related to alcohol abuse as they move into older adulthood. Older adults who have used alcohol in the past without abuse or addiction may experience problems with alcohol consumption as changes occur in their bodies as a result of normal aging (e.g., decreased liver function, changes in body composition) (Morris, 2001).

Assessment. Older adults who abuse alcohol usually display symptoms of anxiety, nervousness, memory impairment, depression, blackouts, confusion, weight loss, and falls. In addition, physical examination of an older adult may indicate the effects of alcohol on the various body systems. Table 18-1 shows age-related and alcohol-related changes in select body systems of older adults. The nurse should assess carefully for the following signs and symptoms: impaired sensations in the extremities, poor coordination, confusion, facial edema, alcohol on the breath, liver enlargement, jaundice, ascites, trembling or fidgeting, lack of attention to personal hygiene, and poor eating habits. Secondary problems may include malnutrition, cirrhosis, compromised hepatic function, osteomalacia as a result of compromised metabolism of vitamin D, cardiomyopathy, atrophic gastritis, and decline in cognitive status, especially in regards to memory and information processing. Laboratory evaluation should include assessment of liver function, electrolytes, glucose, and magnesium, as well as an electrocardiogram study (Videbeck, 2004).

Again, alcohol abuse may not be accurately assessed in older adults because many alcohol abuse symptoms, such as falls, bruises, cardiovascular problems, hypertension, and memory problems, may resemble other medical disease processes. Therefore, if an older adult displays these symptoms, it is imperative that the nurse assess for the possibility of alcohol abuse in addition to medical illness and disease (see Boxes 18-2 and 18-3 for information regarding the medical and psychologic manifestations of substance abuse in older adults).

After obtaining a health history and conducting a physical examination, the nurse should begin to assess specifically for alcohol abuse. The CAGE, MAST, MAST-G, or BMAST screening tools can help the nurse identify the amount of alcohol a client uses and how often the client uses alcohol.

TABLE 18-1 Age- and Alcohol-Related Changes in Body Systems of Older Adults

AGE-RELATED CHANGE	CORRESPONDING ALCOHOL-RELATED CHANGE
Decline in liver function	Hepatotoxicity
Delayed neurologic conduction	Increase of Parkinson's disease symptoms, altered balance
Idiopathic tremors	Tremors related to withdrawal
Predisposition to falls	Predisposition to falls
Loss of short-term memory	Impairment of short-term memory
Decreased glucose tolerance	Inhibition of glucogenesis
Decreased secretion of hydrochloric acid	Impaired absorption of nutrients
Slowed peristalsis	Impaired absorption of nutrients
Decreased saliva production	Impaired absorption of nutrients
Increase in cholesterol levels and cardiovascular disease	Increased plasma triglycerides
Less efficient cardiovascular function	Risk of congestive heart failure
Increased incidence of arthritis and gout	Increased uric acid levels
Decline in immunologic competence	Increased susceptibility to infection

Developed from Coffey CE, Cummings JL: *Textbook of geriatric neuropsychiatry*, Washington, DC, 1994, American Psychiatric Press; Solomon K et al: Alcoholism and prescription drug abuse in the elderly: St Louis University Grand Rounds, *J Am Geriatr Soc* 41:57, 1993.

Input from family and friends should also be obtained. Family and friends may deny the problem; therefore it is imperative that the nurse obtain the alcohol use history in a detailed, nonjudgmental manner (Pokorny, Miller, and Kaplan, 1972; Knight and Mjelde-Mossey, 1995).

The nurse should be able to distinguish alcohol intoxication from alcohol withdrawal to apply the appropriate nursing interventions. Signs associated with alcohol intoxication include the scent of alcohol on the breath, slurred speech, lack of coordination, unsteady gait, nystagmus, impairment in attention or memory, and stupor or coma (APA, 2000). The DSM-IV-TR criteria for alcohol intoxication can be found in Box 18-7. Assessment of the signs and symptoms of alcohol withdrawal is essential to providing the appropriate treatment and preventing DTs and seizures. Indications of alcohol withdrawal are elevated blood pressure, elevated pulse, and autonomic hyperactivity (Box 18-8). In addition, fever; increased hand tremors; insomnia; nausea and vomiting; transient visual, tactile, or auditory hallucinations or illusions; psychomotor agitation; anxiety; and grand mal seizures may occur (APA, 2000). Withdrawal symptoms begin 4 to 12 hours after alcohol use has been stopped or reduced. Symptoms tend to peak 48 to 72 hours after a client's last drink (APA, 2000). It is important to assess older clients for the possibility of alcohol withdrawal if agitation, hallucinations, anxiety, or seizures develop 2 or 3 days after hospitalization (see Emergency Treatment box).

BOX 18-7 DSM-IV-TR Diagnostic Criteria for Alcohol Intoxication

A. Recent ingestion of alcohol
B. Clinically significant maladaptive behavioral or psychologic changes (e.g., inappropriate sexual or aggressive behavior, mood lability, impaired judgment, impaired social or occupational functioning) that developed during or shortly after alcohol ingestion.
C. One (or more) of the following signs, developing during or shortly after alcohol use:
   1. Slurred speech
   2. Incoordination
   3. Unsteady gait
   4. Nystagmus
   5. Impairment in attention or memory
   6. Stupor or coma
D. The symptoms are not a result of a general medical condition and are not better accounted for by another mental disorder.

From American Psychiatric Association: *Diagnostic and statistical manual of mental disorders (DSM-IV), text revision*, ed 4, Washington, DC, 2004, The Association. Reprinted with permission from the Diagnostic and Statistical Manual of Mental Disorders, Copyright 2000. American Psychiatric Association.

Interventions. Nursing interventions for older adult clients who abuse alcohol vary according to whether the client is in detoxification or rehabilitation. Nurses should observe and document signs of withdrawal, provide an environment of low stimulation (e.g., dim lights, quiet atmosphere), and initiate seizure precautions (e.g., padded side rails, bed in lowest position) during the detoxification process. In addition, the nurse should administer prescribed medications that are cross-tolerant to alcohol to minimize the symptoms associated with withdrawal and reduce the potential for seizures. The alcohol-abusing client is withdrawn by the administration of chlordiazepoxide (Librium), lorazepam (Ativan), oxazepam (Serax), or diazepam. Chlordiazepoxide is usually the medication of choice, since the intermediate half-life produces a smooth withdrawal with less sedation. Oxazepam is used in older adults with cirrhosis or those who have compromised

BOX 18-8 DSM-IV-TR Diagnostic Criteria for Alcohol Withdrawal

A. Cessation of (or reduction in) alcohol use that has been heavy and prolonged
B. Two (or more) of the following, developing within several hours to a few days after criterion A:
   1. Autonomic hyperactivity (e.g., sweating or pulse rate greater than 100)
   2. Increased hand tremor
   3. Insomnia
   4. Nausea or vomiting
   5. Transient visual, tactile, or auditory hallucinations or illusions
   6. Psychomotor agitation
   7. Anxiety
   8. Grand mal seizures
C. The symptoms in criterion B cause clinically significant distress or impairment in social, occupational, or other important areas of functioning.
D. The symptoms are not a result of a general medical condition and are not better accounted for by another mental disorder.

From American Psychiatric Association: *Diagnostic and statistical manual of mental disorders (DSM-IV), text revision,* ed 4, Washington, DC, 2004, The Association.

liver function (Fontaine, 2003). Nutritionally compromised older adults may require nutritional supplements; SAMe may reverse the effects of alcoholic hepatitis and cirrhosis (Fontaine, 2003). In alcoholism, acupuncture both relieves the symptoms of withdrawal and decreases the number of relapses (Bernstein, 2000).

During the rehabilitation stage, recommended nursing interventions include education; continued administration of medications; group, individual, and family therapy; and an introduction to the 12-Step Program. The nurse supports the client with education on the harmful effects of alcohol on the body, the effects of alcohol taken with prescription and nonprescription medications (Table 18-2), various methods to overcome potential triggers for future substance abuse, and various plans to maintain sobriety in the community setting. The nurse should also educate family members on the potential changes in family dynamics that may result from the client's sobriety. Encourage the recognition that chemical dependency is a family disease and abstinence is affected by the family process. All family members need relapse prevention education to help identify triggers to relapse and coping strategies for dealing with trigger events (Fontaine, 2003).

Home health nurses can assist older adult clients after discharge by assessing progress and encouraging participation in community activities. Kim A. Pittaway (1998) has developed a social support network exercise that can be helpful in assessing social support. Pittaway encourages clients to draw a circle and put the names of individuals and activities supportive to the client's sobriety inside the circle, then put

EMERGENCY TREATMENT

DELIRIUM TREMENS

The following nursing interventions should be implemented for clients who experience DTs:
1. Vital sign assessment
2. Provision of a safe environment (padded side rails, decreased stimulation)
3. Close observation
4. Administration of prescribed medications such as chlordiazepoxide, lorazepam, and diazepam for symptoms such as agitation; tremors; and increased temperature, blood pressure, and pulse.

names of individuals and activities not supportive to sobriety outside the circle. This exercise enables the client to visually conceptualize the social support network. The nurse should remember that individual, group, and family therapy is conducted by a trained therapist; the nurse may assist as appropriate.

Many pharmacologic interventions have proven to be effective in inhibiting drinking behaviors. Selective serotonin reuptake inhibitors (SSRIs) have been tested extensively for efficacy in alcohol dependence, mostly with disappointing results. If they work at all, they seem to do better in chronic, as opposed to early onset, alcoholics. Studies have shown that opioid antagonists, such as 50 mg of naltrexone (ReVia), work by interfering with reward pathways in the brain; efficacy depends on compliance. Disulfiram (Antabuse) should be used with caution because it interferes with the metabolism of a variety of medications such as warfarin and phenytoin, which may be part of the medication regimen of older adult clients (Finn, 2004).

Evaluation. The evaluation of the treatment of an older adult client who abuses alcohol includes determination of a safe detoxification, adherence to a treatment plan for sobriety, and outpatient support. Safe detoxification consists of weaning from alcohol without seizures, DTs, or other withdrawal complications. The nurse also assesses whether the client is adhering to the sobriety protocol of abstinence, attendance at AA meetings, and individual or family therapy. In addition, a continued relationship with the client's sponsor and the client's progress as reported by home health nurses provide the opportunity for evaluation of the client's transition back into the community (Fontaine, 2003).

Prescription Medications

Prevalence. Abuse of prescription medications among older adults is two to three times higher than in the general population. The number of medications prescribed is directly correlated to the risk of their inadvertent misuse. As a result,

TABLE 18-2 Effects of Alcohol on Selected Prescription Medications

CLASSIFICATION	EFFECTS
ANTIARRHYTHMICS	
Flecainide (Tambocor)	Individuals who have impaired liver function as a result of alcohol abuse require a lower dosage.
ANTIANGINALS	
Nitroglycerin (Nitrostat)	Can cause rapid lowering of blood pressure, resulting in weakness, dizziness, and fainting.
TRICYCLIC ANTIDEPRESSANTS	
Nortriptyline (Pamelor) Amitriptyline (Elavil) Imipramine (Tofranil)	Increases the effects of sedation, confusion, and tremors.
ANTIDIABETICS	
Oral (chlorpropamide [Diabinese])	Flushing of the face and body, as well as breathlessness, throbbing head and neck pain, difficulty breathing, nausea, vomiting, sweating, hypotension, weakness, dizziness, blurred vision, and confusion.
Insulin	Can lower blood sugar; a reduced dosage may be indicated.
BENZODIAZEPINES	
Chlordiazepoxide (Librium) Diazepam (Valium) Lorazepam (Ativan)	If the client uses these as antianxiety medications, alcohol may cause excessive depression, drowsiness, and difficulty breathing.
ANTICOAGULANTS	
Warfarin (Coumadin)	Decreases the effect of warfarin.
NARCOTIC ANALGESICS	
Propoxyphene (Darvon)	Causes drowsiness and sedation.
NONNARCOTIC ANALGESICS	
Acetaminophen (Tylenol)	Increases the probability of liver toxicity.
BRONCHODILATORS	
Theophylline (Bronkodyl)	May decrease the theophylline level.
ANTIHISTAMINES	
Diphenhydramine hydrochloride (Benadryl)	May cause excessive drowsiness and decreased concentration.

From Silverman HM: *The pill book,* ed 6, New York, 1994, Bantam Books.

the possibility of polypharmacy is high (Fig. 18-2) (see Chapter 22). *Polypharmacy* is the prescription, use, or administration of more medications than is clinically indicated. Prescription drugs commonly used by independent older people are cardiovascular medications, benzodiazepines, diuretics, cathartics, antacids, thyroidal medications, and anticoagulants. Benzodiazepine dependence is the most common, and the drugs may have been prescribed for long periods of time (Coogle, Osgood, and Parham, 2000). Because of the cross-tolerance between benzodiazepines and alcohol, there is an increased potential for cross-addiction. Most likely the nurse is the professional who, by taking the client's health history, identifies the possibility of prescription medication abuse. In addition, the rapport between the nurse and client allows the client to feel comfortable discussing medications with this health professional. Therefore it is imperative that the nurse assess for prescription medication abuse in older adults.

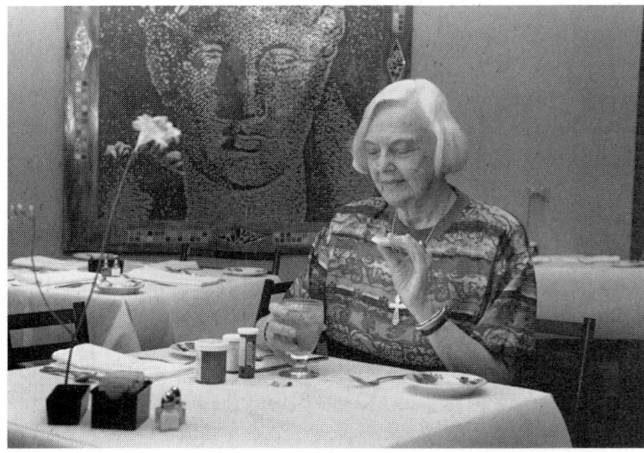

Fig. 18-2 Older adults' concurrent use of many prescription medications can lead to polypharmacy. (Courtesy Loy Ledbetter, St Louis, Mo.)

Assessment. Nursing assessment for prescription drug abuse in older adult clients is similar to the assessment used for alcohol abuse. The nurse should begin the assessment by taking a careful history, using the CAGE, MAST, BMAST, or MAST-G screening tools (Morton, Jones, and Manganaro, 1996). The nurse should remember to substitute the term *prescription medications* for *alcohol*. In addition, the nurse should assess for a tendency to repeatedly lose prescriptions or pills (e.g., "I threw it away by accident," "I didn't think I would use them so I flushed them down the toilet"), prescriptions from multiple physicians, frequent emergency room visits, strong preferences for particular medications (e.g., "Only X medication works for pain for me," "I'm allergic to Y, so I can only take X"), and above-average knowledge about medications, as well as whether the severity of the complaint matches the clinical presentation. Finally, the nurse should assess the client for signs associated with withdrawal, such as anxiety, irritability, insomnia, fatigue, headache, tremors, sweating, dizziness, decreased concentration, nausea, depression, and visual or tactile hallucinations (Fontaine, 2003).

Interventions. The interventions for prescription drug abuse are similar to the interventions associated with alcohol abuse. First, if prescription drug abuse is suspected, the nurse should ask the client or a family member to bring in all medications the client is currently using and inform the physician so a plan for safe detoxification can be established. The client should be informed that by bringing in all medications currently being used, he or she is ensuring that the health care team can develop a comprehensive care plan to address the client's physical needs. In addition, the physician can try to prevent any untoward drug interactions resulting from prescribing a new medication that is contraindicated because of an existing prescription. The nurse should then document any signs of withdrawal, provide an environment of low stimulation, and implement seizure precautions. In addition, the nurse should administer, on a planned reduction schedule, any medications prescribed to minimize withdrawal symptoms. Nutritional support interventions should also be implemented for clients with compromised nutritional status. Finally, after discussion within the multidisciplinary team, concerns about prescription drug abuse and treatment options such as AA, NA, or individual or group therapy should be presented to the client and family members in a client-care conference (Fontaine, 2003).

Evaluation. The evaluation of nursing interventions for an abuser of prescription medication includes assessment of safe detoxification, participation in a rehabilitation treatment plan, and decreased drug-seeking behaviors. The nurse should also observe and document the client's response to any teaching done by the nurse regarding appropriate medication use and the effects of medication misuse on the body.

Nonprescription Medications

Prevalence. Nonprescription medications are consumed by 70% of older adults. Older adults often use nonprescription medications to alleviate ailments because of the prohibitive costs of physician visits and prescription medications. Furthermore, older adult clients may not tell their physicians about the nonprescription medications they are taking; thus physicians may unknowingly prescribe medications that the client already consumes. The addition of nonprescription medications to an existing drug regimen may create serious adverse drug interactions. The nonprescription medications most commonly used by older adults are analgesics, laxatives, antacids, cough preparations, and vitamins (Elseviers and De Broe, 1998). The nurse should also assess older adult clients for the use of natural or herbal remedies because these may also cause serious adverse drug interactions (Nihart, 1998). For instance, a client who is taking an SSRI and is also taking St. John's wort is at increased risk for developing serotonin syndrome.

Assessment, Interventions, and Evaluation. The nurse should begin by assessing a client's nonprescription medication history. Clients should be asked how often they "pick something up at the grocery or drug store" for an ailment. Clients should also be asked what specific nonprescription medications they buy, for what ailment, and how much they use. Furthermore, during the physical assessment the nurse should note any signs of reactions or interactions related to nonprescription medications (Nihart, 1998; Silverman, 1994) (Table 18-3).

Nursing interventions include educating clients about the adverse effects of nonprescription medications. Education regarding the importance of contacting the physician or pharmacist before taking nonprescription medication is essential to reduce the number of unintentional medication interactions. Evaluation of interventions includes determining if the number of nonprescription medications has decreased and assessing the client's understanding of the effects of nonprescription medications (see Client/Family Teaching box).

Nicotine

Prevalence. Tobacco use is the single greatest cause of preventable disease and disability in the United States. Tobacco use is a risk factor in 6 of the 13 leading causes of death for older adults. In the United States alone approximately $50 billion is spent annually on medical costs that are attributed directly to tobacco use. Many tobacco users 50 years and older express a desire to quit; however, only those older adults with chronic illness tend to have the motivation to do so. Older adults who stop tobacco usage can increase life expectancy.

Assessment. The nurse should thoroughly assess a client's tobacco use pattern and also assess for signs of

TABLE 18-3 Reactions and Interactions of Nonprescription Medications in Older Adults

MEDICATION	EFFECTS
Aspirin	Large doses can alter blood coagulation time and cause irritation and bleeding in gastrointestinal system. Laboratory values may be altered. Sodium and chloride excretion can be altered, leading to toxicity. Alone or in combination with other drugs, it can lead to hypothermia. In older adults, lower doses may produce toxic effects, exhibited by confusion, irritability, diarrhea, and hearing and vision disturbances.
Laxatives	Laxatives interfere with absorption of nutrients and fluids and, with habitual use, create bowel dependency, diarrhea, weight loss, weakness, and fluid and electrolyte imbalances.
Antacids	Antacids may increase antibiotic absorption and decrease absorption of digitalis, psychoactive drugs, and nutrients. They interact with iron salts, propranolol (Inderal), and sodium polystyrene sulfonate (Kayexalate) to affect bone mineral metabolism and to cause bone weakening. They may also cause constipation or diarrhea and may delay gastric emptying, which prolongs absorption of medications.
Vitamins	Vitamins containing iron may contribute to constipation. Large amounts of vitamins A and D can cause toxicity. Large amounts of thiamine can adversely affect cardiovascular and nervous systems. Excessive niacin may result in abnormal liver function. Large quantities of vitamin C may cause kidney stones.
Sleeping medications	These may contain bromides, which contribute to confusion and may lead to dependence. Overuse may lead to depression and other neurologic symptoms. Many preparations contain scopolamine and should not be taken by people with glaucoma.
Cough mixtures	These may contain phenylpropanolamine, which may alter blood pressure or precipitate psychiatric symptoms.
Antihistamines	These may cause agitation and excitement.

Developed from Silverman HM: *The pill book,* ed 6, New York, 1994, Bantam Books.

Client/Family Teaching

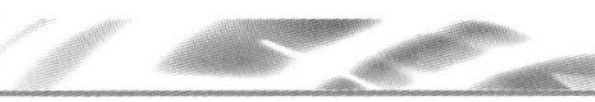

SAFE USE OF MEDICATIONS

Know the name, amount, type, frequency, purpose, and side effects of both the prescription and nonprescription drugs that you are taking.

If you see more than one care provider, always bring all your medications to every provider visit you make.

Never "borrow" medications from anyone else or share your medications with anyone else.

Make sure your family members can safely self-administer medications; adequate vision, memory, judgment, and coordination are all essential.

Supervise medication administration for those people who cannot safely self-administer. Talk to the doctor or advanced practice nurse about simplifying the medication regimen by using a daily dosing schedule set for once or twice a day.

Never mix alcohol with *any* medication.

Use a single pharmacy for filling all prescriptions to reduce the potential for interactions as well as abuse and misuse.

nicotine withdrawal. A helpful assessment tool is the Fagerstorm Nicotine Tolerance Quiz (Box 18-9). The client's responses allow the nurse to plan appropriate interventions. Older adult clients should also be monitored for signs of nicotine withdrawal such as depressed mood, insomnia, irritability, frustration, anger, anxiety, difficulty concentrating, restlessness, decreased heart rate, and increased appetite (APA, 2000). The DSM-IV-TR criteria for nicotine withdrawal can be found in Box 18-10.

Interventions and Evaluation. Nursing interventions for clients who abuse tobacco include monitoring for signs of withdrawal, administration of nicotine replacement, behavior modification, and education. The type of nicotine replacement used is determined by the physician and typically consists of 2 mg nicotine gum, 1 mg/hr nasal spray, or 15 mg nicotine transdermal patches (Fagerstorm et al, 1997). The treatment period lasts from 6 weeks to several months and reduces the craving for cigarettes by weaning the client from nicotine and preventing withdrawal symptoms. Clients who do not tolerate nicotine replacement may respond better to clonidine patches. Clonidine is an antihypertensive that blocks

BOX 18-9 The Fagerström Test for Nicotine Dependence

Question	Answer	Points
1. How soon after you wake up do you smoke your first cigarette?	Within 5 min	3
	6-30 min	2
	31-60 min	1
	After 60 min	0
2. Do you find it difficult to refrain from smoking in places where it is forbidden?	Yes	1
	No	0
3. Which cigarette would you hate most to give up?	The first one in the morning	1
	Any other	0
4. How many cigarettes per day do you smoke?	≤10	0
	11-20	1
	21-30	2
	≥31	3
5. Do you smoke more frequently during the first hours after waking than during the rest of the day?	Yes	1
	No	0
6. Do you smoke if you are so ill that you are in bed most of the day?	Yes	1
	No	0

Comments to Different Degrees of Dependence

POINTS	% SMOKERS	COMMENTS
0-1	20	Very low dependence Few and light withdrawal symptoms Seldomly need help to give up
2-3	30	A big group of smokers A certain degree of dependence Difficult withdrawal symptoms can occur Often manages to give up by themselves Medicines can be of help
4-5	30	A big group of smokers Over average dependence Withdrawal symptoms common Medicines often very helpful Risk for smoking related disorders is real
6-7	15	Strong dependence and withdrawal Likelihood to give up smoking poor High risk for smoking related disorders Medicines important, possibly combinations Higher dose, longer duration may be needed Support treatment important Depression and high alcohol intake common
8-10	5	Small group with extreme dependence Chances to give up are very small Handicapping withdrawal symptoms Support Tx and medicines essential, preferably over long time and in high dose Most will have smoking related disorders Anxiety, depression, pain and alcohol dependence common

the neurologic symptoms that produce nicotine withdrawal. Older adults should be treated with lower dosages than usual as a result of their increased susceptibility to this medication's effects (Cagle, 2004; Epping-Jordan, 1998).

Another medication that has been an effective aid to smoking cessation is 150 mg sustained-release bupropion (Zyban, Wellbutrin SR). The nurse should obtain a detailed client history regarding the existence of any seizure disorder because bupropion is contraindicated in such cases and another medication or technique should be recommended. Furthermore, the nurse must carefully assess the bupropion candidate for any history of alcohol abuse; these clients are at increased risk for seizures (Hurt, 1997; Evans, 2003) (see Research box).

A behavior modification technique that is successful in decreasing tobacco use and helping clients cope with stress is called Postpone/Inhale/Reconsider. The technique requires the client to take a cigarette from a pack, replace it, and wait for 5 minutes. During the 5-minute interval, the client places two

BOX 18-10 DSM-IV-TR Diagnostic Criteria for Nicotine Withdrawal

A. Daily use of nicotine for at least several weeks.
B. Abrupt cessation of nicotine use, or reduction in the amount of nicotine used, followed by four (or more) of the following signs:
   1. Dysphoric or depressed mood
   2. Insomnia
   3. Irritability, frustration, or anger
   4. Anxiety
   5. Difficulty concentrating
   6. Restlessness
   7. Decreased heart rate
   8. Increased appetite or weight gain
C. The symptoms in criterion B cause clinically significant distress or impairment in social, occupational, or other important areas of functioning.
D. The symptoms are not results of a general medical condition and are not better accounted for by another mental disorder.

From American Psychiatric Association: *Diagnostic and statistical manual of mental disorders (DSM-IV), text revision,* ed 4, Washington, DC, 2004, The Association. Reprinted with permission from the Diagnostic and Statistical Manual of Mental Disorders, Copyright 2000. American Psychiatric Association.

fingers to the mouth as if smoking and inhales slowly. After 5 minutes, the entire process is repeated. Clients have reduced smoking by 50% using this technique (Boschert, 2004).

The Nicotrol inhaler uses a plastic cartridge to deliver 4 mg of nicotine through a porous plug. The device is reported to have a 45% quit-rate after 6 weeks (Peck, 2004). The device aids in smoking cessation by an intensive inhalation regimen of 80 deep inhalations over 20 minutes, which releases approximately 4 mg of nicotine to the buccal mucosa, 2 mg of which is systemically absorbed. Box 18-11, based on the clinical practice guidelines developed by the Agency for Health Care Policy and Research (AHCPR), outlines some additional nursing interventions for helping clients quit tobacco use (Fiore et al, 1996). Older adult clients should also be educated on the effects that tobacco has on prescription medications (Table 18-4).

Evaluation of nursing interventions includes assessing for decreased use of tobacco, adherence to a plan to reduce tobacco use, and understanding of the effects that tobacco and nicotine have on the body.

Research

SAMPLE/SETTING

Participants in the study were 615 subjects with a history of smoking from a large Midwestern medical center. Smokers with current depression were excluded, unless they had a history of major depression.

METHODS

A double-blind, placebo-controlled study was conducted. The 615 subjects were randomly assigned to receive placebo, 100 mg bupropion, 150 mg bupropion, or 300 mg bupropion daily for 7 weeks. Follow-up counseling was provided after 8, 12, 26, and 52 weeks.

FINDINGS

The subjects who were continuously abstinent through the 52 weeks showed a mean weight gain inversely proportionate to the drug dose. No effects were observed on depression scores measured by the Beck Depression Inventory. Untoward side effects caused 37 subjects to terminate treatment.

IMPLICATIONS

A sustained-release form of bupropion is effective for smoking cessation and has minimum associated weight gain or side effects. Health care professionals should consider bupropion for smoking cessation treatment of older adult clients who have no comorbid alcohol abuse problems.

Hurt RD et al: A comparison of sustained-release bupropion and placebo for smoking cessation, *N Engl J Med* 337(17):1195, 1997.

Caffeine

Prevalence. Scant literature exists that indicates the exact prevalence of caffeine misuse and abuse among older adults. However, the general effects of caffeine on the major body systems have important implications for older adults. Caffeine stimulates the sympathetic nervous system, pro-

BOX 18-11 Intervention Plan for Clients Who Smoke

Ask every client at every visit about smoking.
Record a client's smoking status and vital signs on the medical chart.
Ask a client about his or her desire to quit and reinforce his or her intentions.
Motivate clients who are reluctant to quit.
Help motivated smokers set a quitting date.
Prescribe nicotine replacement therapy.
Help clients resolve problems that result from quitting; counseling may be helpful.
Encourage relapsed smokers to try quitting again.

Developed from Fiore MC et al: *Smoking cessation: clinical practice guideline no. 18,* AHCPR GPO stock no 017-026-00159-0, Rockville, Md, 1996, Agency for Health Care Policy and Research.

TABLE 18-4 Effects of Tobacco Use on Selected Prescription Medications

CLASSIFICATION	EFFECTS
ANTIARRHYTHMICS	
Flecainide (Tambocor)	Reduces flecainide serum concentrations. Smokers may require increased doses.
TRICYCLIC ANTIDEPRESSANTS	
Nortriptyline (Pamelor) Imipramine (Tofranil) Amitriptyline (Elavil)	May not be as responsive to usual dosages.
ANTIDIABETICS	
Insulin	May increase glucose concentrations. Change in tobacco usage may change insulin dosage.
BENZODIAZEPINES	
Chlordiazepoxide (Librium) Diazepam (Valium)	May be resistant to effects of benzodiazepines. May require larger doses to achieve sedative effects.
ANTICOAGULANTS	
Heparin	May require higher dosages.
NARCOTIC ANALGESICS	
Propoxyphene (Darvon)	May require higher dosages.
BRONCHODILATORS	
Theophylline (Bronkodyl)	May require higher dosages to achieve adequate serum levels, since elimination is increased with tobacco use.

From Hansten PD, Horn JR: *Drug interactions and updates*, Pennsylvania, 1990, Lea & Febiger.

ducing an increase in motor activity, muscle capacity, and alertness; a decrease in fatigue; rapid pulse; and slightly decreased basal metabolism. Therefore the nurse must be aware of signs of caffeine intoxication and caffeine withdrawal so that appropriate nursing interventions can be implemented, and so that symptoms of other physical illnesses are not masked.

Assessment. Caffeine abuse adds to the complexity of assessment of older adult clients. Many symptoms associated with caffeine intoxication mimic gastrointestinal, urinary, cardiovascular, and psychiatric disorders. The DSM-IV-TR criteria for caffeine intoxication are provided in Box 18-12. The assessment of the amount and type of caffeine consumed each day is beneficial in determining the possibility of caffeine abuse in an older adult. Table 18-5 indicates the amount of caffeine in various products. The nurse must also monitor for effects of caffeine withdrawal in older adults. The onset of withdrawal occurs 12 to 24 hours after discontinuation of caffeine use, peaks at 20 to 48 hours, and may last up to 1 week. Symptoms include headache, fatigue, depression, anxiety, nausea, vomiting, and muscle pain and stiffness (APA, 2000). APA studies indicate that caffeine withdrawal can be classified by diagnostic criteria. Box 18-13 provides the research criteria for caffeine withdrawal from the DSM-IV-TR.

Interventions and Evaluation. Nurses should document signs of caffeine withdrawal or intoxication and provide

BOX 18-12 DSM-IV-TR Diagnostic Criteria for Caffeine Intoxication

A. Recent consumption of caffeine, usually in excess of 250 mg (e.g., more than 2 or 3 cups of brewed coffee).
B. Five (or more) of the following signs, developing during, or shortly after, caffeine use:
   1. Restlessness
   2. Nervousness
   3. Excitement
   4. Insomnia
   5. Flushed face
   6. Diuresis
   7. Gastrointestinal disturbance
   8. Muscle twitching
   9. Rambling flow of thought and speech
   10. Tachycardia or cardiac arrhythmia
   11. Periods of inexhaustibility
   12. Psychomotor agitation
C. The symptoms in criterion B cause clinically significant distress or impairment in social, occupational, or other important areas of functioning.
D. The symptoms are not results of a general medical condition and are not better accounted for by another mental disorder (e.g., an anxiety disorder).

From American Psychiatric Association: *Diagnostic and statistical manual of mental disorders (DSM-IV), text revision,* ed 4, Washington, DC, 2004, The Association. Reprinted with permission from the Diagnostic and Statistical Manual of Mental Disorders, Copyright 2000. American Psychiatric Association.

appropriate comfort measures based on the symptoms exhibited. Some physicians may advocate gradual reduction of the use of Excedrin as the client withdraws from caffeine, since Excedrin contains 60 mg caffeine per tablet (see Table 18-5). The nurse may also encourage an older adult to switch from caffeinated to noncaffeinated products. In addition, the nurse should educate the client on the effects of caffeine on medications and should document the client's understanding of any such teaching.

FUTURE TRENDS

Currently little research identifies the prevalence of the abuse of such illicit drugs as cannabis, cocaine, and phencyclidine in the older adult population. There are sporadic case reports of cocaine abuse in older adults, but no studies indicate an exact prevalence. However, as the current middle-aged generation becomes the next older adult population, the prevalence of illicit drug use in this age-group is likely to rise. Therefore research regarding the prevention of illicit drug use and abuse in older adults must be developed now.

BOX 18-13 DSM-IV-TR

RESEARCH CRITERIA FOR CAFFEINE WITHDRAWAL

A. Prolonged daily use of caffeine
B. Abrupt cessation of caffeine use, or reduction in the amount of caffeine used, closely followed by headache and one (or more) of the following symptoms:
   1. Marked fatigue or drowsiness
   2. Marked anxiety or depression
   3. Nausea or vomiting
C. The symptoms in criterion B cause clinically significant distress or impairment in social, occupational, or other important areas of functioning.
D. The symptoms are not a result of the direct physiologic effects of a general medical condition (e.g., migraine, viral illness) and are not better accounted for by another mental disorder.

From American Psychiatric Association: *Diagnostic and statistical manual of mental disorders (DSM-IV), text revision*, ed 4, Washington, DC, 2004, The Association. Reprinted with permission from the Diagnostic and Statistical Manual of Mental Disorders, Copyright 2000. American Psychiatric Association.

TABLE 18-5 Caffeine-Containing Products

PRODUCT	CAFFEINE (mg)
Drip-brewed coffee (6 oz)	90 to 140
Instant coffee (6 oz)	60 to 100
Decaffeinated coffee (6 oz)	2 to 4
Tea (6 oz)	30 to 100
Cola (12 oz)	25 to 50
Hot cocoa (6 oz)	5 to 50
Chocolate bar (1 bar)	25 to 35
Excedrin (1 tablet)	60
Anacin (1 tablet)	30

Developed from Kaplan HI, Sadock BJ, Grebb JA: *Synopsis of psychiatry: behavioral sciences/clinical psychiatry*, ed 7, Baltimore, 1994, Williams & Wilkins.

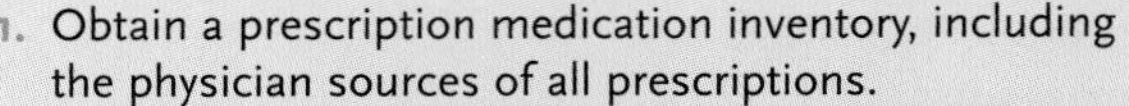

Home Care

1. Obtain a prescription medication inventory, including the physician sources of all prescriptions.
2. Mail-order prescription suppliers send large quantities of drugs to homebound older adults, which predisposes them to drug wasting, overdosing, and other misuse.
3. Assess the number of caregivers involved with medication administration to prevent overdosing and other administration errors.
4. Drug use patterns of homebound older adults, including the administration of prescription drugs, over-the-counter drugs, and home remedies, are influenced by cultural and ethnic health practices.
5. During assessment of homebound older adults, include an inventory of the use of caffeine, nicotine, and alcohol.
6. Assess high risk factors (e.g., social isolation, depression) that may predispose homebound older adults to substance abuse.
7. Assess for signs of substance abuse in homebound older adults.
8. Encourage caregivers to attend support groups such as AA to ease the burden of caring for a homebound older adult with a substance abuse problem.

SUMMARY

The prognosis for untreated substance abuse in older adults is poor because of physiologic and psychologic consequences. It is essential for nurses to identify substance abuse in older adults and to examine their own attitudes about substance abuse in this population. Early identification and intervention are essential to preventing misdiagnosis and ineffective, costly treatments. Nurses should recognize that older adults who abuse substances can be treated effectively. The first step in effective treatment is identification. After a problem is identified, a cost-effective treatment can be initiated to help an older adult return to a healthy lifestyle.

Key Points

- The age-related physiologic changes of altered absorption, distribution, metabolism, and excretion affect drug usage and place older adults at an increased risk for substance abuse and misuse.
- Psychologic changes, primarily a result of the numerous losses older adults may experience in a relatively short

time, place them at an increased risk for substance abuse and misuse.

- Sociologic changes such as decreased finances, transportation, and social support, as well as sociocultural factors such as gender and race, may place older adult clients at risk for substance abuse and misuse.
- The substances most often abused by the older adult population are alcohol, prescription medications, nonprescription medications, nicotine, and caffeine.
- The nurse should assess older adult clients for key medical and psychologic manifestations of substance abuse through their health history. Some of these key manifestations are falls, hypertension, memory loss, depressed mood, and social withdrawal.
- Screening tools such as the CAGE, MAST, MAST-G, and BMAST should be used to obtain a history of substance use in older adult clients.
- Key nursing interventions for substance abuse in older adult clients include assessing for signs of withdrawal; administering appropriate medications to provide safe detoxification; providing a safe environment; educating clients regarding harmful effects; and encouraging clients to participate in AA, NA, or individual, family, or group therapy.

Critical Thinking Exercises

1. Compare and contrast nursing assessment and interventions for prescription drug, nonprescription drug, and alcohol abuse. How are they similar and how are they different? How might assessment techniques be revised for the older adult population?
2. Analyze your own perceptions and attitudes regarding substance abuse in general. How do these perceptions and attitudes differ from those presented here in regard to substance abuse in the older adult population? What factors and assumptions contribute to these perceptions?
3. How might the DSM-IV-TR criteria for substance abuse be revised to specifically address the older adult population?

References

American Psychiatric Association: *Diagnostic and statistical manual of mental disorders, text revision,* ed 4, Washington, DC, 2000, The Association.

Bernstein KS: The experience of acupuncture for the treatment of substance dependence, *J Nurs Scholar* 32(3):267, 2000.

Boschert S: Five a's' in smoking cessation counseling, *Clin Psychiatr News* 32(1):43, 2004.

Brown RP, Gerbarg PL: Integrative psychopharmacology. In Muskin PR, editor: *Complementary and alternative medicine and psychiatry,* Washington, DC, 2000, American Psychiatric Press.

Cagle BB: Kicking butt: a review of smoking cessation strategies, *Adv Nurse Pract* 12(3):61, 2004.

Colyar M: Testing for drugs of abuse, *Adv Nurse Pract* 11(9):30, 2003.

Coogle CL, Osgood NJ, Parham IA: Addictions services, *Community Mental Health J* 36(2):137, 2000.

Eliopoulos C: *Gerontological nursing,* ed 5, Philadelphia, 2001, JB Lippincott.

Elseviers MM, De Broe ME: Analgesic abuse in the elderly: renal sequelae and management, *Drugs & Aging* 12(5):391, 1998.

Epping-Jordan MP et al: Dramatic decreases in brain reward function during nicotine withdrawal, *Nature* 393(6680):76, 1998.

Evans J: Mentholated cigarettes may be harder to quit for some, *Clin Psychiatr News* 31(12):31, 2003.

Fagerstorm KO et al: Aiding reduction of smoking with nicotine replacement medications: hope for the recalcitrant smoker? *Tobacco Control* 6(4):311, 1997.

Finn R: No magic bullets exist for alcohol dependence, *Clin Psychiatr News* 32(1):41, 2004.

Fiore MC et al: *Smoking cessation: clinical practice guideline no. 18,* AHCPR GPO stock no 017-026-00159-0, Rockville, Md, 1996, Agency for Health Care Policy and Research.

Fontaine KL: *Mental health nursing,* Upper Saddle River, NJ, 2003, Prentice Hall.

Hurt RD et al: A comparison of sustained-release bupropion and placebo for smoking cessation, *N Engl J Med* 337(17):1195, 1997.

Knight BG, Mjelde-Mossey LA: A comparison of the Michigan Alcoholism Screening Test and the Michigan Alcoholism Screening Test—Geriatric Version in screening for higher alcohol use among dementia caregivers, *J Mental Health Aging* 1(2):147, 1995.

Mayfield D, McLeod G, Hall P: The CAGE questionnaire: validation of a new alcoholism screening instrument, *Am J Psychiatr* 131:1121, 1974.

Meiner SE: Polypharmacy in the elderly: early intervention can prevent complications, *Adv Nurse Pract* 5(7):28-34, 1997.

Meiner SE: Polypharmacy at the end of life. In Matzo ML, Sherman DW, editors: *Quality nursing care for the older adult at the end of their live,* St Louis, 2004, Mosby.

Mohundro M, Ramsey L: Pharmacologic considerations in geriatric patients, *Adv Nurse Pract* 11(9):21, 2003.

Morris DL: Geriatric mental health: an overview, *J Am Psychiatr Nurses Assoc* 7(6):82, 2001.

Morton JL, Jones TV, Manganaro MA: Performance of alcoholism screening questionnaires in elderly veterans, *Am J Med* 101(2): 153-159, 1996.

Nihart MA: Medication interactions: food, drugs, and liver function, Psychiatric Nursing Conference, 181(a-f), Boston, Apr 16-18, 1998.

Peck P: Smoking cessation program post impressive quit rates, *Clin Psychiatr News* 32(1)41:2004.

Pittaway KA: *Social support network,* personal communication, July 21, 1998.

Pokorny AD, Miller BA, Kaplan HB: The brief MAST: a shortened version of the Michigan Alcoholism Screening Test, *Am J Psychiatr* 129:342, 1972.

Selzer ML: The Michigan Alcoholism Screening Test: the quest for a new diagnostic instrument, *Am J Psychiatr* 127:1653, 1971.

Silverman HM: *The pill book,* ed 6, New York, 1994, Bantam Books.

Videbeck S: *Psychiatric mental health nursing,* Philadelphia, 2004, Lippincott, Williams & Wilkins.

19 Cancer

LINDA L. STEELE, PhD, APRN, ANP-BC, and JAMES R. STEELE, MSN, RN, ANP-C

Learning Objectives

On completion of this chapter, the reader will be able to:

1. Describe the physiologic and environmental factors that contribute to the increased risk of cancer in older adults.
2. Identify the malignancies most commonly found in older adults.
3. Discuss the nurse's role in cancer prevention and early detection.
4. Apply principles of cancer treatment to older adults.
5. Discuss the nursing management of symptoms experienced by older adults receiving cancer treatment.
6. Discuss unique dimensions of psychosocial problems encountered by older adults with cancer.
7. Identify ethical concerns related to the care of older adults with cancer.
8. Identify appropriate resources for older adults with cancer.

Cancer is a disease of aging. The risk of cancer rises steadily beyond middle age and continues to rise thereafter. After heart disease, cancer is the second leading cause of death for adults over 65 years of age. Although individuals over age 65 represented about 12.4% of the population in the year 2000, they accounted for an estimated 60% of all cancer cases and 69% of all cancer deaths; thus a very small percentage of the population bears a disproportionate burden of the disease. In industrialized nations the growth of the older adult population increased sevenfold from 1900 to 1970; in the United States there was a 12% increase in older adults between 1990 and 2000, while the general population increased only 2.5 times. Among the older population, those 85 and over showed the highest percentage increase. By the year 2030, persons over age 65 will represent more than 18% of the population. Since the cancer burden is carried disproportionately by older adults, the incidence can be expected to rise as the population ages (US Census Bureau, 2000).

INCIDENCE

Cancer incidence refers to the number of new cases in a given time period—usually a year—in the general population. The leading types of cancer in men are prostate, lung, and colorectal. The leading types of cancer in women are breast, lung, and colorectal. Incidence differs from mortality. Mortality is the rate of deaths per number of incidences. Many persons survive cancer, and some cancers have relatively high incidence rates and relatively low death rates. For example, the incidence of breast cancer is 13% in women, whereas the death rate is 18% (American Cancer Society, 2004a). In contrast, the incidence of lung cancer in women is 12%, whereas the death rate is 22%. In other words, although more women die from breast cancer overall, fewer women who get lung cancer survive that disease. The National Cancer Institute (2003b) estimates that approximately 7.4 million Americans alive today have a history of cancer. Of the survivors, some may be completely cured, whereas others have some evidence of disease.

Cancer accounts for 22.9% of all deaths. Between 1950 and 2001 death rates from cancer have remained stable (Centers for Disease Control and Prevention, 2004). The incidence of cancer increases continually after the first decade of life; the older a person becomes, the more likely he or she is to develop cancer. Cancer incidence peaks at about 80 years of age, at which time the overall incidence and mortality from all forms of cancer begin to decline for both men and women. This decline after age 80 has been attributed to a variety of influences, including underreporting, underdiagnosing, and natural selection, meaning fewer cancer-prone individuals survive into and beyond the eighth decade (Yancik, 1997).

Racial and Ethnic Patterns

Like the rest of the population in the United States, the aging population is becoming more diverse. In addition to whites of European descent, four other main racial and ethnic groups are present in the American population: African-Americans, Hispanic Americans, Asian/Pacific Islanders, and Native Americans. Cancer affects Americans of all racial and ethnic groups; however, the incidence of cancer does demonstrate patterns according to racial and ethnic origins. African-Americans have higher overall incidence rates than whites, whereas Hispanic Americans and Native Americans have lower incidence rates overall (Tables 19-1 and 19-2).

TABLE 19-1 Cancer Incidence Rates (Number of New Cases Each Year)*

GROUP	BOTH SEXES	MALES	FEMALES
African-American	521.7	696.8	406.3
White	479.8	555.9	431.8
Asian/Pacific Islander	341.7	392.0	306.9
Hispanic/Latino	352.1	419.3	312.2
American Indian/ Alaskan Native	239.6	259.0	229.2

From National Cancer Institute 2003b.
*Statistics are for 1996-2000, are adjusted to the 2000 U.S. standard million population, and represent the number of new cases of invasive cancer per year per 100,000 of both sexes, males, and females, respectively.

TABLE 19-2 Cancer Death Rates (Number of Deaths Each Year)*

GROUP	BOTH SEXES	MALES	FEMALES
African-American	257.1	356.2	198.6
White	199.1	249.5	166.9
Asian/Pacific Islander	124.5	154.8	102.0
Hispanic/Latino	137.9	176.7	112.4
American Indian/ Alaskan Native	138.0	172.3	115.8

From National Cancer Institute, 2003b.
*Statistics are for 1996-2000, are adjusted to the 2000 U.S. standard million population, and represent the number of deaths per year per 100,000 of both sexes, males, and females, respectively.

Racial and ethnic group age cohorts demonstrate different patterns of cancer incidence. Older Japanese immigrant women demonstrate a lower incidence of breast cancer than second- and third-generation Japanese women born in America. Age is an important factor, especially when evaluating environmental influences where persons of the same race and ethnicity had different exposures as children; any examination of patterns of cancer among racial or ethnic groups should include age and environmental considerations.

Because the incidence of cancer has demonstrated patterns by race and ethnicity, both these factors are important in determining which groups are at risk. When examining incidence by race, several cautions are in order. First, race and ethnicity are both prone to misclassification. The U.S. Census Bureau has defined race and ethnicity (Box 19-1), but there is no accepted scientific definition for race. Persons with mixed-race parents lack a single classification. Second, as demonstrated by Freeman (1989) in his landmark investigation of genetics and cancer, there is no known genetic basis to explain the major racial differences in cancer incidence. Third, race and ethnicity may be viewed as a rough indicator for certain lifestyle and environmental factors. Race and ethnicity are highly correlated with socioeconomic status. Persons living in poverty tend to lack education, employment, adequate housing, good nutrition, preventive health practices, and access to health care. Within any one race or cultural group, economic status is the major determinant for cancer risk and outcome. Economic status as a risk factor for cancer is demonstrated globally. For most cancers, there are notable geographic variations in incidence rates that reflect socioeconomic differences, particularly differences between developing and developed countries (Hansen, 1998). Freeman (1989) concluded that correcting poverty among groups of people, regardless of their race or ethnic origin, would lead to decreased cancer incidence and increased survival.

The leading cancers among white men are prostate, lung, colorectal, urinary bladder, and non-Hodgkin's lymphoma. White men have higher urinary bladder cancer incidence rates than men of any other racial or ethnic group, the rates being almost two times higher than those of Hispanic men, who have the second highest rates. U.S. whites had higher rates for cancers of the urinary bladder, brain and central nervous system, and testes and for lymphomas and leukemias. Breast cancer rates among white women are higher than those for women of any other racial or ethnic group. Because most Americans are white, the leading cancer sites for whites are also the leading sites for the United States as a whole (American Cancer Society, 2004a).

African-American men have a higher overall cancer incidence rate than any other racial or ethnic group in America. In addition, African-American men had higher cancer rates than white men for multiple myeloma and for cancers of the lung, oral cavity, prostate, esophagus, stomach, and larynx. Rates for lung and colorectal cancers are higher among African-American women than among women of any other racial or ethnic group except Alaskan Natives. In the United States the incidence rate for all cancers combined was 20% higher among African-American men than white men, whereas the incidence rate for all cancers combined was 5% higher for white women than African-American women (American Cancer Society, 2004a).

Cancer incidence rates vary considerably among the subgroups of Asian/Pacific Islanders. Although Asian/Pacific Islanders experience lower rates overall compared with other groups, they do experience higher death and incidence rates for certain cancers, especially liver and stomach cancer for both sexes. For men, the top three sites among Chinese, Filipinos, Hawaiians, and Japanese are prostate, lung, and colorectal; among Koreans the top sites are lung, stomach, and colorectal; among Vietnamese the top sites are lung, liver, and prostate. Stomach cancer rates among Korean men and liver cancer rates among Vietnamese men are higher than those among men of any other racial or ethnic group. The top three cancer sites among Asian/Pacific Islander women are breast, lung, and colorectal with the following exceptions: the stomach is the leading site among Japanese and Korean women, and the cervix is the leading site among Vietnamese women. Cervical cancer incidence rates among Vietnamese women are more than 21/2 times higher than for any other racial or ethnic group (American Cancer Society, 2004a).

BOX 19-1 U.S. Census Bureau Definitions of Race and Ethnicity

RACE/ETHNICITY	DEFINITION
African-American	Persons having their origins in any of the black racial groups of Africa
Asian/Pacific Islander	Persons having their origins in any of the original peoples of the Far East, Southeast Asia, the Indian subcontinent, or the Pacific Islands. This group is very diverse, including individuals from at least 24 ethnic populations who speak more than 30 major languages or dialects.
Native American	Persons who are American Indians and Alaskan Natives, having their origins in the original peoples of North America, and who maintain cultural identification through tribal affiliations or community recognition. American Indians and Alaskan Natives represent more than 500 tribes, each with unique cultural, genetic, and sociodemographic characteristics.
Caucasian [white]	Persons having their origins in any of the original peoples of Europe, North Africa, or the Middle East. Caucasians are the largest racial group in America.
Hispanic	Persons having their origins in Mexico, Puerto Rico, Cuba, Central or South America, or another Spanish culture, regardless of race. By this definition, Hispanics are present in every racial group.

From US Census Bureau: *Profile of general demographic characteristics,* Washington, DC, 2000, US Department of Commerce.

Information on cancer incidence among Native Americans is only available for Native Americans from New Mexico and for Alaskan Natives. Alaskan Natives have the highest cancer incidence rates among any racial group for the following sites: oral cavity and pharynx, colon and rectum, cervix uteri, and kidney and pelvis. Alaskan Natives have relatively high incidence of cancers of the esophagus, stomach, liver, gallbladder, and pancreas. According to the New Mexico Tumor Registry Surveillance epidemiology and end results program (SEER) data (2003b), American Indians who live in New Mexico and Arizona have excessive incidence rates for stomach, cervix uteri, liver, and gallbladder cancer. American Indians have the highest gallbladder cancer incidence rate of any racial group, such as blacks, whites, or Hispanics (National Cancer Institute, 2003b).

The leading cancer sites for Hispanic men and women are the same as those for whites—prostate, breast, lung, and colorectal. However, incidence rates among Hispanics for each of these cancers are at least 30% lower than the rates for whites. Other cancers commonly diagnosed among Hispanics include cancers of the urinary bladder and stomach in men and cancers of the uterus and cervix in women. Cervical cancer rates among Hispanic women are highest of any group other than Vietnamese women (American Cancer Society, 2004a) (see Cultural Awareness box).

AGING AND ITS RELATIONSHIP TO CANCER

Age is consistently considered the most important determinant of cancer risk. But what is it about the aging process that predisposes a person to cancer?

Biologic aging is a process that occurs naturally in adult life and results in changes in both structure and function. Although it occurs at a variable pace, the aging process creates a pattern of changes that predictably unfolds over a course of time—a biologically programmed life span. Each species has a unique programmed life span. For humans that life span is around 100 years, which is to say that it is biologically improbable that a human will live much beyond 100 years. On the other hand, life expectancy is the number of years an individual can be expected to live, based on averages within a population group born during a particular period and traced through time or cohort. Life expectancy is influenced primarily by external, environmental factors. For example, a cohort of persons living their childhood in conditions of famine and malnutrition might have a different life expectancy from a cohort that did not experience childhood malnutrition. Both biologically programmed life span and environmentally influenced life expectancy are important concepts when considering the relationship between aging and cancer.

The relationship between aging and cancer begins at the cellular level, where two types of cells should be considered: replicating cells and postreplicating cells. Cells show a limited replicating potential—that is, cells divide only a limited number of times before entering a phase in which they can no longer reproduce. At that point, cells survive in a senescent postreplicating state; they continue to metabolize and synthesize nutrients necessary for survival, except deoxyribonucleic acid (DNA) synthesis ceases and replication does not occur. Human cells are estimated to undergo approximately 50 population replications before entering the senescent postreplicating phase. Although cell-replicating capacity generally decreases with age, several age-related processes involve accelerated replication, or hyperproliferation. Prostatic hypertrophy, atherosclerosis, and cancer are examples of disease states among older adults thought to be influenced by accelerated cellular replication.

The aging cell has a tendency toward aberration or abnormalcy as it replicates. Aberrant cell growth is related to failure of growth control mechanisms, which leads to less cell regulation during replication. Cancer occurs more commonly in replicating than in nonreplicating cell groups, which suggests that changes in internal cellular control mechanisms

Cultural Awareness

CULTURAL CONSIDERATIONS IN CANCER

Patterns of cancer distribution among U.S. population groups vary according to racial and ethnic background. These patterns challenge nurses and other health care providers to discover explanations for the large differences in cancer incidence, mortality, and survival among the federally defined minority groups when compared with the white population.

African-Americans have the highest overall rates of cancer incidence and cancer mortality of any U.S. population group. The overall 5-year relative survival rate for cancer in African-Americans is 12% below that of whites. Of the 25 primary cancer sites for which survival data are available, African-Americans have lower survival rates for all but three cancer sites (ovary, brain, and multiple myeloma) (National Cancer Institute, 2003a).

Differences in survival status seem to be substantially based on socioeconomic status and the overrepresentation of an ethnic group in the lower categories of socioeconomic status. Socioeconomic status affects access to health services; nutritional status; immune status and function; educational level; employment; cancer prevention attitudes, awareness, and practices; and acceptance of cancer as a real and potential threat. In turn, all of these affect survival and, ultimately, mortality.

Higher Incidence Rates According to Location of Cancer

AFRICAN-AMERICANS	HISPANICS	ASIAN/PACIFIC ISLANDERS (VARIES BY GROUP)
Prostate	Prostate	Liver
Lung and bronchus	Breast	Stomach
Breast	Colon and rectum	Breast
Colon and rectum	Lung and bronchus	Colon and rectum

NATIVE AMERICANS (HIGHLY VARIABLE AMONG THE GREATER THAN 500 TRIBES)

Lung (Oklahoma Indians)
Gallbladder (Southwest Indians)
Liver (Alaskan Natives)

give rise to cancer. External or environmental factors are believed to contribute to decreased regulation of cell growth by causing cell damage and then promoting the replication of damaged cells (Cohen, 1994).

The process of cancer growth is believed to occur in three stages: initiation, promotion, and progression (Fig. 19-1). *Initiation* results from intense or prolonged exposure to an external agent that causes mutation of genetic material. The mutations are nonlethal, but they are passed on to future cell generations during replication. An initiated cell will continue to produce the mutations with each cell replication; however, the mutations alone are not enough to lead to cancer. Cancerous cell growth begins when an initiated cell encounters a promoting agent; thus the second stage of cancer development is called *promotion*. Promoting agents are external or environmental agents. A number of substances may be considered promoters of cancer in humans; they may come from a variety of sources, including air, water, or soil, and they may be naturally occurring or chemically produced. Promoting agents share the common property of inducing replication of an initiated mutant cell, thus transforming the initiated cell into a cancer cell. The promoting agent cannot cause cellular transformation unless the cell has been initiated, regardless of the intensity of exposure to the promoting agent. Promotion is dose dependent in its effect, and although promotion can transform a cell immediately after initiation, promotion is thought to be most successful when it involves repeated exposure to an initiated cell. Prevailing thought is that initiation is irreversible, whereas promotion is reversible. This belief has been demonstrated clinically in tobacco smokers: once the exposure to the promoter (tobacco) is withdrawn, the incidence of cancer is reduced.

Progression is the third stage of cancer growth. This stage may be subdivided into transformation, clonal progression, and metastasis. Transformation involves conversion of initiated cells to cancer cells. Clonal progression involves further growth of the small cluster of transformed cancer cells. The transformed cells contain mutated genetic material. As the transformed cells replicate, the progeny cells show more and more genetic abnormalities. Unless detected and treated, the cluster of cancer cells will continue to replicate in a somewhat unregulated fashion, ultimately metastasizing. Metastasis involves a change in location of the cancer cells from one organ or part of the body to another that is not directly connected.

Within normal human DNA material are genes that code cell-growth–regulating substances. Oncogenes, thought to be part of normal human DNA material, are genes that produce abnormal codes for growth-regulating substances. Oncogenes are believed to play a role in the development of cancers because, once activated, oncogenes interfere with normal physiologic regulation of cell growth. Oncogene activation is believed to result in excessive production of cell-growth–reg-

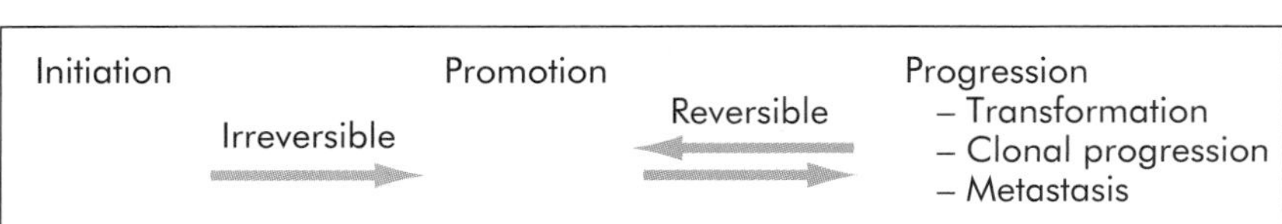

Fig. 19-1 Stages of cancer growth.

ulating substances. Because oncogenes can cause improper regulation of cell growth, they are capable of causing cancerous transformation in normal cells. The mechanism controlling oncogene activation is unclear; however, activation appears to be tightly controlled. The immune system is believed to play an important role in controlling oncogenes.

As a person ages, his or her immune function declines. Although immunogenic tumors can be more aggressive in older adults, solid tumors influenced by hormones are usually less aggressive. Environmental influences over the course of time are likely to have an influence over older adults related to prolonged exposure to carcinogens. Heredity may also contribute to cancer etiology. The older adult may be at increased risk of developing cancer because of mutations in DNA repair or metabolic detoxification, in addition to exposure to environmental carcinogens. Aging may also predispose older adults to increased cancer risks if they have inherited mutated genes. It remains unknown whether cancer in older adults is caused by any one of these factors or a combination of them (Coleman, Hutchins, and Goodwin, 2004).

Several mechanisms have been proposed to explain the way in which the aging process directly influences the cancerous transformation of cells (Box 19-2):

- Aging increases the duration of exposure to substances that may act as promoting agents. Since the effects of promoters are dose dependent, older adults can accumulate a significant dose over the decades. Also, cellular transformations and progression of cancer cells occur over time. Cancer cells grow at various rates, and in some cases significant time is needed for the small cluster of cancer cells to grow large enough to cause signs and symptoms.
- Aging cells demonstrate a tendency toward abnormal growth. Aged cells are more vulnerable to damage; thus aging likely increases the susceptibility of cells to substances that cause genetic mutations.
- Once an aged cell is damaged by an initiating substance, it is more difficult to repair.
- Oncogene activation might be increased in older persons, resulting in increased loss of regulation of cell growth and the development of cancer cells.
- Decreased immune surveillance, or immunosenescence, may contribute to increased development of cancers and their progression, although the evidence on the role of the immune system in the development of cancer is inconclusive (Crawford and Cohen, 1987; Miller, 1991; Pfeifer, 1997a).

BOX 19-2 Stages of Cancer Growth and Influence of Aging on Cancer Development

STAGE OF CANCER GROWTH	INFLUENCE OF AGING ON CANCER DEVELOPMENT
Initiation	Longer time for exposure to agents that may cause cell mutations Aged cells more vulnerable to damage
Promotion	Longer time for exposure to dose-dependent cancer-promoting agents Aged cells less able to repair damage
Progression	Longer time for transformed cells to grow into cancer clusters Aged immune system resulting in decreased surveillance Increased oncogene activation, resulting in greater misregulation of cell growth Continued cluster growth for a time sufficient for development of clinical signs and symptoms

Aging and Cancer Prevention

The risk of cancer, either increased or decreased, frequently reflects changes in the habits of a particular birth cohort. Since most cancers are the result of a lifelong exposure, the risk of developing malignant disease after age 65 is probably already determined by the time one reaches that age. Frequently, cancer risk is similar for a given birth cohort within specific environmental boundaries. Although it appears difficult to undo or reverse the cellular damage sustained in younger years, prolonged exposure to promoting agents is nonetheless needed for the initiated cells to be transformed. If exposure to promoters can be avoided or reduced and antipromoters can be used, then cancerous transformation may not take place or may be delayed.

Interference with the promotion stage of cancer would seem to offer the best prospects for cancer prevention. Only recently has research included the search for interventions that halt the promotion phase. It is currently believed that fresh fruits and vegetables may contain antipromoters. Secondary to this, various vitamins and minerals contained in foods are being examined for their effects on the promotion phase. Older adults should be encouraged to consume the recommended daily requirements of fruits and vegetables, since dietary habits may be beneficial in halting the cancer process. In addition, evaluation of environmental risk factors can lead to specifically targeted education and screening programs among selected high-risk cohorts.

COMMON MALIGNANCIES IN OLDER ADULTS

Breast Cancer

Breast cancer is the most common neoplasm in women, increasing in incidence with advancing age. The incidence of breast cancer is rising, although the death rate has been declining since the early 1990s. The disease will develop in 1 in 8 women who live to be 85, which is an approximate doubling of the incidence since 1970. According to the World Health Organization, more than 1.2 million women were diagnosed with breast cancer worldwide in 2004. The American Cancer Society estimates that in 2004 approximately 215,990 women in the United States were diagnosed with invasive breast cancer. Another 59,390 women were diagnosed with breast cancer in situ. The incidence rate of breast cancer increased by approximately 4% during the 1980s but leveled off to 100.6 cases per 100,000 women in the 1990s. The death rates from breast cancer also declined significantly between 1992 and 2004, with the largest decreases among younger women. Experts attribute this decline in death rates to more effective and earlier screening techniques and advances in the treatment of the disease (American Cancer Society, 2004a).

Of all breast cancer cases, 80% occur in women older than age 50. Breast cancer is the leading cause of death in women ages 55 to 74. Late-stage diagnosis is a serious concern for older adults. The primary presenting symptom is a lump in the breast; however, approximately 10% of women show symptoms of metastasis as the first indication of disease. The lung, liver, bones, and adrenal glands are predominant metastatic sites for breast cancer. Specific symptoms are related to the metastatic site and extent of disease (AGS, 2000).

Although all women are at risk for developing breast cancer, the older a women is, the greater are her chances of developing breast cancer. Breast cancer is more common in white women than in other racial or ethnic groups, but according to the most recent data, death rates are continuing to decline in white women. According to the surveillance, epidemiology, and end results (SEER) program of the National Cancer Institute (2003b), white Hawaiian and African-American women have the highest incidence of invasive breast cancer in the United States. Korean, American Indian, and Vietnamese have the lowest incidence of invasive breast cancer in the United States. African-American women have the highest death rate from breast cancer and are more likely to be diagnosed with a later stage of breast cancer in age-groups 55 to 69. However, in the 70-year-old age-group the death rate is higher for white women than for African-American women (American Cancer Society, 2004a) (see Cultural Awareness box).

Cultural Awareness

CULTURAL CONSIDERATIONS IN BREAST CANCER SCREENING

Mammography screening for early detection of breast cancer has been shown to be an effective method for reducing mortality in older women. Some women from ethnic minority groups have a high prevalence rate, whereas individuals from other groups such as middle-class whites have low prevalence rates. A study of women ages 75 and older by Caplan, Wells, and Haynes (1992) using national data found that 83.5% of African-American women, 93.2% of Hispanic women, and 75% of white women have never had a mammogram.

Among women ages 75 and older, African-American and Hispanic women had markedly lower rates of clinical breast examination in the past year (23.4% and 20.5%, respectively) than white women (35.2%). The most common reasons for not having a mammogram among African-American women ages 65 and older was that the physician or nurse practitioner did not recommend one. For Hispanic and white women in this age-group, the most common reason was that a mammogram was not perceived as necessary.

Barriers to early detection of breast cancer among women from ethnic minority groups were identified as the following: inaccurate knowledge of breast cancer and early screening, low awareness of the necessity for early detection, lack of health insurance to cover screening mammograms, lack of reimbursement to health care providers for clinical breast examinations and health teaching for early detection, and virtually no data on knowledge and attitudes of older adult Asian American and Native American women.

The researchers identified the following strategies to reduce barriers to early detection of breast cancer among older African-American and Hispanic women:

- Educate health care providers about the necessity of early breast cancer detection and their role in recommending it to clients.
- Conduct research to identify culturally appropriate messages and intervention strategies for each of the at-risk groups to influence their early detection behaviors.
- Use the media to increase knowledge and promote positive early detection practices among older women from culturally diverse backgrounds.

Risk Factors. The risk of breast cancer increases with age. Dominant risk factors appear to be related to duration and intensity of exposure to hormonal influences, especially estrogen, and include early menarche (before age 12), late menopause (after age 55), lengthy exposure to post-menopausal estrogen, recent use of oral contraceptives, and never having given birth or having first given live birth at a late age (after age 35) (Reigle, 2000). The highest incidence of breast cancer is in women ages 50 to 59. A first peak of incidence occurs between ages 45 and 49, when women are either premenopausal or menopausal. The high incidence in this age-group is thought to be related to ovarian estrogen. A second peak of incidence occurs in women between ages 65 and 69, most of whom are postmenopausal. The second peak appears to be related to an imbalance of adrenal estrogen. Given these findings, breast cancer appears to be two separate diseases differentiated by menopausal status. Although hormones are not inherently mutagenic, they may act as initiators or promoters by altering cell reproduction and growth (Bergkvist et al, 1989; Pfeifer, 1997a).

A major advance in understanding breast cancer is that the disease has a genetic basis. Approximately 5% to 10% of breast cancers are hereditary. The genes involved in most inherited breast cancers are BRCA1 and BRCA2. These are tumor-suppressor genes that also serve to protect and preserve DNA. Up to 40% of inherited breast cancers are due to mutations in BRCA1, and mutations in BRCA2 are responsible for up to 30% of inherited cancer (Cummings and Olopade, 1998).

High-fat diets and obesity have been suggested as risk factors, although the evidence is inconclusive. In animal studies the proliferation of breast tissue may be altered by changes in estrogen levels and pituitary and thyroid function, which are all sensitive to dietary intake (London and Willett, 1989). The risk associated with obesity may differ according to menopausal status and is thought to be associated with the metabolism of estrogen. Additional risk factors associated with breast cancer include pesticide and other chemical exposure, alcohol consumption, and physical inactivity (Knobf, 1996).

Signs and Symptoms. When a biopsy is performed, the majority of breast lumps are found to be benign. Benign breast lumps are soft, mobile masses with regular borders. Malignant lumps are hard and fixed, with irregular borders, and are sometimes described as frozen peas. Nipple retraction or elevation may be caused by tumor fixation involving underlying tissues. Skin dimpling may also be present, usually because of invasion of the tumor into the ligaments and fixation on the chest wall. Localized erythema and warmth may be present and are related to inflammation. Characteristically, edema appears as "orange peel" skin. Pain is not usually a presenting symptom, unless the disease is locally advanced.

Early Detection. Breast self-examination (BSE) should be performed monthly by all women over age 20. Roughly 90% of all breast lumps are detected by women or their partners. Premenopausal women should perform the examination at each menstrual cycle. Postmenopausal women should select a consistent date, such as the first day of the month. Nurses caring for older women should provide ongoing educational opportunities for women to learn about BSE, and consistent reinforcement to encourage performance. Older women, while having the highest incidence of breast cancer, have been shown to have the least knowledge about the importance of breast examination. The percentage of those women claiming lack of knowledge is highest among minorities. Public and professional education is available from several cancer organizations, including the American Cancer Society and the National Cancer Institute.

Mammography is able to detect breast tumors before they present physical findings. A tumor must be about 10 mm to be palpable. A 10 mm tumor contains about 10^9, or 1 billion cells. Mammography screening can detect 10^7 cells. Mammography screening is more accurate for older women because breast tissue is less dense than that of younger women, making tumors easier to visualize. The American Cancer Society recommends mammography screening every 2 years for women between ages 40 and 49 and annually for women ages 50 and older (American Cancer Society, 2004b). Although Medicare pays for mammography screening every year, the use of mammography by women over age 70 remains low, particularly among minority populations.

Treatment. Breast cancer treatment should be multidisciplinary. Surgery—either lumpectomy or modified radical mastectomy—is indicated for removal of the primary tumor. Because breast cancer metastasizes early in the course of the disease, the ipsilateral (on the same side of the sternum) lymph nodes should be evaluated for the presence of cancer. Follow-up chemotherapy may include antineoplastic agents (usually several in combination) and hormonal therapies. Radiotherapy is indicated postlumpectomy. Postoperative breast irradiation is well tolerated by older women; therefore age is not a contraindication to breast preservation treatment (Wyckoff et al, 1994). In general, older women treated for breast cancer do not experience greater complications or treatment toxicities when compared with younger women (Masetti et al, 1996). Although mastectomy is not the treatment of choice, if mastectomy is done, breast reconstruction is an option, depending on personal preference and the extent of the disease. As with all women, older women should be given information and support to help make treatment decisions. Breast cancer should be treated promptly but is not an emergency. Nurses should provide a supportive atmosphere and encourage family members to participate in treatment decisions.

Survival. Breast cancer survival rates are calculated on averages and depend on tumor characteristics (especially the stage), state of health, genetic background, immune function, levels of stress, and will to live. According to the American Cancer Society, when breast cancer is confined to the breast, the 5-year survival rate is close to 100%. Survival after 20 years is 53% (National Cancer Institute, 2004a).

Lung Cancer

Lung cancer is the most common type of cancer and the leading cause of cancer death in both men and women. The death rate is 32% in men and 25% in women. Lung cancer accounts for 14% of all cancer diagnoses and 32% of all cancer deaths. The incidence of lung cancer has increased steadily in both men and women for several decades, although the increase for women is higher than for men. Since 1987, more women have died of lung cancer than breast cancer, which for more than 40 years was the major cause of cancer deaths in women. Because the majority of women in the United States started smoking later than the average man, lung cancer deaths for women are not projected to peak until the year 2013 (American Lung Association, 2004). Since 1993 the incidence rate for lung cancer in men has been declining, and only recently has the rate begun to decrease for women. There is a sharp increase in lung cancer incidence starting between ages 45 and 50, with the peak incidence between ages 70 and 74 for women and 75 and 79 for men. A close relationship exists between incidence rates and death rates, indicating that most individuals diagnosed with lung cancer die of the disease (American Cancer Society, 2004a).

Risk Factors. Cigarette smoking is by far the most important risk factor in the development of lung cancer, both for active smokers and nonsmokers exposed to environmental, or passive, tobacco smoke (also known as second-hand smoke). Ninety percent of all lung cancer deaths can be attributed to tobacco. Tobacco smoke is considered a cancer promoter demonstrating a *dose-response relationship*; that is, the risk of lung cancer increases with the quantity of cigarettes smoked. The greatest lifetime cumulative exposure to cigarette smoking occurs between ages 70 and 80. It has been known for some time that the risk of lung cancer decreases over time for ex-smokers; about 15 years after the cessation of smoking, their risk is similar to that of lifetime nonsmokers (Wynder and Stellman, 1979).

Other risk factors include exposure to certain industrial substances that act as initiators and promoters, such as arsenic, ether, chromates, coke-oven fumes, nickel, and petroleum products and oils. Organic chemicals linked to a risk of lung cancer include radon and asbestos, with an increased risk for exposed persons who also smoke. Radiation exposure from occupational, medical, and environmental sources is also a risk factor. Air pollution contains several substances that, with repeated exposure, may increase the risk of lung cancer; however, air pollution is only hypothesized, not proven, to increase risk. Close to 342,000 Americans die from lung disease annually. Most lung diseases are chronic and diminish the quality of life for those persons living with the disease (American Lung Association, 2004).

Signs and Symptoms. The presenting signs and symptoms of lung cancer are vague and may be attributed to other problems, especially in older adults who have underlying lung or other chronic illnesses. The classic clinical presentation of lung cancer is persistent cough, sputum streaked with blood, chest pain, and recurring pneumonia or bronchitis. This constellation of symptoms is also associated with cigarette smoking, and their significance as indicators of cancer may be overlooked. Other symptoms include more systemic complaints, such as anorexia, weight loss, and fatigue. Symptoms of local metastasis may include hoarseness in the presence of laryngeal nerve involvement, shoulder pain when the brachial plexus is involved, dyspnea representing esophageal compression or invasion, and head and neck swelling signaling superior vena cava involvement. Older persons more often experience dyspnea and weight loss, while pain is less frequent (DeMaria and Cohen, 1987; Shell, Bulson, and Vanderlugt, 1997).

Early Detection. Lung cancer can grow for years before exhibiting clinical symptoms. Because symptoms often do not appear until the disease is advanced, early detection is difficult. When used in combination, chest x-ray studies and cytologic examination of sputum cells can detect small tumors. Both tests are expensive, requiring special facilities and personnel. The Mayo Lung Project, conducted between 1972 and 1982, examined the benefits of screening for lung cancer and determined that, although screening programs achieved earlier diagnoses and longer survival times, no significant reduction in mortality was demonstrated (Woolner, Fontana, and Cortese, 1984; Woolner et al, 1981). Early detection appears to lengthen the interval between diagnosis and death without increasing total life span (Berlin et al, 1984). Currently, the American Cancer Society does not recommend routine screening for lung cancer in asymptomatic persons. In a retrospective review of lung cancer among male veterans, older men were found to have more local disease at diagnosis than younger men. This finding was attributed to earlier diagnosis in the older group, who likely had lung cancer detected serendipitously by chest radiology used to monitor other chronic conditions such as cardiopulmonary disorders, which were prevalent among the group (DeMaria and Cohen, 1987).

Treatment. Options for treatment include surgery, radiotherapy, and chemotherapy, depending on the type and stage of disease. Lung cancer can be classified into two basic types: small cell cancer (also called oat cell cancer) and non–small cell cancers. Non–small cell cancers are further divided into three types: squamous cell (or epidermoid) cancers, adenocarcinomas, and large cell (also called large cell anaplastic) cancers. These various types of lung cancers have different growth patterns and respond differently to therapy.

Small cell types represent about 20% to 25% of all lung cancers and are strongly associated by dose response with cigarette smoking. Because of small cell cancers' high growth rate and tendency to metastasize early and widely, clients with small cell cancers have a poor prognosis. Small cell lung cancers are very sensitive to both chemotherapy and radiotherapy; in some cases chemotherapy (alone, or in combination with radiation) is used instead of traditional surgery as the treatment of choice. With surgery alone, small cell lung cancers tend to relapse, but with combination chemotherapy and radiotherapy, more persons with small cell lung cancer experience longer periods of remission (American Lung Association, 2004).

Of the non–small cell cancers, the squamous cell type, like the small cell type, is strongly linked by dose response to cigarette smoking. Squamous cell cancers tend to arise in central airways and invade the bronchi; therefore surgery to remove the obstructing tumor is usually the treatment of choice. Adenocarcinomas are the most common lung cancer, first seen as slow-growing masses in peripheral lung tissue. Surgical resection of the lung is the treatment of choice. Because lung cancer has usually metastasized by the time it is discovered, radiotherapy and chemotherapy are also necessary. Evidence has suggested that older adults with non–small cell lung cancers, particularly those individuals over age 75, do not receive the same level of treatment as younger persons, with surgery being omitted more often in older persons. Omission of surgery may reflect age bias, or it may indicate that an older adult is a poor surgical candidate. Guadagnoli et al (1990) noted that older adults who received less aggressive treatment had more comorbid disease. The presence of comorbid disease can increase the demands of illness, which in turn influence not only physical but also psychologic adjustment to lung cancer.

Survival. The survival rate for patients with small cell lung cancer is estimated at 35 weeks with treatment, with a slightly longer survival for limited stage disease. The 5-year survival rate for squamous cell disease is 50% without evidence of spread of the disease. The 5-year survival rate for adenocarcinoma and large cell lung cancer is less than 10%. The United States has the highest survival rate for lung cancer in the world, with only an 8% survival rate in Europe and developing countries (Landis et al, 1999).

Prostate Cancer

Prostate cancer accounts for approximately 23% of all cancer in men in the United States and approximately 12% of all cancer deaths. Prostate cancer is the second most common cancer in American men, and the highest rate of prostate cancer in the world is among African-Americans. Prostate cancer incidence rates are 66% higher for African-American men than for white men, and prostate cancer death rates are more than two times higher for African-American men than for white men. An estimated 220,900 new case of prostate cancer were diagnosed in the United States in 2003 (American Cancer Society, 2004a).

Risk Factors. Prostate cancer is a disease of aging. In a man's fourth decade the risk of developing prostate cancer increases, and every decade after that the probability of developing prostate cancer over each decade is 0.17% for the fourth decade, 2.01% in the fifth decade, and 6.46% in the sixth decade. Approximately 75% of all cases of prostate cancer are diagnosed in men older than 65 years, and 90% of prostate cancer deaths occur in this age-group. Mortality from prostate cancer is 35% lower in non-white Hispanics and 40% lower in Asian Americans and Pacific Islanders. African-American men have a 60% higher incidence rate and a twofold higher mortality from prostate cancer than do white men (American Cancer Society, 2004a).

It is unclear what the exact prostate cancer risk is for men who have a first-generation relative with prostate cancer. Some studies have shown a twofold to elevenfold increase in men with a positive family history (American Cancer Society, 2004a). In the United States men have a 15% life-time risk of a diagnosis of prostate cancer, but only a 3% life-time risk of dying from it (American Cancer Society, 2004a).

Signs and Symptoms. Prostate cancer is asymptomatic in its early stages. Signs and symptoms of cancer are related to the increased growth of the prostate that surrounds the urethra; they include weak or interrupted urine flow; difficulty or inability to begin urine flow; difficulty stopping urine flow; and urinary frequency, especially at night. Additional problems include hematuria; pain or burning during urination; and pain in the lower back, pelvis, and upper thighs. Many of these symptoms are similar to those of infection or benign prostatic hypertrophy.

Early Detection. Annual digital rectal examination (DRE) and prostate-specific antigen (PSA) testing are the two primary screening tests for prostate cancer in the United States. However, only a portion of the prostate can be palpated using the digital technique. Studies suggest that DRE alone detects less than 60% of prostate cancers. Adding PSA testing detects 26% more cancers than PSA testing alone. The American Cancer Society (2004a) recommends that every man over age 40 have a DRE as part of a regular annual physical examination. Ultrasound of the prostate is expensive and to date has not been demonstrated to be more predictive of prostate cancer than DRE. PSA is an immunologically distinct antigen made exclusively by prostate tissue. The American Cancer Society (2004a) recommends that men ages 50 and over have an annual PSA blood test. If either test result—DRE or PSA—is questionable, a complete evaluation is necessary. While the highest rate of prostate cancer is among African-Americans, Collins (1997) found that, when surveyed, only 21% of African-American men correctly identified the screening recommendations and early symptoms of prostate cancer.

Treatment. Four methods of treatment are used, either alone or in combination, to manage prostate cancer: surgery, radiotherapy, endocrine manipulation, and observation. The choice of treatment is determined by the location, stage, and histologic grade or degree of tumor cell differentiation, which is a measure of abnormal cell growth. Well-differentiated, localized prostate cancer grows relentlessly, albeit slowly, and is unlikely to affect survival during the first 7 to 10 years after diagnosis. Because of the slow growth pattern of some prostate cancers, the treatment of choice may be observation, depending on the client's age and the presence of comorbid factors at the time of diagnosis. Treatment may be delayed if life expectancy is estimated to be 10 years or less. Observation is an active process of routinely monitoring the growth of the cancer and evaluating its effect on functional abilities; it should not be confused with "ignoring" the cancer.

Moderately or poorly differentiated localized prostate cancer is rapidly progressive and likely to cause death within 5 years of diagnosis. More aggressive therapy is indicated for moderately or poorly differentiated disease; this may include surgery, radiotherapy, and hormonal manipulation. If the cancer has metastasized, treatment should involve hormonal manipulation to eliminate androgenic influence. Androgenic influence may be removed by using agents that block testosterone influence, such as compounds that contain estrogen, or by orchiectomy, the surgical removal of the testes.

Surgical removal of the cancerous prostate may include either radical prostatectomy or subtotal prostatectomy. Radical prostatectomy is the surgical removal of the entire prostate, including the prostate capsule, the seminal vesicles, and a portion of the bladder neck. Postoperative complications include infection, fecal incontinence from sphincter injury, and thromboembolism, depending on surgical technique. Erectile dysfunction is a common complication of radical prostatectomy, although newer surgical techniques preserve the nerve supply necessary for erection and ejaculation. A subtotal prostatectomy is an enucleative procedure but does not remove the prostate capsule; it is not considered a curative procedure. Subtotal prostatectomy preserves erectile function but results in retrograde ejaculation.

Like surgery, radiotherapy, in the form of either external beam radiation or internal implantation of seeds, can be a primary treatment for prostate cancer. External beam radiation is administered daily in small doses for approximately 40 treatments. Often the radiation treatments are coupled with hormonal therapy with agents such as luteinizing hormone–releasing hormone agonists. The benefits of using accompanying hormone therapy are decreasing the serum testosterone and shrinking the tumor in preparation for radiation (Millikan and Logothelis, 1997). Both surgery and radiotherapy are effective. Convincing proof of the superiority of either approach is not available. The choice of treatment often depends on the presence of comorbidity, availability of treatment facilities, requisite medical expertise, and individual preference. Erectile dysfunction can be a consequence of any of these procedures.

Since treatments can have long-term consequences for sexual performance, the selection of a treatment should include a discussion with the older man and his sexual partner about preservation of sexual function. Age alone does not dictate sexual interest or performance. Some degree of sexual activity is preserved in approximately 75% of persons over age 70. Loss of sexual function may have a serious impact on the quality of life of older adults. Careful consideration of sexual needs should be part of a treatment decision for clients of any age (see Chapter 13).

Survival. Over the past 30 years the survival rate for all stages of prostate cancer combined has increased from 50% to 87%. For localized cancers, the 5-year survival rate is 99% in whites and 65% in African-Americans. Survival rates decline after 5 years; 63% of men diagnosed with prostate cancer survive 10 years; 51% survive 15 years (American Cancer Society, 2004a).

Colorectal Cancer

Colorectal cancer accounts for about 15% of all cancers in both men and women. Colon cancer is the second leading cause of cancer death in America. There were 98,200 new cases of colon cancer and 37,200 cases of rectal cancer diagnosed in 2001. In men prostate and lung cancer incidence exceeds that of colorectal cancer; among women, only breast cancer incidence exceeds colorectal cancer incidence. Incidence rates have declined in recent years for whites and stabilized for African-Americans. Overall mortality rates for colorectal cancer have declined 32% for women and 14% for men over the past 20 years, reflecting decreasing incidence rates and increasing survival rates. Mortality rates for African-American men continue to rise. In 2000 the mortality rate for colorectal cancer was 24.6 per 100,000 in African-Americans and 17.5 per 100,000 for whites (American Cancer Society, 2004a; Bond, 2000).

Risk Factors. A personal or family history of colorectal cancer, polyps, or inflammatory bowel disease has been associated with increased colorectal cancer risk. Diet has been the focus of much research, since ingested foods come into contact with bowel mucosa. Certain foods and the time that they are in contact with the bowel may serve as initiating factors for cancer development by altering the environment of the gut. Colorectal cancer may be associated with a diet low in fiber and high in fat and calories. Research is ongoing in this area. However, high-fiber, low-fat diets have additional health benefits apart from a potential connection to colorectal cancer prevention (National Cancer Institute, 2004b).

Signs and Symptoms. Presenting signs and symptoms are related to the location of the cancer within the colon. In early stages, minor changes in bowel patterns and occasional bleeding may occur. Cancer of the right colon can cause pain, cramping, and appendicitis-like symptoms. Cancers of the transverse colon may cause bloody stool, changes in bowel habits, and obstruction. Cancer on the left side of the colon tends to be constricting, progressively restricting the lumen of the bowel. Because bright red bleeding occurs, left-sided cancers tend to be diagnosed earlier. Rectal cancer presents as a change in bowel habits, with increased frequency of evacuation and bright-red bleeding.

Early Detection. According to the American Cancer Society guideline for the early detection of colorectal cancer, starting at age 50, both men and women should have yearly fecal occult blood tests, and flexible sigmoidoscopy every 5 years, *or* flexible sigmoidoscopy alone every 5 years, *or* fecal occult blood testing yearly, *or* colonoscopy every 10 years, *or* double contrast barium enema every 5 years. An estimated 50% of colorectal cancers are located in the distal 50 cm of the large bowel. Fecal occult blood testing, although inexpensive and low risk, may miss polyps and some cancers and may produce false positive test results; however, it has been proven effective in clinical trails (American Cancer Society, 2004a). Screening is appropriate for individual older adults at high risk, but care should be taken to help clients perform the test properly.

Treatment. Surgery is the treatment of choice for colorectal cancer. The extent of surgery is determined by the location of the cancer and the involvement of lymph nodes. Surgical procedures include removal of the cancer and segments of the major arterial and venous blood suppliers to the affected area. Permanent colostomy is seldom needed for colon cancer. In cases where surgery for colorectal cancer is nonemergent, older adults do not show increased morbidity or mortality compared with their younger counterparts. In addition, the cost of surgical treatment of older persons with colorectal cancer is not significantly higher than for younger persons; therefore there is no financial reason not to treat older adults in the same manner (Audisio et al, 1997).

For localized cancers, surgery is frequently curative. Chemotherapy after surgery is beneficial for clients with spread to the lymph nodes or cancer that has penetrated the bowel wall. Surgery in combination with radiotherapy is the usual treatment for early stages of rectal cancer (American Cancer Society, 2004b). Chemotherapy may be used for advanced disease. Permanent colostomy is infrequently required for rectal cancer. Many lower rectal cancers can be treated radically by proctectomy with total mesorectal excision, followed by colonic J pouch anal anastomosis (CPAA). Functional outcome after CPAA is reported as good to excellent in older persons and compares well with outcomes in younger persons. However, constipation may be more frequent in older adults (Dehni et al, 1998).

Survival. The 5-year survival rate for persons with colorectal cancer is 63% in whites and 53% in African-Americans. When it is discovered before spread, the survival rate is 91%; however, only about 35% of colorectal cancers are detected at this early stage. After the cancer has spread to involve other organs or lymph nodes, the 5-year survival rate drops to 63%. About 50% of all persons diagnosed with colorectal cancer survive 10 years (National Cancer Institute, 2003b).

SCREENING AND EARLY DETECTION: ISSUES FOR OLDER ADULTS

Primary prevention of cancer is most desirable and is affected mainly by changes in lifestyle. Older adults are likely to have had a lifetime of exposure to risk factors, and although changing lifestyles is advantageous for them, the changes may not reverse the effects of exposure. Furthermore, changing habits that have developed over a lifetime is difficult, despite demonstrable benefits. Given the difficulty of cancer prevention, detection of cancer at an early stage can greatly improve survival. Screening asymptomatic persons at risk is feasible in many common malignancies, including breast, cervix, colorectal, and prostate cancer.

When considering a cancer screening program, the health care provider should consider two fundamental questions:

1. Is the screening test sensitive? A sensitive test will correctly identify all screened individuals who have the disease (the true positives).
2. Is the screening test specific? A specific test identifies all individuals who do not have the disease (the true negatives).

Current efforts at advancing the science and technology of screening have resulted in greater accuracy of many screening tests. The accuracy of screening may be increased by the recognition of highly sensitive tumor-specific circulating markers, such as PSA for the detection of prostate cancer; the development of imaging techniques capable of finding smaller lesions, such as refinements in radiographic techniques for mammograms; and the identification of early molecular changes in cancer specimens (e.g., at the cellular level using Pap tests for cervical cancer). Given the limited effectiveness of primary prevention for older adults, screening asymptomatic persons at risk for cancer may be the most promising way to decrease the number of cancer deaths in older adults.

Yet another question to consider with a screening program is the prevalence of the disease in the population. The more prevalent the disease, the more beneficial a screening program will be. Because cancer is more common in older adults, screening is generally beneficial. The incidence of cancer increases with age; thus the positive predictive value of screening tests (i.e., the proportion of persons screened who actually have the disease) is likely to increase. In addition, screening older adults who have comorbid conditions at the time of cancer diagnosis can result in elective treatment at an early stage of disease, thus reducing the possibility of serious treatment-related morbidity and deaths.

Recommendations on planning major screening programs for older adults should be made with caution. Screening guidelines vary greatly among different national organizations. Differences among recommendations are due to the lack of cancer screening trials that include older adults. Since more than 60% of all cancers are diagnosed in those over 65, and 67% of all cancer deaths occur in this age-group, the lack of evidence-based criteria for screening older adults makes choosing screening protocols difficult. A decision-making process that take into account each older adult's personal preference and health should be used rather than relying only on age guidelines for cancer screening and detection methods. Screening should not be conducted if there is no intent or ability to pursue findings with more complete evaluation and treatment.

Screening is costly and useless if there is no follow-up. Other factors that influence the decision to screen an older adult include comorbidity, functional ability, and life expectancy.

Walter and Covinsky (2001) developed a framework for cancer screening in older adults based on the following factors:

- Individualize the decision by conducting a comprehensive geriatric assessment that includes an evaluation of comorbid conditions, polypharmacy, and the presence of dementia or depression.
- Estimate life expectancy. Reducing the risk of dying of a detectible cancer should be the main benefit of cancer screening. Although an exact determination of longevity is impossible, decisions can be made based on understanding the distribution of life expectancies at various ages. The goal of any cancer screening program is to detect those cancers early enough for successful treatment. Therefore a patient with more than 5 years' life expectancy will benefit from a cancer screening program. Although determining life expectancy for a particular individual is difficult, some attempt should be made to correlate life expectancy with the potential for future development of a specific cancer. The decision to screen should consider the treatment implications, but the decisions on treatment and how aggressively to treat are separate and take place after the type and stage of cancer are diagnosed.
- Assess the risk of cancer screening. Certain clinically unimportant cancers increase as people age; therefore older patients are frequently diagnosed with these types of cancer. Older people also have more cognitive and physical conditions that increase their fear of cancer screening.
- Ascertain patient preferences. Consider each older person's approach to health and discuss the risk and benefits of cancer screening tests.
- Consult various cancer screening guidelines. The U.S. Preventive Services Task Force (USPSTF) guidelines are the most widely used and respected; however, these guidelines are very conservative and differ significantly from those of specialty organizations such as the American Cancer Society and the American Geriatric Society. A listing of all USPSTF guidelines can be found at http://www.ahrq.gov/ clinic/uspstfix.htm.

Ideally effective cancer screening programs should lead to an overall reduction of cancer-related deaths, with higher detection rates and prolonged survival times when cancer is diagnosed at an early stage. However, controversy has recently surrounded much of the research that cites the benefits of screening. Several notes of caution should be considered when reviewing the results of screening programs (Yates, 1992):

- Screening programs can sometimes *appear* to prolong survival only because of early detection of a cancer, without any actual extension of life as a result of early treatment. This is known as *lead time bias*; a cancer that has a natural history of 5 years may appear to gain a 2-year survival advantage as a result of diagnosis at year 1 of tumor growth instead of year 3.
- Screening favors the early detection of the more slowly growing and less malignant neoplasms, which leads to the appearance of improved survival, when screening actually only increases the detection of the least aggressive cancers. This is known as *length bias*. Length bias appears to improve survival rates but actually dilutes the real effect of screening programs.
- Of particular importance when screening older adults, screening allows the diagnosis of cancers that would not have become clinically relevant during the person's lifetime. This is known as *overdetection bias*.

These controversies underscore the notion that recommendations for screening require individual consideration.

In addition to the controversies surrounding screening research, other factors may impede screening efforts for older adults. Older adults are often seen for episodic events in the context of chronic illnesses managed by medical specialists. Preventive services may not be appropriate at the time of an acute episode or may not be available within a specialty practice; therefore screening procedures may not be offered. If they are offered, older adults may choose not to participate because they lack information about cancer screening, including the rationale, recommended frequency, and specific procedures. Aging and minority status have been linked to reduced knowledge of and access to cancer screening through mammography, rectal examination, fecal occult blood testing, Pap testing, and proctoscopy (Brant, 1996; Celentano and Klassen, 1992; Kagawa-Singer, 1997; Yates, 1992) (see Research box). In addition to lack of knowledge, older adults may fear the diagnosis of cancer and the associated treatments, or they may be unable or unwilling to pay for health care services.

Nurses working with older adults should examine the role of cancer screening and the potential benefits for the population assigned to their care. The decision to screen or not to screen should be an active one, made after thoughtful consideration within the context of a multidisciplinary health care team. Screening guidelines, individual circumstances, potential complications of aggressive evaluation workups, and associated costs are all factors to consider in deciding to screen older adults.

As a group, older persons generally require more individualized health teaching about cancer risk and detection. Older persons may lack an awareness of the risks of cancer associated with advanced age and may not know the warning signs of cancer. They may be reluctant to report physical complaints that could be indicative of cancer. In addition, many older persons are concerned about, and even fear, the diagnosis of cancer and its effect on their overall well-being and functional status. The nurse should teach older adults the following early warning signs of cancer:

> **Research**
>
> **SAMPLE/SETTING**
>
> The sample consisted of 513 multicultural adults over age 55 (72% women; 68% born in countries other than Canada) living in urban communities in Canada.
>
> **METHODS**
>
> A self-report questionnaire, the Cancer Knowledge Survey for Elders, was administered to participants in their native language (eight different language groups) to identify knowledge levels concerning cancer in older Canadian adults. The questionnaire was distributed by community workers and public health nurses working with older adults.
>
> **FINDINGS**
>
> The largest number of correct responses (87%) was for the item, "Can some cancers be cured if they are discovered early?" The highest number of wrong answers (67%) was for the item, "Can a bump or bruise to the body cause cancer?" About 66% did not consider age a risk factor. For all but three items, the proportion of English to non–English language speakers with correct answers was significant; individuals whose native language was not English were less knowledgeable about cancer.
>
> **IMPLICATIONS**
>
> Public education about the risk factors, signs, and symptoms of cancer is needed, particularly among older adults for whom English is not a native language. Specific information is needed about the increased risk of cancer with advancing age.
>
> Fitch MI et al: Health promotion and early detection of cancer in older adults: assessing knowledge about cancer, *Oncol Nurs Forum* 24:1743, 1997.

- Change in bowel or bladder habits
- A sore that does not heal
- Unusual bleeding or discharge
- Thickening or lump in breast or elsewhere
- Indigestion or difficulty swallowing
- Obvious change in wart or mole
- Nagging cough or hoarseness

MAJOR TREATMENT MODALITIES

Currently, there are four major forms of cancer treatment: (1) surgery, (2) radiotherapy, (3) chemotherapy, and (4) biotherapy. Each form of treatment may be used alone or in combination. Treatment selection is determined by the type and stage of the cancer, the unique biophysiologic characteristics of the cancer cells, and an older client's overall health status at the time of diagnosis. Treatment goals also help determine the type of therapy. Cancer therapies may be directed at *cure,* or elimination of the disease; *control,* or minimization of the disease; or *palliation,* or relief of the symptoms.

Initial large-scale research efforts suggested that age bias is common in the treatment of cancers in older adults (Greenfield et al, 1987; Samet et al, 1986); however, the validity of these studies was subsequently questioned (Patterson, 1992). Currently, researchers and clinicians agree that it is important to raise questions about actual or perceived differences in treatment that may exist among age-groups. Chronologic age is not a major variable in determining a client's ability to tolerate or respond to therapy. Functional status has been reported to be a more important pretreatment variable, influencing both the decision to treat and the type of treatment (Shepherd et al, 1994). In addition, the number of comorbid conditions is a significant predictor of the outcome of an older adult receiving cancer treatment (Yancik, 1997). As with decisions to screen, treatment decisions should consider the individual. Age is but one of many factors that should be considered.

Age-related treatment bias may also occur because of the older adults or their families. Clients or family members may believe a person can be too old to tolerate treatment; thus they choose suboptimum therapies in lieu of more aggressive and curative treatments. Cancer care has changed dramatically over the years; however, many older adults remember friends or relatives who were treated with now-outdated therapies that had devastating side effects. One older woman, for instance, refuses to have follow-up radiotherapy and decides to have a mastectomy when lumpectomy is an option. She remembers her mother's complications related to older methods of cobalt radiotherapy, a delivery method for external beam radiotherapy that has now been greatly improved, and declares, "No one is going to fry me like they did my poor mother." Clients and families need accurate information. Since cancer is so prevalent in older adults, many have some information about cancer, but it is often misinformation. The nurse should be sure that clients and families have accurate information and a clear understanding of the treatment options being offered.

Surgery

Surgery, the oldest method of treating cancer, is indicated for most solid tumors. Initially, using sophisticated biopsy and exploratory techniques, surgery is used to help diagnose the disease, by determining tumor type, and to stage the disease, by determining its extent. The primary treatment goal of surgery is to remove the tumor when localized, thus preventing regional or distant metastasis. Surgery may also be indicated for palliative care to reduce large primary or metastatic tumors, since the size or location of the tumor can create problems such as compression of surrounding tissues and organs, leading to pain, necrosis, or organ failure. Surgery may be indicated for the placement of treatment-related devices such as implanted access devices, shunts, or drains. Surgery may also be indicated for rehabilitation or restorative purposes, such as breast reconstruction after mastectomy. Surgery is not a treatment of choice for disseminated disease, such as when multiple small tumors metastasize in diffuse locations (e.g., when breast cancer metastasizes in the lungs), or for disease that is disseminated from the onset, such as leukemia.

In the past, surgical treatment of cancer involved extensive radical procedures. Such procedures were necessary to treat large, often neglected cancers. Poor understanding of patterns of metastatic spread and little knowledge of the benefits of adjuvant therapy contributed to the focus on radical operations. Greater insight into the pathophysiology of cancer and the development of additional therapies has led to more sophisticated surgical techniques. Early detection of smaller tumors has also contributed to the decline in radical procedures. Less radical procedures result in fewer complications and improved quality of life. Research has demonstrated that older adults with cancer do not have a higher risk or complication rate than age-matched cohorts without cancer (Patterson, 1989).

The curability of cancer in older adults is largely predicted by an individual's ability to tolerate major surgery. Because older adults are at risk for more complications, careful preoperative assessment is critical. In-depth evaluation of respiratory, cardiovascular, hepatic, immunologic, renal, nutritional, and central nervous system status is mandatory. The severity of underlying cancer and comorbid conditions is an important factor to consider in the decision regarding surgical therapy (Pfeifer, 1997b). In addition, a client's rehabilitation potential should be evaluated, particularly if the intended surgery will significantly alter normal physiologic function. Some surgical procedures may produce physiologic alterations that are beyond an older adult's adaptive capabilities. Arthritic changes and diminished visual acuity are two common problems in older adults that can make the management of surgical complications difficult (e.g., after an operation such as a colostomy). In general, older clients have a higher surgical risk than younger clients; however, through careful preoperative assessment to identify risks, older clients can be offered appropriate supportive therapies that minimize complications. Although age alone is not a determinant of surgical risk, data indicate that older adults are less likely to receive surgical therapy than younger persons (Farrow, Hunt, and Samet, 1996).

Postoperative priorities should be preventing respiratory complications and promoting cardiac and renal function. Because of the overall reduced compensatory reserves in these systems, older adults are susceptible to a number of serious complications, including congestive heart failure, electrolyte imbalances, hypoxia, dehydration, and pulmonary embolism. The use of invasive lines and catheters can tax an aging immune system and predispose older clients to sepsis. The overall stress of surgery, including anesthesia and other centrally acting medications, can predispose older adults to the development of delirium. Bowel complications may include paralytic ileus and constipation. Decreased mobility and inadequate nutrition are risk factors for pressure ulcers. Careful, complete, and ongoing assessment of all body systems provides the foundation for the nurse to accurately diagnose, plan, implement, and evaluate nursing care during the postoperative period.

Radiotherapy

Like all cancer therapies, radiotherapy is used for several different purposes. Radiotherapy may be curative for the treatment of several cancers, including skin, prostate, rectal, non–small cell and small cell, cervical, and Hodgkin's cancers. Radiotherapy may also be indicated as an adjuvant therapy to prevent recurrence of breast cancer after lumpectomy. In some cases radiotherapy may be used to control cancers, adding months or years to an individual's life. Radiotherapy and chemotherapy may also be used before surgery to shrink the tumor. Often recurrent breast and lung cancer can be controlled by radiotherapy in combination with chemotherapy and/or surgery. Radiotherapy may also be used for palliative care. Radiotherapy can relieve pain and prevent pathologic fractures associated with bone metastasis of breast, lung, and prostate tumors. Palliative radiotherapy is given for the relief of central nervous symptoms caused by brain metastasis or spinal cord compression. In some cases, palliative radiotherapy may be given before a problem manifests itself, as in the treatment of vertebral lesions when spinal cord compression is eminent. Approximately 60% of all persons with invasive cancer receive radiotherapy at some point in the course of their illness (Iwamoto, 1997).

Not all cancers are sensitive to the effects of radiotherapy, but for other cancers radiotherapy may provide significant advantages over surgical procedures. Radiation can encompass wider areas around the tumor and remove tumors from regions where surgery cannot be effectively performed. The use of radiation can also result in less disability and disfigurement than some extensive surgeries. Radiation also allows simultaneous treatment to multiple metastatic sites (Davis and Lindley, 2004).

Therapeutic doses of radiotherapy are calculated to destroy or to delay the growth of malignant cells without destroying normal tissue. Radiation effects at the cellular level may be either direct or indirect. Direct effects occur when key molecules within the cell—the DNA or ribonucleic acid (RNA)—are damaged. Indirect effects occur when ionization takes place in the tissue surrounding the cellular structures within the cell. Radiation absorbed by tissue water molecules produces free radicals that trigger a variety of chemical reactions, producing new compounds that are toxic to the cell.

The administration of radiotherapy may involve external or internal techniques. External beam therapy, which is radiation from a source at a distance from the body, is administered primarily by linear accelerators and mostly in an outpatient setting. Internal therapy, known as brachytherapy, involves radiation from a source placed within the body or a body cavity. Brachytherapy uses various commercially available instruments or applicators, which are inserted into target areas for a predetermined time. Rotation of either the target site or the radiation beam makes it possible to deliver a high dose to the tumor, with only part of the dose reaching the surrounding noncancerous tissue.

The response of older adults to radiotherapy has not been well evaluated. Several initial reports suggest that there is no difference in response between older persons and any other age-group (Host and Lunde, 1986; Nobler and Venetl, 1985). The Joint Center for Radiation Therapy reported that younger persons (those under 35) treated for breast cancer had higher local recurrence than older persons, implying that radiotherapy may be more effective for older women. Overall, however, both research and clinical data suggest that the response to radiotherapy of cancers in older adults is similar to that of younger ones; therefore decisions to treat using radiotherapy should be based on individual factors (Greenberg and Trotti, 1992).

Radiotherapy's associated side effects are no worse in older adults than in younger ones (Larson et al, 1993). However, older persons have greater difficulty compensating for temporary dysfunction in a single organ or in multiple organ systems. The challenge in treating older adults with radiotherapy is to provide appropriate supportive care to enable the client to complete treatment without any significant alteration in functional status. Age cannot be used as a predictor for how clients will respond to radiotherapy treatment.

Chemotherapy

Since not all cancers can be cured by surgery or radiotherapy, systemic treatment such as chemotherapy may be necessary. Chemotherapy is the use of drugs to destroy cancer cells. Classic chemotherapy kills cancer cells either by damaging DNA, interfering with DNA synthesis, or inhibiting cell division. In contrast to surgery and radiotherapy, which are local therapies, chemotherapy is systemic. Although single-agent chemotherapy may be successful in the treatment of certain types of cancer, most tumors show only a partial response to this type of therapy. In most types of cancer, specifically breast, colorectal, gastric, ovarian, lung, and lymphomas, combination chemotherapy (i.e., with several different drugs given together) is necessary to provide a better chance of long-term, disease-free survival. Broader coverage against cells and cell lines within heterogeneous tumors is provided with chemotherapy combinations (Davis and Lindley, 2004).

The objectives of chemotherapy include cure, control, and palliation. In general, the survival of older persons who receive chemotherapy is significantly longer than that of untreated older persons, even though dose adjustments may be needed to control toxicity. Table 19-3 lists commonly prescribed chemotherapeutic agents by drug classification and mechanism of action.

Pharmacokinetics. *Pharmacokinetics* refers to the activity of drugs in the body, including absorption, distribution, metabolism, and excretion. For oral chemotherapeutic agents, age-related changes in the digestive tract appear to have little effect on the absorptive capacity of the intestine. The exception may be with leucovorin, which, when given in the high doses required by some treatment protocols, may not reach desired blood levels in some older clients (Baker and Grochow, 1997; Einhorn, 1989). Age-related changes in body composition—decreased total body water and increased body fat—can affect drug distribution; however, no consequences for chemotherapeutic agents have been demonstrated (Vestal, 1997). The liver is the main site of metabolism for many chemotherapeutic agents. Liver size decreases by 20% to 40% between the ages of 20 and 80, which may result in reduced hepatic drug clearance in older adults, though for most older persons drug metabolism in the liver appears to be unaffected by age (Baker and Grochow, 1997; Vestal, 1997). Any impairment in drug metabolism is likely related to underlying liver damage, including exposure to environmental toxins or alcohol. Chemotherapeutic agents primarily metabolized by the liver include anthracyclines, mitoxantrone, mitomycin C, and the vinca alkaloids. Biliary excretion of drugs, such as anthracyclines, mitomycin C, and the vinca alkaloids, seems to be unaffected by age (Balducci, Mowrey, and Parker, 1992; Egorin, 1993). Only the age-related decline in kidney function has been demonstrated to have clinical consequences for drug dosing. Toxic drug levels have been demonstrated for those agents which are primarily excreted by the kidney—methotrexate, bleomycin, carboplatin, and cisplatin (Baker and Grochow, 1997). The dosage of these drugs may need to be adjusted to account for age-related changes in the kidney.

Pharmacodynamics. *Pharmacodynamics* refers to the interactions between the chemotherapeutic agents and their cellular targets, including the processes that modulate the activity of the agents. All agents act at the cellular level; however, their mechanisms of action vary, as do their respective administration guidelines and side effect profiles. Nurses caring for clients receiving chemotherapeutic agents should understand the specific actions and side effects of individual agents.

Aging may make cells prone to drug resistance. Synthesis of abnormal proteins in aging cells may interfere with several pharmacodynamic steps, including the availability of membrane receptors for drugs, drug metabolism, and drug-affected enzyme inhibition. Also, aging cells may acquire some ability to repair damaged DNA, resulting in increased drug resistance and offering at least a partial explanation for the clinical observation that cancers in older adults are less

TABLE 19-3 Major Chemotherapeutic Agents

DRUG CLASSIFICATION	MAJOR MECHANISM OF ACTION	DRUGS
Alkylating agents	Alkylating agents are highly reactive compounds that act against already formed nucleic acids by cross-linking strands, thereby preventing RNA transcription and DNA replication. These agents are considered cell cycle nonspecific.	Altretamine Busulfan Carboplatin Carmustine Chlorambucil Cisplatin Cyclophosphamide Dacarbazine Ifosfamide Lomustine Mechlorethamine Melphalan Procarbazine Streptozocin Thiotepa Uracil mustard
Antimetabolites	Antimetabolites are analogs of normal metabolites and act by interfering with synthesis of chromosomal nucleic acid. Some agents block an enzyme necessary for synthesis of essential factors, whereas others are incorporated into RNA or DNA, thus preventing cellular replication. Pyrimidine analogs, purine analogs, and folic acid antagonists are three major subgroups of antimetabolites, which are considered cell cycle specific.	5-Azacytidine 2-Chlorodeoxyadenosine (cladribine) Cytarabine Edatrexate Floxuridine Fludarabine Fluorouracil Mercaptopurine Methotrexate Mitoguazone Pentostatin Thioguanine Trimetrexate
Antitumor antibiotics	Antibiotic agents are natural products of various strains of soil fungus. These agents bind to DNA, preventing RNA and DNA synthesis, and are active in all phases of the cell cycle.	Bleomycin Dactinomycin Daunorubicin Doxorubicin Epirubicin Idarubicin Mitomycin Mitoxantrone PALA Plicamycin
Plant alkaloids	Also called vinca alkaloids, these agents are derived from the periwinkle plant. As a group, the agents are similar in action, binding to proteins within cells and thereby inhibiting mitosis. Since they specifically act during cell division, they are cell cycle specific.	Docetaxel (Taxotere) Etoposide Paclitaxel (Taxol) Teniposide Vinblastine Vincristine Vindesine
Miscellaneous agents	A number of agents have unique mechanisms of action in various phases of the cell cycle.	Amsacrine Asparaginase CPT-11 Mitotane Piroxantrone Suramin Topotecan

susceptible to chemotherapy treatment (Balducci, Mowrey, and Parker, 1992; Kimmick et al, 1997).

Biotherapy

Biotherapy in the field of cancer treatment is relatively new; research and clinical application stepped up in the 1980s. Biotherapy is the use of agents derived from biologic sources or agents that target biologic responses that modify the relationship between tumor and host. The primary mode of action is modification of the host's biologic response to the tumor, thus effecting a therapeutic response. Initial efforts in biotherapy were directed at modifying the immune response and were referred to as *immunotherapy*. But often biologic agents have multiple actions, causing immunologic and other biologic activity. *Biotherapy* is a broader term, and biologic response modifiers (BRMs) refer to biologic agents (Jassak, 1995).

BRMs include interferons, interleukins, hematopoietic growth factors, monoclonal antibodies, and tumor necrosis factor (TNF). Table 19-4 identifies the major agents by classification, area of biologic activity, and indications for use. Although all the agents are considered useful in the treatment of cancers, only some agents are approved by the Food and Drug Administration (FDA) and are commercially available. Research is rapidly expanding knowledge of the agents and testing clinical feasibility.

The most widely used BRMs for the treatment of cancer are the hematopoietic growth factors. Growth factors include erythropoietin to stimulate the production of red blood cells,

TABLE 19-4 Biologic Response Modifiers

AGENT	BIOLOGIC ACTIVITY	INDICATIONS FOR USE
Interferons	High level of antiviral activity interferes with viral protein synthesis and stimulation of cytotoxic T lymphocytes, lysing virally infected cells. Some anticancer activity results from ability to inhibit protein and DNA synthesis.	Chronic myelogenous leukemia Colorectal cancer Hairy cell leukemia Hepatitis Melanoma Multiple myeloma Non-Hodgkin's lymphoma Ovarian cancer Renal cell cancer Squamous cell cancer of skin or cervix T cell lymphoma
Interleukins	As a group of at least 12 different types, actions of interleukins include immunomodulation, promotion of hematopoiesis, and mediation of inflammation.	Interleukin-2 approved by FDA for use for renal cell cancer Clinical trials continue to evaluate use in variety of cancers
Hematopoietic growth factors	These regulate reproduction, maturation, and functional activity of blood cells.	**Erythropoietin**—stimulates production and maturation of red blood cells; indicated for anemia related to chronic renal failure and cancer treatment **GM-CSF**—stimulates production and maturation of neutrophils, eosinophils, monocytes, and basophils; indicated for treatment of acquired immunodeficiency syndrome (AIDS), myelodysplastic syndromes, and myelosuppressive chemotherapy **G-CSF**—stimulates production and maturation of neutrophils; indicated for treatment of granulocytosis secondary to chemotherapy treatment
Monoclonal antibodies (MABs)	This is a passive antibody therapy that may be directed at specific antigens.	MABs used experimentally in cancer treatment; however, have not established a role in standard cancer therapy
TNF	TNF causes necrosis in both tumors and healthy tissue by damaging endothelial lining of blood vessels, causing narrowing or blockage of lumen and intravascular coagulation. It also increases number of white blood cells and generally augments function of the immune system.	TNF used experimentally in cancer treatment; however, has not established a role in standard cancer therapy

and granulocyte-macrophage–colony-stimulating factor (GM-CSF) and granulocyte colony–stimulating factor (G-CSF) to stimulate production of white blood cells. These agents are routinely used to ameliorate the hematopoietic side effects of cancer chemotherapy, and they have greatly decreased infectious complications and increased ability to tolerate therapy (Johnston and Crawford, 1997).

Endocrine Therapy

Certain types of cancer that arise from hormone-sensitive tissues such as the breast, prostate, and endometrium can be treated by the use of endocrine therapy. This type of therapy inhibits tumor growth by blocking the hormone receptor, thereby eliminating endogenous hormones that supply the tumor and aid in its growth. For breast cancer, anti-estrogens such as tamoxifen, toremifene, and fulvestrant or aromatase inhibitors such as anastrozole, letrozole, or exemestane are used.

COMMON PHYSIOLOGIC COMPLICATIONS

Cancer treatments are aimed at destroying cancer cells. Because most treatment pharmacodynamics includes the prevention of cell division, actively dividing cell types are particularly vulnerable and may exhibit side effects. Actively dividing cell types that are most likely to exhibit side effects include those in hematopoietic tissue, the gastrointestinal tract, and hair follicles. Chemotherapy side effects are specific to the type of agent, dosage, and duration of use (see Nursing Care Plan). Radiation-related side effects depend on the location of the radiation field, intensity of the dose, and

Nursing Care Plan
Myelosuppressive Toxicities of Chemotherapy

Clinical Situation: Mr. K is a 69-year-old man recently diagnosed with small cell cancer of the lung. He lives with his wife in a modest home. Mr. K had no functional limitations before his diagnosis of cancer. His oncologist prescribes a chemotherapy regimen of cyclophosphamide (Cytoxan), doxorubicin (Adriamycin), and etoposide (VePesid). As with many chemotherapy regimens, a primary side effect is myelosuppression, resulting in decreased red blood cells, white blood cells, and platelets. Since the therapy is given in the ambulatory care clinic, Mr. K and his wife will need to provide self-care for monitoring and managing the myelosuppressive effects of the agents.

Nursing Diagnosis

Risk for infection related to bone marrow depression (granulocytopenia) secondary to chemotherapy

Potential for injury: bleeding due to bone marrow depression (thrombocytopenia) secondary to chemotherapy

Potential for altered tissue perfusion related to anemia

Outcomes

Client will remain free of infection.

Client will remain free of injury and bleeding incidents.

Client will not experience hypoxia, activity intolerance, or malaise.

Interventions

Monitor complete blood cell count and differential (absolute neutrophil count should remain above 500 cells/mm³).

Instruct the client and family to:

- Maintain client defenses.
  - —Perform frequent oral hygiene using soft bristle toothbrush and low-alcohol mouthwash.
  - —Lubricate dry areas using skin emollients and artificial tears.
  - —Maintain adequate hydration (3000 ml/day is recommended).
- Minimize exposure to potential pathogens.
  - —Restrict visitors with colds or infections.
  - —Avoid large crowds.
  - —Perform routine bathing and perineal hygiene.
- Assess for presence of infection.
  - —Report temperature ≥ 100° F.

Monitor complete blood cell count and differential; platelet count should remain above 50,000 cells/mm³.

Instruct the client and family to:

- Avoid trauma.
  - —Use a soft bristle toothbrush and low-alcohol mouthwash, and avoid flossing and toothpicks.
  - —Avoid tightly fitting or constrictive clothing.
  - —Use a nail file or emery board; avoid clipping or pulling hang nails.
  - —Use an electric razor for shaving.
  - —Prevent constipation; use stool softeners and maintain adequate fluid intake.
- Assess for the presence of bruising or bleeding.
  - —Report minor bleeding such as petechiae, ecchymosis, epistaxis, and occult blood in stool, urine, or emesis.

Monitor complete blood cell count and differential.

- Hematocrit should remain above 25%.

Instruct the client and family to:

- Increase rest and sleep periods.
- Alternate rest and activity periods.
- Incorporate foods into the diet that are high in iron, such as eggs, lean meat, green leafy vegetables, carrots, and raisins.
- Modify roles and responsibilities as needed.

duration of the therapy. In most cases, side effects are reversible.

Bone Marrow Suppression

The most common universal toxicity related to cancer treatment, particularly with chemotherapeutic agents, is myelotoxicity, suppression of the bone marrow. Myelosuppression can result in anemia (decreased red blood cells), neutropenia (decreased neutrophils), and thrombocytopenia (decreased platelets). Older adults with cancer have diminished hematopoietic reserves, which may lead to increased susceptibility to chemotherapy-induced bone marrow suppression. However, older clients have been able to tolerate moderate chemotherapy treatment programs without excessive complications when dosage is adjusted according to level of renal function. Aggressive chemotherapy, such as that used for treating leukemia or in preparation for bone marrow transplantation, may lead to prolonged and severe myelosuppression in older adults (Baker and Grochow, 1997).

Several causes for greater myelosuppression in older clients have been suggested: (1) dosage may not be appropriately adjusted to renal function, (2) preexisting hematopoietic insufficiency may exist due to chronic disease or malnutrition, and (3) chemotherapeutic agents may interact with other prescribed medications that also have myelosuppression as a side effect (e.g., phenytoin) (Baker and Grochow, 1997). Increased risk for myelosuppression is not cause for withholding therapy from older adults. Interventions should be identified that eliminate or reduce the risk. The use of hematopoietic growth factors can greatly enhance an older client's ability to tolerate the myelosuppressive effects of chemotherapy.

Treatment-related anemia is associated with increased fatigue. Fatigue is a complex concept and has been related to other causes besides anemia. However, anemia remains a major contributor to the feelings of tiredness, weakness, and exhaustion that are part of the fatigue syndrome. Erythropoietin or blood transfusions may be administered to increase the red blood cell count. Sleep and rest are recommended. Clients experiencing fatigue should plan periods of rest during the day, but not to the extent that the rest interferes with regular sleep patterns. Activities should be rearranged to allow for periods of rest. Older clients may have less tolerance at baseline; thus they may tire more easily during treatments. Since the sleep cycle changes with age and older persons spend more time in light sleep where they can be easily aroused, the sleeping environment should be as quiet and comfortable as possible. Pain medications should be adjusted to provide the maximum period of uninterrupted, pain-free sleep (see Chapter 11).

Thrombocytopenia predisposes clients to easy bleeding. The risk of spontaneous hemorrhage is considered to be greater when the platelet count is less than 20,000 cells/mm^3. The most common cause of thrombocytopenia in older clients with cancer is decreased platelet production caused by chemotherapy or radiotherapy. In addition, platelet activity may be disrupted by other drugs, including nonsteroidal antiinflammatory drugs, penicillin and cephalosporin antibiotics, phenothiazine, and antidepressants. Platelet counts should be monitored carefully, and clients should be instructed to use precautions during periods of thrombocytopenia. Precautions should be aimed at preventing injury, particularly to the skin and mucous membranes. Clients should be instructed to use electric razors, soft bristle tooth brushes, and nail files instead of clippers for personal hygiene. Enemas, rectal thermometers, and suppositories can traumatize rectal mucosa and should be avoided. In addition to the potential for injury and bleeding, interruptions of skin and mucous membranes predispose the client to infections. Platelet transfusions can be used during periods of thrombocytopenia to avoid bleeding and hemorrhage.

Infection

Older persons receiving cancer treatment are at increased risk for infection. Infection is the major cause of complications and death in those diagnosed with cancer. Infectious processes are implicated in at least 50% of deaths in persons with solid tumors, such as those of the lung, breast, colon, and prostate, and up to 80% in persons with hematologic malignancies, as in leukemia (Camp-Sorrell, 1996).

Several mechanisms have been proposed that explain the introduction of an infectious process in persons with cancer: surgery interrupts the normal protective barrier of the skin; chemotherapy and radiotherapy cause sloughing and interruption of the integrity of the mucous membranes; intravenous delivery systems and treatment-related catheters introduce bacteria; and changes in normal flora predispose clients to serious opportunistic and nosocomial infection. Over 80% of infections developing in persons with cancer arise from endogenous flora, nearly half of which are acquired during hospitalization (Ellerhorst-Ryan, 1993). Chemotherapy and radiotherapy can reduce the number of circulating granulocytes. Persons whose total granulocyte count is less than 1000 cells/mm^3 are considered to be granulocytopenic and at increased risk for infection. When the granulocyte count is less than 500 cells/mm^3, risk is significant. Older adults with cancer and a history of allergy are significantly more likely to have a high risk for infection than those without a history of allergy (Chang, Vredevoe, and Hirsh, 1994).

Nursing care focuses on prevention. Clients and their families should be knowledgeable about self-care measures for the prevention and early detection of infection. Prevention includes good personal hygiene, avoiding crowds, and postponing visits with persons who may have upper respiratory infections. The ability to monitor body temperature using a thermometer is important. Age-related vision changes may make reading a conventional glass thermometer difficult for many older adults. The nurse should evaluate each individual's ability to use a thermometer and experiment with using various digital devices if visual impairment is a problem. Recently, the use of GM-CSF and G-CSF has reduced the risk of infection for many clients. When infection is suspected, it should be considered a potentially life-threatening emergency.

Nausea and Vomiting

Nausea is a subjectively experienced stomach distress that may be described as a heaviness, pressure, or sinking feeling in the epigastric or sternal region. It is often associated with such physical signs as pallor, sweating, and chills. Most often clients are referring to nausea when they describe "feeling sick." *Vomiting* is the ejection of stomach contents through the mouth. Nausea and vomiting are two separate and distinct events, and although they frequently occur together, it is important to distinguish between the two when taking a client history and planning care.

Nausea and vomiting commonly occur with antineoplastic chemotherapy and are among its most distressing side effects. Not all chemotherapeutic agents cause nausea and vomiting, and those which have high emetic potential do not cause equal distress in all persons. Considerable variation exists by client and type of agent. Antiemetic management has changed over the past 10 years with the development of better pharmacologic agents. Before the development of these agents, an estimated 10% of clients refused chemotherapy because of actual or feared nausea and vomiting (Rhodes, Watson, and Johnson, 1985). Since many older adults likely have friends or family members who were treated using older therapies, nurses should reassure clients that management of this side effect has changed for the better.

A number of age-related physiologic changes might be expected to influence the propensity for nausea and vomiting, such as increased taste threshold and decreased gastrointestinal absorption, secretion, and motility; the extent of these influences is unknown. Only a few studies have examined cancer treatment–related nausea and vomiting in older adults. Older adults were found to report less nausea and vomiting within 24 hours of receiving chemotherapy treatments; however, delayed nausea and vomiting are more common and more severe in older persons and are less well managed by pharmacologic interventions (Baker and Grochow, 1997; Balducci, Mowrey, and Parker, 1992; McMillan, 1989).

Nausea can lead to decreased nutritional intake, whereas vomiting can lead to severe metabolic complications, including dehydration. Older adults are less tolerant of dehydration than younger persons and may manifest acute confusion in response. Dehydration can create a metabolic crisis that may necessitate intravenous fluid resuscitation. In addition, chemotherapeutic agents excreted by the kidney may build to toxic levels, leading to increased side effects and renal failure, particularly in the use of agents with known nephrotoxic side effects. Electrolyte imbalances may aggravate cardiac problems and precipitate drug toxicity if a client is taking medication to manage a cardiac condition. Episodes of severe vomiting may require the dosage of drugs to be reduced or treatment to be postponed. Current pharmacologic management of chemotherapy-related nausea and vomiting includes ondansetron and dexamethasone, which in combination have demonstrated effective control of symptoms and become standard therapy.

Nursing care should begin with an in-depth emetic history and a preventive plan. Characteristics that have been linked with chemotherapy-related nausea and vomiting include susceptibility to motion sickness, history of severe nausea during pregnancy, and poor emetic control during prior treatments. Nurses should evaluate the degree and duration of episodes of nausea and vomiting and monitor for signs of dehydration. Long-term nutritional compromise can result from poorly controlled nausea, and consultation with a dietitian may be helpful (see Nutritional Considerations box).

Stomatitis

Stomatitis is caused by the destruction of rapidly proliferating mucosal cells in the oral cavity, which results in inflammation, ulceration, and bleeding. Several chemotherapeutic agents are known to cause severe stomatitis. Evidence suggests that older adults are at increased risk for severe stomatitis related to chemotherapy. The severity of chemotherapy-induced stomatitis in older adults may be caused by delayed and incomplete repair of mucosal injury (Baker and Grochow, 1997; Balducci, Mowrey, and Parker, 1992). Radiotherapy that includes mucosal tissue in the radiation field can lead to dose-related stomatitis, which generally clears when therapy is complete.

Dental and oral care needs should be evaluated by a dentist before treatment begins, and treatment should be delayed until any dental problems are resolved. A client should understand the importance of good oral hygiene and avoid products with alcohol, which can dry the mucous membranes and increase the risk of cracking, bleeding, and infection. Most commercially available mouthwashes contain alcohol. Safer mint-flavored normal saline/hydrogen peroxide products are available at specialty pharmacies. Viscous lidocaine can be used for areas of painful inflammation. Nurses should routinely assess the client's mouth, lips, and tongue for early signs of inflammation. Severe stomatitis can result in decreased oral intake, leading to dehydration and creating a metabolic crisis that may necessitate intravenous fluid resuscitation. Chemotherapeutic agents excreted by the kidney may build to toxic levels, leading to increased side effects and renal failure, particularly in the case of several

Nutritional Considerations

NUTRITIONAL CONSEQUENCES OF CANCER TREATMENT

The nutritional consequences of cancer treatment can be devastating, resulting in an older adult's inability to tolerate treatment and compromising his or her quality of life. Specific consequences are related to the type of treatment. Nurses should be aware of possible nutritional consequences and complete a nutritional assessment early in the course of therapy. Early assessment provides a baseline for persons at high risk. Clients should be weighed at regular intervals. Individuals at the highest risk for nutritional compromise are those experiencing weight losses of 1% to 2% in 1 week, 5 % in 1 month, 7.5 % percent in 3 months, and more than 10% in 6 months.

TREATMENT	POSSIBLE NUTRITIONAL CONSEQUENCES
Chemotherapy	Individual drugs and drug combinations produce taste alterations, notably a decreased tolerance for protein-rich foods. Drugs that cause mucositis and esophagitis (inflammation of the oral cavity) can lead to difficulty chewing and swallowing, resulting in decreased caloric intake and weight loss. Drug-induced nausea and vomiting can result in dehydration, decreased caloric intake, and weight loss. Drugs that cause diarrhea can lead to dehydration, electrolyte imbalance, and bleeding.
Radiotherapy of the head and neck	This can cause taste alterations, xerostomia (dry mouth), mucositis, and esophagitis, leading to difficulty swallowing and decreased appetite.
Radiotherapy of the esophagus	This can cause dysphagia, sore throat, esophagitis, indigestion, and nausea, leading to difficulty swallowing and decreased appetite.
Radiotherapy of the lung	This can lead to shortness of breath, anorexia, and nausea with generalized malaise and decreased appetite.
Radiotherapy of the abdomen	This can cause nausea, vomiting, cramping, gas, and diarrhea, resulting in decreased appetite.
Surgical resection of oropharynx	This surgery can cause postoperative difficulty in chewing and swallowing, changes in taste perception, and loss of appetite, leading to a dependence on tube feedings.
Esophagectomy, esophagogastrectomy, or esophageal reconstruction	This can cause gastric stasis, steatorrhea, and diarrhea, leading to decreased appetite.
Gastrectomy (partial or complete)	These procedures can result in dumping syndrome with symptoms of cramps, fullness, and diarrhea; malabsorption of fats, iron, vitamin B_{12}, and calcium; and early satiety secondary to decreased size of reservoir, with decreased intake of adequate nutrients and calories.
Intestinal resection	This may lead to malabsorption of nutrients, including fat, iron, vitamin B_{12}, fluids, and electrolytes, resulting in weight loss and malnutrition.
Pancreatectomy	This may result in exocrine insufficiency and malabsorption or endocrine insufficiency, leading to diabetes mellitus.

agents with known nephrotoxic side effects. Also, severe stomatitis can result in decreased appetite, which can lead to nutritional compromise and hence decreased ability to tolerate treatment. In general, older persons become less tolerant of dehydration and nutritional depletion with age.

Anorexia

Many clients receiving cancer treatments complain of a general loss of appetite. Contributing factors include chemotherapeutic agents; radiotherapy, especially to the head and neck area; pain medications; and stomatitis. Decreased appetite leads to decreased caloric intake and weight loss. Severe weight loss has been linked to poor outcomes; clients with significant weight loss have more complications and decreased survival rates. Persons over 80 years of age are more vulnerable to increased toxicity from radiotherapy when they are unable to maintain their weight (Zachariah, Casey, and Balducci, 1995). Anorexia can also contribute to decreased immune function, increasing the risk of infectious complications.

Dietary consultation and frequent weight monitoring are necessary to maintain optimum weight. For persons receiving chemotherapy, an increase of 4.4 calories per kilogram of body weight and 2 g of protein per kilogram of body weight should be incorporated into an overall nutritional plan. The nurse should remember that food choices and eating patterns have strong cultural influences, and planning nutritional diets with clients and their families is critical to successful outcomes.

Diarrhea

Diarrhea results from the destruction of the actively dividing epithelial cells of the gastrointestinal tract. When these cells are destroyed, atrophy of the intestinal mucosa occurs, resulting in shortening or denuding of the intestinal villi. When the villi and microvilli become flattened, the absorptive surface area is reduced and intestinal contents move rapidly through the gut, resulting in frequent liquid stools. Absorption of nutrients is decreased, and clients are at risk for dehydration and malnutrition. Circulatory collapse can occur, especially in older adults with cardiac comorbidity. Diarrhea can aggravate perirectal problems such as hemorrhoids and can cause pain, bleeding, and infection. Several chemotherapeutic agents are associated with diarrhea, but 5-fluorouracil is the most common cause.

Assessment of diarrhea includes the number of stools per day, their consistency, and their color. Older clients may be reluctant to discuss diarrhea, ignoring their symptoms until dehydration becomes a problem. Management of diarrhea may be limited to dietary measures, such as a low-residue diet. Anticholinergic drugs such as atropine sulfate reduce gastric secretions and decrease intestinal peristalsis. Opiate agents bind to receptors on the smooth muscle of the bowel, slowing down intestinal motility and increasing fluid absorption. Chemotherapy is usually administered unless diarrhea is severe and dehydration occurs.

Alopecia

Alopecia (hair loss) is a common complication of chemotherapy. Hair loss may range from thinning of scalp hair to total body hair loss, including eyelashes, eyebrows, and pubic hair. The degree of alopecia depends on both the chemical agent and the dose. Chemotherapy-induced hair loss occurs rapidly and becomes apparent over a 2- to 3-week period following initiation of treatment. Chemotherapy-induced hair loss is temporary in most cases, and hair begins to grow back slowly when treatment is completed. Radiation-induced hair loss occurs when the scalp is in the radiation field. Hair loss is permanent if the radiation dose causes irreversible destruction of the hair follicles; otherwise, hair loss is temporary. To date, no type of hair care product or practice has been shown to satisfactorily prevent or reduce hair loss. In addition, practices such as scalp tourniquets and ice caps are not only uncomfortable, but may create a reservoir where cancer cells can hide during therapy to later migrate and grow.

Although the physiologic consequences of alopecia are minimal, the emotional distress can be enormous. Hair greatly contributes to body image and sexuality. Older clients should be informed about the potential for hair loss relative to their individual treatment. Wigs and hair pieces should be purchased *before* total hair loss. Often clients are too embarrassed to shop for hair replacements when they are bald. Once the hair is gone, it may be difficult to match color, texture, or style. The nurse should not assume that hair loss is only an issue for women; men can be equally devastated by hair loss. For instance, an older, completely bald man was mortified when he lost his big bushy eyebrows, but the local university theater created a pair of high-quality stage eyebrows for temporary relief.

OLDER ADULTS' EXPERIENCE OF CANCER

Cancer in older adults has been viewed as aging in the context of cancer, with cancer as the prominent issue. However, cancer for older persons may be more aptly framed as cancer in the context of aging, with aging as the predominant issue. Why focus on aging as the context?

Traditionally, cancer has been viewed from the perspective of younger persons. Attention has been placed on treatments that return persons to precancer functioning and on statistics that highlight survival rates in the years after diagnosis. Successful treatment in this context means that the cancer goes away and stays away for a long time. Although a younger person's cancer experience includes looking beyond the cancer to a disease-free return to a normal lifestyle, an older person has a different experience; older adults with cancer are close to the end of life. For a younger person, cancer may be viewed in the context of a life yet to be lived, whereas for an older person, cancer may be viewed in the context of a life mostly lived (Kagan, 1997).

Quality of Life

Historically, length of survival has been the most important consideration in measuring the outcome of cancer treatment. Recently, efforts have been made to address not only length of life but the circumstances of life—quality as well as quantity. For an older adult experiencing cancer in the context of a life mostly lived, quality is a very—if not the most—important consideration.

Determining quality of life goes beyond evaluating the severity of symptoms (such as nausea, pain, or fatigue) to considering the degree of functional status reflected in the person's ability to perform daily tasks of living. Quality of life is a multidimensional concept that includes not only functional status and severity of symptoms, but also the client's ideas about psychologic development, sociocultural issues, ethical issues, economic issues, and spirituality.

Fig. 19-2 depicts the multidimensional nature of quality of life. Attitudes in three categories—physical well-being, psychologic well-being, and interpersonal well-being—have been demonstrated to be the primary determinants of overall quality of life for older adults (Padilla et al, 1990). Also, in older adults, quality-of-life factors are shown to be rated differently by men and women; for men, vitality and personal

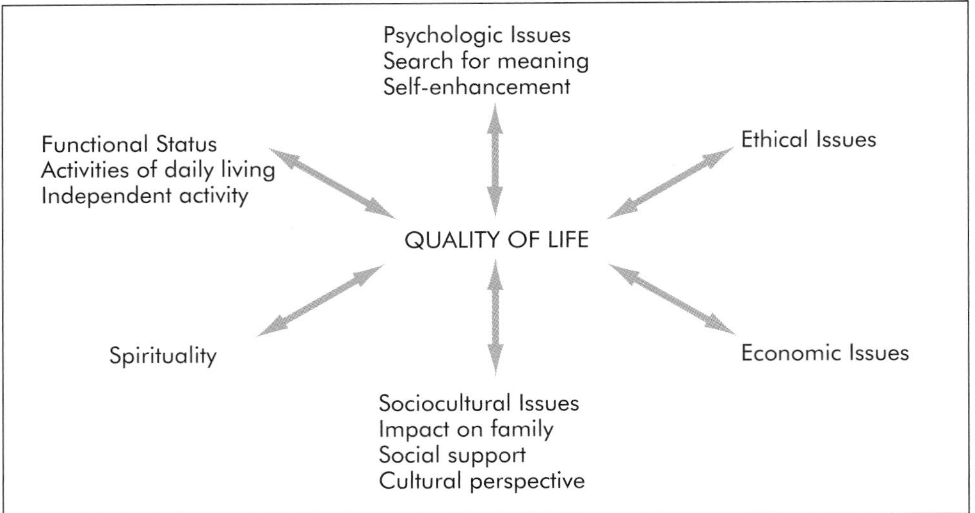

Fig. 19-2 Quality of life as a multidimensional concept.

resources are most important, whereas for women, psychosocial well-being is most important (Dibble et al, 1998).

Quality-of-life evaluation is relevant to both curative and palliative care. In curative care, information obtained from quality-of-life assessment can guide the selection of therapeutic strategies, leading to a more normal life. Older adults may need special quality-of-life consideration when choosing a treatment. A moderate treatment that provides relatively symptom-free disease control may be a better quality-of-life choice for an older adult than a rigorous treatment that statistically offers a prolonged disease-free period. As Yarbro and Ferrans (1998) demonstrated, treatment-related complications influence overall quality of life in older clients (see Research box). In palliative care, quality-of-life assessment can provide insight into areas that may require intervention, such as family counseling, financial planning, and management of depression.

Some measure of a person's quality of life has been included in most studies evaluating treatment modalities or chemotherapeutic agents. Historically, these studies focused on measures of functional status, primarily assessing the ability of clients to perform various activities of daily living (ADLs) using the Karnofsky Performance Index (KPI) (Box 19-3). Although this index continues to be widely used to evaluate the functional status of cancer clients, it has been criticized by both clinicians and researchers. Often newer and better rating scales are used either in place of or in addition to the KPI.

The nurse plays a central role in supporting an older client's quality of life. Nurses manage disease-related symptoms and treatment-related side effects. Few studies have focused on the older adult's perception of health state while receiving cancer treatment. However, Steele and Mills (2004) found that even patients with terminal illness can have a good quality of life when proper resources such as hospice care are initiated (see Research box).

Depression

Few studies have focused on the holistic experience of cancer for older adults. Most insight about older adults' cancer experiences comes from psychologic studies exploring depression among older adults. The association between serious illnesses, such as cancer, and psychologic depression or depressive symptoms has been well documented. Incidences of many illnesses, including cancer, are known to increase with age. The risk of depression does not diminish with age; therefore older adults represent a group at increased risk (see Chapter 14).

The mental health of persons with serious medical diagnoses, including arthritis, diabetes, cancer, renal disease, and nonmelanoma-related dermatologic disorders, has been compared with that of physically healthy outpatients under treatment for depression (Cassileth and Chou, 1992). Both groups were compared with the psychologic status of the general public. Findings suggest that the psychologic status of seriously ill persons approximated that of the public at large, did not differ substantially by diagnosis, and was superior to that of physically healthy psychiatric clients. The researchers concluded that there is no reason to believe that cancer or any other chronic illness leads to mental illness. Most interesting, however, was the finding that older persons consistently displayed a superior psychologic status compared with younger persons, and they expressed strikingly less distress than younger persons in the immediate postdiagnosis period. In general, older clients found the side effects and problems associated with cancer treatment less difficult and coped better than younger clients. Several others studies support these

Research

SAMPLE/SETTING

The sample consisted of 121 men—68 treated by radical prostatectomy and 53 treated with radiotherapy. The setting was a Midwestern community cancer center and teaching hospital.

METHODS

The purpose of this two-group descriptive design was to compare the quality-of-life perceptions of men treated for prostate cancer with surgery and those of men treated for prostate cancer with radiotherapy. The Quality of Life Index (QLI) Cancer Version and the UCLA Prostate Cancer Index were mailed to subjects. The main research variables were quality of life; level of urinary, bowel, and sexual function; and effect of any dysfunction on a client's life.

FINDINGS

No significant differences were found between the groups on the QLI scores, but significant differences were found in urinary, bowel, and sexual function. Urinary function was superior in the radiotherapy group ($p = 0.0002$). Clients who had undergone surgery were more likely to leak urine every day ($p < 0.001$). Only 6% of clients who had undergone radiotherapy needed undergarments for managing incontinence (e.g., pads, diapers), compared with 32% of clients who had undergone surgery ($p = 0.05$). Both groups reported poor sexual function, although it was worse in the surgery group ($p = 0.009$). The study conclusions were that clients treated with surgery had significantly worse urinary and sexual function and better bowel function than those treated with radiotherapy. QLI scores were consistent with these findings, although they did not differ significantly between groups.

IMPLICATIONS

Knowledge of treatment-related problems of survivors of prostate cancer after surgery and radiotherapy and the effect of these problems on quality of life can help nurses support clients in making informed treatment choices. In addition, these findings can help nurses conduct targeted posttherapy assessment and be alert to needs for rehabilitative interventions.

Yarbro CH, Ferrans CE: Quality of life of patients with prostate cancer treated with surgery or radiation therapy, *Oncol Nurs Forum* 25:685, 1998.

results, suggesting that overall adaptation to illness, including cancer, is poorer in younger persons (Ganz, Schag, and Heinrich, 1985; Roberts et al, 1992; Vinokur et al, 1989). These findings suggest the need for more research that focuses on cancer in the context of a life mostly lived.

A note of caution about depressive symptoms in older adults with cancer: depressive symptoms may result from

BOX 19-3 Karnofsky Performance Index

SCORE (%)	STATUS
100	Normal; no complaints; no evidence of disease
90	Able to carry on normal activities; minor signs or symptoms of disease
80	Normal activity with effort; some signs or symptoms of disease
70	Cares for self; unable to carry on normal activity or to do active work
60	Requires occasional assistance, but able to care for most needs
50	Requires considerable assistance and frequent medical care
40	Disabled; requires special care and assistance
30	Severely disabled; hospitalization indicated, although death is not imminent
20	Very sick; hospitalization necessary; active supportive treatment necessary
10	Moribund; fatal processes progressing rapidly
0	Dead

From Karnofsky DA, Burchenal JH: The clinical evaluation of chemotherapeutic agents in cancer, In MacLeod CM, editor: *Evaluation of chemotherapeutic agents,* Washington, DC, 1949, Columbia University Press.

side effects of medications used to control cancer. Depressive symptoms are especially associated with androgen and cortisone medications, two medication groups frequently prescribed for cancer treatment. Also, older adults may have underlying diseases that are controlled by medications. Depressive symptoms are associated with many drugs used to manage chronic illness. In addition, depressive symptoms are known to increase with an increased number of medications taken (see Chapter 22).

Nurses should assess the older adult's risk for depression. Older adults with cancer should be educated about the psychologic implications of having cancer. An understanding of how the experience of cancer can affect such things as feelings of well-being, interpersonal relationships, and self-fulfillment is needed as much as an understanding of the schedule for taking medications. Older clients and their family members should be encouraged to discuss the effects of cancer on family functioning. Individual evaluation of depressive symptoms is needed if an older person is suspected of experiencing depression. Nurses should refer older clients for further psychiatric evaluation when symptoms last longer than a week, worsen rather than improve, or interfere with the ability to carry out daily routines or cooperate with treatment plans. Management of cancer-related depression should be individualized and may include supportive

> **Research**
>
> **SAMPLE/SETTING**
>
> The study was conducted over a three-year period with 129 terminally ill patients enrolled in a home-based hospice program of care in the southeastern United States.
>
> **METHODS**
>
> The purposes of this study were (1) to describe the quality of life of terminally ill patients in a home-based hospice and (2) to examine the relationship between quality-of-life data and symptom distress, patient ability to function, social support, affairs in order, and religious comfort or support as recorded in patient charts. Quality of life was measured by the Missoula Quality of Life Index (MVQOLI), an instrument designed specifically for use with terminally ill patients. The MVQOLI was administered to patients within 20 days of their admission to hospice. A retrospective chart review was conducted to determine levels of symptom distress, patient ability to function, social support, affairs in order, and religious comfort or support.
>
> **FINDINGS**
>
> This study revealed positive scores on the five dimensions of the MVQOLI quality-of-life scale indicating that within 20 days of admission to hospice patients rated their quality of life as good to very good. Data obtained from the chart review also indicated that patients did not experience a great deal of symptom distress (pain, nausea, shortness of breath, and restlessness). There were significant correlations between age and quality of life; interventions count and pain levels; and marital status, well-being, interpersonal relationships, and transcendence. Shortness of breath and well-being were significantly correlated with quality of life. There were no significant correlations between gender, race, or closeness to death and the five dimensions of the MVQOLI and chart review assessments.
>
> Steele LL, Mills B: The quality of life of hospice patients: the relationship of symptom distress to quality of life of hospice patients, *Am J Hospice Palliative Care* 21:884, 2004.

interventions, cognitive intervention, psychotherapy, and psychopharmacology.

Grief and Loss

Grief is a natural and expected human reaction to loss. Grief can be precipitated by a variety of losses. An older adult who is being treated for cancer may experience multiple losses, including loss of energy, loss of a body part, loss of functional ability, loss of self-esteem, and loss of control. The losses associated with cancer may overlap other losses frequently experienced by older adults, such as the loss of a spouse, friends, or family; changes in living arrangements; and physical losses of vision, hearing, or mobility.

Although grief is a universal human reaction, the subject and the intensity of grief are determined by the meaning that an individual places on the loss. Grieving is a human imperative, but how people grieve varies. There is no one way to grieve, and there is no one timetable for grief. People do not "get over" grief. They get through, reconcile with, and learn to live with the loss, but they never get over it; a loss may be mourned forever (Bourne, 1996).

The health care literature often reports that denial is among the initial responses to loss, including losses associated with a diagnosis of cancer. Denial is believed to protect people by providing them with the time needed to assimilate the effect of the diagnosis. Unfortunately, health care providers, including nurses, often haphazardly label a person or family as being in a state of denial. Labels reflect a judgment or conclusion, and conclusions should be supported by evidence. Most persons need some time to allow the diagnosis of cancer to reach conscious awareness. The information about the diagnosis is allowed into the awareness in increments that are tolerable to the person, while at the same time the person is coming to terms with the effect of the diagnosis on his or her life. It may be more reasonable to consider that a client is *titrating information* rather than being in a state of denial. To complicate matters, family members titrate information at different paces as they realize the impact of the diagnosis on their lives. The diagnosis of cancer often leads to a confusing and conflicting experience for the family unit.

Nurses should support older clients and families by patiently repeating information when asked, validating what the family has heard, and determining what the information means to them as individuals and as a family unit. The ongoing process of assessing a client's and family's understanding of the information should spur nursing interventions that are often blocked when nurses judge too quickly. Although clients and families should be allowed to come to their own level of understanding of the diagnosis, the nurse should not support unrealistic ideas about the seriousness of the illness or the benefits of treatment. Interventions may be necessary when a client and family are so threatened by the diagnosis that they are incapable of participating in decision making about the treatment choices. Nurses should validate the client's feelings of grief and loss. Grief cannot be prevented, and nurses should give the individual permission to grieve in reaction to loss.

Older adults experiencing life-changing events generally ask, "What does this mean to me?" as opposed to a younger person who asks, "Who am I?" (Kagan, 1997). Questions of meaning are consistent with identity elaboration and are not to be confused with identity crisis (Moloney, 1995). For older adults, cancer is integrated into an existing life and into patterns of daily living. An older person's life has a long history and a recognized mortality; cancer does not take over life.

Rather, cancer is one of many losses that must be included in daily living (Kagan, 1997).

Social Isolation

Social isolation, the sense of being cut off from people and things of importance, is an experience commonly described by older adults with cancer. Social isolation can be voluntary (i.e., a person seeks disengagement from social interaction) or involuntary (i.e., imposed by others or by circumstances). Choosing to be alone can provide important time for personal reflection, psychologic rebuilding, and renewal. Social isolation, on the other hand, can have negative consequences on psychologic health. Risk factors for social isolation include physical disability or illness, frailties associated with advanced age, psychologic or neurologic disorders, and environmental constraints (e.g., physical surroundings, including diminished personal or material resources that are necessary to access or modify environmental factors) (Tilden and Weinert, 1987).

Voluntary social isolation may result when an older adult with cancer no longer feels comfortable in social settings because of his or her situation, including, for example, changes in body image, energy levels, or interests. Older persons with cancer may withdraw because they perceive that others are uncomfortable in their presence and because they believe, rightly or wrongly, that others are avoiding them because of the cancer diagnosis.

Involuntary social isolation may result from physical changes that prevent a person from continuing with social activities. Treatment-related side effects may interfere with the ability to drive or use public transportation, sit comfortably at a social gathering, or eat politely in public facilities. Special diets, the need to take medications, use of assistive devices, or needs for rest and sleep can interfere with usual social activities.

Older adults experiencing cancer are particularly vulnerable to social isolation. Overall, declining physical health may limit the number or types of social activities available. The availability of social contacts may decline as family members and friends die or relocate. The recent loss of a spouse or partner can lead to social isolation as a person withdraws because of feelings of awkwardness or loneliness. Many older adults feel unsafe going places alone. Social isolation is not reflective of being restricted to a single place, such as a home. Many older adults live a lifetime in a neighborhood only to find that the neighbors have moved, the area has changed and become less safe, and the social network that existed in the neighborhood or town has evaporated slowly over time. Older adults may perceive themselves as disconnected from the unfamiliar people in the neighborhood. Family members may not live in geographic proximity, decreasing the ability to visit or seek assistance. It may be necessary to relocate an older adult during cancer treatment. When an older adult is relocated to live with family or in a residential care facility, he or she needs assistance with developing and maintaining social contacts.

Older adults may substitute interaction with health care personnel for meaningful social interaction. A clinic or home care visit may be an older adult's only social contact for a long time. Nurses should evaluate the older adult's need for social interaction; assess the person's level of social activity before the cancer diagnosis and determine whether it was satisfactory; ask what has changed in regard to social activities since the cancer diagnosis; determine what, if anything, has changed in regard to social activities as the person has gotten older; and work with the client and family to identify strategies for maintaining social activities and contacts. Nurses should explore the importance of various activities described by the older client. Many older adults value religious activities such as church attendance or prayer groups. In addition to meeting social needs, religious activities meet spiritual needs.

Resources and Support

An important component to nursing care of older adults is awareness of resources and referrals to appropriate agencies or support groups. Groups that both cancer patients and their families have found helpful include Make Today Count; I Can Cope; and cancer support groups sponsored by local church groups, hospitals, home health agencies, and hospices. Nurse should have up-to-date listings for the groups in their areas.

Web resources are also being used by older persons. Those related to cancer include:

- National Cancer Institute: http://www.cancer.gov/
- American Cancer Society: http://www.cancer.org
- National Breast Cancer Foundation: http://www.nationalbreastcancer.org
- Prostate Cancer Foundation: http://www.prostatefoundation.org
- American Lung Association: http://www/lungusa.org

SUMMARY

The incidence of most cancers increases with advancing age. However, until recently, little attention was given to the special needs of older adults. The Oncology Nursing Society, in its position statements on cancer and aging, outlines the primary issues nurses should consider in caring for older adults with cancer (Boyle et al, 1992) (Box 19-4). In addition to awareness of personal bias, as listed in the position statement, nurses should be aware of bias in other health care providers, research efforts, family members, and older adults themselves.

Cancer prevention and screening programs for older adults require special attention to ethical issues. Findings may be misleading unless there is attention to specific issues

BOX 19-4 **Oncology Nursing Society Position Statements on Cancer and Aging**

1. It is imperative that oncology nurses recognize personal biases toward aging and older adults that may interfere with the delivery of quality nursing care.
2. It is imperative that oncology nurses advocate cancer prevention and early detection activities for older adults.
3. It is imperative that oncology nurses acknowledge the dynamic and complex interrelationships between cancer and aging that affect nursing care for cancer.
4. It is imperative that oncology nurses intervene to prevent or minimize the unique age-specific sequelae of cancer and its management.
5. It is imperative that oncology nurses integrate comprehensive gerontologic assessment into the nursing care of older adults.
6. It is imperative that oncology nurses assess the availability and capability of the support networks of older adult clients and their significant others.
7. It is imperative that oncology nurses increase communication with colleagues about older adults with cancer to enhance problem solving in a variety of settings and at different points along the cancer continuum.
8. It is imperative that oncology nurses consider age-related factors that affect learning and performance of self-care activities related to the cancer experience.
9. It is imperative that oncology nurses maximize their advocacy role in ethical decision making relative to quality of life of older adults with cancer.
10. It is imperative that oncology nurses recognize the effects of health care policy on the nursing care of older adults who have or who are at risk for cancer.

From Boyle DM et al: Oncology Nursing Society position paper on cancer and aging: the mandate for oncology nursing, *Oncol Nurs Forum* 19:913, 1992.

of length bias, lead bias, and overdetection bias. Decisions to screen older adults should be made on an individual basis.

Older adults are more vulnerable to the development of cancer. Since the aging cell has been exposed to a lifetime of potentially carcinogenic substances, it is more susceptible to damage, and is less able to repair damage. In general, older adults are capable of tolerating cancer treatment when careful attention is paid to dosage adjustments and comorbid factors. The experience of cancer for the older adult is unique. Cancer in the older adult is cancer in the context of a life mostly lived.

Key Points

- The three leading causes of cancer deaths in women between ages 55 and 74 are lung, breast, and colorectal cancer; in men between these same ages, the leading causes of cancer deaths are lung, colorectal, and prostate cancer.
- Aging cells show a tendency toward aberration as they replicate, probably because of the failure of growth control mechanisms. Altered growth control mechanisms make the aging cell more vulnerable to damage, leading to the development of cancer.
- Clinical manifestations of cancer in older adults may be mistakenly attributed to normal, age-related changes. Older adults should be made aware of the warning signs of cancer and report symptoms associated with them to a health care provider.
- Nurses caring for older adults have a major responsibility to recommend strategies aimed at the prevention and early detection of cancer in this age-group.
- The major treatment modalities for cancer include surgery, radiotherapy, chemotherapy, and biotherapy. Therapy with any of these modalities can be used alone or in combination; therapy may be curative or palliative.
- The functional status of an older adult is the most important consideration in selecting a treatment goal and modality. Age alone is not a good predictor of treatment tolerance or response.
- Older adults generally have fewer reserves, and greater attention should be given to the status of major organs, including the kidney, liver, heart, lung, and gastrointestinal

Home Care

1. Instruct homebound older adults and their caregivers to be aware of and report symptoms associated with the warning signs of cancer.
2. Educate older adults about cancer screening and self-examination.
3. Breast cancer is a disease of older women; thus breast screening is a lifelong process. Instruct homebound older women on the American Cancer Society's BSE guidelines.
4. Assess nonspecific symptoms such as indigestion, loss of appetite, and weight loss in both older men and older women. These warning signs are seen in cancer of the stomach, colon, and rectum.
5. Instruct caregivers and homebound older adults with cancer about general comfort measures to promote rest and sleep, with the goal of increasing pain tolerance.
6. Assess for side effects of cancer treatment therapies (e.g., radiotherapy, chemotherapy) and report to a physician as needed for treatment recommendations.
7. Instruct caregivers and homebound older adults on measures to reduce the side effects of cancer treatment therapies.
8. Refer clients to hospice during the last 6 months of terminal illness.

system. Maintenance of fluid, electrolyte balance, and caloric intake is critical to treatment outcomes for older adults.

- Older adults are especially vulnerable to the nephrologic and hematologic toxicity of some chemotherapeutic agents.
- Psychosocial care of older adults with cancer includes addressing issues related to quality of life, depression, loss and grief, and social isolation.
- The experience of cancer for each older adult is unique. Cancer in an older adult is cancer in the context of a life mostly lived.

Critical Thinking Exercises

1. You are asked to make a 30-minute presentation at a senior center on the benefits and risks of cancer screening in older adults. Prepare a topical outline for the presentation.
2. The director of oncology services asks you to develop a procedure for functional assessment of older adults with cancer. Develop the procedure and include any functional assessment parameters and instruments to be used.
3. The family cancer support group has asked you to facilitate a discussion on family considerations when an older family member has cancer. Prepare a list of the points that you would discuss with the group.

REFERENCES

American Cancer Society: *Cancer facts and figures: 2004,* Atlanta, 2004a, The Society.

American Cancer Society: *What are the side effects of chemotherapy?* Atlanta, 2004b, The Society.

American Geriatric Society Clinical Practice Committee: Breast cancer screening in older women. *J Am Geriatr Soc* 48:842, 2000.

American Lung Association Epidemiology and Statistic Unit, Research and Scientific Affairs: *Trends in lung cancer morbidity and mortality,* New York, 2004, The Association.

Baker SD, Grochow LB: Pharmacology of cancer chemotherapy in the older person, *Clin Geriatr Med* 13(1):169, 1997.

Balducci L, Mowrey K, Parker M: Pharmacology of antineoplastic agents in older patients. In Balducci L, Lyman GH, Ershler WB, editors: *Geriatric oncology,* Philadelphia, 1992, JB Lippincott.

Bergkvist L et al: The risk of breast cancer after estrogen and estrogen-progestin replacement, *N Engl J Med* 321:293, 1989.

Berlin NI et al: The National Cancer Institute cooperative early lung cancer detection program, *Am Rev Respir Dis* 130:565, 1984.

Bond J: Colorectal cancer update: prevention screening treatment and surveillance for high risk groups, *Med Clin North Am* 84:1163, 2000.

Bourne V: Grief. In Groenwald SL et al, editors: *Cancer symptom management,* Boston, 1996, Jones & Bartlett.

Boyle DM et al: Oncology Nursing Society position paper on cancer and aging: the mandate for oncology nursing, *Oncol Nurs Forum* 19:913, 1992.

Brant JM: Breast cancer challenges in Native American women. In Dow KH, editor: *Contemporary issues in breast cancer,* Boston, 1996, Jones & Bartlett.

Camp-Sorrell D: Hematologic toxicities. In Liebman MC, Camp-Sorrell D, editors: *Multimodal therapy in oncology nursing,* St Louis, 1996, Mosby.

Caplan LS, Wells BL, Haynes S: Breast cancer screening among older racial/ethnic minorities and whites: barriers to early detection, *J Gerontol* 47:101, 1992.

Cassileth BR, Chou JN: Psychosocial issues in the older patient with cancer. In Balducci L, Lyman GH, Ershler WB, editors: *Geriatric oncology,* Philadelphia, 1992, JB Lippincott.

Celentano DD, Klassen AC: The impact of aging on screening for cervical cancer. In Balducci L, Lyman GH, Ershler WB, editors: *Geriatric oncology,* Philadelphia, 1992, JB Lippincott.

Centers for Disease Control and Prevention: *United States cancer statistics: 2001 incidence and mortality,* Atlanta, 2004, The Agency

Chang BL, Vredevoe D, Hirsh M: Allergy as a risk factor for nursing care problems in the elderly cancer patient, *Cancer Nurs* 18(2):83, 1994.

Cohen HJ: Biology of aging as related to cancer, *Cancer Suppl* 74(7):2092, 1994.

Coleman EA, Hutchins L, Goodwin J: An overview of cancer in the older adult, *Med Surg Nurs* 13(2):75-80, 2004.

Collins M: Increasing prostate cancer awareness in African American men, *Oncol Nurs Forum* 24:91, 1997.

Crawford J, Cohen H: Relationship of cancer and aging, *Clin Geriatr Med* 3(3):419, 1987.

Cummings S, Olopade O: Predisposition testing for inherited breast cancer, *Oncology* 12(8)1227-1241, 1998.

Davis L, Lindley C: *Neoplastic disorders and their treatment: general principles.* In Kimble MA et al, editors: *Applied therapeutics: the clinical use of drugs,* Philadelphia, 2004, JB Lippincott.

Dehni N et al: Effects of aging on the functional outcome of coloanal anastomosis with colonic J-pouch, *Am J Surg* 175:209, 1998.

DeMaria LC, Cohen HJ: Characteristics of lung cancer in elderly patients, *J Gerontol* 42:540, 1987.

Dibble SL et al: Gender differences in the dimensions of quality of life, *Oncol Nurs Forum* 25:577, 1998.

Egorin MJ: Cancer pharmacology in elderly, *Semin Oncol* 20(1):43, 1993.

Einhorn LH: Improvements in fluorouracil chemotherapy? *J Clin Oncol* 7:1377, 1989.

Ellerhorst-Ryan J: Infection. In Groenwald SL et al, editors: *Cancer nursing: principles and practice,* Boston, 1993, Jones & Bartlett.

Elpern EH: Lung cancer. In Groenwald SL et al, editors: *Cancer nursing: principles and practice,* Boston, 1993, Jones & Bartlett.

Farrow DC, Hunt WC, Samet JM: Temporal and regional variability in the surgical treatment of cancer among older people, *J Am Geriatr Soc* 44:559, 1996.

Freeman HP: Cancer in the socioeconomically disadvantaged, *CA-A Cancer J Clin* 39(5):266, 1989.

Ganz PA, Schag CC, Heinrich RL: The psychosocial impact of cancer on the elderly: a comparison with younger patients, *J Am Geriatr Soc* 33:429, 1985.

Greenberg HM, Trotti AM: Radiotherapy of cancer in the older aged person. In Balducci L, Lyman GH, Ershler WB, editors: *Geriatric oncology,* Philadelphia, 1992, JB Lippincott.

Greenfield S et al: Patterns of care related to age in breast cancer patients, *JAMA* 257:2766, 1987.

Guadagnoli E et al: The influence of patient age on the diagnosis and treatment of lung and colorectal cancer, *Arch Intern Med* 150:1485, 1990.

Hansen J: Common cancers in the elderly, *Drugs & Aging* 13:467, 1998.

Host H, Lunde G: Age as a prognostic factor in breast cancer, *Cancer* 57:2217, 1986.

Iwamoto R: Radiation therapy. In Otto S, editor: *Cancer nursing,* St Louis, 1997, Mosby.

Jassak P: An overview of biotherapy. In Rieger PT, editor: *Biotherapy: a comprehensive overview,* Boston, 1995, Jones & Bartlett.

Johnston EM, Crawford J: Hematopoietic growth factors in the reduction of chemotherapeutic toxicity, *Semin Oncol* 25:552, 1997.

Kagan SH: *Older adults coping with cancer: integrating cancer into a life mostly lived,* New York, 1997, Garland Publishing.

Kagawa-Singer M: Addressing issues for early detection and screening in ethnic populations, *Oncol Nurs Forum* 24:1705, 1997.

Kimmick GG et al: Cancer chemotherapy in older adults, *Drugs & Aging* 10(1):34, 1997.

Knobf MT: Breast cancer. In McCorkle R et al, editors: *Cancer nursing: a comprehensive textbook*, Philadelphia, 1996, WB Saunders.

Landis S et al: Cancer statistics, 1999, *CA: Cancer J Clin* 49:8-31, 1999

Larson PJ et al: Influence of age on problems experienced by patients with lung cancer undergoing radiation therapy, *Oncol Nurs Forum* 20:473, 1993.

London S, Willett W: Diet and the risk of breast cancer, *Hematol Oncol Clin North Am* 3(4):559, 1989.

Masetti R et al: Breast cancer in women 70 years of age or older, *J Am Geriatr Soc* 44:390, 1996.

McMillan SC: The relationship between age and intensity of cancer-related symptoms, *Oncol Nurs Forum* 16:237, 1989.

Millikan R, Logothelis C: Update of the NCCN guidelines for treatment of prostate cancer, *Oncology* 11:180-193, 1997.

Moloney MF: A Heideggerian hermeneutical analysis of older women's stories of being strong, *Image J Nurs Schol* 27(4):297, 1995.

National Cancer Institute: *Breast cancer treatment*, Washington, DC, 2004a, US National Institutes of Health.

National Cancer Institute: *Colorectal cancer: who's at risk?* Washington, DC, 2004b, US National Institutes of Health.

National Cancer Institute: *Cancer health disparities*, Washington, DC, 2003a, US National Institutes of Health.

National Cancer Institute: *Surveillance epidemiology and end-results program, 1975-2000*, Washington, DC, 2003b, Division of Cancer Control and Population Sciences.

Nobler MP, Venetl R: Prognostic factors in patients undergoing curative irradiation for breast cancer, *Int J Radiat Oncol Biol Phys* 11:1323, 1985.

Padilla GV et al: Defining the content domain of quality of life for cancer patients with pain, *Cancer Nurs* 13:108, 1990.

Patterson WB: Surgical options in the treatment of cancer: how are they affected by the patient's age? In Balducci L, Lyman GH, Ershler WB, editors: *Geriatric oncology*, Philadelphia, 1992, JB Lippincott.

Patterson WB: Surgical issues in geriatric oncology, *Semin Oncol* 16:57, 1989.

Pfeifer KA: Pathophysiology. In Otto S, editor: *Oncology nursing*, St Louis, 1997a, Mosby.

Pfeifer KA: Surgery. In Otto S, editor: *Oncology nursing*, St Louis, 1997b, Mosby.

Reigle BS: Breast cancer in elderly women. In Luggen AS,Meiner SE, editors: Handbook for the care of the older adult with cancer, Pittsburgh, Pa, 2000, Oncology Nursing Press.

Rhodes VA, Watson PM, Johnson MH: Patterns of nausea and vomiting in chemotherapy patients: a preliminary study, *Oncol Nurs Forum* 12(3):42, 1985.

Roberts CS et al: Psychosocial impact of gynecologic cancer, *J Psychosoc Oncol* 10:99, 1992.

Samet JM et al: Choice of cancer therapy varies with age of patient, *JAMA* 255:3385, 1986.

Shell JA, Bulson BK, Vanderlugt LF: Lung cancers. In Otto S, editor: *Cancer nursing*, St Louis, 1997, Mosby.

Shepherd FA et al: Treatment of small cell lung cancer in the elderly, *J Am Geriatr Soc* 42:64, 1994.

Steele L, Mills B: The quality of life of hospice patients: the relationship of symptom distress to quality of life of hospice patients, *Am J Hospice Palliative Care* 21:884, 2004.

Tilden V, Weinert C: Social support and the chronically ill individual, *Nurs Clin North Am* 22:613, 1987.

US Census Bureau: *Profile of general demographic characteristics*, Washington, DC, 2000, US Department of Commerce.

Vestal RE: Aging and pharmacology, *Cancer* 80:1302, 1997.

Vinokur AD et al: Physical and psychosocial functioning and adjustment to breast cancer, *Cancer* 63:394, 1989.

Walter L, Covinsky K: Cancer screening in elderly adults: a framework of individualized decision making, *JAMA* 285:2750, 2001.

Woolner LB, Fontana RS, Cortese DA: Roentgenographically occult lung cancer: pathologic findings and frequency of multicentricity during a 10 year period, *Mayo Clin Proceed* 59:453, 1984.

Wyckoff J et al: Breast irradiation in the older woman: a toxicity study, *J Am Geriatr Soc* 42:150, 1994.

Wynder EL, Stellman SD: Impact of long term filter cigarette use on lung and laryngeal cancer risk, *J Natl Cancer Institute* 62:471, 1979.

Yancik R: Cancer burden and the aged, *Cancer* 80:1273, 1997.

Yarbro CH, Ferrans CE: Quality of life of patients with prostate cancer treated with surgery or radiation therapy, *Oncol Nurs Forum* 25:685, 1998.

Yates J: Cancer prevention in older persons. In Balducci L, Lyman GH, Ershler WB, editors: *Geriatric oncology*, Philadelphia, 1992, JB Lippincott.

Zachariah B, Casey L, Balducci L: Radiotherapy of the oldest old cancer patients: a study of effectiveness and toxicity, *J Am Geriatr Soc* 43:793, 1995.

20 Loss and End-of-Life Issues

SABRINA FRIEDMAN, MSN, PhD, EdD, FNP

Learning Objectives

On completion of this chapter, the reader will be able to:

1. Distinguish between grief, mourning, and bereavement.
2. Discuss characteristics of grief.
3. State Worden's four tasks of mourning.
4. Identify psychologic, physical, social, and spiritual aspects of normal grief responses.
5. Describe four ways that complicated grief reactions may manifest themselves.
6. Describe nursing care activities that assist grieving older adults.
7. Discuss physical, psychologic, social, and spiritual aspects of dying for older adults.
8. Explain age-related changes that affect older adults who are dying.
9. Describe nursing strategies for assisting dying older adults and their families.
10. Discuss the philosophy of palliative care.

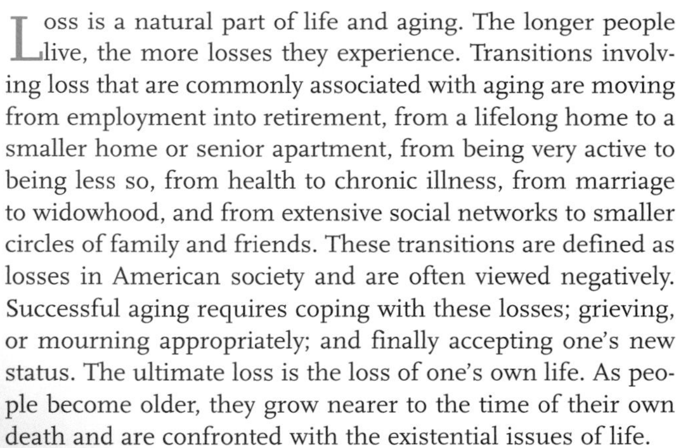

Loss is a natural part of life and aging. The longer people live, the more losses they experience. Transitions involving loss that are commonly associated with aging are moving from employment into retirement, from a lifelong home to a smaller home or senior apartment, from being very active to being less so, from health to chronic illness, from marriage to widowhood, and from extensive social networks to smaller circles of family and friends. These transitions are defined as losses in American society and are often viewed negatively. Successful aging requires coping with these losses; grieving, or mourning appropriately; and finally accepting one's new status. The ultimate loss is the loss of one's own life. As people become older, they grow nearer to the time of their own death and are confronted with the existential issues of life.

The purposes of this chapter are twofold: (1) to provide basic knowledge regarding loss and grief and (2) to discuss the experience of dying among older adults so that nurses can assist the grieving, the dying, and their families during these difficult times. The chapter discusses the nature of life transitions, especially those focused on death and dying; the meaning that these changes may have for older persons and their families; and typical ways in which people respond to such changes. A holistic approach incorporating physiologic, psychosocial, and spiritual aspects is applied, with discussion of the nursing care of older persons and their families throughout this process.

American culture typically defines aging in a negative way, and death and dying are often considered taboo issues. Only recently has research shown that life transitions such as dying can act as catalysts for personal growth. Such intense times of crisis in people's lives have the potential to stimulate spiritual and psychologic growth if the crisis can be successfully managed. A "good death" is defined as one free from avoidable stress and suffering for patients and families and caregivers; in general accord with patients' and families' wishes; and reasonably consistent with clinical, cultural, and ethical standards (Matzo and Sherman, 2001). Nurses often act as guides who accompany older adults and their family members through this final life transition.

LOSS AND LIVING WITH GRIEF

Most of the literature and research on bereavement among older persons focuses on the death of spouses, with less attention on responses to the loss of parents, siblings, adult children, and friends. Other gradual and abrupt life transitions such as retirement, change of residence, ill health, loss of pets, and inability to drive are also viewed as losses that evoke varying degrees of bereavement response. For all types of transition—from moving to a new home to the death of a loved one—people's responses depend on their perception of the events and the meaning of the transition within the context of their lives and their physical, psychosocial, and spiritual life patterns.

Loss of Relationships

The death of one's spouse or life partner is usually the most significant loss that an older person may experience. It involves the loss of a companion who is often one's best friend, sexual partner, and partner in decision making and household management, as well as a source of one's definition of self or identity. Today's older couples often have a sharp division of labor with regard to many of the tasks of daily living. The surviving spouse must take on new responsibilities while coping with the loss of his or her loved one.

Although the bereavement that follows the death of a spouse is a highly stressful process, Lund's (1989) summary of studies of widowed persons concludes that many older surviving spouses are resilient. Although 72% of those studied reported that the spouse's death was the most stressful event they had ever experienced, they also reported high coping abilities. The overall effects of bereavement on the physical and mental health of many older adults were not as severe as expected, with both positive and negative feelings experienced simultaneously. Loneliness and problems associated with tasks of daily living were two of the most common difficulties reported. Although bereaved older adults adjusted in many different ways to the deaths of their spouses, in general the most difficult period occurred in the first several months, improving gradually but unsteadily over time.

Lund's (1989) review also showed that older men and older women are more similar than dissimilar in their bereavement experiences and adjustment. Age, income, education, and anticipation or forewarning of death did not seem to have much effect on future adjustment processes. Religion-related variables also did not contribute much to adjustment. Social support was moderately helpful in the adjustment process, as were internal types of coping resources such as independence, self-efficacy, self-esteem, and competency in performing tasks of daily living.

Older adults' normal grief responses to the loss of a spouse are summarized by Lund (1989). The following conclusions, drawn from his work, speak specifically to the bereavement experiences of older persons:

- Bereavement adjustments are multidimensional in that nearly every aspect of a person's life can be affected by the loss.
- Bereavement is a highly stressful process, but many older surviving spouses are resilient.
- The overall effect of bereavement on the physical and mental health of many older spouses is not as devastating as expected.
- Older bereaved spouses commonly experience both positive and negative feelings simultaneously.
- Loneliness and problems associated with the tasks of daily living are two of the most common and difficult adjustments for older bereaved spouses.
- Spousal bereavement in later life might best be described as a process that is most difficult in the first several months but improves gradually, if unsteadily, over time. The improvement may continue for many years, but for some it may never end.
- There is a great deal of diversity in how older bereaved adults adjust to the death of a spouse.

The deaths of loved ones remind those left behind of their own mortality and evoke significant meaning for those who are grieving. To an adult child, the death of a parent often has many conflicting meanings, depending on the parent-child relationship. Meanings of parental death include being orphaned; becoming the oldest generation, the next in line for death; coming into one's own; changing roles; becoming a role model for one's own aging process; experiencing relief; or losing the opportunity to complete unfinished business (Kowalski, 1986). Often the death of a parent is preceded by an extended period of caregiving, usually by a daughter. Inherent in this caregiving role is a multitude of potential problems. Problems among siblings and feelings of guilt, anger, ambivalence, role reversal, and burden can all influence the bereavement process and adjustment that follows a parent's death.

The death of a sibling is an even more powerful reminder of one's own mortality, since a sibling is of the same generation. Tasks that occur for all siblings include grieving the deceased sibling, coping with family changes, realigning relationships, and attempting to understand the meaning of the tragedy within the family (Matzo and Sherman, 2001).

The death of adult children has received relatively little attention in the literature. Parents usually expect their children to outlive them, so the untimely death of a child, even an adult child, is especially difficult. Feelings of anger and guilt often complicate the grieving process. If the child was the primary caregiver for the parent, the death will directly affect the parent's own living arrangements.

Older persons experience strong emotional reactions on learning of the death of friends and neighbors. Friends are especially important in old age, and contact with close friends is often associated with life satisfaction and mental health. As more friends die, the sense of abandonment may intensify.

Many older adults experience multiple losses with little time for grieving between the losses. The emotional crises imposed by these multiple losses can lead to disorientation, mental confusion, and withdrawal. Individual coping styles, the existence of support systems, the ability to maintain some sense of control, and the griever's health status and spiritual beliefs all influence a person's responses to multiple losses (Garrett, 1987).

Definitions

Grief is defined in this chapter as an acute reaction to one's perception of loss, including physical, psychologic, social, and spiritual aspects. Feelings that may accompany grief include anger, shame, helplessness, sadness, guilt, despair, relief, peacefulness, calm, and release (McCall, 1999). Other characteristics of grief are that (1) it involves many changes over time; (2) it is a natural reaction to all kinds of losses, not just death; and (3) it is based on one's unique perception of a loss (Rando, 1988). Grief responses are characterized in two ways: normal and uncomplicated, or complicated.

Mourning is defined as the long-range process of resolving acute grief reactions; it enables a person to resume a satisfying life. Mourning involves both unconscious and conscious processes that gradually loosen ties to a loved one, that help in adapting to the loss, and that assist in the process of learning to live a healthy life in a world without the loved one (Rando, 1988). The ways in which people mourn are prescribed by social and cultural norms that indicate acceptable coping behaviors in their society (Doka and Davidson, 1998).

Bereavement is defined as the state of having experienced a significant loss. Because it is possible to experience a loss without experiencing an acute grief reaction, the period of bereavement may or may not be accompanied by grief (Fulton and Metress, 1995). Usually the terms *bereavement* and *grief* are used synonymously; however, it is useful to consider them separately to account for experiences where loss is not accompanied by grief.

Perceptions and Meanings

The meaning of loss has been perceived in a variety of ways. Some of the more common meanings attached to illness and loss are punishment by a supreme being, suffering that must be overcome or endured, a normal part of the life experience, and an opportunity for personal growth and transcendence.

Personal beliefs and attitudes, including cultural and religious ones, influence how losses are perceived. For example, a person who views homosexuality as a sin may perceive acquired immunodeficiency syndrome as God's punishment for homosexual individuals. For some, losses are viewed as stressful events that must be overcome to "get on" with life. For others, suffering is considered a virtue, something that may bring a person closer to God. Still others may seek to find meaning in the loss and in life after the loss, transcend the associated suffering, and experience personal growth as a result of the loss. The meaning of a loss to a bereaved person has a significant effect on his or her responses to that loss. For this reason, it is important that caregivers explore the perceptions of the bereaved to understand and assist them in the grieving process.

Responses to Loss

Lindemann's (1944) early study of survivors of the 1942 Coconut Grove fire of Boston identified physical and psychologic symptoms associated with acute grief. The ages of the mourners were not known. Grief reaction can be characterized by time: early, middle, and last phases. In the early phase, shock, disbelief, and denial are common. This phase commonly ends as people begin to accept the reality of the loss after the funeral. The middle phase is a time of intense emotional pain and separation and may be accompanied by physical symptoms and labile emotions. Lastly, reintegration and relief occur as the pain gradually subsides and a degree of physical and mental balance returns (DeSpelder and Strickland, 1992).

Worden (1991) views grief as an active rather than a passive process. He identifies tasks rather than stages and describes the following four tasks of mourning: (1) accept the reality of the loss, (2) work through the pain of grief, (3) adjust to an environment in which the deceased is missing, and (4) emotionally relocate the deceased and move on with life. The first task, accepting the reality of the loss, involves coming to the realization that the person is dead; that he or she will not return; and that reunion, at least in life as we know it, is impossible. The second task, experiencing the pain of grief, is necessary to prevent the pain from manifesting itself in some other symptom or problematic behavior. Sociocultural customs that discourage open expression of grief often contribute to unresolved grief. The third task, adjusting to an environment in which the deceased is missing, involves developing new skills and assuming the roles for which the deceased was responsible. The last task, the withdrawal of emotional energy and the reinvestment in another relationship, entails withdrawing emotional attachment to the lost person and loving another living person in a similar way. For many, this last task is the most difficult.

Worden's tasks of mourning are often a more useful way to think of grief among older persons. Many stage models of grief imply a progression of stages beginning with shock and disbelief, but many older adults do not go through that first stage. They may have expected the death or may be beyond shock and disbelief after having experienced multiple losses in their lifetime. They may also undergo several of the stages at the same time. So concentrating on tasks of grieving may be more helpful for an older person than expecting to progress through stages of grief. Regardless of whether shock or anticipation occurs, the task of accepting the reality of the loss is relevant for all.

It is critical that older persons who have lost loved ones acknowledge that pain is associated with grief and loss and that they must adjust to an environment where the loved one is absent. The expression of pain depends partly on culture and partly on the quality of the relationship with the lost loved one. Guilt often accompanies the pain of grief.

Adjustment to one's environment after the loss of a loved one involves learning new roles, such as those previously assumed by the deceased, and new ways of interacting with others in one's social environment. This adjustment can be especially difficult if a spouse is the loved one lost and the social network consists primarily of other couples.

The final task, emotionally relocating the deceased and moving on with life, gives the bereaved person permission to invest emotionally in others without being disloyal to the lost loved one. Although Worden (1991) pointed out that in one sense mourning is never over, he also stated that in losses that involve a great deal of emotional attachment, the process takes at least 1 year before the wrenching pain subsides. Some older spouses have reported that they feel as though they will never "get over" their loss; instead, they have learned to live with it (Lund, 1989).

Anticipatory grief is defined as grieving that occurs before the actual loss. It includes the processes of mourning, coping, and planning that are initiated when the impending loss of a loved one becomes apparent (Rando, 1986). Anticipatory grief may account for some persons' apparent lack of overt grief reactions after the death of loved ones who experienced long terminal illnesses. Anticipatory grief increases as death becomes eminent and ends when the death occurs. Anticipatory grief does help reduce early shock, confusion, and depression. Survivors who resolve grief before the death of a loved one may be criticized by others or experience self-reproach for lack of a grief reaction to the actual death. These responses can lead to further problems of adjustment.

Normal Grief Responses

Bereavement can have such a profound effect on the bereaved that somatic and psychologic symptoms and illness can occur (see Client/Family Teaching box). It has also been shown to result in a higher death rate in the bereaved. Human beings respond as a whole, manifesting grief physically, psychologically, socially, and spiritually. These different aspects of the whole are discussed in the following section to aid in understanding their nature. The nurse should remember that each aspect is integrated within the whole person. Also, interventions directed at one of these areas will affect the other areas; thus an approach that separates the mind, body, and spirit is not advocated.

Psychologic Responses. Studies of grief responses have consistently identified common psychologic responses. Feelings of sadness are the emotions most often mentioned (Worden, 1991). Other common feelings include guilt, anxiety, anger, depression, apathy, helplessness, and loneliness.

Client/Family Teaching

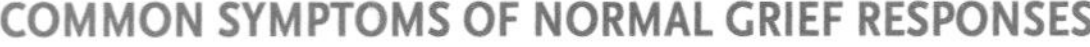

COMMON SYMPTOMS OF NORMAL GRIEF RESPONSES

Grief responses have physical, psychologic, social, and spiritual aspects. The duration and intensity of symptoms are highly variable. Most of the more intense symptoms subside in 6 to 12 months; however, mourning may continue for several years.

Physical symptoms commonly include crying, loss of appetite, decreased energy and fatigue, and sleep difficulties. Psychologic responses commonly include feelings of sadness, guilt, anxiety, anger, depression, helplessness, and loneliness. Social changes following the loss of a loved one depend on the role of the deceased. In widowhood, there is often a loss of social support, an adjustment to living alone, and sometimes an inability to manage tasks of daily living unless new skills are learned. Spiritual responses often lead the bereaved to search for meaning in life and to reexamine his or her faith and belief system.

Guilt and regret regarding one's relationship with the person who has died can be especially troublesome (Landman, 1993). Shock and disbelief may immediately follow the death or loss. The bereaved person may also display diminished self-concern, a preoccupation with the deceased, and a yearning for his or her presence. Some older persons become confused and unable to concentrate after the death of someone significant to them. *Grief spasms*, periods of acute grief, may come when least expected (Rando, 1988). How the grief response manifests itself is individually determined by sociocultural factors in addition to the quality of the relationship between the deceased and the mourner. For some older persons the grief experience may include feelings of relief and emancipation, especially after prolonged suffering or a difficult relationship.

Physical Symptoms. Physical symptoms are commonly associated with acute grief responses. Tearfulness, crying, loss of appetite, feelings of hollowness in the stomach, decreased energy, fatigue, lethargy, and sleep difficulties are common symptoms of grief. Other physical sensations may include tension, weight loss or gain, sighing, feeling something stuck in one's throat, tightness in one's chest or throat, heart palpitations, restlessness, shortness of breath, and dry mouth.

Social Changes. The social changes that follow the loss of a loved one depend on the type of relationship and the definition of social roles within the relationship. Widowhood is the loss that generally has the greatest effect on social role change, but any loss of a person within one's household is especially difficult. In addition to deep psychologic pain, the bereaved person must often learn new skills and roles to manage tasks of daily living. All these social changes occur at a time when withdrawal, a lack of interest in activities, and a lack of energy make decision making and action very difficult. Socialization and interaction patterns also change. If an older couple often socialized together with other couples, widowhood may bring dramatic changes in the type and style of interaction. For others who have strong social support and established patterns of independent interaction outside of the lost relationship, the adjustment process toward creating new social roles and interactions may occur more quickly.

Spiritual Aspects. Lastly, the death of a loved one inevitably causes bereaved people to ponder the existential issues of life and to examine the meaning not only of the lost loved one's life but also of their own. Spiritual issues may surface as the person searches for meaning. Anger at God, sometimes followed by a crisis of faith and meaning, may accompany bereavement. It may be important for the bereaved to view the death of their loved one as a transition to a life with God in the spirit. Meaning in life is highly individualized, but the importance of finding meaning in life is more universal. What a person finds meaningful is not as important as the ability to look back on life and see that it has been meaningful and to understand that life can continue to be meaningful even in its last stages.

Religion and spirituality can provide a stabilizing influence during grief. One's religious institution may provide the sense of belonging to a group of people who support one another in times of need. Some may experience a deep inner sense of peace that they are being cared for by a higher power. For others, however, the grief experience may precipitate a crisis in their beliefs and values. Gender, social class, ethnicity, and culture may influence one's spiritual response to grief (Doka and Davidson, 1998) (see Cultural Awareness box).

Complicated Grief Reactions

The responses described thus far are generally considered to be "normal" or uncomplicated grief reactions. When grief progresses in an unhealthy way and does not move toward resolution, it is called complicated mourning or abnormal grief. The nursing diagnosis for complicated mourning or abnormal grief is "dysfunctional grieving" and shares many of the defining characteristics of normal grief. Dysfunctional grieving occurs for an extended length of time and is severe in its intensity. Nurses need to be familiar with dysfunctional grieving and should refer clients to advanced practice nurses or other health professionals skilled in working with complicated grieving.

Cultural Awareness

LOSS AND END-OF-LIFE ISSUES

In some cultures, people believe that particular omens may warn of approaching death (e.g., some Native-American and Mexican-American groups believe the appearance of an owl and messages in dreams foreshadow death). Research indicates that the desire to be told of one's impending death varies according to culture: 71% of whites, 60% of blacks, 49% of Japanese Americans, and 37% of Mexican Americans want health care providers to tell them if they are dying. Each of these groups indicated that the physician is the most appropriate person to communicate the information, and a family member is the second most appropriate.

Although death is a universal human experience, there are culture-specific considerations concerning attitudes toward the loss of a loved one, including age (e.g., child versus older adult) and cause of death. In many Asian-American cultures the loss of an older adult (perceived as having accumulated years of wisdom and knowledge) may be mourned more than the loss of an infant or child (viewed as having made a lesser contribution to society because of fewer years of life experience). For many whites the reverse may be true; relatively greater sorrow may be expressed over the loss of a younger person (perceived as having been cheated out of achieving his or her fullest potential) than is expressed over the loss of an older individual (perceived as having lived a full and productive life). It should be noted that, regardless of age, human life is valued by all cultures and loss of life is mourned by those who knew and loved the deceased.

Among the Tohono O'odham (Papago Indians of Arizona) the concept of "good" and "bad" death prevails. A good death comes at the end of a full life when a person is prepared, whereas a bad death occurs unexpectedly and violently (e.g., accidents, homicides, suicides) and leaves the victim without a chance to settle affairs or "say good-bye." Some cultural and religious groups consider suicide taboo and may impose sanctions even after death (e.g., burial in church cemeteries may be denied).

Both culture and religion influence postmortem rituals. Muslims have specific rituals for washing, dressing, and positioning the body, whereas some Jewish groups discourage cosmetic restoration or attempts to hasten or retard decomposition by artificial means. Among some Asian-American groups it is customary for family and friends of the same gender to wash and prepare the body for burial or cremation. As part of their lifelong preparation for death, Amish women sew white burial garments for themselves and their family members. Deceased members of the Church of Jesus Christ of Latter Day Saints (Mormons) are dressed in white temple clothing before being viewed by family and friends. Some Native Americans believe that the spirit of the deceased person is contaminated and refuse to touch the body after death. The traditional Navajo is dressed in fine apparel, adorned with expensive jewelry and money, and wrapped in new blankets. Some Navajo believe that the structure in which the person died must be burned.

Often interrelated with religious beliefs and practices, culture influences funeral and burial or cremation practices, as well as what is expected of bereaved family members (e.g., who grieves, for how long, culturally appropriate behaviors during mourning). Among Chinese Americans, five degrees of kinship (*wu-fu*) are recognized, and these determine the severity of mourning that is expected according to the closeness and importance of the deceased to the mourner.

Lastly, the nurse should be aware that culture may influence the choice of a final resting place for the deceased person. For example, the bodies of older Jewish clients may be flown to Jerusalem for burial, Christians may prefer to be buried in ground blessed by a priest or minister, and those who are cremated may have expressed various preferences for the disposition of the ashes. Traditional Chinese Americans may follow a system of double burial: the coffin is initially buried for 7 years, then the remains are exhumed and stored in an urn.

Disenfranchised grief refers to grief that is not or cannot be openly acknowledged (Doka, 1989). This complicates the grieving process both because it cannot be expressed and because social support is not available. Four major situations that cause disenfranchised grief are (1) when a relationship is not recognized by others (e.g., cohabitation, same-sex partners), (2) when a loss is not recognized (e.g., death of a pet), (3) when the griever is not recognized (e.g., very old adults, those with cognitive deficits), and (4) when the death is disenfranchising (e.g., deaths caused by drunk driving or suicide) (Doka, 1997).

Complicated grief reactions may manifest as one of four types: (1) chronic, (2) delayed, (3) exaggerated, or (4) masked. *Chronic grief reactions* are prolonged and never reach a satisfactory conclusion. Since bereaved individuals are aware of their continuing grief, this reaction is fairly easy to recognize. A therapist can assess which tasks of grieving are not being resolved and why. The goal of intervention is to resolve these tasks (Worden, 1991).

In *delayed* or *postponed grief reactions* the griever's response at the time of the loss is either absent or not sufficient to deal with the loss. At some future time the person may experience an intense grief reaction triggered by a subsequent, smaller loss or by any other event that triggers sadness. Feelings of hostility or ambivalence are usually present in this kind of reaction.

Exaggerated grief reactions occur when normal feelings of anxiety, depression, or hopelessness grow to unmanageable proportions. People with exaggerated grief may feel overwhelmed and that they are unable to live without the deceased person. They may lose the sense that the acute grief is transient and may continue in this intense despair for a long time (Worden, 1991).

Lastly, *masked grief reactions* occur when bereaved persons experience feelings related to the loss but do not express or recognize the source of these feelings. This reaction may occur as a self-protective mechanism, since some people may not be able to bear the stress of mourning. This repression of grief responses usually manifests as either a physical symptom, often similar to one that the deceased experienced, or as some type of maladaptive behavior (Worden, 1991).

Factors Affecting Grief Response

Rando (1988) outlines factors that influence how people experience and express their grief. Categories of psychologic factors include the characteristics and meaning of the lost relationship, the personal characteristics of the bereaved, and the specific circumstances surrounding the death (Table 20-1). Social factors include the griever's support system, sociocultural and religious background, education and economic status, and funerary rituals. An individual's physical state also influences the grief response. Important physical factors are the use of drugs and sedatives, nutritional state, adequacy of rest and sleep, exercise, and general physical health. Nurses need to be aware of how all these factors affect dying persons and their families so that they may provide the best care possible.

Nursing Care

The goal of nursing care for older persons who are grieving is not to "make them feel better" quickly, though nurses are often tempted to try to do so. The goal is to assist and support bereaved persons through the grieving process, recognizing that pain is a normal and healthy response to loss and allowing bereaved persons to accomplish the tasks of mourning in their own ways.

Grief counseling is used to facilitate successful progression through the grief process, whereas *grief therapy* is intended for those who are experiencing complicated mourning. Nurses, other health professionals, and specially trained volunteers can provide grief counseling, whereas therapy should be conducted under the guidance of a skilled therapist (Worden, 1991). The following section discusses grief counseling.

TABLE 20-1 Psychologic Factors Influencing Grief Responses

CHARACTERISTICS AND MEANING OF LOST RELATIONSHIP	PERSONAL CHARACTERISTICS OF BEREAVED	SPECIFIC CIRCUMSTANCES OF DEATH
Nature and meaning of loss	Coping behaviors, personality, and mental health	Immediate circumstances of death
Qualities of lost relationship	Level of maturity and intelligence	Timeliness of death
Role and function filled by deceased	Past experiences with loss and death	Perception of preventability
Characteristics of deceased	Social, cultural, ethnic, and religious background	Sudden versus expected death
Amount of unfinished business between bereaved and loved one	Sex-role conditioning	Length of illness before death
Perception of deceased's fulfillment in life	Presence of concurrent stress or crises in life	Anticipatory grief and involvement
Number, type, and quality of secondary losses that accompany the death		

Modified from Rando TA, editor: *Loss and anticipatory grief*, Lexington, Mass, 1986, Lexington Books. Used with permission of Therese A. Rando, PhD.

Worden (1991) suggests four ways that grief counselors can assist grieving persons in the tasks of mourning. They are to (1) increase the reality of the loss, (2) help the counseled person deal with both expressed and latent effects, (3) assist the counseled person in dealing with various impediments to readjustment after the loss, and (4) encourage the counseled person to make a healthy emotional withdrawal from the deceased and to feel comfortable reinvesting that emotion in another relationship.

Nurses working in hospitals encounter clients who are experiencing many different kinds of losses and intense grief reactions on a routine basis. Despite the fact that nurses often have limited time to interact with bereaved clients and family members in the hospital setting, nurses can intervene in many ways. The staff or visiting nurses in nursing facilities or community health settings have repeated encounters with clients and families over a much longer period than do hospital-based nurses; regardless of setting, nurses have contact with at least some of a bereaved person's support systems, which can assist in the mourning process. Nurses are required to recognize grief responses, identify the primary task of mourning for a bereaved person, and intervene using grief counseling principles.

A simple tool to assess progress in bereavement is the 10-Mile Mourning Bridge (Huber and Gibson, 1990) (Fig. 20-1). This tool, useful for both clinical assessment and research purposes, draws on Worden's (1991) work and is conceptualized as a journey across a 10-mile bridge. On the bridge, the 0 represents the time before grief. The 10 reflects Worden's last stage, where clients recover the emotional energy consumed by grieving and reinvest it in their own lives. It is not suggested that people ever "get over" the death of a loved one, but rather that grief can cease to be the primary focus of life. Clients can use the 10-Mile Mourning Bridge as a self-assessment tool with daily or weekly frequency, as determined by the client. Since each person's grief experience is unique, the miles on the bridge are only defined at each end. Use of this instrument can also facilitate client-nurse discussions about grief and progress (Huber and Bryant, 1996).

Worden's (1991) grief counseling principles can be useful in the bereavement process; specifically, they can:

- Help the survivor actualize the loss. Nurses are often the first to initiate this process, especially after the death of a client in a health care institution. Nurses are usually the professionals present to offer details and descriptions of the death or explanations of puzzling situations that family members may not understand. Having information about the death and the events preceding and following it is important in helping to actualize the loss. Survivors may need to be encouraged to talk about the loss, to tell the story of events surrounding the death, and to relate memories of the deceased. This process takes time.

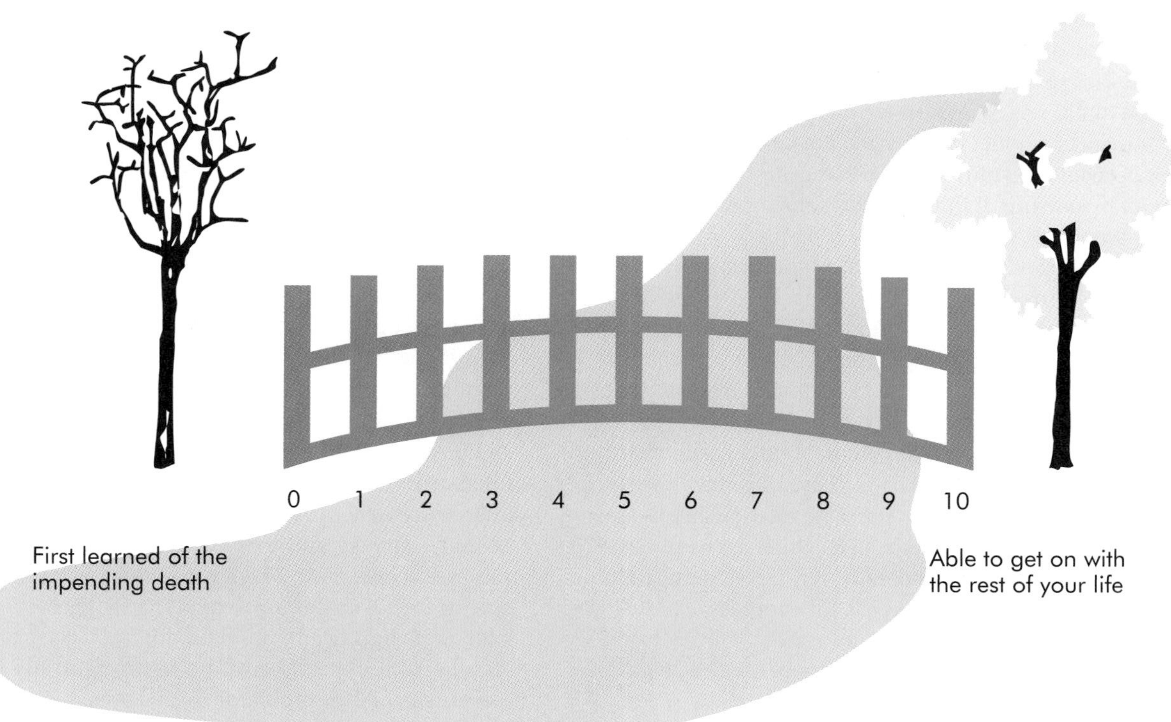

Fig. 20-1 10-Mile Mourning Bridge. (From Huber R, Gibson J: New evidence for anticipatory grief, *Hospice J* 6(1):49, 1990.)

Worden (1991) found that many survivors took up to 3 months before they began to accept the reality that their spouses were dead and not going to return.

- Help the survivor identify and express his or her feelings. Because they are unpleasant, some feelings accompanying bereavement may not be expressed or recognized by the bereaved person. Nurses need to assess a bereaved person's feelings and ask specific questions that encourage expression. Feelings that often go unexpressed include anger, guilt, anxiety, and helplessness (Worden, 1991). Guilt and regret may be recognized and expressed through storytelling, writing in a journal, or writing a letter to the deceased. A ritual such as burying or burning the letter may assist the mourner in resolution. Sometimes, unpleasant emotions are displaced. For example, anger may be directed toward the deceased, toward God, or toward the physician or nurse who helped the family care for the loved one. Such anger may be difficult to understand, but it is helpful for the targets of the anger to detach themselves and not respond defensively. Sociocultural and gender differences influence expression of emotions and need to be taken into account. Older persons may also express their emotions differently than younger ones, especially after dealing with multiple losses; for example, crying may be a less common indicator of sadness among older persons.
- Assist the survivor in living without the deceased. The nurse needs to assess the survivor's daily living situation and identify any existing or potential problems. The roles played by the deceased must now be assumed by the survivor (or someone else) to accomplish tasks of daily living. Knowledge of community resources and teaching of practical skills are necessary to meet this need. In general, survivors should be advised to postpone making major decisions that involve life changes, such as selling property or moving. Calling on the survivor's social support system is also useful.
- Facilitate the survivor's emotional withdrawal from the deceased. The nurse needs to be especially sensitive to when the bereaved should emotionally withdraw from the deceased and begin developing new relationships. This is especially difficult if the relationship lost was that of a spouse. Research has shown that older persons who lose a confidante are less likely than younger persons to replace the confidante. Perhaps they are unwilling to emotionally invest in another intimate relationship when the risk of repeated loss is so high. Other types of relationships such as close friendships may be encouraged to help meet an older person's needs for intimacy.
- Provide the survivor with time to grieve. It used to be believed that after the first anniversary of the death, grief should be resolved. This has been shown to be inaccurate; many factors influence the time for adjustment, as discussed previously. Two points in time seem to be especially critical: 3 months after the death and 1 year after the death (Worden, 1991). Older persons who have experienced multiple losses may need more time. For some, the losses may never be resolved; a person may simply learn to live with the feelings of grief.
- Interpret "normal" behavior for the survivor. It is important that nurses, with a clear understanding of the range of normal grief responses, communicate acceptance and reassurance of the normalcy of a grieving person's responses. Grieving individuals can be reassured that they are not going crazy, that their physical and psychologic responses are normal in the face of significant loss, that grief spasms may occur, and that they will feel better in time.
- Allow for individual survivor differences. Just as nurses must be sensitive to individual differences in styles of grieving, family and friends need to accept differences among themselves in their grief responses. Nurses may need to explain the wide range of responses and assist mourners with allowing one another to grieve in their own ways.
- Provide continuing support for the survivor. Although nurses' interactions with bereaved persons may be brief or intermittent, referrals can be made for outside support. This support may include community resources and support groups. Nurses can also encourage the bereaved to mobilize their own support system of family and friends.
- Examine the survivor's defenses and coping styles. Certain coping behaviors are healthy, whereas others are not. An older person has had a lifetime of experience coping with stressful situations and usually has well-established patterns of coping. Under normal circumstances these defenses and coping mechanisms can often be used successfully; however, they may not be effective in dealing with monumental or accumulated losses. Unhealthy coping mechanisms may lead to destructive behaviors such as alcoholism. Nurses can help the bereaved identify their coping mechanisms, evaluate their effectiveness, and either encourage their continued use or explore other ways of coping more positively.
- Identify pathologic conditions for the survivor and make appropriate referrals. When assistance through grief counseling and professional guidance is not sufficient, additional problems may have arisen that require more intensive help. Nurses need to be particularly alert to serious depressive illness and should refer accordingly. Losing a spouse and living alone puts older persons at risk for depression. Older white men have the highest suicide rate of any group, which may suggest that depression is a significant problem for this age-group. Discussion with older men of the meaning in life may give the nurse clues to problems in this area.

There is a risk of the overuse of sedating and antianxiety medications in treating the symptoms of grief reactions in the elderly. This causes special problems among persons over age 65, who take many more prescription drugs per year than younger persons. Each added drug increases the risk of drug interaction. Also, the risk of side effects and toxic reactions is greater among older adults than among younger persons.

Nurses in all settings are in a position to assist the bereaved at various stages of grief. Nurses are the most effective, however, when they examine their own losses, grief expectations, and patterns of coping with loss. Personal experiences with loss inevitably influence the effectiveness of the help that nurses can give to others who are mourning. A nurse who has successfully worked through a loss—big or small—and has reflected on the experience has valuable insight into the grieving process. On the other hand, a nurse who is grieving may be unable to invest emotional energy in the care of a client who is experiencing acute grief.

APPROACHING DEATH: OLDER PERSONS' PERSPECTIVES

The following section addresses the nature of dying among older persons, including stages of dying; attitudes toward death; and physical, psychosocial, and spiritual responses. Nursing strategies for older persons who are dying, environmental considerations, and family and caregiver perspectives are other important aspects of understanding the nature of dying.

Kübler-Ross, in her classic work on death and dying (1969), identified five stages that have become the basis for practice regarding dying clients. This model purports that dying individual's progress through the stages of denial, anger, bargaining, depression, and finally acceptance of death. All persons may not move through these stages in a sequential and orderly fashion, with some even moving back and forth between stages, but this stage theory has become popular in interpreting the behavior and feelings of dying persons, sometimes to their detriment.

Retsinas (1988) argues for a model of death that takes into account the following factors: (1) that very old persons see themselves as confronting impending death, (2) that they are used to the "sick role" and their gradual decrease of vitality, (3) that roles have already been redefined, and (4) that death may truly be timely for older persons.

Kastenbaum (1978) points to such assumptions as older persons being ready for timely deaths as evidence of our society's ageist attitudes. Although the literature demonstrates that older persons have a variety of attitudes toward death, fear of their own death is relatively rare. Research has generally proven that there is less fear of death among older persons than among younger ones; older adults are also more concerned about being in control and life after death (Thorson and Powell, 1988). Major concerns about dying among older persons are fears about being a burden, suffering, and use of life-prolonging technology (Kohn and Menon, 1988). A person who has had positive experiences of coping and is relatively well adjusted usually approaches the stress of being close to death with adaptation and acceptance. Individual assessments still need to be conducted, however, since older adults have widely varied experiences and attitudes.

Psychologic Aspects

Factors other than age are important in determining an older person's feelings toward his or her own death. Sociocultural and religious background, physical and functional status (especially the degrees of pain and dependency on others), social isolation and loneliness (usually resulting from the death of more than one significant other), and the meaningfulness of everyday life are all important factors in determining one's approach to impending death. These must be considered in the assessment and understanding of an older person's attitudes toward dying and death.

Once people have identified themselves as nearing the end of their lives, they commonly engage in a process called *life review* (Butler, 1963), where they try to make sense of life as a whole. Erikson (1963) identified the last task of life as a psychosocial crisis of integrity versus despair. In this theory, older persons nearing death are expected to review their lives and draw some conclusions about the positive and negative aspects. If they can generally say their life was meaningful and worth living, then a sense of ego integrity emerges. If, however, their lives are evaluated negatively, they may experience a sense of regret or meaninglessness and despair.

Spiritual Aspects

Religious beliefs and spiritual experiences play an important part in older persons making sense of their lives. Faith in a supreme power can give life a transcendent meaning and help people view their lives within the context of a greater purpose or meaning. Sometimes dying or a threat of loss can trigger a crisis of faith, in which people question their previous beliefs in an effort to make sense of the present experience.

Three spiritual needs of dying persons have been identified by Doka (1993): (1) to search for the meaning of life, (2) to die appropriately, and (3) to find hope that extends beyond the grave. These three needs reflect Erikson's developmental task for the last stage of life, as well as other research findings regarding fears associated with dying for older persons. Religious or spiritual beliefs and experiences can be instrumental in helping older persons meet these fears. Assessing clients' desires for religious and spiritual assistance is particularly important when they are dying. Among the many reasons for spiritual care at this time are preparing for death and the afterlife, dealing with anger over dying, seeking forgiveness for past wrongs, searching for peace, and meeting the needs of a family coping with loss (Hall, 1997). Some nurses are comfortable discussing spiritual concerns with clients; those who are not should refer the client to the appropriate clergy or hospital chaplain.

Social Aspects

Once the term *dying* is applied to an individual, role changes are often initiated or reinforced by family and friends. The adoption of the sick role may be accompanied by an acceptance of one's fate. Alternately, dying individuals may adopt a fighting stance, determined to do all they can to outwit or forestall death. Some move ahead with resolve to define themselves as "still living," refusing to accept the label of "dying" and thus living each day as fully as possible. The stance people take toward dying is affected by sociocultural, psychologic, and life history factors. Some of these attitudes toward dying are positive and promote growth; others are negative and difficult to endure, not only for dying persons but also for those around them. For example, it is troublesome when family members want to resolve issues while the client denies that he or she is dying and refuses to discuss matters that need resolution.

Because death and dying have been regarded as taboo topics in American society, most people are uncomfortable, at least initially, when talking about death with someone who is dying. This is partly because of having to confront one's own mortality when facing the death of others. It is fairly easy to live an illusion of stability and immortality when around young, healthy persons. But when a loved one is dying, thoughts turn to one's own mortality and what life will be like without this person. Since these thoughts are uncomfortable for most, one way of relieving this discomfort is to avoid the dying person. Social isolation often results as friends and sometimes family seemingly abandon the dying person. A special concern for older persons results from society's attitude that they are ready to die and therefore have less need to interact with others. It is seen as normal and natural for them to disengage and die quietly. This attitude also fosters social isolation. Thus social isolation, loneliness, and role changes are typical concomitants of dying for older persons.

Physical Aspects

An obvious and sometimes puzzling issue for those working with older persons is when to consider a person to be dying. Is a diagnosis of terminal illness necessary? Are there certain physical signs that must be present? In one respect, all human beings are in the process of dying. But the probable length of time remaining before death occurs or the certainty of a fatal illness generally determines whether one is defined as dying. Life expectancy also enters into people's attitudes about when dying occurs. There is generally a greater expectation of impending death for a frail 100-year-old than for an energetic 75-year-old. The most commonly used definition of a terminal illness is a life expectancy of 6 months or less, which is the length of time determined by Medicare for receipt of hospice benefits. Because there is no clear definition of "dying" for older persons not diagnosed with a terminal illness, this must be explored individually.

Death for older persons usually results from complications from one or more chronic illnesses, rather than from a sudden, unexpected incident or illness. The three leading causes of death, accounting for approximately 70% of deaths among adults over age 65, are heart disease, malignant neoplasms, and cerebrovascular diseases. These are expected to remain the major causes of mortality in the older adult population through the year 2020. Other major causes of death among older adults include chronic obstructive pulmonary disease (COPD), pneumonia and influenza, diabetes mellitus, injury from accidents, renal diseases, septicemia, and complications from Alzheimer's disease (Jackson, 1999).

General Health Care Needs

Regardless of needs that arise from specific diseases and functional problems, dying individuals have general health care needs that nurses help to provide. These general interventions include (1) stabilizing and supporting vital functions and facilitating integrated functioning, (2) determining functional deviation and adjusting treatment, (3) relieving distressing symptoms and suffering, (4) assisting client and family interaction, and (5) supporting a client and his or her family in coping with the realities of death. Common physical problems and symptoms encountered by terminally ill clients include pain, dyspnea, constipation, altered urinary elimination patterns, altered skin integrity, nausea and vomiting, restlessness and agitation, difficulty swallowing, confusion, and nutritional problems (McMillan and Moody, 2003). Family coping and stress, safety needs, and self-care deficits are other important problems (Weitzner, Moody, and McMillan, 2003).

Palliative care refers to the total care of a client whose disease is not responsive to curative treatment, with the goal of achieving the best possible quality of life for the client and family (World Health Organization, 1990). This approach has been successful in guiding the care of dying clients by multidisciplinary health care teams.

Effect of Age-Related Changes

Nursing care aimed at meeting the physical needs of older persons who are dying is no different from the meticulous care needed by any other client with a debilitating condition. However, age-related changes and the effects of long-term chronic illnesses predispose older persons to greater potential for problems in hygiene and skin care, nutrition, elimination, mobility and transfers, rest and sleep, pain management, respiration, and cognitive and behavioral functioning (Sankar, 1991). Only the areas that pose special problems for older persons are discussed in this section.

Age-related changes in the integumentary and vascular systems, coupled with alterations in nutrition, elimination, and mobility, quickly lead to skin breakdown. Loss of the subcutaneous fat layer and a decrease in sebaceous gland activity cause the skin to become thin and dry, making it more susceptible to the hazards of immobility. Pressure ulcers are a problem for older, debilitated clients and are often quick to form and slow to heal. Sometimes even the best skin care and positioning cannot prevent the formation of pressure ulcers.

Rigidity of the chest wall, decreased ciliary activity, and decreased cough and gag reflexes all predispose older persons to respiratory problems, especially pneumonia. Aspiration pneumonia is a common problem for older clients who are unable to feed themselves and who have difficulty maintaining an upright position. The decreased effectiveness of the immune system and the presentation of uncommon symptoms related to pneumonia can make the diagnosis and treatment of pneumonia in older adults more complicated. Shortness of breath and altered respiratory patterns in sleep, such as Cheyne-Stokes respirations or sleep apnea, are more prevalent among older persons and can become problematic if they are seriously ill or dying.

Digestive changes associated with age include decreased amounts of saliva and digestive fluids and enzymes, decreased peristaltic activity, and decreased absorption through the intestinal wall. These changes predispose an older person who is dying to additional problems with maintaining adequate nutritional status and bowel function. These changes are exacerbated by immobility and often contribute to constipation, fecal impaction, and sometimes diarrhea. Although health care professionals often downplay the seriousness of constipation, this problem can cause major discomfort for a dying person and contribute to other life-threatening complications.

Changes in vision and hearing that commonly accompany advancing age reduce the stimulation that older persons receive from the environment. This is complicated by the usual practice of removing eyeglasses and hearing aids from clients who are ill, as well as by providing a quiet, darkened, and peaceful environment. Sensory deprivation can lead to mental confusion among healthy individuals and is of even greater importance among older adults who are dying.

Environmental changes and unfamiliar people and settings also contribute to cognitive impairment among older persons. Because hospitalization or a move to a nursing facility is often a part of the dying experience for older persons, the acute confusion that may result from such a move may be permanent. Institutionalization, even if temporary, may be a rite of passage for an older person and serve as an external indicator that his or her illness is progressing and death is becoming more imminent.

Although it is believed that the experience of superficial pain for older persons is unchanged, many older adults seem to experience less deep pain, such as organ pain associated with terminal illnesses like cancer. On the other hand, older persons reportedly have an increased sense of introspection, which means they have heightened experiences of their internal bodily functions and feelings (Neugarten, 1968). This increased introspection may give rise to more reports (often perceived as complaints) of pain and discomfort, which need to be heeded and validated by the nurse. Nonmedicative interventions for pain relief—such as therapeutic touch, massage acupressure, relaxation, and visualization—need to be used whenever possible.

Age-related changes in pharmacokinetics and pharmacodynamics lead to atypical drug responses. Because drugs are so widely used as an essential part of medical treatment, their effectiveness, side effects, and reactions need to be closely monitored. Physiologic changes associated with dying, such as circulatory changes, increase the difficulty in managing drug regimens. Sleep patterns are also disturbed by physiologic changes, pain, and changes in environment. Medication is the most common answer to dying persons' complaints of an inability to sleep. Although medication may be appropriate in some instances, it needs to be prescribed with caution and monitored carefully. For a dying older person, sleep medications may cause new problems such as incontinence or acute confusion. Nonpharmacologic therapies should be used first. Psychologic causes of sleeplessness should also be explored. For example, if older persons fear dying alone in their sleep and they have unfinished business to resolve with their families, sleep medication is not the best answer. Instead, a careful assessment of the cause of sleeplessness must be followed by appropriate treatment aimed at that cause.

Nursing Care

Excellent nursing care of dying older persons begins with examination of a nurse's own value system regarding older persons in American society. In such a youth-oriented culture, old age is not highly esteemed or valued. The death of older persons greatly benefits a society with a growing problem of overpopulation. An overworked hospital nurse usually has to prioritize; younger clients with greater probability for survival receive more attention than older dying clients who bear the physician orders, "Do not resuscitate; comfort measures only." Sedatives may be administered to make that task easier. The realities of the U.S. health care system and ageist societal values often force nurses to compromise the quality of care they deliver to dying older clients. Death often comes quietly, and the nurse cannot always be present to care for a dying person's physical and emotional needs and share in the wisdom and knowledge that only a lifetime of experience can bring.

Assessment. As with any other nursing care, careful and ongoing assessments must be made of physical, psychosocial, and spiritual needs. Assessment tools for physical needs, described in Chapter 4, are relevant for ill and dying older adults. Special attention, however, needs to be given to potential problem areas such as skin integrity, respiratory status, nutrition, elimination, sensory abilities, cognitive functioning, comfort, and rest.

Psychosocial needs of the dying person, family, and caregivers must also be carefully assessed. This can be a difficult area to approach, especially when time is limited or a client's or family's feelings about the process of dying are unknown. Spiritual and psychosocial needs are often discussed together, since they are interrelated and affect each other. Areas for careful assessment of spiritual needs include searching for meaning in life, dying appropriately, and finding hope that extends beyond the grave (Doka, 1993).

Meaning in life often emerges as a theme among those who are grieving, as well as among those who are dying or nearing the end of their lives. In a study by Burbank (1988) of community-living older adults, leading a meaningful life was associated with both physical health and a lack of depressive symptoms. A series of questions that are useful in assessing the degree of meaning life can be found in Box 20-1.

The hierarchy of a dying person's needs, based on Maslow's hierarchy of needs framework, can assist nurses in identifying a dying older person's specific needs at each level (Ebersole, Hess, and Luggen, 2004) (Fig. 20-2). Careful assessment of the level of a dying person's needs can indicate individualized strategies for meeting those needs.

Strategies. Little difference exists between nursing strategies for younger persons who are ill and those for dying older persons. The same actual interventions may be applied, but older adults require more frequent assessment, application, and evaluation of the effectiveness of nursing strategies. For instance, a debilitated, immobile younger person may require repositioning less often than an older person who is debilitated and immobile. Older persons may suffer from more severe dry mouths than younger persons with the same condition. The nurse needs to ensure that care is not delivered less often because of personal biases and ageist devaluation of older persons. Pacing of care is especially important, with time and patience being given to encourage as much independent functioning as possible.

Particularly difficult problems for older adults who are dying include pain, dyspnea, constipation, urinary incontinence, restlessness, hallucinations and delusions, and nutri-

BOX 20-1 Fulfillment of Meaning Scale

For each of the following statements, circle the response that is most nearly true for you at this time.

1. I feel that I have found a significant meaning or meanings for leading my life.
   Strongly disagree Disagree Uncertain Agree Strongly agree
2. Even though there may be a purpose in my life, I do not try to do much about it.
   Strongly disagree Disagree Uncertain Agree Strongly agree
3. I have a belief or beliefs about life that gives my living significance.
   Strongly disagree Disagree Uncertain Agree Strongly agree
4. Something seems to stop me from doing what I really want to do.
   Strongly disagree Disagree Uncertain Agree Strongly agree
5. I do not value what I am doing in my life.
   Strongly disagree Disagree Uncertain Agree Strongly agree
6. The things that are the most important to me dominate my activities.
   Strongly disagree Disagree Uncertain Agree Strongly agree
7. In thinking of my life, it is hard for me to see a reason for my being here.
   Strongly disagree Disagree Uncertain Agree Strongly agree
8. Basically, I am living the kind of life I want to live.
   Strongly disagree Disagree Uncertain Agree Strongly agree
9. In life, I have no goals or aims at all.
   Strongly disagree Disagree Uncertain Agree Strongly agree
10. My personal existence is purposeful and meaningful.
    Strongly disagree Disagree Uncertain Agree Strongly agree
11. Life seems to be completely routine.
    Strongly disagree Disagree Uncertain Agree Strongly agree
12. Facing my daily tasks is a source of pleasure and satisfaction.
    Strongly disagree Disagree Uncertain Agree Strongly agree

MEANING FRAMEWORK QUESTION

Is there something or things so important to you in your life that they give your life meaning?

Yes No

If no, please describe your life situation at this time.

If yes, please list those things that are currently important to you and that give your life meaning.

From Burbank PM: Assessing the meaning of life among older clients: an exploratory study, *J Gerontol Nurs* 18(9):19-28, 1992.

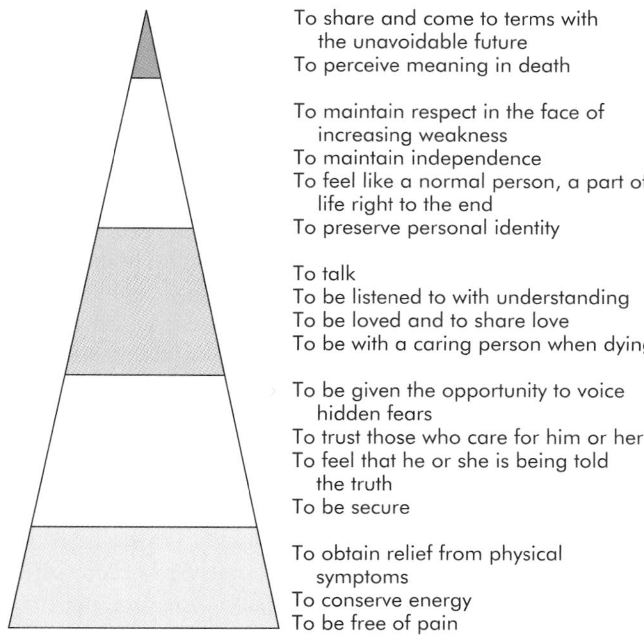

Fig. **20-2** Hierarchy of a dying person's needs. (Modified from Ebersole P, Hess P: *Toward healthy aging,* ed 5, St Louis, 1998, Mosby.)

tional problems. Palliative care measures for these are discussed individually in this section, because they often differ from strategies used with chronically ill older adults who are not close to death.

Pain is prevalent among individuals who are dying and can have a powerful, negative effect on a client's quality of life (Brockopp et al, 1996). The pain experience is complex and its management often difficult. A stepped-care approach is recommended, using aspirin or acetaminophen for mild pain, a moderate opiate such as codeine or oxycodone for more constant pain, and a strong opiate such as morphine for severe pain (Ham and Sloane, 1997). Pain medication should be given around the clock to promote stable blood pressure levels. Nursing responsibilities include careful pain assessment, education of clients and family caregivers regarding pain medication, and close communication with the prescriber for changes in medication as needed. Attention needs to be given to a client's emotional state, since psychosocial factors and emotional pain may accentuate physical pain (Edwards, 1998).

Dyspnea is another common symptom feared by both clients and caregivers. Common causes include hypoxemia, poor handling of secretions, anxiety, bronchospasm, and pain. Elevation of the head of the bed, limitation of activity, a cool room with low humidity (not completely dry), supplemental oxygen, and bronchodilators or analgesics may be sufficient to improve dyspnea. Morphine, which is often the most effective medication to decrease dyspnea, also decreases anxiety. Constipation and depressed respiratory rate are complications of morphine administration.

Constipation is common among older adults who require narcotics for pain and whose diets and activities are restricted. Adding fiber to a client's diet or giving bulk-forming laxatives may not be practical if the person is unable to maintain sufficient fluid intake and diet. Stool softeners and oral cathartics may be more effective, but suppositories, enemas, and manual disimpaction may also be necessary. Bowel evacuation should occur at least every 3 days regardless of intake.

For urinary incontinence an indwelling catheter may be the best intervention. The risk of infection is always a consideration for catheter placement, but for the dying patient with decreased mobility and problems with skin integrity, the benefits outweigh the risks.

Restlessness in a dying client may be caused by constipation, urinary retention, hypoxia, medication, increased pain, or unresolved psychosocial issues. Assessment and treatment of the cause are usually effective. If restlessness continues and is upsetting to the family, sedation may be necessary. The nurse should keep in mind that the palliative care goal is to maintain a level of consciousness that allows for meaningful interactions for as long as possible (March, 1998).

Cognitively impaired older adults who are dying frequently experience hallucinations and delusions. Attempts to confront and reorient the delusional person are usually unsuccessful and may cause additional agitation. A better strategy is to ignore delusional statements and divert the conversation to more neutral topics (Craun, Watkins, and Hefty, 1997). The technique of validation, based on empathic understanding of the emotion and messages behind the confusion, is effective in communicating with those experiencing delusions and hallucinations (Feil, 1993). For instance, if a person, when alone, believes that he or she is talking to his or her mother, asking the client if he or she is feeling lonely or afraid may help the client express underlying emotions and ease some anxiety.

Oral nutrition and hydration should be maintained as long as a client is able to swallow safely. Dehydration and anorexia are often of greater concern to family members than to dying clients who do not ordinarily experience any resulting discomfort. In most cases, intravenous fluids and feedings are not appropriate (see Nutritional Considerations box). Adequate hydration may actually increase respiratory secretions. Nasogastric tube feedings, total parenteral nutrition, and intravenous hydration increase infections and decrease survival time (Storey, 1994; Taylor, 1995). Additional fluids may also contribute to edema caused by impaired circulation in older adults. The only documented side effect of dehydration is dry mouth, which can be relieved by the nurse or caregiver by using saliva substitutes, ice chips, and glycerin swabs, as well as by promoting good mouth care (Taylor, 1995).

Good communication skills are essential in dealing with dying persons and their families. Maintaining eye contact, using touch sensitively, and clarifying statements through reflection (i.e., restating the message as it is understood and asking for verification of its meaning) are important. The

Nutritional Considerations

Loss of appetite frequently accompanies the dying process. Families usually consider providing food as part of basic human caring and something they can do to prolong the client's life. For the dying person, however, eating can be an unpleasant and unwanted experience. Artificial feeding with nasogastric or gastrostomy tubes or intravenous nutrition frequently leads to further complications and earlier death. Since eating and food are often closely tied to many fond memories with loved ones, this is a difficult area and potential source of conflict between clients and their caregivers. Clients and families need to know that anorexia is a normal part of dying and need to have open discussion on the meaning of food and nutrition. Perhaps other meaningful and symbolic ways of providing sustenance can be achieved without artificial feeding.

nurse's awareness of his or her own limitations and strengths is critical because of the level of involvement that can result from interactions with persons confronting death. Once a nurse becomes committed to working with a client and family throughout the dying process, it is important to follow through on that commitment as much as possible.

Another important role of the nurse is to educate and support families and caregivers. Caregivers experience a multitude of problems, including decreased energy levels, health problems, deep grief, and fears associated with life without their loved one. Nurses need to be sensitive to caregiver needs and to provide education, psychologic support, and referrals for additional services.

The role of a social support system is very important during the bereavement process. As a result, it is important that the nurse assess social support networks and help mobilize support for clients and caregivers if necessary.

Nurses as caregivers are not immune to intense feelings of grief after the death of a person for whom they have cared. These feelings can occur whenever close relationships develop between the nurse and clients, especially in long-term care and hospice settings. A dying person may have certain characteristics that invoke memories of previous unresolved losses that the nurse has experienced. Such grief needs to be recognized, accepted, and evaluated, just as any other experience of loss and grief needs to be assessed. The first step is for the nurse to recognize unresolved grief. The next step may be to express his or her thoughts and feelings to a co-worker, friend, or family member. If additional help is needed, sources such as employee assistance programs, clergy, or other counselors can be contacted.

Environment

Most deaths that occur in the United States take place in institutional settings—either hospitals or nursing facilities. This reflects a significant change from the turn of the century, when approximately 75% to 80% of Americans died at home (DeSpelder and Strickland, 1992). Often an older person who is dying moves back and forth, as his or her condition changes, between acute care (hospitalization) and any number of different long-term care settings.

The hospital setting is particularly problematic for dying older persons, since the primary goal in this setting is the restoration of health. Since the implementation of diagnosis-related groups, economic constraints on hospitals force clients to be discharged if they are not receiving active treatment (treatment that cannot be provided in the home or another setting) (Csordas and Kleinman, 1990). Too many times, life-support technology is applied and death becomes even more impersonal.

Nursing facilities and long-term care institutions have different goals and different reimbursement systems. The goal of a nursing facility is to provide a caring environment for those who are unable to care for themselves because of illness, disability, or old age. The emphasis is on care, not cure. Nursing facility settings can foster healthy dying through their primary goal of caring; however, the reality of the situation is that care in many nursing facilities is deficient. Thus compassionate care of the dying is not ensured in either the hospital or the nursing facility setting.

Hospice care was founded on the philosophy of compassionate, humane care of the dying and their families. Although a hospice may be an actual place where dying people go, *hospice* in the United States usually refers to a caring ideology that can be implemented wherever the client may be dying—home, hospital, or nursing facility. A basic goal of hospice is palliative care, helping the dying live as fully as possible with the highest quality of life on a day-to-day basis.

Home care does not necessarily include hospice care. Many older persons die at home, cared for only by their family or sometimes visiting nurses or home health aides. In these situations the goals of caretakers are similar to hospice goals; however, the dying person and family are without the benefit of a multidisciplinary team and an organized approach to follow-up care.

Legislative Initiatives

Legislative initiatives regarding death and dying include the Patient Self-Determination Act, which became law in 1991; it requires all health care facilities receiving Medicare and Medicaid reimbursement to recognize advance directives. These instructions for care (living wills and durable powers of attorney) guide families and health care providers should the client be incapable of decision making. Despite an increased interest in death and dying, the findings of a large study funded by the Robert Wood Johnson Foundation's Program on the Care of Critically Ill Hospitalized Adults are surprising. The majority of seriously ill clients in the study had not completed advance directives, and professional-client communications about advance directives were not as effective in aiding decision making as was hoped (Lo, 1995; SUPPORT Principal Investigators, 1995; Teno et al, 1997).

Nurses caring for very ill older adults need to understand the legal status of advanced directives, living wills, and "Do not resuscitiate" (DNR) orders. As natural extensions of a patient's right to self-determination, the nurse needs to adhere to these preferences (Basanta, 2002).

Other topics relevant to dying and death in the health care system include ethical decisions, euthanasia and assisted suicide, and suicide; however, these topics are so complex that they preclude a cursory treatment in this chapter.

SUMMARY

This chapter covered two major topics: (1) loss and grieving in response to loss and (2) the process of dying. Characteristics of dying or grieving older persons were presented, with a focus on the differences between the experiences of older and younger adults. Lastly, ways of assessing the needs of those who are mourning or dying were described, along with strategies for the nurse to help meet identified needs. Examination of the nurse's own value system and prior experience with loss was emphasized. Health care system approaches to care of the dying have been described.

It is hoped that care and support for dying or grieving older persons will improve with increased knowledge and positive attitudes. This improvement should benefit both older adults and nurses, who have much knowledge and wisdom to gain from those who have the most experience in life.

Home Care

1. Homebound older adults who have lost a spouse or significant other may manifest grief with physical symptoms.
2. Homebound older adults may develop crises of faith and express anger at God. It is important for the home care nurse to avoid being judgmental and to allow an older adult to verbalize anger and grief.
3. Refer to an advanced practice nurse or other health professional skilled in working with complicated grieving if a homebound older adult experiences dysfunctional grieving.
4. Loss of a spouse or significant other, coupled with living alone, puts homebound older adults at risk for depression.
5. Assess a terminally ill homebound older adult's feelings toward his or her own death.
6. Instruct family members and caregivers on the stages of dying and the physiologic changes that accompany them.
7. Use hospice care to help dying homebound older adults live as fully as possible on a day-to-day basis.
8. If hospice care is not available, a home care nurse can assist a homebound older adult in dying.

Key Points

- Grief is the acute reaction to one's perception of loss, mourning is the longer process of resolving acute grief reactions, and bereavement is the state of having experienced a significant loss.
- Grief involves many changes over time, is a natural response to all kinds of losses (not just death), and is based on one's unique perception of a loss.
- Worden (1991) views the grief process as active, involving the following four tasks of mourning: (1) accepting the reality of the loss, (2) working through the pain of grief, (3) adjusting to an environment in which the deceased is missing, and (4) emotionally relocating the deceased and moving on with life.
- Human beings respond as whole people, with grief manifesting in physical symptoms, psychologic responses, changes in socialization patterns, and spiritual issues concerning life's meaning.
- Complicated grief reactions may manifest as one of four types of reactions: (1) chronic, (2) delayed, (3) exaggerated, or (4) masked.
- Nursing care activities that assist in the grieving process include helping the survivor express feelings, providing time to grieve, explaining "normal" grieving behaviors, examining defenses and coping styles, identifying pathologic conditions, and making appropriate referrals.
- Sociocultural and religious background, physical and functional status, social isolation and loneliness, and the meaningfulness of everyday life are all important factors in determining a person's approach to impending death.
- Age-related changes predispose older persons to greater potential problems in areas such as hygiene and skin care, nutrition, elimination, mobility, transfers, rest, sleep, pain, respiratory management, and cognitive and behavioral functioning.
- Nursing strategies for assisting dying older persons include delivering excellent physical care, using good communication skills, conducting a life review, and educating and supporting family caregivers.
- Hospice programs help dying persons live as fully as possible on a day-to-day basis by providing symptom control, addressing psychologic needs of clients, supporting family caregivers, dealing with environmental problems, and assisting clients with spiritual concerns.

Critical Thinking Exercises

1. A 70-year-old woman is admitted to the hospital unit with COPD. She lives alone in a retirement community. Her children live 1 hour away. Her best friend of 40 years recently died, and her husband of 35 years died 1 year ago.

How would you assess and assist this client in coping with multiple losses?

2. An 85-year-old man is dying of terminal lung cancer. He comes from a close-knit family. As the hospice nurse, how do you prepare and help this family work through the anticipatory grief process?

References

Basanta WE: Advance directives and life-sustaining treatment: a legal primer, *Hematol Oncol Clin North Am* 16(6):1381-1396, 2002.

Brockopp DY et al: Elderly hospice patients' perspective on pain management, *Hospice J* 11(3):41, 1996.

Burbank PM: *Meaning in life among older persons*, unpublished doctoral dissertation, Boston, 1988, Boston University.

Butler R: The life review: an interpretation of reminiscences in the aged, *Psychiatry* 26(1):65, 1963.

Craun MJ, Watkins M, Hefty A: Hospice care of the psychotic patient, *Am J Hospice Palliat Care* p 205, July-Aug 1997.

Csordas TJ, Kleinman A: The therapeutic process. In Johnson T, Sargent C, editors: *Medical anthropology: contemporary theory and method*, New York, 1990, Praeger.

DeSpelder LA, Strickland AL: *The last dance: encouraging death and dying*, ed 3, Mountain View, Calif, 1992, Mayfield.

Doka KJ: Disenfranchised grief: an exposition and update. In Morgan JD, editor: *Readings in thanatology*, Amityville, NY, 1997, Baywood.

Doka KJ: The spiritual needs of the dying. In Doka KJ, editor: *Death and spirituality*, Amityville, NY, 1993, Baywood.

Doka KJ: *Disenfranchised grief: recognizing hidden sorrow*, Lexington, Mass, 1989, Lexington Books.

Doka KJ, Davidson JD: *Living with grief: who we are, how we grieve*, Washington, DC, 1998, Hospice Foundation of America.

Ebersole P, Hess P, Luggen AS: *Toward healthy aging: human needs and nursing response*, ed 6, St Louis, 2004, Mosby.

Edwards M: Barriers to effective pain/symptom control, *Am J Hospice Palliat Care* p 107, March-April 1998.

Erikson E: *Childhood and society*, New York, 1963, WW Norton.

Feil N: *The validation breakthrough*, Baltimore, 1993, Health Professions Press.

Fulton GB, Metress EK: *Perspectives on death and dying*, Boston, 1995, Jones & Bartlett.

Garrett JE: Multiple losses in older adults, *J Gerontol Nurs* 13(8):8, 1987.

Hall SE: Spiritual diversity: a challenge for hospice chaplains, *Am J Hospice Palliat Care* p 221, Sept-Oct 1997.

Ham RJ, Sloane PD: *Primary care geriatrics*, ed 3, St Louis, 1997, Mosby.

Huber R, Bryant J: The 10-mile mourning bridge and the brief symptom inventory: close relatives? *Hospice J* 11(2):31, 1996.

Huber R, Gibson J: New evidence for anticipatory grief, *Hospice J* 6(1):49, 1990.

Jackson SA: The epidemiology of aging. In Hazzard WR et al, editors: *Principles of geriatric medicine and gerontology*, ed 4, New York, 1999, McGraw Hill.

Kastenbaum R: Death, dying and bereavement in older age, *Aged Care Serv Rev* 1(3):1, 1978.

Kohn M, Menon G: Life prolongation: views of elderly outpatients and health care professionals, *J Am Geriatr Soc* 36:840, 1988.

Kowalski NC: The older person's anticipation of her own death. In Rando TA, Fulton R, editors: *Loss and anticipatory grief*, Lexington, Mass, 1986, Lexington Books.

Kübler-Ross E: *On death and dying*, New York, 1969, Macmillan.

Landman J: *Regret: the persistence of the possible*, New York, 1993, Oxford University Press.

Lindemann E: Symptoms and management of acute grief, *Am J Psychol* 101:141, 1944.

Lo B: End-of-life care after termination of SUPPORT, special supplement, *Hastings Center Report* 25(6):S6, 1995.

Lund DA: Conclusions about bereavement in later life and implications for interventions and future research. In Lund DA, editor: *Older bereaved spouses: research with practical applications*, New York, 1989, Hemisphere.

March PA: Terminal restlessness, *Am J Hospice Palliat Care* p 51, Jan-Feb 1998.

Matzo ML, Sherman DW: *Palliative care nursing: quality care to the end of life*, New York, 2001, Springer.

McCall JB: *Grief education for caregivers of the elderly*, New York, 1999, Haworth Pastoral Press.

McMillan SC, Moody LE: Hospice patient and caregiver congruence in reporting patients' symptom intensity, *Cancer Nurs* 26(2)113-118, 2003.

Neugarten BL: Adult personality: toward a psychology of the life cycle. In Neugarten BL, editor: *Middle age and aging*, Chicago, 1968, University of Chicago Press.

Rando TA: *Grieving: how to go on living when someone you love dies*, Lexington, Mass, 1988, DC Health.

Rando TA, editor: *Loss and anticipatory grief*, Lexington, Mass, 1986, Lexington Books.

Retsinas J: The theoretical reassessment of the applicability of Kübler-Ross' stages of dying, *Death Studies* 12:207, 1988.

Sankar A: *Dying at home: a family guide for caregiving*, Baltimore, 1991, Johns Hopkins University Press.

Storey P: *Primer of palliative care*, Gainesville, Fla, 1994, Academy of Hospice Physicians.

SUPPORT Principal Investigators: A controlled trial to improve care for seriously ill hospitalized patients, *JAMA* 274(20):1591, 1995.

Taylor MA: Benefits of dehydration in terminally ill patients, *Geriatr Nurs* 16(6):271, 1995.

Teno JM et al: Advanced directives for seriously ill hospitalized patients: effectiveness with the patient self-determination act and the support intervention, *J Am Geriatr Soc* 45:500, 1997.

Thorson JA, Powell FC: Elements of death anxiety and meanings of death, *J Clin Psychol* 44:691, 1988.

Weitzner MA, Moody LN, McMillan SC: Symptom management issues in hospice care, *Am J Hospice Palliat Care* 14(4):190, 2003.

Worden JW: *Grief counseling and grief therapy*, ed 2, New York, 1991, Springer.

World Health Organization: *Cancer pain relief and palliative care: technical report series 804*, Geneva, 1990, The Organization.

21 Laboratory and Diagnostic Tests

SUSAN A. MOORE, PhD, RN

Learning Objectives

On completion of this chapter, the reader will be able to:

1. Identify key laboratory values that increase or decrease with aging.
2. Describe the effect of aging on the erythrocyte sedimentation rate.
3. Name two medications that can interfere with potassium excretion and affect serum potassium levels.
4. Explain the relationship between serum sodium levels and pseudohyponatremia.
5. Explain the difference between serum creatinine concentrations in younger adults and older adults.
6. Explain the relationship between bacteria in the urine and urinary tract infections in older adults.
7. Relate the significance of troponin levels in diagnosing cardiac emergencies.
8. Explain the relationship of the brain natriuretic peptide (BNP) to congestive heart failure.
9. Discuss the role of laboratory tests in determining thyroid function in older adults.
10. Describe the nurse's role in interpreting laboratory values for older adults.

Diagnostic testing in older adults takes on a different meaning than testing in younger adults. The nurse must realize that laboratory values can be classified into three general groups in regard to aging: (1) those which change with aging; (2) those which do not change with aging; and (3) those for which it is unclear whether aging, disease, or both change the values. Researchers are eliminating the term *reference ranges* as it pertains to laboratory test parameters for older adults because it can be difficult to determine whether results are a symptom of a disease or related to normal aging (Sarkozi, 2002).

The gerontologic nurse must consider the effect of laboratory and diagnostic testing on an older adult's overall health and well-being. For example, with aging, subcutaneous tissue is decreased and the fragility of veins increased. Consequently, a frail older adult is more likely to have increased bruising and discomfort after a venous blood drawing than a younger adult. It is also important for the nurse to know what tests have been ordered so that an explanation can be given to an anxious older adult; his or her anxiety may range from concerns about the cost of tests to a concern for privacy to cultural concerns (see Cultural Awareness box). For example, the Chinese and Vietnamese believe that drawn blood is irreplaceable and thus may become upset with repeated blood testing (Burnside, 1988). For other cultural issues, see Chapter 5.

This chapter provides the gerontologic nurse with a basic understanding of the purpose of commonly ordered laboratory and diagnostic tests, the importance of selected hematologic and blood and urine chemistry components in the body's overall function, and the relative "normal" ranges for younger and older adults. These normal ranges may vary from institution to institution, as well as among the literature (Table 21-1). Because of the scant research conducted on older adults, geriatricians and gerontologists may also disagree as to whether changes are related to aging or disease (Beers and Berkow, 2000). However, most aging experts do agree that older adults should be treated as individuals and viewed in terms of symptoms, test results, and overall condition when deciding the best course of treatment.

COMPONENTS OF HEMATOLOGIC TESTING

Blood is a complex connective tissue composed of cells (erythrocytes and leukocytes), specialized cell fragments (platelets), and a fluid matrix called plasma. The cells and cell fragments are suspended in the plasma, which is one of the body's three major fluids (Thibodeau and Patton, 2003).

Red Blood Cells

Red blood cells (RBCs), or erythrocytes, are disk-shaped cells that carry molecules of hemoglobin. The hemoglobin allows the transport and exchange of oxygen and carbon dioxide.

CULTURAL AWARENESS

CULTURAL AND GENDER INFLUENCES ON DIAGNOSTIC AND LABORATORY TESTS

The nurse should be aware that biocultural variations in older adults occur with some diagnostic and laboratory tests, such as measurement of blood glucose and blood analysis of hemoglobin and hematocrit, glucose, and serum cholesterol.

Blacks have average blood pressure readings 5 mm Hg higher than whites; the blood pressure elevation can be less than 5 mm Hg at younger ages but more than 5 mm Hg at older ages. Black women over age 45 have a reading as much as 16 mm Hg higher than white women in the same age-group.

Although healthy older persons have hemoglobin and hematocrit values within the range of younger persons, gender difference in these blood values (i.e., men have higher readings than women) decreases with age. Women experience a rise in the measures up to age 60 and then a slight decline, whereas men show a constant decline from the age of 30 to the end of life. By age 60, men and women have similar blood measures. The racial difference in hemoglobin levels continues into old age. Blacks have lower hemoglobin levels than whites, but they follow the same gender pattern of increasingly similar hemoglobin levels with age.

Whether measured by the glucose tolerance test or by glycosylated hemoglobin determination, the blood glucose level rises with age. The mean blood glucose level after a challenge rises from 99.7 mg/dl at ages 18 to 24 to 166.3 mg/dl at ages 75 to 79. Mean glycosylated hemoglobin determinations are 6.9% at ages 50 to 69 and rise to 8.6% at ages 80 to 89. Women have higher blood levels than men. This gender difference widens with age, showing a difference of 9.5 mg/dl at ages 18 to 24 and 24.1 mg/dl at 75 to 79 years. Blacks have slightly higher levels than whites, but the difference is not apparent between individuals of similar socioeconomic status.

Cholesterol levels rise with age in both men and women, but their patterns of increase differ. In men, peak levels occur at ages 45 to 54 and then decline slightly thereafter. In women, levels continue to rise steadily until the age of 65, when the rise decelerates slightly. Blacks and whites have similar cholesterol levels, but other groups differ substantially. Pima Indians from the Southwest and the Japanese have lower cholesterol levels than blacks or whites. The mean value for Pima Indians is 189 mg/dl; for the Japanese it is 152 mg/dl; whereas blacks and whites have a mean of 223 mg/dl.

From Overfield T: *Biologic variation in health and illness,* Menlo Park, Calif, 1985, Addison-Wesley. Reprinted with permission fromPearson Education, Inc.

Erythrocytes lack a nucleus and other internal cell structures. This not only allows for a greater surface area to carry hemoglobin, but also prevents erythrocytes from reproducing themselves or maintaining function indefinitely. The average life span of an erythrocyte is about 120 days. Although aging does not affect the life span of an erythrocyte, replenishment after bleeding may be delayed (McCance and Huether, 2001).

RBCs are necessary to maintain oxygen and carbon dioxide transport. A reduction in the number of RBCs, or a decrease in quality or quantity of hemoglobin, is classified as anemia. Anemia may be attributed to (1) impaired erythrocyte production, (2) blood loss, (3) increased erythrocyte destruction, or (4) a combination of the above (McCance and Huether, 2001). Signs of anemia may be unnoticed if the anemia is mild, or the client may experience fatigue, shortness of breath, and paresthesia (McCance and Huether, 2001). In addition, clinicians can miss signs of anemia even in markedly anemic older clients (Ham, Sloane, and Warshaw, 2001). The combination of vague symptomatology and clinical presentation may lead the health care provider to attribute an older adult's complaints to "old age" and fail to investigate adequately.

Other conditions involving erythrocytes are related to increased and decreased cell numbers. Increases in RBC count in people living in higher altitudes are known as secondary polycythemia. This occurs as an essential physiologic response to hypoxia encountered at high altitudes and is an example of one of the body's compensatory mechanisms. In sickle cell anemia the RBCs become abnormal in shape and surface composition as a result of a genetic defect in the hemoglobin.

Hemoglobin

Hemoglobin is an important iron-containing protein that is carried on RBCs and makes up about one third of the weight of the RBC. Hemoglobin is necessary for the transport of oxygen. A reduction in hemoglobin can result in a decrease in oxygen content and an increase in fatigue, possibly indicating anemia. Abnormal hemoglobin from mutant genes can cause abnormalities of RBCs, as with sickle cell anemia.

Hematocrit

The hematocrit is the percentage of total blood volume that represents erythrocytes. This is determined in the laboratory by spinning (centrifuging) a sample of blood, causing the heavier red cells to sink to the bottom of the tube while the less dense plasma rises to the top. The percentage of cells to liquid is calculated, giving the hematocrit reading. An increase in the hematocrit can signal volume depletion (Beers and Berkow, 2000). A decrease in hematocrit may be a result of disease or dietary deficiencies (Pagana and Pagana, 2003).

Reported effects of aging on hemoglobin and hematocrit vary among the literature. Hemoglobin has been reported as remaining unchanged (Berghe, Wilson, and Ershler, 2004) or changing slightly, possibly from extrinsic factors rather than

TABLE 21-1 Hematology

TEST NAME	ADULT NORMALS	OLDER ADULT NORMALS	SIGNIFICANCE OF DEVIATIONS
Red blood cells (RBCs)	4.2-6.1 million/unit	Unchanged with aging	*Low:* hemorrhage, anemia, chronic illness, renal failure, pernicious anemia *High:* high altitude, polycythemia, dehydration
Hemoglobin	12-18 g/dl	Values may be slightly decreased	*Low:* anemia, cancer, nutritional deficiency, kidney disease *High:* polycythemia, CHF, chronic obstructive pulmonary disease (COPD), high altitudes, dehydration
Hematocrit	37%-52%	Values may be slightly decreased	*Low:* anemia, cirrhosis, hemorrhage, malnutrition, rheumatoid arthritis *High:* polycythemia, severe dehydration, severe diarrhea, COPD
White blood cells (WBCs) (total)	5.0-10.0 thousand/ mm^3	Unchanged with aging	*Low:* drug toxicity, infections, autoimmune disease, dietary deficiency *High:* infection, trauma, stress, inflammation
Neutrophils	55%-70%	Unchanged with aging	*Low:* dietary deficiency, overwhelming bacterial infection, viral infections, drug therapy *High:* physical and emotional stress, trauma, inflammatory disorders
Eosinophils	1%-4%	Unchanged with aging	*Low:* increased adrenosteroid production *High:* parasitic infections, allergic reactions, autoimmune disorders
Basophils	0.5%-1%	Unchanged with aging	*Low:* acute allergic reactions, stress reactions *High:* myeloproliferative disease
Monocytes	2%-8%	Unchanged with aging	*Low:* drug therapy (predisposition) *High:* chronic inflammatory disorders, tuberculosis, chronic ulcerative colitis
Lymphocytes	20%-40%	Unchanged with aging	*Low:* leukemia, sepsis, systemic lupus erythematosus, chemotherapy, radiation *High:* chronic bacterial infection, viral infections, radiation, infectious hepatitis
Folic acid	5-25 ng/ml	Unchanged with aging	*Low:* malnutrition, folic acid anemia, hemolytic anemia, alcoholism, liver disease, chronic renal disease *High:* pernicious anemia
Vitamin B_{12}	160-950 pg/ml	Unchanged with aging	*Low:* pernicious anemia, inflammatory bowel disease, atrophic gastritis, folic acid deficiency *High:* leukemia, polycythemia, severe liver dysfunction
Total iron binding capacity (TIBC)	250-460 mcg/dl	Unchanged with aging	*Low:* hypoproteinemia, cirrhosis, hemolytic anemia, pernicious anemia *High:* polycythemia, iron deficiency anemia
Iron (Fe)	60-180 mcg/dl	Unchanged with aging	*Low:* insufficient dietary iron, chronic blood loss, inadequate absorption of iron *High:* hemochromocytosis, hemolytic anemia, hepatitis, iron poisoning
Uric acid	4-8.5 mg/dl	May be slightly increased	*Low:* lead poisoning *High:* gout, increased ingestion of purines, chronic renal disease, hypothyroidism
Prothrombin time (PT)	11-12.5 sec	Unchanged with aging	*High:* liver disease, vitamin K deficiency, warfarin ingestion, bile duct obstruction, salicylate intoxication

Continued

TABLE 21-1 Hematology—cont'd

TEST NAME	ADULT NORMALS	OLDER ADULT NORMALS	SIGNIFICANCE OF DEVIATIONS
Partial thromboplastin time (PTT)	60-70 sec	Unchanged with aging	*Low:* early stages of disseminated intravascular coagulation, metastatic cancer *High:* coagulation factor deficiency, cirrhosis, vitamin K deficiency, heparin administration
Platelets	150,000-400,000/ mm^3	Unchanged with aging	*Low:* hemorrhage, thrombocytopenia, systemic lupus erythematosus, pernicious anemia, chemotherapy, infection *High:* malignancy, polycythemia, rheumatoid arthritis, iron deficiency anemia

Adapted from Pagana KD, Pagana TJ: *Manual of diagnostic and laboratory tests,* ed 2, St Louis, 2004, Mosby; Pagana KD, Pagana TJ: *Diagnostic and laboratory test reference,* ed 6, St Louis, 2003, Mosby.

as a result of normal aging (Chatta and Lipschitz, 1999). The hematocrit and hemoglobin decline slightly over the age of 90 (Sarkozi, 2002).

White Blood Cells

White blood cells (WBCs), or leukocytes, are another type of cell present in the blood. Their major function is defense against foreign substances. WBCs function mainly in the interstitial fluid. Leukocytes consist of neutrophils, lymphocytes, monocytes, eosinophils, and basophils. A decrease in leukocytes in older adults may be related to drugs or severe infection (Pagana and Pagana, 2003). Drugs that can cause a decrease in leukocytes include antibiotics, anticonvulsants, antihistamines, antimetabolites, cytotoxic agents, analgesics, phenothiazines, and diuretics (Pagana and Pagana, 2004). An increase in leukocytes is generally seen with infections. However, a white cell count may be only moderately elevated in older adults when an infection, such as pneumonia, is present. Other typical symptoms of infection such as fever, pain, and enlarged lymph glands (lymphadenopathy) may be minimum or absent in older adults with infections (Mouton et al, 2001). Consequently, the nurse must be alert to other signs and symptoms of impending infection, such as the sudden onset of confusion. Pharmacologic agents have also been associated with an increase in leukocytes. These drugs include allopurinol, aspirin, heparin, steroids, and triamterene (Pagana and Pagana, 2003).

Neutrophils, eosinophils, and basophils are produced in the bone marrow and possess similar structures of lobulated nuclei and many membrane-bound granules. Their primary function is phagocytosis (ingestion and destruction of particulate material). In addition, the basophil's cytoplasmic granules contain powerful chemicals such as histamine, bradykinin, and serotonin, which contribute to stimulating the inflammatory response in tissues (McCance and Huether, 2001). The monocyte, the largest of the leukocytes, is produced in bone marrow and differs in appearance from neutrophils, eosinophils, and basophils. The monocyte has a single nucleus and is capable of destroying large bacterial organisms and viral-infected cells by phagocytosis (Thibodeau and Patton, 2003).

Lymphocytes, the smallest of the leukocytes, are classified into two types: B and T. The lymphocytes have a large nucleus and relatively little cytoplasm. Originating in the bone marrow and thymus, lymphocytes are housed in the lymph nodes, spleen, and tonsils. Lymphocytes do not act as phagocytes but rather produce antibodies and other specific defenses against antibodies (Thibodeau and Patton, 2003).

Aging does not appear to affect the function of neutrophils, though there is a reduced effect on the bone marrow to release and store these cells. Lymphocytes of older adults have shown impaired function in vitro and are suspected to be the cause of a reduction in antibody response in later life (Rothstein, 1999). Rothstein (1999) also reports that monocytes in older rodents decline in function; however, these results have not been replicable in older humans. There is suspicion that a decline in monocyte function exists given the increased susceptibility to infections and increased incidence of malignancies in older adults. The remaining leukocytes, eosinophils, and basophils have not been shown to be affected by aging.

The presence and function of leukocytes are necessary for the body's resistance and response to infections, cancers, and other foreign substances. The implications for nurses related to infections and malignancies include recognizing subtle and sometimes altered responses to infections and diseases in older adults. In addition, educating older adults about the importance of participating in cancer screenings and maintaining immunizations throughout life is warranted (see Chapters 8 and 19).

Folic Acid

Folic acid is one of the eight B vitamins that make up the B-complex group. Folic acid is a water-soluble vitamin that functions as a coenzyme, which means it is inactive unless linked to an enzyme. Folic acid is necessary for the normal functioning of RBCs and WBCs. A decrease in folic acid can indicate protein-energy malnutrition, macrocytic anemia, megaloblastic anemia, and liver and renal disease. Alcohol and various other drugs are known to interfere with the absorption of folate. Some drugs have also been shown to decrease folic acid levels. These include anticonvulsants, antimalarials, and methotrexate (Pagana and Pagana, 2003). However, the effect of aging on folate is still debatable because of variance in defining the lower limits of "normal" and the different methods used to determine folate levels (Gilleece and Dexter, 2002).

Because of the relationship of nutrition and alcohol consumption to folic acid levels, it is important for the gerontologic nurse to assess clients regarding their nutritional intake, including habits regarding alcohol consumption. Elevated levels of folic acid may be seen in people with pernicious anemia, who do not have an adequate amount of B_{12} to metabolize folic acid. Therefore the folic acid test should be done in conjunction with assessments for vitamin B_{12} levels (Pagana and Pagana, 2004).

Vitamin B_{12}

Another of the water-soluble vitamins that makes up the B-complex group and acts as a coenzyme is vitamin B_{12}, or cobalamin. Although changes in B_{12} levels are seen in many older adults, some scientists do not believe that aging affects the ileal absorption of B_{12} (Hall and Wiley, 1999). They state that problems with B_{12} tend to be the result of diseases and other conditions such as gastric achlorhydria, pernicious anemia, pancreatic insufficiency, and ileal disease, each of which has much greater impact on B_{12} absorption than aging alone (Hall and Wiley, 1999).

Malabsorption of B_{12} can be caused by the effect of antibodies on gastric parietal cells and a decrease in intrinsic factor, the factor underlying pernicious anemia. The prevalence of pernicious anemia increases significantly with aging (Chatta and Lipschitz, 1999).

B_{12} is important for normal erythrocyte maturation (McCance and Huether, 2001) and acts as a coenzyme with folic acid. The synthesis of nucleic acids, and therefore the structure of deoxyribonucleic acid (DNA), depends on B_{12} containing enzymes (Grodner, Long, and DeYoung, 2004). Vitamin B_{12} deficiency can lead to degeneration of the dorsal and lateral spinal columns, which in turn can lead to paresthesias of the feet and fingers and progress to spastic ataxia (Gaspard, 2002). The combination of vitamin B_{12}, B_6, and folate tends to reduce the levels of homocysteine, thereby decreasing the risk of coronary artery disease (Grodner, Long, and DeYoung, 2004).

Total Iron Binding Capacity

Total iron binding capacity measures the amount of iron and the amount of available transferrin in the serum (McCance and Huether, 2001). Transferrin is a major transport protein responsible for the transport of iron in the body. Transferrin is a protein in the plasma that collects iron and transports it to the bone marrow for incorporation into hemoglobin.

Iron

Iron is found in the hemoglobin of the RBCs. When iron-containing foods are ingested, the iron is absorbed by the small intestine and transported to the plasma (Pagana and Pagana, 2003). Iron is necessary for controlling protein synthesis in the mitochondria and generating energy in the cells (Freedman and Sutin, 2002). Serum iron levels show progressive decreases in both genders with advancing age, although the ability to absorb iron appears to remain intact (Hall and Wiley, 1999). Iron deficiency anemia is the most common form of anemia seen in older adults. However, in spite of the decreases in serum iron levels seen with aging, anemia in older adults is not a normal consequence of aging. The gerontologic nurse should assess older adults for a lack of iron-containing foods in their diets, occult or chronic blood loss, and poor absorption of iron. A deficiency of iron may render older adults more susceptible to infection (Ahluwalia et al, 2004).

Uric Acid

Uric acid is a product of metabolism, specifically purine catabolism. Uric acid is excreted by the kidneys. Age-related changes in uric acid levels are significantly different between the genders. Since estrogen is thought to promote the excretion of uric acid, elevated levels are rarely seen in women before the onset of menopause (McCance and Huether, 2001).

Problems with uric acid may be a result of faulty excretion (e.g., kidney failure), overproduction of uric acid, or the presence of other substances that compete for excretion sites (e.g., ketoacids) (Pagana and Pagana, 2004). Elevated uric acid levels are seen in clients with gout. Gout is a common condition in older adults involving a disturbance in the body's control of uric acid production or excretion. Excess uric acid accumulates in the body's fluids, especially the blood and synovial fluids, forming crystals at high concentrations. These crystals deposit in the connective tissue of the body causing painful, inflamed joints. Thiazide diuretics, caffeine, low-dose aspirin, and antiparkisonian drugs are also a common cause of increased uric acid levels in older adults (Pagana and Pagana, 2004).

Prothrombin Time

Prothrombin is a plasma protein that is converted to thrombin in the first step of the clotting process. Clotting is necessary to prevent the loss of vital body fluids that occurs when blood vessels rupture (Thibodeau and Patton, 2003).

In addition to measuring prothrombin time (PT), health care professionals also measure effectiveness of the activity of fibrinogen and coagulation factors V, VII, and X. The results of the PT laboratory test also reveal how effectively the vitamin K–dependent coagulation factors of the extrinsic and common pathways of the coagulation cascade are performing (McCance and Huether, 2001). An increased PT is seen in liver disease, vitamin K deficiency, bile duct obstruction, and salicylate intoxication. Some medications can also cause an increase in a patient's PT. They are allopurinol, cephalothins, cholestyramine, clofibrate, and sulfonamides (Pagana and Pagana, 2003). Pagana and Pagana (2003) also report that digitalis and diphenhydramine can cause a decreased PT level.

Older adults are often prescribed the drug warfarin (Coumadin) after open-heart surgery and in cases of chronic atrial fibrillation. Warfarin interferes with the production of vitamin K–dependent coagulation factors, thereby decreasing the chance of thrombus formation. Warfarin can interact with many medications, especially those often taken by older adults, such as aspirin, quinidine, sulfa, indomethacin, and nonsteroidal antiinflammatory drugs (NSAIDs) (Pagana and Pagana, 2003). Gerontologic nurses should help clients understand the importance of keeping their appointments for PT checks and consulting their health providers before taking any medications not prescribed. The adequacy of warfarin therapy can be assessed by following a client's PT level. The PT value is traditionally reported in seconds and includes a value called the international normalized ratio (INR). INR is a mathematic "correction" of the results of the one-stage PT and was created to standardize results caused by the variation in reagents. The INR should be between 2.0 and 3.0 for most thrombosis and embolus conditions and between 3.0 and 4.5 for clients with a history of recurrent thromboembolism (O'Neill, 2002) (see Nutritional Considerations box and Chapter 10).

Partial Thromboplastin Time

Partial thromboplastin time (PTT) refers to the measurement of the common pathway of clot formation. Heparin can inactivate prothrombin, so the PTT is a good indicator of whether a client is receiving adequate anticoagulation therapy. The effect of heparin on the body is faster than that of warfarin, but the effects are shorter. Nursing considerations include monitoring for bleeding and correct administration of the heparin dosage.

Nutritional Considerations

Vitamin K is used in emergency situations to counteract the increased anticoagulant times that sometimes occur when clients are receiving heparin or warfarin (Coumadin). The nurse should be aware that foods high in vitamin K can affect clotting times and counteract the prescribed therapy. Food high in vitamin K, such as turnip greens, broccoli, cabbage, spinach, and liver, should be eaten in moderate amounts while receiving anticoagulant therapy (Grodner, Long, and DeYoung, 2004).

Erythrocyte Sedimentation Rate

The erythrocyte sedimentation rate (ESR) test measures the time that RBCs take to settle in normal saline over 1 hour. The measured values are reported in millimeters. The test does not relate to one specific condition or disorder but does indicate the presence of inflammation, so it is useful in monitoring the course of inflammatory activity in commonly occurring rheumatic diseases such as polymyalgia rheumatica, temporal arteritis, and rheumatoid arthritis. In addition, when the test is performed with a white cell count, an elevation can indicate infection. Kane, Ouslander, and Abrass (1999) state that mild elevations of 10 to 20 mm/hr in the ESR may be age related. Other scientists report that elevations as high as 30 to 35 mm/hr above normal adult values may be seen, even though no evidence of inflammatory disorders is present. This makes interpretation of the results of this test in older adults difficult without other clinical data, and also makes it harder to consider differential diagnoses (Calkins, 1999).

C-Reactive Protein

C-reactive protein (CRP) is one of the serum analytes that is present in the acute phase of an inflammatory response (Gambino, 1997). Said to be an earlier indicator than the ESR of any acute processes present in the body (SmithKline Beecham, 1998), CRP is useful to researchers in assessing clients with unstable angina, myocardial infarction, and organ transplants, as well as those recovering from surgical procedures (Gambino, 1997; Oltrona et al, 1997; SmithKline Beecham, 1998). Smith et al (1995) concluded that a persistently high CRP or rising CRP level suggests the failure of antibiotic treatment or the development of a complicated infectious process. Although still a relatively underused and undervalued test to many practitioners, the CRP is now being examined for its value in place of the ESR in detecting many inflammatory conditions (Gambino, 1997; SmithKline Beecham, 1998).

Platelets

Platelets are small, irregular bodies, also known as thrombocytes, which are essential for clotting. They are formed in the red bone marrow, the lungs, and the spleen. When an injury occurs to a blood vessel, platelets are released and become "sticky," forming a plug at the site and helping to trigger a cascade of other clotting functions (Thibodeau and Patton, 2003). Evidence has shown that platelet adhesiveness increases with age, although no changes in platelet numbers or structure have been reported (Adams and Meyet, 1966). Hale and Owen (1999) states that the effect of "age on disorders of hemostasis is at best poorly understood."

Platelets are important for normal body functioning because of their essential part in normal blood clotting. Decreases in platelet counts (to less than 100,000/mm^3) require investigation. In one condition, known as myelodysplastic syndrome (MDS), pancytopenia is noted in more than half the clients diagnosed. Pancytopenia is when the levels of RBCs, WBCs, and platelets are all below normal. Over 50% of the cases found are in adults over the age of 70. Treatment usually consists of transfusions with red cells or platelets, although most clients will die of other disorders rather than MDS. This condition has been known to progress to acute leukemia (Gilleece and Dexter, 2002). At platelet levels below 20,000/mm^3, the nurse should observe for spontaneous bleeding. If the client's levels are 40,000/mm^3 or below, prolonged bleeding after procedures can occur (Pagana and Pagana, 2003).

In assessing clients for potential or hidden blood losses, nurses have traditionally questioned clients about the color and consistency of their bowel movements. The gerontologic nurse, however, must recognize that older adults who take iron supplements have changes in bowel habits and stool color that may not necessarily indicate the passage of occult blood.

COMPONENTS OF BLOOD CHEMISTRY TESTING

Blood chemistry testing involves electrolytes, glucose, and various other blood components. Although many of these tests are done in groups, others may be ordered individually to determine the presence or absence of a particular disorder. Many institutions "package" these chemistries into groups with names, such as "Chem-7," "SMA-16," or "Profile Package," which are only specific within a given institution. Recently laboratories have "repackaged" these groups of tests because of changes in reimbursement from Medicare. The nurse should learn the terminology specific to his or her workplace and be able to identify the individual tests contained in each package.

Electrolytes

Electrolytes are inorganic substances that include acids, bases, and salts. In solutions, electrolytes break up to form positively or negatively charged particles known as ions. Positively charged ions are known as *cations;* negatively charged ions are called *anions*. Compounds that are formed from acids and bases are known as salts. Blood testing can measure the amount of an electrolyte in the circulating blood (extracellular fluid). Although many types of electrolytes can be tested, only the most common are discussed here.

Older adults in particular may have serious problems with electrolyte imbalances. Dehydration is the most common form of electrolyte disorder that occurs in older adults, and it can usually be attributed to excess loss of water or impaired water ingestion. Excess water loss can occur from infections, such as pneumonia and cystitis, or environmental conditions. Impaired water ingestion may be a result of the age-related decrease in thirst sensation in older adults or of decreased functional ability that limits the intake of water (Davis and Minaker, 1999). This includes being bedridden, chemically or physically restrained, or limited by sensory changes.

Sodium. The test for sodium (Na^+) measures the amount of sodium in the circulating blood, but it is actually an index of body water deficit or excess. Sodium regulation is important for the maintenance of blood pressure, transmission of nerve impulses, and regulation of body fluid levels in and out of the cells. This movement of sodium affects blood volume, which is tied to the thirst mechanism and total body fluids (Grodner, Long, and DeYoung, 2004). Although sodium is also present in the intracellular fluid, the majority resides in the extracellular fluid, making it the major cation of the extracellular fluid. The result of sodium testing describes the balance between ingested sodium and that excreted by the kidneys (Pagana and Pagana, 2003). In older adults, kidney changes such as a decrease in the glomerular filtration rate (GFR) and in the number of nephrons do not lead to disability or disease (Beck, 1999). However, these changes could mean that in the presence of crises such as sodium depletion or overload, an older adult may have difficulty in maintaining homeostasis (Table 21-2).

For example, when volume depletion occurs, a younger individual's kidneys adjust for a decrease in sodium by limiting excretion of this electrolyte. In older adults, however, the kidneys, because of sluggish renin-angiotension and aldosterone response, may not respond appropriately and further sodium losses may occur (Beck, 1999). A normal sodium level is necessary for maintaining the extracellular fluid balance (osmolarity).

The occurrence of hyponatremia (a low sodium level) increases with age. The majority of cases are related to the kidneys' inability to excrete free water. Symptoms can be vague, such as malaise, confusion, headache, and nausea, but can also progress to coma and seizures (Davis and Minaker, 1999). It is important, though, to distinguish whether an older adult has a low sodium level but normal osmolarity; this is known as pseudohyponatremia. In these cases the osmolarity remains normal or high as a result of excess amounts of other osmolites, such as glucose, triglycerides, or plasma proteins, in the blood. By determining the underlying cause and providing appropriate treatment, the health care provider can take steps to return the sodium level to normal (Davis and Minaker, 1999).

TABLE 21-2 Blood Chemistry

TEST NAME	ADULT NORMALS	OLDER ADULT NORMALS	SIGNIFICANCE OF DEVIATION
Sodium	136-145 mEq/L	Unchanged with aging	*Low:* decreased intake, diarrhea, vomiting, diuretic administration, chronic renal failure, CHF, peripheral edema, ascites *High:* increased intake, Cushing's syndrome, extensive thermal burns
Potassium	3.5-5 mEq/L	Unchanged with aging	*Low:* deficient intake, burns, diuretics, Cushing's syndrome, insulin administration, ascites *High:* excessive dietary intake, renal failure, infection, acidosis, dehydration
Chloride	98-106 mEq/L	Unchanged with aging	*Low:* overhydration, CHF, vomiting, chronic gastric suction, chronic respiratory acidosis, hypokalemia, diuretic therapy *High:* dehydration, Cushing's syndrome, kidney dysfunction, metabolic acidosis, hyperventilation
Calcium	9-10.5 mg/dl	Tends to stay the same or decrease	*Low:* renal failure, vitamin D deficiency, osteomalacia, malabsorption *High:* Paget's disease of the bone, prolonged immobilization, lymphoma
Phosphorus	3-4.5 mg/dl	Slightly lower	*Low:* inadequate dietary ingestion, chronic antacid ingestion, hypercalcemia, alcoholism, osteomalacia, malnutrition *High:* renal failure, increased dietary intake, hypocalcemia, liver disease
Magnesium	1.3-2.1 mEq/L	Decrease 15% between third and eighth decade	*Low:* malnutrition, malabsorption, alcoholism, chronic renal disease *High:* renal insufficiency, ingestion of magnesium-containing antacids or salts, hypothyroidism
Fasting glucose	70-105 mg/dl	Increase in normal range after age 50	*Low:* hypothyroidism, liver disease, insulin overdose, starvation *High:* diabetes mellitus, acute stress response, diuretic therapy, corticosteroid therapy
Postprandial glucose	Less than 140 mg/dl 2 hr after meal	Less than 160 mg/dl 2 hr after meal	*Low:* hypothyroidism, insulin overdose, malabsorption *High:* diabetes mellitus, malnutrition, Cushing's syndrome, chronic renal failure, diuretic therapy, corticosteroid therapy
Amylase	60-120 Somogyi units/dl	Slightly increased in elderly	*High:* acute pancreatitis, perforated bowel, acute cholecystitis, diabetic ketoacidosis
Glycosylated hemoglobin (Hgb A_{1c})	2.2%-4.8%	Unchanged with aging	*Low:* hemolytic anemia, chronic renal failure *High:* newly diagnosed diabetes, poorly controlled diabetes, nondiabetic hyperglycemia
Total protein	6.4-8.3 g/dl	Unchanged with aging	*Low:* liver disease, malnutrition, ascites *High:* hemoconcentration
Albumin	3.5-5 g/dl	Decrease slightly with aging	*Low:* malnutrition, liver disease, overhydration *High:* dehydration
Blood urea nitrogen (BUN)	7-22 mg/dl	May be slightly higher	*Low:* liver failure, overhydration, malnutrition *High:* hypovolemia, dehydration, alimentary tube feeding, renal disease
Creatinine	0.7 -1.5 mg/dl	Decrease in muscle mass may cause decreased values	*Low:* debilitation, decreased muscle mass *High:* reduced renal blood flow, diabetic neuropathy, urinary tract obstruction

Continued

TABLE 21-2 Blood Chemistry—cont'd

TEST NAME	ADULT NORMALS	OLDER ADULT NORMALS	SIGNIFICANCE OF DEVIATION
Creatinine clearance	87-107 ml/min	Values decrease 6.5 ml/min/decade of life due to a decline in GFR	*Low:* impaired kidney function, CHF, cirrhosis *High:* high cardiac output syndromes
Cholesterol (total)	>200 mg/dl	Increases until about middle age but decreases thereafter (or can increase abruptly in women)	*Low:* malabsorption, malnutrition, cholesterol-lowering medication, pernicious anemia, liver disease, myocardial infarction *High:* hypercholesteremia, hyperlipidemia, hypothyroidism, uncontrolled diabetes mellitus
High-density lipoprotein (HDL)	>45 mg/dl	Unchanged with aging	*Low:* familiar low HDL, liver disease, hypoproteinemia *High:* familiar HDL lipoproteinemia, excessive exercise
Low-density lipoprotein (LDL)	60-180 mg/dl	Increases with aging after menopause	*Low:* hypolipoproteinemia *High:* hypothyroidism, alcohol consumption, chronic liver disease, Cushing's syndrome
Alkaline phosphatase	30-120 U/L	Slightly higher	*Low:* hypothyroidism, malnutrition, pernicious anemia *High:* cirrhosis, healing fracture, Paget's disease
Acid phosphatase	0.13-0.63 U/L	Unchanged with aging	*Low:* thrombosis *High:* heparin administration, cirrhosis, prostate cancer
Aspartate transaminase (AST)	0-35 U/L	Values slightly higher	*Low:* acute renal disease, diabetic ketoacidosis, chronic renal dialysis *High:* myocardial infarction, hepatitis, cirrhosis, multiple trauma, acute hemolytic anemia
Creatinine kinase (CK)	30-170 U/L	Unchanged with aging	*High:* diseases or injury affecting heart muscle, skeletal muscle, and brain

Adapted from Pagana KD, Pagana TJ: *Manual of diagnostic and laboratory tests,* ed 2, St Louis, 2004, Mosby; Pagana KD, Pagana TJ: *Diagnostic and laboratory test reference,* ed 6, St Louis, 2003, Mosby.

The role of the gerontologic nurse for clients with fluid and sodium disorders is to understand the goal of treatment. In clients with fluid deficiencies, the nurse can help identify reasons for a given condition, such as restrictions in mobility, visual disturbances, urinary incontinence, and swallowing disorders. Hypernatremia (a high sodium level) can occur from infusion of high-sodium solute fluids, excess water loss, and excessive diarrhea. Hypernatremia is often seen in hospitalized older adults; some cases are present on admission, whereas some are the consequence of hospitalization. Symptoms are similar to those of hyponatremia, with the neurologic signs of obtundation, lethargy, and coma being the most common. The pathophysiology behind the neurologic signs is thought to be neuronal cell dehydration and brain shrinkage (Beck, 1999). Laxative abuse, usually unreported but often present in older adults, can also lead to hypernatremia (Davis and Minaker, 1999).

Potassium. Potassium (K^+) is another electrolyte that is present in both the intracellular and extracellular fluid. Its presence, however, is opposite that of sodium. The majority of potassium is found within the cell, with minute amounts in the extracellular fluid. This extracellular amount is measured by serum testing. Potassium levels are widely thought to be affected by aging, but conclusive studies have not confirmed this theory (Beck, 1999). However, potassium imbalances in older adults can be caused by the same changes in the renal system mentioned in the section on sodium. Salt substitutes, used by many older adults with hypertension or congestive heart failure (CHF), are high in potassium and should be used with caution. Many medications, such as potassium-sparing diuretics used in conjunction with potassium supplements, can cause hyperkalemia (a high potassium level) in older adults. Also, NSAIDs such as ibuprofen interfere with potassium excretion (Beck, 1999). Hypokalemia (a low potassium level) can be caused by gastrointestinal loss and the use of diuretics. Hypokalemia can predispose older adults to tachyarrhythmias and potentiate digitalis toxicity (Beck, 1999). Since over-the-counter medication use has increased, it is important for the gerontologic nurse to carefully assess an older client's prescription and over-the-counter medication history (see Emergency Treatment box).

Potassium, like sodium, maintains cell osmolarity, muscle function, and the transmission of nerve impulses, and it

EMERGENCY TREATMENT

ABNORMAL LABORATORY VALUES: POTASSIUM

Hypokalemia

If asymptomatic, may repeat test before treatment.

Monitor for possible cardiac arrhythmias (e.g., sinus bradycardia, atrioventricular block, paroxysmal atrial tachycardia).

Observe for signs of digitalis toxicity.

Maximum oral replacement is 40 to 80 mEq/day if renal function is normal.

Maximum safe rate for intravenous replacement is 20 mEq/hr; maximum concentration of 40 mEq/L should be used.

Repeat after replacement therapy (McCance and Huether, 2001).

regulates acid-base balance (Grodner, Long, and DeYoung, 2004). The cardiac muscle is particularly sensitive to serum concentrations of potassium. Hyperkalemia can cause muscle twitching, arrhythmias, and gastrointestinal symptoms (Grodner, Long, and DeYoung, 2004). Hypokalemia can occur because of excessive loss of potassium through the gastrointestinal tract, usually by vomiting. Symptoms include muscle weakness, confusion, and absence of bowel sounds. As noted previously, drugs such as diuretics are also a major source of potassium loss in older adults. When replacing potassium in older adults, the nurse must take care to prevent hyperkalemia.

Chloride. Chloride (Cl^-) is mostly present in the fluid outside the cell; it is the major anion in the extracellular fluid. Chloride is closely tied to sodium, with which it combines to make the salt compound sodium chloride (NaCl). Chloride levels have not been shown to change with aging (see Table 21-2). But since losses and excesses in sodium are closely related to chloride, water balance is also affected (Pagana and Pagana, 2003).

Calcium. Serum calcium (Ca^{++}) level measures only the amount of calcium in the blood, which is about 1% of the body's total calcium. Approximately 99% of the body's calcium is found in the bones and teeth (Grodner, Long, and DeYoung, 2004). There are no age-related increases or decreases in the calcium level, even though there are changes in calcium metabolism with aging. The loss of calcium from bone maintains the normal level of calcium in the blood, but the resulting bone loss secondary to calcium leaching can lead to osteoporosis (Baylink, Jennings, and Mohan, 1999). The circulating calcium in the blood is important in blood clotting, in conduction of nerve impulses, in enzyme activity, and especially in muscle contraction and relaxation (Grodner, Long, and DeYoung, 2004). The calcium levels measure both free calcium and calcium that is protein bound with albumin. Therefore, when calcium levels fall, albumin levels also decrease (Pagana and Pagana, 2004).

Calcium metabolism is one of the factors that determines phosphorus levels; they are inversely related. A decrease in calcium can cause an increase in phosphorus, and vice versa. Parathyroid hormone (PTH) also affects phosphorus levels by affecting the resorption of phosphorus in the kidneys (Pagana and Pagana, 2003). PTH acts on plasma membrane receptors of the nephrons of the kidneys to increase the reabsorption of calcium and to decrease the resorption of phosphorus (McCance and Huether, 2001).

Phosphorus. Phosphorus (phosphate) is a mineral found mostly in bone, in combination with calcium (Grodner, Long, and DeYoung, 2004). Phosphorus is well absorbed, so if malfunctions with absorption occur, it is generally related to a decrease in kidney function or the long-term use of antacids, which bind to the phosphorus (Ott, 1999). Phosphorus plays an important role in the maintenance of homeostasis (as a component in DNA and ribonucleic acid [RNA]); the metabolism of fats, carbohydrates, and proteins; and the transfer of energy stored as adenosine triphosphate (ATP) (Grodner, Long, and DeYoung, 2004). In older adults, phosphorus levels are slightly decreased in comparison with younger adults (see Table 21-2).

Magnesium. Magnesium is a mineral important to enzyme action for the production of energy. The most important sites of function are the muscles (especially the heart) and the nerves. Approximately two thirds of the body's magnesium is contained in the bones (Grodner, Long, and DeYoung, 2004). Magnesium levels have been reported to decrease by 15% between the third and eighth decades (Cavalieri, Chopra, and Bryman, 1992) (see Table 21-2).

Glucose. Glucose, the most common circulating sugar in the blood, is used for energy by the cells (Grodner, Long, and DeYoung, 2004). The result of blood testing for glucose must be evaluated considering the time and circumstances during which the sample was drawn. New criteria for the diagnosis of diabetes mellitus were determined by the Expert Committee on the Diagnosis and Classification of Diabetes Mellitus and began receiving acceptance from the health care community in 1997. Further changes, such as the reference interval for fasting glucose, have begun in laboratories across the nation. The new interpretation of "normal" glucose is those persons with a fasting plasma glucose (FPG) of less than 110 mg/dl and a 2-hour glucose tolerance result less than 140 mg/dl. Impaired fasting glucose is a new category for persons with an FPG ranging from 110 to 126 mg/dl. Impaired intolerance is classified as a 2-hour oral glucose tolerance test (OGTT) ranging from 140 to 200 mg/dl.

Three methods of diagnosing diabetes mellitus are:

1. Symptoms of diabetes plus casual plasma glucose concentration equal to or greater than 200 mg/dl. *Casual* is

defined as any time of day without regard to the last meal eaten. The classic symptoms of diabetes include polyuria, polydipsia, and unexplained weight loss.
2. FPG equal to or greater than 126 mg/dl. Fasting is defined as no caloric intake for at least 8 hours.
3. Two-hour postload glucose equal to or greater than 200 mg/dl during an OGTT. This test should be performed as described by the World Health Organization, using a glucose load containing the equivalent of 75 g anhydrous glucose dissolved in water (Expert Committee on the Diagnosis and Classification of Diabetes Mellitus, 1997).

The principal blood sugar used by the cells for energy is glucose. Glucose must be maintained within a narrow range of 70 to 110 mg/dl. Low blood sugar (hypoglycemia) can cause central nervous system changes such as confusion, which is related to brain cell starvation. Diagnosing and treating hypoglycemia in older adults can be difficult because determining whether a low glucose level is a result of a decrease in glucose metabolism related to aging or the result of noninsulin-dependent diabetes mellitus (type 2) affects the choice of treatment. High blood sugar (hyperglycemia) causes symptoms that include extreme thirst, drowsiness, and frequent urination. More common in older adults than ketoacidosis is hyperosmolar hyperglycemic nonketonic coma, which has a 40% to 70% mortality rate (Halter, 1999).

Amylase

Amylase is an important enzyme in the catabolism of carbohydrates. It is produced by the acinar units of the pancreas and aids the catabolism of carbohydrates in the intestine (Pagana and Pagana, 2003). Amylase levels are primarily tested while trying to rule out pancreatitis. Abnormal levels may be increased or decreased, though they are generally elevated when reported as abnormal. This may be because of damage to or disease of the pancreas or interference in the flow of amylase from the pancreas. Elevated amylase levels also may be seen in nonpancreatic disorders such as perforated ulcer and perforated or necrotic bowel. With aging, amylase may increase slightly (Pagana and Pagana, 2004) (see Table 21-2).

In acute pancreatitis an obstruction causes pancreatic enzymes, including amylase, to "back up" into the pancreas, causing self-digestion of the pancreas. Since amylase plays an important part in the digestion of starches, a decrease can affect digestion. Amylase is needed to convert disaccharides to monosaccharides, and diarrhea can occur when this conversion does not happen as a result of decreased amylase. Amylase is also present in the saliva, where it initiates carbohydrate digestion in the mouth and stomach (Thibodeau and Patton, 2003). Although most older adults experience some decrease in saliva production, others develop a severe dryness of the mouth called xerostomia. The cause of xerostomia is not necessarily a direct result of aging; possible causes include salivary gland dysfunction, medications, and oral and systemic diseases (Ferguson, 2002). The role of the gerontologic nurse is to assist older adults with recognizing the causes of dry mouth and to help identify solutions to cope with the problem, such as eating moist foods, drinking adequate liquids during meals, and using saliva substitutes.

Total Protein

Total protein testing measures the amount of albumin and globulin within the body. Albumin constitutes approximately 60% of the total protein. Globulins are important in the function of antibodies and (to a lesser degree than albumin) in the maintenance of osmotic pressure.

Albumin and Prealbumin

Serum albumin is an indicator of protein nutrition. This test is most useful when used to monitor long-term nutrition changes, since normal values may still be found among patients who are malnourished (Grodner, Long, and DeYoung, 2004). In older adults with impaired skin integrity related to pressure ulcers, the assessment of the albumin level helps determine if the balance is correct for proper wound healing to occur. Clients with low albumin levels need nutritional support to promote healing of wounds. Hypoalbuminemia (a decreased albumin level) is viewed as a significant influence on the lengthening of hospital stays and the increase in hospital mortality in older adults. More recently it has been identified as a risk factor for mortality in community-dwelling older persons. Although albumin levels decrease slightly with age (see Table 21-2), more significant causes of hypoalbuminemia in older adults were linked to tobacco usage, dental illness, lower socioeconomic factors, and gastrointestinal problems (Reuben et al, 1997). Abnormal low values may also be seen in infection, congestive heart failure, fluid overload, and severe hepatic insufficiency. Levels may be affected if a client is experiencing dehydration or has received infusions of albumin, fresh frozen plasma, or whole blood serum albumin (Grodner, Long, and DeYoung, 2004).

Determination of prealbumin levels is also being used to assess an older adult's health and nutritional status. Prealbumin is the measurement of protein status over a short-term period and is a more accurate measurement of malnutrition because of its short half-life of 2 days (Grodner, Long, and DeYoung, 2004). Plasma prealbumin may be useful in evaluating an older adult's response to nutritional supplements (Manning and Shenkin, 1995). A nonnutritional cause of normal values despite patient malnutrition is chronic renal failure. Abnormally low levels of prealbumin have the same causes as high albumin levels (Grodner, Long, and DeYoung, 2004).

Blood Urea Nitrogen

Measurement of the urea in the blood is known as the blood urea nitrogen (BUN) test. Urea is a major waste product of protein catabolism and a result of ammonia conversion in the liver. Urea is excreted from the body by the kidneys. BUN levels are indicative of both liver and kidney function. Values for older men are slightly higher than the adult normal levels of 7 to 22 mg/dl. In older women, BUN levels are also increased, but at lower levels than older men (Pagana and Pagana, 2003) (see Table 21-2).

Creatinine

Creatinine is another end-product of protein metabolism. A rise in a client's BUN and creatinine is indicative of kidney failure (Grodner, Long, and DeYoung, 2004). The physiologic decline in the GFR in older adults does not generally cause a subsequent rise in the creatinine level (Sands and Vega, 1999). This expected rise in the creatinine level does not occur because there is a parallel decrease in mean muscle mass and actual creatinine production with aging (Kane, Ouslander, and Abrass, 1999). An 80-year-old person and a 30-year-old person who have the same creatinine concentrations do not have comparable GFRs. In this example, the older adult has approximately 40% to 50% *less* GFR than the younger adult (Beck, 1999). Therefore a creatinine level in an older adult should not be considered an independent indicator of renal function, as it would be for a younger individual. It should instead be used to calculate the creatinine clearance for a more realistic indication of renal function in older adults.

Creatinine Clearance

Creatinine clearance is the measure of the GFR, estimated from serum creatinine and urine creatinine levels. A 24-hour urine test is required along with a serum level within the same 24-hour period. To allow for changes with aging that are not reflected in the creatinine level, many primary care providers use the Cockcroft and Gault formula to estimate creatinine clearance:

$$\text{Creatinine clearance (ml/min)} = \frac{140 - \text{Age (in years)} \times \text{Weight (in kg)}}{72 \times \text{Serum creatinine (\%mg/dl)}}$$

(For women, multiply final result by 0.85.)

Kane, Ouslander, and Abrass (1999) recommend using this formula for initial estimates of creatinine clearance for drug dosing in older adults, while also considering other factors such as cardiac output and hydration status. The gerontologic nurse should recognize the importance of creatinine clearance as a reflection of an older adult's overall health status. The older adult's response to medications, especially newly prescribed drugs, should be monitored because impaired renal function can precipitate side effects that may be overlooked. The normal reference range is 0.7 to 1.5 mg/dl but may be lower in elderly or clients with low muscle mass (Cook, 1999).

Triglycerides

Triglycerides are the principal lipids (fats) found in circulating blood bound to a protein; they form high-density and low-density lipoproteins (HDLs and LDLs). Triglycerides are produced in the liver from glycerol and fatty acids found in the blood. When the triglyceride level in the blood reaches its peak, the excess is deposited in the fatty tissue (Pagana and Pagana, 2003). The triglyceride level increases with age until about middle age, then decreases thereafter (Hazzard, 1999). However, the increase in triglycerides that happens in women until they reach middle age occurs at a slower rate than in men. Moreover, further changes in triglyceride levels occur in women after the age of 50, when an abrupt increase has been noted related to the decrease in estrogen (Hazzard, 1999).

Total Cholesterol

Cholesterol is a steroid compound that helps stabilize the membranes of the body's cells (Thibodeau and Patton, 2003). It is also the major lipid associated with cardiovascular disease. The liver metabolizes cholesterol and binds it to LDLs and HDLs for transport in the bloodstream (Pagana and Pagana, 2004). Total cholesterol levels are a combination of LDL and HDL levels in the bloodstream. Changes in cholesterol levels with aging mirror changes in triglyceride levels, except that the peak that occurs after women reach age 50 is thought to be mediated by changes in relative body weight (Hazzard, 1999) (see Table 21-2).

High-Density Lipoprotein

HDL, referred to as the "good cholesterol," carries greater amounts of protein and lesser amounts of lipids, hence the term *high density*. Approximately 25% of cholesterol is bound to HDLs. HDLs are thought to help protect against heart disease, but their levels are not affected by diet. Oral estrogen has been shown to increase HDL levels in postmenopausal women, but further studies are needed to determine if this is the only variable in the relationship (Hazzard, 1999).

Low-Density Lipoprotein

The remaining 75% of cholesterol in the bloodstream is bound to LDL (Pagana and Pagana, 2003), known as "bad cholesterol." LDL can be calculated from the total cholesterol level, HDL level, and fasting triglycerides by using the following equation (Lindsey et al, 2004):

LDL cholesterol = Total cholesterol − HDL cholesterol − (Triglyceride level ÷ [5])

When this calculation is compared with the direct LDL, an underestimation of approximately 20 mg/dl was found with the calculated LDL. This resulted in an LDL goal attainment for half of the patients with coronary heart disease or a coronary heart disease risk equivalent (Lindsey et al, 2004).

Age-related changes in HDL and LDL levels differ between the genders. LDL mean levels rise in both genders after puberty, with LDL levels in women rising sharply after menopause, exceeding the levels of men at comparable ages (Hazzard, 1999). (As noted previously, the increase in LDL after menopause is related to decreasing estrogen levels in women.) HDL levels in boys and girls remain similar until puberty, when HDL is noted to decrease in boys. Average levels of HDL in men remain lower than those of women throughout the life span after puberty (Hazzard, 1999).

Brain Natriuretic Peptide

The brain natriuretic peptide is a neurohormone (BNP) secreted from the cardiac ventricles in response to ventricular stretch and pressure overload (Prahash and Lynch, 2004). This new test can help in the diagnosis and treatment of patients with CHF. Several studies have shown that an elevated BNP is highly sensitive and specific for the diagnosis of heart failure. Plasma concentration of BNP reflects the sensitivity of heart failure (Maisel, 2003; Morrison et al, 2002). Plasma levels of BNP are significantly elevated in patients with heart failure and left ventricular dysfunction; however, the values cannot be used to differentiate between systolic and diastolic heart failure (Prahash and Lynch, 2004).

Alkaline Phosphatase

Alkaline phosphatase is an enzyme found in many tissues, although it has its highest concentrations in the liver and bone. Testing for alkaline phosphatase is used to identify liver and bone disorders (Pagana and Pagana, 2004). Testing of the alkaline phosphatase level in older adults is often used in the biochemical assessment of Paget's disease (Lyles, 1999) and other bone diseases. Slight increases in the alkaline phosphatase level accompany aging in both sexes (Pagana and Pagana, 2004) (see Table 21-2).

Acid Phosphatase

Acid phosphatase is also an enzyme, but it is primarily located in the prostate gland. Acid phosphatase levels are used to diagnose prostate cancer and to estimate the extent of the disease. The incidence of prostate cancer increases substantially after age 50, and it is the second most common malignancy in men in the United States (Letran and Brower, 1999). The acid phosphatase level, in addition to assisting with diagnosis, is also helpful in determining whether treatment for prostate cancer has been effective (Pagana and Pagana, 2003). The role of the gerontologic nurse in working with older men is to educate them about the incidence of this disease and to encourage prostate examinations every 2 years after the age of 50.

Aspartate Aminotransferase

Aspartate transaminase (AST) measures the enzyme of the same name, which is found in the heart muscle, skeletal muscle, liver, kidney, and pancreas. Since AST is found in several organs, it may be used to diagnose hepatitis, liver necrosis, and skeletal muscle damage. AST/SGOT levels may be helpful in diagnosing a myocardial infarction but are not as specific as other tests such as the creatinine phosphokinase (CPK) and creatinine phosphokinase-MB (Pagana and Pagana, 2004). In treating tuberculosis in older adults, a threefold to fivefold increase in the SGOT can be indicative of hepatotoxicity from drugs such as isoniazid, rifampin, ethambutol, and pyrazinamide (Rajagopalan and Yoshikawa, 1999). A rise in the AST/SGOT is also seen in renal arterial occlusion, with the increase being noted within 24 hours and decreasing by the fourth day (Sands and Vega, 1999).

Creatinine Kinase

Creatinine kinase (CK) is present in various parts of the body and can be isolated into three isoenzymes to pinpoint the area of the body affected. CK-BB is primarily found in the lungs and brain, whereas CK-MB is associated with cardiac muscle cells. CK-MM is normally found in the circulating blood, and the level rises when there is damage to the skeletal muscles. CK levels rise and peak at specific intervals during myocardial infarction, and these levels are used with lactate dehydrogenase (LDH) and AST/SGOT testing to determine the amount and prognosis of myocardial damage (Siomko, 2000). In older adults, an elevated CK-MB level may be seen in hypothyroidism (Kane, Ouslander, and Abrass, 1999). The nurse should also expect an elevated CK if an older adult has experienced a recent fall or other skeletal muscle trauma.

Lactate Dehydrogenase

LDH, an enzyme found throughout the body, is used in conjunction with CPK and AST/SGOT in assessing myocardial damage. As with CPK, LDH can be isolated into five isoenzymes (CPK only has three). These isoenzymes can clarify the site of release of the LDH and assist the nurse in assessing and monitoring specific complications related to the site of injury. An older adult's condition is monitored by the peaks and duration of elevated levels.

LDH-2 normally has the highest level of the five isoenzymes, originating mainly from the reticuloendothelial system. The origin of LDH-1 lies mainly in the heart and red blood vessels, and its levels are monitored for degree of myocardial activity and damage (Siomko, 2000). In older adults an elevated LDH may be seen in cases of atheroembolic renal disease (Sands and Vega, 1999). In these cases LDH-4 is the most likely elevated portion, since it is found in the kidney.

Troponin

In clients who are first seen with chest pain, the measurement of cardiac myofibrillar proteins in the blood has been a useful tool in determining whether the pain is related to cardiac injury. Two tests, called troponin T and troponin I, may be performed in the emergency department or urgent care center as part of a cardiac diagnostic workup. Specific for necrosis of the cardiac muscle, these indices appear 2 to 8 hours after a decrease in the oxygenation of the heart muscle caused by occlusion of the cardiac vessels. Levels can remain elevated up to 2 weeks following a myocardial infarction (Siomko, 2000).

In clients with recent aggravated unstable angina, slight elevations are rarely noted. Troponin I levels are also not increased with skeletal muscle diseases, severe muscle exertion, or chronic renal failure. Cardiac troponin I has been called a more specific marker for myocardial infarction than CK-MB, with roughly equivalent sensitivity early in the course of infarction (4 to 36 hours); some believe that it may replace the use of LDH isoenzymes for the detection of infarction (Chernecky and Berger, 2001). Normal levels of troponin I are up to 0.60 ng/ml. Higher levels are considered abnormal and indicative of myocardial muscle damage. Elevated levels of cardiac troponin have been reported in patients hospitalized for decompensated heart failure (Hudson et al, 2004).

Thyroid Gland

The thyroid gland has been the focus of many studies on aging. Testing of function includes the assessment of two hormones secreted by the thyroid gland: thyroxine (T_4) and triiodothyronine (T_3). Thyroid-stimulating hormone (TSH), a hormone secreted by the antipituitary gland, is also usually tested when investigating thyroid function. In fact, serum TSH determination has become an excellent means of screening for hyperthyroidism. Its measurement also aids in differentiating primary from secondary hypothyroidism (Table 21-3).

T_4 and T_3 are both responsible for increasing the rate of metabolism. Although T_4 is secreted in larger amounts, scientists now believe that T_3 is the primary thyroid hormone. The rationale is that most of the T_4 in the bloodstream is converted to T_3, and that T_3 binds more easily to target cells than T_4 (McCance and Huether, 2001).

TSH promotes the growth and development of the thyroid gland, as well as the secretion of T_3 and T_4 from the thyroid gland. With normal aging, the secretion of thyroid hormones remains unchanged, although the metabolic clearance rate of these hormones is decreased. Decreased T_4 levels (specifically free T_4) and an elevated TSH are indicative of primary hypothyroidism (Kane, Ouslander, and Abrass, 1999). CPK may also be elevated. T_4, T_3, and radioactive iodine uptake are used in diagnosing hyperthyroidism (Kane, Ouslander, and Abrass, 1999).

The presence of thyroid disease in older adults can be difficult to determine. Classic signs of thyroid disorders seen in younger adults are often absent or clouded because of concomitant illnesses in older adults. Some of the symptoms of thyroid disorders are similar to other complaints common among many older adults, such as anorexia, constipation, lack of energy, mental clouding, cold intolerance, fatigue, and skin dryness and scaling. An older adult may have a feeling that something is not right but may be unable to articulate this feeling. For these reasons, health care professionals may not take an older adult's complaints seriously and may attribute the complaints to the aging process. The gerontologic nurse should be aware that thyroid disease can be present in older adults without any overt symptoms. Assessment of thyroid function should be performed for those adults with vague but persistent symptoms.

TABLE 21-3 Thyroid Testing

TEST NAME	ADULT NORMALS	OLDER ADULT NORMALS	SIGNIFICANCE OF DEVIATIONS
Thyroxine (T_4)	4-12 mcg/dl	Slightly decreased	*Low:* hypothyroidism, malnutrition, renal failure, cirrhosis *High:* hyperthyroidism, hepatitis
Triiodothyronine (T_3)	75-220 ng/dl	Slightly decreased	*Low:* hypothyroidism, pituitary insufficiency, protein malnutrition, renal failure, liver diseases *High:* hyperthyroidism, hepatitis, hypoproteinemia
Thyroid-stimulating hormone (TSH)	2-10 μU/ml	Unchanged with aging	*Low:* pituitary dysfunction, hyperthyroidism *High:* primary hypothyroidism

Adapted from Pagana KD, Pagana TJ: *Manual of diagnostic and laboratory tests,* ed 2, St Louis, 2004, Mosby; Pagana KD, Pagana TJ: *Diagnostic and laboratory test reference,* ed 6, St Louis, 2003, Mosby.

Hypothyroidism results from decreased secretion of thyroid hormones. The decrease in hormone secretion may be a result of an autoimmune response, and it is often idiopathic (Hassani and Hershman, 1999). Symptoms of hypothyroidism in older adults may include confusion, dementia, depression, syncope, seizures, and mild psychotic disturbances. Clients being screened for dementia should have thyroid testing included in the panel of laboratory tests performed. Thyroid testing for the older adult with hypothyroidism usually reveals a combination of a low T_4 and an elevated TSH. The T_3 level is decreased in normal aging and may be seen as "normal" in hypothyroidism. For this reason, T_3 levels are not useful in diagnosing hypothyroidism.

Hyperthyroidism in older adults is more prevalent than scientists originally believed (Hassani and Hershman, 1999). Most symptoms of hyperthyroidism are nonspecific and vague. Younger clients may complain of fatigue, lack of energy, and nervousness, but older adults may not have these symptoms. However, apathy, weight loss, and palpitations commonly appear in both young and old clients with hyperthyroidism. More than 50% of older adults with hyperthyroidism have CHF, which may be initially seen as acute pulmonary edema. Laboratory assessment reveals an elevated T_4 and free T_4 index in most older adults with hyperthyroidism. However, approximately 2% of older adults with the disease have normal T_4 levels and an elevated T_3. But since T_3 is often reported as normal in 30% to 40% of older adults, it is more useful in differentiating the origin of elevated T_4 levels, rather than in the primary diagnosis of hyperthyroidism (Hasssani and Hershman, 1999).

Prostate-Specific Antigen

The use of the prostate specific antigen (PSA) has led to an increase in the detection of prostate cancer in men. Most of the cases are diagnosed in men older than 65 (Hahnfield and Moon, 1999). The PSA is a starting point for the diagnosis of prostate cancer in men. The PSA tends to increase with age. Age specific ranges are 3.5 to 4.5 ng/ml for men ages 60 to 70 and 4.5 to 6.5 ng/ml for men ages 70 to 80 (Hahnfield and Moon, 1999).

URINE CHEMISTRY

Urine chemistry testing includes testing for the presence of protein, glucose, bacteria, blood, ketones, and leukocytes. It also involves studying the sample for properties of specific gravity and pH. Urine is a waste product formed by the kidneys and consists of 95% water. The composition of urine can inform the health professional of the status of many body systems. When blood passes through the kidneys, water, nitrogen compounds, toxins, and electrolytes are filtered, reabsorbed, and secreted. The amounts retained or excreted affect the body's homeostasis.

Protein

Protein in the urine (proteinuria) is usually considered an abnormal finding, and its presence indicates a disruption in normal kidney function, as with diabetes (Table 21-4). Excessive loss of protein from the body can lead to nephrotic syndrome, the result of proteinuria and edema (Pagana and Pagana, 2003). In older adults, however, proteinuria is commonly found and may not be of any clinical significance. Its presence does warrant investigation to rule out urinary tract infection (UTI) or kidney disease.

Glucose

When glucose appears in the urine (glycosuria), it may be an indicator of diabetes, although it may also be seen in cases of normal serum glucose levels. In diabetes the amount of glucose in the filtrate formed by the kidneys exceeds the maximum capacity of the transport system that removes it. Glucose in the urine of older adults may or may not be a sign of diabetes or disease. The reabsorption of glucose diminishes as a normal process of aging; therefore increased glucose may be seen in the urine of older adults even in the absence of disease (McCance and Huether, 2001).

Bacteria and Leukocytes

Although occasional trace amounts of bacteria (bacteriuria) may normally appear in the urine, significant amounts, defined as greater than 10^5 colony-forming units (CFU) per milliliter of urine, indicate infection within the body. If the infection is in the renal system, the site—kidney, bladder, or urethra—must be determined. The gerontologic nurse should assess older adults for symptoms of urinary incontinence, flank pain, fever, frequency, burning, and suprapubic or low back pain. However, common symptoms may be absent in most older adults, and symptoms such as confusion, new onset of incontinence, lethargy, nocturia, and anorexia may be the first indication of an underlying UTI (Duffield, 1997; Riehmann, 1998). Women are more prone to lower UTIs than men because of their shorter urethra and its proximity to the anus. In adults 65 to 70 years of age, bacteria in the urine is found in approximately 15% to 20% of women and 4% to 12% of men; the numbers increase to 20% to 50% of women and 20% of men over the age of 80 (Travis and Lampley-Dallas, 1997). Significant numbers of older adults are asymptomatic, even when bacteria are found in the urine. Pus in the urine (pyuria) is more indicative of a symptomatic UTI, with a level defined as greater than 10 leukocytes/mm^3 of urine on microscopic examination. Recommendations for decreasing the incidence of UTIs in older adults include teaching women to wipe from front to back after voiding and defecation, avoiding bubble baths and sanitary pads, and reducing the use of indwelling catheters

TABLE 21-4 Urine Chemistry

TEST NAME	ADULT NORMALS	OLDER ADULT NORMALS	SIGNIFICANCE OF DEVIATIONS
Color	Yellow; amber	Same	Straw colored urine indicates dilution.
Appearance	Clear	Same	Cloudy urine may indicate presence of pus, casts, blood, and bacteria
Specific gravity	1.005-1.030	Values decrease with aging	*Low:* overhydration, renal failure, diuresis, hypothermia *High:* dehydration, water restriction, vomiting, diarrhea
pH	4.6-8.0	Same	*Acidic urine:* diarrhea, metabolic acidosis, diabetes mellitus, respiratory acidosis, emphysema *Alkaline urine:* respiratory alkalosis, metabolic alkalosis, vomiting, gastric suctioning, diuretic therapy, UTI
Protein	1-8 mg/ml	Same	*Positive:* diabetes mellitus, CHF, systemic lupus erythematosus, malignant hypertension
Glucose	Negative	Same	*Positive:* diabetes mellitus, Cushing's syndrome, severe stress, infection, drug therapy
Ketones	Negative	Same	*Positive:* uncontrolled diabetes mellitus, starvation, excessive aspirin ingestion, high-protein diet, dehydration
Blood	Negative	Same	*Positive:* renal trauma, renal stones, cystitis, prostatitis
Leukocyte esterase	Negative	Same	*Positive:* possible UTI
Bacteria	Negative	May be seen in older adults without symptoms; evaluate for pyuria and symptoms	*Positive:* UTI

Adapted from Pagana KD, Pagana TJ: *Manual of diagnostic and laboratory tests,* ed 2, St Louis, 2004, Mosby; Pagana KD, Pagana TJ: *Diagnostic and laboratory test reference,* ed 6, St Louis, 2003, Mosby.

(Duffield, 1997; Yoshikawa, Nicholle, and Norman, 1996). The addition of cranberry juice or cranberry pills in the diet to reduce bacterial adherence to the bladder wall has been studied, but its significance is still controversial (Yoshikawa, Nicholle, and Norman, 1996) (see Research box).

Ketones

The presence of ketones, the result of fatty acid breakdown, in the urine is another abnormal finding. When overaccumulation of ketones occurs in the blood, the excess is excreted in the urine. Causes of ketones in the urine include a high-protein diet, starvation or fasting, and ingestion of isopropyl alcohol (Pagana and Pagana, 2003).

pH

The pH of the urine sample indicates the acid or base value of the urine, which reflects the body's homeostatic state. The normal range for urine pH is 4.6 to 8.0. Some drugs can cause the urine to be alkaline or acidic. Renal calculi are acid or base in origin, depending on the underlying substances that form the stones. Prevention and treatment of calculi are aimed at changing the urine to the reverse pH of the stone's composition (Pagana and Pagana, 2003). When collecting a urine specimen, the health care professional must cover the sample, since urine left uncovered can change its pH.

Blood

The presence of blood in the urine (hematuria) is always an abnormal finding. The cause may be renal obstruction from calculi, trauma to the kidney, inflammation, infection, or malignancy. The blood may be grossly apparent or occult, giving the urine a cloudy or pink hue on visual inspection.

COMPONENTS OF ARTERIAL BLOOD GAS TESTING

Arterial blood gas (ABG) testing involves drawing a sample of blood from an artery, usually from the radial or brachial artery. Components of ABG testing are pH, oxygen, and carbon dioxide content, oxygen saturation, and bicarbonate level (Table 21-5). It is important that the primary care provider and laboratory personnel be aware of the conditions of a client's oxygenation when the blood was drawn (e.g., client

Research

SAMPLE/SETTING

Subjects included 153 volunteer women with a mean age of 78.5 years. Subjects were randomly assigned to drink 300 ml of cranberry juice or a similar tasting placebo substance per day. Sixty-five female subjects were nursing facility residents in the Midwestern United States who were incontinent for at least 2 weeks, according to nursing facility administrators.

METHODS

Baseline urine samples and six clean-voided samples were collected at 1-month intervals and quantitatively tested for bacteriuria and WBCs.

FINDINGS

Subjects consuming the cranberry juice had odds of bacteriuria, defined as equal to or greater than 10^5 mL, with pyuria at only 42% of the odds of the control group. The odds of remaining bacteriuric-pyuric were 27% of the control group, assuming they were bacteriuric-pyuric the month before.

IMPLICATIONS

The study findings suggest that the ingestion of cranberry juice by older women decreases the frequency of bacteriuria.

Avorn J et al: Reduction of bacteriuria and pyuria after ingestion of cranberry juice, *JAMA* 271(10):751, 1994.

on room air, amount of oxygen support, type of oxygen delivery device). Pulse oximetry is a reliable alternative to ABG testing when seeking the oxygen saturation percentage of the blood. The use of pulse oximetry is less painful and less expensive, and the results are immediately available (Pagana and Pagana, 2003).

Oxygen

Oxygen (Pao_2) levels have been shown to decline significantly with age (Cavalieri, Chopra, and Bryman, 1992). Age-related changes such as a decrease in chest wall recoil, decrease in alveolar surface area, and less effective oxygen-to–carbon dioxide (CO_2) exchange all contribute to this change in the oxygen level. In the absence of disease, older adult respiratory function remains adequate. However, changes in Pao_2 should be considered in view of a client's age. The Pao_2 decreases approximately 25% between the ages of 30 and 80 years (Cavalieri, Chopra, and Bryman, 1992). The following formula for arterial oxygen may be used in calculating age-appropriate PO_2 levels (Cavalieri, Chopra, and Bryman, 1992):

$$Pao_2 \text{ (mm Hg)} = 100.1 - (0.325) \text{ (Age)}$$

pH of the Blood

The pH of the blood is a measure of alkalinity and acidity, which is inversely related to the concentration of hydrogen ions (Pagana and Pagana, 2004). No significant changes in the pH of the arterial blood are seen with aging (Cavalieri, Chopra, and Bryman, 1992). The normal adult values for blood pH are 7.35 to 7.45 (see Table 21-5).

Carbon Dioxide

No significant changes in the carbon dioxide ($Paco_2$) level are seen with aging (Cavalieri, Chopra, and Bryman, 1992). The normal adult range for carbon dioxide is 35 to 45 mm Hg.

Oxygen Saturation

Oxygen saturation (O_2 sat %) refers to the binding of oxygen onto molecules of hemoglobin. The saturation of venous blood is approximately 75%, with a Pao_2 of 40 mm Hg. In the arterial blood the saturation is approximately 97%, with a

TABLE 21-5 Arterial Blood Gases

TEST NAME	ADULT NORMALS	OLDER ADULT NORMALS	SIGNIFICANCE OF DEVIATION
pH	7.35 – 7.45	Same	*Low:* respiratory or metabolic acidosis *High:* respiratory or metabolic alkalosis
Pao_2	80-100 mm Hg	Decreases 25% between 30 and 80 years old	*Low:* cardiac or respiratory disease
$Paco_2$	35-45 mm Hg	Same	*Low:* respiratory alkalosis *High:* respiratory acidosis
O_2 saturation	95%-100 %	95%	*Low:* impaired gas exchange
HCO_3	21-28 mEq/L	Same	*Low:* metabolic acidosis *High:* metabolic acidosis

Adapted from Pagana KD, Pagana TJ: *Diagnostic and laboratory test reference,* ed 6, St Louis, 2003, Mosby; and Pagana KD, Pagana TJ: *Manual of diagnostic and laboratory tests,* ed 2, St Louis, 2004, Mosby.

Pao_2 of 100 mm Hg. The normal adult value for oxygen saturation is greater than 97%. Some researchers, however, believe that the normal value of an older adult's oxygen saturation (95%) is slightly lower than that of a younger adult (Ogburn-Russell and Johnson, 1990; Pagana and Pagana, 2003).

Bicarbonate

Bicarbonate (HCO_3) is a buffer present in the blood that plays an important role in acid-base balance. When the acidity of the blood increases, the kidneys conserve bicarbonate in an effort to regain proper acid-base balance. When the blood is alkalotic, the kidneys increase excretion of bicarbonate. Bicarbonate levels in the blood are unchanged with aging (Pagana and Pagana, 2004).

BLOOD LEVEL MONITORING

Three other blood tests performed on older adults receiving drug therapy that requires monitoring are for digoxin, theophylline, and phenytoin levels. Digoxin (Lanoxin) is a drug used to control ventricular response in chronic atrial fibrillation (Goroll, May, and Mulley, 2000). The normal therapeutic range is 0.9 to 2.0 ng/ml, with toxicity occurring above 3.0. However, in older adults, toxicity can occur at the upper, and sometimes even the lower, levels of the normal range. The nurse should be aware of a client's own level of "normal," where the heart rate is controlled but signs and symptoms of toxicity, such as confusion and diarrhea, are absent.

Phenytoin (Dilantin) has normal level ranges between 10 and 20 mcg/ml, with toxicity occurring at levels of 30 mcg/ml or greater. In older adults, signs of toxicity can sometimes appear at values slightly above 20 mcg/ml; signs may include confusion and lethargy. Phenytoin and digoxin levels should be taken at least 4 hours after a dose is given.

Theophylline is a drug often given to clients with pulmonary disease to improve respiratory muscle strength. The side effects of theophylline may prohibit its use in some older adults, since its plasma concentrations must be at the upper limits of normal to produce any significant benefit (Connolly, 2002). Side effects include nausea, restlessness, increased respirations, and diuresis (Beers and Berkow, 2000). More serious side effects include ventricular arrhythmias and seizures. This level should be obtained 4 hours after a dose of the drug is given. As with the previous drugs, the therapeutic range of theophylline can be narrow for some older adults. The normal range for a therapeutic level is 10 to 20 mcg/ml, with toxicity at levels greater than 20 mcg/ml.

SUMMARY

Aging today is vastly different from aging in previous generations. Health care researchers and scientists have traditionally used young or middle-age men for studies, generalizing findings and results to both genders and a variety of age-groups. But researchers are now beginning to realize that older adults have different "normals" than younger adults, as well as complex health histories that can affect their body's overall responses to stressors and disease. Consequently, older adults are now being included in research studies aimed at determining the effects of interventions based on age.

In providing age-specific and age-appropriate health care, providers must recognize that individuals do not respond in the same way to similar experiences. Although many laboratory values are being rewritten to compensate for age-related changes in older adults, many questions remain unanswered. An older adult must be considered within the total context of a person with unique responses to disease. Laboratory tests and their results should be considered as an adjunct to the detection and treatment of illness, not in isolation from the presenting clinical picture.

The gerontologic nurse plays an important role in promoting the well-being of older adults by reviewing and reporting laboratory values. Awareness of the changes in laboratory and diagnostic test values as a result of age can augment the management of older adults' health problems. The gerontologic nurse may need to serve as an advocate for older adults when repeated symptoms and concerns are not addressed by the primary care provider, but are instead attributed to the complaints of "old age." As always, appropriate assessments must be carried out, supplemented by laboratory testing, before establishing nursing interventions.

Home Care

1. The home care nurse must know the purpose of the tests ordered and must explain the reasoning for the tests to both caregivers and homebound older adults.
2. The nurse should assess the homebound older adults' cultural values and beliefs regarding diagnostic testing.
3. Home care nurses must realize that laboratory values in homebound older adults may be altered because of aging or medication regimens.
4. Home care nurses must be able to differentiate normal versus abnormal laboratory results for homebound older adults, and the nurses must know when to notify a physician.
5. The nurse should instruct caregivers and homebound older adults about activities required before laboratory testing (e.g., nothing by mouth from midnight the night before until the procedure).

Key Points

- The ESR rises approximately 10 to 20 mm in older adults; this is considered a normal age-related change.

- Potassium-sparing diuretics and NSAIDs can interfere with potassium excretion.
- Older adults may have hyponatremia in the presence of normal osmolarity, indicating the presence of other osmolarities in excess in the blood.
- Renal and hepatic system functioning can be reflected in the BUN level.
- Hypokalemia can potentiate digitalis toxicity in older adults.
- Comparable serum creatinine levels in younger adults and older adults are not indicators of comparable kidney function.
- Urine testing for glucose in older adults is considered unreliable in view of age-related changes in renal function.
- Thyroid disease can be present in older adults without the overt symptoms typically seen in younger adults with thyroid disorders.
- Older adults may be asymptomatic in the presence of bacteriuria.
- Pyuria is more indicative of a symptomatic UTI than the presence of bacteria in the urine of older adults.
- The "normal" oxygen saturation in older adults may be 95% or greater in the arterial blood.

Critical Thinking Exercises

1. When evaluating the laboratory data for a 74-year-old man, you note that his ESR and serum creatinine are slightly elevated and his serum magnesium is decreased. What conclusion, if any, can be drawn from these findings? Should the data be reported to the physician?
2. You are making home visits to an 81-year-old woman who is recovering from a fractured femur. During your last three visits she has consistently complained of being cold, even though it is summer and her house is very warm. In addition, she has had frequent complaints of constipation, not feeling like eating, and being tired. She has a bottle of hand lotion next to her chair for her dry skin. What is your assessment, and is any action warranted on your part?

References

Adams EB, Meyet FG: Hypochromic anaemia in chronic infections, *South African Med J* 40, 1966.

Ahluwalia N et al: Immune function is impaired in iron deficient homebound, older women, *Am J Clin Nutr* 79(3):516, 2004.

Avorn J et al: Reduction of bacteriuria and pyuria after ingestion of cranberry juice, *JAMA* 271(10):751, 1994.

Baylink DJ, Jennings JC, Mohan S: Calcium and bone homeostasis changes with aging. In Hazzard WR et al, editors: *Principles of geriatric medicine and gerontology*, ed 4, New York, 1999, McGraw-Hill.

Beck LH: Aging changes in renal function. In Hazzard WR et al, editors: *Principles of geriatric medicine and gerontology*, ed 4, New York, 1999, McGraw-Hill.

Beers MH, Berkow R: *The Merck manual of geriatrics*, Rahway, NJ, 2000, Merck.

Berghe C, Wilson A, Ershler WB: Prevalence and outcomes of anemia in geriatrics: a systemic review of the literature, *Am J Med* 116(7):3, 2004.

Burnside IM: *Nursing and the aged*, ed 3, New York, 1988, McGraw-Hill.

Calkins E: Autoimmune rheumatic diseases in the older patient. In Hazzard WR et al, editors: *Principles of geriatric medicine and gerontology*, ed 4, New York, 1999, McGraw-Hill.

Cavalieri TA, Chopra A, Bryman PN: When outside the norm is normal: interpreting lab data in the aged, *Geriatrics* 47:66, 1992.

Chatta GS, Lipschitz DA: Anemia. In Hazzard WR et al, editors: *Principles of geriatric medicine and gerontology*, ed 4, New York, 1999, McGraw-Hill.

Chernecky CC, Berger BJ: *Laboratory tests and diagnostic procedures*, ed 3, Philadelphia, 2001, Saunders.

Connolly MJ: Respiratory diseases. In Tallis RC et al, editors: *Brocklehurst's textbook of geriatric medicine and gerontology*, ed 6, Edinburgh, 2002, Churchill Livingstone.

Cook L: The value of lab values, *Am J Nurs* 99(5):66, 1999.

Davis KM, Minaker KL: Disorders of fluid balance: dehydration and hyponatremia. In Hazzard WR et al, editors: *Principles of geriatric medicine and gerontology*, ed 4, New York, 1999, McGraw-Hill.

Duffield P: Urinary tract infections in the elderly: a common complication of aging, *Adv Nurse Pract* 5:30, 1997.

Expert Committee on the Diagnosis and Classification of Diabetes Mellitus: Report of the Expert Committee on the Diagnosis and Classification of Diabetes Mellitus, *Diabetes Care* 20:7, July 1997.

Ferguson MWJ: Aging and the orofacial tissues. In Tallis RC et al, editors: *Brocklehurst's textbook of geriatric medicine and gerontology*, ed 6, Edinburgh, 2002, Churchill Livingstone.

Freedman ML, Sutin DG: Blood disorders and their management. In Tallis RC et al, editors: *Brocklehurst's textbook of geriatric medicine and gerontology*, ed 6, Edinburgh, 2002, Churchill Livingstone.

Gambino R: C-reactive protein—undervalued, underutilized, *Clin Chem* 43:2017, 1997.

Gaspard KJ: The red blood cell and alterations in oxygen transport. In Porth CM: *Pathophysiology: concepts of altered health states*, ed 6, Philadelphia, 2002, JB Lippincott.

Gilleece MH, Dexter TM: Aging and the blood. In Tallis RC et al, editors: *Brocklehurst's textbook of geriatric medicine and gerontology*, ed 6, Edinburgh, 2002, Churchill Livingstone.

Goroll AH, May LA, Mulley AG: *Primary care medicine*, ed 4, Philadelphia, 2000, JB Lippincott.

Grodner M, Long S, DeYoung S: *Foundations and clinical applications of nutrition: a nursing approach*, St. Louis, 2004, Mosby.

Hahnfield LE, Moon TD: Prostate cancer, *Med Clin North Am* 83(5):1231, 1999.

Hale LP, Owen J: Thrombotic and hemorrhagic disorders in the elderly. In Hazzard WR et al, editors: *Principles of geriatric medicine and gerontology*, ed 4, New York, 1999, McGraw-Hill.

Hall KE, Wiley JW: Aging of the gastrointestinal system. In Hazzard WR et al, editors: *Principles of geriatric medicine and gerontology*, ed 4, New York, 1999, McGraw-Hill.

Halter JB: Diabetes mellitus. In Hazzard WR et al, editors: *Principles of geriatric medicine and gerontology*, ed 4, New York, 1999, McGraw-Hill.

Ham RJ, Sloane PD, Warshaw GA: *Primary care geriatrics*, ed 4, St Louis, 2001, Mosby.

Hassani S, Hershman J: Thyroid diseases. In Hazzard WR et al, editors: *Principles of geriatric medicine and gerontology*, ed 4, New York, 1999, McGraw-Hill.

Hazzard WR: The gender differential in longevity. In Hazzard WR et al, editors: *Principles of geriatric medicine and gerontology*, ed 4, New York, 1999, McGraw-Hill.

Hudson M et al: Implications of elevated cardiac troponin T in ambulatory patients with heart failure: a prospective analysis, *Am Heart J* 147(3), 2004.

Kane RL, Ouslander JG, Abrass IB: *Essentials of clinical geriatrics*, ed 4, New York, 1999, McGraw-Hill.

Letran JL, Brower MK: Disorders of the prostate. In Hazzard WR et al, editors: *Principles of geriatric medicine and gerontology,* ed 4, New York, 1999, McGraw-Hill.

Lindsey C et al: A clinical comparison of calculated version and direct measurement of low density lipoprotein cholesterol level, *Pharmacotherapy* 24(2):167-172, 2004.

Lyles KW: Hyperparathyroidism and Paget's disease of bone. In Hazzard WR et al, editors: *Principles of geriatric medicine and gerontology,* ed 4, New York, 1999, McGraw-Hill.

Maisel AS: The diagnosis of acute congestive failure: role of BNP measurements, *Heart Failure Rev* 8(4):327-334, 2003.

Manning EM, Shenkin A: Nutritional assessment in the critically ill, *Crit Care Clin* 11(3):603, 1995.

McCance KL, Huether SE: *Pathophysiology: the biologic basis for disease in adults and children,* ed 4, St Louis, 2001, Mosby.

Morrison LK et al: Utility of a rapid B-natriuretic peptide assay in differentiating congestive heart failure from lung disease in patients presenting with dyspnea, *J Am Coll Cardiol* 39(2):202-209, 2002.

Mouton CP et al: Common infections in older adults, *Am Fam Phys* 63(2), 2001.

Ogburn-Russell L, Johnson JE: Oxygen saturation levels in the well elderly: altitude makes a difference, *J Gerontol Nurs* 16:10, 1990.

Oltrona L et al: C-reactive protein elevation and early outcome in patients with unstable angina pectoris, *Am J Cardiol* 80:1002, 1997.

O'Neill PA: Venous thrombotic disease and varicose ulcers: In Tallis RC et al, editors: *Brocklehurst's textbook of geriatric medicine and gerontology,* ed 6, Edinburgh, 2002, Churchill Livingstone.

Ott S: Osteomalacia and osteoporosis. In Hazzard WR et al, editors: *Principles of geriatric medicine and gerontology,* ed 4, New York, 1999, McGraw-Hill.

Pagana KD, Pagana TJ: *Manual of diagnostic and laboratory tests,* ed 2, St Louis, 2004, Mosby.

Pagana KD, Pagana TJ: *Mosby's diagnostic and lab test reference,* ed 6, St Louis, 2003, Mosby.

Prahash A, Lynch T: B-type natriuretic peptide: a diagnostic, prognostic, and therapeutic tool in heart failure, *Am J Crit Care* 13(1):46, 2004.

Rajagopalan S, Yoshikawa T: Tuberculosis. In Hazzard WR et al, editors: *Principles of geriatric medicine and gerontology,* ed 4, New York, 1999, McGraw-Hill.

Reuben DB et al: Correlates of hypoalbuminemia in community-dwelling older persons, *Am J Clin Nutr* 66:1, 1997.

Riehmann M: Urinary tract infections in the elderly, *Clin Geriatr* 6:16, 1998.

Rothstein G: White cell disorders. In Hazzard WR et al, editors: *Principles of geriatric medicine and gerontology,* ed 4, New York, 1999, McGraw-Hill.

Sands JM, Vega SR: Renal disease. In Hazzard WR et al, editors: *Principles of geriatric medicine and gerontology,* ed 4, New York, 1999, McGraw-Hill.

Sarkozi L: Biochemical tests. In Tallis RC et al, editors: *Brocklehurst's textbook of geriatric medicine and gerontology,* ed 6, Edinburgh, 2002, Churchill Livingstone.

Siomko AJ: Demystifying cardiac markers, *Am J Nurs* 100(1):36, 2000.

Smith RP et al: C-reactive protein: a clinical marker in community-acquired pneumonia, *Chest* 108:1288, 1995.

SmithKline Beecham: *SmithKline Beecham Laboratories update,* Chicago, July 1998.

Thibodeau GA, Patton KT: *Structure and function of the body,* ed 12, St Louis, 2003, Mosby.

Travis SS, Lampley-Dallas VT: Nursing management of elderly patients with asymptomatic bacteriuria, *Geratr Nurs* 18(3):103-106, 1997.

Yoshikawa TT, Nicholle LE, Norman DC: Management of complicated urinary tract infection in older patients, *J Am Geriatr Soc* 44:1235, 1996.

22 Pharmacologic Management

CHRISTOPHER BENJAMIN, MSN, RN, FNP,
and KATHLEEN FLETCHER, MSN, RN, APRN-BC, GNP, FAAN

Learning Objectives

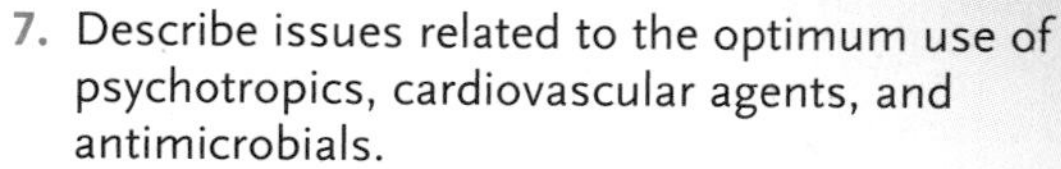

On completion of this chapter, the reader will be able to:

1. Describe the characteristics of medication use in older adults.
2. List medications that are best avoided in older adults.
3. Identify potential risk factors for adverse drug reactions.
4. Describe the pharmacokinetic and pharmacodynamic changes associated with aging and the implications for drug therapy.
5. Recognize significant drug-drug, drug-food, and drug-disease interactions, giving specific examples of each.
6. State the impact that drugs may have on an older adult's quality of life.
7. Describe issues related to the optimum use of psychotropics, cardiovascular agents, and antimicrobials.
8. Anticipate the effects of increased availability of nonprescription and herbal remedies on client self-management.
9. Identify risk factors for noncompliance, and suggest strategies to improve compliance.
10. Describe the general principles of prescribing for older clients and the systemwide approaches to improving medication use.

Medicating the older adults is both a blessing and a curse. Drugs are powerful tools designed to improve the consumer's health, yet all too often they cause or contribute to premature frailty. The prescription of multiple concurrent medications in older clients is often necessary to effectively manage multiple chronic conditions, which become more common with age. Minimizing adverse drug effects while achieving the cure or optimum management of a chronic illness requires a unique knowledge of drug responses in older adults.

The knowledge deficit in this arena is reflected in the fact that inappropriate prescribing for older adults is alarmingly high. Recent prevalence studies estimate that it is 20% among community-dwelling older adults and a stunning 40% among nursing home residents (Liu and Christensen, 2002). Further evidence demonstrates that 40% of all serious adverse drug events that occur in the older adults are preventable (Gurwitz et al, 2003).

This chapter provides insights for those who prescribe, administer, or consume drugs into the principles and practices of medication use in older adults. The nurse's role in assessing and analyzing the client's medication regimen and determining the relative risk for an adverse drug event is emphasized.

A special thanks for foundational work done by June Felice Johnson.

OVERVIEW OF MEDICATION USE AND PROBLEMS

Demographics of Medication Use

The pharmaceutic needs of the aging population are significant. Persons 65 and older are prescribed the highest proportion of medication in relation to their percentage in the population. Currently elders make up 13% of the population yet consume 30% of all prescribed and nonprescribed medications (Novelli, 2003).

Drugs remain the mainstay of treatment for existing acute and chronic disease and additionally are often used to prevent disease in those determined to be at risk. Consequently, older adults, being most vulnerable to disease, use more drugs than any other age-group. In the United States, of individuals over age 65, 90% use at least one medication per week, 40% use five or more medications per week, and 12% use 10 or more different medications per week (Kaufman et al, 2002).

Frail older clients use the most drugs, with drug use in hospitals and nursing homes being more common than that in the community. The types of medications used by older adults also vary with the setting. Community-dwelling older adults use analgesic, diuretic, cardiovascular, and sedative-hypnotic drugs most often, whereas nursing home residents use antipsychotics and sedative-hypnotics most often, followed by diuretics, antihypertensives, analgesics, cardiovascular drugs, and antibiotics (Abrams and Berkow, 2000).

This disproportionate medication burden places the older population at high risk for adverse medication events (see Research box). Inappropriate prescribing, although it is considered a dominant reason, is not the only influence on medication errors in older adults. The following section illustrates the broader context of the problem.

Medication Error: Human and Economic Burdens

An error, as defined by the Institute of Medicine (IOM, 1999), is the failure of a planned action to be completed as intended or the use of a wrong plan to achieve a desired outcome. Medication errors may be related to prescribing, dispensing, administering, or monitoring a drug. Root causes of medication-related errors have been attributed to human knowledge–based deficiencies and a lack of sophisticated systems to support prescribing and monitoring drug therapy (Gurwitz et al, 2003; Leape et al, 1995; Lesar, Lomaestro, and Pohl, 1997). The types of error might include omitting a drug that was ordered; administering a drug to the wrong patient, in the wrong drug strength, or at the wrong time, route, or dosage form; using the wrong technique; giving it at the wrong rate of infusion or duration; committing a monitoring error (allergy, drug-drug interaction, drug-food interaction, drug-disease interaction); or administering an expired drug.

Two important distinctions in medication error language include the adverse drug reaction (ADR) and the adverse drug event (ADE). The ADR is any unintended response to a drug that occurs when drugs are used to diagnose, treat, or prevent disease. These include predictable events (drug inherent property) and unpredictable events (idiosyncratic reaction). An ADE is any injury that results when medications are used, and this includes both ADRs and medication errors that lead to an ADR.

The human and economic burden associated with medication errors is staggering. One third of all hospital admissions in older patients have been linked to drug-related problems, many of which are drug-drug interactions that could have been avoided (Juurlink et al, 2003). In addition, medication-related problems that occur in the combined ambulatory, hospital, and nursing home settings come with a $200 billion dollars of additional health care expenditures (Juurlink et al, 2003).

Health care providers working with older clients, as well as the older clients themselves and their caregivers, make daily decisions about what constitutes appropriate drug therapy. Multiple medications and complex drug schedules may be justified in some circumstances. The use of too many or the wrong types of medications increases the risk of both an ADE and nonadherence.

Polypharmacy is a major concern in geriatric care, with the risk of an adverse drug event increasing incrementally with the number of drugs consumed. Certain drugs are considered riskier than others. The most common medication categories associated with preventable ADRs in ambulatory elders were cardiovascular drugs, diuretics, nonopiod analgesics, hypoglycemics, and anticoagulants (Gurwitz et al, 2003). The most common ADRs that resulted in hospitalizations of nursing home residents included the nonsteroidal antiinflammatory drugs (NSAIDs), psychotropics, digoxin (Lanoxin), and insulin (Cooper, 1999). Recommendations include targeting the high-risk older population—including individuals who have multiple conditions and take multiple medications—to reduce the risk of an adverse drug event (Field et al, 2004).

Problems with medication use in the nursing facility have prompted federal legislation—the Nursing Home Reform Amendments of the Omnibus Budget Reconciliation Act of 1987 (OBRA). These amendments affected pharmacy practice in nursing facilities by providing guidelines for the use of specific drug categories and by requiring implementation of

Research

SAMPLE/SETTING

The sample consisted of data in the National Ambulatory Medical Care Survey and the National Hospital Ambulatory Medical Care Survey on elderly persons' office-based or outpatient visits from 1995 to 2000.

METHODS

Trends in the prevalence of potentially inappropriate drug prescribing at ambulatory care visits were examined. Explicit criteria were used to identify potentially inappropriate prescribing. Multivariate regression was used to identify related factors.

FINDINGS

During the defined interval at least one drug considered inappropriate by the Beers expert panel was prescribed at 7.8% of ambulatory care visits by elderly patients. At least one drug classified as never or rarely appropriate by the Zhan expert panel was prescribed at 3.7% of these visits. Pain relievers and central nervous system acting drugs were the main offenders. The odds of potentially inappropriate prescribing were highest for women and those taking multiple drugs.

IMPLICATIONS

Potentially inappropriate prescribing at ambulatory care visits by elderly patients is a substantial problem. Interventions targeting more appropriate drug selection and administration, particularly with pain relievers, anxiolytics, sedatives, and antidepressants, are indicated.

Goulding MR: Inappropriate medication prescribing for elderly ambulatory care patients, *Arch Intern Med* 164:305, 2004.

pharmacist recommendations during drug regimen reviews. Federal guidelines outlining accepted indications and dosing of antipsychotics were implemented in October 1990. Similar guidelines for anxiolytics and sedatives were established in 1992 (Avorn and Gurwitz, 1995). More recently the Center for Medicare and Medicaid Services (CMS) developed surveyor guidelines for potentially inappropriate medications in long-term care residents based on the Beers's criteria (Beers, 1997).

The Beers list of inappropriate drugs to give to older adults was first developed by six experts and examined in the nursing home population using explicit criteria. The results of this initial study revealed that nearly half of the nursing home residents (40.3%) received at least one inappropriate drug, 10.4% had two or more inappropriate drugs, and 1.3% had three or more inappropriate drugs prescribed (Beers et al, 1992). An updated Beers list was developed for all older patients (Beers, 1997). Further refinements were made when Zahn categorized the 1997 Beers list of drugs as drugs that should always be avoided, were rarely appropriate, or had some indications for use in older patients but were often misused. Zahn and colleagues applied the Beers list to ambulatory older adults and found that 2.6% of those ages 65 and older took a drug that should never be used in this age-group, 9.1% used drugs judged to be rarely appropriate, and 13.3% were using drugs with minimum benefit that should generally be avoided in older adults (Zahn et al, 2001). Table 22-1 reflects modifications of the Beers list and includes drugs that should be avoided by older adults and justification for nonselection. It is important to keep in mind that there may be times where these drugs might be given, but they are never first-line therapy; if the choice is made, the specific indication should be explicit in the patient's record, and the patient should be monitored carefully for a potential adverse effect, with documentation reflecting the patient's response to therapy. In summary, then, the Beers list is a helpful general guide regarding potentially inappropriate medications for older adults, but it must be used in conjunction with a patient-centered care process. Ultimately decisions about medication prescribing must be clinically based and consider the patient's total clinical picture.

Data on the overuse or inappropriate choice of a medication are relatively easy to collect, document, and report. However, health care providers must also recognize clients who experience an adverse medical outcome in cases where they are *not* prescribed a medication that may be needed to enhance quality of life or prevent disease. Underuse of indicated therapy is a medication error as well.

Daily low-dose (81 to 325 mg) aspirin has been demonstrated to reduce long-term mortality in post–myocardial infarction (MI) clients. Yet only 76% of older adults surveyed in four states who had no contraindications to aspirin were prescribed aspirin on hospital discharge after an MI (Krumholz et al, 1996). The American Diabetes Association (ADA) recommends low-dose aspirin in clients with diabetes for secondary prevention of heart disease if they have large-vessel disease and for primary prevention in clients who are cigarette smokers or who have hypertension, obesity, albuminuria, hyperlipidemia, or a positive family history of coronary heart disease (ADA, 1998). Unfortunately, this therapy is often omitted from the medication regimen of older diabetic clients.

Although cardiovascular disease remains the leading cause of death for older persons, after MI use of beta-blockers is less likely in the elderly (Krumholz, 1998), less aggressive treatment of systolic hypertension has been reflected (Williams, 2002), and older clients with atrial fibrillation appear to have the lowest rate of anticoagulation (Gage et al, 2000). Lipid lowering with statin therapy has been demonstrated to be cost-effective in those ages 75 and older (Prosser et al, 2000), yet the statins continue to be underused in this age-group.

Pain continues to be undertreated, as evidenced by a study of older adult nursing facility cancer patients in five states. The study found that as many as 38% of patients continued to experience daily pain, and 26% of patients received no analgesic agent at all (Bernabei et al, 1998).

A final example of the underuse of preventive treatment relates to vaccinations. Only 52% of those ages 65 and older received an annual influenza vaccination, and only 28% had ever received a pneumococcal vaccine (Sisk et al, 1997). These figures are in stark contrast to the recommendations of the Advisory Committee on Immunization Practices of the Centers for Disease Control and Prevention (CDC, 1997).

Clearly there are knowledge, system, and policy-related barriers to reducing ADEs and improving therapeutic outcomes. Fragmentation of the health care system increases the likelihood that older adults may not have their care coordinated by a single health care professional. Obtaining and maintaining a complete and current medication profile is complicated by several factors, including multiple prescribers for any one patient; self-medication with over-the-counter, herbal, and nutritional products; and pharmacy shopping for the best price, drug availability, or convenience. In addition, medication expense is often a major deterrent to compliance in older clients. Generic equivalents may not be available for recently marketed medications. It is not unusual for clients taking multiple cardiac medications along with a proton pump inhibitor such as omeprazole (Prilosec) or a new NSAID to be faced with a monthly prescription cost of $200 or more if they do not carry prescription coverage. Overcoming these barriers requires the efforts of all health care providers, as well as policy makers and health care system administrators.

Changes in Drug Response With Aging

In addition to medication errors, other factors that contribute to the increased risk of adverse drug events in older adults include altered pharmacokinetics and pharmacodynamics

TABLE 22-1 Inappropriate Medications for Older Adults—Beers List*

APPLICABLE MEDICATIONS†	PRESCRIBING CONCERNS	SEVERITY RATING
Propoxyphene (Darvon); combination products (Darvon with ASA, Darvon-N, Darvocet-N)	Generally avoid in older adults. Offers few analgesic advantages over acetaminophen, yet has side effects of other narcotic drugs.	Low
Indomethacin (Indocin, Indocin SR)	Of all available NSAIDs, produces the most CNS side effects. Avoid in older adults.	High
Pentazocine (Talwin)	A narcotic analgesic that causes CNS side effects, including confusion and hallucinations, more commonly than other narcotic drugs. Additionally, it is a mixed agonist and antagonist. Avoid in older adults.	High
Trimethobenzamide (Tigan)	One of the least effective antiemetic drugs, yet can cause extrapyramidal side effects. When possible, avoid in older adults.	High
Muscle relaxants and antispasmodics: methocarbamol (Robaxin); carisoprodol (Soma), chlorzoxazone (Paraflex); metaxalone (Skelaxin); cyclobenzaprine (Flexeril); oxybutynin (Ditropan). Do not consider extended release Ditropan.	Most are poorly tolerated by older adults, leading to anticholinergic side effects, sedation, and weakness. Questionable effectiveness at doses tolerated by older adults. Although beneficial in some circumstances, whenever possible avoid in older adults.	High
Flurazepam (Dalmane)	Extremely long half-life in older adults (often days), producing prolonged sedation and increasing incidence of falls and fractures. Medium- or short-acting benzodiazepines preferred.	High
Amitriptyline (Elavil); chlordiazepoxide-amitriptyline (Limbitrol); perphenazine-amitriptyline (Triavil)	Strong anticholinergic and sedating properties, so rarely antidepressant of choice for older adults.	High
Doxepin (Sinequan)	Strong anticholinergic and sedating properties, so rarely antidepressant of choice for older adults.	High
Meprobamate (Miltown, Equanil)	Highly addictive and sedating anxiolytic to be avoided in older clients. Prolonged usage may lead to addiction and necessitate slow withdrawal.	High
Doses of short-acting benzodiazepines: lorazepam (Ativan), 3 mg; oxazepam (Serax), 60 mg; alprazolam (Xanax), 2 mg; temazepam (Restoril), 15 mg; zolpidem (Ambien), 5 mg; triazolam (Halcion), 0.25 mg	With increased sensitivity to benzodiazepines in older adults, smaller doses effective and safer. Total daily doses should rarely exceed suggested maximums.	High
Long-acting benzodiazepines: chlordiazepoxide (Librium); chlordiazepoxide-amitriptyline (Limbitrol); clidinium-chlordiazepoxide (Librax); diazepam (Valium); quazepam (Doral); halazepam (Paxipam); chlorazepate (Tranxene)	Long half-life in older adults (often several days), producing prolonged sedation and increasing risk of falls and fractures. Short- and intermediate-acting benzodiazepines preferred if a benzodiazepine is required.	High
Disopyramide (Norpace, Norpace CR)	Of all antiarrhythmic drugs, the most potent negative inotrope and therefore may induce heart failure in older adults. Also strongly anticholinergic. When appropriate, use other antiarrhythmic drugs.	High
Digoxin (Lanoxin)	Decreased renal clearance, so doses in older adults should rarely exceed 0.125 mg/day.	Low
Short-acting dipyridamole (Persantine). Do not consider long-acting dipyridamole (which has better properties than the short acting in older adults) except for patients with artificial heart valves.	May cause orthostatic hypotension in older adults. Has been proven beneficial only in clients with artificial heart valves. Whenever possible, avoid use in older adults.	Low
Methyldopa (Aldomet); methyldopa and hydrochlorothiazide (Aldoril)	May cause bradycardia and exacerbate depression in older adults. Alternate treatments for hypertension generally preferred.	High

TABLE 22-1 Inappropriate Medications for Older Adults—Beers List*—cont'd

APPLICABLE MEDICATIONS†	PRESCRIBING CONCERNS	SEVERITY RATING
Reserpine at doses >0.25 mg	Imposes unnecessary risk in older adults, inducing depression, impotence, sedation, and orthostatic hypotension. Safer alternatives preferred.	Low
Chlorpropamide (Diabinese)	Prolonged half-life in older adults and can cause prolonged and serious hypoglycemia. Additionally, the only oral hypoglycemic agent that causes SIADH. Avoid in older adults.	High
GI antispasmodic drugs: dicyclomine (Bentyl); hyoscyamine (Levsin, Levsinex); propantheline (Pro-Banthine); belladonna alkaloids (Donnatal and others); clidinium-chlordiazepoxide (Librax)	Highly anticholinergic and generally produce substantial toxic effects in older adults. Questionable effectiveness at doses tolerated by older adults. Best avoided in older adults, especially for long-term use.	High
All nonprescription and many prescription antihistamines, such as single and combination preparations containing chlorpheniramine (Chlor-Trimeton); diphenhydramine (Benadryl); hydroxyzine (Vistaril, Atarax); cyproheptadine (Periactin); promethazine (Phenergan); tripelennamine; dexchlorpheniramine (Polaramine)	Potent anticholinergic properties. Cough and cold preparations without antihistamines are safer substitutes in older adults.	High
Diphenhydramine (Benadryl)	Potently anticholinergic and usually should not be used as hypnotic in older adults. When used to treat or prevent allergic reactions, use in smallest possible dose and with great caution.	High
Ergot mesyloids (Hydergine); cerebral vasodilators; cyclospasmol	Not shown to be effective, in doses studied, for treatment of dementia or any other condition.	Low
Iron supplements >325 mg	Rarely need doses exceeding 325 mg of ferrous sulfate daily. With higher doses, total absorption not substantially increased, but constipation more likely.	Low
All barbiturates (except phenobarbital) except when used to control seizures	More side effects than most other sedative or hypnotic drugs in older adults. Highly addictive. Should not be started as new therapy in older adults except when used to control seizures.	High
Meperidine (Demerol)	Not an effective oral analgesic in doses commonly used. May cause confusion and has many disadvantages compared with other narcotic drugs. Avoid in older adults.	High
Ticlopidine (Ticlid)	Has been shown to be no better than aspirin in preventing clotting and is considerably more toxic. Avoid in older adults.	High
Ketorolac (Toradol)	Avoid immediate and long-term use in older persons, since many have asymptomatic GI pathologic conditions.	High
Amphetamines and anorexic agents	May cause dependence, hypertension, angina, and myocardial infarction.	High
Long-term use of full dosage, longer half-life, non-COX-selective NSAIDs: naproxen (Naprosyn, Anaprox, and Aleve); oxaprozin (Daypro); piroxicam (Feldene)	May produce GI bleeding, renal failure, high blood pressure, and heart failure.	High
Daily fluoxetine (Prozac)	Long half-life and risk of producing excessive CNS stimulation, sleep disturbances, and increasing agitation.	High
Long-term use of stimulant laxatives: cascara sagrada, bisacodyl (Dulcolax); Neoloid except in the presence of opiate analgesic use	May exacerbate bowel dysfunction.	High
Amiodarone (Cordarone)	Associated with QT interval problems, presents risk of provoking torsades de pointes, and lacks efficacy in older adults.	High

Continued

TABLE 22-1 Inappropriate Medications for Older Adults—Beers List*—cont'd

APPLICABLE MEDICATIONS†	PRESCRIBING CONCERNS	SEVERITY RATING
Orphenadrine (Norflex)	Causes more sedation and anticholinergic adverse effects than safer alternatives.	High
Guanethidine (Ismelin)	May cause orthostatic hypotension.	High
Guanadrel (Hylorel)	May cause orthostatic hypotension.	High
Cyclandelate (Cyclospasmol)	Lack of efficacy.	Low
Isoxsuprine (Vasodilan)	Lack of efficacy.	Low
Nitrofurantoin (Macrodantin)	Potential for renal impairment.	High
Doxazosin (Cardura)	Potential for dry mouth, hypotension, and urinary problems.	Low
Methyltestosterone (Android, Virilon, Testred)	Potential for prostatic hypertrophy and cardiac problems.	High
Thioridazine (Mellaril)	Greater potential for CNS and extrapyramidal adverse effects.	High
Mesoridazine (Serentil)	CNS and extrapyramidal adverse effects.	High
Short-acting nifedipine (Procardia, Adalat)	Potential for hypotension and constipation.	High
Clonidine (Catapres)	Potential for orthostatic hypotension and CNS adverse effects.	Low
Mineral oil	Potential for aspiration and adverse effects. Safer alternatives available.	High
Cimetidine (Tagamet)	CNS adverse effects, including confusion.	Low
Ethacrynic acid (Edecrin)	Potential for hypertension and fluid imbalances. Safer alternatives available.	Low
Desiccated thyroid	Concerns about cardiac effects. Safer alternatives available.	High
Amphetamines (excluding methylphenidate hydrochloride and anorexics)	CNS stimulant adverse effects.	High
Estrogens only (oral)	Evidence of carcinogenic potential (breast and endometrial cancer) and lack of cardioprotective effect in older women.	Low

Modified from Beers MH: Explicit criteria for determining potentially inappropriate medication use by the elderly, *Arch Intern Med* 157:1531, 1997; Fick MF et al: Updating the Beers criteria for potentially inappropriate medication use in older adults, *Arch Intern Med* 163:2716, 2003.

SIADH, Syndrome of inappropriate antidiuretic hormone; *COX*, cyclooxygenase; *NSAIDs*, nonsteroidal antiinflammatory drugs; *CNS*, central nervous system; *GI*, gastrointestinal.

*Most package circulars produced by drug manufacturers do not include language identical to the statements presented herein. Although adverse effects that these drugs can produce are generally listed in the package circulars, these as well as warnings and contraindications must be approved by regulatory agencies and in general are not based on consensus or surveys.

†Dose limits are total daily dose.

and medication adherence problems. Physical aging changes occur over time that influence the dynamic process that drugs undergo to produce therapeutic effects. These changes involve the process of pharmacokinetics (what the body does to the drug) and pharmacodynamics (what the drug does to the body). These processes are described in the following section.

Pharmacokinetic Changes: What the Body Does to the Drug

An altered and sometimes unexpected drug response in older clients may be related to different pharmacokinetics with aging—that is, changes in drug absorption, drug distribution or protein binding, hepatic metabolism, and renal excretion. These changes can be reflected in serum drug levels. If these pharmacokinetic changes result in excessive serum concentrations at doses similar to those used in younger persons, a greater response with attendant increase in drug toxicity may be experienced unless adjustments are made in drug dosage or interval. The *degree* of change may vary greatly among older adult clients (i.e., among the young-old [65 to 74 years old] versus the oldest-old [greater than 85 years old], or among healthy older adults versus those with multiple chronic illnesses or multiorgan failure). Other influences on drug disposition include interacting medications; nutritional status; intake of caffeine, tobacco, and alcohol; and exposure to environmental substances. These variables must be kept in mind when extrapolating study results to a specific population of older adults. Table 22-2 summarizes and gives examples of age-related changes in pharmacokinetics (Hammerlein, Derendorf, and Lowenthal, 1998).

Age-related changes in drug absorption do not usually contribute to a significantly altered drug response and are generally thought to have a less significant impact on pharmacokinetics than does drug distribution, metabolism, or excretion. There is a particular need, however, for studies

TABLE 22-2 Age-Related Changes in Pharmacokinetics

VARIABLE	CHANGE	EXAMPLE
ABSORPTION		
Gastric pH	Increased	Calcium carbonate: decreased dissolution
Acid secretory capacity	Decreased	Calcium carbonate: decreased dissolution
GI blood flow or gastric motility	Diminished	Analgesics: delayed onset of effect Naproxen, salicylates: increased free concentration
DISTRIBUTION		
Plasma albumin	Diminished	Meperidine: increased free concentration caused by decreased binding to red blood cells
Protein affinity	Diminished	Propranolol: reduced unbound fraction
Alpha-1-acid glycoprotein	Increased	Psychotropics: increased distribution into fat; potential accumulation
Body fat	Increased	Long-acting benzodiazepines, tricyclic antidepressants, beta-blockers, narcotic analgesics: higher concentrations from decreased metabolism
METABOLISM		
Size of liver	Decreased	Long-acting benzodiazepines, tricyclic antidepressants, beta-blockers, narcotic analgesics: higher concentrations from decreased metabolism
Hepatic blood flow	Decreased	Long-acting benzodiazepines, tricyclic antidepressants, beta-blockers, narcotic analgesics: higher concentrations from decreased metabolism
RENAL FUNCTION		
Glomerular filtration rate	Decreased	Allopurinol, cephalosporins, chlorpropamide, ciprofloxacin, digoxin, H_2-receptor blockers: higher concentrations due to reduced renal clearance
Renal plasma flow	Decreased	Allopurinol, cephalosporins, chlorpropamide, ciprofloxacin, digoxin, H_2-receptor blockers: higher concentrations due to reduced renal clearance

From Hammerlein A, Derendorf H, Lowenthal DT: Pharmacokinetic and pharmacodynamic changes in the elderly: clinical implications, *Clin Pharmacokinet* 35(1):49, 1998.

examining the influences of age on absorption of medications given by various routes of administration such as rectal, pulmonary, intramuscular, or dermal routes. Additional factors that influence absorption of drugs include the presence of pain, the concurrent use of anticholinergic medications, and coexisting metabolic disease such as thyroid disease or diabetes. Still another consideration is whether the medication actually passes through the esophagus so that it can be properly absorbed. The older adult who does not take (or is not given) adequate fluids with the drug has an increased risk for esophageal damage from dissolution of drugs in this area. Drugs that are particularly caustic to the esophagus include alendronate, quinidine, potassium, and tetracycline.

Drug distribution into the peripheral circulation and tissues is altered as a function of age. A decrease in plasma albumin levels with age may result in decreased binding of drugs that are mainly bound to serum albumin. Since it is the unbound fraction of a drug that is available to create the desired pharmacologic effect or toxicity, an increase of unbound drug with age (resulting from decreased serum albumin binding) may result in exaggerated pharmacologic effects or side effects. Along with aging itself, disease states, gender, coadministration of other drugs, acute illness, and nutritional status may influence serum protein binding. Cultural differences may also be a factor (see Cultural Awareness box).

Changes in body composition, which differ between men and women, may influence drug distribution. A decrease in total body water and intracellular water volumes may lead to an increased serum concentration of water-soluble drugs such as lithium or alcohol. An increase in body fat may increase the distribution of fat-soluble medications such as benzodiazepines into fatty tissue, resulting in prolonged half-lives and drug accumulation. A decrease in lean body mass may cause an increased serum concentration of drugs such as digoxin, warfarin (Coumadin), or meperidine. Distribution changes are significant in the patient who is malnourished and dehydrated.

Drug distribution also relies on the bioavailability of the drug. The amount of the drug that reaches the systemic circulation may be increased or decreased depending on certain factors such as the route of administration (inhalants are typically the fastest); the solubility of the drug (aqueous solutions are available more quickly than oily ones); and general circulation to the site of drug administration (blood flow increases with heat, massage, or the presence of an occlusive dressing).

Age-related changes in hepatic drug metabolism are not easily measured. Biotransformation occurs in all body tissues but primarily in the liver, where enzymatic activity (cytochrome system) alters and detoxifies the drug to prepare it for excretion. Although a reduction in liver size and hepatic blood flow has been observed with age, results of liver function tests are

CULTURAL AWARENESS

ETHNOPHARMACOLOGY

Metabolic, Genetic, and Environmental Factors

Numerous researchers have identified cultural differences in drug response and metabolism. The majority of studies providing evidence for transcultural differences in the pharmacokinetic and pharmacodynamic properties of various drugs have compared individuals of Asian, black, Hispanic, and Native-American descent to whites.

Differences in pharmacokinetics may be genetic or a result of environmental influences.

Misdiagnosis or Underdiagnosis

Individuals of different culture may have different degrees of access to health care resources. Health disparities clearly exist. Consequently underdiagnosis and misdiagnosis may occur, and undertreatment or inappropriate drug treatment may be the result.

Culture and Level of Medication Adherence

Cultural influences may account for a significant degree of "nonadherence." Members of some cultural groups may perceive that medication should have a short-term effect and are not culturally conditioned to continue medication that does not produce an immediate response.

A less empirical but real consideration is the client's confidence and trust in the health care provider. For example, based on a combination of historic fact and myth, some Hispanic clients do not have confidence or trust in white health care providers. Other cultural considerations such as traditional beliefs and practices; advice of traditional, folk, or indigenous healers; and religious beliefs undoubtedly influence adherence with drug regimens prescribed by health care professionals.

not useful in predicting the extent of changes in metabolism. In addition, hepatic drug metabolism is influenced by a host of variables, including concurrent disease states; gender; genetic determinants; nutritional status; lifelong environmental exposure to various chemicals; activity levels; and caffeine, tobacco, and alcohol intake.

It has been observed that drugs which undergo phase I metabolism (oxidation or reduction to more polar compounds), such as long-acting benzodiazepines (like diazepam) or tricyclic antidepressants, are more likely to have a reduced hepatic clearance and an increased half-life in older clients. On the other hand, those drugs undergoing phase II metabolism (conjugation to a more water-soluble molecule), such as acetaminophen or short-acting benzodiazepines like lorazepam or oxazepam, are more likely to be cleared by older clients in a manner similar to younger clients and may not need a dose adjustment (Hammerlein, Derendorf, and Lowenthal, 1998). Decreased blood flow to the liver may slow the metabolism of drugs such as lidocaine, propranolol, and meperidine. It is also important to consider the potential for drug interactions. Unfortunately, since the net effects of hepatic drug metabolism are impossible to predict accurately, nurses must rely on their assessment of pharmacologic or toxicologic effects in a given client. Screening the prescription orders to ensure that the lowest effective dose is being prescribed and alerting the prescriber if problems are suspected will reduce the chance of a future ADE.

The most important pharmacokinetic parameter that changes with age is the renal excretion of drugs, which may result in significant decreases in renal elimination for drugs primarily eliminated by the renal route. Although the change in renal function is extremely variable, the majority of older adults, especially those with hypertension, diabetes, and multiple medical problems, have a decline in kidney function. This may require a decreased dose or extension of the dosing interval for certain drugs.

Serum creatinine may be used as an indirect estimate of renal function by calculating creatinine clearance:

$$\text{Creatinine clearance (ml/min)} = \frac{140 - \text{Age (in years)} \times \text{Weight (in kg)}}{72 \times \text{Serum creatinine (mg/dl)}}$$

(For women, multiply final result by 0.85.)

Creatinine clearance is an estimate of glomerular filtration rate (GFR) and decreases with age. Even if an older adult has a serum creatinine value that is "within normal limits" by laboratory standards, this does *not* mean that creatinine clearance is normal. This is because of decreased muscle mass and muscle metabolism, which is normally responsible for decomposition of creatine to creatinine. For example, an 80-year-old woman who weighs 50 kg and has an apparently normal serum creatinine of 1 mg/dl has a calculated creatinine clearance of 35 ml/min, a dramatic reduction from the normal range of 70 to 120 ml/min. Examples of drugs that would need downward dose adjustments because of reduced renal function include allopurinol, digoxin, many cephalosporins, ciprofloxacin, and histamine receptor antagonists (e.g., cimetidine [Tagamet], ranitidine, famotidine).

Pharmacodynamic Changes: What the Drug Does to the Body

Much less information is available on age-related pharmacodynamic changes because of the difficulty in measuring the time course and effect of drugs on the cellular and organ function. Aging may result in different responses for older adults to the same drug concentrations at the site of action compared with those observed in younger adults. For example, an older person may have an exaggerated depressant response to central nervous system depressants, even when serum concentrations are similar to those of a younger person. The clinical implications for anticipating this response are important when benzodiazepines are used, and downward dose adjustments are made to prevent excessive sedation. These changes may be due to altered receptor number or affinity, altered cellular responses, organ pathologic condition, or altered homeostatic mechanisms (Abrams and Berkow, 2000). Box 22-1 reviews age-related changes in physiology that can result in altered drug response.

Drug Interactions

The altered pharmacokinetics and pharmacodynamics associated with aging must always be considered when reviewing medication therapy. In addition, the potential for drug interactions (drug-drug, drug-food, and drug-disease) must be explored.

Drug-Drug Interactions

An interaction between one drug and another can result from altered pharmacokinetics or pharmacodynamics. It is now largely thought that alterations in hepatic metabolism are specifically responsible for drug-drug interactions. Biotransformation of drugs is catalyzed by a variety of liver enzymes, the most common being the cytochrome P-450 system. A new field of pharmacogenetics is emerging as researchers are studying each of the 400 genes in an individual that produce these enzymes, which determine how any one individual will metabolize drugs. This new information is expected to result in individually tailored drug therapy. Drug interactions are commonly encountered in older clients as a result of polypharmacy. However, even taking two medications concurrently can result in a drug-drug interaction if the inhibition or induction of drug metabolism is influenced by the combination. Drugs may have opposing or antagonistic actions, may have similar actions, or may have a similar side effect profile. These interactions are often considered great “masqueraders,” because they may be mistaken for drug toxicity, an increase in disease severity, suboptimum treatment, or an apparently unrelated event. The consequences of an unrecognized drug interaction include client injury, additional office or emergency department visits, unnecessary invasive testing, weakening of the client-prescriber relationship, and inappropriate medication or dose changes. Table 22-3 lists examples of significant drug-drug interactions.

BOX 22-1 Age-Related Changes in Physiology That Impact With Kinetic Changes on Pharmacodynamic Responses

ALTERATIONS IN BODY COMPOSITION	
Body fat	Increased
Lean body mass	Decreased
Total body water	Decreased
CHANGES IN CARDIOVASCULAR FUNCTION	
Resting heart rate	Decreased
Stroke volume	Slightly decreased
Cardiac output	Slightly decreased
CENTRAL NERVOUS SYSTEM FUNCTION	
Blood supply to the brain	Diminished
REFLEX RESPONSES	
Baroreceptor reflex activity	Diminished
RENIN-ANGIOTENSIN-ALDOSTERONE SYSTEM	
Plasma renin	Diminished
Urine aldosterone	Diminished
Sympathetic innervation to juxtaglomerular cells	Diminished

From Hammerlein A, Derendorf H, Lowenthal DT: Pharmacokinetic and pharmacodynamic changes in the elderly: clinical implications, *Clin Pharmacokinet* 35(1):49, 1998.

Drug-Food Interactions

The effect of a drug or food can be influenced by their combined actions. This is a relatively new area of study with only limited evidence-based research. Table 22-4 lists examples of drug-food interactions.

Drug-Disease Interactions

Certain disease states may be exacerbated by specific drug therapies, and these drugs may be contraindicated in patients with a coexisting underlying disease. The significance of these potential interactions is unclear at this time. Table 22-5 lists examples of drug-disease interactions.

TABLE 22-3 Common Drug-Drug Interactions in Older Adults

DRUG-DRUG COMBINATION	POTENTIAL EFFECT
Warfarin and aspirin	Increased risk of bleeding
Warfarin and chloral hydrate	Increased risk of toxicity
Digitalis and quinidine	Increased risk of toxicity
Cimetidine and propranolol	Decreased clearance, increased bradycardia
Thiazides and longer acting antidiabetics	Increased risk of hypoglycemia
Levodopa and clonidine	Decreased antiparkinsonian effect
Diuretics and NSAIDs	Renal impairment
Lithium and diuretics	Increased risk of toxicity
Lovastatin (Mevacor) and gemfibrozil (Lopid)	Toxic liver effect
Prednisone and barbiturates	Decreased steroid effect
St. John's wort and pseudoephedrine	Increased blood pressure
Ginkgo with aspirin	Increased bleeding risk

TABLE 22-4 Common Drug-Food Interactions in Older Adults

FOOD	DRUG	POTENTIAL EFFECT
Caffeine	Theophylline	Increased potential for toxicity
Fatty food	Griseofulvin	Increased absorption of drug
Blue cheese	Penicillin	Antagonistic action
Fiber	Digoxin	Absorption of drug into fiber, reducing drug action
Vitamin K foods: cabbage, greens, egg yolk, fish, rice	Warfarin	Decreased effect of drug, inhibiting anticoagulation
Food	Many antibiotics	Reduced absorption rate of drug
Mineral oil	Oil-soluble vitamins	Fat solubles dissolve in oil; deficiency possible
Tyramine foods: aged cheese, wines, pickled herring, chocolate	MAO inhibitors (phenelzine [Nardil], tranylcypromine [Parnate]), St. John's wort	May precipitate hypertensive crisis
Vitamin B_6 supplements	Levodopa-carbidopa	Reverses antiparkinsonian effect
Grapefruit juice	Cisapride, calcium channel blockers, quinidine	Altered metabolism and elimination can increase concentration drug level
Citrus juice	Calcium channel blockers	Gastric reflux exacerbated

TABLE 22-5 Common Drug-Disease Interactions in Older Adults

DISEASE	DRUG	POTENTIAL EFFECT
Atrophic gastritis	Aspirin, NSAIDs	GI hemorrhage
Sinus or atrioventricular note disease	Digitalis, verapamil	Bradycardia
Venous insufficiency	Calcium channel blockers or beta-blockers	Edema, intermittent claudication
Cataracts	Corticosteroids	Accelerated cataract formation
Unstable bladder	Diuretics	Incontinence
Prostatic hypertrophy	Anticholinergics	Urinary retention
Parkinson's disease	Metoclopramide, neuroleptics	Parkinson's syndrome
Renal impairment	NSAIDs, contrast material, aminoglycosides	Acute renal failure
Chronic obstructive pulmonary disease	Beta-blockers	Bronchoconstriction
	Opiates	Respiratory depression
Hypokalemia	Digitalis	Cardiac toxicity
Osteopenia	Corticosteroids	Fracture risk
Orthostatic hypotension	Diuretics, psychotropics, antihypertensives	Increased fall risk
Depression	Central acting antihypertensives, alcohol, antianxiety drugs, corticosteroids	Exacerbation of depression

Medications and Quality of Life

Traditionally outcomes such as a cure for a disease or a reduction in surrogate end points, such as blood pressure, have been viewed as measurements of successful pharmacotherapy. However, these outcomes may not reflect influences of pharmacotherapy on a client's quality of life. A quality-of-life assessment is a summary of the individual's ability to participate fully in and enjoy life. A variety of tools exist to measure both general quality of life and specific areas such as physical or cognitive function.

Medications from diverse categories may have detrimental effects on cognition, emotional status, ambulation, continence, and maintenance of posture. These negative effects on an older client's quality of life must be carefully considered when selecting certain medications and dosages. In assessing a client, the nurse must consider whether functional or cognitive deficits or changes are related to drug therapy and discuss these concerns with the prescriber. The nurse should also consider the client's personal goals regarding his or her quality of life because, for example, some clients might agree to decreased function in exchange for improved pain relief.

COMMONLY USED MEDICATIONS

Psychotropics

Psychotropic medications, which include antipsychotics (neuroleptics or major tranquilizers), antidepressants, and sedative-hypnotics (anxiolytics), are often prescribed in the older adult population. Psychotropics are likely to be prescribed for behavioral problems in nursing facility populations, where it is not uncommon for some residents to have either a psychiatric diagnosis or a mental disorder. Some general problems with psychotropic prescribing that have been reported in older adults include (1) overprescribing of anxiolytics and hypnotics, often at doses that are too high and for extended, rather than short-term, periods; (2) underprescribing of antidepressants and maintenance of subtherapeutic doses that may cause side effects without providing maximum therapeutic benefit; and (3) both underprescribing and overprescribing of antipsychotics, potentially denying benefit to some and causing side effects without therapeutic benefit in others. However, improved prescribing patterns in part as a result of the OBRA legislation were reported in a 1996 survey of 30 long-term care facilities, which found a decrease in the use of sedative-hypnotics and an increase in use of antidepressants compared with usage in 1992 (Sandberg, 1998).

Anxiolytics and Hypnotics

Anxiety can be a significant problem in older persons and is often associated with depression and dementia. Proper diagnosis and treatment of any underlying causes (e.g., depression, medication side effects, dementia, hypothyroidism) can decrease the inappropriate use of anxiolytic medications.

One anxiolytic agent, buspirone (BuSpar), can be an effective agent for the older adults without many of the adverse effects and dependence potential of the benzodiazepines. In addition, buspirone is not a controlled substance and does not require the same medication "counting" procedures in nursing homes that the benzodiazepines (and other controlled substances) require. Compared with the benzodiazepines, buspirone is also less likely to attract the attention of state surveyors during the nursing home inspection process.

According to the Beers list, benzodiazepines with long half-lives should be avoided because of the likelihood of accumulation of the parent drug and its active metabolite, resulting in increased toxicity, impaired memory, decreased psychomotor performance, and balance disturbances (Beers, 1997; Fick et al, 2003). However, the study by Wagner and colleagues (2004) reveals that even short-acting benzodiazepines place the older person at high risk of a devastating hip fracture (Box 22-2). Overall avoidance of benzodiazepines is advised if possible. If a benzodiazepine is required, then start with the smallest dose possible and monitor closely for side effects. Periodic evaluation of the need for anxiolytics or hypnotics is necessary, since only a small subset of clients require chronic treatment. Benzodiazepines should not be used for extended periods. Table 22-6 reviews comparative profiles of these agents.

Barbiturates are not recommended for older adults because of their narrow margin of safety, potential for significant drug interactions, and dependence liability.

Antihistamines have sometimes been used for nonallergic indications such as treatment for insomnia and anxiety. Antihistamines are now considered inappropriate for use in older adults for nonallergic indications because of significant anticholinergic adverse effects such as dry mouth, urinary retention, sedation, and delirium.

Other hypnotics such as zolpidem (Ambien) have become popular medications for treating insomnia. Their use in older adults should be limited, though, because of the potential for confusion and sedation despite their relatively short half-life. Nonpharmacologic treatment for insomnia is initially preferred

BOX 22-2 Benzodiazepine Use and Hip Fractures in the Elderly

Benzodiazepines have disadvantages when used in the elderly. According to a study by Harvard Medical School researchers, benzodiazepine use increased the rate of hip fractures 24% in a study of 125,203 people (Wagner et al, 2004). The study also found that short-life, half-potency benzodiazepines, used mainly as sleep aids, led to twice the likelihood of a hip fracture than longer-life benzodiazepines. The fracture rate was the highest in the two weeks after starting the medication.

TABLE 22-6 Benzodiazepines: Comparative Profiles

DRUG	HALF-LIFE	ACTIVE METABOLITES	SPEED OF ONSET
Alprazolam (Xanax)	Intermediate	Yes	Intermediate
Chlordiazepoxide (Librium)	Long	Yes	Intermediate
Clonazepam (Klonopin)	Long	No	Intermediate
Clorazepate (Tranxene)	Long	Yes	Fast
Diazepam (Valium)	Long	Yes	Very fast
Halazepam (Paxipam)	Intermediate	Yes	Slow
Lorazepam (Ativan)	Intermediate	No	Intermediate
Oxazepam (Serax)	Intermediate	No	Slow
Triazolam (Halcion)	Short	No	Fast

From *Drugs facts and comparisons,* ed 59, St Louis, 2005, Facts & Comparisons.

in older adults. If pharmacologic sleep aids are necessary, very low dose (25 mg) trazodone (Desyrel) may be preferable on an as needed basis (Reuben et al, 2004). At this dosage, it is unlikely to cause a serotonin syndrome reaction even if the patient is concurrently taking another serotonin selective reuptake inhibitor (SSRI) medication for depression. Caution is still advised with low-dose trazodone, since sedation is still a risk.

Antidepressants

All antidepressants are generally equally effective and typically take effect in 2 to 4 weeks. Selection of an antidepressant is based on side effect profiles, which differ among available agents (Table 22-7). For instance, in Table 22-7 you will notice that mirtazapine (Remeron) has more potential for sedation than most of the SSRI antidepressants. Although not indicated in the table, it can also reduce anxiety and increase appetite. If the patient suffers from depressive symptoms of anxiety, insomnia, and lack of appetite, then mirtazapine may be an appropriate choice at bedtime to help the patient sleep, increase appetite, and reduce anxiety. On the other hand, a patient exhibiting depressive symptoms like increased sleepiness, decreased affect, and decreased socialization may benefit from a more stimulating antidepressant like sertraline (Zoloft) or venlafaxine (Effexor). Thus you can use the side effect profile of an antidepressant to your advantage depending on the depressive symptom pattern.

Older antidepressants (e.g., tricyclic antidepressants) have been used to treat depression, insomnia, and neuropathic pain. As an antidepressant, however, significant side effects occur even in low doses and well before therapeutic levels are reached. As a treatment for insomnia, the tricyclic antidepressants are generally too sedating and can cause daytime somnolence. If a tricyclic antidepressant is needed to treat neuropathic pain, desipramine may be preferred due to its

TABLE 22-7 Antidepressants: Comparative Profiles

DRUG	AVOID IN OLDER ADULTS	ANTICHOLINERGIC SIDE EFFECTS	SEDATION	ORTHOSTATIC HYPOTENSION
TRICYCLICS: TERTIARY AMINES				
Amitriptyline	✓	++++	++++	++
Clomipramine	✓	+++	+++	++
Doxepin	✓	++	+++	++
Imipramine	✓	++	++	+++
Trimipramine	✓	++	+++	++
TRICYCLICS: SECONDARY AMINES				
Amoxapine	✓	+++	++	+
Desipramine	✓	+	+	+
Nortriptyline	✓	++	++	+
Protriptyline	✓	+++	+	+
PHENETHYLAMINES				
Venlafaxine (Effexor)		o	o	o
TETRACYCLICS				
Maprotiline	✓	++	++	+
TRIAZOLOPYRIDINES				
Trazodone (Desyrel)		+	++	++
AMINOKETONES				
Bupropion (Wellbutrin)		++	++	++
SELECTIVE SEROTONIN REUPTAKE INHIBITORS				
Fluoxetine (Prozac)		o/+	o/+	o/+
Paroxetine (Paxil)		o	o/+	o
Sertraline (Zoloft)		o	o/+	o
Citalopram (Celexa)		o/+	o/+	o/+
Escitalopram (Lexapro)		o/+	o/+	o/+
Fluvoxamine (Luvox)		o/+	o/+	o
MISCELLANEOUS				
Nefazodone (Serzone)		o/+	++	+
Mirtazapine (Remeron)		++	+++	++

From *Drug facts and comparisons*, ed 59, St Louis, 2005, Facts & Comparisons.

improved side effect profile compared with others in this class.

Overall, tricyclic antidepressants should be avoided in the older patient because of their anticholinergic and sedative side effect profile. The newer SSRIs are often considered the first choice for antidepressants in older adults because of their lack of tricyclic-associated side effects. However, they are more likely to cause dose-related gastrointestinal disturbances and central nervous system arousal effects. Fortunately, most of the side effects of the SSRIs last only a few days.

Antipsychotics

Antipsychotics should be prescribed only when valid and clear documentation of need exists, since many side effects occur with use of these agents. Nursing assessment of reversible or treatable causes of psychotic symptoms, along with interventions to modify behavior, should always be initiated before prescribing antipsychotics. Appropriate indications for antipsychotic prescription include schizophrenia, paranoid states, and symptoms of psychosis such as hallucinations and delusions. Insomnia and dementia are not acceptable diagnoses for antipsychotic use. One author has suggested that, in accordance with OBRA guidelines, the presence of the following "three Ds" may justify antipsychotic use: (1) danger to the resident or others, (2) distress for the resident, and (3) dysfunction of the resident, including interference with basic nursing care (Drinka, 1993).

Generally high-potency, low-dose drugs such as haloperidol (Haldol) are chosen because of their safer cardiovascular profile, lower adverse sedative and anticholinergic effects, and minimum orthostasis (Table 22-8). Haloperidol is also popular because it is one of the few antipsychotics that can be given intramuscularly in emergent situations. However, even small doses of these drugs may cause excessive sedation, which may impair function for days in sensitive older clients, and they are more frequently associated with extrapyramidal

TABLE 22-8 Antipsychotic Agents

DRUG	SEDATION	EXTRAPYRAMIDAL SYMPTOMS	ANTICHOLINERGIC EFFECTS	ORTHOSTATIC HYPOTENSION	WEIGHT GAIN
PHENOTHIAZINES					
ALIPHATIC					
Chlorpromazine	+++	++	++	+++	
Promazine	++	++	+++	++	
Triflupromazine	+++	++	+++	++	
Piperazine					
Fluphenazine	+	++++	+	+	
Perphenazine	++	++	+	+	
Trifluoperazine	+	+++	+	+	
PIPERIDINES					
Mesoridazine	+++	+	+++	++	
Thioridazine	+++	+	+++	+++	
THIOXANTHENES					
Thiothixene	+	+++	+	++	
PHENYLBUTYLPIPERADINES					
Haloperidol	+	++++	+	+	
Pimozide	+	+++	++	+	
DIHYDROINDOLONES					
Molindone	++	++	+	++	
Ziprasidone	++	++	+	++	+
DIBENZEPINE					
Loxapine	+	++	+	+	
NOVELS (ATYPICAL AGENTS)					
Clozapine	+++	o	+++	+++	++++
Olanzapine	++	+	++	++	++++
Quetiapine	++	o	o/+	++	+++
Risperidone	+	++	o/+	++	+++
QUINOLINONE					
Aripiprozole	++	o	o/+	+	+++

From *Drug facts and comparisons,* ed 59, St Louis, 2005, Facts & Comparisons.

side effects such as tremors, akinesia, akathisia, and rigidity. All the antipsychotics have been reported to cause tardive dyskinesia (TD) with the chronic use of even small doses. Nursing assessment for the abnormal involuntary movements associated with antipsychotic use is essential in caring for this population of patients.

The newer atypical antipsychotic medications (e.g., olanzapine [Zyprexa], risperidone [Risperdal]) offer a lower risk of extrapyramidal side effects and perhaps a better overall side effect profile. However, the risk of developing or aggravating diabetes mellitus is significant with these drugs, so blood glucose levels need to be monitored. The atypical antipsychotics can also aggravate lipid levels and cause weight gain (Henderson, 2002). Increased risk of stroke in older clients who use the atypical antipsychotics is also a new concern. In 2004 warnings were published regarding a potential increase in stroke risk for older clients. The risk level is not well defined at this time, but the practitioner should try to use alternative medications in patients with previous stroke or at risk for stroke (Herrmann, Mamdani, and Lanctôt, 2004; Rosack 2004).

Cardiovascular Medications

The Seventh Report of the Joint National Committee on Prevention, Detection, Evaluation, and Treatment of High Blood Pressure (JNC 7, 2003) recommends lifestyle modification as a primary method for preventing and treating hypertension. In older adults weight loss, reduced sodium intake, and exercise can be especially beneficial in preventing or reducing hypertension (JNC 7, 2003).

If a pharmacologic agent is needed to treat hypertension, the JNC 7 recommends thiazide diuretics (alone or in combination with other drugs) as first-line therapy based on outcomes data from clinical trials that show unsurpassed ability to prevent the cardiovascular complications of hypertension (e.g., kidney disease, stroke, coronary artery disease, irreversible white matter brain changes on magnetic resonance imaging, and dementia) (JNC 7, 2003).

Older adults tend to have isolated systolic hypertension (ISH) where the systolic blood pressure is elevated but the diastolic measurement remains near normal. The JNC 7 recommends the same methods of treatment for older adults as the younger population. However, since older adults are likely to have more comorbidities (e.g., diabetes, reduced kidney function, heart disease), JNC 7 recommends selecting hypertensive treatment based on comorbid conditions or compelling indication (JNC 7, 2003) (Table 22-9). For example, a 70-year-old patient with hypertension and diabetes would benefit from thiazide-type diuretics and an angiotensin-converting enzyme inhibitor (ACEI) or angiotensin II receptor blocker (ARB) because the combination can further reduce blood pressure and help prevent microalbuminuria and the kidney disease that is common in diabetic patients. On the other hand, if the patient had ischemic heart disease as well, adding a beta-blocker to the regimen would be helpful. Because the hypertensive older adult is likely to have other chronic comorbidities, it may be necessary to treat the hypertension with multiple medications that can assist in treatment of those other conditions. One advantage to multidrug treatment is that it allows you to use smaller doses of each individual drug and, therefore, reduce the adverse effects from any single drug. On the other hand, multidrug treatment can increase the cost of therapy and may require more blood testing to monitor for adverse effects.

The ACEIs and ARBs have demonstrated value in decreasing cardiac mortality in clients with heart failure (Cohn, 1996; JNC 7, 2003; Schaefer and Porter, 1996), as well as conferring renal protection, particularly for those with diabetes (JNC 7, 2003; Redon, 1997). The advantages these agents have for older adults are improved tolerability; improved quality of life compared with that associated with other antihypertensives; lack of central nervous system–mediated effects (e.g., drowsiness, impotence); and lack of adverse metabolic effects on electrolytes, glucose, lipids, and uric acid (Small et al, 1997).

The long-acting calcium channel blockers (CCBs), while not first-line therapy, may be reasonable alternatives for older

TABLE 22-9 Compelling Diagnoses for Prescribing Specific Antihypertensive Drug Classes

	RECOMMENDED DRUGS*					
COMPELLING INDICATION	DIURETIC	BB	ACEI	ARB	CCB	ALDOANT
Heart failure	✓	✓	✓	✓		✓
After myocardial infarction		✓	✓			✓
High coronary disease risk	✓	✓	✓		✓	
Diabetes	✓	✓	✓	✓	✓	
Chronic kidney disease			✓	✓		
Recurrent stroke prevention	✓		✓			

Derived from Joint National Committee: The Seventh Report of the Joint National Committee on the Prevention, Detection, Evaluation, and Treatment of High Blood Pressure, 2003. Accessed at website: http://www.nhlbi.nih.gov/guidelines/hypertension/index.htm.
BB, Beta-blocker; *ACEI*, angiotensin-converting enzyme inhibitor; *ARB*, angiotensin II receptor blocker; *CCB*, calcium channel blocker; *ALDOANT*, aldosterone antagonist.
*For initial drug therapy recommendations and references, see *2005 Physicians' Desk Reference*, ed 59, Montvale, NJ, 2004, Thomson PDR.

clients because they do not cause the metabolic abnormalities commonly seen with diuretics or the fatigue associated with beta-blockers. Lower doses are often effective in older adults because of a decrease in first-pass hepatic metabolism, which results in increased serum concentrations. The type 1 agents (verapamil and diltiazem) are more prominent in slowing atrioventricular conduction, whereas the type 2 agents (such as nifedipine) are potent vasodilators, resulting in different side effects profiles. Short-acting CCBs are not advised in treating hypertension.

The main concerns with the use of cardiovascular medications in older adults are an increased risk of orthostatic hypotension and dehydration, especially with volume-depleting agents and vasodilators. Dehydration is common among older people and is a frequent reason for admission to the hospital. The aging person has reduced kidney function and decreased ability to maintain fluid and electrolyte balance. In addition, some older patients may have decreased appetite and sense of thirst and subsequent decreased oral intake of food and fluids and increased risk of dehydration. Assessing for the adverse effects of antihypertensive treatment is essential in maintaining the health of the older patient and reducing devastating complications and hospitalizations.

Antimicrobials

Infections in older adults can be devastating health events because of generally decreased physiologic reserves. Urinary tract infections (UTI) and respiratory infections (especially pneumonia and exacerbations of chronic lung diseases) are common and often lead to hospital admissions. For example, a frail older person with a UTI can experience significant mental status changes, weakness, and sepsis and may require extended hospitalization and weeks of rehabilitation to return to baseline functional status. However, a UTI in a young person is more often an annoyance (potentially dangerous nonetheless) than a serious illness.

Pharmacologic treatment of infections has the potential to effect cures, but a number of barriers may contribute to antibiotic treatment failures. It has been estimated that as few as 25% of clients given an antibiotic prescription will actually have it filled, particularly in the case of expensive antibiotics (*Antibiotic update 1998*, 1997). Even clients who fill their prescriptions may not comply with the regimen because of the frequency of daily dosing, long duration of therapy, and adverse effects. In addition, close to 40% of older adults showed limited or global misunderstanding of their medicines or adherence to the medication regimen (Spiers, Kutzik, and Lamar, 2004). Cost of medications can also be a significant factor for older adults. Until 2004, Medicare did not cover the cost of outpatient medications. The Medicare Modernization Act (http://www.cms.hhs.gov/medicarereform/), signed into law in 2003, has mandated a measure of Medicare drug coverage to be fully implemented by 2006.

Antibiotic resistance is becoming increasingly problematic in all health care settings. Examples of resistant organisms include methicillin-resistant *Staphylococcus aureus* (MRSA), vancomycin-resistant enterococci (VRE), penicillin- and cephalosporin-resistant pneumococci, and beta-lactamase–producing *Haemophilus influenzae*, as well as nosocomial isolates such as multiple-antibiotic–resistant gram-negative bacilli (*Antibiotic update 1998*, 1997; Gaynes, 1997). Overuse of broad-spectrum and expensive antibiotics is a significant contributing factor to these resistance patterns. The newer generation cephalosporins, quinolones, and macrolides have the advantages of an extended spectrum of activity and improved pharmacokinetic profiles, which offer infrequent daily dosing and better side effect profiles (*Antibiotic update 1998*, 1997; Bartlett et al, 1998). However, the trade-offs are a higher cost and greater selective pressure for the emergence of resistant organisms.

Dosing of antibiotics may need to be altered in older clients because of reduced renal elimination. Many easily accessed drug references, such as the *2005 Physicians' Desk Reference* (2004), include recommendations for dose adjustment related to renal impairment.

Nonprescription Agents

Of all drugs purchased in the United States, 60% are nonprescription or over-the-counter, and 85% of Americans believe access to over-the-counter medications is important in relieving minor problems (*From Rx to OTC: more drugs make the switch*, 1997; Nordenberg, 1996).

Factors cited as contributing to growing availability of over-the-counter products are (1) the self-care movement to increase clients' involvement in their own care; (2) increasing health care costs; (3) the advancing age of many consumers; and (4) interest by pharmaceutic manufacturers in broadening the market for their products, especially when patents near expiration. The Food and Drug Administration's (FDA's) Division of Over-the-Counter Drug Evaluation considers three main criteria when reviewing a request to switch a prescription product to over-the-counter status. First, a record of established safety data for the prescription product is necessary. Second, the drug's expected use should be appropriate for over-the-counter treatment—that is, the problem should be able to be readily identified and managed without physician intervention. Finally, the drug should lack undesirable properties and not require special precautions when used without physician oversight (*From Rx to OTC: more drugs make the switch*, 1997; Nordenberg, 1996).

Many prescription drugs have been reclassified to over-the-counter status in the past 30 years, including a number of NSAIDs, histamine receptor antagonists, topical antifungals, smoking cessation aids, and antihistamines. Potential advantages to the growth in over-the-counter products include greater access, choice, and convenience for clients; improved use of the physician's time for more serious illnesses; extension of marketing time and improved sales volume for manufacturers; and savings to the health care system from lower rates of office visits and fewer or eliminated pharmacy dispensing fees. Potential disadvantages are mainly associated with the consumer: greater out-of-pocket expense, problems with readability and package labeling, delays in seeking effective care when over-the-counter products fail, and a lack of safety monitoring (Jacobs, 1998).

The challenge for health care professionals will be to remain informed regarding *all* medications clients are currently taking and to caution clients against certain products that may interact negatively with their particular medical conditions or other medications.

Herbal Remedies

The use of herbal remedies, or dietary supplements as they are legally classified by the FDA, appears to be more than just a passing fad. Nearly one in five individuals taking prescription medications also was taking herbs, high-dose vitamin supplements, or both (Eisenberg et al, 1998). Persons with chronic conditions such as human immunodeficiency virus, cancer, epilepsy, and bone and joint disorders, and the caregivers of persons with Alzheimer's disease, frequently use alternative therapies (Abdel-Rahman and Nahata, 1997). Yet, in one survey, more than 70% of those using alternative therapies had never discussed this with their physicians (Eisenberg, 1997). Furthermore, health care professionals are not uniformly well prepared to answer questions from clients because many professional schools do not require instruction on herbal products (Miller and Murray, 1997).

There are a number of concerns regarding the use of herbal medications. Since these products are classified as dietary supplements, they are not regulated for safety and efficacy by the FDA, as are prescription (legend) drugs, which undergo a rigorous drug approval process. Manufacturers of herbal products are authorized only to describe the product's effects on structure and function. Medical claims, such as effectiveness in the diagnosis, treatment, cure, or prevention of specific diseases, are prohibited. The use and safety of these products in special populations, such as in pregnant or lactating women, children, or frail older adults with multiple organ dysfunction, have not been studied. Lack of predictable product quality, variability in actual versus labeled potency, and adulteration are all ongoing problems. An excellent source for updated information on product quality or safety concerns is the FDA's web site at www.fda.gov/medwatch.

Toxicity, including carcinogenicity, has been reported with herbs such as comfrey, colt's foot, life root, sassafras bark, calamus, gerrymander, apricot kernels, and rue. Ginkgo and ginseng have also been associated with increased bleeding tendency. On the other hand, those herbs which appear to offer some therapeutic benefit are saw palmetto for mild prostatism, garlic for mild lipid disorders, ginkgo for circulation, and St. John's wort (hypericum) for depression (Croom and Walker, 1995; Tyler, 1995).

Health care providers must educate themselves about herbal medications and include questions on their use in intake assessments of clients. One resource, the *PDR for Herbal Medicines,* would be a valuable addition to an office library and could assist practitioners in these efforts.

CLIENT EDUCATION AND ADHERENCE

Assessing Risk Factors for Nonadherence

Nonadherence may contribute significantly to increased morbidity in older clients. It is estimated that 125,000 deaths and 300,000 hospitalizations each year are the result of nonadherence with cardiovascular drug regimens alone.

Many factors may place older clients at risk for noncompliance. Living alone without social supports, especially if depression or cognitive impairment is present, may lead clients into a declining pattern of self-care. Visual or auditory impairments may distort an older client's perception of information given by a health care professional or may simply make the medication label itself hard to read and interpret.

The use of multiple health care providers and multiple pharmacies, along with a large medication burden or complex medication regimen, is a recipe for trouble. The increasing use of alcohol with advancing age may lead to nonadherence. Lack of knowledge about the purpose of medications, instructions for their use, and management of their side effects also contributes to adherence problems. Socioeconomic factors, such as inadequate insurance or high deductibles or copayments, may force clients to choose between housing, food, and medication. Certain dosage forms, such as unpalatable bulk powders or large tablets, may act as barriers to client adherence. The presence of arthritis may cause pain and hinder a client's ability to open child-proof caps.

The interchangeability of trade and generic names is a common source of client confusion. A pharmacy's substitution of one generic brand with another that is chemically identical but different in shape or color may increase the likelihood of medication error. The presence of learning barriers, such as low literacy, limits a client's ability to organize thoughts and perceptions concerning medication instructions.

Strategies for Improving Adherence

A complete client assessment during an intake interview by the nurse is essential in determining the risk factors present in a particular client. The following key questions should be asked:

- What were the prescription and nonprescription medications and regimens used just before the office or hospital visit? Can office records, prescription vials, a written list from home, or pharmacy files be used to help verify this information?

- Who prescribed the medications? When were they started? Were there any recent changes, and why were these made?
- Does the client understand the purpose of each medication and benefits to be gained?
- Does the client know what side effects to expect? What would the client do if one were experienced?
- What would the client do if a dose was missed?
- Does the client have any memory aids for assistance (e.g., written list, medication calendar, pill box)?
- Does the client have any psychiatric diagnosis or symptoms that may affect learning and memory? (This can be obtained from the client's chart or caregiver.)
- What is the client's living situation? Is the client taking the medications alone, or does someone assist?
- How does the client pay for his or her medication? How much, if any, has to be paid out of pocket per month? Does the client sometimes need to stretch the medications to save money?
- What is the client's perception (e.g., on a scale of 1 to 5) of the value of medication? Has the client felt better or worse since the medication was started?

Once this assessment is completed, a number of approaches can be taken to improve adherence based on a client's unique risk profile. If knowledge deficits are a problem, the nurse should provide verbal education reinforced with written instructions and allow time for client feedback. The nurse should also maintain a log of these sessions, along with currently prescribed medications, in an easily accessible part of the client's medical record. Reinforcement and review at subsequent visits strengthens a client's understanding and allows the opportunity for clarification if needed. The nurse should encourage a client who "pharmacy shops" to have prescriptions filled at the same pharmacy each time. The nurse should also provide a client with specific cues to assist in remembering to take medications (e.g., when brushing teeth, removing glasses, cleaning dentures) and tailor the medication regimen to the client's home schedule to cause the least disruption in daily life and give him or her a sense of control over the medications. The regimen should be simplified as much as possible, avoiding multiple daily doses where appropriate and feasible.

The nurse should test a client's functional ability to take the medication by ensuring that the client can actually read the prescription label, open and close the cap, remove a specified number of pills, distinguish between the color of various oral dosage forms, and correctly interpret instructions (e.g., "If your doctor told you to take this three times a day, when would you take it?"). Although this process may initially be time consuming, the investment should pay off in improved client understanding and compliance.

Clients should be just as informed about their nonprescription medications as they are about their prescribed medications. Unfortunately, they often find themselves surrounded by a confusing array of nonprescription choices in the pharmacy. Even if a client requests help, the pharmacist may be unaware of certain aspects of a client's medical history that could significantly affect any recommendation. An ideal time to assist a client is while he or she is in the office so that the health care provider most familiar with the client's unique medical history may assist with making the best choice. A "safe over-the-counter medication" list may be a useful tool for health care providers to review with patients before completing the office visit (Table 22-10).

TABLE 22-10 Your Safe List for Over-the-Counter Medications

IF YOU HAVE	GENERALLY AVOID OVER-THE-COUNTER MEDICINES CONTAINING	EXAMPLES	BECAUSE	SAFER ALTERNATIVES
Asthma or lung disease	Ephedrine Epinephrine Extra theophylline Pseudoephedrine Caffeine	Bronkaid Primatene Bronkaid Sudafed NoDoz, DeWitt's pills	May cause insomnia, nervousness, irregular heartbeats, especially when taking prescription asthma medicines	Ask your doctor
	Aspirin/salicylates (if you have aspirin allergy)	Ecotrin	May cause allergic reaction (e.g., wheezing, itching, hives)	Acetaminophen (Tylenol)
	NSAIDs (if you have aspirin allergy)	Nuprin		
Blood clots (and are taking blood thinners)	Aspirin/salicylates	Ecotrin, Vanquish, Alka Seltzer, Pepto-Bismol	May cause bleeding	Acetaminophen Kaopectate
NSAIDs	Nuprin	May cause bleeding		

Continued

TABLE 22-10 Your Safe List for Over-the-Counter Medications—cont'd

IF YOU HAVE	GENERALLY AVOID OVER-THE-COUNTER MEDICINES CONTAINING	EXAMPLES	BECAUSE	SAFER ALTERNATIVES
Heart problems (high blood pressure, heart failure, abnormal heartbeat)	Sodium, salt Phenylpropranolamine Ephedrine Epinephrine Pseudoephedrine Caffeine	Alka-Seltzer, antacids Dexatrim Bronkaid Primatene Sudafed No-Doz	May worsen your condition	Acetaminophen, nasal sprays, nonmedicated throat lozenges
Diabetes	Liquid or syrups containing alcohol or sugar	Emetrol, many cough or cold syrups	May alter blood sugar	Sugar-free, sugarless, or alcohol-free liquids
	Phenylpropanolamine Ephedrine Epinephrine	Dexatrim Acutrim Bronkaid, Primatene	May increase blood sugar	Nonmedicated nose sprays, throat lozenges
	Aspirin/salicylates	Ecotrin, Pepto-Bismol	May decrease blood sugar if taking oral diabetes pills to lower sugar	Kaopectate, acetaminophen
Seizures	Aspirin/salicylates		May change levels of prescription seizure medicines	Acetaminophen
	Antihistamines (depressant medicine)	Benadryl, Unisom	May add to drowsiness caused by prescription seizure medicines	Ask your doctor
	Theophylline	Bronkaid Ecotrin	May change levels of prescription seizure medicine	
Stomach ulcers	Aspirin/salicylates NSAIDs Theophylline	Nuprin Bronkaid	May worsen your ulcers May have more side effects from theophylline if on certain prescription ulcer medicines	Acetaminophen Ask your doctor

These are general suggestions and should be discussed with your doctor. He or she may want to change this list or may add suggestions to fit your individual needs. *Always* read the label on nonprescription (over-the-counter) medicines before purchasing, and have a pharmacist assist you if you're not sure what choice to make.

Reviewing Medication List for Problems

Nurses confronted with a complex medication regimen for an older client should determine the answers to the following:

- Is there a documented and appropriate indication for the medication? For example, is omeprazole prescribed for a client without documentation of gastroesophageal reflux disease or peptic ulcer disease?
- Is a medication dosage appropriate for the client's age, weight, and renal or liver function? Digoxin at 0.25 mg/day is not acceptable in a cachectic 92-year-old woman with renal insufficiency.
- Does the client have a documented drug allergy to a medication? For example, is a client allergic to penicillin currently receiving ampicillin?
- Are doses of medication being scheduled appropriately? For example, is furosemide (Lasix) being taken at 10 PM instead of 10 AM?
- Is the duration of treatment appropriate? For example, is an antibiotic for an uncomplicated infection being prescribed for more than 2 weeks?
- Is a chosen medication the best one for the client (i.e., the most effective with the least side effects)? For example, would the depressed patient be better treated with an SSRI rather than the prescribed amitriptyline (Elavil)?
- Are two or more similar drugs prescribed (i.e., therapeutic duplication)? For example, is an H_2 receptor antagonist being combined with omeprazole?
- Is the client experiencing an adverse drug reaction? For example, is there a dramatic increase in weight or fluid

retention in a client with congestive heart failure who is started on an NSAID?

- Is there a drug-drug interaction? For example, is the client receiving both theophylline and full doses of cimetidine?
- Is there a medical indication for use of a medication when none is currently prescribed? For example, is a client with osteoporosis receiving no treatment for this?
- Is the client using over-the-counter medications inappropriately? For example, is the client receiving warfarin and also taking a cough and cold combination containing aspirin?

Home Care

1. During each home visit, assess both the prescription and nonprescription medications being taken by the homebound older adult.
2. Document and notify the primary health care provider of the homebound older adult's medication regimen and of multiple physician sources for medications.
3. Teach the complications and interactions of all over-the-counter medications to homebound older adults and their caregivers.
4. Collaborate with social workers to identify community resources for financial assistance with pharmaceutic needs.
5. Use laboratory parameters to monitor overuse and underuse of medications, as well as interactive states of medications.
6. Monitor urinary output status of clients, since changes in renal excretion may require a decrease or increase in drug dosage.
7. Teach the homebound older adult to set up a daily or weekly schedule for medications using a method or tool that fosters safe, independent administration.
8. Reduce the chance of medication error by labeling or color coding medication bottles.
9. Keep an accurate record of the homebound older adult's weight, since many medication dosages are calculated by body weight.
10. Teach drug safety in the home environment by instructing clients to do the following:
    - Keep drugs in original, labeled container.
    - Dispose of outdated medications in a sink or toilet only; never dispose of them in the trash within reach of children.
    - Never "share" drugs with friends or family members.
    - Always finish a prescribed medication; do not save it for a future illness.
    - Read labels carefully and follow all instructions.
11. Instruct older adults who have difficulty opening child-proof containers to request their health care providers ask for nonchild-proof containers when writing prescriptions.

- What herbal or alternative therapies is the client using? Is the client's health care provider aware of these?
- Is the client adherent? For example, are blood levels subtherapeutic at doses appropriate for the client's condition?

GENERAL PRESCRIBING PRINCIPLES

MASTER Rules for Rational Drug Therapy

It may be helpful to remember this mnemonic, based on the word *master,* when using medications in older clients:

- **M**inimize number of drugs used. Use the fewest number of drugs possible.
- **A**lternatives should be considered. Alternative therapy, drugs, and dosage forms should be considered for older adult clients.
- **S**tart low, and go slow. Start with lowest dosage and increase gradually.
- **T**itrate therapy. Adjust initial dosage according to individual characteristics, and readjust dosage to optimize the monitored plasma levels and clinical response.
- **E**ducate the client. To increase compliance and decrease side effects, instruct the client, family, or significant other about the need for and potential problems of therapy.
- **R**eview regularly. Monitor response regularly, and reevaluate the client's need periodically.

SUMMARY

Achieving positive therapeutic outcomes and reducing ADEs requires a knowledge of changes in drug response and of use patterns in normal and frail, chronically ill older adults. Health care professionals must accept this responsibility if improved client outcomes are to be realized.

Key Points

- Older adults consume a large proportion of pharmaceutic products. Use of inappropriate medications results in significant morbidity and mortality, as well as adding an economic burden to clients and health care systems.
- Older clients may be at risk for adverse drug reactions because of changes in drug disposition with age, multiple chronic illnesses, polypharmacy, dysfunctional prescribing, client demands and expectations, deficits in adherence and education, fragmentation of health care, and medication expense.
- Reduction of drug dosage is often required for older clients in whom renal or hepatic function and the ability to eliminate medications are reduced.
- Knowledge of clinically important drug interactions is essential in planning alternate medication regimens and preventing potentially serious ADEs.

- Medication problems should always be suspected in clients experiencing overt or subtle changes in cognitive or physical function.
- Psychotropics should be used judiciously in older adults; agents with the lowest side effects profiles should be preferred.
- Newer cardiac medications may offer opportunities for an improved quality of life for older clients.
- The nurse can play a key role in assessing clients for risk factors that may reduce compliance and developing strategies to reduce or to eliminate these risks.
- Start low, go slow, and periodically review medication regimens.

Critical Thinking Exercises

1. An 82-year-old man with a history of congestive heart failure is taking a number of prescription medications, including Metamucil, Lanoxin, Dilantin, and Tagamet. He is 5 foot, 9 inches tall and weighs 139 pounds. Based on potential drug interactions, identify the relevant assessment priorities. What factors place this client at risk for drug toxicity?
2. A home care nurse is seeing an 81-year-old man who is on a complex medication regimen. He cannot remember when he last took several of his medications, and his wife states she is confused by the recent switch of several drugs to other generic brands. What questions should the nurse ask to establish the client's risk for noncompliance?
3. A client's daughter wonders if she should use ginkgo and other herbals to help with her dad's Alzheimer's disease. How would you advise her?

References

Abdel-Rahman SM, Nahata MC: Perspective on alternative medicine, *Ann Pharmacother* 31:1397, 1997.

Abrams WB, Berkow R: *The Merck manual of geriatrics*, ed 3, Rahway, NJ, 2000, Merck.

American Diabetes Association: Aspirin therapy in diabetes, *Diabetes Care* 21(suppl 1):S45, 1998.

Antibiotic update 1998: Outcome-effective treatment guidelines for bacterial infections managed in the primary care and emergency department settings, *Emerg Med Rep* 18(26):1, 1997.

Avorn J, Gurwitz JH: Drug use in the nursing home, *Ann Intern Med* 123:195, 1995.

Bartlett JG et al: Community-acquired pneumonia in adults: guidelines for management, *Clin Infect Dis* 26:811, 1998.

Beers MH: Explicit criteria for determining potentially inappropriate medication use by the elderly, *Arch Intern Med* 157:1531, 1997.

Beers MH et al: Inappropriate medication prescribing in skilled-nursing facilities, *Ann Intern Med* 117(8):684, 1992.

Bernabei R et al: Management of pain in elderly patients with cancer, *JAMA* 279:1877, 1998.

Centers for Disease Control and Prevention: Prevention of pneumococcal disease: recommendations of the Advisory Committee on Immunization Practices (ACIP), *Morbid Mortal Weekly Rep* 46 (No RR-8):1, 1997.

Cohn JN: The management of chronic heart failure, *N Engl J Med* 335(7):490, 1996.

Cooper JW: Adverse drug reaction–related hospitalizations of nursing facility patients: a 4-year study, *South Med J* 92(5):485, 1999.

Croom EM, Walker L: Botanicals in the pharmacy: new life for old remedies, *Drug Topics* 84, Nov 1995.

Drinka P: OBRA-1987 nursing home regulations, *J Am Geriatr Soc* 41(4):466, 1993.

Drugs facts and comparisons 2005, ed 59, St Louis, 2005, Facts & Comparisons.

Eisenberg DM: Advising patients who seek alternative medical therapies, *Ann Intern Med* 127:61, 1997.

Eisenberg DM et al: Trends in alternative medicine use in the United States, 1990-1997, *JAMA* 280:1569, 1998.

Fick MF et al: Updating the Beers criteria for potentially inappropriate medication use in older adults, *Arch Intern Med* 163:2716, 2003.

Field TS et al: Risk factors for adverse drug events among older adults in the ambulatory setting, *J Am Geriatr Soc* 52(8):1349, 2004.

From Rx to OTC: more drugs make the switch, *JAMA* 278(2):103, 1997.

Gage BF et al: Adverse outcomes and predictors of underuse of antithrombotic therapy in Medicare beneficiaries with chronic atrial fibrillation, *Stroke* 31(4):822, 2000.

Gaynes R: The impact of antimicrobial use on the emergence of antimicrobial-resistant bacteria in hospitals, *Infect Dis Clin North Am* 11(4):757, 1997.

Goulding MR: Inappropriate medication prescribing for elderly ambulatory care patients, *Arch Intern Med* 164:305, 2004.

Gruenwald J, editor: *PDR for herbal medicines*, ed 3, Stamford, Conn, 2004, Thomson Healthcare.

Gurwitz JH et al: Incidence and preventability of adverse drug events among older persons in the ambulatory care setting, *JAMA* 289(9):1107, 2003.

Hammerlein A, Derendorf H, Lowenthal DT: Pharmacokinetic and pharmacodynamic changes in the elderly: clinical implications, *Clin Pharmacokinet* 35(1):49, 1998.

Henderson DC: Atypical antipsychotic-induced diabetes mellitus: how strong is the evidence? *CNS Drugs* 16(2):77, 2002.

Herrmann N, Mamdani M, Lanctôt KL: Atypical antipsychotics and risk of cerebrovascular accidents, *Am J Psychiatry* 161:1113, 2004.

Institute of Medicine Committee on Quality of Health Care in America. In Kohn LT, Corrigan JM, Donaldson MS, editors: *To err is human: building a safer health care system*, Washington, DC, 1999, Committee on Quality of Healthcare in America, Institute of Medicine, National Academies Press.

Jacobs LR: Prescription to over-the-counter drug reclassification, *Am Fam Phys* 57(9):2209, 1998.

Joint National Committee: *The Seventh Report of the Joint National Committee on the Prevention, Detection, Evaluation, and Treatment of High Blood Pressure*, 2003. Accessed on website: http://www.nhlbi.nih.gov/guidelines/hypertension/index.htm.

Juurlink DN et al: Drug-drug interactions among elderly patients hospitalized for drug toxicity, *JAMA* 289(13):1652, 2003.

Kaufman DW et al: Recent patterns of medication use in the ambulatory adult population of the United States: the Slone survey, *JAMA* 287(3):337, 2002.

Krumholz HM et al: National use and effectiveness of beta-blockers for the treatment of elderly patients after acute myocardial infarction, *JAMA* 180:623-629, 1998.

Krumholz HM et al: Aspirin for secondary prevention after acute myocardial infarction in the elderly: prescribed use and outcomes, *Ann Intern Med* 124:292, 1996.

Leape LL et al: Systems analysis of adverse drug events: ADE Prevention Study Group, *JAMA* 274(1):35, 1995.

Lesar TS, Lomaestro BM, Pohl H: Medication-prescribing errors in a teaching hospital: a 9-year experience, *Arch Intern Med* 157(14):1569, 1997.

Liu GG, Christensen DB: The continuing challenge of inappropriate prescribing in the elderly: an update of the evidence, *J Am Pharm Assoc* 42:847, 2002.

Miller LG, Murray WJ: Herbal instruction in United States pharmacy schools, *Am J Pharm Educ* 61:160, 1997.

Nordenberg T: Now available without a prescription, *FDA Consumer* 30:6, Nov 1996.

Novelli WD: Health care in the 21st century, 2002, AARP. Accessed March 2005 from website: http://www.aarp.org/Articles/a2003-01-07-21century.html

Prescriber's Letter 5(9):51, 1998.

Prosser LA et al: Cost-effectiveness of cholesterol-lowering therapies according to selected patient characteristics, *Ann Intern Med* 132:769, 2000.

Redon J: Treatment of patients with essential hypertension and microalbuminuria, *Drugs* 54(6):857, 1997.

Reuben DB et al: *Geriatrics at your fingertips*, ed 6, Malden, Mass, 2004, Blackwell Publishing.

Rosack J: Olanzapine gets warning for use in elderly, *Psych News* 39(8), April 2004.

Sandberg A: Changes in psychoactive drug prescribing over 4 years in 30 nursing facilities, *Consult Pharm* 1:77, 1998.

Schaefer KL, Porter JA: Angiotensin II receptor antagonists: the prototype losartan, *Ann Pharmacother* 30:625, 1996.

Sisk JE et al: Cost-effectiveness of vaccination against pneumococcal bacteremia among elderly people, *JAMA* 278:1333, 1997.

Small RE et al: Evaluation of the total cost of treating elderly hypertensive patients with ACE inhibitors: a comparison of older and newer agents, *Pharmacotherapy* 17(5):1011, 1997.

Spiers MV, Kutzik DM, Lamar M: Variation in medication understanding among the elderly, *Am J Health-System Pharmacists* 61(4):373, 2004.

2005 Physicians' Desk Reference, ed 59, Montvale, NJ, 2004, Thomson PDR.

Tyler VE: Herbal remedies, *J Pharm Technol* 11:214, 1995.

Wagner AK et al: Benzodiazepine use and hip fractures in the elderly: who is at greatest risk? *Arch Intern Med* 164:1567, 2004.

Williams CM: Using medications appropriately in older adults, *Am Fam Phys* 66(10):1917-1924, 2002.

Zhan C et al: Potentially inappropriate medication use in the community-dwelling elderly: findings from the 1996 Medical Expenditure Panel Survey, *JAMA* 286(22):2823, 2001.

23 Cardiovascular Function

LYNN FEREBEE, MSN, RN, FNP

Learning Objectives

On completion of this chapter, the reader will be able to:

1. Explain the age-related changes in the structure and function of the cardiovascular system.
2. Identify contributing risk factors for cardiovascular disease.
3. Explain the pathophysiology and treatment regimen for cardiovascular conditions common in older adults.
4. List nursing interventions for older clients with cardiovascular conditions.
5. Implement the nursing process for older adults with cardiovascular conditions.

The leading cause of death in the United States for both men and women is cardiovascular heart disease, accounting for approximately 650,000 Americans having their first coronary attack in 2001. Older adults account for half of these deaths. Medications such as statins have reduced cardiovascular heart disease by 25% to 60%; however, the target goals established by the National Cholesterol Education Program have not been met (Mola and Lloyd, 2002). This chapter examines the age-related changes of the cardiovascular system and the common problems and conditions that affect older adults.

AGE-RELATED CHANGES IN STRUCTURE AND FUNCTION

Aging alters the cardiovascular system both structurally and physiologically. However, there is increasing evidence that lifestyle and diet can modify some of these age-related changes. Older adults who stay physically fit have twice the work capacity and lower body fat than sedentary older adults (Abrams and Berkow, 2000).

As people age, changes occur within the heart. The overall heart size decreases in the absence of clinical disease. Heart rate decreases, and the left ventricular wall thickens. There may be as much as a 25% thickening of the wall by age 80 (Burrell, Gerlach, and Pless, 1997), as well as increased collagen and decreased elastin in the heart muscle and vessel walls. These changes decrease myocardial muscle contraction and thus cardiac output and cardiac reserve. It is estimated that between ages 20 and 80 cardiac output decreases by 1% each year (Burrell, Gerlach, and Pless, 1997). An S_4 heart sound commonly occurs in older adults and may indicate decreased left ventricular compliance (Seidel et al, 1999).

Heart valves in older adults may be thicker and stiffer as a result of lipid accumulation, collagen degeneration, and fibrosis. These changes occur more in the mitral and aortic valves. Systolic ejection murmurs may be found on assessment of older adults.

Conduction System

The sinoatrial node becomes fibrotic with aging. The number of pacemaker cells located in the sinoatrial node decreases with age. By age 75, 10% of the normal number of pacemaker cells may remain (Lewis, Collier, and Heitkemper, 1996). This can cause sinus node dysfunction, resulting in sinus bradycardia.

Electrocardiogram (ECG) changes that are considered normal for an older adult include increased PR, QRS, and Q-T intervals. Decreased amplitude of the QRS complex occurs secondary to left ventricular wall thickening (Lewis, Collier, and Heitkemper, 1996). Atrial fibrillation can occur from fibrosis and cellular alteration (Seidel et al, 1999).

Vessels

Calcification of vessels occurs, making them tortuous. The elastin in the vessel wall decreases. This causes thickening and rigidity, especially in the coronary arteries (Seidel et al, 1999). This increases the risk of atherosclerotic buildup, especially in those individuals with adverse lifestyle practices.

Systolic blood pressure (SBP) is increased in older adults because of a loss of arterial distensibility. The diastolic blood pressure (DBP) remains the same or may be elevated slightly; thus the pulse pressure widens.

Older adults are less sensitive to the baroreceptor regulation of blood pressure. This causes fluctuation in blood pressure and contributes to increased SBP. Isolated systolic hypertension (ISH) is common in the older adult population.

Response to Stress and Exercise

Decreased cardiac output and cardiac reserve decrease the older adult's response to stress. Decreased distensibility of the vessel walls, decreased heart rate, and decreased myocardial contractility affect the response to exercise. An older adult's heart rate does not increase as quickly with exercise and does not decrease as rapidly after exercise. However, this does not exclude older adults from participating in exercise programs.

COMMON CARDIOVASCULAR PROBLEMS

Cardiovascular disease (CVD) is the leading cause of death for both men and women in the United States. One out of two women will die of CVD (Jensen and King, 1997). In addition, CVD accounts for more hospital admissions than any other disease or condition. Changes in the cardiovascular system from advancing age predispose older adults to a variety of problems and conditions such as coronary heart disease (ischemic heart disease), hypertension, pump failure, arrhythmia (particularly heart block), valvular conditions, and peripheral vascular disease (PVD).

The aging process varies among individuals, which may be attributed to factors of heredity. In addition, the effects of advancing age on cardiovascular structure and function are influenced by the presence of noncardiovascular disease and variations in lifestyle. It may not always be clear which changes in the cardiovascular system are from the normal aging process and which are caused by lifestyle (Burrell, Gerlach, and Pless, 1997). Many forms of CVD can be accelerated by unhealthy lifestyle choices such as smoking, physical inactivity, high-risk dietary behaviors, obesity, stress, and hormonal use by females. Chronic diseases such as hypertension and diabetes mellitus also play a role in accelerating changes.

Contributing Factors to Heart Disease

Risk factors are classified as nonmodifiable and modifiable (Box 23-1). Age, gender, and family history are risk factors that cannot be modified. Smoking, high blood pressure, a high-fat diet, obesity, physical inactivity, and stress are amenable to change. Research has demonstrated that the adoption of a healthier lifestyle has the potential to reduce or prevent the incidence of morbidity and death from ischemic heart disease and stroke. Health promotion and disease prevention are discussed in Chapter 8.

BOX 23-1 Risk Factors for Cardiovascular Disease

NONMODIFIABLE

- Age
- Gender
- Family history

MODIFIABLE

- Hypertension
- Smoking
- Elevated blood cholesterol levels
- Diabetes mellitus
- Sedentary lifestyle
- Obesity
- Stress
- Hormonal use
- Alcohol intake

Blood Pressure. High blood pressure, or hypertension, is a major modifiable risk factor that contributes to the incidence of coronary artery disease (CAD) and stroke. It also contributes to the development of congestive heart failure (CHF), renal failure, and PVD. More than 50 million Americans, or approximately 25% of the population, have hypertension. There is a 90% lifetime risk for hypertension for people with normotensive ranges at age 55 (Joint National Committee [JNC 7], 2003).

ISH occurs more commonly in the older adult population. The Systolic Hypertension in the Elderly Program study found that pharmacologic treatment for individuals with ISH over age 60 decreased the incidence of cardiovascular events by 32% within 5 years and decreased nonfatal myocardial infarction (MI) and coronary events by 27%. It has also been demonstrated that 80% of older adults with an SBP of 140 to 159 mm Hg will develop an SBP greater than 160 mm Hg (Sadowski and Redeker, 1996). This has changed the theory of treating older persons more cautiously for hypertension; they should receive the same treatment as others to prevent complications.

Diet. An elevated serum cholesterol level is a major risk factor for coronary heart disease in both men and women. A total cholesterol level of 150 mg/dl is where atherosclerosis begins to accelerate. The average American's cholesterol level is around 200 to 210 mg/dl (LaRosa, 1996). As the cholesterol level rises, so does cardiac risk for the individual. It has been shown that for every 1% reduction of total cholesterol, there is a 2% reduction in cardiac risk (Arnstein et al, 1996). A cholesterol level below 200 mg/dl is optimum. A woman has a nine times greater chance of experiencing a recurrent MI with a cholesterol level of 275 mg/dl or higher than with a cholesterol level below 200 mg/dl. In the Framingham Heart Study, men had a four times greater risk of developing a second MI if their cholesterol levels were above 275 mg/dl (LaRosa, 1996). Even if symptoms of atherosclerosis and coronary heart disease are evident, lowering cholesterol levels is beneficial. Lowering cholesterol in these individuals can reduce the chance of another coronary event as much as by one third (LaRosa, 1996).

The serum levels of low-density lipoprotein (LDL) and high-density lipoprotein (HDL) are also important to monitor. LDL carries cholesterol to the walls of the arteries (a positive risk factor), and HDL represents the cholesterol being carried from the cells (a negative risk factor). An optimum LDL level is below 130 mg/dl; an optimum HDL level is over 45 mg/dl for men and 55 mg/dl for women (McDonald, 2003).

The Third National Health and Nutrition Examination Survey (NHANES III) found that over one third of Americans between ages 65 and 74 have total cholesterol levels of 240 mg/dl or higher. However, a high cholesterol level in later life may not be a good indicator of cardiac risk. The highest mortality in older women was found in those with total cholesterol levels below 200 mg/dl. The Framington study indicates that the cholesterol level at age 50 is a better predictor of cardiac disease at age 70 than the cholesterol level at age 70 (Grandjean and Talbott, 1997).

Decreasing fat content in the diet is the first step in reducing cholesterol levels. The American Heart Association's (AHA's) Step I diet provides 30% or less total calories from fat. No more than 10% of calories should originate from saturated fat, and no more than 300 mg of cholesterol per day should be consumed. More stringent restrictions may decrease an older person's consumption of adequate minerals and vitamins and usually are not recommended.

Smoking. Smoking continues to be a major risk factor in the development of heart disease. Although there has been a decline in the use of tobacco, largely as a result of health promotion campaigns, clean air environments, and peer pressure, 30% of all deaths are still attributed to smoking. Cigarette smokers have twice the chance of contracting CAD and four times the chance of sudden death compared with nonsmokers (Keller and Lemberg, 1996). Smoking increases platelet aggregation and causes coronary artery spasm. Nicotine increases blood pressure and cardiac demands. Carbon monoxide in tobacco smoke decreases the oxygen-carrying capacity of the blood. Smoking is a significant cardiac risk factor.

Smoking a few cigarettes a day greatly increases cardiac risk. The Nurse Health Study found that nurses who smoked one to four cigarettes a day had 2.5 times the risk of fatal coronary heart disease and nonfatal MI (Keller and Lemberg, 1996). Smoking cessation decreases the risk of MI. After 10 years of abstinence, an individual's risk is the same as for a nonsmoker. Smoking cessation should be encouraged at every encounter. The Agency for Health Care Policy and Research has established recommendations for smoking cessation (see Chapter 24 for smoking cessation information).

Physical Activity. A sedentary lifestyle is another modifiable cardiac risk factor. A sedentary lifestyle accounts for more than 25,000 deaths per year (Maron and Rader, 1998). Aerobic exercise such as brisk walking raises HDL levels, lowers LDL levels, decreases blood pressure, increases well-being, and decreases stress (Halm and Penque, 1999). The AHA recommends 30 minutes of moderate-intensity exercise four or five times a week. Health care professionals should encourage clients to exercise and promote ways to increase activity with daily routines, such as parking the car a little farther from the store, using the stairs to go up or down one floor, or walking to the post office if it is close enough. It is recommended that anyone beginning an exercise program should first consult a physician for guidelines.

Older adults should begin an exercise program with a 10- to 15-minute warm-up to achieve 75% of their maximum heart rate safely. Too many people want to progress too quickly, which increases their chance for injuries. Walking is the best aerobic exercise for older adults. They can set their own pace, decide the location, and avoid injuries. When beginning an exercise program, older adults should start with 5 to 10 minutes 2 or 3 times a week and gradually increase to the recommended 30 minutes 4 or 5 times a week (Stone, Wyman, and Salisbury, 1999).

Obesity. Obesity is another modifiable cardiac risk factor. Obesity is usually associated with a sedentary lifestyle and a high-fat diet, which add to the individual's cardiac risk profile. The HANES III data show that more than 65 million Americans have a body mass index (BMI) over 25. BMI is calculated by kg/m^2. Recommended guidelines are a BMI of 21 to 25. A BMI of 25 to 30 is considered overweight, and a BMI over 30 is considered obese (Maron and Rader, 1998). Weight reduction aids in decreasing blood pressure, an added benefit for a hypertensive adult.

Diabetes. In the Framingham study, individuals with diabetes mellitus were twice as likely to die from cardiovascular causes. The study also showed that those with diabetes mellitus had more extensive cardiac disease at a younger age than those without (Burrell, Gerlach, and Pless, 1997). Silent MI is more common in individuals with diabetes mellitus and in older adults. Thus older adults with diabetes should be monitored closely for other symptoms of CVD.

Stress. At one time, stress was thought to be associated with the type A behavior of the goal- and task-oriented high achiever. This belief is now being modified, and researchers are examining the individual's adaptation to stress from other perspectives, such as anger control; support by family, friends, and significant others; and the means by which individuals cope with stress.

There are many ways of decreasing stress, and much literature is available on the topic. Yoga, meditation, relaxation tapes, visualization, and physical activity are a few of the methods used. It is imperative that research continue to examine the effects of stress on those ages 65 and older and that nurses examine factors in the client's environment that are amenable to change. For example, an older client may not be able to prepare meals because of physical limitations or safety reasons. Referral to a Meals on Wheels program or a community-based program in which individuals share meals is just one example of simple modification. Older individuals living in an apartment, sharing their meals, and dividing tasks of shopping, meal preparation, and clean-up are other popular concepts. This way, older clients can maintain balanced diets and enjoy the companionship of peers.

Hormone Usage. The effects of estrogen on the development of heart disease are still being debated in the literature. Studies have shown the benefit of hormone replacement therapy in postmenopausal women for protection against osteoporosis. The Women's Health Initiative results (http://www.nhlbi.nih.gov/whi/index.html) showed that combination hormone replacement therapy increased the risk of ischemic stroke and coronary heart disease. Other findings include more cases of breast cancer that is at an advanced stage at the time of diagnosis. Hormone replacement therapy is effective for short-term use for management of moderate to severe symptoms of menopause, primarily hot flashes, night sweats, and vaginal dryness. Nurses play an essential role in educating clients regarding risk factors and lifestyle changes (Aschenbrenner, 2004) (see Research box).

Research

SAMPLE/SETTING

Five hundred participants from a telemetry unit were randomly assigned to an intervention group (247 subjects) or a control group (253 subjects).

METHODS

During the initial hospitalization the control group was given the standard discharge instructions of medication information and follow-up appointment without additional teaching. The intervention group was given the standard discharge instructions and viewed a video with written information and a copy of the patient's latest ECG. The patients were given instructions to place the information near their phone and to bring their ECG to their next follow-up visit or emergency department visit.

FINDINGS

The researchers found no significant difference for the three outcome variables between the control and intervention group. The three outcome variables were percentage of patients who came during the first hour from symptom onset, percentage of patients using emergency medical services, and the median time interval from symptom onset to emergency department arrival during the return visit.

APPLICATIONS

Patient teaching should be a continuous process rather than a one-time event, such as at the time of hospital discharge. Teaching should be reinforced at every opportunity. The goal of patient teaching should be to provide information and change behavior.

Blank FS, Smithline HA: Evaluation of an educational video for cardiac patients, *Clin Nurs Res* 11(4):403, 2002.

Hypertension

Hypertension has been termed the *silent killer,* since much of the population with high blood pressure is unaware of having this condition, despite the availability of advanced screening programs. The detection and treatment of hypertension have increased over the years. But in spite of this, the incidence of complications of hypertension has not decreased. These complications include stroke, end-stage renal failure, and heart failure (Miller, 1999).

Prevention of hypertension is a realistic goal, based on improving the average blood pressure in the general population. The tools available to accomplish this lifesaving goal are contained in a large body of evidence, which has increased greatly in the past two decades and implicates key aspects of modern lifestyle in the epidemic of hypertension. Adoption of a healthier lifestyle, starting in childhood and youth, can prevent and reverse abnormal blood pressure patterns.

Hypertension is the most commonplace CVD in the United States today. Blood pressure and pulse pressure increase progressively with age. According to Framingham data, adults at age 55 with normal blood pressures have an estimated 90% lifetime risk for developing hypertension (Vasan et al, 2002). Blood pressure screening must be done during every health care encounter with an older adult to detect hypertension and prevent its complications.

Hypertension stage 1 is classified as SBP of 140 to 159 mm Hg and DBP of 90 to 99 mm Hg; it indicates the necessity of taking antihypertensive medications. The JNC (2003) has adopted hypertension guidelines and reclassified the disease into several categories (Table 23-1).

The diagnosis is made after at least two subsequent visits after the initial visit. Blood pressure is measured with the client supine or sitting, and then standing (except for those clients whose SBP is greater than 210 mm Hg and DBP is greater than 120 mm Hg; these individuals are deemed to have high blood pressure after one visit).

The JNC (2003) recommends that blood pressure be monitored as follows:

- In 1 week if the client is in stage 2 hypertension
- In 1 month if the client is in stage 1 hypertension
- In 1 year if SBP is 120 to 139 mm Hg and DBP is 80 to 89 mm Hg, which is considered the prehypertension stage
- In 2 years if SBP is below 120 mm Hg and DBP is below 80 mm Hg, which is considered normal

ISH is more common in older adults, as SBP rises disproportionately to DBP because of increased arterial stiffness and rigidity. In the past, it was argued that hypertension was a normal process of aging and did not require therapy. However, data from the Framingham Heart Study confirm that cardiovascular risk escalates dramatically in older adults. The addition of risk factors such as smoking, glucose intolerance, hypercholesterolemia, and left ventricular hypertrophy significantly elevates risk.

TABLE 23-1 Classification of Blood Pressure

CATEGORY	SYSTOLIC (mm Hg)		DIASTOLIC (mm Hg)
Normal	<120	and	<80
Prehypertension	120–139	or	80–89
Stage 1 hypertension	140-159	or	90-99
Stage 2 hypertension	≥160	or	≥100
Stage 3	>180	or	>110

From Joint National Committee: *The seventh report of the Joint National Committee on the Prevention, Detection, Evaluation, and Treatment of High Blood Pressure,* 2003. Accessed on website: http://www.nhlbi.nih.gov/guidelines/hypertension/index.htm.

The phenomenon of pseudohypertension—falsely elevated blood pressure—is found in the older adult population. Pseudohypertension is a result of the calcification and thickening of the arterial wall. Rigidity in the brachial artery leads to ineffective compression of the brachial artery with a sphygmomanometer. Pseudohypertension may be suspected without evidence of target organ damage despite elevated blood pressure readings, or if hypotensive symptoms develop with therapy while blood pressure readings remain high. Osler's maneuver is a screening test for pseudohypertension. It is performed by palpating the brachial or radial artery after inflating the sphygmomanometer above the systolic pressure. A positive Osler's reveals a palpable pulse (Lookinland and Beckstrand, 2003).

Hypertension has been classified into two types: primary and secondary. Primary hypertension is the most common form. Although the exact cause is unknown, the contributing factors are family history, age, race, diet (e.g., foods high in saturated fats and salt; decreased potassium, magnesium, and calcium intake), smoking, stress, alcohol and drug consumption, physical activity, and hormonal intake.

Secondary hypertension refers to elevated blood pressure caused by underlying disease such as renal artery disease, renal parenchymal disorders, endocrine and metabolic disorders, central nervous system (CNS) disorders, coarctation of the aorta, and increased intravascular volume.

All prescription and over-the-counter medications need to be assessed for possible causes of elevated blood pressure. Drug-induced hypertension has occurred with the administration of amphetamines and glucocorticoids. Decongestants, phenobarbital, rifampin, and nonsteroidal antiinflammatory drugs (NSAIDs) may adversely affect the action of some medications for hypertension. NSAIDs have been found to cause elevated blood pressure in normotensive older adults (Tucker, 2003). Many older adults are taking NSAIDs for various musculoskeletal problems. These individuals should have their blood pressure closely monitored.

A positive correlation exists between obesity and high blood pressure. Advancing age is associated with a loss of lean body mass and an increase in adipose tissue. Excess fat in the upper body or a waist circumference of 35 inches or greater in women or 40 inches or greater in men increases the risk for hypertension. Metabolic syndrome includes abdominal obesity, glucose intolerance, high triglycerides, and a low HDL. A 10% reduction of total weight will decrease blood pressure in many overweight individuals. This factor has significance, since it underscores the importance of weight reduction in the older adult population (JNC 7, 2003).

Research data have correlated increased sodium intake and high blood pressure. It has been shown that a reduction in sodium to 100 mmol/day may reduce SBP 2 to 8 mm Hg. The DASH diet can reduce systolic blood pressure 8 to 14 mm Hg. These results were higher in older adults and those with increased blood pressure (JNC 7, 2003).

The pathophysiology of hypertension is complex, since various environmental, structural, renal, hormonal, and homeostatic mechanisms contribute to blood pressure maintenance, especially in the aging population. A detailed description of the mechanisms involved is outside the scope of this text.

Hypertension has been associated with arteriolar thickening, vascular smooth muscle constriction, and elevated vascular resistance. With age, peripheral vascular resistance elevates significantly. It is also possible that functional changes in the vascular smooth muscle contribute to these changes. The alpha-adrenergic responsiveness of the vascular smooth muscle does not change with age; however, the beta-adrenergic responsiveness declines with age with a consequent decrease in the relaxation of the vascular smooth muscle. There also appears to be increased renal vascular resistance and lower renal blood flow. Left ventricular hypertrophy occurs as an adaptation to longstanding hypertension and may lead to CHF. Once this occurs, there is a significant increase in cardiovascular risk, particularly for ventricular arrhythmia and sudden death.

In mild to moderate hypertension the client may be asymptomatic. As the disease progresses, the client may experience fatigue, dizziness, headache, vertigo, and palpitations. In severe hypertension the client may experience throbbing occipital headache, confusion, visual loss, focal deficits, epistaxis, and coma.

It is imperative that the practitioner assess for other target organ damage and symptoms. Hypertension may lead to damage in various organs, resulting in the following conditions:

- Heart: CHF, ventricular hypertrophy, angina, MI, sudden death
- CNS: transient ischemic attack, stroke
- Peripheral vessels: PVD, aneurysm
- Renal: serum creatinine greater than 133 mmol/L (1.5 mg/dl), proteinuria, microalbuminuria
- Eye: hemorrhage or exudates, with or without papilledema

The diagnostic tests and procedures search for secondary causes of hypertension and assess for end-target organ damage. In assessments for comorbidity, older adults are likely to have coexisting cardiac, vascular, and renal disease.

The health care provider should obtain a history regarding lifestyle factors and conduct an in-depth physical examination. The following tests should be included: hemoglobin and hematocrit to exclude anemia or polycythemia; urinalysis to investigate for proteinuria or other signs of renal failure; serum sodium, potassium, and creatinine; fasting plasma glucose, since diabetes mellitus is a cardiac risk factor that maybe affected by antihypertensive therapy; serum total cholesterol and HDL to assess for hyperlipidemia; ECG; chest x-ray study; and possibly echocardiogram to assess left ventricular function and hypertrophy.

The physical examination should include examination of the following: neck to detect carotid bruits, jugular vein distention, or enlarged thyroid; heart to detect abnormalities in rate and rhythm, heaves, lifts, murmurs, and third or fourth heart sounds; lungs to detect rales; abdomen to detect bruits, masses, and aortic pulsations; and extremities to detect peripheral pulses and edema.

Pharmacologic Treatment. One of the most important considerations in drug therapy in older adults is that blood pressure should be lowered gradually, beginning with low doses of a single agent. The various steps involved in treatment of blood pressure include:

1. Use nonpharmacologic interventions and lifestyle modifications. Older adults respond to modest sodium reduction and weight loss.
2. Select an appropriate agent with consideration for comorbidity. Diuretics and beta-blockers are first-line medications based on clinical trials.
3. Increase the dose of the first drug, and then add a second drug of a different class or substitute a drug from another class.
4. Continue adding agents from other classes. Consider referral to a hypertensive specialist.

The general principles for managing high blood pressure in older clients include the following:

- The goal of treatment is a blood pressure less than 120/80 mm Hg. For those with significant systolic hypertension, an interim goal of less than 160/90 mm Hg may be necessary. (The results of the Hypertensive Optimal Treatment Study were released after the JNC's *Seventh Report on Prevention, Detection, Evaluation, and Treatment of High Blood Pressure.*)
- ISH (SBP over 160 mm Hg and DBP of 85 to 90 mm Hg) should be treated.
- Older adults are more likely to experience an orthostatic drop in blood pressure than younger adults. Blood pressure should always be taken with the client both sitting and standing.
- When pharmacologic therapy is used, the initial daily dose should be half that recommended for middle-aged adults.
- Thiazide diuretics or beta-blockers in combination with a thiazide (e.g., atenolol [Tenormin] with hydrochlorothiazide) are recommended because they decrease morbidity and mortality.
- Diuretics are preferred for ISH.
- The choice of an alternative first- or second-step drug should be based on the client's individual characteristics.
- After blood pressure has been controlled for 1 year, the dosage of the drug should be stepped down if possible.

The use of antihypertensive drugs has been shown to be effective and well tolerated in older adults. The prescription is "to proceed slowly and with caution" and to monitor for adverse reactions. If this principle is adhered to, older adults can be treated with minimal side effects. Table 23-2 provides the classifications of antihypertensive drugs, their adverse effects, and the nursing implications.

Diuretics. The thiazide diuretics hydrochlorothiazide and chlorthalidone continue to be the most commonly prescribed antihypertensive agents for older adults. The initial dosage should be 12.5 to 25 mg/day. Loop diuretics, such as furosemide, are not used unless the client has renal impairment or CHF.

The primary concern related to diuretic therapy is hypotension or hypokalemia. Clients should be carefully monitored for hypokalemia. If hypokalemia becomes difficult to manage, an alternate antihypertensive agent is indicated. Hypomagnesemia, hyperglycemia, and increased uric acid may also occur. Increases in blood glucose are generally minor with low doses of a thiazide diuretic.

Beta-Blockers. Beta-blockers are effective in lowering morbidity and mortality in older adults. Beta-adrenergic blockage decreases heart rate and contractility. This decreases cardiac output and is cardioprotective. Atenolol and metoprolol are beta-blockers that are cardioselective. They may be better tolerated in older adults with lung disease or PVD.

Angiotensin-Converting Enzyme Inhibitors. Angiotensin-converting enzyme inhibitors (ACEIs) inhibit the converting enzyme that is responsible for the formation of angiotensin II, a potent vasoconstrictor that stimulates the release of aldosterone. These drugs decrease mortality in older adults with decreased left ventricular function and preserve renal function in those with diabetes mellitus. Side effects of these drugs include rash, cough, taste disturbance, neutropenia, and proteinuria. ACEIs should not be used if acute renal failure or bilateral renal artery stenosis is suspected.

Calcium Channel Blockers. Calcium channel blockers inhibit the inward movement of calcium across the cell membrane of the vascular smooth muscle, which results in vasodilation of peripheral, coronary, and renal arteries. They may cause orthostatic hypotension in older adults. These drugs typically have vasodilator effects such as headache, flushing, dizziness, and weakness. Constipation may also occur. Calcium channel blockers are useful agents in the treatment of older adults and can be used when diuretics are not tolerated or are contraindicated.

Prognosis. Hypertension, if unrecognized and untreated, significantly increases the risk of coronary disease, heart and renal failure, and stroke. Risk increases with smoking, glucose intolerance, hyperlipidemia, left ventricular hypertrophy, male

TABLE 23-2 Classification of Antihypertensive Drugs, Adverse Effects, and Nursing Implications

ANTIHYPERTENSIVE DRUG	ADVERSE EFFECTS	NURSING IMPLICATIONS
DIURETICS		
Thiazides		
Chlorothiazide (Diuril) Chlorthalidone Hydrochlorothiazide (Microzide, HydroDIURIL) Polythiazide (Renese) Indapamide (Lozol) Metolazone (Zaroxolyn)	Hyperglycemia Hypokalemia Hypomagnesemia Hyponatremia Hyperuricemia Hypercholesterolemia Sexual dysfunction Photosensitivity Hypersensitivity to sulfonamides	Diabetics may require an increase in insulin. Encourage clients to restrict sodium intake and eat foods high in potassium. Check baseline and later levels of LDL and HDL, cholesterol, and triglycerides. Report dry mouth, muscle weakness, cramps, drowsiness, and loss of appetite, which may be indicative of electrolyte imbalance. Be cautious in sunlight.
Loop Diuretics		
Bumetanide (Bumex) Furosemide (Lasix) Torsemide (Demadex)	Fluid electrolyte imbalance Diuresis leading to hypovolemia, hypotension, and shock May cause thromboembolism in older clients	Observe for signs of dehydration and acid-base imbalance. Monitor blood pressure to detect signs and symptoms of shock. Observe for signs and symptoms of thromboembolism.
Potassium-Sparing Diuretics		
Amiloride (Midamor) Triamterene (Dyrenium)	Hyperkalemia May cause breast pain and amenorrhea in women May cause renal calculi Impotence, sexual dysfunction	Monitor serum potassium levels. Potassium supplements should be discontinued when these drugs are added to sulfonamide diuretic regimen. Triamterene should be given cautiously to clients taking indomethacin.
Aldosterone Receptor Blockers		
Eplerenone (Inspra) Spironolactone (Aldactone)	Hyperkalemia GI bleeding or ulceration	Monitor electrolytes. Use K diuretics sparingly. Do not give NSAIDs.
BETA-BLOCKERS		
Atenolol (Tenormin) Betaxolol (Kerlone) Bisoprolol (Zebeta) Metoprolol (Lopressor) Metoprolol extended release (Toprol XL) Nadolol (Corgard) Propranolol (Inderal) Propranolol long-acting (Inderal LA) Timolol (Blocadren)	Cardiac effects, including bradycardia and heart block Dizziness and fainting Fatigue, weakness, lethargy, depression, disorientation, and hallucinations Sexual dysfunction Nausea, vomiting Bronchospasm in clients with asthma May mask hypoglycemia May aggravate peripheral vascular insufficiency	Report bradycardia and episodes of dizziness and syncope. Do not administer drugs to clients in heart failure or with advanced degrees of heart block. Observe client for any changes in physical and mental status. Check LDL and HDL, triglyceride, and cholesterol levels. Instruct clients to never abruptly discontinue the drug.
BETA-BLOCKERS WITH INTRINSIC SYMPATHOMIMETIC ACTIVITY		
Acebutolol (Sectral) Penbutolol (Levatol) Pindolol	Fatigue, dizziness, headache, urinary frequency May mask hypoglycemia or hyperthyroidism Constipation, diarrhea Insomnia Safety concerns Bradycardia, edema, weight gain, hypotension, syncope, atrioventricular block Diarrhea, nausea, hyperglycemia, abnormal vision, dyspnea	Avoid abrupt discontinuation of medication Monitor weight, blood sugar, and vital signs.

TABLE 23-2 Classification of Antihypertensive Drugs, Adverse Effects, and Nursing Implications—cont'd

ANTIHYPERTENSIVE DRUG	ADVERSE EFFECTS	NURSING IMPLICATIONS
COMBINED ALPHA- AND BETA-BLOCKERS		
Carvedilol (Coreg) Labetalol (Normodyne, Trandate)	Fatigue, dizziness, postural hypotension, muscle weakness, diarrhea or constipation	Avoid driving during initial administration. Take with food. Report any new cough that continues. Report any unusual swelling of extremities.
ACEIs		
Benazepril (Lotensin) Captopril (Capoten) Enalapril (Vasotec) Fosinopril (Monopril) Lisinopril (Prinivil, Zestril) Moexipril (Univasc) Perindopril (Aceon) Quinapril (Accupril) Ramipril (Altace) Trandolapril (Mavik)	Tickle in throat or hacking cough Hyperkalemia Rash Reversible renal failure in clients with proteinuria or renal artery stenosis Dizziness, headache, diarrhea, and fatigue Impaired sense of taste and sexual dysfunction rare	Observe clients for cough. Check electrolytes for increase in potassium. Observe for rash. Check for increase in BUN or serum creatinine. Observe for signs of dizziness, headache, and diarrhea.
ANGIOTENSIN II ANTAGONISTS		
Candesartan (Atacand) Eprosartan (Tevetan) Irbesartan (Avapro) Losartan (Cozaar) Olmesartan (Benicar) Telmisartan (Micardis) Valsartan (Diovan)	Dizziness, cough, upper respiratory infection, diarrhea, fatigue, and headache Edema, flushing, palpitations, and dizziness Safety concerns May increase angina or myocardial infarction	Monitor renal function. Instruct client to avoid alcohol, barbiturates, and narcotics. Adjust insulin and antidiabetic medications, which potentiate hydrochlorothiazide, headaches, and dizziness. Potentiated by grapefruit juice. Avoid beta-blockers, digitalis, and diuretics. Do not crush. Monitor liver studies in older clients.
CALCIUM CHANNEL BLOCKERS		
Nondihydropyridines		
Diltiazem extended release (Cardizem CD, Cardizem LA, Dilacor XR, Tiazac) Verapamil immediate release (Calan, Isoptin) Verapamil extended release (Calan SR, Isoptin SR) Verapamil–Coer (Covera-HS, Verelan PM)	Headache, dizziness, flushing, and weakness Bradycardia Edema Nausea Constipation (especially with verapamil) Gingival hyperplasia	Monitor heart rate. Monitor blood pressure during dose adjustment. Check laboratory results to assess liver and kidney function.
Dihydropyridines		
Amlodipine (Norvasc) Felodipine (Plendil) Isradipine extended release (DynaCirc CR) Nicardipine sustained release (Cardene SR) Nifedipine long-acting (Adalat CC, Procardia XL) Nisoldipine (Sular)	Edema, fatigue, palpitations, dizziness, abdominal pain, GI upset, flushing Drowsiness	Monitor for hepatic dysfunction, CVD, and/or aortic stenosis

Continued

TABLE 23-2 Classification of Antihypertensive Drugs, Adverse Effects, and Nursing Implications—cont'd

ANTIHYPERTENSIVE DRUG	ADVERSE EFFECTS	NURSING IMPLICATIONS
ALPHA$_1$-BLOCKERS		
Doxazosin (Cardura) Prazosin (Minipress) Terazosin (Hytrin)	Syncope with first dose, dizziness, fatigue, edema, rhinitis, tinnitus, epistaxis, sexual dysfunction, polyuria, urinary incontinence, ataxia, leucopenia, neutropenia, arrhythmia, somnolence, rash, red eyes, dry mouth	Impaired liver function, dose changes Check orthostatic blood pressure Limit ETOH Pregnancy
CENTRAL ALPHA$_2$-AGONISTS AND OTHER CENTRALLY ACTING DRUGS		
Clonidine (Catapres) Clonidine patch (Catapres-TTS) Methylodopa (Aldomet) Reserpine Guanfacine	Dry mouth, drowsiness, dizziness, weakness, constipation, rash, myalgia, urticaria, nausea, insomnia, agitation, orthostatic hypotension, impotence, arrhythmias	Severe coronary disease Recent MI CVD, renal failure Taper Do not stop abruptly
DIRECT VASODILATORS		
Hydralazine (Apresoline) Minoxidil (Loniten)		

Adapted from Joint National Committee: *The seventh report of the Joint National Committee on the Prevention, Detection, Evaluation, and Treatment of High Blood Pressure*, 2003. Accessed on website: http://www.nhlbi.nih.gov/guidelines/hypertension/index.htm; and Tierney LM, McPhee SJ, Papadakis MA: *Current medical diagnosis and treatment*, ed 43, New York, 2004, McGraw-Hill.

gender, black race, and increasing age. With an individual pharmacologic and nonpharmacologic treatment program based on assessment of total cardiovascular risk, the risk of cardiovascular-related death from stroke and heart attack can be reduced. The degree of end-organ damage affects overall morbidity and mortality (JNC, 1997).

NURSING MANAGEMENT

 Assessment

The majority of clients with hypertension are asymptomatic. Symptoms that do occur are variable depending on the progression of disease on target organs. Vague discomfort, fatigue, headache, epistaxis, and dizziness may be early indicators. Severe hypertension may result in a throbbing occipital headache—particularly prevalent in the morning but disappearing several hours later—as well as confusion, vision loss, focal deficits, and coma. Symptoms of heart failure, such as dyspnea, may be present. If the kidneys are affected, hematuria or nocturia may occur.

Objective data include a thorough assessment of blood pressure on three separate occasions. Blood pressure readings, both sitting and standing, should be recorded. The client's arms should be bared and supported at heart level. The nurse should instruct the client not to ingest caffeine or smoke for 30 minutes before the blood pressure reading. The proper cuff size must be used. The bladder of the cuff should surround a minimum of 80% of the arm. Many older individuals will require a large cuff. If these steps are not taken, blood pressure readings may be inaccurate.

 Diagnosis

Nursing diagnoses for an older adult client with hypertension include:

- Knowledge deficit: hypertension and self-care management related to new diagnosis and interventions
- Ineffective individual coping related to perceived limitations of diagnosis
- Ineffective management of therapeutic regimen related to lack of knowledge of diagnosis
- Altered nutrition: more than body requirements related to high fat, caloric, and sodium intake

Planning and Expected Outcomes

Expected outcomes for an older client with hypertension include:

1. Client will identify personal risk factors.
2. Client will explain the disease process and its effects on health and well-being.
3. Client will incorporate nonpharmacologic treatment measures into daily living.
4. Client will verbalize purpose, dose, action, and significant and reportable side effects of medications prescribed for hypertension.
5. Client will increase social interaction, as evidenced by participation with others in activities outside the home 2 or 3 times a week.
6. Client will eat a low-fat, low-cholesterol, and reduced-calorie diet, as evidenced by weight loss of 1 to 2 lb a week.

Intervention

Knowledge levels vary among hypertensive clients. The teaching plan should incorporate an explanation of the disease process and therapeutic (nonpharmacologic and pharmacologic) interventions. An explanation of the physical examination and appropriate tests should be given to allay anxiety. Anxiety, depression, denial, and fear are often involved with a chronic condition. Although these emotions diminish as the condition is controlled, the client's ability to absorb this information and make the required changes is initially hampered because the client may still be in denial. For older adults, participation in a Hearts for Life program using videotapes and handouts with large print may be beneficial.

Client education includes providing information regarding the disease process; signs and symptoms of hypertension; treatment regimen; medications and their actions and side effects, including sexual impotence; and the need for frequent monitoring of blood pressure and risk factors. The nurse should explain the importance of a low-sodium, high-potassium, low-fat, reduced-calorie diet. Weight loss should be encouraged if indicated. A dietitian may assist with meal planning, preparation, and label reading. Foods are healthier if prepared by baking, broiling, or steaming. The nurse should also discuss the importance of alcohol restriction and smoking cessation; explain the relationship between stress, anxiety, anger, and hypertension; identify stressful situations at the client's home and work; and teach meditation and relaxation techniques. Exercise is beneficial for weight and stress reduction. Initially, the client should walk 10 to 15 minutes a day, gradually increasing to 1-hour walks 3 or 4 times a week. Other activities include mall-walking and water aerobics. Encourage the client to reduce or eliminate smoking through a smoking cessation program. Therapeutic medications and aids are available. Other alternatives for smoking cessation include hypnotism or behavior modification. Positive reinforcement should be provided whenever possible.

Evaluation

Evaluation consists of determining the client's achievement of the expected outcomes. The client's blood pressure should decrease and return to optimum levels. The client should be able to maintain the treatment plan without side effects and demonstrate no evidence of complications. Outcome measures related to quality of life are also important because of the chronic nature of hypertension. The nurse must determine the client's perception of any change in quality of life resulting from the prescribed therapeutic regimen. Documentation includes accurate records of blood pressure, weight, exercise, and activity patterns; 24-hour dietary intake; cholesterol levels; and any blood pressure monitoring results outside of the clinical encounter.

Coronary Artery Disease

CAD, or ischemic heart disease, refers to a broad group of conditions that partially or completely obstruct blood flow to the heart muscle. Obstruction of coronary arteries can result in ischemia (an imbalance between the oxygen supply and demands of the heart) or infarction (death or necrosis) of the myocardium. Ischemia and infarction occur when the oxygen supply is unable to meet the demands of the heart. Atherosclerosis is the usual cause of CAD; angina, MI, and sudden death may be the final outcomes.

Atherosclerosis usually begins in childhood and is characterized by a local accumulation of lipid and fibrous tissue along the intimal layer of the artery. Lipids accumulate and infiltrate the area, forming a raised fibrous plaque over the site. Eventually the plaque becomes calcified, which causes the vessel to lose its elasticity and dilatory qualities. Progressive narrowing of the artery occurs, resulting in compromised blood flow to the area of myocardium supplied by that vessel. In advanced stages of the disease, hemorrhage into the atheromatous plaque, thrombus formation, embolization of a thrombus or plaque fragment, and coronary arterial spasm can cause additional insult to the body. Although the development of atherosclerosis appears to be a normal process of aging, the severity of this process can be accelerated with the adverse lifestyle behaviors of smoking, physical inactivity, and obesity, as well as elevated serum cholesterol levels, hypertension, and diabetes mellitus. Promoting healthy lifestyles in younger and older individuals is an important aspect of care in the prevention of CAD. The adoption of healthier lifestyles by an older adult may be difficult because of long-term habits; however, healthy behavior changes can slow or halt the progression of the disease.

CAD is the major cause of morbidity, disability, and mortality in the older adult population. Coronary alterations are more likely to create a "cardiac cripple" in the older adult than other disease processes (Ebersole, Hess, and Luggen, 2004).

Angina is caused by an inadequate blood flow to the myocardium. The classic symptom is chest pain with activity that is relieved with rest or nitroglycerin. MI is caused by total disruption of blood flow to the myocardium; it is characterized by more severe, more intense chest pain for a longer time than that associated with angina. Other symptoms that may accompany MI include nausea, diaphoresis, shortness of breath, dizziness, and weakness.

An older adult may not exhibit CAD and its sequelae like younger adults. Many times an older adult does not have the typical chest pain. Diminished activity level compared with younger adults is one reason for this. Neuropathies and changes in pain recognition in older adults also limit the use of chest pain as a diagnostic sign for older adults (Stone, Wyman, and Salisbury, 1999). However, other symptoms may occur as the initial symptoms in older adults (Box 23-2). Women, especially older women, may not exhibit the classic

BOX 23-2 Symptoms Associated With Atypical Presentation of Coronary Artery Disease in Older Adults

Shortness of breath
Fatigue
Syncope
Confusion
Abdominal or back pain

signs of CAD, and the nurse needs to be aware of this to adequately assess female clients.

Because symptoms of angina or MI may be vague and atypical of "textbook" symptoms, older adults may not recognize their seriousness and may not seek medical attention as soon as they should. Their family may not think the symptoms are as serious as they are. This may cause a delay in seeking medical attention. Unrecognized MI may cause cardiac damage and precipitate complications of heart failure and pulmonary edema (Stone, Wyman, and Salisbury, 1999).

Diagnostic Tests and Procedures. Diagnosis is based on client history, alterations on the ECG, and serum cardiac enzyme levels.

- Serum cardiac enzymes of creatinine phosphokinase (CPK). Serum CPK values rise shortly after infarction as a result of myocardial damage, peak at 24 hours, and return to normal levels within 72 hours (Murphy and Berding, 1999). Cardiac-specific isoenzymes confirm a diagnosis of MI.
- Cardiac troponin levels (a component of the myocardium). Levels elevate when infarction causes cell membrane permeability changes. Cardiac troponin T increases 3 to 5 hours after MI and remains elevated for 14 to 21 days. Cardiac troponin I elevates within 3 hours, peaks at 14 to 18 hours, and remains elevated for 5 to 7 days (Murphy and Berding, 1999).
- ECG to obtain information on rate, rhythm, hypertrophy, and myocardial injury (ischemia or infarction); and to assess for Q waves, ST segment elevation, ST segment depression, and T wave inversion.
- Complete blood count (CBC) to determine whether angina is caused by anemia.
- Serum electrolytes, particularly sodium, potassium, and calcium. Elevated or reduced levels of these electrolytes can lead to fluid imbalance, ventricular arrhythmias, or asystole.
- Chest x-ray examination to determine overall size, shape, and position of the heart. In older adults, however, an echocardiogram may be superior in assessing cardiac chamber size and ventricular function.
- Myocardial imaging (using thallium), multiple-gated acquisition cardiac pool imaging, or digital subtraction angiography to evaluate myocardial perfusion or ventricular abnormalities.
- Cardiac catheterization to detect the presence, location, and extent of lesions in coronary arteries.
- Exercise stress test to determine activity tolerance. Stress tests can be combined with myocardial imaging to identify changes in myocardial perfusion during exercise. An exercise stress test can be troublesome for older adults with coexisting diseases such as arthritis, PVD, and chronic obstructive pulmonary disease (COPD). Pharmacologic stress tests may be a better choice in these older individuals (Flack et al, 1998).
- Holter monitor or echocardiogram for older adults who may not tolerate test completion because of debilitating conditions such as musculoskeletal or CNS impairments (Stone, Wyman, and Salisbury, 1999).

Pharmacologic Treatment. Treatment is directed toward restoring the balance between myocardial oxygen demand and oxygen supply for the prevention of CAD. Pharmacologic agents play a major role. Normal changes with aging (e.g., alterations in body mass, water composition, liver size, renal system, and plasma protein concentration) tend to increase the concentration and prolong the excretion of standard drug doses, so smaller doses are generally prescribed for older adults (Flack et al, 1998).

Nitrates. Nitrates are used for the prevention and termination of anginal attacks and for reducing the pain associated with myocardial ischemia. These agents decrease the preload and afterload of the circulatory system, which reduces the myocardial demand for oxygen because of the vasodilating effects on coronary arteries and peripheral vessels. Intravenous, sublingual, and aerosol preparations have a rapid onset of action (1 to 3 minutes) and are used to prevent or terminate an anginal attack. Daily doses of oral or dermal preparations have a prolonged and continual onset of action and are used to prevent anginal attacks; however, tolerance to these preparations reduces drug effectiveness, and periods of discontinuation are recommended. Headache, flushing, dizziness, hypotension, syncope, and tachycardia are side effects attributed to the vasodilating effects. Nitrates are effective in older adults; however, aggressive therapy to reduce the preload and afterload may trigger reflex tachycardia and severe orthostatic hypotension. Older adults should take rapid-acting nitrates in the sitting or lying position to prevent falls (Lehne et al, 1998). Older adults with predictable angina (i.e., with a specific activity) can take sublingual nitroglycerin before the activity to increase exercise capacity (Flack et al, 1998).

Beta-Blockers. Beta-blockers are used to prevent attacks in clients with stable angina or to reduce the size of infarction and complications of MI. Reduced heart rate, stroke volume, and contractility and decreased myocardial requirements are attributable to decreased sympathetic nervous stimulation through blockage of the beta-adrenergic receptors in the heart. Side effects include bradycardia, hypotension, dyspnea, dizziness, syncope, gait difficulties, impotence, CHF, heart block, bronchoconstriction, and depression. For clients with lung disease, metoprolol and atenolol are safer medications. Sudden cessation of therapy may induce myocardial ischemia. Older adults are more sensitive to decreased heart rate. This can decrease exercise performance and cause syncope. Older adults should start at a low dose and gradually increase (Flack et al, 1998).

Calcium Channel Blockers. Calcium channel blockers are used to treat stable and variant angina and to increase coronary perfusion, reduce blood pressure, and decrease myocardial contractility in individuals with MI. These drugs decrease the myocardial oxygen demand and increase coronary perfusion by blocking the entry of calcium ions into vascular muscle cells. Adverse reactions are bradycardia, hypotension, flushing, dizziness, syncope, headaches, dyspnea, palpitations, and peripheral edema. Verapamil and diltiazem are not recommended for older adults because they decrease heart rate and increase the incidence of heart block. Amlodipine (Norvasc) is recommended for older adults because of once daily dosing and because it has good blood pressure–lowering properties and is safe in heart failure (Flack et al, 1998).

Fibrinolytics, Anticoagulants, Antiplatelets. These agents are used to prevent, reduce, and dissolve thrombi around atherosclerotic plaques by altering blood-clotting mechanisms. Fibrinolytic or thrombolytic agents are given intravenously within 6 hours of the onset of symptoms. Clients must be observed for arrhythmia, allergic reaction, and bleeding. Older adults have an increased risk for bleeding with fibrinolytics; adults 65 to 75 years of age are considered to be within the upper limits of the appropriate client population (Buhse, 1998). Heparin followed by oral anticoagulation should be administered after cessation of fibrinolytic therapy to prevent secondary clot formation.

Heparin and warfarin (Coumadin) are anticoagulants used to prevent the enlargement of existing thrombi and new clot formation following MI. Therapeutic effects of heparin are monitored by partial thromboplastin times (PTTs); the antidote is protamine sulfate. Warfarin is monitored by the international normalized ratio (INR); the antidote is vitamin K. Clients who initially receive heparin for anticoagulation and who need oral anticoagulation for maintenance usually take both forms of medication for 3 to 5 days to develop therapeutic blood levels. Bleeding is a complication. Clients need to be taught bleeding precautions.

Studies have shown that aspirin decreases the mortality rate of acute MI. It inhibits platelet aggregation and facilitates fibrinolysis. Its effects on platelets occur within 20 minutes of administration. About 160 to 325 mg should be given on admission and daily indefinitely thereafter (Buhse, 1998). Aspirin is also given to prevent angina.

Antihyperlipidemics. Antihyperlipidemics are used to lower serum lipid levels by preventing absorption of cholesterol and promoting its secretion. A common side effect is gastrointestinal upset. Older adults are prone to constipation. These agents are given to prevent CAD and should be prescribed if dietary and activity measures are ineffective. Older adults can benefit from cholesterol-lowering treatment.

Nonpharmacologic Treatment. Older adults with risk factors of inactivity, obesity, and smoking should be encouraged to eliminate or reduce these factors and to control the comorbid conditions of diabetes mellitus and hypertension. Elimination of these factors has the potential to reduce the progression of CAD by half.

Invasive and Surgical Procedures. Older adults who are healthy are candidates for invasive treatment. Age is not an excluding factor (Flack et al, 1998).

Percutaneous Transluminal Coronary Angioplasty (PTCA). PTCA involves the insertion of a specially designed balloon-tipped catheter under fluoroscopy through advancement from the femoral or brachial artery. When situated over the stenotic or occluded area, the balloon is inflated to compress the obstructing plaque, resulting in a larger vessel lumen and improved blood flow to the myocardium.

Stents. A stent is made of stainless steel. It is placed in the obstructed artery after PTCA is performed. This keeps the vessel open and maintains blood flow through the artery.

Coronary Artery Bypass Graft (CABG). CABG is a surgical procedure that grafts portions of the saphenous vein or internal mammary artery to sites above and below the obstructed coronary artery to bypass the stenotic vessel and supply blood to the ischemic myocardium.

Prognosis. Age-related physiologic changes, long duration of adverse lifestyle behaviors, and the presence of other disease conditions in older adults can complicate the progress and treatment of CAD; however, advances in the medical and surgical treatment of CAD and the adoption of healthier lifestyles have the potential to influence the course and outcome of this disease in older adults.

CAD is the leading cause of death and disability in women over 40 years old. It is estimated that every minute in the United States a women dies from heart disease (Holcomb, 2004). Women have smaller coronary arteries that occlude more easily. Women have a lower hematocrit and blood volume, which decreases the oxygen-carrying capacity of the blood. Women also have a higher heart rate at rest, higher stroke volume at rest, and lower left ventricular end diastolic pressure than men. These findings contribute to a higher incidence of false positive stress tests. Women experience more epigastric pain and shortness of breath than they do typical chest pain.

Differences in treatment between women and men with CAD include the following: Women experience a longer interval between emergency room admission and an echocardiogram. Women are less likely to be admitted to an intensive care unit. Women are less likely to receive thrombolytic therapy. Women have a higher incidence of total occlusion after PTCA. Women have an increased incidence of CABG after PTCA. Women experience more recurrent angina, heart failure, recurrent infarction, and strokes after MI. Women are referred less often to cardiac rehabilitation. Women have poorer attendance at cardiac rehabilitation if they are referred. Women typically are 10 years older than men when diagnosed with cardiac disease and experience worse outcomes than men (Tecce, Dasgupta, and Doherty, 2003).

NURSING MANAGEMENT

Assessment

Assessment of an older adult with CAD begins with a complete health history and physical examination. Complaints of dyspnea, fatigue, syncope, vertigo, and confusion warrant further investigation. Subjective data may have to be collected when vital signs are stable and discomfort is relieved (Box 23-3).

Specific health questions during the assessment (e.g., "Are you able to shop for groceries?") may elicit more detailed responses than open-ended questions (e.g., "Do you have any difficulties with activities at home?"). When gathering objective data on older adults, the nurse should remember that slower heart rates, irregular heart rhythms, the presence of a third or fourth heart sound, systolic ejection murmurs, higher SBPs, and wider pulse pressures may be a result of the normal aging process, not the current ischemic episode (Seidel et al, 1999).

BOX 23-3 Assessment of Clients with Chest Pain

SUBJECTIVE DATA

Chest pain (location, intensity, radiation, onset, and duration)
Precipitating factors (activity, emotions, rest, hot or cold exposure, and eating)
Associated symptoms (diaphoresis, dyspnea, vomiting, weakness, palpitations, and indigestion)
Relieving symptoms (rest and nitrates)
Prior hospitalization (for angina, MI, and other disorders)
Medications
Family history (parents or siblings with CAD onset before age 50)
Modifiable cardiac risk factors (smoking, high cholesterol level, hypertension, diabetes mellitus, obesity, and physical inactivity)
Psychosocial state (denial, anxiety, fear, or anger)
Activity levels
Support systems

OBJECTIVE DATA

Behaviors (nervous, lethargic, rubbing chest, or grimacing)
Changes in vital signs
Changes in cardiac rhythm
Associated symptoms (diaphoresis, pallor, or cold and clammy skin)
Peripheral pulses (radial, femoral, and pedal)
Heart sounds and murmurs
Respiratory rate and breath sounds
Jugular vein distention
Diagnostic test results (cardiac enzymes, ECG, chest x-ray study, CBC, and electrolytes)

Diagnosis

Nursing diagnoses common for an older client with CAD include:

- Pain related to imbalance between oxygen need and supply
- Risk for decreased cardiac output related to decreased pumping ability of the heart
- Activity intolerance related to decreased cardiac output
- Knowledge deficit: CAD related to new diagnosis and treatment plan
- Anxiety related to fear of death

Planning and Expected Outcomes

As with all clients, older adults with CAD should be included in the planning of care. Family should also be included in the planning process; however, older adults should be consulted to determine the extent of the family involvement. Discharge planning should begin on admission to the hospital, with special attention given to the necessary support services in the home.

Expected outcomes for an older client with CAD include:

1. Client will verbalize pain relief, as evidenced by reduction in anginal episodes.
2. Client will maintain adequate circulation, as evidenced by stable vital signs, mental alertness, urine output greater than 30 ml/hr, no ECG changes, and clear breath sounds.
3. Client will tolerate activity, as evidenced by stable vital signs and no chest pain or dyspnea.
4. Client will explain the disease process and therapeutic plan, including causes and risk factors for CAD; precipitating and alleviating factors for angina; and names, dosages, actions, and side effects of medications.
5. Client will describe actions to take in the event of chest pain.
6. Client will express fears and have reduced anxiety.

Intervention

Interventions for an older adult with CAD focus on relieving pain, improving myocardial blood flow, decreasing myocardial workload, and educating the client.

Cardiovascular, respiratory, renal, and neurologic assessments should be conducted on a regular basis to detect progress and prevent complications. Diagnostic tests (especially of potassium, since older clients are prone to hyperkalemia) should be conducted and evaluated daily, and any adverse changes in client status should be reported to the physician.

Older adults and their family members may express concern about emergency measures such as resuscitation or life support. The nurse should be sensitive to these needs and initiate discussion with the client, family, and physician to establish a plan of action.

Older adults should be encouraged to participate in cardiac rehabilitation programs to restore their physical and mental health to the highest level of function. Cardiac rehabilitation promotes restoration; diminishes the effects of disease; and encourages optimum physical, psychologic, and social functioning. Cardiac rehabilitation consists of three phases. Phase 1 begins in the hospital and includes early ambulation and client and family education. Phase 2 lasts about 12 weeks and takes place in a supervised outpatient setting. Phase 3 is a maintenance phase that lasts indefinitely; it includes counseling, exercise, education, and socialization (Barker, Burton, and Zieve, 1999).

Exercise should be gradually increased during recovery. Older adults should be taught to monitor their pulse rate to evaluate tolerance to activity. Walking, with a progressive increase in duration and frequency, is recommended. Heavy lifting should be avoided. Activities should be paced throughout the day. Older adults may benefit from a written plan of progressive activities. Properly designed exercise programs for older adults incorporate longer times for the return to a resting heart rate after exercise. Orthostatic hypotension is more common in the older population because of decreased baroreceptor sensitivity. Thermoregulation is impaired; thus exercise must be reduced in hot and humid environments. A heart rate of 50% to 70% of the maximum heart rate achieved at exercise testing with no discomfort during exercise is recommended (Ebersole, Hess, and Luggen, 2004).

Activities that are encouraged should be those that build endurance and self-reliance to increase the level of self-care and quality of life. Activities that can be suggested include walking, swimming, water aerobics, bowling, and dancing.

Older adults with unstable angina should not exercise. Those who require cardiac monitoring during rehabilitation include those who have an ejection fraction of less than 39%, a resting complex ventricular arrhythmia, or decreased blood pressure during exercise. They also include survivors of sudden death, survivors of MI (complicated by heart failure or shock), and those who demonstrate inability to self-monitor their heart rates because of physical or intellectual impairment (Lomacher, 1998).

In spite of the documented benefits of cardiac rehabilitation programs, compliance with them remains low. About 50% of clients drop out before completing the program. Reasons for this include other medical problems, lack of transportation, personal and financial factors, and conflicts with work schedules (Barker, Burton, and Zieve, 1999). Women have been documented as having the poorest adherence to the program (Ebersole, Hess, and Luggen, 2004). The interdisciplinary team should recognize these issues and make every effort to assist clients with these problems.

The resumption of sexual activity should be discussed with older adults. It is generally safe to resume sexual activity within 4 to 6 weeks of MI, as long as an older adult is symptom free during his or her usual daily activities. The equivalency or expenditure of energy for sexual activity correlates with the same energy expenditure required for climbing a flight of stairs or walking around the block. Coitus has accounted for less than 1% of sudden deaths. These deaths usually involve extramarital affairs or alcohol consumption (Barker, Burton, and Zieve, 1999). A pamphlet, *Sex and Heart Disease,* available through the AHA, can be used to supplement counseling. If a stable older adult develops angina during sexual activity, prophylactic sublingual nitroglycerin can be given (Barker, Burton, and Zieve, 1999).

Visiting nurse programs can provide education, support, and supervised activities in the home environment if older clients are unable to attend outpatient services. Home care services are usually available to assist older clients with activities of daily living (ADLs). Both programs may require physician referral.

Local heart associations are excellent sources for learning materials and community programs on CAD. Some heart associations offer educational and support programs for clients recovering from CAD (e.g., Heart to Heart) or surgery (e.g., Mended Hearts), and they can usually provide direction for community programs on risk factor reduction, cardiopulmonary resuscitation (CPR), and mall-walking.

Evaluation

Evaluation and documentation of the progress of an older client with CAD focus on the achievement of goals outlined in the planning process. Older adults should demonstrate adequate circulation, ability to perform ADLs, and control of symptoms. Documentation should focus on the older adult's risk factor profile and progress, with measures aimed at reducing risks, since a reduction of behaviors associated with the identified risks will reduce morbidity and mortality (see Nursing Care Plan).

Arrhythmia

Arrhythmia is an abnormal heart rate or rhythm caused by a disturbance in automaticity, conductivity, or both. Arrhythmias can originate in the atria, ventricles, or atrioventricular junctions, and can result in decreased cardiac output and impaired perfusion of coronary arteries.

Older adults can develop any type of arrhythmia; however, atrial fibrillation, sick sinus syndrome, and heart block occur more often in the older population because of fewer pacemaker cells and extensive deposits of fat and fibrous tissue throughout the conduction system (Lewis, Collier, and Heitkemper, 1996; Seidel et al, 1999). The incidence of atrial

Nursing Care Plan
Myocardial Infarction

Clinical Situation: Mrs. S is an 83-year-old widow who was admitted to the hospital from a nursing facility with complaints of fatigue, weakness, and vertigo. Staff at the nursing facility became concerned after two episodes of syncope. Mrs. S suffered a stroke 4 years ago that left her with severe weakness in her left arm and left leg. She was unable to care for herself at home; her daughter encouraged her to enter the nursing facility. She has been following a diet low in saturated fat and cholesterol and takes enteric-coated aspirin daily, as well as levothyroxine (Synthroid) for hypothyroidism. Mrs. S is mobile with the use of a walker.

A routine ECG showed pathologic Q waves. Cardiac enzymes were tested. CPK levels were normal, but lactate dehydrogenase was elevated. She was diagnosed with an inferior MI. Since she did not meet the time criteria for fibrinolytic therapy, the physician instituted prophylactic measures with oral anticoagulants on a daily basis. Mrs. S developed occasional premature contractions and periodic bouts of atrial fibrillation. Digoxin and nitroglycerin were added to her regimen. She became agitated in the coronary care unit about being a burden to her family and declined invasive treatment procedures. The nurse organized a meeting with the physician, daughter, and client to discuss her anxiety, and a "no resuscitation" order was written. Lorazepam 1 mg as needed three times a day was added to the protocol.

Currently, Mrs. S denies having chest pain and can walk short distances with her walker. She follows a low-cholesterol/low–saturated fat diet, and she is scheduled for an echocardiogram later in the week. Her blood pressure is in the low to normal range, and her pulse is irregular at 102 beats/min. Atenolol has been added to the regimen to reduce her heart rate.

Nursing Diagnoses

Anxiety related to threat of death and change in health status

High risk for chest pain related to alteration in cardiopulmonary perfusion

Decreased cardiac output related to electrical dysfunction

Activity intolerance related to imbalance of myocardial oxygen supply and demand and left peripheral limb weakness

Knowledge deficit: disease process and treatment plan related to lack of exposure

Outcomes

Client will verbalize reduced anxiety as evidenced by slower heart rate, reduced apprehension, and participation in self-care.

Client will obtain pain relief as evidenced by verbal statements.

Client will maintain adequate circulation as evidence by stable vital signs, mental alertness, clear lung sounds, and urine output greater than 30 ml/hr.

Client will tolerate activity as evidenced by stable vital signs; absence of pain, weakness, fatigue, and vertigo; and participation in activity.

Client will demonstrate knowledge of disease process and symptoms of ischemia with appropriate response and treatment plan, as evidenced by explanation of and participation in plan.

Client will demonstrate accurate pulse-taking method.

Interventions

Explain equipment, procedures, and unit routine.

Encourage verbalization of feelings.

Teach relaxation techniques and guided imagery to alleviate anxiety.

Supervise tolerance to visitation.

Offer lorazepam as needed.

Encourage participation in care, and emphasize improvements in health status.

Encourage relaying of pain sensations to nurse.

Explain how sensations of fatigue, weakness, and vertigo may be symptoms of ischemia and need to be reported to nurse.

Encourage client to take nitroglycerin at onset of chest pain or at sensations of ischemia.

Obtain vital signs during episodes, and contact physician if medication is ineffective.

Offer oxygen if needed.

Monitor therapeutic effects of nitrates and atenolol, observing for hypotensive effects.

Measure blood pressure, apical pulse, and rhythm every 4 hours. Auscultate heart and lungs every 8 hours.

Monitor ECG for reversion to normal sinus rhythm, INR, digoxin levels, and electrolytes.

Administer and evaluate the effects of warfarin, digoxin, and atenolol.

Observe for signs of hemorrhage, shock, heart failure, and emboli.

Assist with ADLs as needed.

Remind client to perform leg exercises every hour and range-of-motion exercises. Apply antiembolic stockings.

Before ambulation, encourage client to do leg exercises and sit at bedside for 3 to 5 minutes before standing.

Gradually increase distance and frequency of walking.

Monitor vital signs before and after activity.

Offer nitroglycerin and oxygen if needed.

Keep call bell and walker within reach.

Encourage client to wear shoes with good support and to walk in lighted areas.

Balance activity with rest.

Teach client to count own pulse.

Encourage client to recognize sensations of ischemia and cease activity when they occur.

Include daughter in teaching sessions.

Describe the disease and healing process of MI using pictures, models, and large printed material.

Nursing Care Plan
Myocardial Infarction—cont'd

- Describe the client's sensations of ischemia, and teach appropriate use of nitrates and rest.
- Discuss and provide written information for medication dosage, purpose, side effects, and special precautions for warfarin, digoxin, and atenolol.
- Encourage progressive increase in activity.
- Assess emotions and reassure client that depression is common.
- Teach client to take radial pulse and to monitor before, during, and after activity.

fibrillation increases with age and is the most common contributing factor for ischemic stroke in older adults. This is caused by an embolus from the heart that occludes a cerebral vessel. The 5-year incidence of stroke from atrial fibrillation is 44% in clients ages 60 to 70, 80% in clients ages 71 to 80, and 63% in clients ages 81 to 90 (Chrzanowski, 1998). Atrial fibrillation is characterized by chaotic depolarization within the atria of 400 to 700 beats/min and an irregular ventricular response. Older adults need increased diastolic filling pressures to compensate for structural changes within the heart and to maintain cardiac output, so chaotic or quivering depolarization within the atria diminishes this atrial kick needed for adequate ventricular filling (Seidel et al, 1999). Atrial fibrillation can occur during intense emotional stress, exercise, or alcohol intoxication. Chronic atrial fibrillation tends to occur in clients with hypertension, CAD, rheumatic heart disease, cardiac valve disease, CHF, pericarditis, COPD, and cardiomyopathy; it increases the risk for pulmonary, peripheral, and cerebral thromboembolism. Thyroid disorders can also precipitate atrial fibrillation (Chrzanowski, 1998).

Sick sinus syndrome is characterized by alternating episodes of bradycardia (less than 60 beats/min), normal sinus rhythm (60 to 100 beats/min), tachycardia (greater than 100 beats/min), and periods of long sinus pause that fail to stimulate the atria or ventricles. Sick sinus syndrome tends to occur in clients with CAD, rheumatic heart disease, and hypertension.

Heart block is characterized by delayed or blocked impulses between the atria and ventricles and is classified as first-, second-, or third-degree heart block, each respective classification increasing in severity. First-degree block is common in older adults with or without CAD and is a common complication of MI. Digitalis preparations may also cause first-degree heart block. Second- and third-degree block can be caused by degeneration within the conduction system, ischemia, enhanced vagal tone, electrolytes, and effects of drugs (e.g., digoxin, beta-blockers), which are common conditions and treatments associated with aging (Barker, Burton, and Zieve, 1999).

Symptoms of arrhythmia are weakness, fatigue, forgetfulness, palpitations, dizziness, hypotension, bradycardia, and syncope, all of which predispose older clients to falls and injuries. Clients with first-degree block and fibrillation may have no symptoms, whereas clients with atrial fibrillation have an irregular pulse.

Diagnostic Tests and Procedures. Arrhythmias are diagnosed by ECG evaluation. When an arrhythmia is diagnosed, a variety of tests may be performed to determine a causative factor. Continuous ECG monitoring provides the most efficient and reliable method of detection. A Holter monitor is also often used.

Treatment. Treatment should be limited to symptomatic clients with significant arrhythmias. Antiarrhythmic medications should be avoided when possible (Barker, Burton, and Zieve, 1999).

Atrial Fibrillation. The treatment of atrial fibrillation has two objectives: (1) control rate with maintenance anticoagulation therapy and (2) convert the rhythm to a normal sinus rhythm. The most commonly used drugs for rate control with exercise and at rest include the beta-blockers atenolol and metoprolol, and the calcium channel blockers diltiazem and verapamil. Digoxin (Lanoxin) is only effective at rest and is not considered a drug of choice. Half the usual dose should be given to older adults with renal insufficiency. The risk of digitalis toxicity increases with renal insufficiency and hypokalemia. Elective cardioversion should be used if pharmacologic treatment is not effective. Oral anticoagulants are prescribed to reduce the risk of thromboembolic events. If arrhythmia is severe, a pacemaker may be inserted to control ventricular response (Snow et al, 2003).

Sick Sinus Syndrome. Treatment may include the administration of vagolytic agents such as atropine to block vagal impulses, resulting in an increased heart rate. A pacemaker is the treatment of choice for symptomatic clients (Adan and Crown, 2003).

Heart Block. Treatment for first-degree heart block includes observation to prevent deterioration into severe heart block, as well as correction of the causative factor (e.g., electrolyte imbalance, drug toxicity). With second- and third-degree block, vagolytic and sympathomimetic agents are usually employed to increase heart rate and conduction. Pacemakers may also be inserted to correct arrhythmia.

Prognosis. Older adults with the arrhythmias of sick sinus syndrome or heart block have an excellent prognosis when these arrhythmias are corrected. Clients with atrial fibrillation have ischemic stroke as a complication.

NURSING MANAGEMENT

Assessment

Older adults should be assessed for a history of CAD, heart failure, hypertension, cardiac valve disease, and current medications (e.g., cardiac, diuretic, supplemental electrolyte), which may be causative factors of arrhythmias. Symptoms of weakness, forgetfulness, palpitations, dizziness, and syncope should be investigated for frequency, length, precipitating factors, and home treatment remedies.

Objective data include heart rate and rhythm, blood pressure, peripheral pulses, urine output, and sensorium. Measuring the apical pulse for 60 seconds yields the most accurate measurement of heart rate. Apical and radial rates should be compared to assess peripheral perfusion. Electrolyte, hemoglobin, and hematocrit values should be assessed for imbalances and anemia.

Diagnosis

Nursing diagnoses common for an older client with arrhythmia include:

- Decreased cardiac output related to altered heart rate and rhythm
- Activity intolerance related to altered heart rate and cardiac output
- High risk for injury related to potential thrombus and emboli formation
- Knowledge deficit: disease process, medications, and treatment plan related to lack of information

Planning and Expected Outcomes

The overall goals for a client with arrhythmia are to maintain ADLs and adequate heart rate, sustain cardiac output, and prevent complications. Expected outcomes include:

1. Client will maintain an adequate cardiac output, as evidenced by heart rate and rhythm within normal range, stable blood pressure, adequate peripheral pulses, mental alertness, urine output of 30 ml/hr, and clear breath sounds.
2. Client will tolerate activity, as evidenced by stable vital signs and no complaints of dizziness, fatigue, or syncope.
3. Client will remain free from injury.
4. Client will verbalize increased knowledge about diagnosis, treatment plan, and health maintenance behaviors.

Intervention

Vital signs should be monitored every 15 to 60 minutes if the client's condition is acute and every 4 hours if it is stable. Heart rate and rhythm should be monitored continuously with a telemetry unit or Holter monitor. The client should be encouraged to promptly report symptoms of weakness, dizziness, and palpitations to the nurse for comparison with electrical cardiac activity. Cardiovascular, respiratory, and neurologic systems, as well as intake and output measurements, should be assessed on a regular basis. Benefits and adverse reactions of prescribed drugs should be evaluated. Older clients with slow or fast ventricular responses to atrial fibrillation, long periods of sinus arrest with sick sinus syndrome, and second- or third-degree heart block are at risk for asystole and sudden death, so the nurse should be prepared to administer CPR.

Sensations of weakness, fatigue, dizziness, or dyspnea affect a client's tolerance of activity. The nurse can assist clients with the identification of factors that increase or decrease activity tolerance, and he or she can develop activity patterns that are spaced with adequate rest. Physiologic responses to activity should be monitored.

Tachycardia, bradycardia, and long periods of sinus pause reduce cardiac output and place clients at a higher risk for fainting and falls. Interventions to prevent injury include (1) having the client sit for 3 to 5 minutes before an activity and (2) protecting the client from objects with sharp or protruding edges by rearranging or padding objects in the client's environment.

The disease process and the dosage and side effects of all medications should be reviewed with the client. Older clients taking anticoagulants should be taught ways to prevent injury, such as not going barefoot, using a soft toothbrush, shaving with an electric razor, having blood drawn at the proper times, and taking medication at the same time every day.

If older clients anticipate difficulty with home recovery, a home health agency may be consulted. Heart associations are excellent sources for information and community programs. The family or significant others should be encouraged to attend CPR programs. All clients should be encouraged to wear medical-alert bracelets to identify the arrhythmia, the use of a pacemaker, and any medications they use (see Client/Family Teaching box).

Evaluation

Older adults with arrhythmias or pacemakers should maintain a cardiac rhythm that supports adequate cardiac output. An ability to resume ADLs, knowledge of the therapeutic plan, and achievement of expected outcomes define an older adult's readiness for independence in his or her care. Documentation focuses on a client's response to the treatment plan, specifically, how well symptoms are controlled. Hemodynamic stability is reflected in documented trends in the client's vital signs.

Orthostatic Hypotension

Orthostatic hypotension is a major risk factor for syncope and falls in older adults. Orthostatic hypotension is defined as a drop in blood pressure of 10 to 20 mm Hg with upright posture. After changing from a lying to a standing position, approximately 300 to 800 ml of blood moves into the lower

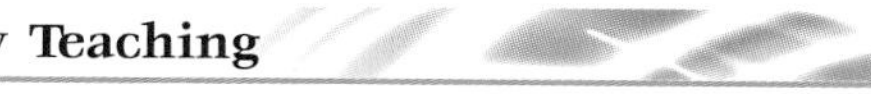

Client/Family Teaching

PACEMAKER

Maintain follow-up care with the health care provider to evaluate pacemaker function.

Watch for signs of infection at the incision site (e.g., redness, swelling, drainage). Report these to the health care provider.

Avoid activities that would cause direct blows to the generator site (e.g., contact sports, use of a rifle).

Avoid close proximity to high-output electrical generators or to large magnets such as magnetic resonance imaging (MRI) scanners. These devices can reprogram the pacemaker.

Microwave ovens are safe to use and do not threaten pacemaker function.

Travel without restriction is allowed. The metal case of a small implanted pacemaker rarely sets off airport security alarms.

Take the radial pulse daily. Contact the health care provider if the rate is below the setting of the pacemaker.

Carry a pacemaker identification card at all times. Information should include the type and brand of pacemaker, Inter-Society Commission on Heart Disease code, and settings.

From Lewis S, Collier I, Heitkemper M: *Medical-surgical nursing: assessment and management of clinical problems*, ed 4, St Louis, 1996, Mosby.

extremities (Bradley and Davis, 2003). It is even more common among persons with certain risk factors such as autonomic dysfunction, low cardiac output, and hypovolemia. The use of certain medications, such as sedatives, antihypertensives, vasodilators, and antidepressants, also predisposes older adults to orthostatic hypotension. A drop in SBP is sometimes more pronounced on arising in the morning because of diminished baroreceptor function after prolonged recumbence (Besdine, Bubenstein, and Snyder, 1996). Orthostatic hypotension in older adults can be caused by an increase in sedentary activity and blunting of autonomic reflexes (Barker, Burton, and Zieve, 1999).

NURSING MANAGEMENT

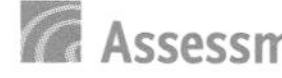

Assessment

Assessment of an older client begins with a complete health history and physical examination. Reports of syncope, falls, and near falls should be investigated in relation to meals, medications, and environmental factors. Hydration status should be evaluated along with a CBC and serum glucose. Dehydration, anemia, and hypoglycemia can also cause syncope and falls.

To assess for orthostatic blood pressure changes, the nurse should first determine the blood pressure of the client in a recumbent position. Then the nurse should help the client to a sitting position, with feet dangling or flat on the floor, and repeat the blood pressure reading. Then, if the client can stand, the nurse should auscultate a third blood pressure in this position, noting the differences in the blood pressures and recording all three in the client's record.

All prescribed and over-the-counter medication and herbal preparations should be reviewed carefully. Special attention should be given to medications known to induce hypotension in older adults, such as amitriptyline, antidepressants, antihypertensives, bromocriptine, alpha- and beta-blockers, diphenhydramine, diuretics, insulin, marijuana, minor tranquilizers, monoamine oxidase inhibitors, narcotics or sedatives, nitrates, phenothiazines, sildenafil, sympatholytics, sympathomimetics (with prolonged use), tricyclic antidepressants, vasodilators, and vincristine (Bradley and Davis, 2003).

Diagnosis

Nursing diagnoses common for an older adult with orthostatic hypotension include:

- Risk for injury related to transient hypoperfusion of brain
- Knowledge deficit: techniques to lessen the impact of orthostatic hypotension related to lack of previous exposure
- Impaired physical mobility related to the fear of falling

Planning and Expected Outcomes

Expected outcomes for an older adult with orthostatic hypotension include:

1. Client will remain free of injury.
2. Client will verbalize and correctly demonstrate measures to prevent symptoms of orthostatic hypotension.
3. Client will verbalize fears and identify coping measures.

Intervention

The nurse should teach an older adult at risk for or with orthostatic hypotension to move from a recumbent position to a sitting position slowly. The client should then remain sitting for several minutes before attempting to stand.

Exercising the lower legs and ankles facilitates venous return and raises the blood pressure. Elastic stockings help in the same way. In some instances a higher salt diet may increase blood volume and ameliorate orthostatic changes. The nurse should work with the client and physician to eliminate unnecessary medications that can contribute to orthostatic hypotension; the nurse should also encourage the client to limit alcohol intake, avoid large meals, and monitor and control diabetes mellitus, which is associated with peripheral autonomic dysfunction.

Environmental safety remains important. Grab bars, nonskid surfaces, and an uncluttered living space can minimize injuries. In long-term care settings, low beds are sometimes used for cognitively impaired individuals with orthostatic hypotension and a history of falls.

Postfall syndrome produces fear that frequently causes older adults to limit activity. In addition, caregivers may also fear injury for an older adult and feel compelled to limit the older person's freedom. This leads to a cycle of disuse, atrophy, and increased frailty, with a concomitant increased risk of injury. Educating the client on the proper technique of standing can aid in alleviating this fear. Encouragement and support are also important means for relieving fear.

Evaluation

Evaluation is based on achievement of the expected outcomes and the safe performance of ADLs. Documentation of the client's blood pressure trends in the three positions aids in evaluating the effectiveness of the recommended treatments.

Syncope With Cardiac Cause

Syncope is a transient loss of consciousness with spontaneous recovery. Syncope accounts for approximately 3% of emergency room visits and 6% of general hospital admissions (Pavri and Ho, 2003). Syncope usually results from acutely diminished cerebral blood flow. Causes of syncope can be broadly grouped into the categories of neurologic, cardiac, neurocardiogenic, and psychiatric disease (Hauer, 2003). Cardiovascular causes of syncope are more prevalent in older adults, and vasovagal syncope is more prevalent in younger person. The most frequent cardiovascular causes of syncope in older adults are cardiac arrhythmias, sick sinus syndrome, atrioventricular block, carotid hypersensitivity, aortic stenosis, and postprandial and orthostatic hypotension (Pavri and Ho, 2003).

Vasovagal syncope occurs when fright, pain, or nauseous stimuli stimulate the vagus nerve. Signs and symptoms include nausea, diaphoresis, anxiety, and a feeling of warmth. These same signs can also be part of the atypical presentation of MI in an older adult. Vasovagal syncope can also be caused by straining with bowel movement and by pushing up in bed without assistance. Vasovagal attacks usually occur in upright positions, and the client regains consciousness when he or she lies down. There is usually a prodromal period where the older adult may feel dizzy or flushed, experience mild nausea, and occasionally experience palpitations and tightness in the throat (Barker, Burton, and Zieve, 1999).

Cardiac arrhythmias often are first seen as a loss of consciousness without warning. Ectopic beats, whether supraventricular or ventricular, increase in frequency with age. Specific arrhythmias include supraventricular and ventricular tachycardias and a variety of bradyarrhythmias.

Atrial fibrillation is a supraventricular arrhythmia recognized by the lack of a clear P wave on the ECG and an irregular ventricular rate. Because atrial fibrillation is associated with an increased risk of cerebral embolism, anticoagulation should be considered in any older adult with this arrhythmia (Abrams and Berkow, 2000). Atrial fibrillation can cause syncope if the ventricular rate becomes too fast for adequate ventricular filling during diastole. Also, with this type of arrhythmia the loss of atrial kick, which accounts for 30% of ventricular filling, can be enough to cause lower cardiac output and thus syncope.

Ventricular tachycardia is a medical emergency. It is usually seen as a regular tachycardia with a wide QRS complex—often up to rates of 300 beats/min. Again the problem is inadequate ventricular filling during diastole, leading to very diminished cardiac output and syncope if not quickly treated. Ventricular tachycardia associated with hypotension or syncope requires immediate electrical cardioversion (Abrams and Berkow, 1995). Long-term control of this type of arrhythmia is accomplished through medication and implantable automatic defibrillators.

Bradyarrhythmias are more common in older adults because of intrinsic conduction system disease and a higher prevalence of acute illness, such as MI and digitalis toxicity. Bradyarrhythmias that require pacemakers are Mobitz type II, third-degree heart block, and sick sinus syndrome if the bradycardia is symptomatic (Abrams and Berkow, 2000). Structural problems in the heart, such as aortic stenosis, cardiomyopathy, and acute MI, can also cause syncope.

NURSING MANAGEMENT

Assessment

The assessment of an older client with syncope begins with a complete history and physical examination. Family members or other witnesses to the client's syncopal episode should be asked to describe what the client was doing just before losing consciousness. A witness may describe the older adult as having cold hands and pale skin just before the loss of consciousness. After syncope, a client often becomes flushed (Barker, Burton, and Zieve, 1999). A 12-lead ECG should be examined for evidence of acute infarction and arrhythmias. The carotid arteries should be auscultated for bruits. Blood work should include CBC, electrolytes, and glucose (Abrams and Berkow, 2005).

Diagnosis

Nursing diagnoses for an older adult with syncope include:

- Decreased cardiac output related to inadequate left ventricular filling, arrhythmia, or orthostasis
- Anxiety related to near or full loss of consciousness

Planning and Expected Outcomes

Syncope with cardiac causes is often an emergency situation requiring sophisticated intensive care for the older client. It is hoped that a health care proxy is available if the client can no longer speak for himself or herself. In any event, communication with the medical team and family or other caregivers is very important.

Expected outcomes for an older client with syncope include:

1. Client will regain normal range of cardiac output as demonstrated by stable vital signs and alert and oriented sensorium.
2. Older adult and family will verbalize understanding of the cause of syncope and the therapeutic treatment plan.

Intervention

Emergency measures to correct life-threatening arrhythmias, such as CPR and defibrillation, should be employed when needed. Oxygen should be applied, and oxygen saturation should be evaluated.

The nurse needs to help older adults identify causes of syncope, such as straining with bowel movement. Constipation is a common complaint among older adults. Measures to avoid constipation include an increase in fiber, adequate fluid intake, and exercise. The nurse should instruct the client to lie down if he or she becomes dizzy or experiences other prodromal symptoms. Psychologic and spiritual care can become especially important when clients are faced with the possibility of death from their condition.

Evaluation

Evaluation is based on achievement of the expected outcomes and a positive change in the clinical picture of the older adult. Older adults should be able to identify the cause of their syncope and methods of prevention, including methods of preventing injury if syncope occurs.

Valvular Disease

Valvular disease occurs when the cardiac valves do not completely open (stenosis) or close (regurgitation insufficiency), which prevents efficient circulation of blood through the heart and increases the myocardial workload. Valvular disease is more common in the mitral and aortic valves.

Stenosis of the mitral valve impedes blood flow from the left atrium to the ventricle during diastole. With time, the left atrium becomes accustomed to increasing volumes and pressure, causing dilation and hypertrophy. Stenosis of the aortic valve obstructs blood flow from the left ventricle to the aortic arch during systole. With time, hypertrophy of the left ventricle occurs as a result of increased pressures and volumes. Both stenotic conditions can eventually lead to hypertrophy of pulmonary vessels and decreased cardiac output.

Mitral regurgitation allows ejected blood to flow back into the left atrium from the ventricle during systole, resulting in dilation and hypertrophy of the left atrium and ventricle. Aortic regurgitation allows ejected blood to flow back into the left ventricle from the aorta during diastole, leading to volume overloads in dilation and hypertrophy of the left ventricle. Mitral valve prolapse (a form of valvular insufficiency) occurs when one or both cusps prolapse into the left atrium during ventricular systole. The prolapse is normally benign but can progress to severe regurgitation with ventricular dilation.

Rheumatic fever is the most common cause of valvular disease, although the incidence of rheumatic fever has declined since the introduction of antibiotics. Inflammatory, infective connective tissue disorders and atherosclerosis are other causes. Mitral regurgitation and aortic stenosis can also be attributed to degeneration or calcification of valves.

Aortic insufficiency, mitral stenosis, and mitral valve prolapse are more common in younger individuals than in older ones. Pulmonary and tricuspid valvular disorders do not often occur in older individuals. In older adults, aortic stenosis and mitral regurgitation are more common as a result of the degenerative process.

Individuals with valvular disease may be asymptomatic for many years, but with the deterioration of the valves and hypertrophic changes in the atria or ventricles, symptoms become evident (Box 23-4). Exertional dyspnea is frequently the initial symptom. Other symptoms include dizziness, fatigue, weakness, and palpitations. Atrial fibrillation is often associated with mitral disorders from distention of the left atria, and symptoms of angina are more common with aortic disorders because of decreased cardiac output. Symptoms of valvular disease may be difficult to recognize in older adults because symptoms can mimic those of CAD, which is common in the older adult population.

BOX 23-4 Clinical Manifestations of Valvular Heart Disease

MITRAL STENOSIS

Dyspnea on exertion, orthopnea, fatigue, loud accentuated S_1, opening snap, low-pitched rumbling diastolic murmur heard at apex

MITRAL REGURGITATION

Weakness, fatigue, dyspnea, palpitations, soft S_1, S_3 often present, high-pitched pansystolic murmur with a harsh, blowing quality that radiates to the axilla

AORTIC STENOSIS

Angina, syncope, heart failure, soft S_1, prominent S_4, crescendo-decrescendo harsh ejection systolic murmur that radiates to carotids

AORTIC REGURGITATION

Exertional dyspnea; orthopnea; nocturnal angina; soft or absent S_2, S_3, or S_4; soft decrescendo high-pitched diastolic murmur; wide pulse pressure

From Davey P, editor: *Medicine at a glance,* Oxford, 2002, Blackwell Science.

Diagnostic Tests and Procedures. A chest x-ray examination and ECG are initial diagnostic tests that may suggest valvular disease or evaluate damage to the heart from valvular problems. An echocardiogram with Doppler and ultrasound provides the most detailed information on the valve's structure, function (abnormal cusp movement), and chamber enlargement. Cardiac catheterization may be done to assess the severity of the valve disorder (i.e., valve size, pressure changes within the chamber, pressure gradients across valves) and additional effects on the heart. Exercise tests may also be conducted to evaluate the client's symptomatic response to exertion and the heart's capacity to function (Segal, 2003a).

Treatment. Treatment is directed toward the management of presenting symptoms and correction of the cause of the valvular disorder. Treatment for symptoms of heart failure consists of digoxin therapy, diuretics, vasodilating agents, restricted sodium intake, and oxygen therapy. Symptoms of decreased cardiac output related to atrial fibrillation are treated with digoxin, beta-blockers, calcium channel blockers, cardioversion, or anticoagulant therapy. Symptoms of decreased cardiac output related to ischemia are treated with vasodilating agents. Prophylactic antibiotics before invasive procedures (e.g., surgery, invasive tests, and dental work) are recommended for all clients with valve replacement to prevent infective endocarditis. For clients with valvular disorders resulting from degenerative processes, medical treatment of symptoms tends to be unsuccessful over time and surgical repair or replacement of diseased valves may be necessary.

Prognosis. Mortality and morbidity rates are higher for older adults requiring valve surgery. This is because older adults often have more advanced disease and more coexisting chronic diseases. Valvular surgery on older adults has steadily increased during the past decade; this has increased the quality of life for older adults (Segal, 2003b).

NURSING MANAGEMENT

Assessment

Assessment should include the history of prior episodes of rheumatic fever, infective endocarditis, staphylococcal and streptococcal infections, and family history of cardiac disease. Symptoms of valvular disease (e.g., fatigue, dyspnea, palpitations, dizziness, weakness, syncope, peripheral edema, distended neck veins, periods of memory loss or confusion, chest pain) or related complications (e.g., arrhythmia, angina, heart failure) should be noted, as well as the client's level of fatigue, toleration of activity, and current medications.

Objective data should be obtained primarily from the cardiovascular and respiratory assessment. Cardiovascular data include blood pressure, pulse pressure, heart rate and rhythm, weight loss or gain, peripheral pulses, presence of peripheral edema, neck vein distention, and heart sounds. Different heart sounds can be heard with each valvular disorder, and these sounds should be auscultated for abnormalities or changes. Respiratory data include rate, depth, and breath sounds.

Aortic stenosis is the most common valvular disorder among older adults because of calcification of the valve with aging. Stenosis of this valve tends to occur without fusion of the cusps, resulting in a spray of blood through the valve rather than forceful propulsion. Physical examination may reveal softer and more musical heart murmurs that can be confused with the normal aging process rather than a valvular disorder. Older adults may require diagnostic testing to support a diagnosis of valvular disease.

Diagnosis

Nursing diagnoses common for an older client with valvular disease include:

- Decreased cardiac output related to altered blood flow through the heart
- Activity intolerance related to decreased cardiac output
- Anxiety related to diagnosis, treatment plan, and uncertain outcome
- Knowledge deficit: disease process, medications, and treatment plan related to lack of previous exposure to information

Planning and Expected Outcomes

Expected outcomes for an older client with valvular disease depend on the severity and extent of the disease. Outcomes include:

1. Client will maintain adequate cardiac output, as evidenced by stable vital signs, mental alertness, urine output of 30 ml/hr or greater, and clear breath sounds.
2. Client will tolerate usual level of daily activity, as evidenced by stable vital signs and no dyspnea.
3. Client will experience reduced anxiety, as evidenced by verbalization of decreased anxiety, the ability to express specific fears, and stable vital signs.
4. Client will correctly explain the disease process, therapeutic plan, and preventive precautions.

Intervention

Cardiovascular and respiratory assessments should be conducted on a regular basis to detect progress and to prevent complications. The nurse should monitor clients for therapeutic and adverse reactions to the medications prescribed; monitor blood pressure, heart rate, respirations, heart sounds, breath sounds, and cardiac rhythm; maintain the client on bedrest when ordered and perform range-of-motion exercises to prevent complications; elevate the head of the bed to maximize thoracic excursion; and administer oxygen as prescribed.

The nurse should also assess a client's activity level and balance activity with rest periods; organize care to provide rest periods and advance activity according to client's tolerance; and assist the older adult with ADLs to prevent fatigue. Older adults are more prone to dizziness with position changes because of decreased sensitivity of baroreceptors (Seidel et al, 1999). The client should rise slowly and stay in a sitting position for a few minutes before standing. Older adults require secure footwear and handrails for support.

Older clients should understand the disease process and treatment plan and should recognize the signs and symptoms of heart failure and when to notify a health care provider. The client's low-sodium diet should be reviewed, as should bleeding precautions if the client is on anticoagulant therapy. Antibiotics for invasive procedures, including all dental work, should be discussed. Appropriate oral hygiene should be explained to older clients to prevent trauma and infective endocarditis.

For clients who do not respond to medical treatment, valvular surgery may be necessary to improve cardiac performance. Older clients benefit more from surgery when their condition is stabilized and the procedure is performed on an elective basis. Clients scheduled for valvular surgery are subjected to extensive diagnostic tests and blood studies, which should be explained to the client and family to alleviate anxiety. The client and family should also be oriented to the intensive or coronary care unit and the equipment that will be used postoperatively. Postoperative assessment activities and treatments should be explained.

After surgery, older clients should be monitored closely for complications of MI, heart failure, thromboembolism, hemorrhage, arrhythmia, and infection. Older clients have a greater risk for complications than younger individuals. Older adults are also prone to the development of acute confusion or delirium following surgery because of multiple factors, including the stress of the procedure, drug and other treatment modalities, and environmental alterations. The presence of the family and familiar belongings and the use of personal hearing aids or eyeglasses may alleviate episodes of delirium.

Recovery from valvular surgery is generally complete within 6 to 8 weeks; however, recovery may be delayed in older adults as a result of a higher incidence of complications. Exercise and ADLs should be gradually resumed during the first 6 weeks of recovery. Clients should be taught to monitor their pulse and respiratory rate to evaluate tolerance to activity. Walking with a progressive increase in duration and frequency is recommended, and clients should avoid lifting heavy objects. Driving a car may impede the healing of the sternal incision. Prophylactic use of antibiotics should be explained to the client. Anticoagulants may be prescribed for clients with prosthetic valves, and special precautions should be explained. Signs, symptoms, and complications of valvular disease should be reviewed with the client, since clients may develop deteriorating symptoms that necessitate valve replacement, and clients with valve replacement may need new valves inserted over time.

Evaluation

Evaluation of an older client with valvular disease focuses on achievement of the expected outcomes. Older adults should demonstrate adequate cardiac output, the ability to perform ADLs within limitations, and control of symptoms. The nurse should also note the client and family's ability to manage the care requirements and resolve any problems appropriately. Documentation should accurately reflect the care delivered in the preoperative and postoperative periods, as well as the older adult's response. Assessment of the progress toward self-care and the degree of functional ability must also be documented on an ongoing basis, since the older adult's recovery depends in large part on returning to the prior level of functioning.

Congestive Heart Failure

CHF is the leading cause of hospitalization in the older adult population (Miller, 1997). Approximately 5 million Americans, primarily older ones, have been diagnosed with CHF. CHF occurs in less than 1% of adults in their 50s, and the incidence doubles every decade after age 50 (Aronow et al, 1998). In the Framingham study the majority of adults diagnosed with CHF did not survive for more than 5 years (Ebersole, Hess, and Luggen, 2004).

CHF is the inability of the heart to pump an adequate cardiac output to meet the body's metabolic demands (Ebersole, Hess, and Luggen, 2004). CHF is not a disease in itself, but it has several precipitating factors. Some of these contributing factors include age; hypertension; CAD; rheumatic heart disease; valvular heart disease; arrhythmias; renal disease; diabetes mellitus; thyrotoxicosis; MI; cardiomyopathy; pulmonary embolism; infection; anemia; liver disease; emotional stress; and other factors related to biologic, socioeconomic, iatrogenic, and lifestyle considerations.

Age-associated cardiovascular and renal changes that affect the clinical course of CHF and responses to treatment include decreased renal and systemic blood flow, increased arterial stiffness and peripheral resistance, reduced ventricular compliance, and reduced maximum aerobic capacity. In older adults the inability to maintain function because of pulmonary and systemic congestion can create a cycle of decreased activity that leads to a decreased ability to provide self-care (Stone, Wyman, and Salisbury, 1999).

Diagnostic Tests and Procedures. The AHCPR has established the following guidelines for testing: ECG to detect MI and arrhythmia, CBC to rule out anemia, urinalysis and serum creatinine and blood urea nitrogen (BUN) to rule out renal disease, serum albumin to differentiate edema caused by hypoalbuminemia, serum brain natriuretic peptide (90% specificity and sensitivity for heart failure), thyroid tests to rule out thyroid disease, and echocardiogram to determine left ventricular ejection fraction (Shamsham and Mitchell, 2000).

Treatment. Management of CHF in older adults requires careful control of precipitating factors, pharmacologic therapy (Table 23-3), a low-sodium diet, restriction of fluids, and appropriate rest and exercise. The American College of Cardiology (ACC) and the AHA collaborated and produced guidelines for the treatment of systolic and diastolic CHF (ACC and AHA, 1996).

Systolic CHF. ACEIs are first-line therapy; these are generally given in large doses as long as the client can tolerate them. Diuretics are used with the ACEIs. Sodium restriction

TABLE 23-3 Selected Medications for Congestive Heart Failure

DRUG CLASSIFICATION	ADVERSE REACTIONS	PRECAUTIONS
ACEIs		
Captopril (Capoten) Enalapril (Vasotec) Lisinopril (Zestril) Quinapril (Accupril) Ramipril (Altace) Trandolapril (Mavik)	Cough, skin rash, hypotension, taste disturbance, angioedema	Monitor renal function. Avoid sudden changes in position.
ALDOSTERONE ANTAGONIST		
Spironolactone (Aldactone)	GI bleeding, impotence, fever, uticaria, confusion, ataxia	Monitor for fluid and electrolyte imbalance. Monitor renal and hepatic levels.
BETA-BLOCKERS		
Bisoprolol (Zebeta) Carvedilol (Coreg) Metoprolol (Lopressor) Metoprolol extended release (Toprol-XL)	Bradycardia, shortness of breath, fatigue, dizziness, depression, diarrhea, pruritus, rash, arthralgia May mask symptoms of hyperthyroidism and hypoglycemia.	Monitor heart rate. Monitor for signs of hyperglycemia.
DIURETICS		
Thiazides		
Hydrochlorothiazide (Hydrodiuril, Esidrix) Metolazone (Zaroxolyn)	Electrolyte depletion, hypovolemia, hyperglycemia, gastric irritation	Monitor electrolytes, especially potassium. Monitor urine output.
Loop Diuretics		
Furosemide (Lasix) Bumetanide (Bumex) Ethacrynic acid (Edecrin) Torsemide (Demadex)	Electrolyte depletion, anorexia, diarrhea, malaise, mental confusion, ototoxicity A dramatic increase occurs in urine output	Monitor electrolytes, especially potassium. Monitor hearing.
CARDIAC GLYCOSIDES		
Digoxin (Lanoxin)	Altered color perceptions, visual disturbances, confusion, headache, muscle weakness, nausea, anorexia, arrhythmias, bradycardia	Monitor potassium levels. Use with caution in clients with idiopathic hypertrophic subaortic stenosis (IHSS). Monitor vital signs.
SYMPATHOMIMETICS		
Dopamine (Intropin)	Headache, tachycardia, arrhythmias, hypertension	Contraindicated in clients with IHSS or sensitivity to any sulfite.
Dobutamine (Dobutrex)	Headache, nausea, hypotension	Contraindicated in clients with IHSS or hypersensitivity to metabisulfite.
Amrinone (Inocor)	Headache, anorexia, hepatotoxicity, thrombocytopenia, hypotension	Use with caution in clients with CAD or recent MI. Contraindicated in clients with metabisulfite hypersensitivity.

Data from Lehne R et al: *Pharmacology for nursing care,* ed 3, Philadelphia, 1998, Saunders; and Chavey WE et al: Guideline for the management of heart failure caused by systolic dysfunction, part 2, Treatment, *Am Fam Phys* 64(6):1045, 2001.

is critical. Digoxin is effective for moderate to severe CHF. Low-dose dobutamine infusion may benefit clients with refractory CHF. Anticoagulation is indicated if atrial fibrillation is present. Exercise as tolerated is also encouraged.

Diastolic CHF. The goal is to reduce ventricular filling pressure and control symptoms. Diuretics and nitrates are first-line therapy. Calcium channel blockers, beta-blockers, and ACEIs may be beneficial. Because its positive inotropic effects also increase myocardial oxygen demand, digoxin is not used

ACEIs. These drugs inhibit the progression of heart failure and reduce mortality in older adults. They are also associated with decreased hospitalizations for clients (Aronow et al, 1998). They block the conversion of angiotensin I into angiotensin II, a potent vasoconstrictor that also promotes the release of aldosterone. These drugs decrease afterload and preload.

Diuretics. Diuretics reduce preload; they reduce the symptoms associated with pulmonary and systemic vascular congestion. Loop diuretics are the most commonly prescribed and provide predictable and controllable diuresis in severe heart failure. Hypokalemia needs to be monitored, especially if a client is also taking digoxin. Older clients with early, mild CHF characterized by normal renal function and only minimal ankle edema might do well with a thiazide diuretic.

Digitalis. Systolic dysfunction and atrial fibrillation are the principal indicators for digitalis in the older client. Digoxin is used when ACEIs are used at maximum doses and more relief is needed. The Digitalis Investigation Group study concluded that digitalis had no effect on survival (Aronow et al, 1998). Therapeutic serum levels must be closely monitored in older adults to prevent toxicity because of older adults' decreased lean body masses and reduced glomerular filtration.

Beta-Blockers. These drugs have generated increased use in the treatment of CHF. Carvedilol, a nonselective beta-blocker, is used for the treatment of CHF. It has demonstrated a reduction in mortality and need for hospitalization in class II and III CHF clients (Aronow et al, 1998). Beta-blockers decrease the sympathetic stimulation to the heart that is believed to aid in the progression of the disease. As a class, beta-blockers exert negative inotropic effects (slowing of heart rate), so caution should be used if they are given with agents that also depress contractility (e.g., calcium channel blockers, antiarrhythmics).

Sympathomimetics. These medications mimic the sympathetic nervous system. They increase the force of myocardial contraction, which is the rationale for their use with CHF. Tachycardia may occur.

Prognosis. The Framington study has associated CHF with a poor prognosis. The probability of surviving 5 years after the onset of CHF was 38% for men and 58% for women (Burrell, Gerlach, and Pless, 1997). The prognosis varies with the cause of CHF. Valvular disease that is surgically corrected has a better prognosis than CHF caused by cardiomyopathy.

Classifying CHF can be done in several ways. The categories for CHF are:

1. **Right or left failure**—Although left ventricle failure is more prevalent, a number of individuals, especially those with chronic disease, experience failure in both ventricles. In left ventricle failure, the left ventricle fails to pump an adequate stroke volume. This leads to pulmonary congestion, and pulmonary symptoms predominate. Generally, right ventricle failure is caused by increased pulmonary pressure that results from left ventricle failure. This prevents the right ventricle from pumping adequately, causing generalized systemic symptoms to appear. Older adults with chronic CHF tend to exhibit signs of both left-sided and right-sided heart failure.
2. **Acute or chronic failure**—Acute heart failure results from a sudden reduction in cardiac output and inadequate organ perfusion; it may lead to pulmonary edema and circulatory collapse. Compensatory mechanisms do not activate. Chronic heart failure occurs slowly, often as a result of hypertension, valvular or ischemic heart disease, or chronic lung disease. Hypervolemia occurs, sodium and water are retained, and the ventricle dilates and hypertrophies. The heart may be able to activate compensatory mechanisms to minimize clinical symptoms (Thelan et al, 1998).
3. **Systolic or diastolic failure**—Systolic heart failure is caused by decreased left ventricular contractility. Cardiac output decreases, and the ventricle hypertrophies. CAD is a cause for this type of heart failure. Diastolic heart failure is caused by decreased compliance of the ventricle; it becomes stiffer and cannot accept adequate blood volume. As a result, stroke volume and cardiac output decrease. Hypertension is a cause for this type of heart failure (Box 23-5).

BOX 23-5 New York Heart Association Functional Classification of Heart Failure

CLASS	DEFINITION
I	Asymptomatic: Normal daily activity does not initiate symptoms.
II	Moderate daily activity initiates onset of symptoms of shortness of breath or fatigue, but is comfortable at rest.
III	Very mild activity initiates symptoms; usually symptom-free at rest.
IV	Client is exhausted, and any type of activity initiates symptoms; symptoms are present at rest: sitting still or lying down.

From Rittenhouse SK: Spironolactone for heart failure: a worthy addition to therapy, *Adv Nurse Pract* 9(1):35, 2001. This table has been reprinted with permission from ADVANCE Newsmagazines.

NURSING MANAGEMENT

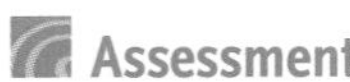

Assessment

Older adults should be assessed for history of CAD, rheumatic heart disease, hypertension, cardiac valve disease, infection, and current medications. The initial physical evaluation of an older adult suspected of having CHF includes measurement of blood pressure, evaluation for pitting edema of the legs and ankles, assessment of jugular venous pressure, heart and lung auscultation, and percussion of the lung for effusions. Orthopnea, fatigue at rest, paroxysmal nocturnal dyspnea, nocturnal urination, and edema are also important to assess. Assessment of how symptoms have affected ADLs is also important for older adults (Box 23-6).

Diagnosis

Common diagnoses for an older adult client with CHF include:

- Decreased cardiac output related to decreased contractility and increased preload
- Impaired gas exchange related to pulmonary venous congestion
- Fluid volume excess related to increased sodium and water reabsorption
- Anxiety related to perceived threat to self
- Activity intolerance related to decreased cardiac output and fatigue
- Ineffective individual coping related to knowledge deficit and fear of uncertain outcome
- Sleep pattern disturbance related to nocturnal dyspnea
- Knowledge deficit: disease process, medications, and treatment plan related to lack of previous exposure

BOX 23-6 Congestive Heart Failure

SYSTOLIC HEART FAILURE

Dyspnea initially on exertion, but as the CHF worsens, also at rest
Orthopnea
Paroxysmal nocturnal dyspnea
Weakness and fatigue
Diminished exercise tolerance
Crackles on auscultation of the lungs
S_3 gallop
Pulsus alternans (alternating intensity of the pulse)

DIASTOLIC HEART FAILURE

Fatigue with a low exercise tolerance
Edema that worsens in dependent position and subsides with rest and elevation; usually occurs in lower extremities and is bilateral
Weight gain
Extra heart sounds: S_3 and S_4
Nausea, anorexia, and abdominal distention
Hepatomegaly
Nocturia
Jugular vein distention

Adapted from Bollinger K, Sadar AM: Care and management of the patient with right heart failure secondary to diastolic dysfunction: an advanced practice perspective and case review, *Crit Care Nurs Q* 26(1):22, 2003.

Planning and Expected Outcomes

Expected outcomes are aimed at maximizing myocardial function and assisting with the lifestyle modifications and emotional adjustments imposed by the disease. Expected outcomes for an older adult with CHF include:

1. Cardiac output will be maximized, as evidenced by vital signs within acceptable range, no arrhythmia, adequate cardiac output, urine output greater than 30 ml/hr, and alert mental state.
2. Gas exchange will be improved, as evidenced by decreased or no reported dyspnea, normal respiratory rate, lungs clear to auscultation, no evidence of central or peripheral cyanosis, and a client report of improved activity tolerance.
3. Excess fluid volume will be reduced, as evidenced by reductions in water weight, dependent edema, and abdominal girth.
4. Client will experience less anxiety, as evidenced by communication of fears to nurse and self-report of use of coping skills.
5. Activity will be restored to its level prior to illness, as evidenced by fewer or no reports of fatigue with usual activities and no reports of symptoms induced by select activities.
6. Client will experience adequate coping, as evidenced by the naming of two coping skills used in the past and a self-report of feeling positive about the future.
7. Client will experience an acceptable sleeping pattern, as evidenced by reports of sleep uninterrupted by dyspnea and a feeling of being rested on awakening.
8. Client will demonstrate adequate knowledge level, as evidenced by ability to correctly state information about disease process; treatment plan; and medication indication, dosage, frequency, and side effects.

Intervention

It is essential that the nurse assess blood pressure, apical pulse, heart rate, heart and lung sounds, and peripheral edema to detect early signs and symptoms of decreased cardiac output. The intake and output and daily weights should be monitored and recorded. The client should be weighed at the same time daily to monitor accurately for fluid loss or retention. The nurse should increase the client's activity according to tolerance and provide time for rest; while in bed, the client should maintain a Fowler's position. The client may need more than one pillow to sleep with at night. The nurse should instruct the client to take his or her diuretic in the morning so sleep is not disturbed. The nurse should encourage the client to take slow deep breaths during dyspneic episodes and maintain a calm environment.

The nurse should instruct the client on a restricted sodium and fluid intake. A dietitian may be consulted. Older adults should be instructed to avoid canned foods and prepared foods from the frozen food section and to use salt sparingly. A weight gain of 3 lb in 48 hours and a return of any symptoms should be reported to the health care provider immediately. Electrolyte levels, especially potassium, and signs and symptoms of electrolyte imbalance should be monitored.

Older adults need to be given instructions on their condition, procedures, diet, and risk factors in a clear, simple manner, using proper language, reading level, and cultural considerations. The nurse should maintain an environment that is as relaxed and quiet as possible, explain all procedures before beginning, and answer questions clearly and concisely. The nurse should also provide opportunities for older clients and family members to verbalize their concerns.

Referral to a home health agency for assistance with ADLs and referral to Meals on Wheels may be necessary for some individuals. The client may wish to enter a cardiac rehabilitation program to monitor activity tolerance in a secure environment.

Evaluation

Older adults should demonstrate that ventricular function is improved through unlabored respirations, no peripheral edema, no cough or orthopnea, and a normal urine output. The client should increase activity without experiencing dyspnea and should demonstrate an ability to return to usual ADLs. Documentation of trends is critical for older adults with heart failure, especially in regard to assessment findings and treatment responses (see Nursing Care Plan).

Nursing Care Plan

Congestive Heart Failure

Clinical Situation: Mr. H, an 82-year-old man who is widowed and lives alone, arrives in the emergency room complaining he has had difficulty breathing, especially at night, associated with nausea, for the past week. He states that he must sleep with two pillows to breathe more easily at night and still does not get a good night's rest. He also complains of a cough that is worse at night and relieved by nothing. Mr. H is concerned he has pneumonia. Assessment of Mr. H reveals the following:

- Vital signs: temperature, 98° F; apical heart rate, 86 beats/min and irregular; respiratory rate, 36 breaths/min and labored; and blood pressure, 170/96 mm Hg
- Skin—pale, cool, and diaphoretic
- Inspiratory bibasilar crackles that do not clear with coughing
- S_3 heart sound on auscultation
- Visible jugular vein distention
- 3+ bilateral pedal edema

A 12-lead ECG and a chest x-ray examination are ordered. An intravenous line is started at a "keep vein open" (KVO) rate. Oxygen via mask is administered. Intravenous furosemide is given, and Mr. H is admitted with a diagnosis of CHF.

Nursing Diagnoses

Decreased cardiac output related to ineffective myocardial contractility

Fluid volume excess related to sodium and water retention

Impaired gas exchange related to increased fluid in pulmonary vasculature

Knowledge deficit: disease process and treatment plan related to lack of previous exposure

Outcomes

Cardiac output is maximized as evidenced by vital signs within acceptable limits, controlled arrhythmias, clear breath sounds, fewer dyspneic episodes, and alert mental status.

Client will demonstrate normal fluid balance, as evidenced by clear breath sounds, reduced pedal and pretibial edema, an intake greater than output, and a loss of water weight with a stable dry weight.

Client will correctly verbalize prescribed sodium and fluid restrictions.

Client will demonstrate improved gas exchange as evidenced by activity tolerance, absence of shortness of breath and nocturnal dyspnea, and clear breath sounds.

Client will describe CHF and reasons for limitations, identify own risk factors, and explain techniques to initiate lifestyle changes.

Client will participate in treatment plan.

Interventions

Monitor and document heart rate, rhythm, blood pressure, respirations, and lung and heart sounds hourly and as needed.

Assess for edema and jugular vein distention every 2 to 4 hours.

Monitor intake and output hourly.

Assess skin temperature and color, and assess for the presence of diaphoresis at regular intervals.

Provide a restful environment.

Administer cardiac medications as ordered; document client's response.

Monitor intake and output hourly.

Weigh daily, using the same scale at the same time of day.

Continued

Care Plan
Congestive Heart Failure—cont'd

Interventions—cont'd

Administer diuretics as ordered; document client's response.
Assess electrolytes, BUN, and creatinine, as well as symptoms of imbalance.
Instruct client to elevate extremities when sitting.
Instruct client on sodium and fluid restrictions.
Assess respiratory status hourly and as needed (rate, rhythm, use of accessory muscles, and lung sounds).
Maintain client in semi- or high-Fowler's position to aid breathing.
Administer oxygen as ordered, monitoring oxygen saturation.
Instruct client to avoid strenuous and taxing activities and to take advantage of peak energy periods.
Discuss normal function of heart and how CHF alters this.
Discuss diet and fluid restrictions and medications.
Discuss specific risk factors and the client's role in modifying them.
Review signs and symptoms that need to be immediately reported to a health care provider.
Provide an environment that allows client to verbalize feel ings and ask questions.
Discuss the benefits of increased activity (e.g., walking program).
Refer client to community resources and support groups.
Encourage client to obtain annual flu immunization.

Peripheral Artery Occlusive Disease

Peripheral artery occlusive disease (PAOD) is any disturbance in the systemic arteries that impairs tissue perfusion. Arteriosclerosis (hardening or thickening of arterial wall) and atherosclerosis (the usual cause of arteriosclerosis, involving plaque formation within the arterial wall) are common disturbances affecting the arterial vasculature. Atherosclerosis is the most common cause of arteriosclerosis obliterans, which is the narrowing or obstruction of arterial walls. Although the exact cause of atherosclerosis is unknown, several risk factors have been identified. These include smoking, elevated serum cholesterol, hypertension, diabetes mellitus, physical inactivity, obesity, and family history.

Atherosclerosis involves the development of atheromatous plaques on the intimal layer of arterial vessels. These lesions progressively narrow the artery lumen and lead to the formation of thrombi and aneurysms.

Arteriosclerosis obliterans is a chronic occlusive disease of the arteries caused by plaque formation. As the lumen narrows, partial or complete obstruction can occur, leading to inadequate tissue perfusion beyond the lesion and ischemia. Common sites for atherosclerotic lesions are the aortoiliac vessels, femoral-popliteal vessels, and popliteal-tibial arteries. Symptoms appear when the artery is unable to supply the tissues with adequate oxygenated blood flow.

Thrombi that develop at the site of the atherosclerotic lesion or within arterial aneurysms can break loose and circulate through the arterial system. Thromboemboli also originate in the heart as a result of atrial fibrillation, MI, or mitral stenosis. Thromboemboli tend to block arteries at bifurcation points of the femoral and popliteal arteries. Impaired blood flow and ischemia occur at sites distal to the occlusion.

As the atheromatous plaque progresses, the medial layer of the wall calcifies and loses elasticity, which weakens the arterial wall. As the vessel wall weakens, pouches or aneurysms form. Pressure within the arteries, especially in the presence of hypertension, can further dilate the aneurysm until it ruptures. Aneurysms commonly occur in large arteries such as the abdominal aorta. Multiple aneurysms can develop in the popliteal artery. Thrombi can form within the aneurysm and circulate to smaller distal vessels in the arterial system.

Signs and symptoms of arterial insufficiency depend on the site, extent of occlusion, and degree of collateral circulation. Collateral circulation often develops with the gradual elevation of plaque formation.

Intermittent claudication (muscle ischemia) is one of the initial symptoms with atherosclerosis obliterans. Pain in the foot or calf is experienced with exercise and subsides with rest. As the disease progresses, the distance walked becomes shorter before pain is felt. Burning pain in the foot at rest or during sleep indicates a severe form of the disease. Cold, numbness, and tingling may accompany the pain. The foot appears pale when elevated and red in dependent positions. Dry skin, thickened toenails, loss of pedal hair, and cool skin can result from poor circulation. Painful arterial ulcers may be noticed on the toes, between the toes, or on the upper aspect of the foot. Cold extremities with mottling, delayed filling of capillaries, and absent pedal pulses are indicative of acute arterial insufficiency and should be treated immediately. Care should be taken to examine both extremities for comparison. Advanced stages of ischemia lead to necrosis, ulceration, and gangrene of the toes.

The pain with arterial emboli is sudden and severe. The affected extremity appears pale and cool, and distal pulses are absent. Impaired motor and sensory function is evident. Shock can develop if large arteries are occluded.

With abdominal and peripheral aneurysms, there are usually no overt signs and symptoms until rupture or acute thrombosis. A pulsating mass may be palpated in the abdominal area with aortic aneurysms, and clients may sense abdominal or back pain.

Diagnostic Tests and Procedures. Routine screening for PAOD in asymptomatic patients is not recommended in the U.S. Preventive Services Task Force guidelines (Kuznar, 2004).

Doppler ultrasound detects and measures the velocity of blood flow through the arterial segments and grafts. Duplex imaging uses a Doppler system that maps a region of an artery in which blood is flowing. Radionuclide scanning consists of the injection of dye and scanning at intervals to determine radionuclide accumulation in the damaged vessel. Blood flow through the vessel and graft can be assessed, perfusion pressures can be calculated, and the vascular system can be visualized. Arteriography is performed to determine the exact location and extent of arterial occlusion. Contrast material is injected into the arterial system through a specialized catheter inserted into the brachial or femoral artery, and a series of x-ray studies trace the dye through the arterial system.

Treatment. The first line of treatment includes aspirin, 81 to 325 mg/day with food. Antiplatelet medications such as aspirin inhibit the adherence and aggregation of platelets along damaged vessels. Ticlopidine (Ticlid) and clopidogrel (Plavix) are antiplatelet drugs that decrease platelet activity. Pentoxifylline (Trental) reduces blood viscosity, enhances the flexibility of red blood cells (RBCs), and improves tissue perfusion. Cilostazol (Pletal) reduces platelet activity and is an arterial vasodilator. These prophylactic drugs may help reduce blood viscosity. Thrombolytics are also used for acute conditions (Kuznar, 2004).

Surgical Procedures. Percutaneous transluminal angioplasty involves gaining access to the arterial system with a specialized balloon-tipped catheter. The catheter is advanced under fluoroscopy to the atherosclerotic lesion and inflated over the site to compress the plaque and improve blood flow. Arterial bypass and reconstruction may be performed to increase blood flow. Intravascular stents keep the vessel open. Endarterectomy is the opening of the artery and removal of the plaque. Advanced cases of atherosclerosis and gangrene of the extremities necessitate amputation of the limb.

Prognosis. Pharmaceutic agents are not particularly effective in the treatment of PAOD; surgical interventions, however, have been more successful. The key to preventing or halting the progression of PAOD and subsequent complications appears to be controlling the risk factors for atherosclerosis. Death seldom results from PAOD (see Client/Family Teaching box).

NURSING MANAGEMENT

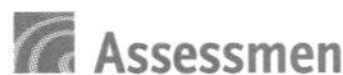

Assessment

Assessment of an older adult with PAOD begins with a complete history and physical examination. Subjective and objective assessment of a client with PAOD is outlined in Box 23-7.

Client/Family Teaching

PERIPHERAL ARTERY OCCLUSIVE DISEASE (PAOD)

Prevention is the key to management of PAOD.

Control risk factors: stop smoking; lose weight; control hypertension and diabetes mellitus; eat a low-fat, low-cholesterol diet; and exercise daily with walking.

Do not cross legs while sitting; do not stand or sit for long periods.

Do not wear constricting garments.

Foot care is essential. Inspect the feet daily and keep them clean and dry. After bathing, dry well between the toes; lubricate feet with lotion daily. Avoid walking barefoot and wear proper-fitting footwear that is flexible yet protective.

Notify the health care provider immediately of changes in color, temperature, or sensation of the affected area, or of a break in skin integrity.

From Kuznar K: Peripheral arterial occlusive disease: evaluation and management in the primary care setting, *Adv Nurse Pract* 12(2):36, 2004.

BOX 23-7 Assessment of Older Adults with Peripheral Artery Occlusive Disease

SUBJECTIVE DATA

Pain in extremity (location, intensity, onset, and duration)

Precipitating factors (activity or rest)

Relieving factors (activity or rest and position)

Presence of intermittent claudication (frequency and distance)

Modifiable risk factors (smoking, high cholesterol levels, hypertension, diabetes mellitus, obesity, and physical inactivity)

Personal and family history (of CAD and PAOD)

Psychosocial state (anxiety, fear, or depression)

OBJECTIVE DATA

Skin changes (color, temperature, appearance, and sensations)

Condition of nails

Circulation (peripheral pulses, bruits, and capillary filling)

Muscle tone

Assessment data should reflect the presence of acute or chronic arterial insufficiency.

Diagnosis

Nursing diagnoses for older adults with PAOD include:

- Altered peripheral tissue perfusion related to decreased arterial blood flow
- Activity intolerance related to imbalance between tissue need and blood supply

- Risk for impaired skin integrity related to decreased tissue perfusion and sensation
- Knowledge deficit: disease process, medication, and treatment plan related to lack of previous exposure

Planning and Expected Outcomes

Older clients with PAOD and their family members should be included in the planning of care. Discharge planning should begin as soon as an older client is admitted to the hospital, since this type of client typically needs additional support services during home recovery.

Expected outcomes for an older client with PAOD include:

1. Client will manifest reduced signs and symptoms of arterial insufficiency, as evidenced by warm skin temperature over affected area, presence of pedal pulses, and decreased claudication in affected extremities.
2. Client will successfully participate in activities within limits imposed by disease.
3. Client will demonstrate protective behavior and self-care measures to prevent injury to skin.
4. Client will correctly describe the disease process and treatment plan, including medication action, dosage, and side effects.
5. Client will identify personal risk factors and methods to reduce these factors.

Intervention

Nursing interventions include the initiation of a graduated, regular exercise program to enhance collateral circulation. Clients should be encouraged to balance activities with rest and may need assistance to develop a schedule of paced activities. Client education is also important to prevent injury.

Evaluation

Evaluation of an older client with PAOD focuses on achievement of expected outcomes. Short-term evaluation focuses on those interventions aimed at reducing risk factors. Long-term evaluation is based on trends in progress toward improving tissue perfusion and viability. An older adult and family's willingness to participate is a crucial factor in achieving a successful outcome over time (see Nursing Care Plan).

Venous Disorders

PVD is any disturbance that impairs tissue perfusion. The most common underlying causes of PVD are (1) varicose veins, (2) deep vein thrombosis, and (3) venous ulceration.

Varicose veins of the leg occur particularly in women and may be divided into primary and secondary varicose veins. Primary varicose veins are more common, and the varicosity, which occurs in the wall of the vein, may be related to weakness of the wall or to incompetent valves of the saphenofemoral junction or perforating veins. Underlying causes include obesity, estrogenic hormones, and, in older adults, a previous occupation that required long periods of standing. Secondary varicose veins are the result of thrombosis in the deep system, which may subsequently occur with obstruction of the valves. The signs and symptoms of varicose veins are protrusion of veins on the legs, aching, ankle swelling, night cramps, skin changes such as itching, varicose eczema, and (in extreme cases) hemorrhage. The majority of cases may be treated with conservative therapy, including the use of elastic support bandages, regular exercise, and weight reduction. In more severe cases, surgical intervention such as sclerotherapy and ligation may be required.

Deep vein thrombosis is a common and serious disorder and has been associated with 600,000 hospitalizations each year in the United States. Approximately 60,000 to 200,000 individuals die each year as a result of pulmonary embolism. Immobility (prolonged bedrest), advancing age (over age of 45), obesity, hormonal usage, and cigarette smoking are contributing factors. Medical conditions predisposing individuals to deep vein thrombosis include blood dyscrasias, cancer, systemic infection, dehydration, heart disease, stroke, inflammatory bowel disease, and incompetent venous valves. Clients at highest surgical risk are those undergoing knee or hip surgery; 10% to 40% of these clients develop thrombosis (Crowther and McCourt, 2004).

Venous ulceration occurs in clients who have chronic venous insufficiency. The superficial system is subjected to high pressure, which results in poor tissue oxygenation of the lower limbs. Venous ulcers occur on the medial side of the lower half of the leg. The ulcer is usually painful, may easily be infected, and, if left untreated, may involve the circumference of the leg. The management of venous ulceration depends on relieving the hypertension occurring in the superficial system through bedrest, elevation of the limb, and compression bandaging. A characteristic brownish discoloration of the skin develops from deposits of melanin and hemosiderin. Older adults often complain of heaviness in the legs.

Diagnostic Tests and Procedures. Indirect methods to detect obstruction include Doppler ultrasound, plethysmography, venous duplex ultrasonography, and contrast venography. Doppler ultrasound measures venous obstruction and reflux of blood by changes in the frequency of sound waves. Laboratory work includes a platelet count, prothrombin time, PTTs, and INR.

Treatment. The therapeutic aim for the treatment of PVD is to preserve not only the limb, but also its function. Interventions range from palliative measures to ease symptoms to the use of pharmacologic and surgical strategies to enhance blood flow and prevent clot formation.

Nursing Care Plan
Peripheral Artery Disease

Clinical Situation: Mrs. A, a 70-year-old woman, is complaining of decreased activity level because of pain in her right leg when walking. This has been getting worse over the past few months, and it is now difficult for her to go to her mailbox without pain. She states that sometimes her toes tingle at night. She does not complain of chest pain or shortness of breath. She denies smoking and takes amlopidine for high blood pressure and aspirin as needed for arthritis.

Assessment of Mrs. A reveals:

- Vital signs: temperature, 98.4° F; heart rate, 84 beats/min and regular; respiratory rate, 16 breaths/min and not labored; blood pressure, 160/84 mm Hg
- Height, 5 ft, 6 in; weight, 164 lb
- Skin: warm and dry
- Right foot pale and cooler than left
- Pedal pulse: right foot 1+; left foot 2+
- Femoral pulse: 2+ bilateral
- Able to move toes equally

Pentoxifylline (Trental) is ordered, and an exercise program is prescribed. Doppler studies are scheduled.

Nursing Diagnoses

Activity intolerance related to pain when walking

Risk for impaired skin integrity related to decreased circulation

Potential altered health maintenance related to lack of knowledge of disease and treatment plan

Outcomes

Client will identify factors that cause pain.

Client will participate in a plan to increase activity and decrease claudication.

Client will demonstrate no sign of skin breakdown or impairment of skin integrity.

Client will identify the risk factors of the disease, describe lifestyle changes, and participate in the treatment plan.

Interventions

Plan activities to include walking program.

Increase walking regimen daily, up to 30 minutes per day.

Have the client walk until experiencing pain, rest until pain abates, and then walk again.

Encourage client and give reassurance that activity does not harm painful tissue.

Assist client in identifying, reducing, and eliminating risk factors (e.g., reducing weight, controlling hypertension).

Assess for ischemic ulcers.

Have client report ulcers or darkened areas on skin to health care provider.

Teach foot care measures, including daily inspection, daily washing using mild soap, and drying well; client may use lotion but should avoid use between the toes.

Teach client to cut nails straight across; wear proper-fitting shoes; avoid going barefoot; avoid sandals; always wear socks with shoes; and eat a well-balanced diet that is low in saturated fat.

Explain the importance of pertinent risk factors (e.g., smoking, high cholesterol, obesity, hypertension).

Explain the importance of walking; help develop a walking program.

Instruct client to keep extremity warm but not to use heating pads and hot water bottles.

Explain medications and when to call the health care provider.

Identify available community resources.

Palliative measures are important for maintaining comfort. Preservation of skin integrity is of prime importance in maintaining the overall health of the limb. Pharmacologic intervention is directed at increasing blood flow and preventing clot formation. Specifically, anticoagulation therapy—with heparin and warfarin—is used to prevent further clot formation. For prophylaxis, rather than treatment during the acute phase, low–molecular weight heparins such as enoxaparin sodium (Lovenox) are used for their antithrombi action. This class of medication has a lower risk of bleeding and does not require laboratory monitoring for therapeutic doses. Typically, low–molecular weight heparins are given subcutaneously once or twice a day. A variety of surgical procedures can be performed to reduce the effects of PVD. Surgical procedures include those involving the superficial venous system and the deep venous system, as well as surgery for venous obstruction (Crowther and McCourt, 2004).

Prognosis. The prevalence, risk factors, and mortality rate for PVD in the older adult population have received limited attention in the literature, but varicose veins are known to be one of the most prevalent conditions in this population. Deep vein thrombosis is diagnosed in 2.5 million people per year; 200,000 are first-time episodes. It is estimated that the mortality rate from deep vein thrombosis is 13% to 21% for a lower extremity and 48% for an upper extremity (Crowther and McCourt, 2004). Prevention, awareness, and immediate treatment are essential to avoid complications or death (Day, 2003).

NURSING MANAGEMENT

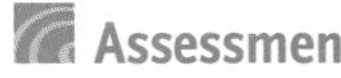

Assessment

Assessment of an older adult with PVD begins with a complete history and physical examination. Subjective data include pain in the extremity, precipitating factors, relieving factors, modifiable risk factors, and personal and family history. Objective data include skin color, hair distribution, atrophy, edema, varicosities, petechiae, lesions, and ulcerations. Table 23-4 provides more information for the assessment for peripheral arterial and venous disease.

Diagnosis

Nursing diagnoses for an older adult with PVD include:

- Risk for impaired skin integrity related to venous stasis and fragility of small blood vessels
- Altered tissue perfusion related to interruption of venous flow
- Pain related to inflammatory process

Planning and Expected Outcomes

Expected outcomes for an older client with PVD include:

1. Skin integrity will be maintained or improved.
2. Client will exhibit no ulceration or signs of the inflammatory process.
3. Tissue perfusion will be improved, as evidenced by decreased edema and fewer complaints of discomfort.

Intervention

Nursing interventions for an older client with venous disease include assessment of skin integrity (e.g., skin texture, skin temperature, pain, color, edema, pulses). The nurse should use a Doppler sensor if pulses seem absent. The affected extremity should be elevated to facilitate venous circulation, and the size of the affected limb should be measured and recorded at least daily. Elastic compression stockings may also be ordered; it is helpful to demonstrate their application and removal and require a return demonstration to assess the client's ability. Devices are available through medical supply companies for assistance with application if necessary. Stockings should be replaced every 3 to 6 months if there is no evidence of excess wear.

If a client has a deep vein thrombosis, bedrest is usually prescribed for several days. An older adult is at even greater risk for development of the complications associated with bedrest, so the nurse must implement measures based on the client's individual risk factors to prevent the hazards of immobility. The client and family should be reassured that the activity restrictions are for a limited period.

Managing venous stasis ulcers involves healing the ulcers and preventing recurrence (see Chapter 30 for a full discussion of ulcer treatment options). Prevention of ulcer formation is of prime importance. The nurse should encourage ambulation to enhance collateral circulation. In fact, a progressive exercise program should be prescribed. Clients should be instructed to wear elastic or support stockings before walking and to avoid standing for prolonged periods. Instruction on foot care is an important part of the prevention plan. The skin should be inspected daily and washed gently in tepid water with a neutral soap

TABLE 23-4 Differentiating Arterial and Venous Insufficiency

ASSESSMENT	ARTERIAL DISEASE	VENOUS DISEASE
Pain		
Acute	Sudden and severe	Little or no pain; tenderness along inflamed vein
Chronic	Intermittent claudication; rest pain	Heaviness; fullness
Hair	Hair loss distal to occlusion	No hair loss
Nails	Thick and brittle	Normal
Sensation	Possible paresthesia	Normal
Skin texture	Thin, dry, shiny	Stasis dermatitis; veins may be visible; skin mottled
Skin color	Pallor or reactive hyperemia (pallor when limb is elevated; rubor when limb is dependent)	Brawny (reddish brown); cyanotic if dependent
Skin temperature	Cool	Warm
Skin breakdown (ulcers)	Severely painful; usually on or between toes or on upper surface of foot over metatarsal heads or other bony prominence	Mildly painful, with pain relieved by leg elevation; usually in ankle area
Edema	None or mild, usually unilateral	Typically present (usually foot to calf); may be unilateral or bilateral
Pulses	Diminished, weak, or absent	Normal

From Lewis S, Collier I, Heitkemper M: *Medical-surgical nursing: assessment and management of clinical problems,* ed 4, St Louis, 1996, Mosby.

and patted dry, with special attention to adequately drying between the toes. Lubricant should be applied after washing to aid in retaining moisture. A professional should perform nail care. Shoes should fit well and provide good support.

Evaluation

Evaluation focuses on the client's progress in improving skin integrity and venous circulation and reducing pain and discomfort, measured by a decrease in signs and symptoms. If skin is intact and edema is minimal, education has been successful. Documentation emphasizes accurate recording of the skin assessment, including measurements of the affected extremity.

Anemia

Anemia is defined as a low RBC count, decreased quantity of hemoglobin, and decreased hematocrit. Anemia is not a diagnosis but a condition caused by some other pathologic condition. Since oxygen is carried on the hemoglobin molecule, anemia causes a decreased oxygen-carrying capacity of the blood. The severity of the symptoms of anemia depends on the ability of compensatory mechanisms to respond. If the blood count drops quickly, these mechanisms are unable to fully correct the situation. The body adjusts by increasing cardiac output and respirations, increasing the release of oxygen from hemoglobin, and redistributing blood to the vital organs (Tefferi, 2003). An older adult's compensatory mechanisms may be slower to respond because of coexisting chronic disease, which then causes symptoms of anemia to appear more quickly.

Anemias are classified according to the changes in the RBCs. *Microcytic* and *macrocytic* are terms that describe the size of the RBC: microcytic cells are smaller than normal, and macrocytic cells are larger than normal. *Chromic* is a term that describes the color of the cell: hypo cells are pale. There are three major classes of anemia: normocytic normochromic, macrocytic normochromic, and microcytic hypochromic.

In normocytic normochromic anemia the size of the RBCs and the amount of hemoglobin they contain are normal. Acute blood loss and anemia of chronic disease are examples. In macrocytic normochromic anemia the RBCs are large with normal amounts of hemoglobin. Vitamin B_{12} and folic acid deficiencies cause this type of anemia. In microcytic hypochromic anemia the RBCs are smaller than normal with a decreased amount of hemoglobin. Iron deficiency causes this type of anemia.

Symptoms vary in frequency and severity. Fatigue is a frequent complaint of older clients with anemia. Pallor is another common sign. Skin color is not a good indicator of pallor because of varying pigmentation. Oral mucous membranes, as well as conjunctivae and nail beds, are better indicators. Headache, dyspnea, and dizziness are other common symptoms of anemia. Older adults may exhibit symptoms of anemia (e.g., fatigue, dizziness) but attribute these to the aging process or to other chronic diseases. The nurse should be aware of this so detection and treatment can be initiated as soon as possible.

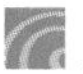

Anemia of chronic disease and nutritional anemias are common in older adults. Altered iron metabolism, deficiency of erythropoietin, and a shortened life span of RBCs are causes of anemia from chronic disease. Nutritional deficits and blood loss (commonly gastrointestinal) cause iron-deficiency anemia. Inadequate intake or inadequate absorption of folic acid and altered absorption of vitamin B_{12} are causes of macrocytic anemias.

Diagnostic Tests, Procedures, and Treatment. With iron-deficiency anemia (microcytic hypochromic) the CBC with differential has decreased mean corpuscular volume (MCV) and mean corpuscular hemoglobin concentration (MCHC). The iron and ferritin levels are decreased. The stool is tested for occult blood and is positive with anemia caused by gastrointestinal blood loss. The treatment includes dietary or supplemental intake of iron. Ferrous sulfate (325 mg) is given three times a day. Iron therapy should be given for 3 to 6 months to rebuild the iron stores.

With anemia of chronic disease (normocytic normochromic) the CBC with differential has normal MCV and MCHC. The iron level is decreased with a normal or increased ferritin level. The treatment is to treat the underlying disease. Blood transfusion for low hemoglobin is determined by the client's condition and coexisting diseases (Chernecky and Berger, 2001).

With folic acid deficiency the CBC with differential has an elevated MCV. The serum B_{12} level is normal. The folic acid level is decreased. The gastric analysis reveals the presence of free gastric acid. The treatment includes an increased dietary intake of folic acid; alcoholics usually require a higher dose of folic acid.

With pernicious anemia the CBC with differential has an elevated MCV. The serum B_{12} level is normal. The gastric analysis shows no free gastric acid, and with gastroscopy the gastric mucosa appears pale and gray. The treatment is vitamin B_{12} (cyanocobalamin) given intramuscularly for life.

Prognosis. The prognosis for anemia depends on the cause. With medications and dietary changes, prognosis is usually good. In the early stages any anemia can appear to be normocytic (Basch et al, 2002).

NURSING MANAGEMENT

Assessment

The assessment of an older adult with anemia focuses on the underlying cause and its effects on functional ability (Box 23-8).

BOX 23-8 Assessment of Older Adults with Anemia

SUBJECTIVE DATA

History (gastric surgery, liver or renal disease, recent blood loss, or trauma)
Current medications (over-the-counter vitamins and minerals, NSAIDs)
Nutritional habits
Alcohol intake
Change in bowel habits (color, consistency)
Weight loss
Complaints (fatigue, palpitations, dyspnea, paresthesia, painful tongue, dizziness, headache, or tinnitus)

OBJECTIVE DATA

Pallor (of nail beds, conjunctivae, or oral mucous membranes)
Tachycardia
Tachypnea
Syncope
Systolic murmur
Confusion
Unsteady gait
Stomatitis
CHF (severe anemia)
CBC values

Diagnosis

Nursing diagnoses for an older adult with anemia include:

- Activity intolerance related to imbalance between oxygen supply and demand
- Altered nutrition: less than body requirements related to malabsorption or decreased intake of vitamins, minerals, and nutritious foods
- Knowledge deficit: condition and treatment plan related to lack of exposure to information

Planning and Expected Outcomes

Expected outcomes for the older adult include:

1. Client will experience increases in activity without dyspnea or other previous symptoms over a period of 3 to 6 weeks.
2. Client will consume a well-balanced diet with foods high in minerals and vitamins, as evidenced by weight increases of 1 lb per week.
3. Client will verbalize an understanding of the cause of anemia, as well as of the treatment plan.

Intervention

Nursing interventions for an older adult with anemia focus on dietary management, a balance of rest and activity to support functional ability, and education about the condition. Environmental safety issues are also important for an older client experiencing symptoms that increase the risk of injury.

The client and family should be instructed about appropriate food selection and meal preparation to promote RBC formation. The nurse should provide a list of foods high in iron, folic acid, and vitamin B_{12} to incorporate into the daily meal plan. The physician or nurse practitioner may order supplemental iron preparations and, if so, should assess the client's tolerance of the preparation. Side effects include gastrointestinal upset, constipation or diarrhea, and green or black stools. It may be helpful to recommend taking the iron preparation after meals to minimize gastrointestinal upset.

In addition to dietary recommendations, the gerontologic nurse should ensure that the client has adequate income to purchase necessary foods; the functional ability to purchase and prepare foods; and adequate oral health, including properly fitting dentures. The nurse should also be alert to the presence of other variables that may adversely affect the older adult's ability to eat, such as loneliness, grief, depression, or alcoholism.

Nutritional Considerations

DASH Diet

DAILY FOOD GROUP	SERVINGS	NUTRIENTS SUPPLIED
Grains	7 to 8	Energy and fiber
Vegetables	4 to 5	Potassium, magnesium, and fiber
Fruits	4 to 5	Potassium, magnesium, and fiber
Low-fat or nonfat dairy foods	2 to 3	Calcium and protein
Meats, poultry, and fish	Less than 2	Protein and magnesium
Nuts, seeds, and legumes	4 to 5 per week	Energy, magnesium, potassium, protein, and fiber

From Joint National Committee: The sixth report of the Joint National Committee on the Prevention, Detection, Evaluation, and Treatment of High Blood Pressure, *Arch Intern Med* 157:2413, 1997.

Home Care

1. Homebound older adult clients, spouses, family, significant others, and caregivers should be included in all aspects of the care planning process in the home setting.
2. Clients value education in the home care setting, and this should continue as an important focus of care after hospitalization.
3. Clients dealing with chronic disease management in the home setting often experience anxiety, frustration, and depression. This factor should be taken into consideration when providing home care services, and appropriate interagency referrals should be initiated.
4. The fear of dying is often a major factor for homebound older adults with cardiovascular disease, particularly CHF. Counseling and referral to agencies should be provided.
5. Homebound older adults have a high anxiety level about needing help and not being able to obtain it. Establishing a link with an emergency community service, such as a lifeline program, may alleviate some anxiety.
6. The nurse should direct teaching of homebound older adults toward the anatomy and physiology of the heart, modifiable risk factors, medication regimen (especially in regard to dose and side effects), exercise tolerance, daily weight monitoring, and dietary factors (e.g., low sodium, low fat, fluid restriction).
7. Caregivers need to be educated about signs that suggest deterioration in status.
8. Assistance with ADLs may be required, especially for those homebound older adults who live alone or are responsible for household tasks. Often these clients do not request assistance, so the nurse should offer these services where appropriate.
9. Participation in a cardiac rehabilitation program or activities such as walking or swimming should be encouraged by the home care nurse.
10. Homebound older adult clients should be encouraged to wear medical-alert bracelets that identify their condition and medications.

Older clients and their families should also be instructed about balancing rest and activity. It is helpful for older adults to identify peak energy periods during waking hours and carry out desired or important activities during those times. However, clients should not carry out activities to the point of fatigue or dyspnea; rather, they should rest at intervals until activities are completed. Refer to Chapter 12 for interventions related to the safety of older adults who experience falls as a result of anemia.

Evaluation

Evaluation focuses on the client's progress toward meeting the expected outcomes. Specifically, the client should have fewer complaints of dyspnea, fatigue, and dizziness, and weight should be within the established norm for the client. Normal values of the client's hemoglobin, hematocrit, and RBC count indicate the success of interventions. The client's symptoms, weight trends, and activity levels are documented, along with any client and family teaching.

SUMMARY

CVD remains the leading cause of death in the United States. In the older adult population it is often difficult to clearly distinguish between CVD and normal aging. The presentation and effects of CVD can vary widely from person to person. Older adults many times display atypical symptoms of CVD and allow the disease process to advance before treatment is initiated. The challenge for the nurse is to obtain an accurate and complete assessment of an older adult client that allows the planning and initiation of the appropriate physical and psychosocial care. The nurse should focus on assisting older clients in modifying risk factors and optimizing health status.

Key Points

- CVD is the leading cause of death for both men and women.
- For those over age 65, mortality rates for CVD rise sharply, and it is anticipated that the actual number of deaths resulting from CVD will escalate as the proportion of the older adult population increases.
- Older adults who stay physically fit have twice the work capacity and a lower amount of body fat than older adults who are sedentary.
- Smoking cessation in older adults significantly reduces the risks of coronary events and of cardiac death within 1 year of quitting. The risk continues to decline gradually for many years thereafter.
- Smokers have twice the chance of developing CAD and 4 times the chance of sudden death compared with nonsmokers.
- It is estimated that more than 45% to 50% of the population over age 65 has high blood pressure, and the consequences are the most common causes of morbidity and mortality, including MI, CHF, and PVD.
- Older adults may have difficulty adopting healthier lifestyles because of long-term habits; however, healthy behavior changes can slow or halt the progression of the disease.
- Older adults have more atypical signs of CAD.
- Older adults may not recognize the onset of ischemia. Initial symptoms may consist of sudden dyspnea, confusion, fatigue, weakness, vertigo, syncope, vomiting, and exacerbation of heart failure.
- The incidence of atrial fibrillation increases with age and is the most common contributing factor to ischemic stroke in older adults.

- Atrial fibrillation, sick sinus syndrome, and heart block appear more often in the older adult population as a result of fewer pacemaker cells and extensive deposits of fat and fibrous tissue throughout the conduction system.
- Orthostatic hypotension is a major risk factor for syncope and falls in older adults.
- Older adults are prone to dizziness with position changes, resulting from decreased sensitivity of baroreceptors.
- CHF is the leading cause of hospitalization in the older adult population.
- Older adults may exhibit symptoms of anemia that are attributed to the aging process or to a variety of chronic diseases.
- Nursing interventions (e.g., education on the role of cardiovascular risk factors, preventive measures, treatment regimens) can enhance the quality of life of older clients, reduce hospitalization, and positively affect the cost-effectiveness and efficiency of cardiovascular programs.

Critical Thinking Exercises

1. You are preparing to teach an 83-year-old woman about the actions and side effects of nitroglycerin for the treatment of angina. What aspects of teaching would you emphasize, given the client's age?
2. A 76-year-old woman has a longstanding history of atrial fibrillation. She takes Lanoxin (0.125 mg) and warfarin (2.0 mg) daily. She recently read of the advantages of taking aspirin and started taking 4 tablets daily. How would you intervene in this situation and why?
3. What specific assessment findings indicate that an older adult client being treated for CHF is not responding to digoxin, Lasix, and vasodilator therapy? How would you differentiate between expected, adverse, and toxic side effects?

References

Abrams WB, Berkow R: *The Merck manual of geriatrics,* ed 3, Whitehouse Station, NJ, 2000, Merck.

Adan V, Crown LA: Diagnosis and treatment of sick sinus syndrome, *Am Fam Phys* 67(8):1725, 2003.

American College of Cardiology, American Heart Association: ACC/AHA collaborate on guidelines for the evaluation and management of heart failure, *Am Fam Phys* 53(6):2196, 1996.

Arnstein P et al: Women and heart attacks: prevention, diagnosis, and care, *Nurs Pract* 21(5):57, 1996.

Aschenbrenner DS: HRT reconsidered what should you tell patients about it now? *Am J Nurs* 104(6):51-53, 2004.

Aronow W et al: Treatment priorities for heart failure, *Patient Care* 32(10):68, 1998.

Barker L, Burton J, Zieve O: *Principles of ambulatory medicine,* ed 5, Philadelphia, 1999, Williams & Wilkins.

Basch EM et al: *The MGH primer of outpatient medicine,* ed 1, Philadelphia, 2002, Lippincott Williams and Wilkens.

Besdine RW, Bubenstein LZ, Snyder L: *Medical care of the nursing home resident: what physicians need to know,* Philadelphia, 1996, American College of Physicians.

Bradley JG, Davis KA: Orthostatic hypotension, *Am Fam Phys* 68(12):2393, 2003.

Buhse M: Quick thinking needed for early management of acute myocardial infarction, *Adv Nurs Pract* 6(8):29, 1998.

Burrell L, Gerlach MJ, Pless B: Adult nursing: acute and community care, ed 2, Stamford, Conn, 1997, McGraw Hill.

Chernecky CC, Berger BJ: *Laboratory tests and diagnostic procedures,* ed 3, Philadelphia, 2001, Saunders.

Chrzanowski D: Managing atrial fibrillation to prevent its major complication: ischemic stroke, *Nurs Pract* 23(5):26, 1998.

Crowther R, McCourt K: Get the edge on deep vein thrombosis, *Nurs Manage* 35(1):21, 2004.

Day M: Recognizing and managing deep vein thrombosis, *Nursing 2003* 33(5):36, 2003.

Ebersole P, Hess P, Luggen, AS: *Toward healthy aging: human needs and nursing response,* ed 6, St Louis, 2004, Mosby.

Flack J et al: Four commonly seen cardiovascular diseases, *Patient Care* 32(9):98, 1998.

Grandjean A, Talbott S: Hypercholesterolemia in elderly adults, *Adv Nurs Pract* 5(10):63, 1997.

Halm M, Penque S: Heart disease in women, *Am J Nurs* 99(4):26, 1999.

Hauer KE: Discovering the cause of syncope: a guide to the focused evaluation, *Postgrad Med* 113(1):31-38, 95, 2003.

Holcomb SS: Prevent cardiovascular disease in women, *Nurse Pract* 29(7):6-11, 2004.

Jensen L, King K: Women and heart disease: the issues, *Crit Care Nurs* 17(2):45, 1997.

Joint National Committee: The sixth report of the Joint National Committee on the Prevention, Detection, Evaluation, and Treatment of High Blood Pressure, *Arch Intern Med* 157:2413, 1997.

Joint National Committee: *The seventh report of the Joint National Committee on the Prevention, Detection, Evaluation, and Treatment of High Blood Pressure,* 2003. Accessed on website: http://www.nhlbi.nih.gov/guidelines/hypertension/index.htm.

Keller K, Lemberg L: Smoking: a burden to patient and society, *Am J Crit Care* 5(4):314, 1996.

Kuznar K: Peripheral arterial occlusive disease: evaluation and management in the primary care setting, *Adv Nurse Pract* 12(2):36, 2004.

LaRosa J: Does reducing cholesterol improve CAD survival? *Patient Care* 30:61, 1996.

Lehne R et al: *Pharmacology for nursing care,* ed 3, Philadelphia, 1998, WB Saunders.

Lewis S, Collier I, Heitkemper M: *Medical-surgical nursing: assessment and management of clinical problems,* ed 4, St Louis, 1996, Mosby.

Lomacher MC: Exercise and rehabilitation in women, *Cardiol Clin* 1(16), 1998.

Lookinland S, Beckstrand RL: Evidence-based treatment of hypertension, JNC7, guidelines provide an updated framework, *ACV Nurse Pract* 11(9):32-40, 2003.

Maron D, Rader D: Current strategies for the primary prevention of CAD, *Patient Care* 32(19):19, 1998.

Mola A, Lloyd M: Time for results: a better way to reduce cardiovascular risk, *Adv Nurse Pract* 10(4):34-41.

McDonald K: Lipid-lowering strategies: today's therapies and co-therapies can reduce CHD risk, *Adv Nurs Pract* 11(12):24, 2003.

Miller S: Hypertension update, *Adv Nurs Pract* 7(1):53, 1999.

Miller S: Congestive heart failure: clinical assessment and pharmacologic management, *Adv Nurs Pract* 5(6):17, 1997.

Murphy M, Berding C: Use of measurements of myoglobin and cardiac troponins in the diagnosis of acute myocardial infarction, *Crit Care Nurs* 19(1):58, 1999.

Pavri BB, Ho RT: Syncope: identifying cardiac causes in older patients, *Geriatrics* 58(5):26, 2003.

Rittenhouse SK: Spironolactone for heart failure: a worthy addition to therapy, *Adv Nurs Pract* 9(1):35, 2001.

Sadowski A, Redeker N: The hypertensive elder: a review for the primary care provider, *Nurs Pract* 21(5):99, 1996.

Segal B: Valvular heart disease, part 1, *Geriatrics* 58(9):31, 2003a.

Segal B: Valvular heart disease, part 2, *Geriatrics* 58(10):26, 2003b.

Seidel H et al: *Mosby's guide to physical examination*, ed 4, St Louis, 1999, Mosby.

Shamsham F, Mitchell J: Essentials of the diagnosis of heart failure, *Am Fam Phys* 61:1319, 2000.

Snow V et al: Management of newly detected atrial fibrillation: a clinical practice guideline from the American Academy of Family Physicians and the American College of Physicians, *Ann Intern Med* 139:1009, 2003.

Stone J, Wyman J, Salisbury S: *Clinical gerontological nursing: a guide to advanced practice*, ed 2, Philadelphia, 1999, WB Saunders.

Tecce MA, Dasgupta I, Doherty JU: heart disease in older women, *Geriatrics* 58(12):33-38, 2003.

Tefferi A: Anemia in adults: a contemporary approach to diagnosis, *Mayo Clin Proc* 78:1274, 2003.

Thelan L et al: *Critical care nursing: diagnosis and management*, ed 5, St Louis, 2005, Mosby.

Tucker CA: Hidden dangers of self-medication by hypertension patients, *Adv Nurse Pract* 12(11):61-63, 2003.

Vasan R et al: Residual lifetime risk for developing hypertension in middle-aged women and men, *JAMA* 287:1003-1010, 2002.

24 Respiratory Function

LYNN FEREBEE, MSN, RN, FNP

Learning Objectives

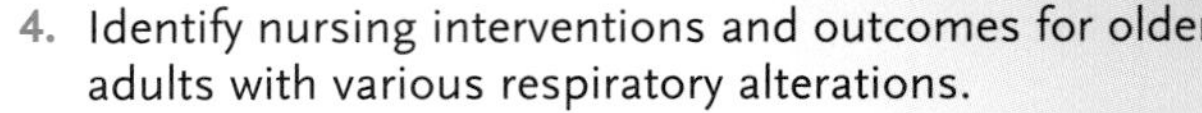

On completion of this chapter, the reader will be able to:

1. Describe anatomic changes in the lungs resulting from the normal aging process.
2. Describe age-related changes in ventilation.
3. List nursing diagnoses for older adults with respiratory diseases.
4. Identify nursing interventions and outcomes for older adults with various respiratory alterations.
5. Discuss smoking cessation methods and interventions.
6. Identify risk factors for the development of tuberculosis in older adults.
7. List the benefits of pulmonary rehabilitation for older adults with chronic obstructive pulmonary disease.

The respiratory system is responsible for gas exchange between the environment and the lung parenchyma and for respiration between oxygen molecules and the cells at the cellular level. Respiration is achieved through the coordination of neurochemical control and the muscles of respiration. Extrapulmonary factors, such as the thoracic cage and the muscles of the thorax and upper torso, as well as the intrapulmonary factor of the lung parenchyma, affect respiratory system functions.

AGE-RELATED CHANGES IN STRUCTURE AND FUNCTION

Normal aging results in changes to the ribs and vertebrae. The ribs become less mobile, and the compliance of the chest wall decreases. Osteoporosis and calcification of the costal cartilage lead to increased rigidity and stiffness of the thoracic cage. If an older adult has kyphosis or scoliosis, degeneration of the intervertebral discs occurs, resulting in a shorter thorax with an increased anteroposterior diameter. Advanced cases may result in marked limitation of thoracic movement because of the rib cage resting on the pelvic bones. In addition, a reduction in maximum inspiratory and expiratory force occurs as a result of a decrease in the breathing efficiency. Table 24-1 summarizes various changes in the aging respiratory system.

Respiratory muscles weaken with aging, as do all other muscles in the body. Inspiratory and expiratory forces are decreased because of less forceful contractions. Older adults require increased effort to breathe. Breathing is less efficient because of the increased stiffness of the chest wall and the decreased muscle strength. The diaphragm, the major muscle of respiration, does not lose mass with aging; however, it may flatten and become less efficient in clients with advancing chronic obstructive pulmonary disease (COPD) as the chest takes on a barrel-shaped configuration. Because of this, older adults use the less efficient accessory muscles of respiration such as the abdominal, sternocleidomastoid, and trapezius muscles.

Breathing patterns of older adults are more dependent on intraabdominal pressure changes. Positioning and increased abdominal pressure can greatly affect their breathing patterns. Respiratory rates are generally higher in older adults, with a normal rate of 16 to 25 breaths/min. The increase in the respiratory rate does not alter the arterial carbon dioxide pressure ($Paco_2$) because of a decrease in tidal volume (V_T). The distribution of ventilation is also affected by positioning. Shallow breathing patterns of older clients may result in hypoxemia and hypercapnia as the alveoli at the base of the lungs are underventilated. This results in a decreased ventilation/perfusion ratio and ineffective alveolar gas exchange. Age-related reductions in cardiac output and mixed venous oxygen content compound the effect of ventilation/perfusion imbalance in older adults. The less uniform ventilation/perfusion matching leads to an increase in physiologic dead space and a compensatory increase in resting minute ventilation, which is of no clinical significance.

In healthy older adults the number of alveoli changes little; however, the structure is altered. With age, the functional alveoli decrease in number, as is seen in emphysema. The supporting structures of the alveoli deteriorate, which leads to a progressive loss of the intraalveolar septum. The walls of the alveoli become thinner and contribute to a loss of alveolar septal tissue; fewer capillaries are available for gas

TABLE 24-1 Age-Related Changes in the Respiratory System

RESPIRATORY FUNCTION	PATHOPHYSIOLOGIC CHANGES	CLINICAL PRESENTATION
Mechanics of breathing	Increased chest wall compliance Loss of elastic recoil Decreased respiratory muscle mass and strength	Decreased vital capacity Increased reserve volume Decreased expiratory flow rates
Oxygenation	Increased ventilation/perfusion mismatch Decreased cardiac output Decreased mixed venous oxygen Increased physiologic dead space Decreased alveolar surface area available for gas exchange Reduced CO_2 diffusion capacity	Decreased PaO_2 Increased A-a oxygen gradient
Control of ventilation	Decreased responsiveness of central and peripheral chemoreceptors to hypoxemia and hypercapnia	Decreased V_T Increased respiratory rate Increased minute ventilation
Lung defense mechanisms	Decreased number of cilia Decreased effectiveness of mucociliary clearance Decreased cough reflex Decreased humoral and cellular immunity Decreased IgA production	Decreased ability to clear secretions Increased susceptibility to infection Increased risk of aspiration
Sleep and breathing	Decreased ventilatory drive Decreased upper airway muscle tone Decreased arousal	Increased frequency of apnea, hypopnea, and arterial oxygen desaturation during sleep Increased risk of aspiration Snoring Obstructive sleep apnea
Exercise capacity	Muscle deconditioning Decreased muscle mass Decreased efficiency of respiratory muscles Decreased reserves	Decreased maximum oxygen consumption Breathlessness at low exercise levels
Breathing pattern	Decreased responsiveness to hypoxemia and hypercapnia Change in respiratory mechanics	Increased respiratory rate Decreased V_T Increased minute ventilation

Modified from Pierson DJ, Kacmarek RM, editors: *Foundations of respiratory care,* New York, 1992, Churchill Livingstone.

exchange; and the alveoli enlarge because of dilation of the proximal bronchioles. The net result is a decrease in the surface area available for gas exchange from the normal 80 m^2 at age 20 to about 65 to 70 m^2 by age 70.

Older adults have a decrease in the number and effectiveness of cilia in the tracheobronchial tree, which results in increased difficulty in clearing secretions and increased risk for the development of respiratory tract infections. With repeated respiratory tract infections or smoking, the effectiveness of the ciliary action and number of cilia are significantly decreased, resulting in an ineffective mucociliary escalator. Changes in the alveoli result in less surface area for gas exchange to take place, contributing to the overall reduction in partial pressure of arterial oxygen (PaO_2). The increase in physiologic dead space is seen as the capillary structures surrounding the alveoli diminish.

Production of surfactant in the lung does not appear to decrease with aging. However, the production of type II alveolar cells, those responsible for surfactant production, is diminished. Alveolar macrophage activity is defective in older clients, especially those who smoke. Older clients have decreased immunoglobulin A (IgA), which is found in the nasal respiratory mucosal surface that neutralizes viruses.

One of the primary functions of the respiratory system is gas exchange. PaO_2 falls at a rate of 4 mm Hg per decade of life. A normal PaO_2 for a 70-year-old is between 75 and 80 mm Hg. The mnemonic "70 at 70" refers to the absolute lower limit of normal PaO_2 in older adults. Most healthy older adults have levels well above 70 mm Hg at sea level. A fall in PaO_2 is most likely caused by an increased closing volume during tidal breathing.

The oxygen-carrying capacity (hemoglobin $\times$ 1.34) of the blood is reduced with age. Hemoglobin, which is responsible for the transport of oxygen from the lung to the peripheral tissue, is diminished in older adults. The alveolar-arterial (A-a) oxygen gradient (the difference between the amount of oxygen in the alveoli and the amount that actually reaches the arterial blood) is 25 mm Hg in octogenarians. The A-a oxygen gradient widens with advancing age, most likely because of ventilation/perfusion mismatch. An increase in right to left shunting of blood occurs, most likely as a result of a reduction in mixed venous oxygen content, which is related to a decrease in cardiac output and an increase in postpulmonary shunting through the bronchial veins. The arterial pH of the older person remains within the normal adult range of 7.35 to 7.45, unless influenced by an acute illness. $Paco_2$ remains unchanged with advancing age. Despite the increase in physiologic dead space seen in the older adult, $Paco_2$ does not increase because of the increased ventilation. The response of older adults to hypoxemia or hypercapnia appears to be blunted. The normal clinical response to hypoxemia is an increase in the rate and depth of respiration, as well as an increase in heart rate and blood pressure. Older clients show less increase in heart rate and a lower response to increasing carbon dioxide (CO_2). Ventilatory responses to hypoxia and hypercapnia may be diminished by as much as 50% in comparison with adults in their 20s. The blunted response in older clients is the result of reduced sympathetic nervous system response. The most sensitive clinical indicator for hypoxia and hypercapnia in older clients is mental status changes and complaints of occipital headache or forgetfulness that are not otherwise explained. A minor increase in oxygen demand can result more quickly in hypoxic symptoms in older adults.

Respiratory system compliance decreases with advancing age because of a progressive loss of elastic recoil of the lung parenchyma and conducting airways and reduced elastic recoil of the lung and the opposing forces of the chest wall. The lung becomes less elastic as collagenic substances surrounding the alveoli and alveolar ducts stiffen and form cross-linkages that interfere with the lungs' elastic properties. The result is an increase in lung tissue compliance that partially compensates for the decrease in the chest wall compliance, reducing the work required of the weakened respiratory muscles to move the stiffened chest wall.

Changes in pulmonary functions in older adults are related to the changes in elastic recoil and musculoskeletal changes of the chest wall. Table 24-2 lists the lung volumes measured, the normal findings, and alterations related to aging. The ability to determine accurate pulmonary function test (PFT) results relies on the client's complete cooperation. An older client may not be able to perform an accurate test because of musculoskeletal changes and therefore may require an extended time to complete the testing.

Total lung capacity (TLC) changes little with age. However, the components change dramatically. V_T is decreased in older adults. Vital capacity (VC) is decreased as a result of decreased mobility of the chest wall and altered inspiratory and expiratory capabilities. The rate of reduction of VC is greater in older men than in older women. Decreased compliance of the thorax accounts for the increase in residual volume (RV) and expiratory reserve volume (ERV). The inspiratory capacity of older adults is affected by the decreased ability to take a deep breath. The reduction in muscle strength and a shallow breathing pattern contribute to the increase in RV. Functional dead space ventilation is increased from one third to as much as one half of each breath, resulting in a decrease in the volume of air that can participate in gas exchange.

Airflow in the tracheobronchial tree is affected by four factors: (1) size of the airway, (2) resistance in the airway, (3) muscle strength, and (4) elastic recoil. When measured in

TABLE 24-2 Pulmonary Function Changes in Older Adults

	DESCRIPTION	AVERAGE VALUE: ADULT MALE	AVERAGE VALUE: OLDER CLIENT
LUNG VOLUME			
Tidal volume (V_T)	Volume of air inhaled or exhaled per breath	5 to 10 ml/kg	Decreased
Inspiratory reserve volume (IRV)	Volume of air inhaled in addition to normal V_T	3000 ml	Decreased
Expiratory reserve volume (ERV)	Maximum volume of air that can be exhaled in addition to normal V_T	1200 ml	Decreased
Residual volume (RV)	Volume of air left in lungs after maximum exhalation	1200 ml	Increased by as much as 25%
LUNG CAPACITY			
Functional residual capacity (FRC)	Volume of air left in lung after a normal exhalation (RV + ERV)	2400 ml	Increased
Residual volume/total lung capacity (RV/TLC)	Ratio of RV to TLC expressed as percentage	33%	Increased
Vital capacity (VC)	Volume of air exhaled after maximal inhalation (IRV + V_T ERV)	4800 ml	Decreased by as much as 25%
Total lung capacity (TLC)	Total volume of air in lungs following maximum inhalation (IRV + V_T + ERC + RV)	6000 ml	Unchanged

the older client, all of these indices are decreased. Forced expiratory volume in 1 second (FEV_1) is reported to drop between 25 and 30 ml per year after age 30. Changes in the airflow measures are related to the stiffness of the chest wall and the loss of elastic recoil of the lung. The decrease in thoracic muscular strength contributes to the decreased force of the air moved. The older client can demonstrate as much as a 50% reduction in the maximum voluntary ventilation and FEV between ages 30 and 90.

Early airway closure is seen in older clients as a result of increased compliance of the lung. At low V_Ts small airways tend to close early because of the loss of elastic recoil and decreased flow rates caused by increased airway resistance, trapping air in the alveoli. In addition, the closing capacity (CC)—the lung volume at which smaller airways close during forced exhalation—contributes to early airway closure and increased ventilation/perfusion mismatch. CC increases with age, and by age 65 it exceeds functional residual capacity (FRC) when in the upright position. This contributes to early airway closure. Other factors contributing to early airway closure include increased time in a supine position, advanced age, and shallow breathing.

In younger adults, pulmonary vascular circulation is a relatively low-pressure system with high distensibility and low resistance. As adult ages, the vessels become less distensible and more fibrous. The pulmonary artery increases in diameter, as does the thickness of the vessel wall. This results in an increased pulmonary vascular resistance and increased pulmonary artery pressure. The alveolar capillary membrane thickens, affecting the surface area available for gas exchange. The number of functional capillaries declines, resulting in decreased alveolar vascularity. Combined with a diminished cardiac output, there is a decrease in pulmonary capillary blood flow.

FACTORS AFFECTING LUNG FUNCTION

Exercise and Immobility

Exercise has a positive effect on the respiratory and cardiovascular systems. The capacity of older clients to perform exercise is affected by the changes in cardiac output, skeletal muscle and joint function, and overall muscle power and coordination. In addition, older clients may have cardiovascular and respiratory illness. Increased oxygen demands during exercise periods may exceed the abilities of older clients. For those with COPD, activity intolerance is a major concern. The older client's strength and endurance may be reduced, leading to increased immobility and increased breathlessness when activity is attempted. Older clients with COPD and immobility may benefit from a program of regular exercise to increase strength and endurance and decrease breathlessness as the respiratory muscles are trained (see Research box).

Research

SAMPLE/SETTING

The sample consisted of 41 hospitalized subjects with COPD from an urban medical center in the northeastern region. The average age of the subjects was 70 years, with a range from 43 to 89 years old.

METHODS

The subjects were all asked five questions about dyspnea by the nurses, who recorded the subjects' responses verbatim. The last question asked the subjects to numerically rate their level of dyspnea during their acute attack using the Modified 0-10 Borg Scale.

FINDINGS

Common themes from the subjects' answers to question 1 included fear, helplessness, and urgency. Question 2 theme was presence. Question 3 theme was of legitimacy and preoccupation with breathing. Question 4 theme was of external demands. The range of scores for the dyspneic episode was a 7 (very severe breathlessness).

IMPLICATIONS

To help nurses address the subject's pathophysiologic components and the psychologic components that accompany dyspnea.

Heinzer MM, Bish C, Detwiler R: Acute dyspnea as perceived by patients with chronic obstructive pulmonary disease, *Clin Nurs Res* 12(1):85, 2003.

Smoking

Smoking has long been known to damage the lungs. Recently prolonged exposure to secondhand smoke has been shown to damage the lungs of nonsmokers. Heavy smokers may demonstrate a ninefold increase in the reduction of FEV_1 over normal expected reductions. Cilia, which are paralyzed by nicotine, are unable to clean the lung. Tobacco smoke increases the goblet cell's production of mucus. Cigarette smoke causes bronchoconstriction, increased airway resistance, and increased closing volumes. Older clients who did not smoke but were exposed to prolonged inhalation of secondhand smoke may show similar changes in the lung. Smoking interferes with gas exchange because the carbon monoxide byproduct competes with oxygen for the hemoglobin molecule. Bedrest compounds gas exchange in the older smoker. Many medications are affected by smoking, decreasing clearance and increasing serum drug levels. Some drugs altered by smoking include antidepressants, propranolol, theophylline, aminophylline, insulin, erythromycin, and lidocaine.

Smoking Cessation. Smoking cessation is imperative. The five components of smoking cessation consist of the

5 As: ask, advise, assess, assist, and arrange. At each encounter the patient is *asked* about tobacco use. This gives the health care worker an opportunity to *advise* and discuss the health benefits and promote smoking cessation. When speaking to older adults, the nurse should use strong, clear, and personalized language. The nurse should *assess* older adults for willingness to give up smoking and determine how soon they are ready to start the process. Then the nurse *assists* older adults with smoking cessation by encouraging them to set a quit date, reviewing preparations for quitting (e.g., removing associated objects like ashtrays), recommending nicotine replacement therapy, providing advice on successful quitting (e.g., avoid constant exposure to other smokers), providing supplemental educational materials, and offering appropriate skills training and support. Finally, the nurse *arranges* for follow-up (Agency for Health Care Research and Quality [AHCRQ, 2000).

Many new treatments are available to assist older smokers in quitting. These include the use of bupropion hydrochloride, nicotine gum, nicotine patches, and nicotine inhalation systems. Bupropion hydrochloride is given for 3 days at 150 mg per day and then increased to 150 mg twice a day, with doses 8 hours apart and the first dose in the morning. Older clients are encouraged to smoke during the first week of treatment and to set a quit-smoking date before the end of the first 14 days of treatment. Nicotine inhalation systems, gums, and patches are used to replace the client's need for nicotine. While using these nicotine substitutes, the client should not smoke. Gradually over a 6- to 8-week period, the frequency of usage is decreased.

Obesity

Obesity results in a decrease in chest wall compliance and reduction in FRC, VC, and ERV. In older clients with already decreased chest wall mobility and stiffening of the chest, added weight greatly reduces pulmonary functions and increases breathlessness. Ventilation at the bases of the lungs may be diminished because of the client's inability to take a deep breath. Coupled with immobility, the risk of the older obese client developing atelectasis and upper and lower respiratory tract infections is increased. Early airway closure may also be associated with underventilation of the lower lobes of the lungs.

Sleep

Increased sleep time of older adults increases the risk of aspiration and oxygen desaturation during sleep. Older adults have diminished ventilatory drive and a loss of upper airway tone that predisposes them to apnea, hypopnea, and nocturnal oxygen desaturation. Diminished cough and arousal reflexes increase the likelihood of aspiration during sleep.

Anesthesia and Surgery

An older client undergoing surgery has an increased risk of aspiration as a result of loss of laryngeal reflexes. If surgery is an emergency, risk is increased because of the older client's delayed gastric emptying and the potential for a full stomach. Incisions, pain, and decreased postoperative deep breathing increase the older client's chance of developing postoperative atelectasis. Subsequent immobility decreases ventilation and effective airway clearance. Hypovolemia contributes to thickened secretions. Because older clients have a less effective cough, a painful incision further diminishes the likelihood of effective airway clearance. Promotion of deep breathing, adequate hydration, frequent position changes, and early mobility will decrease the risk of developing atelectasis.

RESPIRATORY SYMPTOMS COMMON IN OLDER CLIENTS

Respiratory symptoms common in older clients include alterations in breathing patterns, dyspnea, and coughing. Normally, older clients have an elevated respiratory rate of 16 to 25 breaths/min and decreased V_T and minute ventilation. Abnormal breathing patterns in older clients can be indicative of other metabolic and respiratory illnesses. One of the first signs that an older client is having respiratory problems is a change in mental status. Older clients' responses to hypoxemia and hypercapnia are blunted. Changes in heart rate, respiratory rate, and blood pressure may be delayed. Mental status changes may include subtle increases in forgetfulness and irritability. Older clients may complain of an occipital headache or confusion when awakening from sleep. If these signs persist, a more in-depth evaluation of the client's respiratory status is indicated.

Complaints of dyspnea or breathlessness in older clients are often associated with respiratory and cardiac disease. Dyspnea is a perception of breathlessness that is difficult for the older client to quantify; dyspnea may therefore be dismissed, especially when no clinical evidence can be attributed to the complaint. Older clients most often describe their breathlessness as a sensation of an inability to get enough air, difficulty taking a deep breath, breathing rapidly, or a choking or smothering feeling. Dyspnea at rest is most often associated with an acute respiratory or cardiac illness, whereas dyspnea on exertion may be related to immobility and respiratory muscle deconditioning. Older clients with COPD may experience dyspnea on exertion initially and dyspnea at rest as the disease progresses. Dyspnea is a common complaint in older clients with pulmonary disease. However, older clients usually do not complain of dyspnea until it begins to interfere with their activities of daily living (ADLs), and then only if those activities are important to them. For example, it may become difficult to use the stairs. An older client may simply choose the elevator or escalator and not consider reporting the shortness of breath associated with stair climbing. It is important to determine which ADLs an older client no longer participates in and why.

The cough mechanism in older clients is altered because of the loss of elastic recoil, decreased respiratory muscle strength, and decreased V_T. Causes of coughing in older clients include postnasal drip, chronic bronchitis, acute respiratory tract infections, aspiration, gastroesophageal reflux, congestive heart failure (CHF), interstitial lung disease, cancer, and angiotensin-converting enzyme inhibitor medications for hypertension and CHF. Because of the age-related changes that affect an older client's cough mechanism, it is important to recommend cough suppressants with caution. Suppression of the cough and depression of any respiratory function could lead to retention of pulmonary secretions, plugged airways, and atelectasis.

RESPIRATORY ALTERATIONS IN OLDER CLIENTS

Recent health statistics indicate that respiratory disorders in the United States account for $36 billion per year in direct health care costs. The indirect health care costs are estimated at $72 billion per year. In the United States approximately 17 million Americans have COPD, the fourth leading cause of death (Mannino, 2002). Prevention of respiratory illness is a crucial part of care (see Health Promotion box).

Chronic respiratory disease affects not only older clients, but also their families. Many clients with respiratory illness feel a loss of control over their lives because of breathlessness on exertion and at rest. They may become demanding and controlling in dealing with their families and friends. The quality of the older clients' life depends on their feelings about and control of the disease. Support groups sponsored by the American Lung Association and local hospitals are available to help clients and families deal with anger, loss of control, and hopelessness. The family or a significant other needs to be included in all aspects of planning and care for an older client with respiratory illness. The client's success in complying with the medical recommendations may depend on assistance he or she receives in getting to the physician's office, getting to the pharmacy for medications, administering medications, and performing ADLs. Older clients with respiratory disease need a good family support system and a team of caregivers to support both them and their families.

Respiratory disease is divided into two categories: (1) obstructive pulmonary disease and (2) restrictive pulmonary disease. Obstructive lung diseases are characterized by changes in expiratory airflow rates and obstruction of the airway. The lumen of the airway can be decreased by mucus; edema of the airway lining; or constriction of the muscles surrounding the airway, causing bronchoconstriction. Restrictive lung disease is characterized by a decreased ability to expand the chest, impaired inhalation, and decreased lung volumes. Changes in the chest wall, lung parenchyma, pleural space, and extrapulmonary factors such as body mass can result in restrictive lung disease. Examples of these diseases include bronchogenic carcinoma and tuberculosis. Other respiratory diseases seen in older clients include bronchopulmonary infections, pulmonary edema, and pulmonary emboli.

Health Promotion/Illness Prevention

The Respiratory System

- Avoidance of cigarette and secondhand smoke
- Avoidance of environmental and air pollutants
- Healthy diet and exercise plan
- Immunizations
- Avoidance of allergens
- Use of mask, scarves, and filters to protect against community-acquired illnesses
- Stress management and relaxation for breathing control
- Early diagnosis and treatment of respiratory tract infections
- Careful monitoring and adherence to medical regimen for chronic respiratory illnesses
- Maintenance of a clean environment (e.g., dusting regularly, changing air filters in furnace every 3 months, changing toothbrush every 3 to 4 months and after an illness)
- Maintenance of adequate hydration (at least 64 ounces of water daily)

OBSTRUCTIVE PULMONARY DISEASE

Asthma

Asthma is a chronic inflammatory disease that affects the airways and is characterized by reversible airway obstruction, airway inflammation, and increased airway responsiveness to a variety of stimuli. Airway inflammation contributes to airway hyperresponsiveness; airflow limitations, including acute bronchoconstriction, airway edema, and mucous plug formation; airway wall remodeling; respiratory symptoms; and disease chronicity (National Heart, Lung, and Blood Institute [NHLBI], 1997). Inflammation causes recurrent episodes of wheezing, breathlessness, chest tightness, and coughing, often at night or early in the morning. Recent evidence suggests that persistent abnormalities in lung function are associated with subbasement membrane fibrosis in some clients. Asthma accounts for more than 100 million days of restricted activity, 470,000 hospitalizations, and 5000 deaths annually (NHLBI, 1997).

An asthma attack can be precipitated by exposure to allergens or irritants such as changes in weather, odors, or stress. In older clients asthma is often associated with viral respiratory infection. Signs and symptoms include dyspnea, audible wheezing, palpitations, increased respiratory rate, use of accessory muscles of respiration, tachycardia, pulsus paradoxus, diaphoresis, and chest hyperinflation. Initially a client may hyperventilate and effectively blow off increasing CO_2. Falling PaO_2 and pH with rising $PaCO_2$ are indicative of imminent respiratory failure. The increasing $PaCO_2$ is a result of the client's exhaustion and inability to hyperventilate. Cigarette smoking is the single most important factor that exacerbates chronic bronchitis. Chronic bronchitis is associated with right-sided heart failure (cor pulmonale), polycythemia, hypoxemia, and respiratory insufficiency. Clinical symptoms include persistent cough, dyspnea on exertion, purulent sputum, cyanosis, crackles on auscultation, tachycardia, pedal edema, unexplained weight gain, and decreased PaO_2 with normal or elevated $PaCO_2$.

Prognosis. The prognosis for an older adult with asthma is good. Success is based on a partnership between the client and the caregiver to properly use prescribed medications, avoid asthma triggers, and maintain a healthy lifestyle.

Treatment. The goals of asthma therapy are the prevention of chronic and troublesome symptoms, maintenance of normal pulmonary functions, maintenance of normal activity levels, prevention of exacerbations, and satisfaction of the client's and family's expectations of asthma care (NHLBI, 1997). The NHLBI (1997) recommends a stepwise approach to pharmacologic management. Medications are classified into two categories: long-term-control medications and quick-relief medications.

Long-Term Control Medications. Long-term control medications are taken on a daily basis and include antiinflammatory agents, long-acting bronchodilators, and leukotriene modifiers. Corticosteroids are the most potent and effective long-term–control medications in the treatment of mild, moderate, or severe persistent asthma. They are well tolerated and safe when used at the recommended dosage. The clinical response to corticosteroids is a reduction in airway inflammation, improvement in PEFR, diminished airway hyperresponsiveness, prevention of exacerbations, and possible prevention of airway wall remodeling. Corticosteroids are generally inhaled twice a day.

Long-acting $beta_2$ agonists act by relaxing the smooth muscle of the airways and stimulating $beta_2$-receptors to increase cyclic adenosine monophosphate. Duration of action is 12 hours for a single dose. These medications are not indicated for acute exacerbation. An example of these medications is inhaled salmeterol (Serevent Diskus).

The newest medications are the leukotriene antagonists. Leukotrienes are potent biochemical mediators that are released from mast cells, eosinophils, and basophils. They act on the lung, causing airway smooth muscle contraction and increased mucous secretion; they also attract and activate inflammatory cells in the airways. Leukotriene antagonists improve lung function, diminish symptoms, and reduce the need for short-acting $beta_2$ agonists. An example of a leukotriene antagonist is montelukast (Singulair).

Quick-Relief Medications. Quick-relief medications are used to reverse acute symptoms such as chest tightness, cough, and wheezing. This group of medications includes short-acting $beta_2$ agonists, anticholinergics, and systemic corticosteroids. Short-acting $beta_2$ agonists provide smooth muscle relaxation within 30 minutes and are the drug of choice for treating acute asthma symptoms (NHLBI, 1997). Clients who use more than one canister per month do not have adequate control and need additional antiinflammatory therapy. Daily use of short-acting $beta_2$ agonists is not recommended.

Anticholinergics, such as ipratropium bromide (Atrovent), may provide an additive benefit to inhaled $beta_2$ agonists in treatment of severe exacerbation. Systemic corticosteroids are used in the treatment of moderate to severe asthma exacerbations. The onset of action is more than 4 hours. They act by preventing progression of the exacerbation, speeding recovery, and preventing early relapse (NHLBI, 1997).

Asthma Medications Administered Through a Stepwise Approach.

Step 1: No daily medication indicated. Short-acting $beta_2$ agonists are used as required (prn). If they are used more than two times a week, consider long-term control therapy.

Step 2: Daily antiinflammatory, such as inhaled corticosteroid. A leukotriene modifier may be added at this step. Short-acting $beta_2$ agonists are used prn. If they are used daily or there is an increase in use, add additional long-term control therapy.

Step 3: Daily antiinflammatory: inhaled corticosteroid (medium dose) or an inhaled corticosteroid (low-medium dose) and a long-acting bronchodilator. Short-acting $beta_2$ agonists are used prn. If they are used daily or there is an increase in use, add additional long-term control therapy.

Step 4: Daily antiinflammatory (high dose), a long-acting bronchodilator, and a trial of other bronchodilators. Short-acting $beta_2$ agonists are used prn. If they are used daily or there is an increase in use, add additional long-term control therapy.

Asthma management in older adults may coexist with management of chronic bronchitis or emphysema. A trial of systemic corticosteroids is useful in determining the presence of reversible airflow obstruction (NHLBI, 1997). An older adult may have medical conditions such as cardiac disease and osteoporosis that are aggravated by asthma medications. Older adults with ischemic heart disease may be more sensitive to $beta_2$ agonist side effects such as tremors and tachycardia; medications may need to be adjusted. Corticosteroids may cause confusion, agitation, and changes in glucose metabolism in older adults. The use of inhaled corticosteroids in older adults may predispose them to a reduction in bone mineral content, especially if there is preexisting osteoporosis, changes in estrogen levels affecting calcium utilization, and a sedentary lifestyle. NHLBI (1997) recommends calcium and vitamin D supplements, as well as estrogen replacement therapy when appropriate. There is also an increased risk for adverse drug and disease interactions: asthma may be exacerbated by the use of nonsteroidal antiinflammatory agents for arthritis, nonselective beta-blockers for hypertension, or glaucoma eyedrops that contain beta-blockers.

NURSING MANAGEMENT

Assessment

Evaluation of respiratory symptoms includes effect on ADLs, quantity of breathlessness on a scale of 1 to 10 (Gift and Narsavage, 1998), presence of asthma triggers, and frequency of the need for bronchodilator therapy. Physical assessment includes inspection of the chest for shape and symmetry, respiratory rate and pattern, body position, use of accessory muscles of respiration, and amount and color of sputum production. Palpation and percussion of the chest are indicated to assess for increased tactile fremitus, chest wall movement, and diaphragmatic excursion. When the chest wall is auscultated, the older adult should be given enough time to take deep breaths comfortably without becoming dizzy. Determine the presence of any wheezing, the phase of respiration in which it occurs, and whether it is present during a forced expiratory maneuver. Determination of the peak expiratory flow rate (PEFR) with a peak expiratory flow meter (PEFM) is important in determining trends of airway resistance (Fig. 24-1).

Diagnosis

Nursing diagnoses common for an older client with asthma include (Gordon, 2002):

- Ineffective airway clearance related to tracheobronchial obstruction
- Impaired gas exchange related to alveolar-capillary membrane changes
- Knowledge deficit: asthma related to lack of previous exposure

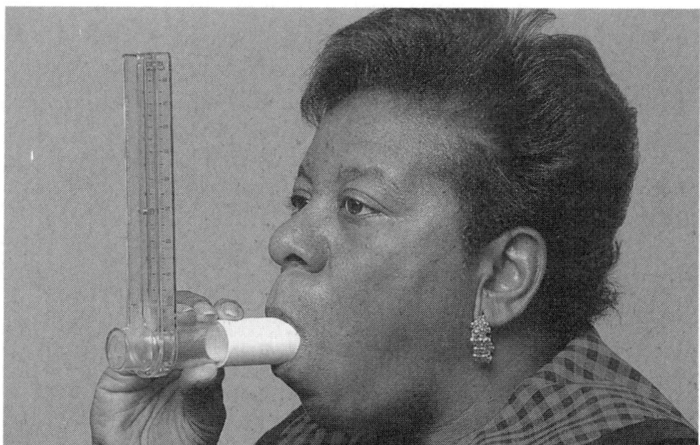

Fig. 24-1 Using a peak expiratory flow meter. (From Perry AG, Potter PA: *Clinical nursing skills and techniques*, ed 4, St Louis, 1998, Mosby.)

The diagnosis of asthma is based on episodic symptoms of airflow obstruction that are partially reversible. Key indicators for the diagnosis of asthma include (1) wheezing; (2) a history of cough that is worse at night; (3) recurrent difficulty breathing and chest tightness; (4) variation in PEFR of 20% or more; and (5) symptoms that worsen during exercise; with viral infection; in the presence of environmental irritants such as animal fur, dust mites, mold, smoke, pollen, changes in weather, airborne chemicals, or dust; during menses; or with strong emotional expression (NHLBI, 1997).

PFTs are used to measure the presence and amount of airway obstruction. An FEV_1/forced vital capacity (FVC) ratio of less than 65% indicates obstruction of airflow. Measurements of FEV_1, FVC, and the FEV_1/FVC ratio before and after inhaled short-acting bronchodilators are recommended. Other diagnostic procedures include methacholine; histamine or exercise challenge; chest x-ray studies; allergy testing; ear, nose, and throat evaluation for nasal polyps and sinus disease; evaluation for gastroesophageal reflux; a 1- to 2-week evaluation of diurnal variation in PEFR; and evaluation for vocal cord dysfunction (NHLBI, 1997).

The diagnosis and management of asthma in older clients is more difficult than in younger clients. The symptoms of asthma mimic other conditions such as myocardial ischemia or pulmonary embolus (NHLBI, 1996). Asthma may appear as late as the eight or ninth decade of life. Older adults with asthma may not show allergic skin sensitivity, and therefore serum immunoglobulin E and eosinophil levels can be more predictive. Incomplete reversibility of airflow obstruction is increasingly common (NHLBI, 1996). Older adult clients with asthma may only achieve a 12% improvement in their FEV_1, even with optimum inhaled bronchodilators (NHLBI, 1996). In older clients with heartburn, cough, nocturnal symptoms occurring early in the night, and resistance to routine therapy, gastroesophageal reflux disease should be considered (NHLBI, 1996).

Asthma is classified in four steps by the severity of symptoms, frequency of nighttime symptoms, and lung function (Table 24-3). Asthma also occurs as seasonal asthma, cough variant asthma, and exercise-induced asthma.

Planning and Expected Outcomes

Older clients with asthma and their families should be included in care planning (NHLBI, 1996). It is important to incorporate the changes in ADLs that are required for ongoing monitoring and maintenance of clients with asthma. Expected outcomes include (Johnson and Maas, 1997):

1. Client will maintain a patent airway.
2. Client will maintain arterial blood gas (ABG) values at baseline.
3. Client will be able to demonstrate proper use of the PEFM.
4. Client will be able to demonstrate relaxation techniques to control breathing.
5. Client will be able to list the significant and reportable signs and symptoms.

TABLE 24-3 Asthma Severity Classification

STEP	SYMPTOMS	NIGHTTIME SYMPTOMS	LUNG FUNCTION
I Mild Intermittent	≤2 times per week Asymptomatic and normal pulmonary expiratory force between exacerbations Brief exacerbations	≤2 times per month	FEV_1 or PEF ≥ 80% predicted PEF variability <20%
II Mild Persistent	>2 times per week, <1 time per day Activity affected by exacerbations	>2 times per month	FEV_1 or PEF ≥ 80% predicted PEF variability 20% to 30%
III Moderate Persistent	Daily Daily use of short-acting $beta_2$ agonists Activity affected by exacerbations Exacerbations ≥ 2 times per week; may last days	>1 time per week	FEV1 or PEF 60% to <80% predicted PEF variability >30%
IV Severe Persistent	Continual Limited physical activity Frequent exacerbations	Frequent	FEV_1 or PEF ≤60% predicted PEF variability >30%

Adapted from National Heart, Lung, and Blood Institute: *Clinical practice guidelines; guidelines for the diagnosis and management of asthma,* NIH Publication No 97-4051, 1997.
PEF, Pulmonary expiratory force; *FEV,* forced expiratory volume.

Intervention

Interventions for clients with asthma include health maintenance and lifestyle changes, administration of medications at designated time intervals, exercise, and promotion of hydration and good nutrition (McCloskey and Bulechek, 1996). The nursing care for a client with asthma focuses on development of a partnership between the care providers and the client. Education is started at the time of diagnosis and integrated into every aspect of care. Emphasis is placed on asthma self-management; basic facts about asthma; roles of medications; environmental control measures; the use of inhalers, spacers, and PEFMs; and a daily written action plan for management of exacerbations (NHLBI, 1997). Additional topics include smoking cessation, weight gain or loss, exercise requirements, and breathing retraining.

Evaluation

Evaluation is based on the client's success in following through with the self-management plan. It is important to determine how often the client is using the rescue inhaler, how successful he or she is at avoiding triggers, and how well he or she is able to monitor and address lifestyle changes. These changes may initially be difficult for older adults; however, after they understand the need for the lifestyle changes, older adults are more likely to make permanent changes rather than temporary adjustments. Regular follow-up with the primary care provider is critical for assessment of a client's success. Providing written material, pictures, and time for return demonstration will increase the success rate.

Chronic Bronchitis

Chronic bronchitis is a clinical syndrome characterized by excessive mucous production with chronic or recurrent cough on most days for a minimum of 3 months of the year for at least 2 consecutive years. There is hypertrophy of the bronchial mucous gland, an increase in the number of goblet cells, and a decrease in the effectiveness of the mucociliary escalator, usually as a result of repeated infections.

Emphysema

Emphysema usually occurs between ages 60 and 70 and is characterized by progressive destruction of the alveoli and their supporting structures. The alveoli distal to the terminal bronchioles become enlarged. Loss of connective tissue supporting the alveoli leads to permanent obliteration of the peripheral airways. Physical signs include the classic barrel chest appearance with use of accessory muscles of respiration. Emphysema is often associated with clients who have a history of smoking. Clinical presentation includes dyspnea on exertion or at rest; decreased weight; chronic cough with little sputum production; digital clubbing; chest hyperresonant to percussion; elevated hemoglobin; crackles and wheezes on auscultation; and abnormal PFTs with decreased VC, increased TLC, increased FRC, and decreased FEV_1.

Chronic Obstructive Pulmonary Disease

COPD is characterized by airway obstruction and decreased expiratory flow rate. The two reversible components in COPD are airway diameter and expiratory flow rate. Emphysema, chronic bronchitis, and bronchiectasis are often referred to as

COPD. Asthma may also be included in COPD, especially if there is a component of airway hyperreactivity. COPD is a progressive and ultimately fatal disease. The fatality rate for COPD is more than two times as high in men as in women between the ages of 65 and 74 and three times as high between the ages of 75 and 84. There has been an increase in the number of women with COPD since 1991 (NHLBI, 2001). This is most likely a result of the increased number of women who smoke. Risk factors for COPD include age, male gender, reduced lung function, air pollution, exposure to secondhand smoke, familial allergies, poor nutrition, and alcohol intake. COPD is often a comorbid factor in deaths from pneumonia and influenza, and it accounts for increased physician visits (Mannino, 2002).

Symptoms of COPD vary, depending on whether emphysema or chronic bronchitis is the predominant factor. Symptoms include dyspnea (especially on exertion), cough, sputum production, weight loss, and fatigue. Diagnosis is based on client history and alterations in the PFTs (NHLBI, 2001).

Diagnostic Tests and Procedures. The diagnosis of COPD is made based on a history exposure to tobacco smoke; occupational dusts and chemical; smoke from home cooking and heating fuels; and progressive dyspnea, chronic cough, and chronic sputum production, usually in the morning. PFTs or simple spirometry is used for the initial diagnosis of airflow obstruction. A resting ABG measurement and a standard baseline posteroanterior chest x-ray study are also obtained. The blood hemoglobin level is obtained to assess for the presence of polycythemia, which is an indicator of prolonged hypoxemia. COPD is staged based on the percent of the predicted value of FEV_1.

STAGE	DEGREE VALUE	% PREDICTED FEV_1
0	At risk	Normal spirometry Chronic symptoms (cough, sputum production)
I	Mild	≥ 80%
II	Moderate	< 80%
III	Severe	<30%

From National Institutes of Health, National Heart, Lung and Blood Institute: *Global initiative for chronic obstructive lung disease (GOLD)*, NIH pub. No. 2701, Bethesda, Md, 2001, The Institute.

Treatment. Treatment is focused on symptom management through education about the disease and active engagement of the older client in care management. Aspects of management include smoking cessation; a stepwise approach to pharmacotherapy; and a healthy lifestyle, including regular exercise, weight control, and limited occupational exposure to toxins and air pollution. Proper nutrition is essential to promoting efficient respiratory muscle work. Adequate nutrition maintains muscle mass, muscle function, and immunologic competence. Pneumococcal and annual influenza vaccination is recommended for older clients. During peak influenza season, older clients with COPD should avoid crowds to decrease the risk of contracting influenza.

The single most important intervention is smoking cessation. Although smoking prevalence has decreased steadily, 25% of the United States population still smokes (American Cancer Society [ACS], 1998). Smoking cessation has been shown to improve FEV_1 and relieve symptoms. If an older client with COPD is a smoker, it is critical he or she stop smoking. Benefits to smoking cessation include reduction in the number of respiratory infections, improvement in the function of the mucociliary clearance of the lungs, decreased cough and dyspnea, increased appetite, and decreased sputum production. Older clients with COPD should also avoid secondhand smoke; it can cause bronchospasm and coughing.

Pharmacotherapy is recommended in a stepwise approach based on the severity of airway obstruction and client symptoms. Medication includes the use of bronchodilators, beta-adrenergic drugs, anticholinergic drugs, corticosteroids, and oxygen therapy. Inhaled $beta_2$ agonists are used in mildly to moderately obstructed clients with intermittent symptoms. For patients with persistent symptoms or poor response to $beta_2$ agonists, ipratropium bromide is the drug of choice. If symptoms persist or become severe, theophylline is added. For acute exacerbations, oral corticosteroids and antibiotics may be added.

$Beta_2$ Agonists. These sympathomimetic drugs work by stimulating the $beta_2$ receptors in the lung. This results in bronchial dilation, increased mucociliary clearance, and possibly increased diaphragmatic function. The drugs may be administered by metered-dose inhaler (MDI) with a spacer or by aerosolized therapy (Fig. 24-2). Oral sympathomimetics are available but are associated with more systemic side effects, tremors, and cardiac arrhythmias. $Beta_2$ agonists should be used with caution in the older client with ischemic heart disease. Examples of $beta_2$ agonists include albuterol (Proventil, Ventolin), metaproterenol sulfate (Alupent, Metaprel), and pirbuterol acetate (Maxair).

Anticholinergics. Inhaled anticholinergics—ipratropium bromide or oxitropuim bromide—are used to treat chronic bronchitis. They work by inhibiting vagal stimulation of the lung, preventing contraction of the smooth muscle, and decreasing mucous production.

Steroids. Oral steroids may be used in clients who have a reversible component. The dosage is guided by improvement in spirometry and client symptoms. Steroid therapy may not be well tolerated in older clients.

Oxygen Therapy. Supplemental oxygen therapy is indicated for clients with a resting Pao_2 less than or equal to 55 mm Hg and a saturation of less than or equal to 88% by pulse oximetry (Fig. 24-3). Oxygen therapy may also be indicated if the client's Pao_2 is between 55 and 60 mm Hg and there is evidence of right-sided heart failure or secondary polycythemia (hematocrit 56%). Oxygen desaturation associated

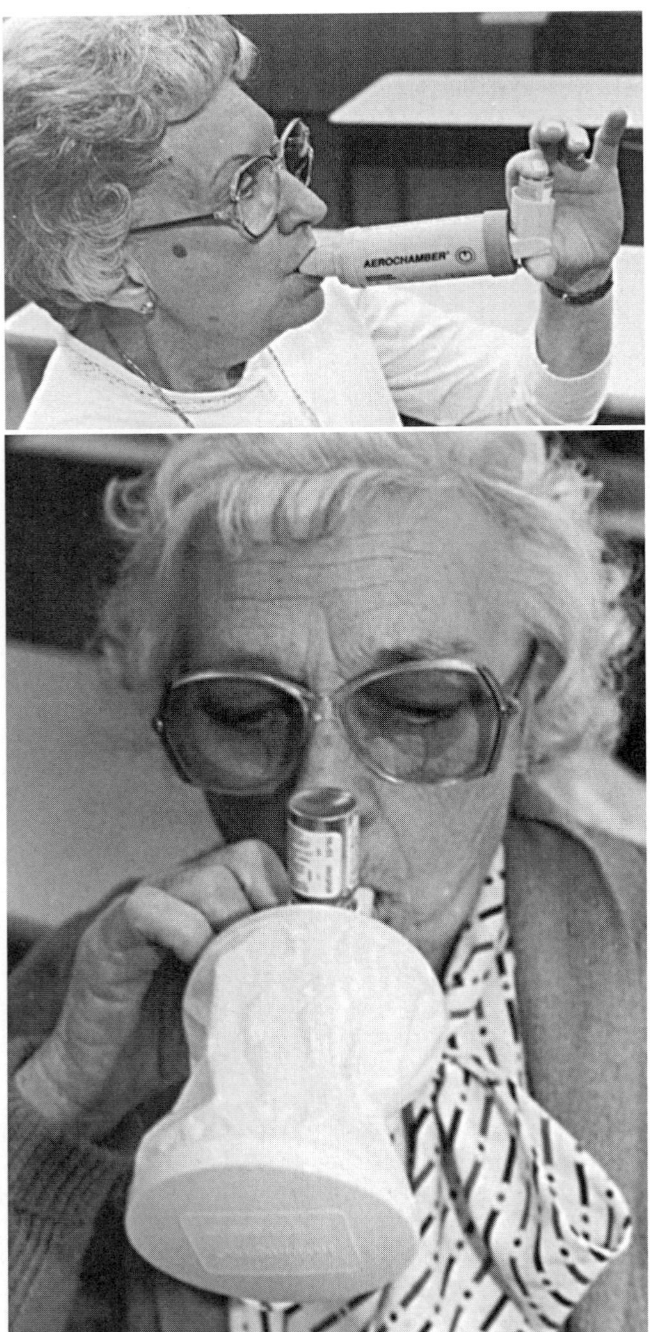

Fig. 24-2 Commercial spacers for MDIs: *Top,* AeroChamber; *bottom,* InspirEase. (From Dettenmeier P: *Pulmonary nursing care,* St Louis, 1992, Mosby.)

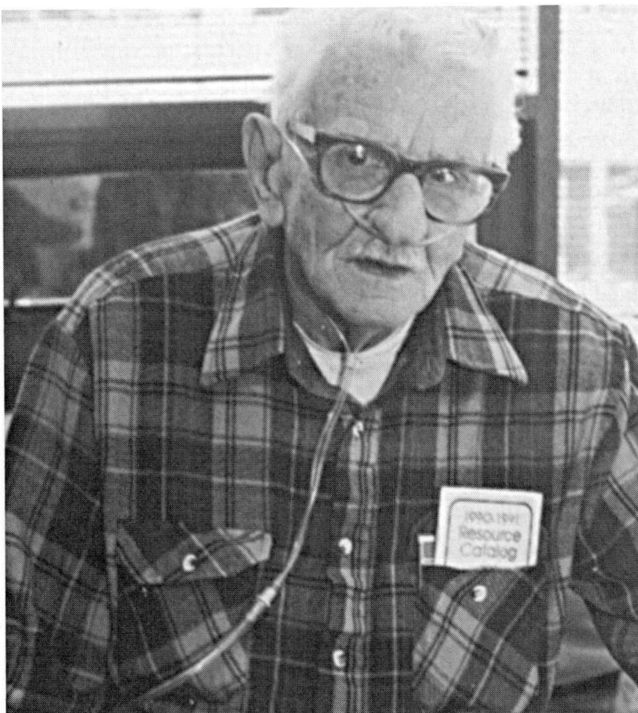

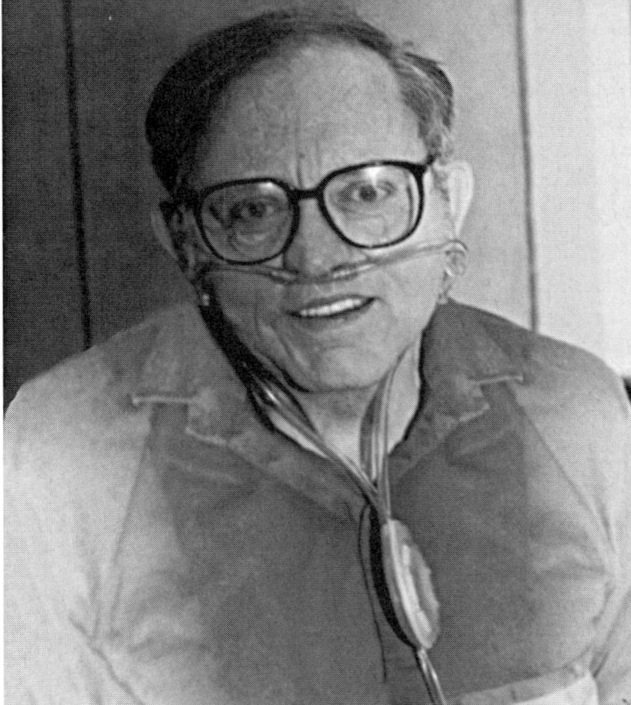

Fig. 24-3 Nasal cannula oxygen delivery device. (From Dettenmeier P: *Pulmonary nursing care,* St Louis, 1992, Mosby.)

with sleep or exercise is also an indication for supplemental oxygen therapy. These criteria are used by third-party payers in determining whether to cover oxygen therapy.

Antibiotics. Antibiotics are used when there is a concomitant bacterial infection. The choice of antibiotic is based on the infecting organism, with therapy lasting from 7 to 14 days.

Surgical Options. Surgical options consist of a bullectomy, removing the bullae, which reduces dyspnea and improves lung function by allowing previously compressed lung tissue to reexpand. A lung volume reduction surgery is considered a controversial surgical option. The final option is a lung transplantation, which often improves functional capacity and improves the patient's quality of life.

NURSING MANAGEMENT

Assessment

Evaluation of respiratory symptoms includes assessing their effect on ADLs, quantifying breathlessness on a scale of 1 to 10, and identifying environmental and social factors that may be contributing to the symptoms. The nurse also identifies the type of onset of the symptoms—whether sudden or insidious—and any precipitating factors such as exercise, temperature changes, and stress. Physical assessment includes assessment of the shape and symmetry of the chest; respiratory rate and pattern; body position; use of accessory muscles of respiration; color, temperature, and appearance of extremities; and sputum color, amount, consistency, and odor.

To assess cyanosis in darkly pigmented older adults, the nurse should examine the client with favorable lighting conditions (e.g., use overbed light or natural sunlight). Be attentive to factors that may mask cyanosis by causing vasoconstriction. These include environmental conditions (e.g., air conditioning, mist tents) and client behaviors (e.g., smoking, medications causing vasoconstriction). Examine the usual places in which cyanosis is found, that is, the lips, nail beds, circumoral region, cheek bones, and earlobes. Be aware that the darker skin may mask the underlying cyanosis, and that the region around the mouth is often darker in people of Mediterranean descent. When cyanosis is questionable, apply light pressure to create pallor. In cyanosis, tissue color returns slowly from the periphery to the center. Normally color returns in 1 second, from below the pallid spot as well as from the periphery. Cyanosis of an extremity may become more recognizable if the position of the extremity can be changed from elevated to dependent or vice versa.

Observe for other clinical manifestations of decreased oxygenation of the brain. These include changes in level of consciousness, increased respiratory rate, use of accessory muscles of respiration, nasal flaring, and positional changes and other manifestations of respiratory distress.

Palpation and percussion of the chest are indicated to assess for increased tactile fremitus, chest wall movement, and diaphragmatic excursion. When auscultating the chest wall, the nurse must give an older adult enough time to take deep breaths comfortably without becoming dizzy.

Diagnosis

Nursing diagnoses common for an older client with COPD include (Gordon, 2002):

- Ineffective airway clearance related to retained secretions
- Impaired gas exchange related to altered oxygen supply
- Altered health maintenance related to ineffective individual coping
- Risk for infection related to inadequate primary and secondary defenses and chronic disease
- Knowledge deficit: COPD related to lack of previous exposure
- Inadequate nutrition related to inability to digest or ingest food or to absorb nutrients
- Altered role performance related to change in self-perception and changes in physical capacity to resume role
- Ineffective breathing pattern related to musculoskeletal impairment and decreased energy or fatigue
- Inability to sustain spontaneous ventilation related to respiratory muscle fatigue
- Activity intolerance related to imbalance between oxygen supply and demand

Planning and Expected Outcomes

As with all clients, older clients with COPD should be included in the care planning. It is important to include the spouse or significant other, family, and any other caregivers in the planning process. Discharge planning should begin as soon as an older client is admitted to the hospital. If an older client requires special equipment for home care, such as supplemental oxygen therapy or aerosolized therapy, the client and family can benefit from learning the new skills in the acute care setting. Expected outcomes for the older client with COPD include (Johnson and Maas, 1997):

1. Client will maintain a patent airway.
2. Client will maintain a stable weight.
3. Client will maintain ABG values at baseline.
4. Client will maintain a balanced intake and output.
5. Client will be able to effectively clear secretions.
6. Client will be able to demonstrate diaphragmatic and pursed-lip breathing.
7. Client will be able to demonstrate relaxation techniques to control breathing.
8. Client will maintain a respiratory rate between 16 and 25 breaths/min.
9. Client will be able to list significant and reportable signs and symptoms.

Intervention

Interventions for clients with COPD include maximizing the effects of bronchodilator therapy; administering medications at designated intervals; and promoting hydration, good nutrition, and increased mobility (McCloskey and Bulechek, 1996). The majority of nursing care for the client with COPD involves extensive education. Topics include normal respiratory anatomy and changes associated with the disease; medical intervention, including tests and medications; and lifestyle changes such as smoking cessation, weight gain or loss, exercise, and breathing retraining (see Nursing Care Plan).

Nursing Care Plan

Chronic Obstructive Pulmonary Disease

Clinical Situation: Mr. W is an 80-year-old retired truck driver admitted to the medical ICU for exacerbation of his COPD. He lives with his wife, who is 78 years old. Mr. W continues to smoke one to two packs of cigarettes per day, as he has done since the age of 15.

Over the past week, Mrs. W has noticed a decrease in Mr. W's activity level and attention span. He has a productive cough of thick tenacious sputum, averaging 1 cup per day. Over the past week the sputum has become yellow. His appetite has decreased, and he has difficulty sleeping at night, often awakening and gasping for breath. Mr. W is having increasing difficulty in bathing and dressing.

Physical examination reveals a thin man with weight of 138 lb. He has a barrel chest and uses his accessory muscles of respiration to breathe. Auscultation of the chest reveals diminished breath sounds with scattered coarse crackles bilaterally and no wheezes. Mr. W's blood pressure is 138/68 mm Hg, his pulse is 92 beats/min, and his respiratory rate is 35 breaths/min. His oral temperature is 38.3° C (101° F).

Laboratory tests show ABG measurements to be pH of 7.40, $Paco_2$ of 41 mm Hg, Pao_2 of 55 mm Hg, Sao_2 of 90%, and bicarbonate (HCO_3) of 28. Mr. W has a white cell count of 12,000. Sputum cultures reveal *Haemophilus influenzae*. A diagnosis of *H. influenzae* pneumonia is made.

Because of increasing shortness of breath and decreasing oxygenation, Mr. W is intubated and placed on mechanical ventilation according to the couple's wishes. Intravenous antibiotic therapy is started, and bronchodilator therapy is initiated to reduce airway resistance and promote pulmonary hygiene. Mr. W remains on mechanical ventilation for 6 days until he is successfully weaned and transferred to the medical division.

He remains in the medical division for 10 additional days. Mr. W is sent home on home oxygen therapy, bronchodilators, and absolutely no smoking.

Nursing Diagnosis

Activity intolerance related to decreased strength and endurance
Ineffective airway clearance related to retained secretions
Impaired gas exchange related to alveolar hypoventilation
Inability to sustain spontaneous ventilation related to infection and decreased respiratory muscle endurance
Impaired verbal communication related to endotracheal intubation
Knowledge deficit: home oxygen therapy and smoking cessation related to inexperience with concepts

Outcomes

Client will be able to safely and comfortably perform ADLs.
Client will be able to effectively clear secretions with coughing or suctioning.
Client will maintain ABG levels at baseline, as evidenced by the ability to adhere to techniques and perform activities that maximize ventilation/perfusion matching.
Client will be able to maintain spontaneous ventilation without mechanical assistance.
Client will be able to effectively communicate with caregivers and family.
Client and family will be able to demonstrate use of the home oxygen equipment.
Client and family will be able to verbalize oxygen safety measures.
Client and family will be able to verbalize the need to quit smoking and techniques for achieving success.

Interventions

Provide active and passive range-of-motion exercises to maintain mobility.
Assess the need for supplemental oxygen to enhance activity tolerance.
Arrange for physical and occupational therapy consultation.
Pace activities to provide rest and decrease episodes of breathlessness.
Teach client to reduce activities that exacerbate fatigue.
Provide suctioning as needed based on assessment findings.
Provide CPT to promote secretion removal and chest expansion as tolerated.
Provide hydration to maintain fluid volume status and to decrease viscosity of secretions.
Turn every 2 hours to promote ventilation and to help drain pulmonary secretions.
Monitor ABGs as ordered.
Monitor pulse oximetry continuously.
Provide mechanical ventilation during acute phase.
Suction as needed based on assessment findings; maintain patent airway.
Monitor peak airway pressure every 2 hours.
Monitor ventilator settings every 2 hours.
Provide reassurance for the client and family.
Provide oral care every 2 hours.
Provide rest periods.
Schedule care activities based on the client's energy level.
Provide an alternative method of communication such as a picture board, talking board, or alphabet board.
Speak in clear, short sentences and ask questions that only require a short response.
Provide the client and family with information about home oxygen therapy, liter flow, and equipment for home use. Provide instruction about oxygen safety.
Instruct the client and family in smoking cessation techniques and how this relates to oxygen safety.
Provide information about local smoking cessation programs.

Pulmonary Rehabilitation. Clients with COPD need to be taught how to breathe effectively and how to adapt their lifestyles and ADLs. Pulmonary rehabilitation programs are designed to provide the client with supervised exercise, breathing retraining, adaptation of ADLs, education about the disease, smoking cessation assistance, medications, nutrition, and exercise. A newer component of pulmonary rehabilitation includes 20 to 30 minutes of exercise 3 to 5 times a week with moderate intensity and strength training. Pulmonary rehabilitation can help reduce health care costs by reducing the frequency of hospitalizations and helping older clients and their families learn to cope with the disease process (Covey and Larson, 2004).

Smoking Cessation. Older clients with COPD who continue to smoke increase their risk of repeated respiratory infections and progression of the underlying disease process. Older clients should be encouraged to stop smoking. It is important to provide support for older clients attempting to quit smoking. Success depends in part on the support of family and friends. Many older clients find it impossible to stop smoking completely. They should be encouraged to reduce the amount and frequency of their smoking. Although smoking reduction is not ideal, it may help decrease some of the symptoms associated with respiratory illness. Programs are available through the American Lung Association, ACS, and many community hospitals.

Nutrition. Older clients need to be instructed on the benefits of eating nutritious meals. Adequate nutrition is often difficult to maintain in older clients (see Chapter 10). Clients with COPD have the additional problem of breathlessness, which makes eating difficult. The client should be instructed to eat frequent small meals, avoid gas-producing foods, reduce carbohydrates to only 50% of the diet (the breakdown of carbohydrates has been shown to increase the CO_2 load and thereby increase the work of breathing, especially in those with CO_2 retention), eat high-protein foods, and reduce the intake of fat (see Nutritional Considerations box).

Breathing Retraining. The goals of breathing retraining include decreasing the work of breathing, improving oxygenation, increasing the efficiency of breathing patterns, and promoting client control of breathing. Two of the most commonly taught techniques are diaphragmatic breathing and pursed-lip breathing (Boxes 24-1 and 24-2; Figs. 24-4 and 24-5). Diaphragmatic breathing increases client awareness of breathing patterns and improves the efficiency of breathing. Pursed-lip breathing increases expiratory pressure, improves oxygenation, helps prevent early airway closure, increases exhalation time, reduces the respiratory rate, and allows clients to slow their breathing.

Chest Physiotherapy. Chest physiotherapy (CPT) includes chest percussion, postural drainage (PD), and vibration and rib shaking. CPT is used for clients who have difficulty clearing their own secretions. Contraindications include hemoptysis, pulmonary emboli, osteoporosis, and bleeding disorders. PD consists of positioning the client in a head-down position after CPT to facilitate drainage of pulmonary secretions. Older clients may not tolerate the head-down position of PD or the percussion of CPT. The nurse should explain to clients that they may experience increased breathlessness as a result of the mobilization of secretions and increased coughing as they try to clear their airways. To help decrease discomfort

Nutritional Considerations

Respiratory System

Nutrient requirements for clients with respiratory disease are:

Calories—25 to 35 kcal/kg of body weight for maintenance; 35 to 40 kcal/kg for replacement and building

Protein—1 to 1.5 g/kg of body weight for maintenance; 1.5 to 2 g/kg for replacement and building; 25%-50% of caloric intake

Carbohydrates—50% of caloric intake; the breakdown of carbohydrates increases the CO_2 load and may increase the work of breathing, especially in older clients with CO_2 retention

Fats—20% to 25% nonprotein calories

BOX 24-1 Diaphragmatic Breathing

1. Lie in a supine or semi-Fowler's position.
2. Place one hand on the middle of the stomach below the sternum.
3. Place the other hand on the upper chest.
4. Inhale slowly through the nose. The stomach should expand. (Note the movement of the hand over the stomach.)
5. Exhale slowly through pursed lips. The stomach should contract.
6. Rest.
7. Repeat.

BOX 24-2 Pursed-Lip Breathing

1. Assume a comfortable position.
2. Inhale slowly through the nose, keeping the mouth closed.
3. Remember to use the diaphragmatic breathing technique.
4. Pucker the lips as if blowing out a candle, kissing, or whistling.
5. Exhale slowly, blowing through pursed lips (exhalation should be at least twice as long as inhalation).
6. Rest.
7. Repeat.

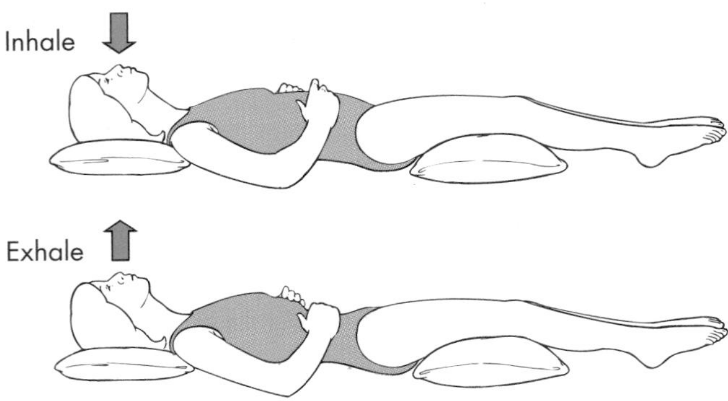

Fig. 24-4 Diaphragmatic breathing.

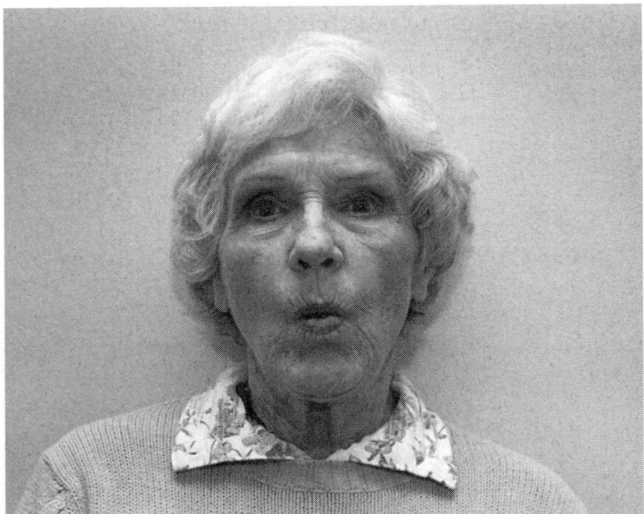
Fig. 24-5 Pursed-lip breathing. (Courtesy Ursula Ruhl, St Louis.)

associated with chest percussion, the nurse should place a bath towel over the area being percussed.

Pulmonary Hygiene. Pulmonary hygiene consists of hydration, deep breathing exercises, and cough techniques (Box 24-3). Older clients are prone to dehydration and therefore are at risk for airway plugging. The nurse should encourage a volume of oral fluids of 4 to 6 quarts a day, if not contraindicated by cardiovascular disease; he or she should also instruct older clients to sip fluids all day to decrease the chance of feeling full by drinking a large amount at one time, and teach older clients the signs and symptoms associated with a respiratory infection; these include sputum color changes, fever, chills, and a change in breathing pattern.

Medications. Client education regarding medications includes the purpose of the medication, dosage, side effects, and schedule of administration. Medications are administered by mouth, MDI (Box 24-4), or nebulizer.

BOX 24-3 Effective Cough Techniques

CASCADE COUGH

1. Take a deep breath and hold it for 1 to 3 seconds.
2. Cough out forcefully several times until all air is exhaled (usually two to six coughs).
3. Inhale slowly through the nose.
4. Repeat once, if necessary.
5. Rest.
6. Repeat as needed.

HUFF COUGH

1. Take a deep breath and hold it for 1 to 3 seconds.
2. Keeping glottis open, cough out several times until all air is exhaled (usually two to six coughs). Sometimes it helps to say the word "huff" while coughing.
3. Inhale slowly through the nose.
4. Repeat as necessary.

END-EXPIRATORY COUGH

1. Take a deep breath and hold it for 1 to 3 seconds.
2. Exhale slowly.
3. At the end of the exhalation, cough once.
4. Inhale slowly through the nose.
5. Repeat as necessary.
6. Follow with a cascade or huff cough, in which secretions are moved from smaller to larger airways.

AUGMENTED COUGH

1. Take a deep breath and hold it for 1 to 3 seconds.
2. Perform one or more of the following maneuvers:
   a. Tighten knees and buttocks to increase intraabdominal pressure.
   b. Bend forward at the waist to increase intraabdominal pressure.
   c. Place hand flat on the upper abdomen just under the xiphoid process and press in and up abruptly during the cough or exhalation, or place hands on the lateral rib cage and quickly press in and release with each cough (this is called rib springing).
   d. Keep hands on the chest wall and press inward with each cough.
3. Inhale slowly through the nose.
4. Rest, if necessary.
5. Repeat as needed.

From Dettenmeier P: *Pulmonary nursing care,* St Louis, 1992, Mosby.

Inhaled medications are only as effective as the delivery. Simple human errors that affect delivery of inhaled medications include failure to shake the inhaler before use, failure to exhale slowly before inhaling, lack of mechanical coordination of compression of inhaler and inhaling, rapid inhalation or lack of deep inhalation, not waiting at least 30 seconds between puffs, failure to clean MDI periodically, holding the MDI upside down, and failure to remove the cap before spraying the medication (Self, Kilgore, and Sheldon, 2003).

BOX 24-4 Using a Metered-Dose Inhaler

1. Select the appropriate canister of medication.
2. Shake the inhaler 15 to 20 times.
3. Hold the inhaler directly in front of the mouth about 2 to 3 inches from the lips. When a spacer is used, place the inhaler in the spacer and place the mouthpiece directly into the mouth.
4. Take a deep breath and exhale completely.
5. Open the mouth wide. When a spacer is used, seal the lips around the mouthpiece.
6. Activate the inhaler.
7. Inhale slowly and deeply.
8. Hold breath for a count of 10.
9. Exhale slowly.
10. Wait 1 to 5 minutes between puffs. Repeat the steps for each puff ordered.

Exercise. Exercise training is an important component of pulmonary rehabilitation. Regular exercise of 20 to 30 minutes of moderate intensity 3 to 5 days a week reduces cardiovascular disease risks, improves musculoskeletal functioning, helps control weight or promote weight loss, and may help prevent bone loss in older clients (Covey and Larson, 2004). One of the best exercises is walking or using a treadmill. It strengthens both the legs and the upper body, especially if the arms are used. Exercise on a stationary bicycle is also useful, but it does not have the benefit of overall body conditioning that can be achieved with walking. Older clients with COPD may start a program in small increments, such as walking or biking for 3 to 5 minutes daily. It is important to develop an exercise program that is achievable for an older client. Targets are based on desired outcomes. The appropriate exercise intensity for health benefit is maintaining heart rate of at least 55% of the maximum rate for a client's age (i.e., a rate of 88 beats/min for a 60-year-old and 80 beats/min for a 75-year-old).

One benefit of a formal pulmonary rehabilitation program is the social aspect. The classes and exercise times usually allow many clients to participate at once. This helps motivate older clients, provides emotional support, and offers them an opportunity to get out of the home. The exercise sessions are often mini–support groups. As a client progresses, 1- to 2-pound weights may be added while walking to help strengthen the upper body.

Home Oxygen Therapy. Oxygen therapy decreases morbidity and mortality for clients with COPD when used more than 18 hours a day. A client's acceptance of oxygen therapy and attitude about the disease determine the level of compliance with treatment. Oxygen therapy is considered a medication and should be treated as such. Clients and families need to be taught proper liter flow, the times that oxygen is to be used, and the proper use of the equipment.

Home oxygen therapy is available in E-cylinder, concentrators, and liquid systems. A liquid oxygen system with portability is the most easily transported and may provide older clients with more mobility; however, it is the most expensive. The concentrator is a machine about the size of small bedside table. It is stationary and usually accompanied by an E-cylinder for limited portability. The E-cylinder, a small green tank that can be pulled on a cart similar to a luggage rack, is economical though a little less portable because of its size.

All the persons involved in a client's care—client, family, physician, and nurse—should discuss the client's level of activity and select the right system to support his or her lifestyle. Social workers can be helpful in determining the amount and type of insurance coverage the client has available for home oxygen therapy. Many third-party payers do not cover liquid oxygen systems unless the client is active and spends a good portion of the day out of the home. If an older client is homebound, only leaving the home for medical appointments, the most economical system is the concentrator with an E-cylinder.

Evaluation

Evaluation of an older client with COPD focuses on the ability to return to ADLs, control of symptoms, and achievement of the expected outcomes. Older clients may need additional caregivers in the home, since the spouse or significant other is most likely of a similar age and thus may have chronic health problems as well. Evaluation should include monitoring functional ability throughout the disease process. The nurse should determine if an older client can use the adaptive and energy-conserving techniques to reduce breathlessness and fatigue that are taught in pulmonary rehabilitation. Older clients may need more time to learn the educational materials; however, once taught, they should have a good understanding and be able to adapt these techniques to their lifestyle.

RESTRICTIVE PULMONARY DISEASE

Restrictive lung disease results in loss of functioning alveoli, loss of lung volume, and decreased chest wall compliance. Restrictive lung disease can be the result of extrapulmonary factors such as excessive weight and muscle mass, a chest splint, or restrictive dressing. Mechanisms of restrictive lung disease include pleural-based diseases, impaired lung expansion, impaired neuromuscular contraction, and thoracic deformities.

Lung Carcinoma

Lung cancer is the leading cause of cancer deaths, accounting for 28% of cancer deaths. In 2003 over 157,200 deaths resulted from lung cancer (Baldwin, 2003). It is rare in clients less than 40 years of age but increases in incidence between ages 60 and 70 (National Cancer Institute [NCI], 1998). The 5-year survival rate is 14%, or 49% if diagnosed before there is lymph node involvement. The increase in smoking by women has raised their death rate from lung cancer to the point that it now exceeds the rate of breast cancer.

Risk factors for development of lung cancer include tobacco use; marijuana use; recurring inflammation; asbestos, talcum powder, or mineral exposure; and less frequently radon exposure, heredity, vitamin A deficiency, and air pollution. The leading cell types of lung cancer include (1) small cell lung carcinoma (SCLC), which accounts for 20% of cases; (2) non–small cell lung carcinoma (NSCLC), including squamous cell carcinoma and adenocarcinoma, which accounts for 30% to 40% of cases; (3) alveolar cell and large cell undifferentiated carcinoma, which account for 10% of cases; (4) bronchoalveolar carcinoma; and (5) terminal arborization of bronchi. Rare types of lung cancer include carcinoid tumors (typical and atypical), adenoid cystic carcinoma, mucoepidermoid carcinoma, pulmonary blastoma, pulmonary sarcoma, and lymphoepithelial carcinoma (Baldwin, 2003; NCI, 1998). The most common and lethal type of lung cancer is SCLC, which usually has a life expectancy of less than 1 year. SCLC is an aggressive cancer that metastasizes to the central nervous system, bones, and liver. NSCLC is a slower growing and less aggressive cancer.

Diagnostic Tests and Procedures. Diagnosis is based on the clinical history and chest radiography. Initial workup includes a complete blood count (CBC), carcinoembryonic antigen, chest x-ray study, computed tomographic (CT) scan, ABG measurements, PFTs, and an electrocardiogram (ECG). Sputum cytology is used to determine cell type. If metastasis is suspected, additional diagnostic tests include magnetic resonance imaging of the brain, a bone scan, exercise PFTs, a quantitative ventilation/perfusion scan, a treadmill exercise test, a Doppler echocardiogram, and carotid Doppler ultrasound. A fiberoptic bronchoscope is used to obtain tissue confirmation of the diagnosis. Surgical diagnosis includes cervical mediastinoscopy, mediastinotomy, and thoracotomy. PFTs are used to determine impairment in ventilation and help predict functionality if surgery is a consideration.

In 1997 the NCI established new staging for lung cancer. Stage I is NSCLC, stage II is NSCLC with lymph node or chest wall invasion, stages III A and III B consist of further chest wall invasion that requires resection of the lung and ribs, and stage IV involves distant metastasis.

Treatment. Treatment is based on lung cancer staging. Stage I is treatable with surgery. Options include lobectomy; segmental, wedge, or sleeve resection; radiotherapy; and adjuvant chemotherapy. Stage II treatment options comprise all options from Stage I, as well as curative radiotherapy, radiotherapy with curative surgery, and adjuvant chemotherapy. Stage IIIA treatment includes surgery, chemotherapy, surgery, and postoperative radiotherapy. Treatment options for Stage IIIB include radiotherapy, chemotherapy, chemotherapy and radiotherapy, or radiotherapy and resection. Stage IV treatment is palliative and includes radiotherapy, chemotherapy, and endobronchial laser therapy for obstructive lesions (NCI, 1997). Non–small cell cancers are usually treated with surgical resection, followed by radiotherapy and chemotherapy. If an older client has significant lung disease, resection of the lung or segmental resection may not be possible. The decision to perform a surgical resection depends on the amount of functional lung tissue that would remain after the surgery.

Careful management of pain, symptoms such as nausea and vomiting, and chemotherapy-related side effects is important for providing as much comfort as possible for the client and family. Older clients may not be able to tolerate a complex medical regimen, especially if there is other organ involvement or underlying disease processes.

Prognosis. The survival rate for clients with lung cancer is 14% at 5 years. Stage I NSCLC has a 60% to 80% curative rate with surgery and 15% to 25% curative rate with radiotherapy. If peripheral nodule removal for SCLC and adjuvant chemotherapy are used, there is a 35% curative rate. Stage II NSCLC has a 30% to 45% curative rate with surgery. The death rate for older adults undergoing surgical resection of the lung is 10% to 14% (ACS, 1998; NCI, 1998).

NURSING MANAGEMENT

Assessment

Assessment includes the identification of risk factors for lung cancer. The clinical presentation of lung cancer can easily be mistaken for other chronic lung diseases such as chronic bronchitis. Many times there are no symptoms, or symptoms are ignored or attributed to smoking or a preexisting lung disease. Common early signs include cough, chest pain, and hemoptysis.

Diagnosis

Nursing diagnoses for lung cancer include (Gordon, 2002):

- Impaired gas exchange related to altered blood flow and alveolar-capillary membrane changes
- Ineffective coping related to situational crises and perceived vulnerability
- Hopelessness related to failure or deterioration of physiologic condition and long-term stress
- Chronic pain related to physical disability

Planning and Expected Outcomes

Planning includes developing interventions and expected outcomes for the client that focus on improving gas exchange and promoting airway clearance and comfort. Expected outcomes include (Johnson and Maas, 1997):

1. Client will be able to maintain ABG values at baseline.
2. Client will be able to sustain spontaneous respiration.
3. Client and family will be able to verbalize their feelings related to the diagnosis of lung cancer.
4. Client's pain will be controlled.
5. Client will report a decrease in the number of episodes of breathlessness.
6. Client's lungs will be clear on auscultation.
7. Client will maintain a stable weight.
8. Client will report feeling a decrease in fatigue.
9. Client will maintain a realistic level of activity.

Intervention

Nursing care of an older client with lung cancer includes relief of pain, emotional support, counseling, and discussion of options and alternatives. The older client may have few friends and family members for support if losses have been numerous. Interventions include providing factual information concerning the diagnosis, treatment, and prognosis; encouraging an attitude of realistic hope as a way of dealing with feelings of helplessness; acknowledging the client's spiritual and cultural background; and encouraging verbalization of feelings, perceptions, and fears (McCloskey and Bulechek, 1996). The nurse needs to be sensitive to the values of older clients and how they see the diagnosis affecting their quality of life. Many older clients may be more concerned about immediate survival and quality-of-life issues than the 5-year postoperative survival rate.

Evaluation

Symptom management is evaluated by assessing how often symptoms occur, how the client has been able to incorporate changes into his or her lifestyle, and how the symptoms alter the client's ADLs. The nurse should determine the success of pain management and the level of client comfort. Older adults may not have the same tolerance for pain and discomfort as younger clients. The nurse should help clients quantify their pain on a scale from 1 to 10 (see Chapter 15). This will help both nurse and client monitor the effectiveness of pain management. The nurse should also evaluate the older adult's use of pain medication. Many older adults are concerned about becoming addicted to their pain medication and may not use it as prescribed. In addition, many older adults may become depressed after a diagnosis of cancer and should be monitored for signs of depression.

Tuberculosis

Tuberculosis (TB) is caused by the *Mycobacterium tuberculosis* organism. TB is most often seen in populations living in close quarters and those with little or no health care or preventive care. It is the number one fatal and communicable disease in the United States. TB is transmitted by inhalation of infected droplets aerosolized in the air from the cough or sneeze of an infected person. TB is divided into primary and active varieties. Primary TB is contracted by inhalation of infected droplets and deposits into the upper lobes of the lung, since the organism is aerobic and seeks the greatest ventilation. The body's immune system responds to the local inflammation by walling off the bacteria. Active TB presents symptoms. Inflammation of the airway leads to the development of a lesion and necrosis of the tissue. TB can remain inactive in the body for decades. Active TB can be present in any patient admitted with pneumonia, pleural effusion, human immunodeficiency virus (HIV) or acquired immunodeficiency syndrome (AIDS), weight loss, cancer, or alcohol or substance abuse (Sibilano, 1996).

In an older client the presence of TB may be a reactivation of a dormant organism that has been present in the individual for some time; changes in an older client's immune system increase the risk for the reactivation of TB. Medical risk factors that substantially increase the risk of TB include silicosis; gastrectomy; jejunal bypass; weight more than 10% below ideal body weight; chronic renal failure; diabetes mellitus; and hematologic disorders such as leukemia, lymphomas, and other malignancies. Residents of nursing and other long-term care facilities for older adults are at increased risk of developing TB, with a 2 to 7 times greater incidence of the disease than in demographically similar persons in other settings.

TB incidence is higher in adults over 65 years of age than in any other population. Many older adult clients have underlying lung disease, and more than 50% have sputum smears that test positive for acid-fast bacilli (AFB), which are capable of transmitting the infection to other persons. Older adults represent most of the nation's nursing facility residents while constituting a large repository of *M. tuberculosis*. These concentrations of older adults, many of whom are infected and some of whom are immunocompromised, create high-risk situations for transmission of TB. The incidence of TB among nursing facility residents is 39.2 per 100,000 population (CDC, 1997c).

Diagnostic Tests and Procedures. Tuberculin skin testing in older clients is an unreliable indicator of TB. Older clients often display a false negative skin test result because of reduced immune system activity. If skin testing is used, it is recommended that the standard 5 tuberculin unit (TU) Mantoux test be given and then repeated to create a booster effect. The second test may be a 5 TU or a second strength 250 TU test.

Older clients with any of the following symptoms should alert the practitioner to a high probability of TB: night sweats, atypical pneumonia, low-grade fever, nonproductive cough, hemoptysis, anorexia, and weight loss. A purified protein derivative (PPD) is then used. If the size of the induration is equal to or greater than 10 mm (or equal to or greater than 5 mm in an HIV-positive client), the PPD is positive. In the event of a positive PPD with symptoms, a chest x-ray study is recommended within 72 hours.

A positive chest x-ray study with infiltration in the posterior and apical segments of the upper lobes or in the superior segments of the lower lobes; cavitation, nodular infiltrates, atelectasis, and fibrotic scarring with retraction of the hilum; and deviation of the trachea strongly indicate TB. TB in older adults may show lower lobe nodular infiltrates without cavitation. Diffuse, finely nodular, uniformly distributed lesions characterize hematogenous TB. Any persistent infiltrate in older clients must be suspected as TB. Although the aforementioned radiographic changes are most common, TB can produce almost any form of pulmonary radiographic abnormality. Older clients should be questioned about potential exposure to TB; tested for HIV infection; and screened for other symptoms such as chronic osteomyelitis, chronic urinary tract infections, and any of the aforementioned symptoms not present on initial examination. If a client has a positive PPD and is asymptomatic, prophylaxis with isoniazid for 6 months is indicated.

For older clients with a positive PPD, symptoms, and a positive chest x-ray study, a number of additional laboratory tests and referrals are indicated. These include a CBC, erythrocyte sedimentation rate, chemistry panel, sputum test for AFB × 3, and a bone marrow biopsy. A referral to an infectious disease specialist is also recommended, especially if the client has been determined to have multiple drug–resistant-TB (MDR-TB).

Treatment. Treatment with the standard four-drug anti-TB therapeutic regimen will cause a rapid reduction in the number of viable mycobacteria (CDC, 1998a). Reduction in viable organism load is seen within 2 weeks. Cultures will convert to negative within 3 months in clients compliant with their therapy. Medications include a combination of bactericidal drugs. The most common drugs are isoniazid, rifampin, ethambutol, streptomycin, and pyrazinamide (CDC, 1998a). Other drugs used in the treatment of TB include ethionamide, kanamycin, paraaminosalicylic acid, cycloserine, and rifabutin. Fluoroquinolones, such as ciprofloxacin, are also being used to treat TB.

Monitoring of liver function on a monthly basis is recommended, since older adults are at greater risk of developing hepatitis. Isoniazid can lead to toxic hepatitis and peripheral neuropathy, especially in malnourished or diabetic older adults.

The incidence of MDR-TB rose 6.8% between 1993 and 2002. From 1993 to 1996 there was a relatively stable level of resistance to isoniazid and a reduction in MDR-TB (CDC, 1997c). The CDC recommends anti-TB drug–susceptibility testing on initial *M. tuberculosis* isolated from all TB patients. MDR-TB is more common in clients who have spent time with someone with MDR-TB; those who do not take their medicine regularly or do not take all their prescribed medication; those who redevelop TB after having been treated; and those who come from areas high in MDR-TB incidence, such as Mexico (25.6%), Philippines (11.6%), Vietnam (8.4%), India (7.7%), and China (4.8%) (CDC, 1998b). Resistance to treatment with isoniazid and rifampin extends the usual 6-month treatment to 18 to 24 months with only a 60% cure rate.

The greatest effect on the prevalence of TB could come from the development of a new vaccine (CDC, 1998a). In 1997, 40% of the new TB cases in the United States occurred in foreign-born persons. There has been widespread use of bacille Calmette-Guérin (BCG) vaccine in Europe and other foreign countries with little effect on the disease. In some cases it has worsened the disease (CDC, 1998b). The BCG vaccine has never been widely used in the United States because of questions about its efficacy and because it may induce dermal hypersensitivity to PPD tuberculin in most recipients (CDC, 1998a). Therefore it is necessary to look to a new vaccine to reduce the current pandemic of TB.

Prognosis. The prognosis for an older client with TB is good if the client follows the medical regimen and maintains good nutrition. The greater risk is the side effects of isoniazid.

NURSING MANAGEMENT

Assessment

Signs and symptoms include fatigue, weight loss, weakness, night sweats, low-grade fever, purulent sputum, and sputum positive for AFB. Older adults may not manifest all the classic symptoms of TB. The nurse should suspect TB when an older client complains of weight loss and chronic cough. If the disease has progressed, the client may have hemoptysis, lung consolidation, crackles and wheezes on auscultation, upper-lobe patchy infiltrates, and cavitation on chest radiography. Sibilano (1995) developed a Tuberculosis Index of Suspicion Tool (TIST) to assist in the assessment of clients at risk for TB. The tool includes assessment of symptoms, high-risk group assessment, and diagnostic workup.

Diagnosis

Nursing diagnoses for an older client with TB include (Gordon, 2002):

- Knowledge deficit: TB related to lack of previous exposure
- Altered health maintenance related to lack of material resources
- Noncompliance with treatment regimen related to client's value system
- Social isolation related to altered state of wellness

Planning and Expected Outcomes

Planning for older clients with TB must include the client and family. If a client is a resident in a nursing or extended care facility, the medical and nursing directors need to be included in planning as well. Expected outcomes include (Johnson and Maas, 1997):

1. Client will be able to demonstrate safe coughing techniques.
2. Client and family will be able to verbalize the medication regimen.
3. Client and family will be able to verbalize the side effects of the anti-TB medications.
4. Client will be able to verbalize the need for continued medication.
5. Client and family will be able to state how TB is transmitted.
6. Client will be able to verbalize feelings related to social isolation.

Intervention

Nursing measures for clients with TB include education about TB and how it is transmitted. Clients and families should be educated about the measures necessary to prevent further TB transmission, the importance of continued medication administration, and good nutrition. Table 24-4 lists the most common drugs used to treat TB, their dosages, adverse reactions, and nursing considerations. The nurse should instruct the client and family on the side effects of isoniazid: hepatotoxicity, psychotic reactions, coordination difficulties, muscle twitching, memory impairment, loss of self-control, dizziness, stupor, tinnitus, peripheral neuritis, agranulocytosis, aplastic anemia, hemolytic anemia, epigastric distress, dry mouth, nausea, vomiting, urinary retention, metabolic acidosis, hyperglycemia, lack of appetite, yellowish skin or eyes, fever for 3 or more days, abdominal pain, and tingling in the fingers and toes. If a client experiences any of these, he or she should call the doctor or nurse immediately. Clients should not drink alcohol while taking isoniazid.

Other TB drug side effects to report to the health care practitioner include skin rash, easy bleeding, aching joints, dizziness, tingling or numbness around the mouth, easy bruising, blurred or changed vision, ringing in the ears, and hearing loss. Rifampin can turn urine, saliva, or tears orange; make the client more sensitive to the sun; and make birth control pills and implants less effective (CDC, 1994).

Older adults may view a diagnosis of TB as a socially bad disease. They remember the stigma of TB in the early 1900s, a disease that required separation from family and friends and placement in sanatoriums. The nurse must address the need for psychosocial interaction and support.

TABLE 24-4 Antituberculosis Medications

MEDICATION	DOSAGE	ADVERSE REACTIONS	NURSING CONSIDERATIONS
Isoniazid	**Primary therapy:** 5 mg/kg po daily up to 300 mg/day Intramuscular—same as po	Anemia, hepatitis, hypersensitivity, peripheral neuritis, seizures, and systemic lupus erythematosus	Therapy lasts for 6 to 9 months and is used in conjunction with other antituberculosis medication. Instruct client to avoid alcohol.
Rifampin (Rifaden, Rofact)	10 mg/kg body weight (maximum 600 mg)	Decreased effectiveness of oral contraceptives, hemolysis, hepatic toxicity, increased metabolism of hepatically excreted drugs, induction of methadone withdrawal, renal failure, thrombocytopenia, orange body fluids, and rash	Monitor hepatic, renal, and hemolytic parameters. Give 1 hour before or 2 hours after meals. Monitor hepatic function (urine may become red-orange). Instruct client to avoid alcohol. Usually used with one other drug. Monitor platelet count and CBC.
Pyrazinamide (PZA)	20-35 mg/kg/day up to 3 g/day	Anorexia, arthralgia, gout (rare), hepatitis, hyperuricemia, nausea, renal failure (rare), and vomiting	Have client take medication with meals or snack to reduce gastric irritation. Instruct client to report any problems with urination. Monitor liver function tests. Instruct client regarding signs of thrombocytopenia, such as unexplained bleeding or bruising, appearance of petechiae, and nosebleeds.

po, By mouth.

Evaluation

Evaluation of an older client with TB includes assessment of compliance with the medication regimen; older adults may find it difficult to adhere to a medication regimen. The nurse should evaluate compliance with public health measures such as wearing a mask in public. Evaluation also includes monitoring of hepatic and renal function and repeated sputum cultures for AFB. The client's mood should be evaluated for depression because of social isolation.

BRONCHOPULMONARY INFECTION

Influenza

Older clients are prone to complications from the influenza virus, especially if they have underlying chronic illness. Changes related to the normal aging process decrease an older adult's ability to clear secretions and to protect the airway. Older clients account for 80% to 90% of all influenza-related deaths. The influenza season in the United States is from November until April, with peak activity between January and March (CDC, 1997b). It takes about 1 to 2 weeks to develop antibody protection after receiving the influenza vaccine. Persons ages 65 and older, residents of nursing and other chronic care facilities, and adults with COPD or cardiac disease should receive an annual influenza vaccine. Because of normal changes in an older adult's immune system, older adults have a decreased response to influenza immunization (NHLBI, 1996).

Diagnostic Tests and Procedures. Diagnosis includes obtaining a history of fever, chills, anorexia, and general malaise, which may be blunted or atypical in older adults.

Treatment. Much of the illness and death associated with influenza can be prevented with annual influenza vaccination. The vaccine is recommended for all clients ages 65 and older and for clients with any chronic diseases, immunosuppression, or severe forms of anemia (CDC, 1997b). In older clients and those with chronic medical conditions, the vaccine is mostly effective in reducing the severity of the illness and the risk of serious complications and death (CDC, 1997b).

Treatment includes rest, fluid, hydration, and careful monitoring for progression to a more serious illness. Antibiotics are often used to prevent a secondary bacterial infection, especially in older clients with underlying respiratory and cardiac disease (Holman, 2003).

The use of antiviral agents such as amantadine, rimantadine, or the use of a neuraminidase inhibitor (oseltamivir [Tamiflu]) can reduce the severity and shorten the duration of influenza A in healthy adults when administered within 48 hours of onset. It is unknown whether either of these antivirals will prevent complications in high-risk groups. Side effects of amantadine and rimantadine include behavioral changes, delirium, hallucinations, agitation, and seizures. They are associated with high plasma drug concentration, which occurs most often in older adult clients and clients with renal insufficiency. Side effects of Tamiflu include gastrointestinal upset, bronchitis, headache, insomnia, vertigo, and fatigue. This medication is used with caution with clients who have hepatic impairment or chronic cardiac or respiratory disease.

Prognosis. Of all influenza-related deaths, 80% to 90% occur in the older adult population (CDC, 1997b).

NURSING MANAGEMENT

Assessment

It is difficult to recognize infection in older clients. The signs associated with infection may be subdued or absent. Changes in mental status, exacerbation of underlying chronic conditions, and subnormal temperature may indicate infection in older clients. Subnormal temperature accompanied by hypotension; rapid pulse; and cool, clammy skin are signs of sepsis in older clients. General fatigue, malaise, and decreased appetite and fluid intake may indicate influenza in older clients. The nurse should examine a client's chest for decreased breath sounds, wheezing, and clinical signs of pneumonia; he or she should also assess tissue turgor and oral mucosa to determine whether an older client is dehydrated.

Diagnosis

Nursing diagnoses for clients with influenza include (Gordon, 2002):

- Ineffective breathing pattern related to decreased energy or fatigue
- Fatigue related to increased energy requirements for ADLs
- Risk for fluid volume deficit related to altered intake and factors influencing fluid needs
- Pain related to physical injury factors

Planning and Expected Outcomes

Planning for an older adult with influenza must include the client and family. If the client is a resident in a nursing or extended care facility, the medical and nursing directors need to be included in developing a plan to prevent transmission to other residents. Expected outcomes for an older client with influenza include (Johnson and Maas, 1997):

1. Client will maintain a patent airway.
2. Client will have a decrease in complaints of fatigue.
3. Client will have clear lungs on auscultation.
4. Client will be able to effectively clear secretions.
5. Client will be able to rest without body aches or pain.
6. Client will maintain adequate hydration with a fluid intake of 4 to 6 ounces per hour.

Intervention

Nursing care includes hydration, rest, and symptomatic relief. Nonsteroidal antiinflammatory drugs are used to treat muscle aches and fever. These should be given with food or milk to prevent gastrointestinal upset in older adults. One of the greatest risks is dehydration. Older clients should be encouraged to drink eight 8-ounce glasses of water per day, which many find difficult. Encouraging older adults to drink small glasses of water when passing the sink may help in ensuring an adequate intake. Other sources of fluids include juices, Jell-O, popsicles, and replacement drinks such as Gatorade. The nurse should also monitor the older client's mucous membranes, skin turgor, thirst, intake and output, presence or absence of vertigo on rising, blood pressure, heart rate, and weight during the acute phase and recovery period (McCloskey and Bulechek, 1996).

During peak influenza season, older clients should avoid crowds to decrease the risk of contracting influenza. The nurse should encourage clients to do shopping and other errands early in the morning when it is less crowded, or to have someone else shop for them. The older adult should be alerted to the fact that the holidays are particularly problematic with regard to crowds. The use of a scarf across the nose and mouth can help reduce transmission of airborne viruses.

Evaluation

Evaluation is based on the improvement of the clinical picture and the resolution of symptoms. The nurse should monitor older adults for improvement in their condition. Failure to improve may indicate the development of a secondary bacterial infection such as pneumonia. The nurse should monitor hydration by evaluating vital signs, weight, and skin turgor. The development of congestion, crackles, or dullness on chest percussion should alert the nurse to possible pneumonia.

Pneumonia

Pneumonia is an inflammation of the lung parenchyma, usually associated with the filling of the alveoli with fluid. Pneumonia can be viral, be bacterial, or be caused by aspiration, which is often found in older adults. Pneumonia is a particularly serious illness in older clients, often resulting in death. The serious nature of the illness is related to the normal age-related deterioration of the immune system, underlying chronic illnesses, weakened cough reflex, and decreased mobility. The diagnosis of pneumonia may be missed because symptoms are obscured by coexisting disease or the use of corticosteroids or antiinflammatory drugs. An older client may manifest altered mental status, dehydration, and a failure to thrive (Fielden, 1998). The client may require hospitalization and admission to the intensive care unit (ICU) with subsequent intubation and mechanical ventilation. The incidence of pneumonia in older adults in chronic care institutions is 2 to 3 times higher than among older adults in the community (CDC, 1997a).

Community-Acquired Pneumonia. Community-acquired pneumonia (CAP) accounts for approximately 6% of all Medicare discharges (Lave et al, 1996). There is increased morbidity and mortality in older clients, especially in the presence of other chronic diseases (Fielden, 1998). Factors that may contribute to increased mortality in older adult clients include advanced age, absence of chest pain, tachypnea, diastolic hypotension, confusion, elevated blood urea nitrogen (BUN), leukocytosis, leukopenia, and digitalis toxicity (Fielden, 1998). Pleuritic chest pain or chills have been associated with a lower mortality rate (Marrie, 2003).

Classic symptoms of community-acquired or bacterial pneumonia include fever, cough, sputum production, general feelings of fatigue and malaise, and shortness of breath. Older clients do not always exhibit fever and cough, often having symptoms of dehydration, confusion, and a respiratory rate greater than 26 breaths/min. Other signs include tachycardia, chest discomfort, dyspnea, headache, nausea, vomiting, myalgia, arthralgia, fatigue, weakness, abdominal pain, diarrhea, and anorexia (Hannaford and Mann, 2000). In multiple lobe pneumonia, a chest x-ray study may show incomplete consolidation of the lung. Some older clients manifest dramatic symptoms, resembling septic shock or adult respiratory distress syndrome (ARDS).

Streptococcus pneumoniae is the leading cause of CAP in older adults, accounting for approximately 25% of pneumonia cases, with a death rate of 30% to 40% among older adults (CDC, 1997a). About 5% to 15% of cases are caused by *H. influenzae, Moraxella (Branhamella) catarrhalis,* and *Legionella pneumophila*.

Nosocomial Pneumonia. *Staphylococcus aureus, Klebsiella pneumoniae, Pseudomonas aeruginosa,* and *Escherichia coli* most often cause nosocomial pneumonia. Older clients have an incidence of nosocomial pneumonia 3 times higher than younger clients. This is because of the age-related decline in the immune system and a high incidence of coexisting disease. In addition, older adults are more likely to be in high-risk areas such as residential centers, hospitals, and extended care facilities for other coexisting diseases.

Viral Pneumonia. Viral pneumonia in older clients is most often associated with a history of the influenza A virus. Older adults are especially susceptible to secondary bacterial infections such as *S. aureus* and *H. influenzae*.

Aspiration Pneumonia. Aspiration pneumonia is commonly associated with clinical situations such as stupor, coma, cardiopulmonary resuscitation, alcohol or drug intoxication, neurologic illness, nasogastric feeding, and general anesthesia. Aspiration of gastric contents into the airway may result in obstruction, chemical pneumonitis, or infection. Older adults are especially prone to aspiration pneumonia because of decreased cough and gag reflexes. In addition, positioning, feeding, and the use of a feeding tube places older clients at increased risk for aspiration pneumonia. The use of narcotic medications, alcohol, and sedatives increases the risk of aspiration.

Diagnostic Tests and Procedures. The diagnosis of pneumonia is made based on a history of colds and influenza and the clinical presentation. Signs and symptoms include fever, chills, pleuritic chest pain, crackles on auscultation, and a productive cough with purulent sputum. Atypical pneumonia is first seen with fever, constitutional symptoms, dry cough, and headache. Laboratory sampling includes total white blood cell (WBC) count, blood cultures, Gram stain, and sputum culture. Of older clients, 20% to 25% fail to demonstrate leukocytosis, and about one third are unable to produce a sputum sample. A chest x-ray study (posterior, anterior, and lateral) is obtained to identify infiltrates and assess for complications such as effusions or lung abscess. The chest x-ray is the gold standard for diagnosis. If the client is dehydrated, infiltrates may not be evident even if they are present (Hannaford and Mann, 2000).

Treatment. Treatment consists of administration of the appropriate antibiotics, hydration, good nutrition, and rest. Length of treatment with antibiotics can range from 10 to 14 days, depending on the causative organism. The initial management of immunocompetent clients with CAP is an emphasis on empiric treatment instead of extensive testing because of the difficulty in determining the etiologic pathogen in the disease.

Severity of illness, site of acquisition (e.g., community or nursing facility), age, and comorbid illness are all considerations in determining initial antibiotic therapy. Therapy is aimed at pneumococcal disease and atypicals. Antibiotics used include macrolides such as azithromycin and clarithromycin for outpatients. For clients with advanced age and comorbidity, a second-generation cephalosporin such as cefuroxime or a combination agent such as trimethoprim-sulfamethoxazole is added. If an older client is hospitalized, a second-generation or third-generation cephalosporin or a beta-lactam/beta-lactamase inhibitor is used in combination, with or without a macrolide. Clients with resistant or severe CAP may need an aminoglycoside, an antipseudomonal agent, or quinolone (Hannaford and Mann, 2000).

The American Thoracic Society Criteria for Assessing Pneumonia Severity established guidelines for ICU admission of older clients. To qualify for admission, the client must meet at least three criteria, including a respiratory rate of 30 beats/min or less; Pao_2/fractional concentration of oxygen in inspired gas (Fio_2) of 250 mm Hg, or Pao_2 of 60 mm Hg or less; bilateral or multilobe infiltrates on chest x-ray; and systolic blood pressure of 90 mm Hg or less, or diastolic blood pressure of 60 mm Hg or less (Marrie, 2003). Risk factors for hospitalization include an age greater than 65 years, presence of coexisting illness, altered mental status, chronic alcohol abuse, dehydration, malnutrition, nursing facility residency, aspiration, history of cigarette smoking, recent upper respiratory tract infection or influenza, and previous hospitalization within 1 year (Fielden, 1998). Clinical signs include unstable vital signs, extrapulmonary involvement, leukopenia, hypoxemia, and Pao_2 of 60 mm Hg or less.

Prognosis. Pneumonia remains the most common cause of death in older adults because of altered immune response related to aging, underlying chronic disease, and a diminished cough reflex.

NURSING MANAGEMENT

Assessment

A history of generalized fatigue, malaise, decreased appetite and fluid intake, or a recent viral infection may indicate a bronchopulmonary infection in an older adult. Fever, chills, shortness of breath, sputum production, and an abnormal chest examination suggest pneumonia. The nurse should examine the chest for decreased breath sounds, wheezing, dullness to percussion, egophony, and increased vocal and tactile fremitus. The nurse should also assess for symptoms of dehydration and confusion and other signs and symptoms such as tachycardia, tachypnea, chest discomfort, dyspnea, headache, nausea, vomiting, myalgia, arthralgia, fatigue, weakness, abdominal pain, diarrhea, and anorexia.

The nurse must be alert to signs and symptoms suggestive of increasing severity of illness and a potential need for intensive care. These include tachypnea (30 to 35 breaths/min or more); severe respiratory failure (Pao_2/Fio_2 of 250 mm Hg or less); shock (diastolic hypotension of 60 mm Hg or systolic hypotension of 90 mm Hg or less); fever (temperature over 39.3° C); decreased urine output (20 ml/hour); and abnormal laboratory values for BUN (over 20 mg/dl), creatinine (over 1.2 mg/dl), WBCs (4000 or over 30,000), hemoglobin (9 g/dl), Pao_2 (60 mm Hg), or $Paco_2$ (over 50 mm Hg) (Fielden, 1998). Another sign is a rapid change in chest x-ray studies, consisting of spreading infiltrates and extrapulmonary sites of infection. An older client with such indications needs close monitoring, ongoing nursing care, and possibly even short-term mechanical ventilation for respiratory support.

Diagnosis

Nursing diagnoses for a client with bronchopulmonary infection include (Gordon, 2002):

- Ineffective airway clearance related to decreased energy and tracheobronchial infection, obstruction, and secretions
- Impaired gas exchange related to altered oxygen supply and alveolar-capillary membrane changes

- Ineffective breathing pattern related to respiratory muscle fatigue
- Risk for fluid volume deficit related to altered intake and factors influencing fluid needs

Planning and Expected Outcomes

Planning for an older adult with pneumonia should include the client and family. It is important to focus on supporting respiratory function, promoting good pulmonary hygiene, and maintaining adequate oxygenation. Expected outcomes for an older client with a bronchopulmonary infection include (Johnson and Maas, 1997):

1. Client will maintain a patent airway.
2. Client will maintain a Pao_2 of 80 mm Hg by ABG or arterial oxygen saturation (Sao_2) greater than 90% by pulse oximetry.
3. Client will have decreased complaints of fatigue.
4. Client will have clear lungs on auscultation.
5. Client will be able to clear secretions effectively.
6. Client will be able to sleep through the night without episodes of breathlessness or coughing.
7. Client will maintain baseline vital signs and weight.

Intervention

Nursing management of an older client with a bronchopulmonary infection includes maintenance of hydration, promotion of effective airway clearance, and proper positioning (McCloskey and Bulechek, 1996). Other interventions include monitoring fluid status (see Intervention under the heading of Influenza), monitoring vital signs and oxygenation parameters, maintaining a clean environment, and assisting the client with airway clearance by encouraging coughing or by suctioning (McCloskey and Bulechek, 1996). Because of ventilation/perfusion imbalance in the lung, it is important to position the client with the "good lung down." This promotes drainage of secretions from the lung with the pneumonia and increases the perfusion of the good lung, resulting in improved oxygenation. It may be a challenge to keep the older client positioned on the appropriate side (McCloskey and Bulechek, 1996).

The key to pneumonia prevention is early vaccination. Antibodies to most pneumococcal vaccine antigens remain elevated in healthy adults for at least 5 years. Antibody declines have been shown in older adults after 5 to 10 years (CDC, 1997a). Therefore all persons ages 65 and older should receive the pneumococcal vaccine, including all persons who have not previously been vaccinated and those who have not received the vaccination within 5 years and were 65 or younger at the time of their last vaccination (CDC, 1997a). Vaccination is recommended for all persons with unknown vaccination status (CDC, 1997a). Revaccination is recommended for immunocompromised clients ages 65 and older, including those with HIV infection, leukemia, lymphoma, Hodgkin's disease, generalized malignancy, chronic renal failure, and organ or bone marrow transplantation and those taking long-term systemic corticosteroids or undergoing immunosuppressive chemotherapy (CDC, 1997a; *Clinical update: pneumococcal vaccine: an immunization update*, 1997).

Nursing care planned to prevent aspiration focuses on careful assessment of residual volumes of feedings and proper positioning of the older client during and after eating.

Evaluation

Evaluation includes achievement of the expected outcomes, return of sputum to preinfection color and consistency, and return to baseline respiratory status. The nurse should monitor the client for adequate hydration by assessing vital signs, body weight, and tissue turgor. Dehydration contributes to secretion retention and an inability to clear the airways. The effectiveness of an older adult's cough should be monitored; ineffective coughing can contribute to fatigue and can result in aspirated secretions. The nurse should also monitor the client's lungs for adventitious lung sounds and the respiratory pattern for effective breathing and use of accessory muscles of respiration.

OTHER RESPIRATORY ALTERATIONS

Severe Acute Respiratory Syndrome

The first outbreak of severe acute respiratory syndrome (SARS) occurred in 2003 initially in China and spread to Canada. SARS-associated coronavirus has recently moved from the animal kingdom to the realm of humans. The client's history of foreign travel is imperative to determine if he or she had exposure or close contact within 10 days of symptoms with a person known to have or suspected of having SARS (Dreher et al, 2004). The client may be asymptomatic or have a mild respiratory illness. The signs and symptoms of moderate respiratory illness include temperature over 100.4° F, cough, shortness of breath, difficulty breathing, or hypoxemia. Severe respiratory illness includes the ladder and radiographic evidence of pneumonia or ARDS.

The detection of antibody to SARS-coronavirus (CoV) drawn during the acute illness or after 21 days after the onset of illness confirms diagnosis (Marthaler, Keresztes, and Tazbir, 2003). Other diagnostic tests include chest x-ray, CBC, ABG analysis, pulse oximetry values, clotting profile, respiratory viral panel for influenza and syncytial viruses, metabolic profile, C-reactive protein test and *Legionella* and pneumococcal urinary antigen testing. The client should wear a mask, universal precautions should be observed, and clients and exposed staff should be quarantined. Researchers are developing a vaccine for SARS (Simmerman, Chu, and Chang, 2003).

Cardiogenic and Noncardiogenic Pulmonary Edema

Pulmonary edema is an abnormal increase in the amount of extravascular fluid in the lungs and may be cardiogenic or noncardiogenic in origin. The most common form of pulmonary edema is a result of left ventricular failure. Left ventricular failure commonly occurs in older adults, especially in those ages 85 and older, because of coronary artery disease, mitral stenosis and insufficiency, and aortic stenosis. Cardiogenic pulmonary edema is the most common form of pulmonary edema and is caused by the increased capillary hydrostatic pressure that results from myocardial infarction, mitral stenosis, decreased myocardial contractility, left ventricular failure, or fluid overload. Other predisposing factors include CHF, infusion of excessive volumes or an overly rapid infusion of intravenous fluids, impaired pulmonary lymphatic drainage from Hodgkin's disease or obliterative lymphangitis after radiation, inhalation of irritating gases, left atrial myxoma, pneumonia, and pulmonary venoocclusive disease. A rise in the pulmonary capillary pressure occurs as a result of elevated left ventricular end-diastolic filling pressure, elevated left atrial pressure, and elevated pulmonary venous pressure.

Clinical presentation of acute cardiogenic pulmonary edema includes acute shortness of breath; orthopnea; frothy, blood-tinged sputum; cyanosis; diaphoresis; and tachycardia. Auscultation of the lungs reveals crackles in the bases, fremitus, and dullness to percussion

Noncardiogenic pulmonary edema results from a variety of noncardiac causes. Examples of noncardiogenic pulmonary edema include ARDS, reexpansion pulmonary edema, and neurogenic pulmonary edema.

Cardiogenic Pulmonary Edema

Diagnostic Tests and Procedures. Diagnosis is based on clinical presentation. ABG measurements are drawn to determine arterial Po_2, arterial Po_2 saturation, and pH. Hemodynamic measurements reveal decreased cardiac output, increased pulmonary artery pressure, and right-sided heart pressure in biventricular failure. Because older clients have difficulty maintaining normal hemoglobin levels, it is important to take blood samples judiciously.

Treatment. Treatment includes improvement of gas exchange with supplemental oxygen, improvement of myocardial function by reducing preload and afterload, and correction of the underlying process if possible. If pulmonary edema is extensive, an older client may require transfer to the ICU, initiation of mechanical ventilation, and insertion of a pulmonary artery catheter.

Prognosis. The prognosis for a client with cardiogenic pulmonary edema is good when symptoms are easily reversed and cardiac complications are controlled. However, older adults usually have comorbidity, such as underlying cardiac or lung disease, which increases their risk for complications. With extensive rehabilitation and physical therapy, older adults may be able to return to independent living and baseline ADLs.

Noncardiogenic Pulmonary Edema: Adult Respiratory Distress Syndrome

Diagnostic Tests and Procedures. The most commonly used test is the ABG to determine the degree of hypoxia. Other tests include chest x-ray study, CT scan, CBC, and hemodynamic measurements. Older clients may need intubation and mechanical ventilation. In addition, the placement of an arterial line and pulmonary artery catheter may be indicated to monitor oxygenation and cardiopulmonary hemodynamics.

Treatment. Treatment consists of supplemental oxygen therapy, ventilation support, and maintenance of hemodynamics. Neuromuscular blocking agents, sedatives, and narcotics may be used to reduce anxiety, decrease the work of breathing, decrease oxygen consumption, and increase oxygen delivery. Positive end-expiratory pressure may be added to mechanical ventilation to improve oxygenation.

A pulmonary artery catheter is used to monitor fluid volume status. Fluids and vasopressors may be indicated to maintain adequate blood pressure. If a bacterial infection is evident, antibiotic therapy can be added. Corticosteroids are reserved for ARDS caused by a chemical injury or fatty emboli.

Prognosis. The prognosis is fair to poor with mortality rate of approximately 30% to 60%. Comorbidity, frailty, and nosocomial infections put older adults at increased risk for complications. If an older adult does not require mechanical ventilation, the prognosis is good to fair, depending on underlying disease states and complications. Extensive rehabilitation, physical therapy, and retraining of ADLs may be necessary to return the older adult to independent living (Davey, 2002).

NURSING MANAGEMENT

Assessment

The nurse should determine through the health history whether the client has risk factors for the development of pulmonary edema. Assessment begins with the evaluation of respiratory and cardiac status. The nurse should observe the older client for signs and symptoms of pulmonary edema. Nonspecific signs may include insomnia, wandering, anorexia, nausea, delirium, weakness, and weight gain.

Assessment for noncardiogenic pulmonary edema includes identifying predisposing factors, which include aspiration of gastric contents, pneumonia, thoracic injury, pulmonary contusion, smoke inhalation, multiple blood transfusions, uremia, cardiopulmonary bypass surgery, fracture of long bones, and sepsis. Clinical presentation of noncardiogenic pulmonary edema includes refractory hypoxemia, crackles on auscultation, hypotension, cyanosis, tachypnea, hyperventilation, and increased tracheobronchial secretions.

Diagnosis

Nursing diagnoses for an older client with pulmonary edema include (Gordon, 2002):

- Ineffective breathing pattern related to decreased energy
- Impaired gas exchange related to alveolar-capillary membrane changes and altered blood flow
- Ineffective airway clearance related to decreased energy and tracheobronchial obstruction
- Excess fluid volume related to compromised regulatory mechanism
- Inability to sustain spontaneous ventilation related to metabolic factors and respiratory muscle fatigue
- Risk for infection related to inadequate primary and secondary defenses
- Activity intolerance related to generalized weakness and imbalance of oxygen supply and demand
- Knowledge deficit: cardiogenic pulmonary edema or noncardiogenic pulmonary edema related to lack of previous experience

Planning and Expected Outcomes

Planning includes developing interventions and expected outcomes for older clients that focus on restoration of the oxygen supply and demand balance. The client and family must be included to help the client achieve the expected outcomes. It is important that both the client and family know the expected outcomes and what interventions may be necessary, such as oxygen or mechanical ventilation. Expected outcomes include (Johnson and Maas, 1997):

1. Client will maintain ABG values within normal limits.
2. Client will maintain oxygenation within normal values.
3. Client will have a cardiac output within normal values.
4. Client will be able to verbalize feelings related to the illness.
5. Client will maintain a patent airway.
6. Client will maintain a balanced intake and output.
7. Client will have an alternative method of communication if on mechanical ventilation.
8. Client will maintain skin integrity.
9. Client will be able to sustain spontaneous ventilation without mechanical ventilation.
10. Client will have stable hemodynamics.

Intervention

The effect of pulmonary edema can be severe for older adults because of its associated functional disability secondary to activity intolerance, drug therapy, and frequent rehospitalization. The nurse should be alert to these factors and plan interventions that include daily weight assessments, energy-conserving ADLs, elevation of the feet and legs, reduction in or elimination of sodium intake, and use of diuretics. The nurse should assess the client for adventitious lung sounds, respiratory muscle fatigue and use of accessory muscles of respiration, and airway patency. The client should be positioned to facilitate ventilation/perfusion matching and to minimize respiratory efforts; this can be accomplished by adding pillows at the back and under the arms and encouraging the client to sit up straight with legs and feet elevated. The client should be encouraged to cough effectively; change positions frequently; and practice slow, deep breathing (McCloskey and Bulechek, 1996).

Inpatient interventions for pulmonary edema include positioning the client to improve ventilation by elevating the head of the bed 30 degrees. If the client is producing large amounts of frothy sputum, he or she should be turned to the side to facilitate drainage. The nurse should reassure the client and family or significant other and, if necessary, prepare them for intubation and mechanical ventilation. This can be particularly frightening for an older client. The nurse should provide frequent suctioning to remove secretions.

An integral part of planning nursing care for older clients requiring intensive care is a discussion about the client's wishes in regard to high-technology medical care. The client and family should be asked if they have any advance medical directives (AMDs) or durable powers of attorney in case the older client becomes unable to speak. If the client is unaware of AMDs but expresses an interest, a family conference including the physician, nurse, social worker, and pastoral caregiver should be planned to help the older client express his or her wishes. If the older client has an AMD or a durable power of attorney, a copy should be filed in the medical record and reviewed with the older client, family, physician, and any other caregivers. It is important to understand and respect the wishes of older clients and families before initiating high-technology medical care (see Chapter 3).

Interventions include supplemental oxygen, mechanical ventilation, and nursing measures to promote oxygen balance. Nursing care is planned to provide adequate rest periods. Monitoring Pa_{O_2} saturation helps the nurse determine which activities deplete oxygen saturation. Interventions such as suctioning, turning, and positioning have been well documented as increasing oxygen consumption and decreasing arterial and mixed venous oxygen levels. The nurse should plan care to decrease the number of interventions performed at one time. This helps minimize oxygen consumption and decrease the stress on the client. It is important to provide an alternative means of communication for older clients receiving mechanical ventilation. If a client has a hearing aid, it may be difficult for him or her to hear over the noise of the technology in the intensive care setting (McCloskey and Bulecheck, 1996).

Older clients in the ICU often need to be reoriented to time. The ICU does not acknowledge day and night. Older clients are particularly sensitive to continuous stimuli in the unit—sound, sights, smells, and textures—and may become confused and combative. The nurse should try to establish a regular nighttime routine with older clients, such as vital sign assessment, oral care, and toileting. The lighting should then be reduced as low as possible to promote rest and sleep while allowing for safe care. This helps older clients establish a routine or pattern they are able to recognize as "time to sleep."

Evaluation

Evaluation is based on improvement in the clinical picture and resolution of symptoms. The nurse should monitor the client's vital signs, cardiac function, and oxygenation status for stability and improvement. The nurse should also monitor the older adult's reaction to therapies and interventions, which can be frightening and invasive. Older adults need continual reassurance and information to reduce their anxiety. The nurse should monitor the airway for effective clearance of secretions. Careful evaluation of daily weight and the client's intake and output will help determine whether the client is retaining additional fluids. The nurse should monitor the client's subjective measure of dyspnea using the dyspnea scale.

Pulmonary Emboli

A pulmonary embolus, an obstruction of the pulmonary artery bed, is most often the result of a deep vein thrombosis in the older client. The thrombosis breaks loose, becoming an embolus, and travels to the lungs through the venous system, where it is trapped in a small vessel of pulmonary circulation. Occlusion of the lung with a large embolus causes pulmonary infarction, which results in necrosis of the lung tissue. The embolus, which is composed of platelets, red blood cells, and WBCs, releases vasoactive substances that cause bronchial constriction, ventilation/perfusion mismatch, and hypoxia. The amount of physiologic dead space—ventilation in excess of perfusion—is increased, leading to an increase in intrapulmonary shunt and hypoxia.

Risk factors for the development of pulmonary emboli include an age greater than 40 years, immobility, recent surgery, lower limb fracture and a history of vascular disease, COPD, heart disease, diabetes mellitus, malignancy, and previous pulmonary emboli. Thromboembolism is more common in older clients who are naturally hypercoagulable (Davey, 2002).

Clinical presentation includes coughing, dyspnea at rest, hypotension, hypoxia, hemoptysis, tachycardia, anginal or pleuritic chest pain, decreased Pao_2, and S_3 or S_4 gallop (Koschel, 2004).

Diagnostic Tests and Procedures. Diagnosis is based on a ventilation/perfusion lung scan or pulmonary angiography. ABG measurements may reveal hypoxemia with Pao_2 between 60 and 80 mm Hg. An ECG may show a right axis deviation, right bundle branch block, tall peaked P waves, depressed ST segment, and supraventricular tachycardia if the emboli are extensive. Massive pulmonary emboli may result in electromechanical dissociation, in which electrical conduction continues without heart muscle response or cardiac output.

The chest x-ray examination may reveal an elevated hemidiaphragm, atelectasis and/or consolidation, and a pleural effusion.

Treatment. Heparin is the drug of choice for treatment of pulmonary emboli (Davey, 2002). Heparin is administered subcutaneously or intravenously to achieve a protime of 1.5 to 2.5 times control. Thrombolytic therapy such as the use of streptokinase, urokinase, or recombinant tissue plasminogen activator is used in clients with extensive pulmonary emboli that exhibit unstable hemodynamic situations. Although this therapy is useful, there are little data showing a reduction in mortality or morbidity in older clients (Shua-Haim and Gross, 1997). Clients with a likelihood of recurring pulmonary emboli are treated long-term with warfarin (Coumadin) and monitoring of their INR. The goal range of the INR is 2.5 to 3.0. Clients with recurrent pulmonary emboli are candidates for Greenfield vena cava filters.

Prognosis. Prognosis for pulmonary emboli is guarded. Older adults are at increased risk for deep vein thrombosis and pulmonary emboli because of decreased mobility. Many times the diagnosis is made on postmortem examination.

NURSING MANAGEMENT

Assessment

Assessment begins with the identification of risk factors for the development of pulmonary emboli. In older adults, dehydration and immobility are leading causes. If an older client has a history of recent fracture of a long bone or a pelvic fracture secondary to falling, fat emboli should be suspected. Clinical signs and symptoms include sudden dyspnea; chest pain; restlessness; weak, rapid pulse; tachypnea; and tachycardia.

Diagnosis

Diagnoses for an older client with pulmonary emboli include (Gordon, 2002):

- Impaired gas exchange related to altered blood flow and oxygen supply
- Altered cardiopulmonary tissue perfusion related to interruption of arterial flow
- Inability to sustain spontaneous ventilation related to metabolic factors

Planning and Expected Outcomes

Planning includes developing interventions and expected outcomes for the older client that are aimed primarily at improving oxygenation and reducing pain. Expected outcomes include (Johnson and Maas, 1997):

1. Client will maintain ABG values within normal limits.
2. Client will maintain adequate respiratory muscle function.
3. Client will be able to sustain spontaneous ventilation without mechanical ventilation.
4. Client will maintain adequate oxygenation.
5. Client will have adequate pain control.
6. Client will maintain adequate cardiac output.
7. Client will maintain adequate vital signs.

Intervention

Maintaining effective oxygenation and ventilation is paramount. The nurse should monitor tissue oxygen delivery, signs and symptoms of respiratory failure, laboratory values for changes in oxygenation or acid-base balance, and hemodynamic parameters and respiratory pattern for symptoms of respiratory difficulty (McCloskey and Bulechek, 1996). Oxygen therapy is administered to improve oxygenation and decrease breathlessness. Heparin therapy is initiated to prevent formation of future clots. Older clients need reassurance and careful monitoring of vital signs. Sedation relieves pain and anxiety and reduces oxygen consumption. If an older client is dehydrated or hypotensive, intravenous fluids are administered. The nurse may use vasopressors if hypotension cannot be reversed with fluids.

The client needs to be monitored for complications of anticoagulant therapy. The nurse should observe the urine for color changes; check the stool for occult blood; and monitor for other complications, including bruising, gastric bleeding, hemorrhage, and cerebrovascular accident.

Since immobility is a risk factor for the development of pulmonary emboli, it is important to promote mobility as soon as medically possible. The nurse should use antiembolic stockings and passive and active range-of-motion exercises during the acute phase. The older client should be encouraged to move about as soon as is medically feasible.

Education topics for the older client and his or her family include signs and symptoms of pulmonary emboli, anticoagulant therapy, and the importance of exercise and mobility. Education on anticoagulant therapy includes elimination of aspirin or nonsteroidal antiinflammatory medications, elimination of green leafy vegetables, cautionary use of over-the-counter medications that potentiate the anticoagulation effect, and prompt reporting of any bleeding. An electric razor is recommended for male clients. The nurse must also help the client understand the importance of regular monitoring of the INR and of taking anticoagulation medication at the same time every day.

Evaluation

Evaluation is based on successful achievement of the expected outcomes. The nurse should monitor the older client's response to oxygen therapy and respiratory support. The nurse should monitor the older adult for effective pain management and relief by using a pain scale. The nurse should also monitor the client for follow-up care with INR blood draws, dietary restrictions, and medication compliance. The nurse should evaluate the client's ability to recall the signs of over-anticoagulation.

Obstructive Sleep Apnea

Obstructive sleep apnea syndrome (OSAS) is the result of upper airway closure, obstruction in the pharynx, and an imbalance between the forces that dilate the pharynx and the forces that promote pharyngeal closure. Obstruction of airflow results when the soft palate and tongue fall backward and partially or completely obstruct the pharynx (Woods, Higgins, and Dowdy, 2001). OSAS produces adverse physiologic and neurobehavioral effects. Pathogenic factors include intermittent hypoxemia or hypercapnia, mechanoreceptor activation during obstructed efforts, chemoreflex activation through chronic body and central nervous system excitability, and arousal that results from abnormal breathing (Strohl, 1998). These changes result in partial awakening of the client with a startle response of snorts and gasps, which move the tongue and soft palate and relieve the obstruction. This cycle of apnea and arousal can occur as many as 200 to 400 times in 8 hours of sleep (Hoffman and Manzetti, 1996). Chronic effects on the cardiovascular system are a result of increased sympathetic nervous system activity. During obstructive apnea, large fluctuations in intrathoracic pressure occur, causing changes in venous return, left ventricular filling, cardiac output, baroreflex, and release of volume-regulatory peptides (Strohl, 1998).

Obesity is the dominant risk factor for OSAS in both men and women. OSAS is twice as common in men as in women. Other risk factors include family history; genetic syndrome; smoking; alcohol use; employment requiring shift rotation or sleep restrictions; medications; and ethnicity—blacks, Hispanics, and Pacific Islanders have a higher incidence of OSAS than whites (Woods, Higgins, and Dowdy, 2001).

Diagnostic Tests and Procedures. The diagnosis of OSAS is made on the basis of the history and objective measurement of sleep and breathing variables in the sleep laboratory. The peak prevalence of OSAS is between 30 and 60 years of age (Woods, Higgins, and Dowdy, 2001). Diagnostic criteria include complaints of excessive daytime sleepiness, frequent episodes of obstructed breathing during sleep, loud snoring, morning headaches, and dry mouth on awakening. Sleep study criteria include more than five episodes of obstructive apnea longer than 10 seconds in duration per hour of sleep and one or more of the following: frequent arousal from sleep, bradycardia, tachycardia, and arterial oxygen desaturation associated with apneic episodes (Phillips, 1998). It is important to differentiate between sleepiness and fatigue or tiredness, which does not always predispose a person to sleep (Phillips, 1998). Clients with OSAS often report falling asleep while driving.

Treatment. The first line of treatment for clients with OSAS is nasal continuous positive airway pressure (CPAP). It provides immediate prevention of upper airway collapse and leads to correction of ABG derangements, improved sleep continuity, improved cognition, and reduction of sleepless symptoms (Woods, Higgins, and Dowdy, 2001). The most critical factor in the use of nasal CPAP is the client's level of compliance. Some studies have shown a compliance rate of 46% for use of CPAP for 4 hours, 5 nights a week. Alternatives to nasal CPAP include weight reduction; sleep position training; and avoidance of alcohol, sedative-hypnotic and narcotic medications, cigarette smoking, and sleep deprivation (Epstein, 1998).

Adjunct therapy includes humidification to prevent nasal dryness and nasal steroids or decongestant to relieve nasal congestion (Woods, Higgins, and Dowdy, 2001). In milder cases of OSAS weight loss is encouraged and mandibular devices are used (Davey, 2002). Surgical interventions include tracheotomy or uvulopalatopharyngoplasty (UVPP). The goal of UVPP is to remove obstructing tissue of the soft palate, uvula, and posterolateral pharynx, thereby eliminating obstruction. The procedure may eliminate snoring but not reduce the apneic episodes (Woods, Higgins, and Dowdy, 2001).

Prognosis. Prognosis for a client with OSAS is good. Client commitment to medical management, such as weight loss and daily use of nasal CPAP, is essential to a good outcome. Older adults may have difficulty with weight reduction. They may also find the nasal CPAP machine annoying and disruptive to their sleep and therefore not wear it consistently at night. Although surgery may be an option, comorbidity may preclude its use in some older adults.

NURSING MANAGEMENT

Assessment

The nurse should assess the client for the presence of chronic loud snoring, gasping or choking episodes during sleep, excessive daytime sleepiness (especially when driving), automobile or work-related accidents attributed to fatigue, and personality changes or cognitive difficulties. Clinical signs include obesity, systemic hypertension, nasopharyngeal narrowing, and, in rare cases, pulmonary hypertension and cor pulmonale (Phillips, 1998).

Diagnosis

Nursing diagnoses for a client with OSAS include (Gordon, 2002):

- Fatigue related to increased energy required for ADLs
- Sleep pattern disturbance related to sensory alterations
- Ineffective breathing pattern related to decreased energy or fatigue
- Altered nutrition related to excessive intake in relationship to metabolic need

Planning and Expected Outcomes

Expected outcomes for an older client with OSAS include (Johnson and Maas, 1997):

1. Client will verbalize a feeling of rest and well-being.
2. Client will verbalize an improvement in quality of life.
3. Client will report an absence of sleepy episodes during the day.
4. Client will have increased ability to concentrate.
5. Client will have increased endurance, as evidenced by ability to participate in ADLs.
6. Client will maintain adequate vital signs.
7. Client will maintain adequate oxygenation and ventilation during sleep, as evidenced by continuous pulse oximetry monitoring.
8. Client will achieve or maintain appropriate body weight.

Intervention

Interventions for a client with OSAS include monitoring the client's sleep pattern; noting physiologic and psychologic circumstances that interrupt sleep; and implementing sleep-promoting therapies such as massage, lifestyle changes, bedtime routines, and use of CPAP (Fig. 24-6). The nurse should assist the client with nutrition counseling, weight reduction, and exercise plans. Exercise may be especially difficult for older adults with underlying orthopedic problems and decreased activity. Exercise programs that incorporate water aerobics can be helpful for older adults with joint problems. The nurse should encourage older adults to eat more fresh fruits and vegetables and less processed and prepackaged foods. Again, this may be difficult for older adults who live alone and do not cook often.

Evaluation

Evaluation is based on achievement of the expected outcomes and improvement in the client's perception of sleep. The nurse should evaluate the client's daytime somnolence and ability to complete ADLs; note the frequency of naps; and monitor for lower extremity edema, fluid retention, and weight gain.

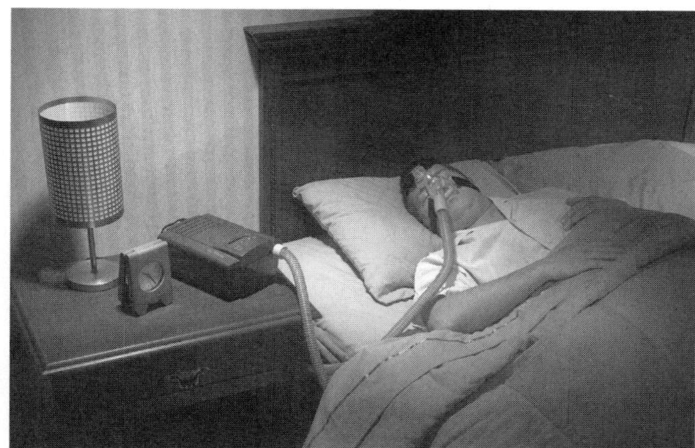

Fig. 24-6 Management of sleep apnea often involves sleeping with a nasal mask in place. The pressure supplied by air coming from the compressor opens the oropharynx and nasopharynx. Patient is using a REMstar® Pro with a Comfort Classic™ face mask. (Courtesy Respironics, Inc, Murrysville, Pa, and its affiliates. ©2005. All rights reserved. In Lewis SM, Heitkemper MM, Dirksen S: *Medical-surgical nursing: assessment and management of clinical problems*, ed 6, St Louis, 2004, Mosby.)

SUMMARY

Neurochemical control and the respiratory muscles are involved in the process of respiration. The structures of the lungs include upper and lower airways, as well as extrapulmonary and intrapulmonary structures. Age-related changes in pulmonary structure and function include elastic recoil and musculoskeletal changes of the chest wall and decreased compliance of the thorax. Asthma, chronic bronchitis, emphysema, and pneumonia are respiratory conditions common in older adults. Chronologic age and tobacco use put older clients at risk for bronchogenic carcinoma. Nursing management of older clients with respiratory alterations focuses on a complete and accurate physical assessment; minimization of risk factors for disease development; development of partnerships with the client to successfully implement lifestyle changes and treatment regimens; and, most important, pulmonary hygiene and airway patency.

Home Care

1. Encourage homebound older adult clients with respiratory disease to drink 8 to 10 glasses of water a day, if not contraindicated.
2. Encourage homebound older adult clients with respiratory disease to exercise within their capacity to promote thoracic muscle conditioning.
3. Monitor homebound older adult clients for smoking and exposure to secondhand smoke. Encourage family members to not smoke in the presence of the client.
4. Encourage homebound older adult clients to use pursed-lip breathing to control breathlessness and improve oxygenation.
5. Monitor pulse oximetry to assess oxygenation.
6. Encourage frequent small meals to reduce breathlessness associated with eating.
7. If a client is using home oxygen, assess the home environment for potential safety hazards, including the possibility of the client tripping over oxygen tubing.
8. Assess clients for confusion, occipital headaches, and forgetfulness. These symptoms may be indicative of CO_2 retention. Teach family caregivers these signs as well.

Key Points

- Changes in lung function that are associated with the aging process, in the absence of primary pulmonary disease, are not associated with decreased activity or increased breathlessness.
- Older adults with chronic lung disease can lead active lives with proper medical and nursing management.
- Breathing retraining (e.g., pursed-lip breathing, diaphragmatic breathing) can result in decreased breathlessness and increased oxygenation.
- It is important to include the family in planning care for an older adult with chronic lung disease.
- An older client with chronic lung disease may demonstrate unacceptable behavioral patterns because of the loss of control experienced with chronic illness.
- Smoking cessation may not be achievable for some older clients; interventions for these clients should focus on reducing the number of cigarettes smoked.
- Exercise plays an important part in overall lung function and has been shown to improve breathing in older clients.
- Care planning that includes the use of mechanical ventilation or other high technology should include the client and family.
- Primary nursing diagnoses for the older client with respiratory disease focus on increasing airway clearance, decreasing breathlessness, and improving oxygenation.

Critical Thinking Exercises

1. How might pulmonary hygiene measures be revised for a frail older adult with a history of CHF and osteoporosis?
2. You are caring for a 70-year-old man who has a 75 pack–per-year history of smoking. He has COPD but continues to smoke, stating it would be impossible to quit now and besides, “It’s too late.” How would you assist this client?
3. Think about your own personal views regarding advanced life-support measures for the older adult population. What are the ethical implications of placing (or not placing) an 80-year-old person on mechanical ventilation for acute

respiratory failure? How would you assist clients and family members faced with decisions of this nature?

References

Agency for Health Care Research and Quality (AHCRQ): *You can quit smoking: consumer guide,* Silver Springs, Md, 2000, The Agency.

American Cancer Society: *Cancer facts and figures: 1998,* Atlanta, 1998, The Society.

Atlas of pathophysiology, Springhouse, Penn, 2002, Springhouse.

Baldwin PD: Lung cancer, *Clin J Oncol Nurs* 7(6):699, 2003.

Celli BR: Standards for the optimal management of COPD, *Chest* 113(4):283, 1998.

Centers for Disease Control and Prevention: Development of new vaccines for tuberculosis: recommendations for the Advisory Council for the Elimination of Tuberculosis (ACET), *Morbid Mortal Weekly Rep* 47(RR-13), 1998a.

Centers for Disease Control and Prevention: Recommendations for prevention and control of tuberculosis among foreign-born persons, *Morbid Mortal Weekly Rep* 47(RR-16), 1998b.

Centers for Disease Control and Prevention: Prevention of pneumococcal disease, *Morbid Mortal Weekly Rep* 46(RR-8), 1997a.

Centers for Disease Control and Prevention: Recommendations for the prevention and control of influenza, *Morbid Mortal Weekly Rep* 46 (RR-9), 1997b.

Centers for Disease Control and Prevention: *Tuberculosis surveillance report,* 1997c. Accessed at website: http:/www.cdc.gov.

Centers for Disease Control and Prevention: *Questions and answers about TB,* Atlanta, 1994, US Department of Health and Human Services.

Clinical update: pneumococcal vaccine: an immunization update, *Clin Rev* 7(9):1115, 1997.

Covey MK, Larson, JL: Exercise and COPD, *Am J Nurs* 104(5):40, 2004.

Davey P, editor: *Medicine at a glance,* Malden, Mass, 2002, Blackwell Science.

Dreher HM et al: What you need to know about SARS now, *Nursing 2004* 34(1):58, 2004.

Epstein LJ: Non-surgical alternatives to continuous positive airway pressure, *Respir Care* 43(4):370, 1998.

Fielden NM: Community-acquired pneumonia, *Perspect Respir Nurs* 9(1):1, 1998.

Gift AG, Narsavage G: Validity of the numeric rating scale as a measure of dyspnea, *Am J Crit Care* 7(3):200, 1998.

Gordon M: *Manual of nursing diagnosis,* ed 10, St Louis, 2002, Mosby.

Hannaford MM, Mann S: Lower respiratory tract infections, *Adv Nurse Pract* 8(12):30, 2000.

Hoffman LA, Manzetti JD: Respiratory system. In Lewis SM, Collier IC, Heitkemper MM, editors: *Medical-surgical nursing: assessment and management of clinical problems,* ed 4, St Louis, 1996, Mosby.

Holman JR: Influenza: are you ready for the upcoming season? *Consultant* 43(12):1437, 2003.

Johnson M, Maas M: *Nursing outcomes and classification,* St Louis, 1997, Mosby.

Koschel MJ: Pulmonary embolism, *Am J Nurs* 104(6):46, 2004.

Lave JR et al: Hospitalized pneumonia: outcomes, treatment patterns, and cost in urban and rural area, *J Gen Int Med* 11(7):415, 1996.

Mannino DM et al: Chronic obstructive pulmonary disease surveillance—United Stated, 1971-2000, *Morbid Mortal Weekly Rep Surveillance* 52(6):1, 2002.

Marrie TJ: Assessing and treating community-acquired pneumonia, *Emerg Med* 11(20):20, 2003.

Marthaler M, Keresztes P, Tazbir J: SARS: what have we learned? *RN* 66(8):59, 2003.

McCloskey JC, Bulechek GM: *Nursing interventions classification,* St Louis, 1996, Mosby.

National Cancer Institute: Lung cancer, 1998. Accessed at website: http:/www.NCI.NIH.gov.

National Heart, Lung, and Blood Institute: *Clinical practice guidelines; guidelines for the diagnosis and management of asthma,* NIH Publication No 97-4051, 1997.

National Heart, Lung, and Blood Institute: *National asthma education and prevention program working group report: considerations for diagnosing and managing asthma in the elderly,* NIH Publication No 96-3662, 1996.

National Heart, Lung, and Blood Institute/World Health Organization, GOLD Workshop Panel: *Global strategy for the diagnosis management and prevention of chronic obstructive pulmonary disease, NHLBI/WHO Workshop Report,* NIH Publication No 2701, Bethesda, Md, 2001, The Institute.

Phillips BA: Clinical diagnosis of sleep apnea, *Respir Care* 43(4):288, 1998.

Self TH, Kilgore K, Shelton V: Pitfalls in prescribing, *Consultant* 43(6):702, 2003.

Shua-Haim JR, Gross JS: Pulmonary embolism: a medical emergency frequently underdiagnosed in older patients, *Geriatrics* 52(7):77, 1997.

Sibilano H: TB or not TB: the tuberculosis index of suspicion nursing assessment tool, *Perspect Respir Nurs* 7(3):1, 1996.

Sibilano H: Clinical dimensions of TB: nursing management. In Cohen F, Durham J, editors: *Tuberculosis: a source book for nursing practice,* New York, 1995, Springer.

Simmerman JM, Chu D, Chang H: Implications of unrecognized severe acute respiratory syndrome, *Nurse Pract* 28(11):21, 2003.

Strohl KP: Consequences of sleep-disordered breathing, *Respir Care* 43(4):277, 1998.

Woods DL, Higgins LJ, Dowdy S: Sleepwalking through life: identifying and treating obstructive sleep apnea syndrome, *Adv Nurse Pract* 9(5):31, 2001.

Website

www.ahrq.gov/consumer/tobacco/quits.htm

25 Endocrine Function

CATHERINE HILL, MSN, RN, GNP-C

Learning Objectives

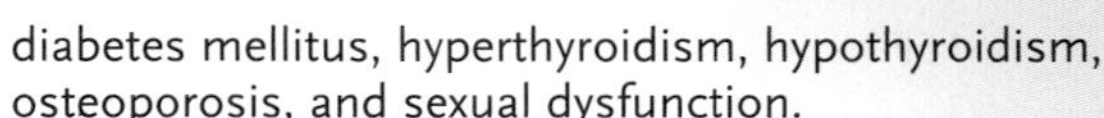

On completion of this chapter, the reader will be able to:

1. Discuss the normal age-related physiologic changes that occur in the endocrine system.
2. Describe the major characteristics of common endocrine diseases in older adults: metabolic syndrome, type 2 diabetes mellitus, hyperthyroidism, hypothyroidism, osteoporosis, and sexual dysfunction.
3. Apply the nursing process in caring for an older adult with an endocrine disorder.

Previously dominated by diabetes and thyroid disease, gerontologic endocrinology has recently stepped into the limelight, redefining itself through the use of innovative insights developed from the mapping of the human genome (Veldhuis, 2000). Our knowledge of aging endocrine physiology and genetic influences (Wu and Yu, 2004) has begun to grow at a very fast pace (DeGroot, 2001). By the year 2000 the "Endocrinology of Aging" (Veldhuis, 2000), as a subspecialty, had accumulated enough significant scientific advances to warrant its own symposium in Tempe, Arizona. Andropause, circadian dysrythmias, dehydroepiandrosterone (DHEA) replacement, erectile dysfunction, glycagon-like peptide 1 replacement, male osteoporosis, menopause, metabolic syndrome, and metabolic presbycusis joined the traditional topics of diabetes and thyroid disease in the newly emerged subspecialty.

Endocrinology's new "ensemble view of neuroendocrine aging" was discussed in terms of decreased estrogen production in women (menopause), decreased testosterone production in men (andropause), decreased adrenal function (adrenopause), and decreased growth hormone–insulin-like growth factor (somatopause) (Veldhuis, 2000). Endocrinologic aging is now viewed as an increased molecular disorderliness of the endocrine regulatory mechanisms that result in reduced vitality of the overall person. This molecular dysregulation of neurohormones from or with the central nervous system (CNS) is believed to be one of the earliest measurable characteristics of endocrine aging. Notable in the current literature is the consensus on the limited role of genetics in the aging process and the predominant (although not exclusive) focus on diminished (rather than excessive) hormone levels. These "new" views on aging may contribute to a dichotomy among biologists, researchers, and health care providers. Many believe natural endocrine aging is not a "disease" to be "cured" (Walker, 2002); others believe that our knowledge can provide important "antiaging" therapies that benefit humans as a whole.

ENDOCRINE PHYSIOLOGY IN OLDER ADULTS

Composed of ductless glands (Fig 25-1, *A*), which secrete 40 major hormones (Copstead and Banasik, 2005) that control numerous processes throughout the body (Table 25-1), the endocrine system uses a delicate balance of chemical messengers in the bloodstream to excite and regulate mood, growth, organ function, metabolism, and sexual activity (Thomas, 1979). Dependent on a complex interplay of factors, many hormones are secreted in a cyclic pattern of minutes, hours, days, or months (Rubin and Levin, 1994). Feedback control processes (Fig. 25-1, *B*) of these intricate gland-hormone-organ-tissue systems depend on secretion and degradation of hormones classified by chemical structure and cell receptor type (Copstead and Banasik, 2005).

Apoptosis (cell death) is a theme that has dominated cellular research on the physiology of aging and some age-related diseases since 1972 (Perez and Tilly, 1997). Three basic categories are used to classify endocrine pathology—hyposecretion, hypersecretion, and hyporesponsiveness—an elaborate system that increases in complexity with the aging processes (Table 25-2). In addition, clinical manifestations in the older persons may be exacerbated by disease processes in other body systems such as in the syndrome of inappropriate antidiuretic hormone secretion, which occurs with many types of tumors. Therefore this chapter discusses the typical aging changes of menopause, andropause, adrenopause, and somatopause physiology before moving on to specific pathophysiologic states superimposed over typical aging changes.

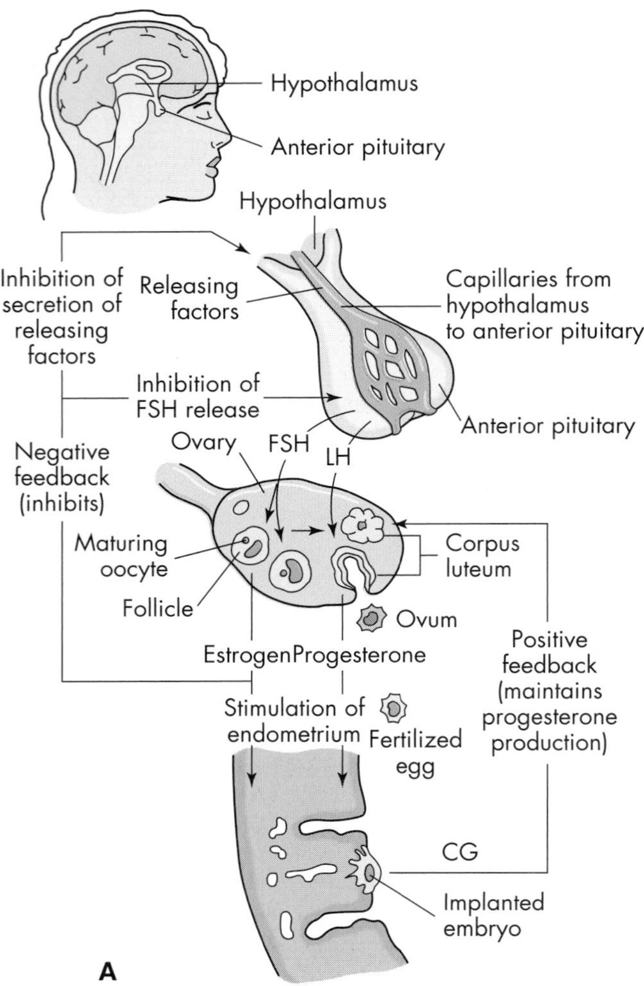

Fig. 25-1, A Endocrine feedback loops involving the hypothalamus–pituitary gland and end organs (endocrine regulation). (From Phipps W, Sands J, Marek J: *Medical-surgical nursing*, ed 6, St Louis, 1999, Mosby.)

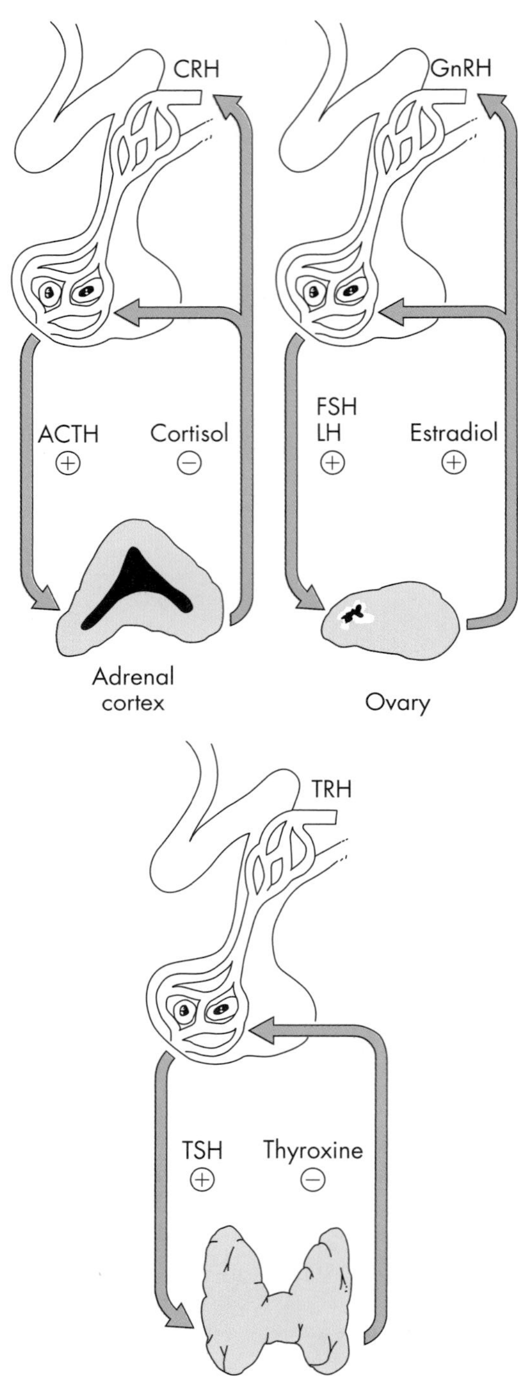

Fig. 25-1, B Feedback-regulating systems where the target gland hormone feeds back to the hypothalamus. Pituitary release of the tropic hormone follows. *Top left,* Corticotropin-releasing hormone (CRH). *Top right,* Gonadotropin-releasing hormone (GnRH). *Bottom,* TSH-releasing hormone (TRH). *ACTH,* Adrenocorticotropic hormone; *FSH,* follicle-stimulating hormone; *LH,* luteinizing hormone; *TSH,* thyroid-stimulating hormone (thyrotropin). (From Price SA, Wilson LM: *Pathophysiology,* ed 5, St Louis, 1997, Mosby.)

Andropause and Menopause

Older men (Gould, Petty, and Jacobs, 2000) and women (Cufson and Meuleman, 2000) experience a decline in the biosynthesis of their dominant sex hormones from the cholesterol precursor as they age. In both genders the hypothalamus–anterior pituitary–testes/ovary system declines, although the timing is gender specific (Tenover, 1997; Vetrosky and Aliabadi, 2002). Both genders may experience hot flashes, night sweats, depression, and sexual dysfunction in response to age-related declines in androgen (Morales, Heaton, and Carson, 2000) or estrogen (Women's Health Initiative, 2002). In contrast to the previous gender similarities in symptoms, laboratory values to determine the endocrine decline are unique to each sex, with luteinizing hormone (LH) and testosterone of primary importance in

TABLE 25-1 Principal Endocrine Glands

NAME	LOCATION	FUNCTION	AGING ENDOCRINE DISORDER
Thyroid	Anterior aspect of neck	Basal metabolic rate growth, nutrition	Marasmus, kwashiorkor, obesity, hyperthyroidism, hypothyroidism, autoimmune thyroiditis, Graves' disease, euythroid sick syndrome, thyrotoxicosis, thyroid storm, multinodular toxic goiter
Parathyroid	Near thyroid	Calcium and phosphorus metabolism, muscular irritability	Osteoporosis, osteomalacia, Paget's disease, hypocalcemia, hypercalcemia, hypophosphatemia, hyperphosphatemia, hypomagnesemia
Adrenal cortex	Above each kidney	Carbohydrate metabolism, salt/water balance, some sexual characteristics	Addison's disease, Cushing's syndrome, dehydration, hyponatremia, hypernatremia, hyperkalemia, hypokalemia
Adrenal medulla	Embedded in kidney, surrounded by cortex	Sympathetic nervous system, carbohydrate metabolism	Acidosis, alkalosis
Anterior pituitary	Base of brain	Growth, sexual development, skin pigmentation, thyroid function, adrenocortical function (indirectly)	Hypopituitarism
Posterior pituitary	Attached to anterior pituitary	Uterine contraction, water balance	Dehydration, diabetes insipidus
Testes	Scrotum	Secondary sexual characteristics and function, metabolism	Andropause
Ovaries	Pelvic cavity	Secondary sexual characteristics and function, metabolism	Menopause
Pancreas	Abdomen	Sugar metabolism	Diabetes type 1 or type 2, hypoglycemia
Pineal gland	Center of brain	Daily biologic clocks	Sleep disturbance
Thymus	Chest cavity	Influences immune system response	Immune senescence: reduced response to immunization, cancer, monoclonal gammopathy, increased autoantibodies
Hypothalamus	Brain	Regulates autonomic nervous system; influences hormone production, sleep, and appetite	Kwashiorkor, obesity, hypothermia, hyperthermia, sleep disturbance

Data taken from Beers MH, Berkow R, editors: *Merck manual of geriatrics,* 2000-2005, Merck. Accessed Oct 16, 2004, from website: http://www.merck.com/mrkshared/mm_geriatrics/home.jsp. Copstead LE, Banasik JK: *Pathophysiology: biological and behavioral perspectives,* ed 2, Philadelphia, 2000, WB Saunders.

males, whereas follicle-stimulating hormone (FSH) and estrogen are of primary importance in females.

Hormone replacement therapy, in both genders, is a hotly debated topic among intelligent providers, since risks and benefits are under intense research scrutiny. Ongoing debate over whether "aging" is a disease contributes to the controversy. Those who advocate testosterone replacement cite the benefits of improvements in relation to arthralgia, bone density, libido, muscle mass, strength, visuospatial skills, depression, fatigue, hot flashes, irritability, mood, and sleep (Vetrosky and Aliabadi, 2002). Testosterone replacement in andropause is complicated by adverse lipid effects, risk of promoting prostate cancer, worsening of sleep apnea, potential hepatotoxicity, increased aggressive behavior, and risk of erythrocytosis. Menopausal and postmenopausal hormone replacement practices continue to change based on larger, more rigorous research studies (Women's Health Initiative, 2002).

TABLE 25-2 Aging Changes in Endocrine System

HYPORESPOSIVENESS	HYPOSECRETION	DEGRADATION CHANGES	HYPERSECRETION
Increased connective tissue, pigment, and structure changes in target tissue Decreased receptor-ligand binding	Plasma insulin-like growth factor T3 Aldosterone Active renin Calcitonin Arginine vasopressin Growth hormone	Thyroid hormones Cortisol Aldosterone Inactive to active renin conversion Norepinephrine clearance	Norepinephrine Parathyroid hormone Atrial natriuretic peptide Insulin Glucagon

The presence or absence of a uterus continues to guide clinicians on the types of hormones used in menopausal and postmenopausal women. In 2002 and 2003 the Women's Health Initiative, funded by the National Institutes of Health, revealed new information about the benefits and risks associated with hormone replacement therapy. Scientists found that, for every 10,000 women taking a pill containing conjugated equine estrogen and medroxyprogesterone acetate each year, there would be (1) eight additional cases of breast cancer, (2) seven more cases of heart disease, (3) eight more cases of stroke, (4) eight more cases of blood clots in the lungs, and (5) double the risk of dementia. The benefits of combined hormone replacement included five fewer cases of hip fracture. Recently conjugated equine estrogen has been identified as less desirable than esterified estrogens for women without a uterus (Smith et al, 2004).

Adrenopause

Weighing approximately 4 g, the adrenal glands sit on top of the kidneys (Guyton, 1986). The adrenal medulla influences the sympathetic nervous system through the secretion of epinephrine and norepinephrine, whereas the adrenal cortex secretes mineralocorticoids, glucocorticoids, and androgenic hormones. A total loss of adrenocortical function causes death within days; however, age-related changes are usually manifested by changes in body composition, skeletal mass, muscle strength, body weight, and metabolism (Veldhuis, 2000). Current research suggests the ability of the adrenal zona fasciculata to secrete cortisol is preserved, while mineralocorticoid and glucocorticoid receptors are down regulated. Age-related decreases in DHEA and norepinephrine can produce fluid and electrolyte imbalances and changes in glucose, protein, and fat metabolism. The decline of DHEA with age parallels that of growth hormone, so by age 65 your body makes only 10 to 20 percent of what it did at age twenty." The mechanism of these declines has yet to be identified (Veldhuis, Iranmanesh, and Mulligan, 1999), but they closely parallel declines in the growth hormone–insulin-like growth factor 1 axis, a process now referred to as somatopause (Veldhuis and Iranmanesh, 1999).

Somatopause

Somatopause is often spoken of from a neuroendocrine point of view, since certain neurons in the hypothalamus secrete hormones (neurosecretion). Somatopause focuses on the neuron-hypothalamus-pituitary axis and has not been systematically evaluated in various ethnic populations (Lamberts, van den Beld, and van der Lely, 1997). The failure of CNS integration of the endocrine and nervous systems somehow relates to peripheral endocrine gland insufficiency, contributing to a disrupted feedback axis in aging. Specifically, somatotropin secretion from the hypothalamus-pituitary axis influences many age-related changes such as nutrition, metabolism, body temperature, and circadian dysrythmias (Van Cauter et al, 1998), circulation, salt/water balance, growth, and reproduction (Veldhuis, Iranmanesh, and Mulligan, 1999). Recent research has focused on various secretagogue compounds that stimulate pulsatile growth hormone secretion and increase insulin-like growth factor 1 in the older adults to levels approximating those found in young adults (Arvat et al, 1999).

COMMON ENDOCRINE PATHOPHYSIOLOGY IN OLDER ADULTS

Metabolic Syndrome

Pathophysiology. Over 40% of elders have metabolic syndrome, and this figure is projected to increase as the U.S. population ages (Ford, Giles, and Dietz, 2002). The root causes of this syndrome are improper nutrition, inadequate physical activity, and obesity. Recent epidemiologic research has identified, defined, and measured the metabolic syndrome as a significant antecedent to American illness trends in diabetes (Kreier et al, 2003) and heart disease (National Health and Nutrition Examination Survey [HANES], 1999). Considered by many as a continued refinement of earlier ideas on insulin resistance and syndrome X, the metabolic syndrome is a "cluster of common metabolic abnormalities associated with increased risk of type 2 diabetes and atherosclerotic cardiovascular disease" (Arauz-Pacheo, 2004).

Signs and Symptoms. Clinical criteria as established by the World Health Organization (1999) include (1) insulin resistance, plus any two of the following: (2) elevated blood pressure (over 139/89 mm Hg), (3) plasma triglycerides over 149 mg/dl, (4) high-density lipids less than 35 mg/dl in men or less than 40 mg/dl in women, (5) body mass index over 30 kg/m^2, or (6) urinary albumin over 20 mg/min. Current therapeutic approaches to metabolic syndrome focus on the treatment of insulin sensitivity and obesity (NHLBI/NIDDK Obesity Education Initiative, 2004). The cardiologists have adopted a variation of the World Health Organization criteria that used waist circumference of over 102 cm in men and 88 cm in women in place of the body mass index criteria (Third Report of the National Cholesterol Education Program, Expert Panel on Detection, Evaluation and Treatment of High Blood Cholesterol in Adults, 2001).

Medical Management. Weight loss is the primary therapeutic objective in metabolic syndrome (Blackburn and Bevis, 2003). Weight loss, therapeutic lifestyle changes, pharmacotherapy, and surgical therapy are included in the medical approach to the primary objective. Modest weight loss of 5% to 10% of initial body weight is associated with significant clinical improvement (Goldstein, 1992). Therapeutic lifestyles changes (TLC) adapted for metabolic syndrome are detailed in Box 25-1. The physician or nurse practitioner should offer practical and specific recommendations such as (1) reduce calories by 500 per day with portion-controlled foods or meal replacements, (2) gradually increase physical exercise or activity by 10 to 20 minutes per day until 300 minutes per week are achieved, and (3) keep a record of all food intake and physical activity. Medications such as sibutramine, phentermine, and orlistat can be prescribed as an adjunct to diet and exercise when patients have a body mass index of 27 kg/m^2 or greater and no specific contraindications. When used as monotherapy, antiobesity medications have not been particularly effective (Wadden et al, 2001). Surgical therapy is the most effective treatment modality in terms of amount and duration of weight loss in selected patients with a body mass index over 40 kg/m^2 (Pratt and Blackburn, 2003).

BOX 25-1 Steps Every 6 Weeks in Therapeutic Lifestyle Changes

Visit 1: Begin weight reduction, encourage physical activity, refer to dietitian.
Visit 2: Evaluate weight, waist circumference, low-density lipoprotein (LDL), high-density lipoprotein (HDL-C), triglycerides, blood pressure, and fasting glucose. Reinforce TLC. Consider meal replacements.
Visit 3: Evaluate weight, waist circumference, LDL, HDL-C, triglycerides, blood pressure, and fasting glucose. Reinforce TLC. Consider meal replacements.
Visit 4: Evaluate weight, waist circumference, LDL, HDL-C, triglycerides, blood pressure, and fasting glucose. Reinforce TLC. Consider meal replacements
If no improvement in parameters, consider drug therapy.
Intensify weight management and physical activity.
Visit 5: Monitor adherence to TLC and medications if used.

TLC, Therapeutic lifestyle changes.

Nursing Process Applied to Metabolic Syndrome. The nursing process is applied to the metabolic syndrome by initially focusing on the root causes of improper nutrition and inadequate physical activity, as detailed in Table 25-3.

Type 2 Diabetes Mellitus

Pathophysiology. The hyperglycemic state that results from defects in insulin secretion, insulin action, or both constitutes the group of metabolic diseases known as diabetes mellitus. Diabetes is one of the most common chronic conditions affecting the older adult population, and the incidence is expected to rise. The disease ultimately produces dysfunction and failure of various organs such as the heart, kidneys, nerves, eyes, and blood vessels. Endocrine disease may manifest in the form of hormone resistance instead of absence, a condition in which tissue response to hormones is inadequate. The cause of type 2 diabetes mellitus is unknown, but it is theorized that both genetics and the environment play important roles. The most important variables associated with type 2 diabetes mellitus are obesity and insulin resistance. Insulin resistance is thought to be related to at least two factors: hyperglycemia and obesity. Obese clients with type 2 diabetes have high levels of endogenous insulin (hyperinsulinemia), which in turn causes a reduction in the number of insulin receptors on target tissues. It is as though the body attempts to compensate for glucose not entering the cell by increasing insulin production. Thus the basic pathophysiologic defects in type 2 diabetes are impaired insulin secretion and insulin action. Insulin levels may be normal, elevated, or decreased in type 2 diabetes. Insulin resistance is common but is often treatable.

The NHLBI/NIDDR's Expert Committee on the Diagnosis and Classification of Diabetes Mellitus (2004) recognizes five classifications of diabetes mellitus based on etiology. In 1999 the committee eliminated the terms *insulin-dependent* and *non–insulin-dependent* diabetes; instead it classifies the disease by treatment method rather than by cause. Clients are now classified as type 1, type 2, or other. Type 1 diabetes is a condition of absolute insulin deficiency; type 2 diabetes is a condition of relative insulin deficiency. Type 1 always requires exogenously administered insulin for blood glucose control because insulin-producing cells of the pancreas have been destroyed to such an extent that the insulin-secreting ability of the gland is negligible or completely absent (Fig. 25-2). Individuals with type 2 diabetes have defects of insulin secretion, but many retain the ability to produce insulin in normal or supernormal levels. The central issue for most people with

TABLE 25-3 Metabolic Syndrome

ASSESSMENT	DIAGNOSIS	PLANNING	INTERVENTION	EVALUATION
NUTRITION 1. Mini Nutritional Assessment 2. Body mass index 3. Overweight: >10% over ideal 4. Obese: >20% over ideal 5. Triceps skin fold: >15 mm in men or >25 mm in women 6. Lifetime weight trends 7. Thyroid function 8. Medications 9. Nutrition knowledge 10. Cultural issues 11. Comorbidities 12. Medications 13. Social support network	1. Imbalanced nutrition: more than body requirements	1. Use calorie count and dietary log. 2. Use satiety and emotional scale. 3. Adjust seasonings prn. 4. Introduce behavior modification techniques. 5. Provide teaching on medication and Dietary Recommendations of National Research Council Report for adults over 65 years.	1. Review log and weight weekly. 2. Eat only at kitchen table. 3. Drink 8 oz of water before meal. 4. Limit fat, sweets, and alcohol. Eat low-calorie snacks. 5. Control portions, eat slowly, wait 15 seconds between bites.	1. Client is able to list dietary rules and reasons. 2. Client demonstrates slow, steady weight loss toward goal. 3. Client lists medication effects and dietary implications.
ACTIVITY 1. Respiratory system 2. Cardiovascular system 3. Musculoskeletal system 4. Developmental status 5. Comorbidities 6. Medications 7. Cultural issues 8. Social support network	1. Activity intolerance 2. Ineffective health maintenance 3. Ineffective coping	1. Accommodate comorbidities, sensory deficits, safety concerns, financial aspects. 2. Address motivation, lifestyle, and environmental barriers. 3. Provide role models and social support. 4. Include aerobic and strength training.	1. Assess resting vital signs and 3 minutes after activity. 2. Reduce intensity or duration of activity if pulse takes longer than 3-4 minutes to return within 6 beats of baseline. 3. Begin with active range-of-motion exercises twice a day; add isometrics. Gradually increase tolerance from 15 minutes. 4. Provide support, safety, and fall protection. 5. Use personal incentives such as playing with grandchildren, returning to work, or going fishing. 6. Teach primary and secondary prevention related to aging and sensory deficits. 7. Teach stress-related signs and symptoms.	1. Client will progress to specified activity level. 2. Client is able to verbalize and engage in health maintenance behaviors. 3. Client will make decisions and follow through with appropriate actions.

Data from Carpenito-Moyet LJ: *Nursing diagnosis: application to clinical practice,* ed 10, Philadelphia, 2004, JB Lippincott.
prn, As needed.

type 2 diabetes is that without treatment (i.e., diet, exercise, and medication) the insulin produced is not effective in controlling blood glucose levels. Insulin, if prescribed, is not essential to life as in type 1 diabetes.

Pathophysiology of the type 2 diabetes resistance state often involves defects in the cell membrane, receptors, or intracellular pathways (Figs. 25-2 and 25-3). Although recent basic research indicates a unique role of glucagon-like peptide 1 in seniors with type 2 diabetes (Meneilly et al, 2003), the American Diabetes Association (ADA) recently presented in vivo and in vitro evidence on glucose metabolism and transport that supports the importance of visceral obesity, rather than aging per se, as the primary pathophysiology of type 2 diabetes (Imbeault et al, 2003).

In type 2 diabetes an individual may have some defective insulin receptors on target tissues. Consequently, abnormally high levels of insulin and hyperglycemia result from the body's inability to use insulin effectively. In hormone resistance states such as insulin resistance the individual's blood levels of insulin may be increased, but the main symptoms are those of a hypofunctioning state. Resistance often results in the need for more than the usual hormone replacement. Obese clients with type 2 diabetes have high levels of endogenous insulin (hyperinsulinemia), which in turn causes a reduction in the number of insulin receptors on target tissues. It is as though the body attempts to compensate for glucose not entering the cell by increasing insulin production.

In type 2 diabetes it is common for an individual to have insulin receptor defects that result in underuse or ineffective use of the hormone insulin. In addition, antibodies to insulin may be present that destroy insulin once secreted and make it impossible to achieve normal blood glucose control. Some individuals with type 2 diabetes actually produce decreased or inadequate amounts of insulin. Thus three possible types of defects may be present in type 2 diabetes mellitus: (1) abnormal receptors, (2) insulin antibodies, and (3) decreased insulin secretion. It is possible for disturbances at any level of a system to disrupt the entire system, resulting in metabolic derangement.

Signs and Symptoms. At the time of diagnosis (Box 25-2), uncontrolled type 2 diabetes may be associated with symptoms of excessive thirst, hunger, and urination (i.e., polydipsia, polyphagia, and polyuria, respectively). However, too

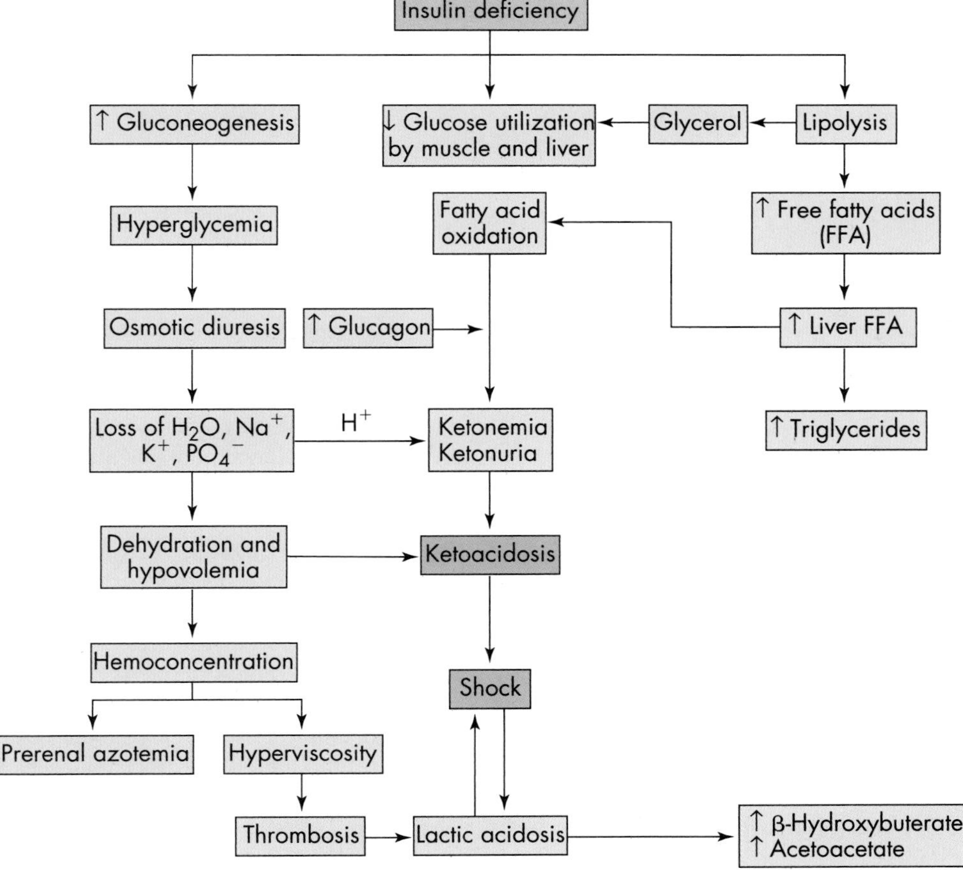

Fig. 25-2 Pathophysiology of insulin deficiency. (From Phipps W, Sands J, Marek J: *Medical-surgical nursing*, ed 6, St Louis, 1999, Mosby.)

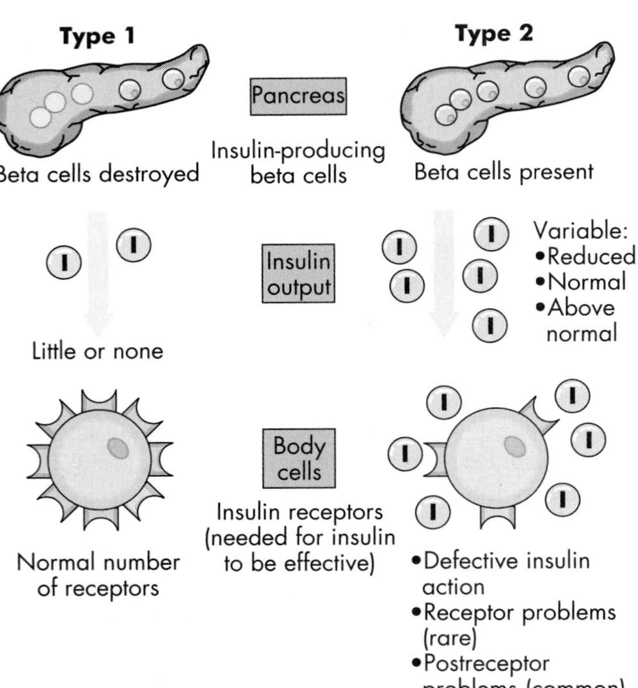

Fig. 25-3 Insulin defects in type 1 and type 2 diabetes mellitus. (From Phipps W, Sands J, Marek J: *Medical-surgical nursing*, ed 6, St Louis, 1999, Mosby.)

BOX 25-2 American Diabetes Association 2004 Diagnostic Criteria for "Prediabetes" and Type 2 Diabetes

Any one of the following:

PREDIABETES

Impaired glucose tolerance: 2-hour value on a 75 g glucose tolerance test 140-199 mg/dl

Impaired fasting glucose: fasting plasma glucose 100-125 mg/dl

TYPE 2 DIABETES

Fasting plasma glucose ≥126 mg/dl noted on two occasions

2 hour postload 75 g glucose level ≥ 200 mg/dl noted on two occasions

Random plasma glucose level ≥ 200 mg/dl associated with symptoms (polyuria, polydipsia, weight loss) noted on two occasions

often the older individual with type 2 diabetes does not have classical symptomology and will not complain of weight loss or fatigue along with these classic symptoms (Colleen, 2003). Clinical signs and symptoms can range from asymptomatic to comatose. Often a newly diagnosed older individual will describe symptoms of fatigue, blurred vision, weight change (gain or loss), and infections. When questioned, both men and women attribute these changes to "aging." Individuals are often diagnosed with diabetes with a concurrent infection, such as a major foot or leg wound, vaginitis, or urinary tract infection; or they may be seen with impotence, numbness of extremities, or changes in vision.

Medical Management. Current medical management focuses on the disease process, not just the glucose levels (Wyne and Bell, 2004), using several new classes of medications. Data from recent research indicate sulfonylureas, insulin, and biguanides do not prevent a loss of beta cell function, so current therapy recommendations use drug combinations that include thiazolidinediones to preserve beta cell function while controlling serum glucose (Fig. 25-4). Five different oral drug classes are currently available and used in diabetes management (Box 25-3). Some medications prescribed for comorbid problems can make glucose control more difficult.

NURSING MANAGEMENT

The nursing process in type 2 diabetes addresses the core defects of impaired insulin secretion and insulin action, as well as prevention of vascular and microvascular complications of the eye, heart, kidneys, and feet (see Fig. 25-3).

Assessment

Comprehensive nursing assessment of an individual at risk for diabetes includes a thorough review of medical and family history, since type 2 diabetes commonly crosses generations. The nurse should ask a client about current medications, particularly diuretics, beta-blockers, anticonvulsants, antihypertensives, and steroids. Requesting that clients bring in their prescription and over-the-counter medications can help the nurse assess for potential problems related to drug interactions or for drugs that alter blood glucose.

For clients already diagnosed with diabetes and being treated with oral agents or insulin, the nurse should determine the medication's name, type, dose, and schedule; if possible, the nurse should try to observe medication administration. Self-care abilities or restrictions, self-monitoring of blood glucose, and any history of hypoglycemia or hyperglycemia should be assessed.

Nutritional assessment includes a current weight measurement and recent patterns of loss or gain, typical dietary patterns, changes in sense of taste or smell, dentition, and ability to shop for and prepare foods. Because uncontrolled diabetes affects fluid and food balance, it is important to assess clients for signs and symptoms of nausea, vomiting, hunger, and thirst, keeping in mind that hyperglycemia may produce subtle symptoms in older adults.

Assessment of elimination in an older adult with diabetes includes obtaining a history of urinary incontinence, urinary

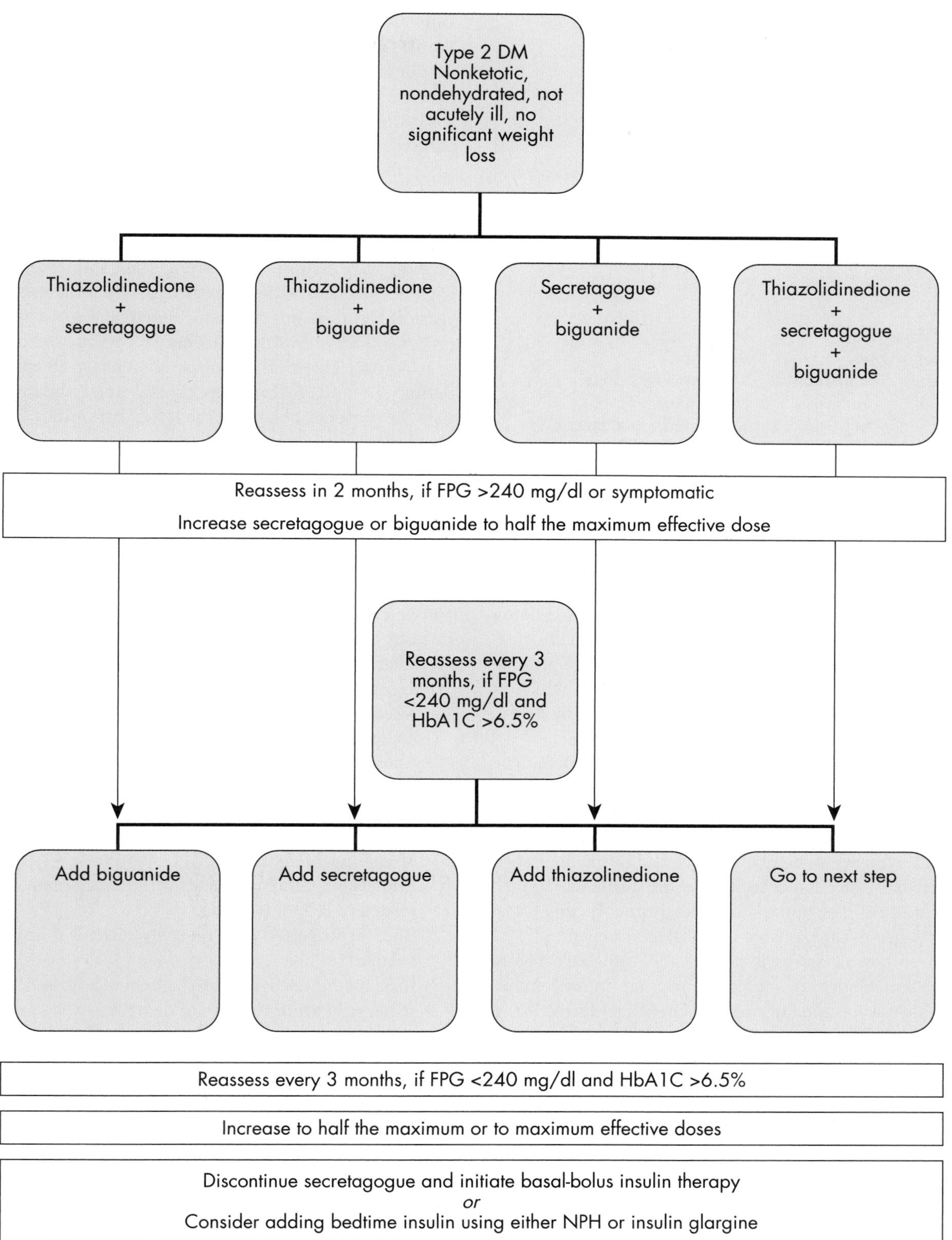

Fig. 25-4 Medical management of type 2 diabetes. *DM*, Diabetes mellitus; *FPG*, fasting plasma glucose; *HbA1C*, hemoglobin A_{1c}.

BOX 25-3 Oral Antidiabetic Agents

CLASSIFICATION	MEDICATIONS
Thiazolinediones	Rosiglitazone
	Pioglitazone
Biguanides	Metformin
	Metformin extended release (Fortamet)
Alpha-glucosidase inhibitors	Acarbose
	Miglitol
Sulfonylureas	Chlorpropamide
	Glipizide
	Glimepiride
Nonsulfonylurea secretagogues	Nateglinide
	Repaglinide
Fixed-dose combinations	Metformin/glyburide
	Metformin/glipizide
	Metformin/rosiglitazone

Data from Wyne KL, Bell DSH: An algorithm for managing type 2 diabetes: a focus on the disease process, not just the sugar, *Clin Geriatr* Aug 2004.

frequency, nocturia, polyuria, impotence, and pain on urination. The nurse should evaluate for the presence of bowel incontinence, constipation, and diarrhea. When assessing elimination in an older adult, the nurse should obtain the medical and surgical history, including problems with the prostate gland, urethra, and bladder. Stress incontinence, which is more common in older adults, may be intensified by hyperglycemia.

Assessment of current living conditions is essential. The nurse should ask if the individual lives alone or with others, if living arrangements afford the ability to prepare food, and if there are adequate financial resources for food and shelter. Older adults who live alone may eat little and be malnourished because of social isolation or functional impairments (Funnell and Merritt, 1998). The nurse should determine whether transportation to health care services is available to a client.

It is important to assess a client's ability to learn before assessing knowledge of diabetes and its management. Learning styles vary, and knowing the client's preferred learning style facilitates education. Some individuals prefer to learn by visual methods, others by listening, and still others by experiencing contact in a "hands-on" approach.

Type 2 diabetes is associated with increased depression and memory problems in older adults. These problems are often aggravated by uncontrolled diabetes or hyperglycemia. It is important for the nurse to evaluate current and past blood glucose results. The nurse should assess the client's ability to remember simple facts, mood, and level of anxiety. For example, the nurse can ask a client to explain content that was just presented. If the client cannot recall, the nurse needs to determine whether there is a learning or memory problem. Memory testing can be accomplished simply by asking clients to repeat number sequences, or by making a short- or long-term memory assessment (see Chapter 4). The nurse should ask the client about neurologic symptoms such as numbness; tingling; blurred vision; headaches; and inability to sense temperature, especially in the feet.

The nurse should assess the client's skin condition, paying particular attention to the skin on the feet, legs, and elbows, since these areas are at greatest risk for skin breakdown because of pressure. The nurse should assess skin for intactness, color, presence of swelling, discharge, odor, turgor, dryness, peeling, and lesions. Skin in the perianal area may provide information on current skin status and general hygiene practices. Clients with hyperglycemia are prone to yeast and fungal infections in this area. Poor hygiene may predispose an individual to urinary or vaginal infections.

To assess circulation, the nurse should take an apical pulse, noting rate and rhythm; check pedal pulses bilaterally; and note the presence of hair on the lower extremities. The nurse should take blood pressure measurements with the client in both recumbent and sitting positions; note any dizziness associated with a change of position; and assess respiratory rate, depth, and chest sounds.

Diagnosis

Nursing diagnoses for a client with type 2 diabetes mellitus include:

- Altered nutrition: more than body requirements related to overeating habits or lack of regular exercise pattern
- Altered nutrition: less than body requirements related to inadequate intake of nutrients or metabolic imbalance
- Altered tissue perfusion related to decreased or interrupted arterial flow
- Sexual dysfunction related to metabolic alterations
- Altered thought processes related to metabolic alteration or feelings of distress
- Knowledge deficit: diabetes self-management and skills related to lack of exposure
- Risk for impaired skin integrity related to impaired circulation
- Risk for ineffective individual coping related to lack of social support or feelings of distress

Planning and Expected Outcomes

The goal of nursing management for the older adult with diabetes mellitus is the achievement and maintenance of desired blood glucose control, prevention of symptoms and complications, and self-care management, when feasible. Expected outcomes for the plan of care include:

1. Client follows the plan of care by taking action on the basis of professional advice as evidenced by:
   a. Reports of following prescribed regimen
   b. Correct modification of the regimen as directed by a health professional
   c. Performance of self-screening currently and routinely

2. Client shows evidence of successful individual coping as evidenced by:
   a. Verbalization of sense of control
   b. Verbalization of acceptance of the situation
   c. Use of available social support
3. Client demonstrates increased knowledge of ADA diet, as evidenced by:
   a. Verbalization of rationale for prescribed diet
   b. Setting of goals for diet
   c. Selection of foods recommended in diet
4. Client demonstrates understanding of medication administration as evidenced by:
   a. Statement of correct medication name, dose, and schedule
   b. Correct demonstration of drawing up and self-injection of insulin
   c. Description of side effects of medication
5. Client maintains peripheral circulation as evidenced by:
   a. Pink, warm extremities without lesions or ulcers
   b. Verbalization of need for daily skin and extremity inspections
6. Client correctly demonstrates foot care regimen of foot cleansing and inspection techniques.
7. Client verbalizes satisfaction with degree of sexual functioning and ability.

The family or significant others should be involved in the care planning, since they so often provide the support and reinforcement needed for long-term management of such a chronic condition.

Intervention

The nursing care of an older adult client with type 2 diabetes is often complex. Usually many issues must be dealt with; therefore it is important to prioritize client problems. In general, emergent issues or life-threatening crises such as severe hyperglycemia, hypoglycemia, and sepsis are top priorities. Once crises are resolved, the nurse can provide education to support diabetes management.

Education. The nurse provides or coordinates education on a variety of recommended diabetic topics such as medication, pathophysiology of diabetes, monitoring of blood glucose and urine ketones, hypoglycemia and hyperglycemia, sick-day management, foot care, eye care, complications, the diabetic diet, product supplies, and instructions on when to contact the health care team. Teaching is facilitated if older clients and significant others are actively involved in learning (e.g., having clients demonstrate glucose monitoring or insulin injection techniques to the nurse). Teaching aids such as booklets and handouts can enhance learning. Resources for client educational handouts may be obtained from the ADA, the National Diabetes Information Clearinghouse, and commercial sources.

Diet. Although diet is the cornerstone of therapy for diabetes, it may be difficult to persuade an older adult to change his or her dietary pattern. Other factors that may affect dietary adherence include limited finances, social isolation, and lack of motivation (Le and Tuck, 1994). Dietary planning with a registered dietitian may be helpful in achieving dietary goals. Dietary goals include achieving good nutrition and reaching or maintaining ideal body weight while decreasing the risk of hyperlipidemia, atherosclerosis, and hypertension. When a diet plan is established, nursing interventions are directed at supporting the dietitian's recommendations through assessment of the client's understanding of and adherence to the plan (see Nutritional Considerations box).

Nutritional Considerations

Nutritional Goals for Client with Diabetes Mellitus

CALORIES

Based on achievement and maintenance of ideal body weight

PROTEIN

Approximately 12% to 20% of total calories
Recommended daily allowance: 0.8 g per kg of body weight for adults (Most adults eat twice as much protein as needed.)

CARBOHYDRATES

Approximately 45% to 60% of total calories
Emphasis placed on total carbohydrate intake rather than eliminating simple sugars
Modest sucrose intake perhaps acceptable based on metabolic control
Consistent mealtime carbohydrate intake

FATS

No more than 30% of total calories
May need further reduction depending on lipid profile
Polyunsaturated fats: 6% to 8%
Saturated fats: 10%
Monounsaturated fats: remaining percentage

FIBER

25 g/1000 kcal for low-calorie intake
Up to 40 g/day

SODIUM

3000 mg/day or less
May be reduced for medical conditions such as hypertension, CHF, and edema

VITAMINS AND MINERALS

No specific recommendations

Modified from Phipps W et al: *Medical-surgical nursing*, ed 7, St Louis, 2003, Mosby.

Insulin and Other Medications. An older client's cognitive function, vision, motivation, ability to accurately draw up and self-administer insulin, access sites, and family support need to be considered before insulin therapy is initiated (Funnell and Merritt, 1998). Written instructions about the medication regimen should be provided for a client and his or her significant other. The nurse should explain that Humulin insulin is not equivalent to beef insulin. Injecting Humulin insulin and then switching to beef or pork insulin alters the time of insulin action initiation, peak insulin action, and duration of insulin action. Therefore it is important that a client verbally state the type of insulin ordered and identify the notation on the insulin bottle that indicates the type of insulin prescribed.

The nurse should observe the client and his or her significant other preparing the prescribed insulin dosages; observe the client actually injecting insulin; and note if the client draws up an accurate amount of insulin, injects it into an appropriate site, and discards the sharp needle in a puncture-proof container. Vision or manual dexterity problems common among older adults that may interfere with proper insulin delivery can be identified through observation. Aids are available to assist visually impaired clients with insulin administration (Box 25-4).

Sometimes an older adult client is placed on a sliding scale of insulin. This system of insulin dosage indicates specific blood glucose ranges and doses of regular insulin. For example, the instructions to the client may be to give 4 U of regular insulin for blood glucose values ranging from 250 to 300 mg/dl. But for blood glucose values between 301 and 350 mg/dl, the client may be instructed to give 6 U of regular insulin.

Older clients often require two insulin injections a day to adequately control blood glucose levels. Splitting the intermediate insulin dose or adding a short-acting insulin may help prevent hypoglycemia and offer flexibility for older adults with eating pattern variations or decreased renal function. Home care or visiting nurse services may be useful to older adults in the initial phases of insulin therapy (Funnell and Merritt, 1998).

Oral hypoglycemic agents (OHAs), such as the sulfonylureas, are frequently used to lower blood glucose concentrations in older adults with type 2 diabetes. Glyburide and glipizide are well tolerated by older adults, but the long-acting drug chlorpropamide increases the risk of hypoglycemia, which does not respond well to simple carbohydrates (Funnell and Merritt, 1998). Recent studies indicated that a newer drug, metformin, classified as a biguanide, may be the drug of choice for overweight clients. Side effects such as anorexia, nausea, and abdominal discomfort may, however, limit its use in older adults (Wallace, 1999).

OHAs act by stimulating the secretion of insulin and the insulin-producing ability of the pancreas, which increases the sensitivity of the body to the effects of insulin and decreases the production of glucose by the liver. These drugs are totally ineffective in clients with type 1 diabetes, since these clients have lost the ability to produce insulin. OHAs are more readily accepted by clients than is insulin administration. More than 60% of all individuals with type 2 diabetes are, at least initially, candidates for OHAs. Table 25-4 lists common oral medications for type 2 diabetes.

It is important for the nurse to teach clients who are taking OHAs about the potential for drug interactions. All OHAs bind to serum proteins, but first-generation OHAs, compared with second-generation OHAs, have a higher incidence of interacting with other drugs that bind with albumin (e.g., anticoagulants, hydantoin, salicylates). Because some over-the-counter drugs interact negatively with OHAs, it is important for clients who take OHAs to check with their health care provider before taking any new drugs. Older adults are more likely than younger adults to have many drugs ordered concurrently with an OHA.

Since hypoglycemia is the major complication of OHA therapy, clients should be instructed about this complication. OHAs are associated with other adverse effects such as rashes, itching, nausea, vomiting, liver damage, and increased urinary frequency and urgency. Routine medical visits that include laboratory testing for complications are important. Alcohol ingestion may be contraindicated in people receiving chlorpropamide therapy, since alcohol use can cause an "Antabuse effect," in which facial flushing, headaches, and dizziness occur. Nursing interventions for clients taking OHAs include teaching clients to abstain from alcohol consumption and to be aware of the potential for side effects and complications such as hypoglycemia.

Clients taking medications that lower glucose levels should recognize the symptoms of mild hypoglycemia and test their blood glucose accordingly; if the result is abnormal, they should ingest a source of rapid-acting carbohydrate, such as 4 oz of orange juice. The early recognition and treatment of mild hypoglycemia prevents the more serious neuroglycopenic symptoms associated with moderate and severe hypoglycemia. Unrecognized and untreated hypoglycemia puts an individual with diabetes at risk for seizures and even death.

BOX 25-4 Diabetic Aids for the Visually Impaired

- Insulin syringe magnifiers
- Use of smaller dosed syringes
- Blood glucose meters that talk, display results in large type, and are easy to use
- Syringe-filling devices with dose gauges
- Needle and syringe holders

Modified from Beaser R et al: Buyer's guide to diabetes supplies, *Diabetes Fore* 46(10):48, 1993.

Emergency Identification. Clients should be advised to carry medical emergency identification. In the event that an

TABLE 25-4 Common Oral Medications for Type 2 Diabetes Mellitus

PARAMETER	METFORMIN	TROGLITAZONE	SULFONYLUREAS	ACARBOSE
Mode of action	Decreased hepatic glucose Increased skeletal muscle glucose utilization	Decreased hepatic glucose Increased skeletal muscle glucose utilization	Increased insulin secretion Decreased hepatic glucose production	Alpha-glucosidase inhibition Decreased carbohydrate digestion and absorption from gastrointestinal tract
Glucose effects	Fasting and postprandial	Fasting and postprandial	Fasting and postprandial	Postprandial
Hypoglycemia as monotherapy	No	No	Yes	No
Weight gain	No	Possible	Yes	No
Insulin levels	Decreased	Decreased	Increased	Decreased
Side effects	Gastrointestinal (self-limiting symptoms of nausea, diarrhea, anorexia)	None; equal to placebo	Potential allergic reaction if client has sulfa allergy Potential drug interactions (first-generation agents) Syndrome of inappropriate antidiuretic hormone	Gastrointestinal (flatulence, abdominal distention, diarrhea)
Lipid effects	Decreased	Decreased	Increased or decreased	Decreased
Starting dose for a 70 kg man	500 mg bid with meals	200 mg qd with breakfast	Varies with each agent: Glyburide 2.5 mg qd Glipizide extended release (Glucotrol XL) 5 mg qd Glyburide (Glynase) 3 mg qd Glimeperide (Amaryl) 2 mg qd	25 mg tid with first bite of each meal
Maximum dose	850 mg tid with meals	600 mg qd with breakfast	Varies with each agent: Glyburide 10 mg bid Glucotrol XL 20 mg qd Glyburide (Glynase) 6 mg bid Amaryl 8 mg qd	100 mg tid with first bite of each meal
Contraindications	Type 1 diabetes Renal dysfunction Hepatic dysfunction History of alcohol abuse Chronic conditions associated with hypoxia (asthma, chronic obstructive pulmonary disease, congestive heart failure [CHF]) Acute conditions associated with potential for hypoxia (surgery, acute myocardial infarction, CHF) Situations associated with potential renal dysfunction (e.g., intravenous contrast media)	Type 1 diabetes	Type 1 diabetes Hepatic dysfunction	Type 1 diabetes Inflammatory bowel disease Bowel obstruction Cirrhosis Chronic conditions with maldigestion or malabsorption

bid, Twice a day; *qd,* every day; *tid,* three times a day.

individual who takes OHAs experiences a major complication such as severe hypoglycemia, medical emergency identification facilitates treatment of the condition by health care workers or others (Table 25-5).

Monitoring. Monitoring blood glucose is recommended for older clients with type 2 diabetes because they tend to have higher renal thresholds. Blood glucose monitoring is used to achieve and maintain desired glucose goals; detect complications such as hyperglycemia and hypoglycemia; and educate clients about the effects of diet, medications, activity, and stress (Funnell and Merritt, 1998). Blood glucose monitoring is particularly important for individuals on medications that lower blood glucose (e.g., oral hypoglycemic agents, insulin). Glucose monitoring devices are generally easy to use and reliable; however, practicing the glucose-monitoring technique is important to ensure the accuracy of test results.

Exercise. Exercise is a strategy for decreasing insulin resistance and hyperglycemia. It is beneficial for older adults from both physiologic and psychologic perspectives. The assumption that older persons are not physically capable of or willing to exercise may result in neglect of this important aspect of care. Once the client's capabilities and limitations are considered, an exercise program is personalized to the client. Older adults may derive the greatest benefit from morning exercise because that is the time of greatest insulin resistance (Funnell and Merritt, 1998). Teaching topics should include the safety rules of exercising, which include wearing a medical-alert bracelet, checking blood glucose before exercise, identifying signs and symptoms of hypoglycemia, carrying a source of carbohydrate, and avoiding dehydration. Older adults should be advised to avoid exercise when blood glucose levels exceed 250 mg/dl. With inadequate insulin, exercise causes an escalation of hyperglycemia and increased production of free fatty acids and ketones. Inadequate insulin levels also promote the release of glucose from the liver by gluconeogenesis and glycogenolysis. Exercise should be resumed only when blood glucose levels are in the normal range.

Exercise-related complications or injuries are more likely to occur in this population as a result of preexisting conditions such as cardiac, musculoskeletal, and ophthalmic diseases. Precautions and exercise modifications for older adults are therefore indicated to help prevent problems.

Lifestyle Changes. Lifestyle changes are required for individuals with diabetes. It is difficult to manage a chronic illness that affects diet, exercise, weight, medication, sexuality, and finances. Proper management of diabetes requires knowledge, skills, and the organization of a team of experts that includes the client as the core of the team. Avoidance of smoking and alcohol is believed to improve diabetes management. An older client's ability to adapt to lifestyle changes needs to be evaluated frequently so that additional support can be provided when needed.

Sick-Day Management. Older adults have a high incidence of chronic illness, and those with diabetes need to take special measures for "sick days." Sick days are generally defined as illness days that necessitate an alteration of typical treatment strategies (e.g., increasing medications [insulin doses], meals, and fluids) or the initiation of medical interventions (e.g., antibiotics for infections). For example, when an individual with diabetes becomes ill with a "stomach flu," the stress of even this common illness may precipitate severe hyperglycemia. The individual may detect significant hyperglycemia during routine blood glucose testing and should contact the health care provider for specific instructions on how to increase insulin dosage. Individuals with nausea and vomiting are generally instructed to take 8 oz of fluids (nondiet beverages) hourly and increase monitoring of blood glucose and urine ketones. Instructions from the provider usually indicate the levels of blood glucose and ketones that require an immediate call to the provider or a visit to the emergency room (see Emergency Treatment box).

Skin Alterations. Lower extremity amputations are a tragic yet preventable problem for individuals with diabetes. About 50% to 70% of all amputations of the feet are performed on individuals with diabetes (Fig. 25-5). Prevention of foot ulcers is the key to proper foot management in older clients with diabetes. This is achieved through daily cleansing of the feet with nondrying agents, inspection of the feet, and prompt treatment of problems (see Client/Family Teaching box). When older adult clients are unable to inspect their own feet

TABLE 25-5 Hypoglycemia Levels, Symptoms, Treatment

HYPOGLYCEMIA LEVEL	SYMPTOMS	TREATMENT
Mild	Hunger, diaphoresis, nervousness, shakiness, tachycardia, and pale skin	15 g of carbohydrate 4 oz of juice (no sugar added)
Moderate	Headache, irritability, fatigue, blurred vision, and mood changes	15 g of carbohydrate; may repeat
Severe	Unresponsiveness, confusion, coma, and convulsions	Glucagon; intravenous glucose

EMERGENCY TREATMENT

SICK-DAY MANAGEMENT FOR THE INDIVIDUAL WITH DIABETES MELLITUS

Sick days for individuals with diabetes are episodes of acute illnesses involving complications such as nausea, vomiting, and diarrhea. Illnesses trigger stress hormone production and result in hyperglycemia. With the onset of gastrointestinal symptoms, individuals with diabetes become easily dehydrated. If the client's meal plan cannot be tolerated, easily digested foods such as regular soda, soups, popsicles, and crackers are taken instead. This diet can be supplemented with noncaloric liquids like water or diet sodas to keep up with fluids lost from vomiting or diarrhea.

Individuals with diabetes must continue taking prescribed medications such as insulin or oral hypoglycemic agents, ensure adequate hydration, and test urine and blood more often. Urine should be tested for ketones whenever the blood glucose is greater than 240 mg/dl. Other recommendations include taking temperature and weight and recording all values and interventions. Clients with diabetes should contact their health care provider whenever they have unanswered questions or concerns or the treatment regimen is not working, which can be evidenced by worsening fever, decreasing alertness or ability to think, vomiting more than once, diarrhea that persists for 6 or more hours, blood glucose values of 250 mg/dl or greater despite additional insulin, or moderate or large ketones in the urine.

Sick-day management is important in individuals with type 2 diabetes, since untreated illness may lead to a complication called hyperglycemic hyperosmolar nonketotic coma (HHNC). This hyperglycemic condition is more common in older clients with type 2 diabetes, whereas clients with type 1 diabetes are more likely to experience diabetic ketoacidosis. HHNC is characterized by severe dehydration and hyperglycemia (blood glucose values 600 mg/dl or greater, and hyperosmolarity of the blood [340 or greater mOsm/L of water]). Treatment for this condition consists of insulin, intravenous fluids, and identification and treatment of the precipitating event (e.g., infection, cardiovascular problems) in an intensive care setting of a hospital.

because of mobility or vision problems, significant others should be taught how to perform thorough inspections.

Foot care is the same for older adults as for other persons with diabetes. Daily cleansing of the feet with nondrying agents is important to free the feet of potential infectious organisms. Lubrication of the feet (but not between the toes, where heat and lotions may be trapped and lead to infections) with unscented lotions is often needed to help decrease skin dryness and cracking. Appliances such as corn pads and drying agents such as alcohol should be avoided because they impair the integrity of the skin. New shoes need to be tested for good fit and gradually broken in. Individuals or others should cut nails straight across to prevent complications. Individuals with diabetes should seek care from their provider whenever wounds exhibit tenderness, swelling, or leakage of fluids. Individuals with diabetes who have neuropathy of the feet, significant hyperglycemia (blood glucose values of 250 mg/dl or greater), or a history of foot infections should seek care at the first sign of a foot infection.

Wound Infections. Older adults with diabetes are at a higher risk for complications of the feet than those without diabetes because of changes in nerves and blood vessels. The phrase *diabetic foot syndrome* has evolved, since these foot problems are so common, to describe the vascular and neurologic pathologic condition associated with diabetes. Inadequate blood flow to the feet and nerve damage contribute to the development of ulcers and infections. Hyperglycemia also plays a role in foot problems, since blood glucose levels of 200 mg/dl or greater are associated with an altered immune system leukocyte response.

The clinical symptoms of foot infections vary from no symptoms to fever, erythema, warmth, discharge with ulceration, and leukocytosis (Genuth, Palmer, and Zimmerman, 1999). The skin over and around the infection may appear to be white, pink, red, or shades of blue. Blood vessels may be distended and pronounced over the infection site. Nail beds may be pale and show slowed capillary refilling when pressed. The shape of the foot may be altered by infection as a result of significant soft tissue swelling. Lesions may drain or may be dry. Superficial inspection of a lesion may be deceptive because the outside appearance often does not reflect the extent of the problem beneath the skin surface. For example, when an older individual with diabetes has a grossly swollen but nondraining lesion on the sole of the foot, it is common for the infected fluids to be trapped below the lesion. If a foot looks swollen and red despite the absence of discharge, it is likely that the infection is deeper.

Wound infections in older adults with diabetes are common and serious events that require immediate attention. Infections may manifest symptoms, such as pain, swelling, and redness, or may be symptom free and go undetected until they are at an advanced stage. Significant delays can occur before the health care provider is contacted and treatment is initiated, and infection can spread from the skin to fat, muscle, fascia, and bone.

Specific causal agents of diabetic foot infections include proteus, *Klebsiella* and *Enterobacter* organism, pseudomonads, *Escherichia coli*, staphylococci, *Streptococcus epidermis*, corynebacteria, *Bacteroides fragilis*, and clostridia. Polymicrobial wound infections are common in older clients with diabetes. Individual wounds may be infected with gram-positive cocci, gram-negative rods, and anaerobic bacteria. The rates of recovery from infections vary according to the time of treatment initiation, the treatment form, and the client's condition.

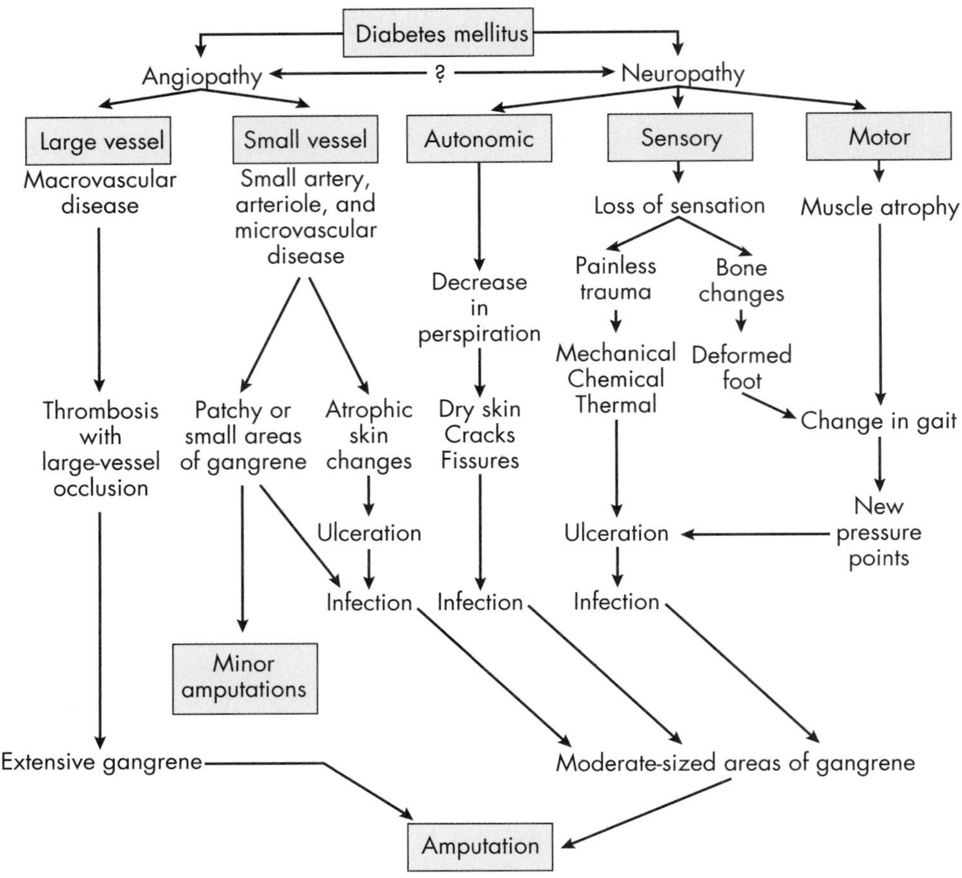

Fig. 25-5 How foot lesions of diabetes can lead to amputation. (In McCance KL, Huether SE: *Pathophysiology*, ed 3, St Louis, 1998, Mosby; from Levin ME, O'Neal LW, Bowker JH: *The diabetic foot*, ed 5, St Louis, 1993, Mosby.)

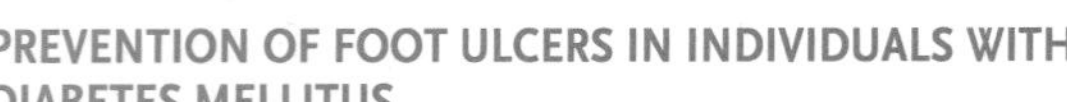

Client/Family Teaching

PREVENTION OF FOOT ULCERS IN INDIVIDUALS WITH DIABETES MELLITUS

- Perform daily foot inspection.
- Perform daily foot hygiene using warm (not hot) soapy water to wash feet; pat feet dry.
- Gently apply mild skin cream to feet if dry or rough; do not apply between toes.
- Keep toenails trimmed straight across.
- Wear proper-fitting shoes and do not go barefoot.
- Break in new shoes gradually.
- Do not wear tight shoes or stockings that bind.
- Exercise regularly and maintain ideal body weight.
- Avoid smoking, since it impairs circulation to the feet.
- Seek early interventions to problems (e.g., tenderness, redness, swelling, leakage of fluid).

Another foot problem associated with diabetes is the loss of the ability to sweat, which leads to dry skin. Untreated dry skin can progress to cracked skin, which allows for entry of organisms and subsequent infections (see Nursing Care Plan).

Evaluation

The nurse evaluates the effectiveness of the care plan for an older client with diabetes by frequently measuring the achievement of established specific outcomes. For example, for nutritional outcomes the client is encouraged to select foods consistent with the prescribed meal plan. Achievement of weight change goals is measured over time with weight graphs. The client can log exercise accomplishments so that progress with activity is clearly displayed. Medication administration is observed and, when needed, critiqued by the nurse. When insulin is used, injection sites are checked for complications reflecting overuse of sites or local irritation. The client can log blood glucose values, which can be compared with corresponding laboratory results. Clients are examined to see if they are wearing or carrying medical-alert bracelets or other emergency information. Clients can be asked to review their recent experiences with sick days and their management of fluids, nausea, vomiting, medication, and testing.

A principle of diabetes management is having the client "take control" of the diabetes. Self-care activities such as daily

Nursing Care Plan
Diabetes Mellitus With Foot Infection

Clinical Situation: Mr. J notices that his right foot aches slightly. Taking off his shoe, he can see that his foot is red and swollen with a small amount of purulent fluid draining from a lesion on his small toe. He can even see the indentations from his shoes on the skin of his feet. He is surprised that his foot looks this bad when he had no problems earlier. He makes an appointment with his primary care physician. The appointment is 2 days after he first noticed the problem. During those 2 days Mr. J becomes increasingly tired. Despite drinking fluids nonstop, he is thirsty all the time. At the visit with his physician, Mr. J is found to have 3+ edema in the affected foot, a temperature of 101° F, and a blood glucose level of 250 mg/dl. He is diagnosed with a diabetic foot infection. Mr. J first learns of his diagnosis of diabetes mellitus at this time.

The physician sends Mr. J to the local community hospital for inpatient admission. Hospitalization is necessary to treat the foot infection and his newly diagnosed diabetes.

Nursing Diagnoses

Impaired skin integrity related to altered metabolic state
Pain related to treatments for foot ulcer (e.g., biopsy, currettage, and debridement)
Knowledge deficit: newly diagnosed diabetes mellitus related to new experience
Knowledge deficit: foot care management related to new experience

Outcomes

Wound healing will occur, as demonstrated by decreasing size of wound and less purulent drainage, as well as laboratory values of complete blood count with differential and electrolytes within normal limits.
Circulation to affected area will be maintained, as evidenced by normal skin color and temperature, presence of pedal pulses, and no evidence of edema.
Client will verbalize comfort following debridement procedures.
Client will maintain stable vital signs before, during, and after procedure.
Client will verbalize and demonstrate understanding of diabetes and diabetes management as evidenced by making appropriate diet selections, correctly and safely administering medications, and accurately testing blood glucose.
Client will verbalize appropriate sick-day management regimen.
Client will demonstrate daily foot care regimen of inspecting, cleansing, and using emollients.
Client will verbalize when to contact physician for complications.
Client will achieve optimum level of physical mobility as evidenced by ability to safely meet self-care needs.
Client will protect affected extremity as evidenced by ability to adhere to weight-bearing restriction.
Client will verbalize reduced levels of anxiety with increasing knowledge and skill acquisition.

Interventions

Assess wound at each dressing change for wound stage, epithelialization, color, edema, and discharge.
Assess vital signs.
Administer antibiotics as prescribed.
Provide physician-ordered intravenous fluids, insulin, and medications.
Notify physician of signs and symptoms of increased pain, swelling, drainage, or fever.
Change linens as needed to maintain clean wound environment.
Provide pain control during debridement by medicating before procedures.
Assess client's vital signs and level of consciousness before administering medications.
Assess pain level, vital signs, and level of comfort and sedation after medication.
Document client tolerance of procedure.
Assess client understanding of condition.
Monitor readiness and determine best methods for teaching and learning.
Provide diabetes teaching, including topics such as type 2 diabetes; ADA diet; exercise; medications; sick-day management; monitoring; lifestyle factors (e.g., smoking and alcohol); complications, especially of hypoglycemia and hyperglycemia; and eye, kidney, nerve, foot, and vessel problems.
Provide proper foot care teaching with demonstration, including topics such as daily inspection and cleansing, wearing shoes, avoidance of tape and drying chemicals, use of proper foot gear, applying emollients, keeping feet dry, and safe nail cutting.
Have client give a return demonstration.
Instruct client on reportable signs and symptoms such as fever, pain, swelling, redness, and breaks in skin integrity.
Instruct client not to bear weight on infected foot.
Set up room to maximize client independence in ADLs.
Assess client mood and coping mechanisms.
Allow client to verbalize feelings about diagnosis of chronic disease of diabetes.
Support client in self-care and management of diabetes by (1) encouraging involvement in self-care activities, (2) providing environment conducive to relaxation, and (3) reassuring client when he or she safely or accurately performs self-care skills and techniques.

inspection of the feet with basic diabetic foot care support this self-care approach. The nurse can help a client evaluate the effectiveness of self-care activities by direct examination and through interview techniques.

The nurse should positively reinforce effective diabetes management strategies used by an older client. For example, when an older client improves in foot care or the technique for insulin injections, the nurse needs to acknowledge the client's skill. If a client does not comply with management strategies, the situation needs to be reassessed so that adaptations can be made. It may be that an older client has financial or social support problems that are obstacles to compliance.

Documentation of assessments, including client response to treatment measures, client comprehension of teaching, and client ability to self-manage treatment measures and diet, as well as other nursing interventions, is an essential component of care for older adult clients with diabetes.

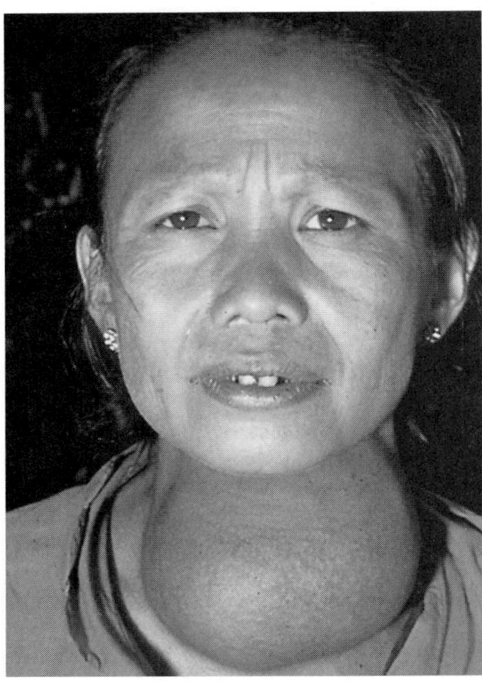

Fig. 25-6 Simple goiter. (Courtesy Bergman LV and Associates, Cold Spring, NY. In Phipps W et al: *Medical-surgical nursing*, ed 7, St Louis, 2003, Mosby.)

Hyperthyroidism

Pathophysiology. A *hyperfunctioning* endocrine state results from excessive secretion of hormones. For example, primary hyperthyroidism involves hypersecretion of thyroid hormones, which is usually associated with an enlarged thyroid gland. In the absence of coexisting systemic illness or pharmacologic drug interference, a low or suppressed thyroid-stimulating hormone (TSH) level is diagnostic of hyperthyroidism (Walfish, 1996). Although hyperthyroidism is most commonly a condition of young adulthood and middle age, 10% to 15% of persons with hyperthyroidism are over age 60 (Kennedy and Caro, 1996). Hyperthyroidism in seniors is often caused by multinodular and uninodular toxic goiter rather than Graves' disease, which is the most common cause in younger adults (Beers and Berkow, 2000-2005). Thyroid nodules are identified in 5% of people over age 60, with 90% of nodules being benign (Fig. 25-6). Iodine-induced hyperthyroidism is another common type of hyperthyroidism among older patients using amiodarone, a cardiac drug containing iodine that deposits in tissue and delivers iodine to the circulation over long periods of time.

Subclinical hyperthyroidism, a condition in which an otherwise healthy, asymptomatic client has a suppressed serum TSH level with normal thyroxine (T_4) and triiodothyronine (T_3) levels, has been associated with an increased incidence of atrial fibrillation and decreased bone mineral density. Thyroid storm is a life-threatening syndrome consisting of fever, severe tachycardia, altered mental status, dehydration, and irritability. It is most commonly seen in persons with Graves' disease, but it can occur from other causes of hyperthyroidism. It can be precipitated by a concurrent illness, withdrawal from antithyroid drugs, or treatment with radioactive iodine (Singer et al, 1995).

Signs and Symptoms. In younger patients hyperthyroidism produces a complex of signs and symptoms, such as palpitations, heat intolerance, insomnia, breathlessness, increased bowel movements, light menstrual flow, trembling, weight loss, weakness, fatigue, and hair loss. Such signs often indicate a need to run thyroid function laboratory tests. Although some of these signs may appear in the senior population, the classic presentation includes tachycardia, weight loss, and fatigue (Beers and Berkow, 2000-2005). An enlarged, palpable goiter is present in 60% of seniors with hyperthyroidism. The most common complication, occurring in 27% of geriatric hyperthyroid patients, is atrial fibrillation that does not convert back to sinus rhythm when a euthyroid state is achieved.

Medical Management. Treatment of subclinical hyperthyroidism in older adults is controversial unless established heart disease or osteoporosis exists (Ringel and Cooper, 1996). The treatment of choice for hyperthyroidism in older adults is generally radioactive sodium iodine. It is safe and simple to use but not particularly suited in cases of toxic goiter (Beers and Berkow, 2000-2005). Clients must be rechecked every 6 months after initial treatment for the rest of their lives. In clients with toxic goiter, surgery is preferred for those clients at low risk of postoperative complication because of the slow and prolonged treatment regimen needed for radioactive sodium iodine. Propranolol or other beta-blockers are frequently used to manage hyperthyroid-induced tachycardia.

NURSING MANAGEMENT

Assessment, diagnosis, planning, intervention, and evaluation in hyperthyroidism focus on the primary human response to the hypersecretion of thyroid hormone, as detailed in Table 25-6.

Hypothyroidism

Pathophysiology. A common *hypofunctioning* endocrine state that results from inadequate thyroid hormone function is hypothyroidism. Diagnosis is based on precise, reliable assays of serum TSH and T_4 levels. The most sensitive indication of hypothyroidism caused by primary thyroid gland failure is a marked elevation of serum TSH. The most specific test finding is a subnormal serum free T_4 level, since it corrects for abnormalities in the T_4-binding proteins. As the thyroid gland ages, it develops moderate atrophy, fibrosis, colloid nodules, and lymphocyte infiltration (Beers and Berkow, 2000-2005). The production of T_4 decreases by about 30% between young adulthood and advanced age, but serum levels are usually maintained because of the body's decreased use of T_4 as a correlate to the age-related decline in lean body mass. Hypofunctioning thyroid states may result from defects in hormone production, target tissues, or receptors. When the defect involves a hypofunctioning peripheral gland like the thyroid, it is called primary hypothyroidism. If the hypothyroid state is a result of a nonfunctional anterior pituitary gland, the condition is called secondary hypothyroidism. Tertiary hypothyroidism results from a defect in the hypothalamus.

An aging thyroid gland consistently recognizes and synthesizes TSH despite a decrease in size as a result of cellular atrophy, which is most notable in women over age 70. Changes in thyroid function that naturally occur with aging include slowing of T_4 secretion and degradation; decline in plasma levels of T_3, especially in men; reduced conversion of T_4 to T_3; increased metabolic half-life of T_4; and overall reduced TSH secretion (McCance and Huether, 1998). Thyroglobulin binding remains unchanged except when polypharmacy occurs, since many drugs interfere with protein binding of T_4 and T_3.

Research studies report that elevated TSH levels were found in 17.4% of women older than age 75, compared with 7.5% of women overall, and in 3.5% of men older than age 75, compared with 2.8% overall (Felicetta, 1996). Autoimmune thyroiditis is the most common cause of primary hypothyroidism in older persons. It is diagnosed in 5% of older women and 2% of men of the same age. Drug-induced hypothyroidism can occur with the use of lithium carbonate, amiodarone, and iodine. Other causes of hypothyroidism include ablation of the thyroid gland with radioiodine or surgery for the treatment for hyperthyroidism, and postsurgical or radiation treatment of head and neck cancer. Hypothalamic

TABLE 25-6 Hyperthyroidism

ASSESSMENT	DIAGNOSIS	PLANNING	INTERVENTION	EVALUATION
1. Weight loss trends over 3 and 6 months 2. Body mass index 3. Serum albumin and TSH 4. Mini Nutritional Assessment 5. MiniMental State Examination 6. Dysphagia 7. Manual dexterity 8. Financial resources 9. Dentition 10. Comorbidities 11. Medications 12. Social support 13. Cultural influences 14. Tachycardia defined a >90 beats/min 15. Fatigue as mentioned in Box 25-4	1. Imbalanced nutrition: less than body requirements 2. Potential complication: decreased cardiac output 3. Fatigue	1. Teach disease, treatment and monitoring. 2. Teach Dietary Recommendations of the National Research Council Report for those over 65 years old. 3. Add 250- to 300-calorie snacks to increase body weight slowly. 4. Refer to Meals on Wheels, consultations, or other community resources as needed. 5. Monitor cardiovascular status.	1. Explain hyperthyroidism, complications, testing techniques, activity restrictions, dietary measures, medications, radioactive iodine therapy (if needed), surgery (if needed), eye care for exophthalmos (if needed). 2. Facilitate specific meal plans, procurement, preparation, and social support. 3. Monitor for pulse rate <90 beats/min, respiratory rate <22 breaths/min, normal blood pressure, bibasilar crackles, decreased urine output, mentation changes, cool or mottled skin, distended neck veins, decreased Sao_2.	1. Client will increase intake as evidenced by gradual weight gain to normal range of body mass index. 2. Client will maintain adequate cardiac output.

Data from Carpenito-Moyet LJ: *Nursing diagnosis: application to clinical practice,* ed 10, Philadelphia, 2004, Lippincott.

or pituitary problems are rarely originating causes (Wallace and Hofmann, 1998).

Aged thyroid glands are more susceptible to the destructive autoimmune effects of Hashimoto's disease than are those of younger persons (Beers and Berkow, 2000-2005). Thyroid antibodies appear more often in women who are older than age 60 than in men or younger women. This condition of autoimmune thyroiditis can be triggered by a virus or by treatment of Hodgkin's disease, for instance, which in turn manifests lymphocyte and plasma cell infiltrates and leads to atrophy of thyroid tissue. Antithyroid antibodies can block the TSH receptors and cause a thyroid-deficient state.

Signs and Symptoms. The clinical symptoms of hypothyroidism in older people are atypical compared with those of younger adults. Almost all cases (99%) of hypothyroidism in older adults are subclinical, are inconspicuous, and progress slowly toward thyroid failure. Since the condition is insidious, the symptoms are often attributed to "old age." Most older clients are seen with nonspecific complaints such as confusion, anorexia, weight loss, falling, incontinence, and decreased mobility (Beers and Berkow, 2000-2005). Arthralgia complaints occur often, but arthritis is rare. Muscular aches and weakness can mimic polymyalgia rheumatica or polymyositis, and occasionally an elevated creatine phosphokinase level may occur. Signs that are frequently linked to hypothyroidism in older adults include an unexplained elevation in triglycerides or plasma cholesterol, mild cognitive impairment, slow metabolism, cardiovascular changes, fecal impaction, macrocytic anemia, and depression with underlying apathy and withdrawal (Felicetta, 1996) (Table 25-7).

Decreased appetite and weight loss are common but may be overlooked. Decreased calorigenesis (production of heat) contributes to symptoms of cold intolerance. Cardiovascular symptoms in both genders, when they occur, include bradycardia and angina pectoris. Neuromuscular and neurosensory symptoms may include syncope, seizures, muscle cramps, numbness and weakness of the hands, and unsteadiness of gait (Thyroid Foundation of America, 1999). Mild macrocytic anemia is commonly identified with hypothyroidism and occurs as a result of bone marrow hypoplasia or iron deficiency.

Medical Management. Serum TSH screening every 5 years is recommended for all men over 65 years old and for all women over 35 years old (Beers and Berkow, 2000-2005). The treatment of choice is T_4 replacement with levothyroxine sodium at an average dosage for senior patients of 0.075 to 0.1 mg/day by mouth. Medication is increased by 0.0125 mg/day every 2 weeks or by 0.025 mg/day every 4 weeks. One

TABLE 25-7 Hypothyroidism

ASSESSMENT	DIAGNOSIS	PLANNING	INTERVENTION	EVALUATION
1. Fatigue on a scale of 1 to 10 2. Onset, pattern, and aggravating and relieving factors of fatigue 3. Effects of fatigue on activities of daily living (ADLs), instrumental ADLs (IADLs), mood, accident proneness, concentration, motivation, leisure activities, and libido 4. Depression Scale 5. MiniMental State Examination 6. Laboratory values of TSH, hemoglobin, and hematocrit 7. Comorbidities 8. Medications 9. Social support network 10. Weight as detailed in Table 25-3	1. Fatigue	1. Identify client's energy patterns and teach energy conservation. 2. Facilitate prioritization and delegation of tasks. 3. Teach disease pathophysiology, medication management, and monitoring. 4. Facilitate appropriate community and financial resource use.	1. Explain client's type of hypothyroidism, symptoms, complications, diagnostic tests, activity restrictions, dietary guidelines, lifelong therapy, and symptoms of accidental thyroid hormone overdose. 2. Work with client to target ADLs and IADLs for client performance, health care surrogate, and community services assistance.	1. Client will achieve a balance of activity and rest. 2. Client can verbalize pathophysiology, medication use, and monitoring required.

Data from Carpenito-Moyet LJ: *Nursing diagnosis: application to clinical practice,* ed 10, Philadelphia, 2004, Lippincott.

to two months after reaching a dose of 0.075 mg/day, the client should have his or her serum TSH level measured by a second- or third-generation TSH assay.

NURSING MANAGEMENT

Assessment, diagnosis, planning, intervention, and evaluation in hypothyroidism focus on the human age–related response to the core defect of decreased thyroid hormone, as detailed in Table 25-8.

Primary Osteoporosis

Pathophysiology. Osteoporosis is a legitimate concern for postmenopausal women (Seeman, 2000) and andropausal men (Bain, 2001) because of the influence of systemic sex hormones on bone. Found 6 times more frequently in women, osteoporosis is a disease characterized by low bone mass leading to fragile, easy to break bones (Black, 2000). The geriatric skeleton is a metabolically active organ that experiences continuous remodeling, which provides structural integrity, support to the body, protection of vital organs, and a reservoir of calcium and other minerals (Beers and Berkow, 2000-2005). Low bone mass can result from a failure to reach peak bone mass as a young adult, from increased bone resorption, or from decreased bone formation; all three of these mechanisms are believed to play a role in the osteoporosis found in today's older adults. Recently researchers have suggested that 50% to 80% of peak bone mass is genetically determined, which supports the importance of family history in determining an individual's risk.

Menopausal and senescent bone losses have different features (Box 25-5). Sex steroids influence skeletal development and adult remodeling by altering the activity of osteoclasts and osteoblasts (Manolagas, 2000). Parathyroid hormone has also been shown to increase skeletal resorption in estrogen-deficient menopausal women (Masiukiewicz et al, 2000); this same mechanism is believed to influence male osteoporosis (Falahati, Riggs, and Atkinson, 2000). In addition, low vitamin D status in older persons contributes to bone loss mediated by the aging parathyroid gland, low daily exposure to

BOX 25-5 Comparison of Menopausal and Senescent Bone Loss

MENOPAUSAL BONE LOSS	SENESCENT BONE LOSS
High remodeling rate	Low remodeling rate
Loss of trabecular bone	Loss of cortical bone
Increased risk of wrist and vertebral fracture	Increased risk of hip and vertebral fracture
Increased osteoblast formation	Decreased osteoblast formation
Increased osteoclast formation	Decreased osteoclast formation

Data taken from Beers MH, Berkow R, editors: *Merck manual of geriatrics,* 2000-2005, Merck. Accessed Oct 16, 2004, from website: http://www.merck.com/mrkshared/mm_geriatrics/home.jsp.

TABLE 25-8 Osteoporosis

ASSESSMENT	DIAGNOSIS	PLANNING	INTERVENTION	EVALUATION
1. Use of hormone replacement 2. Calcium and vitamin D intake 3. Exercise habits 4. Alcohol, caffeine, and protein intake 5. Current or past use of corticosteroids 6. History of thyroid, bowel, kidney, or liver disease 7. Use of excessive thyroid replacement 8. Weight as listed in Box 25-1 9. Comorbidities 10. Medications 11. Social support. 12. Cultural influences	1. Ineffective health maintenance	1. Teach disease and medical management and Dietary Recommendations of the National Research Council Report for those over 65 years old. 2. Therapeutic lifestyle changes. 3. Ensure safety and fall awareness.	1. Teach pathophysiology, testing, medications, monitoring, complications, sources of support and information, and fall precautions. 2. Provide for supervised meal planning, encourage food label reading, and calcium and vitamin D supplementation. 3. Have client undergo postural retraining and weight-bearing exercises.	1. Client will have an absence of fractures, no falls, and improved bone mass density.

Data from Carpenito-Moyet LJ: *Nursing diagnosis: application to clinical practice,* ed 10, Philadelphia, 2004, JB Lippincott.

natural sunlight, and reduced dietary intake (New, 2000). The primary role of calcium alone in maintaining bone mass in older persons continues to spur controversy (Heaney, 2000; Speaker, 2000). However, milk products have been shown to improve bone density to a greater extent then calcium alone (Devine, Prince, and Bell, 1996), presumably because of their interactions with insulin-like growth factor 1.

Osteopenia precedes osteoporosis, which is defined as bone mass less than 2.5 standard deviations below that of a young control population (New, 2000). Osteoporosis generally occurs in those in the sixth decade or older. Divided into primary and secondary types based on etiology, osteoporosis involves both the appendicular and axial skeleton (Black, 2000). Other endocrine disorders such as parathyroid disease, Cushing's syndrome, hypogonadism, alcohol abuse, liver disease, and amenorrhea can cause secondary osteoporosis. Osteoporosis is diagnosed by dual x-ray absorptiometry (DEXA) of the proximal femur and lumbar spine, since these scans are sensitive to subtle changes in mineral density.

Signs and Symptoms. Spontaneous fractures or those caused by minimum trauma in addition to loss of height should trigger DEXA scanning in older clients because of the high incidence of occult osteoporosis. Ultrasound densitometry, because of its low cost and portability, is frequently used on the heel; however, it is not considered as reliable as DEXA scanning. History of fracture after a person is 40 years old, family history of osteoporosis, cigarette smoking, and low body mass index have been shown to correlate strongly with osteoporosis. Dorsal kyphosis, chronic back pain, and loss of height are common signs of primary osteoporosis in the older persons (Beers and Berkow, 2000-2005).

Medical Management. Calcium and vitamin D supplementation, exercise, and antiresorptive therapy are the cornerstones of medical therapy in primary osteoporosis (Beers and Berkow, 2000-2005). The recommended intake for older Americans is at least 1200 mg/day of elemental calcium and at least 400 IU/day of vitamin D in two divided doses to maximize gastrointestinal absorption. Weight-bearing and muscle-strengthening exercises add minimally to bone density, but the benefit in improved posture, balance, and reduced falls is considerable. Estrogens, biphosphonates, selective estrogen receptor modulators, and calcitonin are used in antiresorptive therapy based on the older client's risk profile. In addition, some physicians choose a thiazide diuretic for those with hypertension as a comorbidity, since it decreases urinary calcium excretion, slowing bone loss.

NURSING MANAGEMENT

Assessment, diagnosis, planning, intervention, and evaluation in osteoporosis focuses on the response to the core defect of decreased bone mass, as detailed in Table 25-8.

Sexual Dysfunction

Erectile dysfunction (ED) and female sexual dysfunction (FSD) have garnered increased interest and research dollars in recent years as many older people strive to retain the vitality of their younger years. Previously, sexual dysfunction was discreetly minimized or overlooked in the geriatric professional literature. FSD is an ill-defined, rapidly growing subspecialty medicine that has drawn considerable attention from health care providers and the public (Berman et al, 2000). Sildenafil (Viagra) provided a simple and effective treatment for male ED, which produced a demand for an equally simple and effective treatment for women.

Pathophysiology. Hormonal changes associated with ED begin at 40 years old in the aging man and include decreased testosterone, decreased bioavailability of testosterone, increased sex hormone–binding globulin, decreased DHEA, mildly increased estradiol-17-beta, decreased melatonin, and decreased growth hormone and insulin-like growth factor 1 (Porst, 2002).

The female sexual response cycle is a neuroendocrine-mediated vascular and nonvascular smooth muscle relaxation, which results in increased pelvic blood flow, vaginal lubrication, and clitoral engorgement. Similar to males, these mechanisms are mediated by a combination of neuromuscular and vasocongestive events. More urologists are seeing women with FSD. In a multidisciplinary evaluation of a cohort with FSD, the mean age of presentation was 43 ± 11 years; the mean duration of symptoms was 9 ± 9 years; and many were receiving antidepressants, oral contraceptives, or estrogen/progesterone replacement (Talakoub et al, 2001). Some researchers think that androgen deficiency or relative inactivity of the adrenal enzyme 17,20-lyase in women is the pathophysiologic entity responsible for FSD, which is often characterized by diminished libido, diminished arousal and orgasmic capabilities, and deficient androgen levels. Researchers in Boston (Munarriz, Talakoub, and Lahey, 2001) treated 32 women with androgen deficiency by administering DHEA 50 mg/day for 6 months with significant benefits such as increased spontaneity, decreased time to achieve arousal, return of sexual fantasies, and increase in desire. Adverse effects were mild and limited to acne and breast tenderness.

Signs and Symptoms Erectile dysfunction (ED) is the persistent inability to achieve or sustain an erection firm enough for sexual intercourse and penetration (Rosen et al, 2003). ED ranges from mild to severe and occurs in 50% of 65-year-old men, and 75% of men 80 years or older. The word *impotence* should be used to describe other problems that interfere with sexual intercourse and reproduction, such as lack of sexual desire and problems with ejaculation or orgasm.

FSD is a sexual arousal disorder that may develop as women age. Menopause and declining estrogen produce a thin and dry vaginal vault. As a result, the ability to become aroused may decline due to painful sexual intercourse. In addition, in FSD neuroendocrine physiologic impairments interfere with the normal female sexual response and frequently bring about complaints of diminished sexual arousal, libido, genital sensation, and ability to achieve orgasm. Other physical contributors to FSD include vaginitis, cystitis, endometriosis, hypothyroidism, and diabetes mellitus. Drugs such as oral contraceptives, hormone replacement, antihypertensives, antidepressants, or sedatives can cause a sexual arousal disorder as a side effect.

Medical Management. Medications for other medical problems often contribute to ED in older men (Rosen et al, 2003). Patients who are taking antihypertensives, antidepressants, sedatives, cimetidine, digoxin, lithium, and antipsychotics are warned of ED as a possible side effect. Often these medications must continue to be taken and additional medicine is added to address ED. Sildenafil, phentolamine, yohimbine, testosterone, and alprostadil are a few of the medications prescribed to increase blood flow to the penis and correct ED.

Most men with ED can achieve erections by using a constriction device with or without a vacuum device (Rosen et al, 2003). These devices are among the least expensive treatments for ED, and they enable a man to avoid the side effects that can occur with drug treatment. Constriction bands or rings made of metal, rubber, or leather are placed at the base of the penis to slow the outflow of blood. A constriction band used alone may produce an erection in a man with mild ED, especially if the problem is erection maintenance. When that doesn't work, a constriction device can also be used in combination with a vacuum device. Vacuum devices consist of a hollow chamber attached to a source of suction that fit over the penis, creating an air seal. Then suction applied to the chamber draws blood into the penis, producing an erection; a binding device can then be applied to maintain the erection. Surgical implantation of firm rods or pump-operated devices is an option for men with a low risk of postoperative complication, who find the 3-day hospital stay and 6-week recovery acceptable. Recently sensate focus psychotherapy has enjoyed some popularity because of its ability to mitigate compounding psychologic factors that may overlay physiologic ED.

Medical management of FSD includes watchful waiting, dose reduction of offending medication, bupropion, buspirone, sildenafil, testosterone replacement, and sensate focus psychotherapy (Quan, 2004).

NURSING MANAGEMENT

The nursing process in sexual dysfunction requires a biopsychosocial approach to the issues in ED and FSD, as detailed in Table 25-9.

TABLE 25-9 Sexual Dysfunction

ASSESSMENT	DIAGNOSIS	PLANNING	INTERVENTION	EVALUATION
1. Genital anatomy 2. Sexual identity and sexual behaviors 3. Sex drive 4. Fatigue 5. Emotional lability 6. Painful intercourse 7. Cultural influences 8. Partner availability 9. Available private time 10. Baseline function 11. Couple's connectedness 12. Erectile dysfunction, ejaculatory dysfunction, or anorgasmia 13. Depression 14. Comorbidities 15. Fears related to sexually transmitted disease 16. Medications	1. Ineffective sexuality patterns	1. Explore client's patterns of functioning. 2. Discuss relationship between sexual functioning and life stressors. 3. Reaffirm need for candid discussion between partners. 4. Identify and problem solve acute or chronic illness and other contributing factors.	Use the PLISSIT model: 1. **P**ermission: convey a willingness to discuss sexual matters. 2. **L**imited **i**nformation: provide some information on likely situations and treatments. 3. **S**pecific **s**uggestions: offer some specific instructions based on client's acknowledged situation. 4. **I**ntensive **t**herapy: refer client to appropriate therapist, counselor, or physician.	1. The client will achieve satisfactory sexual function.

Continued

TABLE 25-9 Sexual Dysfunction—cont'd

ASSESSMENT	DIAGNOSIS	PLANNING	INTERVENTION	EVALUATION
17. Job or financial worries 18. Values or relationship conflicts 19. Alcohol or drug use 20. Energy level 21. Laboratory abnormalities				

Data from Carpenito-Moyet LJ: *Nursing diagnosis: application to clinical practice*, ed 10, Philadelphia, 2004, JB Lippincott.

Home Care

1. Regularly assess homebound older adults diagnosed with endocrine disorders for signs and symptoms indicating exacerbation or instability.
2. Instruct caregivers and homebound older adults about reportable signs and symptoms related to the endocrine problems being monitored and about when to report these changes to the home care nurse or health care provider.
3. Instruct caregivers and homebound older adults on types, dosage, and technique of administering insulin. Have caregivers and homebound older adults do a return demonstration of this skill. Ensure that they receive written instructions to assist them in the learning process.
4. Instruct caregivers and homebound older adults about laboratory indications used to evaluate endocrine disorders. Inform them of the results of the tests after the health care provider has been notified.
5. Instruct caregivers and homebound older adults on safety tips related to insulin injection. Injecting Humulin insulin and then switching to beef or pork insulin without a physician order results in altering the times of insulin action, initiation, peak insulin action, and duration of insulin action.
6. Instruct caregivers and homebound older adults on diabetes management.
7. Instruct caregivers and homebound older adults on the proper dosage of medications used to treat hormone imbalances associated with endocrine disorders.

SUMMARY

This chapter discussed endocrine aging as an increased molecular disorderliness of the regulatory mechanisms, which results in reduced vitality of the overall person. It described a new "ensemble view" in terms of decreased estrogen production in women (menopause), decreased testosterone production in men (andropause), decreased adrenal function (adrenopause), and decreased growth hormone–insulin-like growth factor 1 (somatopause). The chapter scanned the current literature on aging endocrine physiology and discovered a vast horizon of new knowledge. Finally, the nursing process was applied to some of the most common endocrine diseases affecting older adults.

Key Points

- The endocrine system is regulated by feedback systems that involve a chemical connection between structures of the brain, peripheral glands, and hormones. The feedback loops regulate hormone production.
- A hypo functioning state is one that results from inadequate endocrine secretions.
- A hyper functioning state is one that results from excessive secretion of hormones.
- Endocrine pathology may also be manifested in the form of hormone resistance, a condition in which there is an inadequate tissue response to hormones. Resistance can be caused by a genetic defect or can be acquired, as in the case of type 2 diabetes mellitus.
- Older adults experience andropause and menopause as a decline in biosyntheses of their dominant sex hormones occurs.
- Adrenopause and somatopause are changes that occur as the result of aging.
- Metabolic syndrome is rapidly increasing in the older population. It is caused by improper nutrition, inadequate physical activity, and obesity.
- Type 2 diabetes mellitus is very common in the older population.
- The most important variables associated with type 2 diabetes mellitus are obesity and insulin resistance.
- Older individuals with type 2 diabetes mellitus should strive for proper control of their blood glucose to reduce the risk for potential complication.
- A comprehensive nursing assessment of older clients with type 2 diabetes mellitus includes assessment of the client's feet, knowledge of diabetes management (e.g., of diet,

desirable weight, exercise, medications, and treatment of hypoglycemia and hyperglycemia), learning styles, and emergency identification.

- Management of serious wounds in older clients with diabetes optimally needs to involve a multidisciplinary health team.

  Thyroid disorders are more common among persons and more difficult to diagnose than in the younger population.

- Primary hypothyroidism in older persons may often be unnoticed or indiscernible. Symptoms of mild depression, apathy, decreased appetite, weight loss, and weakness should be investigated.
- Thyroid homone replacement should always be carefully monitored; follow-up appointments are essential for incremental dosing over several weeks.
- Hyperthyroidism may have an atypical presentation in older adults. Symptoms often include apathy, tiredness, weakness, anorexia, weight loss, angina heart failure, atrial fibrillation, and absence of thyroid changes.
- Older adults need to be taught the actions and side effects of prescribed medications and the need for lifelong monitoring of thyroid status.

Critical Thinking Exercises

1. Compare the endocrine gland function of a 70-year-old man with that of a 30-year-old man.
2. A 64-year-old woman was recently diagnosed with metabolic syndrome. She is sedentary, has a BMI of over 30, and has abdominal obesity. What three issues would you prepare to teach the client about her condition?
3. A 72-year-old man was recently diagnosed with insulin-dependent diabetes mellitus. While teaching him to administer 70/30 Humulin insulin, you note that he is unable to draw up the correct number of units into a syringe. What further information do you need about your client before proceeding with your teaching plan?

References

American Diabetes Association: Diagnosis and classification of diabetes mellitus, *Diabetes Care* 27:S5, 2004.

Arauz-Pacheo C: Dealing with global risks in a shrinking world: detabolic syndrome, *Primary Care Update,* Presbyterian Hospital of Dallas, 2004.

Arvat E et al: Neuroendocrinology of the human growth hormone–insulin-like growth factor I axis during aging, *Growth Hormone IGF Research* 9:111, 1999.

Bain J: Andropause: testosterone replacement therapy for aging men, *Canadian Fam Phys* 47:91, 2001.

Beers MH, Berkow R, editors: *Merck manual of geriatrics,* 2000-2005, Merck. Accessed on Oct 16, 2004, from website: http://www.merck.com/mrkshared/mm_geriatrics/home.jsp.

Berman JR et al: Clinical evaluation of female sexual function: effects of age and estrogen status on sexual arousal responses in 60 women, abstract 651. In *Program and abstracts of the American Urological Association 95th Annual Meeting,* April 29–May 4, 2000, Atlanta.

Black D: Bone density, bone quality and fracture risk. In 22nd Annual Meeting of the American Society for Bone and Mineral Research, 2000. Accessed Oct 4, 2004, from website: http://www.medscape.com/viewprogram/.

Blackburn GL, Bevis LC: *The obesity epidemic: prevention and treatment of the metabolic syndrome, 2003.* Accessed Oct 1, 2004, from website: http://www.medscape.com/viewprogram/2015_pnt.

Carpenito-Moyet LJ: *Nursing diagnosis: application to clinical practice,* ed 10, Philadelphia, 2004, JB Lippincott.

Colleen S: *Screening for common endocrine disorders in the primary care setting,* presentation at Endo 2003: the Endocrine Society 85th Annual Meeting, June 19-22, 2003, Philadelphia.

Copstead LE, Banasik JK: *Pathophysiology,* ed 3, St Louis, 2005, Elsevier.

Cufson TM, Meuleman E: Managing menopause, *Am Fam Phys* 61(5):1391, 2000.

DeGroot LJ: Treatment of multimodular goiter by surgery, *J Endocrinol Investigations* 24(10):820-822, 2001.

Devine A, Prince RL, Bell R: Nutritional effect of Ca supplementation by skim milk powder or Ca tablets on total nutritional intake in post-menopausal women, *Am J Clin Nutr* 64:731, 1996.

Falahati A, Riggs BL, Atkinson EJ: Estrogen, but not testosterone, prevents the increase in bone resorption following induction of hypogonadism and aromatase inhibition in normal elderly men, *J Bone Mineral Res* 15(suppl 1):S148, 2000.

Felicetta JV: The aging thyroid: its effects—and how it affects diagnosis and therapy, *Consultant,* April 1996.

Ford ES, Giles WH, Dietz WH: Prevalence of the metabolic syndrome among US adults: findings from the Third National Health and Nutrition Examination, *JAMA* 287(3):356-359, 2002.

Funnell MM, Merritt JH: The older adult with diabetes, *Nurse Pract* 9(2)98-107, 1998.

Genuth S, Palmer J, Zimmerman B: New diagnostic criteria for diabetes, *Patient Care for the Nurse Pract* February 1999.

Goldstein DJ: Beneficial health effects of a modest weight loss, *Int J Obesity* 16:397, 1992.

Gould DC, Petty R, Jacobs HS: For and against: the male menopause—does it exist? *Br Med J* 320:858, 2000.

Guyton AC: *Textbook of medical physiology,* Philadelphia, 1986, WB Saunders.

Heaney RP: There should be a dietary guideline for calcium, *Am J Clin Nutr* 71:658, 2000.

Kennedy JW, Caro JF: The ABCs of managing hyperthyroidism in the older patient, *Geriatrics* 51(5), May 1996.

Imbeault P et al: Aging per se does not influence glucose homeostasis, *Diabetes Care* 26(2):480, 2003.

Kennedy JW, Caro JF: The ABCs of managing hyperthyroidism in the older patient, *Geriatrics* vol 15, no 5, May 1996.

Kreier F et al: Hypothesis: shifting the equilibrium from activity to food leads to autonomic imbalance and the metabolic syndrome, *Diabetes* 52(11):2652, 2003.

Lamberts S, van den Beld A, van der Lely A: The endocrinology of aging, *Science* 278:419, 1997.

Le CM, Tuck ML: Diabetes mellitus: how it differs in the elderly, *Consultant,* 1994.

Manolagas SC: Birth and death of bone cells: basic regulatory mechanisms and implications for the pathogenesis and treatment of osteoporosis, *Endocrinol Rev* 21:115, 2000.

Masiukiewicz US at al: Interleukin-6 mediates increased skeletal sensitivity to parathyroid hormone in postmenopausal women, *J Bone Mineral Res* 15(suppl 1):S148, 2000.

McCance KL, Huether SE: *Pathophysiology,* St Louis, 1998, Mosby.

Meneilly GS et al: Effects of 3 months of continuous subcutaneous administration of glucagon-like peptide 1 in elderly patients with type 2 diabetes, *Diabetes Care* 26(10):2835, 2003.

Morales A, Heaton JP, Carson CC: Andropause: a misnomer for a true clinical entity, *J Urol* 163:705, 2000.

Munarriz R, Talakoub L, Lahey N: Hormone, sexual function and personal sexual distress (SDS) outcomes following dehydroepiandrosterone (DHEA) treatment for female sexual dysfunction (FSD) and androgen deficiency syndrome (ADS), abstract 1116. In *Program and abstracts of the 96th Annual Meeting of the American Urological Association*, June 2-7, 2001, Anaheim, Calif.

National Health and Nutrition Examination Survey, 1999. Accessed on Jan 9, 2003, from website: http://www.nhlbi.nih.gov/guidelines.

National Heart, Lung, and Blood Institute/National Institute on Diabetes and Digestive and Kidney Diseases (NHLBI/NIDDK)

www.niddk.nih.gov/federal/dmicc/grundy.ppt

New SA: *Dietary and nutritional influences on skeletal health—a review of current knowledge and future perspectives*, presentation at 22nd Annual Meeting of the American Society for Bone and Mineral Research, 2000. Accessed on Oct 4, 2004, from website: http://www.medscape.com/view program/.

Perez G, Tilly J: Cumulus cells are required for the increased apoptotic potential in oocytes of aged mice, *Human Reprod* 12:2781, 1997.

Porst H: (2002). *Expanding treatment options for erectile dysfunction*, presentation 4th Congress of the European Society for Sexual and Impotence Research (ESSIR), Oct 2, 2001, Rome. Accessed Oct 4, 2004, from website: http://www.medscape.com.

Pratt JSA, Blackburn GL: Surgical approaches to the treatment of obesity: a practical guide for the covering physician. In Bray GA, editor: *Office management of obesity*, ed 1, Philadelphia, 2003, Elsevier.

Quan MA: PriMed presentation Working toward the three "Rs" for managing depression: managing sexual dysfunction, Oct 17, 2004, Dallas. Risks and benefits of estrogen plus progestin in healthy postmenopausal women: principal results from the Women's Health Initiative randomized controlled trial, *JAMA* 288(3):321, 2004.

Ringel MD, Cooper DS: Detection and management of hyperthyroidism: special considerations, *Hosp Med* 32(6), June 1996.

Rosen R. et al: Lower urinary tract symptoms and male sexual dysfunction: the multinational survey of the aging male, *Eur Urol* 44:637, 2003.

Rubin SA, Levin ER: The endocrinology of vasoactive peptides: synthesis to function, *J Clin Endocrine Metab* 78(1):6, 1994.

Seeman E: *Treatment for osteoporosis: new drugs and new data on old drugs*, presentation at 22nd Annual Meeting of the American Society for Bone and Mineral Research, 2000. Accessed Oct 4, 2004, from website: *http://www.medscape.com/viewprogram/*.

Singer et al: Treatment guidelines for patients with hyperthyroidism and hypothyroidism, *JAMA* 273(10), March 8, 1995.

Smith NL et al: Esterified estrogens and conjugated estrogens and the risk of venous thrombosis, *JAMA* 292(13):1581, 2004.

Speaker BL: Should there be a dietary guideline for calcium intake? No, *Am J Clin Nutr* 71:661, 2000.

Talakoub L et al: Multidisciplinary evaluation of female sexual dysfunction, abstract 1110. In *Program and abstracts of the 96th Annual Meeting of the American Urological Association*, June 2-7, 2001, Anaheim, Calif.

Tenover JL: Testosterone and the aging male, *J Andrology* 18:103, 1997.

Third Report of the National Cholesterol Education Program (NCEP): Expert panel on detection, evaluation, and treatment of high blood cholesterol in adults (adult treatment panel III), NIH Pub No 01-3670, Bethesda, Jd, 2001, NHLBI Health Information Center.

Thomas CL: *Taber's cyclopedic medical dictionary*, Philadelphia, 1979, Davis.

Thyroid Foundation of America: Thyroid disease in the elderly, 1999. Accessed via website http://www.clark.net/pub/tfa/brochure/ brochure-elderly.html.

Van Cauter E et al: Alteration of circadian rhythmicity and sleep in aging: endocrine consequences, *Hormone Res* 49:147, 1998.

Veldhuis JD: *Endocrinology of aging*, conference report, 2000. Accessed Oct 4, 2004, from website: http://www.medscape.com/viewarticle/407921.

Veldhuis JD, Iranmanesh A: Pathophysiology of impoverished growth hormone secretion in aging. In *Toward a healthier old age: biomedical advances from basic research to clinical science*, Barcelona, 1999, Prous Science Publishers.

Veldhuis JD, Iranmanesh A, Mulligan T: Current insights into hypothalamo-pituitary mechanisms of reproductive aging in men. In *Toward a healthier old age: biomedical advances from basic research to clinical science*, Barcelona, 1999, Prous Science Publishers.

Vetrosky DT, Aliabadi Z: The andropause debate: aging process or disease state? *Clin Rev* 12(3):78, 2002.

Wadden TA et al: Benefits of lifestyle modification in the pharmacologic treatment of obesity: a randomized trial, *Arch Intern Med* 161:218, 2001.

Wallace JI: Management of diabetes in the elderly, *Clin Diabetes* 17(1), 1999.

Wallace K, Hofmann MT: Thyroid dysfunction: how to manage overt and subclinical disease in older patients, *Geriatrics* 53(4), 1998.

Walfish PG: *Health guides on thyroid disease #10: thyroid disease in later life*, 1996, Thyroid Foundation of Canada.

Walker RF: *Is aging a disease?* A review of the Serono Symposia Workshop held under the auspices of the Third World Congress on the Aging Male, Feb 9, 2002, Berlin.

Women's Health Initiative: *www.nhlbi.nih.gov/whi/index.html*, Washington, DC, 2002, The Agency

World Health Organization: *Definition, diagnosis and classification of diabetes mellitus and its complications: report of a WHO consultation*, Geneva, 1999, The Organization.

Wu CJ, Yu ZR: Effects on blood glucose, insulin, lipid, and proatherosclerotic parameters in stable type 2 diabetic subjects during an oral fat challenge, *Lipids Health Dis* 3:17, 2004.

Wyne KL, Bell DSH: An algorithm for managing type 2 diabetes: a focus on the disease process, not just the sugar, *Clin Geriatrics* Aug 2004.

Helpful Resources

American Association of Clinical Endocrinologists
http://www.aace.com/serv/other

American College of Obstetricians and Gynecologists
www.acog.com

Human Genome Project Information
http://www.ornl.gov/TechResources/Human_Genome/home.html

Menopause
www.menopause.com

National Institute of Diabetes and Digestive and Kidney Disease of the National Institutes of Health
http://www.niddk.nih.gov/

Nutrition and Your Health: Dietary Guidelines for Americans—USDA
http://www.health.gov/dietaryguidelines/

Office of Disease Prevention and Health Promotion
http://odphp.osophs.dhhs.gov/

Physical Activity Readiness Questionnaire (PAR-Q)
www.d.umn.edu/student/loon/soc/phys/par-q.html

The Practical Guide: Identification, Evaluation and Treatment of Overweight and Obesity in Adults
http://www.nhlbi.nih.gov/guidelines/obesity/practgde.htm

26 Gastrointestinal Function

LINDA A. STAMM, APRN, BC, CON, and
ROBYN A. LEVY, MSN, RN, BC, ANP

Learning Objectives

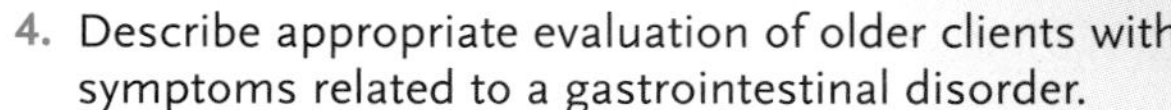

On completion of this chapter, the reader will be able to:

1. Describe the age-related physiologic and functional changes in the gastrointestinal system.
2. Explain primary and secondary preventive care related to the gastrointestinal tract for older clients and the rationalizations for such care.
3. Discuss the alterations of normal structure and function accompanying common gastrointestinal diseases of older adults.
4. Describe appropriate evaluation of older clients with symptoms related to a gastrointestinal disorder.
5. Describe the cause, incidence, and pathophysiology of the various types of gastrointestinal disorders, including cancer and liver disease.
6. Discuss the nursing management of gastrointestinal disorders in older adults.
7. Write an appropriate care plan for an older client with a gastrointestinal disorder.

The gastrointestinal (GI) system, including the accessory organs of digestion, functions in the ingestion, digestion, and absorption of nutrients essential for life and growth, as well as in the excretion of solid wastes from the body. GI system– related symptoms and complaints are common with advancing age, and the nurse is often the first health care provider to identify and to acknowledge these. Therefore knowledge of normal, age-related changes in the GI system and appropriate management methods is essential.

AGE-RELATED CHANGES IN STRUCTURE AND FUNCTION

Although many health-related complaints from older adults pertain to the GI system, these complaints are rarely responsible for death. Older individuals are usually very aware of alterations in GI function, and many of these changes can be ameliorated through appropriate self-care practices. Some changes in the GI tract are due to normal aging; however, poor habits such as drugs, stress, poor nutrition, and poor hygiene all contribute to the problem (Bottomley and Lewis, 2003; Lewis, Heitkemper, and Dirksen, 2004). Just as often, misinformation about GI changes can lead to more complex problems because of failure to seek health care or engage in appropriate treatment measures. The nurse has the responsibility for teaching prevention and self-management strategies to these clients.

Many of the systemic changes in the functions of digestion and absorption of nutrients result from changes in older clients' cardiovascular and neurologic systems, rather than their GI systems. For example, arteriosclerosis and other cardiovascular problems may cause a decrease in splanchnic and mesenteric blood flow, leading to a decrease in absorption in the small intestine. Additionally, the motility of the entire GI system is affected by the central and peripheral nervous systems, and any change there may alter peristalsis, thereby reducing or increasing transit time. Chronic illnesses that involve the neurologic system may also have GI complications such as increased gastric reflux and fecal incontinence. For example, the peripheral neuropathy associated with diabetes predisposes older adults to gastroparesis (Lewis, Heitkemper, and Dirksen, 2004).

Oral Cavity and Pharynx

Changes in the oral cavity have an effect not only on an older person's well-being, comfort, and health, but also on overall nutrition and digestion. The most obvious change in the mouth is the loss of teeth. It is suggested that about half the people in the United States who are 65 years or older wear dentures. Many other older clients are edentulous (without teeth), and the teeth that are present are often diseased or decayed. A common cause of loss of teeth in older adults is periodontal disease, which damages the tissue surrounding the teeth and supporting bones. The surface of the teeth may also be mechanically worn down (Coleman, 2002).

Taste buds may atrophy with age, resulting in an inability to discriminate among flavors, especially salty and sweet. This may contribute to decreases enjoyment of food, resulting in poor eating habits and nutritional deficiencies (Miller, 2004).

The amount of saliva produced does not significantly decrease in healthy older adults, but medications and disease processes do cause 30% of adults to experience xerostomia (dry mouth) (Ghezzi et al, 2000; Ship, Pillemer, and Baum, 2002).

Healthy People 2010 reflects on the importance of oral health as an integral component of healthy life. Poor oral health and disease conditions have a significant impact on the older adult's feelings of self-esteem and depression. One of the goals of *Healthy People 2010* is the access to preventive and early intervention to oral care for older adults (US Department of Health and Human Services, 2000).

Esophagus

Many of the age-related changes in the esophagus result in a decline in its motility. Degenerative changes in the smooth muscle lining the lower esophagus may contribute to a change in the amplitude of contractions, an increased resting pressure, and increased numbers of disordered contractions. This decrease in intensity of propulsive waves and increase in frequency of nonperistaltic waves may result in a condition known as presbyesophagus (Miller, 2004). Whether this is a clinically significant problem is still being debated. Neurogenic, hormonal, and vascular changes may also contribute to a decrease in esophageal motility. These changes may lead to complaints of dysphagia, heartburn, or vomiting of undigested foods; these symptoms may lead to poor nutrition, dehydration, and decreased food intake as a result of a fear of the recurrence of symptoms.

Stomach

Age-related changes in the stomach include degeneration of the gastric mucosa, decreased secretion of gastric acids and digestive enzymes, and decreased motility (Lewis, Heitkemper, and Dirksen, 2004). Researchers agree that when large amounts of food are consumed by the older adult, gastric emptying is slowed. Early satiation (feeling full with less food intake) is common in older adults and may be explained by delayed gastric emptying (Morley, 2002).

By the age of 60, gastric secretions decrease to 70% to 80% of those of the average adult. A decrease in pepsin may hinder protein digestion, whereas a decrease in hydrochloric acid and intrinsic factor may lead to malabsorption of iron, vitamin B_{12}, calcium, and folic acid. This, combined with atrophy of the mucosa and a decrease in protective juices, increases the incidence of pernicious anemia, peptic ulcer disease (PUD), and stomach cancer.

Small Intestine

Age-related changes in the small intestine include atrophy of the muscle and mucosal surfaces, thinning of the villi, and a decrease in epithelial cells. This results in some decrease in the absorption of fats and vitamin B_{12}; however, there do not seem to be significant alterations in digestion and absorption of nutrients (Miller, 2004). Since these age-related changes in the small intestine are usually not enough to cause any significant impairment, any change in function reported by older adults should be addressed seriously in the search for an underlying pathologic inflammation or infection.

Large Intestine

Age-related changes in the large intestine include a decrease in mucous secretion and in the elasticity of the rectal wall, but no documented changes in motility. The tone of the internal anal sphincter decreases, which may lead to incontinence or incomplete emptying of the bowel. Nerve impulses that usually indicate the need to defecate may be dulled. This may account for the increased incidence of constipation (Lewis, Heitkemper, and Dirksen, 2004). In addition, the incidence of diverticula increases, which may or may not cause symptoms.

Gallbladder

The gallbladder and bile ducts are unaffected by aging. However, the incidence of gallstones does increase with age (Lewis, Heitkemper, and Dirksen, 2004). Bile may become more lithogenic with advancing age, possibly because of an increase in biliary cholesterol related to diet and hormonal changes that affect cholesterol metabolism. The bile salt pool also decreases as a result of a decrease in bile salt synthesis. These predispositions for stone development, along with a tendency for dehydration in older adults, explain the increased incidence of cholelithiasis and cholecystitis in older adults. The complications of cholelithiasis in older adults include empyema, perforation, and choledocholithiasis, which are seen in persons over age 65 and those with diabetes (Lyder and Moloney, 2003).

Pancreas

The pancreas shows some age-related changes, such as fibrosis, fatty acid deposits, and atrophy, but size is not affected (Lewis, Heitkemper, and Dirksen, 2004). However, the volume of pancreatic secretions declines after the age of 40, and enzyme output diminishes with advancing age. This decrease in enzyme activity affects the digestion of fats and may account for a vague intolerance of fatty foods in older adults. There is increased incidence of pancreatic cancer in older adults, as well as increased incidence of pancreatitis.

Liver

The liver is a sturdy organ and retains most of its functions throughout the life span. After age 50, as the lean body mass decreases, so does the size of the liver. A decline in cardiac output associated with aging contributes to a decrease in hepatic blood flow. As hepatic blood flow slows, there is a reduced drug metabolism and slow clearance of hepatitis B surface antigen (Smeltzer and Bare, 2004). Some evidence suggests that normal aging may adversely affect liver tissue regeneration. The mechanism of this effect is not fully known, but it may be a result of a generalized slowing of repair or an inadequate response to regeneration of liver tissue.

PREVENTION

Although some changes in the GI system are associated with aging, there are strategies for both primary and secondary prevention of problems associated with aging (Boxes 26-1 and 26-2). Nurses caring for older clients should include instruction regarding these strategies in their care plan, and should reinforce and remind clients on an annual basis.

BOX 26-1 Gastrointestinal Primary Prevention Strategies for Older Adults

ORAL HYGIENE AND PREVENTIVE DENTAL CARE

- Daily flossing and brushing
- Semiannual, professional dental care
- Properly fitting dentures

NUTRITION

- Foods that are low in fat and high in fiber
- Small portions
- Variety of food textures, odors, and colors
- Basic food groups (see the Food Guide Pyramid in Chapter 10)
- Change in recommended daily allowances for older adults:
  - — Decrease in calories
  - — Decrease in amount of B vitamins
  - — Decrease in iron for postmenopausal women
  - — Increase in calcium
- Avoidance of spicy or irritating foods (e.g., hot pepper, coffee)
- Maintenance of daily fluid intake of 2000 ml (unless cardiac status contraindicates it)

HABITS

- Avoidance of tobacco products (e.g., cigarettes, pipe or cigar smoking, chewing tobacco)
- Avoidance of large amounts of alcohol

ELIMINATION

- Maintenance of regular bowel routines
- Not avoiding the urge to defecate
- Avoidance of laxatives, suppositories, and enemas

SLEEP AND REST

- Maintenance of activity level
- Adequate sleep

Compiled from Miller C: *Nursing for wellness in older adults: theory and practice*, ed 4, Philadelphia, 2004, Lippincott Williams & Wilkins.

COMMON GASTROINTESTINAL SYMPTOMS

No clear-cut GI diseases can be attributed directly to the aging process. However, many conditions show a higher incidence in older adults and have a greater effect on older clients, physical and social well-being. These complaints can be related to normal physiologic changes with aging but must be

BOX 26-2 Gastrointestinal Secondary Prevention and Early Detection Strategies for Older Adults

AMERICAN CANCER SOCIETY RECOMMENDATIONS FOR SCREENING FOR COLORECTAL CANCER (2004)

Adults at average risk should begin colorectal cancer screening at age 50, using one of the following options for screening:

1. Annual fecal occult blood test
2. Flexible sigmoidoscopy every 5 years
3. Annual fecal occult blood test plus flexible sigmoidoscopy every 5 years
4. Double-contrast barium enema every 5 years
5. Colonoscopy every 10 years

The American Cancer Society recommends more intensive surveillance for:

1. Persons at increased risk due to a history of adenomatous polyps
2. Persons with a history of curative-intent resection of colorectal cancer
3. Persons with a family history of either colorectal cancer or colorectal adenomas diagnosed in a first-degree relative before age 60 years
4. Persons at significantly higher risk due to a history of inflammatory bowel disease of significant duration
5. Persons at significantly higher risk due to a family history of or genetic testing indicating the presence of one hereditary syndrome

OTHER "RED FLAGS" REQUIRING MEDICAL FOLLOW-UP:

Mouth

Sore that does not heal
Any lump
Persistent red or white patch
Difficulty or pain with chewing or swallowing

Stomach

Persistent indigestion or heartburn
Abdominal pain
Persistent nausea or vomiting

Elimination

Any change in bowel habits
Presence of any blood in stool; black stool

From Lewis S, Heitkemper M, Dirksen S: *Medical-surgical nursing: assessment and management of clinical problems*, ed 6, St Louis, 2004, Mosby; Smith R, Cokkinides V, Eyre H: American Cancer Society Guidelines for the Early Detection of Cancer, *Cancer J Clin* 54:41, 2004.

distinguished from the pathologic problems that increase in frequency in older adults.

Older adults may complain of symptoms related to the GI tract that have not yet been related to a diagnosis. Any symptom reported by an older client needs to be thoroughly assessed, whether or not it has a known or probable cause. The following are a few of the common GI symptoms experienced by older adults; the sections include information on definition, assessment, nursing interventions, and self-care measures. (For more on nursing assessment as it relates to various cultures, see Chapter 5.)

Nausea and Vomiting

Vomiting is controlled through a central vomiting center in the medulla. This center is close to the pain and respiratory centers; it is also near the centers that control vestibular and vasomotor function. Occasionally stimuli from one center spill over to another and symptoms may become mixed. No distinct nausea center exists; however, the symptom of nausea may result from early stimulation of the vomiting center (Fig. 26-1).

Nausea may be difficult for clients to describe; many use the phrase "I feel sick" to convey the symptom of nausea. It is important to keep in mind that although nausea usually precedes vomiting, it may also be a freestanding symptom. In general, nausea in the absence of vomiting is of central, rather than peripheral, origin (i.e., the symptom is initiated centrally in the brain rather than peripherally in the GI tract). Central nausea is usually a response to a metabolic disorder.

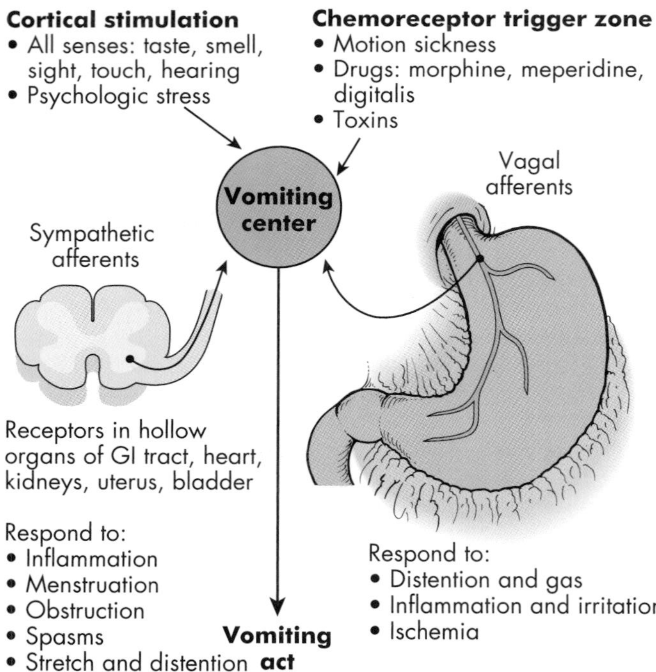

Fig. 26-1 Stimuli involved in the act of vomiting. (From Lewis S, Heitkemper M, Dirksen S: *Medical-surgical nursing: assessment and management of clinical problems*, ed 6, St Louis, 2004, Mosby.)

It is important to obtain a detailed description of events surrounding a complaint of nausea and vomiting. Data should be elicited about precipitating factors (e.g., the relationship of nausea and vomiting to food intake, medications, and activity). The client should be questioned about the presence of nausea and vomiting, as well as diarrhea or constipation. It is important to obtain information about the amount and characteristics of the emesis and whether the vomitus contained food particles, bile, or blood (bright red or "coffee grounds" color). Other symptoms such as fever, sweating, pallor, dizziness, and pain should be determined. Since older adults are at particular risk for dehydration and electrolyte imbalances, it is essential to establish the frequency and amount of emesis and to examine clients for signs and symptoms of fluid and electrolyte imbalances.

Nursing interventions include many self-help measures, including dietary changes such as drinking clear liquids; progressing from eating bland foods to solid foods; and small, frequent feedings. If vomiting occurs, fluid replacement should be a priority. Sips of soda every 15 minutes until more can be tolerated may decrease episodes of dehydration. Older adults are at high risk for aspiration, and they should be placed in a semi-Fowler's or side-lying position when drinking liquids. For older clients, instruction concerning the signs and symptoms of dehydration and electrolyte imbalances, as well as when to seek medical care, is important. Any episodes of prolonged nausea or vomiting require careful evaluation by a health care provider.

Anorexia

Anorexia as a symptom should not be confused with anorexia nervosa, which is an eating disorder of psychiatric significance. The term *anorexia* literally means "lack of appetite." Hunger and appetite are not synonymous; hunger is related to the physiologic need for food. It is important for the nurse to ascertain whether the decreased food intake is truly because of a loss of appetite. Once that is determined, the nurse must ask questions regarding other symptoms, including weight loss, nausea, vomiting, abdominal pain, diarrhea, and constipation. In addition, psychosocial factors such as stress, grief, pain, and concomitant illnesses may also need to be assessed.

Nursing interventions for older clients with anorexia include monitoring of intake, output, and weight. It is important to acknowledge a client's symptoms and provide gentle encouragement for him or her to eat for nutritional purposes. Small, frequent feedings may be helpful. Encouraging older clients to seek medical attention for anorexia is also important because clients may not be aware it is a problem.

Abdominal Pain

The symptom of abdominal pain is often difficult to assess fully. With older adults, it can be even more difficult, even for a skilled clinician. The assessment of pain can be made easier by thinking in terms of the three pathways for pain impulses. The first types are the visceral pain pathways, which are activated by receptors in the wall of the abdominal viscera and develop from stretching or distending the abdominal wall or from inflammation. This pain is often diffuse; is poorly localized; and has a gnawing, burning, or cramping quality. The second types are somatic or parietal pathways, which are activated by receptors in the parietal peritoneum and other supporting tissues. This type of pain is usually sharp, more intense, constant, and better localized than visceral pain. The third types are referral pathways, which account for referred pain (i.e., pain felt at a different site than the source of the pain, but sharing the same dermatome). This pain is usually sharp and well localized; it may resemble somatic pain (Fig. 26-2).

In assessing any type of pain, the nurse should elicit information about its duration, location, mode of onset, intensity, character, rhythm, relationship to food, alleviating and aggravating factors, and accompanying symptoms. Vague abdominal symptoms seen in older adults should be monitored closely to promote early recognition of emergent or atypical presentations (Lyder and Molony, 2003).

Nursing interventions include measures to increase comfort and pain relief. Again, the nurse should encourage older clients to see their health care provider for a complete evaluation of the abdominal pain. Abdominal pain that is severe is often known as an acute abdomen. Nursing procedures commonly done for an acute abdomen include (1) start intravenous fluids as ordered; (2) place a nasogastric tube for decompression of the stomach; (3) monitor and record vital signs and report abnormal findings; (4) monitor intake and output frequently and record accurate amounts hourly; (5) complete an assessment on the onset of pain, presence of vomiting or diarrhea, presence of fever, and an accurate medical and surgical history.

Gas

Complaints come in the form of belching, bloating, or fullness, and flatus. About 99% of the gas present in the GI tract of adults comprises five gases: nitrogen, oxygen, hydrogen, carbon dioxide, and methane. The percentage of each individual gas depends on the source; these sources include swallowing, diffusion of gas from the bloodstream to the intestinal lumen, and processing of food. All these gases are odorless; the unpleasant odor associated with flatus is probably a result of hydrogen sulfide that is metabolized from sulfur-containing foods. A frequency of 7 to 20 gas passages a

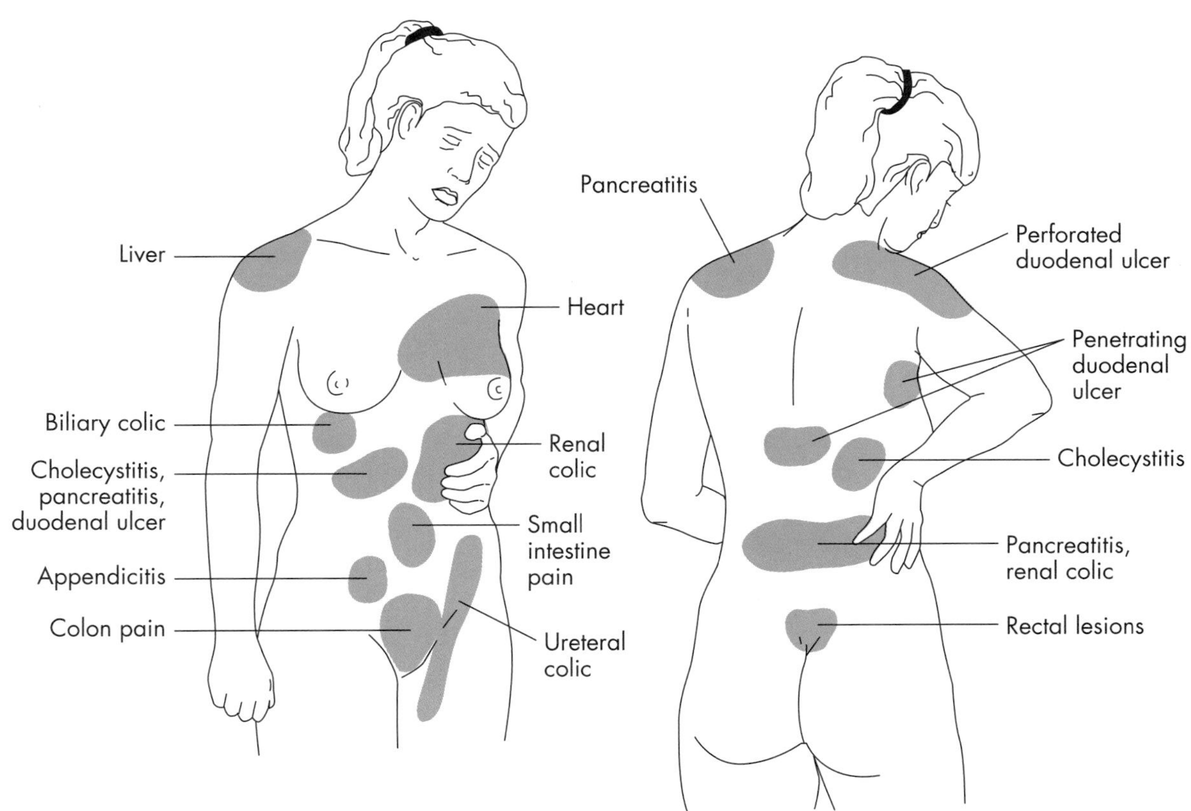

Fig. 26-2 Common sites of referred abdominal pain. (From Phipps W et al: *Medical-surgical nursing: health and illness perspectives*, ed 7, St Louis, 2003, Mosby.)

day is considered normal. Intestinal gas is frequently accompanied by intense abdominal pain, which may be relieved by positioning or walking.

Although belching primarily comes from the unconscious swallowing of air, it is important to assess clients for other symptoms suggestive of gastritis or PUD. Many complaints of bloating and fullness are related to a motility disorder or malabsorption, but in older adults the complaints must be taken more seriously. Further assessment is required, such as questioning about changes in bowel function, pain, and other GI tract symptoms.

Although the expulsion of flatus is a normal event, excessive flatus may have several causes. Some clients form more gas within the gut, some swallow a lot of air, and others may have excessive flatus because of the nature of the foods consumed. Frequent offenders are air-containing foods such as whipped foods, carbonated beverages, and certain fruits; gas-forming foods such as beans and legumes; and sulfur-containing foods such as eggs. In addition, clients who are lactose intolerant may produce more gas (see Chapter 10). Careful questioning may reveal one or a combination of these causes.

Nursing interventions focus on client education about the cause and nature of intestinal gas. The keys to treatment are changes in dietary factors (e.g., focusing on eating more slowly, avoiding gas-producing foods) and a routine exercise plan.

Diarrhea

Diarrhea is an increase in the frequency of stools, but many definitions also include a change in consistency (e.g., watery stools). Diarrhea may be due to increased bowel motility or interference in the normal absorption of water and nutrients in the bowel. When an older client complains of diarrhea, it is important to ascertain exactly what is meant. In addition, the description of the diarrhea may be useless unless a client's normal bowel habits are known.

Questions to ask when assessing a client with diarrhea include those regarding onset (recent or acute), precipitating events (travel out of the country, eating at a restaurant), timing (intermittent or continuous), associated factors (fever, weight loss, abdominal pain, vomiting, dietary or medication changes, any systemic diseases), characteristics of the diarrhea (frequency, consistency, volume, foul smell, presence of mucus or blood, incontinence, awakening from sleep [e.g., nocturnal diarrhea usually points to an organic cause rather than a functional or infectious cause]). All these questions help assess the diarrhea further to aid in determining the cause.

Nursing care focuses on maintaining adequate hydration and nutrition, assessing for complications, and providing emotional support as necessary. Usual water loss in stools is 150 ml/day; severe diarrhea can account for up to 5 to 10 L of water loss daily. Therefore assessing for signs and symptoms of dehydration and volume depletion in older clients is important. Clients and their families need to learn to report complications, such as increased thirst, weakness, dizziness, palpitations, and fatigue. If fluid and electrolyte imbalances occur, either oral or parenteral treatment may be required, since diarrhea in older adults can be life threatening. Nursing interventions should also be aimed at identifying and correcting the cause. Depending on the causative factor, antispasmodic and antidiarrheal medications may be used. Education of clients and their families should also include dietary changes such as avoiding gas-forming foods, vegetables, spices, and milk products (for chronic diarrhea) and eating bland foods, such as the BRAT (*b*ananas, *r*ice, *a*pplesauce, *t*oast) diet and clear liquids (for acute diarrhea).

Constipation

Constipation has been broadly defined as an abnormally infrequent or difficult passage of hard, dry feces. Failure to relieve the constipation may result in a fecal impaction. Constipation can be acute or chronic in onset and either intermittent or constant in frequency. Constipation is not a disease, but a symptom with an underlying cause (Lyder and Molony, 2003).

Another aspect of this problem is that older clients may define constipation differently than their health care providers (Rao, 2003). For example, a client may have the misperception that one bowel movement a day is necessary for good health.

Common causes of constipation include diet (decreased fiber), medications (aluminum- and calcium-based antacids, iron preparations, anticholinergics, narcotics, antidepressants, antipsychotics, and overuse of laxatives), metabolic abnormalities (diabetes, hypothyroidism), motility abnormalities, inflammation, mechanical obstruction (fecal impaction, cancer), environmental changes (inability to reach toilet, lack of privacy), and depression (Miller, 2004; Smeltzer and Bare, 2004). Perhaps the most widespread cause of constipation in older adults is diet. It is usually a lack of certain foods, rather than the addition of certain foods, that leads to the problem. For example, many foods, such as fresh fruits and vegetables, contain natural laxatives, although older adults may have difficulty eating these foods because of dental problems. A second dietary cause of constipation is the lack of fiber or bulk and a decrease in fluid intake. In general, unrefined foods have more fiber than the refined foods that are popular in American society.

It is important to keep in mind that constipation can be a result of overuse or improper use of laxatives because of excessive concern about the frequency of bowel movements. In this instance the nurse can reinforce with a client and his or her family that as long as the consistency is normal and the bowel movements occur at regular intervals, there is no reason to take laxatives.

Constipation is treated through dietary measures such as increasing fluid intake and increasing fiber, combined with light exercise and development of a regular toileting routine that includes responding to the urge to defecate. In teaching older adults about dietary changes, the nurse can instruct them that fiber need not be a "medicine"; it can be a "food."

Multiple medications are available to treat constipation, and many of them are available over the counter. Laxatives are defined as drugs used to facilitate or stimulate the passage of feces and are classified as bulking agents (bran, psyllium), surfactants (stool softeners), emollients (mineral oil), contact stimulants (cascara, castor oil, bisacodyl), saline cathartics (magnesium hydroxide [Milk of Magnesia], citrate, sodium or potassium phosphate), and osmotic agents (lactulose, sorbitol). Laxatives may also be categorized by speed of action: group I drugs (castor oil, saline laxatives in high doses) act in 2 to 6 hours and produce watery stool; group II drugs (other contact stimulants, low-dose saline laxatives) act in 6 to 12 hours and produce a semiformed stool; and group III medications (bulking agents, surfactants, lactulose) produce soft stools in 1 to 3 days.

In addition to oral laxatives, several rectal agents are available. Enemas provide immediate relief but should be limited in their use for long-term treatment. Soap suds enemas should never be used because they lead to mucosal irritation. Small-volume enemas such as Fleets are the easiest to use. Rectal suppositories (bisacodyl, glycerin) may also be used, but they must be retained for 20 to 30 minutes for optimum results, and so may be more difficult for older clients to use.

Fecal Incontinence

Fecal incontinence, the involuntary passing of stool, may be acute or chronic, and it demands evaluation. For older adults the loss of bowel control is devastating and may significantly alter the quality of life. Fecal incontinence may be a result of colorectal lesions (perianal disease, proctitis, and tumors), neurologic problems (neuropathy, spinal cord lesions), laxative abuse, impaction, chronic diarrhea, stress, medications, or a general decline in muscle tone.

Nursing interventions focus on education concerning the prevention and treatment of incontinence in older adults. Examining the cause of the incontinence is important for the nurse, client, and family. Laxative abuse is completely preventable and treatable simply with education and reassurance to the client that one or two bowel movements a day are not necessary to be "regular."

Regardless of the cause, an older client who is aware of and distressed by incontinence can usually be helped by a program of bowel control (see Client/Family Teaching box). It is important to reassure older clients that control and retraining are achievable, since many older adults believe that fecal incontinence is the first step on the road to permanent institutionalization. Other nursing interventions include methods to deal with the embarrassment of the incontinence, ways to decrease fecal odor, use of adult diapers, and skin care. Maintenance of skin integrity is important to prevent skin breakdown (Hill, 2004).

Client/Family Teaching

BOWEL TRAINING PROGRAM

Provide a private, stress-free atmosphere.
Include family and older client in all teaching.
Explain the importance of responding to the urge to defecate.
Have client determine a specific time each day for bowel evacuation (e.g., after breakfast or dinner).
Have client sit on toilet or commode for evacuation.
Encourage high-fiber diet.
Encourage client to increase fluids to 2 L/day.
Avoid long-term or habitual use of laxatives; instead, use stool softeners, laxatives, suppositories or enemas only as needed.
Use psyllium seed bulking agents on a regular basis if dietary measures are not adequate.
Encourage light activity on a regular basis if possible.
If necessary, use digital stimulation to promote defecation, and massage the left lower quadrant of the abdomen while on the toilet.

From Hill C: Hemorrhoids and problems of the anus and rectum. In Meiner S, editor: *Care of gastrointestinal problems in the older adult,* New York, 2004, Springer.

COMMON DISEASES OF THE GASTROINTESTINAL TRACT

The following is an overview of common GI disorders seen in older clients, including the related nursing care. Box 26-3 provides an explanation of the diagnostic tests used in this section.

Gingivitis and Periodontitis

The gingivae, or gums, are subject to localized and systemic diseases, problems caused by drug therapy, poor oral hygiene, and poor nutrition. Gingivitis, an inflammation of the gums surrounding the teeth, may result in pain and bleeding; it can lead to periodontitis, a spread of the inflammation to the underlying tissues, bones, or roots of the teeth. This is the most common reason for tooth loss with advancing age. Gingivitis resulting from overgrowth of the gingivae may occur in people taking phenytoin (Dilantin) on a long-term basis.

Candida albicans, or thrush, is an infection causing white lesions in the oral mucosa. It is often seen in persons with compromised immune systems and those with suppressed immunity such as individuals taking immunosuppressant drugs and antibiotics.

NURSING MANAGEMENT

Assessment

Assessment begins with a good history of dental care and dental hygiene practices. A complete health history focusing

BOX 26-3 Radiologic and Diagnostic Tests and Procedures

Plain film of abdomen, kidneys, ureter, and bladder—Simple x-ray of the abdomen requiring no preparation; should include supine and erect views when an obstruction is suspected.

Upper GI/barium swallow—X-ray using an opaque contrast medium (barium) to examine the structure and motility of the upper GI tract, including the pharynx, esophagus, and stomach. May be extended (small bowel follow-through) to examine the duodenum and small bowel. Preparation is nothing by mouth (NPO) after midnight the night before the test. Client must increase fluids after examination to facilitate the evacuation of the barium, which colors stool white.

Upper endoscopy—Endoscopic examination of the upper GI tract allowing for direct visualization through a lighted fiberoptic tube that contains a lens, forceps, and brushes for biopsy. Preparation is similar to that for the upper GI. Sedation is required. The procedure is performed by the gastroenterologist in the procedure suite or at the bedside.

Barium enema—X-ray using an opaque contrast medium to examine the lower GI tract. Preparation includes NPO status after midnight the night before the procedure, as well as a bowel prep to clean out the large intestine before the procedure.

Ultrasound—Radiologic technique used to examine abdominal and other organs and tissues that does not use ionizing radiation. It cannot be used on organs that contain air because the ultrasound waves cannot penetrate air. Preparation depends on the organ being examined and may require the client to be NPO for up to 12 hours before the procedure.

Colonoscopy—Endoscopic examination of the colon with use of a colonoscope, which is inserted through the rectum. Preparation is similar to that for the barium enema. Sedation is required. The procedure is conducted by the gastroenterologist in the GI procedure suite.

Flexible sigmoidoscopy—Endoscopic examination of the interior of the sigmoid colon (does not examine as much of the colon as a colonoscopy). The procedure is performed by the gastroenterologist in the GI procedure suite. Preparation is similar to that for the barium enema.

Endoscopic retrograde cholangiopancreatography (ERCP)—Fluoroscopic upper endoscopic examination through the esophagus and duodenum into the common bile duct, used to examine structures in the biliary tree. Sedation is required. The client must be NPO for 8 to 13 hours before the procedure, which is performed in the GI procedure suite by a gastroenterologist.

Nuclear medicine studies—Radionucleotide imaging using an injection of an isotope that concentrates at the site to be examined (e.g., HIDA scan, DISIDA scan, and liver scan). No sedation is necessary. Preparation is NPO status after midnight the night before the test, which is performed in the nuclear medicine section of the radiology department.

Computed tomography (CT) scan—CT scan is used to produce pictures of internal organs of the body and allow visualization and identification of both normal and abnormal structures. It may be performed with or without a contrast material. Preparation varies from NPO status 8 to 12 hours before the procedure to no preparation, depending on the type of CT scan ordered. It is completed in the radiology department.

From Lewis S, Heitkemper M, Dirksen S: *Medical-surgical nursing: assessment and management of clinical problems,* ed 6, St Louis, 2004, Mosby.

on other illnesses and concomitant medications, as well as a physical assessment of the mouth, is necessary.

Diagnosis

The most common nursing diagnoses for an older client with gingivitis or periodontitis include:

- Impaired oral mucous membrane
- Impaired dentition
- Ineffective health maintenance
- Altered nutrition: less than body requirements related to pain

Planning and Expected Outcomes

An older adult must understand the relationship between oral health and overall health and well-being. The nurse must determine a client's feelings and attitude about performing the self-care necessary to achieve the desired goals.

Expected outcomes for an older client with gingivitis or periodontitis include:

1. Client will maintain a comfortable and functional oral cavity.
2. Client will establish and maintain a mouth care routine, including regular professional dental care.
3. Client will maintain normal body weight and nutritional status.

Intervention

Nursing management of an older client with gingivitis or periodontitis includes promotion of regular oral hygiene, regular preventive dental care, and maintenance of nutritional status. In addition, assessing the client's knowledge of the importance of oral hygiene and frequently reinforcing oral hygiene practices are important roles for the nurse. Oral hygiene includes flossing regularly, brushing teeth or dentures, and using saline mouth rinses as needed. Professional dental care should be sought routinely every 6 months or more often as needed. Proper fit of dentures initially and at all subsequent visits to both the dentist and the primary health care provider is also encouraged. Pain relief to ensure adequate nutrition can be managed by nonnarcotic pain medications (acetaminophen, aspirin), frequent mouth rinses, and a liquid or soft diet.

The key to treatment of gingivitis and periodontitis is prevention. Although good oral hygiene needs to begin early in life, it is never too late for an older client to begin routine dental care and oral hygiene. The nurse should discuss with the client the use of nutritional foods that are nonirritating, such as soft foods like pudding and custards, and the use of nutritional supplements like Ensure.

Evaluation

Evaluation includes documentation of achievement of the expected outcomes, establishment and maintenance of regular dental care and oral hygiene practices, and prevention of infection. Evaluation focuses on an older adult's ability to carry out the recommendations and whether any changes in self-care have occurred as a result. Findings of an oral cavity inspection should be noted, as should any instructions or explanations given to the client. The client's response to recommended treatment measures should also be documented.

Dysphagia

Dysphagia, or difficulty swallowing, is a symptom with many underlying causes, including stroke and other neurologic conditions, local trauma and tissue damage, achalasia, and tumors that obstruct the passage of food and liquids. Symptoms of dysphagia range from mild discomfort, such as the feeling of a lump in the throat, to a severe inability to swallow. Odynophagia, or severe pain while swallowing, may be present.

These abnormalities cause food and liquids to accumulate in the distal end of the esophagus and may cause the esophagus to become greatly dilated. The absence or ineffectiveness of peristalsis of the distal esophagus, with failure of the esophageal sphincter to relax in response to swallowing, is achalasia (Smeltzer and Bare, 2004). Symptoms of achalasia include progressive dysphagia, vomiting of food, nausea, and weight loss. The dysphagia progresses from solid foods to liquids. Pain occurs in only about one third of cases. Nocturnal aspiration can often occur, leading to infections by unusual organisms (mycobacteria). The onset of symptoms is insidious, and delay in diagnosis is common. However, food irritation and erosions can lead to cancer of the esophagus in some cases (Price and Wilson, 2003).

NURSING MANAGEMENT

Assessment

Assessment begins with an accurate and precise history that focuses on whether the dysphagia occurs with liquids, solids, or both, as well as the time frame for the progression of the dysphagia. Physical examination may be unremarkable.

Diagnosis

Nursing diagnoses for an older client with dysphagia include:

- Altered nutrition: less than body requirements
- Risk for aspiration related to abnormal swallowing
- Acute pain related to odynophagia
- Fear related to diagnosis and prognosis

Planning and Expected Outcomes

It is essential to determine whether an older client is ready to learn the self-care measures necessary to reduce the symptoms. Determining the extent of a client's specific fears created by learning of the palliative nature of interventions is important, since the type and degree of fear affects the nurse's specificity in intervention strategies.

Expected outcomes for an older client with dysphagia include:

1. Client will maintain weight within 10% of ideal body weight.
2. Client will remain free from aspiration.
3. Client will learn techniques to swallow that minimize pain.
4. Client will be free of epigastric discomfort.
5. Client will be able to verbalize fears related to diagnosis and prognosis.

Intervention

Nursing management of an older client with dysphagia includes maintenance of hydration and nutritional status, prevention of aspiration, and provision of emotional support and information regarding diagnosis and prognosis. Additionally, the nurse provides support and reassurance directed at a client's fear of eating related to the pain, difficulty in swallowing, and frequent regurgitation. Optimizing nutritional status and preventing weight loss are important, since fear of eating may lead to chronic weight loss. Instruction regarding eating habits and maintaining weight and nutrition is important. For example, small, frequent meals; pureed or soft foods; and high-protein, high-calorie foods are helpful. The nurse should instruct the client to elevate the head of the bed to prevent nocturnal aspiration.

Evaluation

Evaluation includes documentation of achievement of the expected outcomes, prevention of aspiration, and maintenance of nutrition. Evaluation of how the client is coping with the diagnosis may be assessed through a client's resumption of activities and ability to verbalize feelings. Additionally, evaluation focuses on a client's ability to satisfactorily incorporate and adhere to the dietary recommendations, as well as to modify behaviors and lifestyle to reduce symptoms.

Gastroesophageal Reflux and Esophagitis

Gastroesophageal reflux is the movement of gastric contents back up into the esophagus. Aging increases the incidence of reflux (Smeltzer and Bare, 2004). Normally, pressure on the lower esophageal sphincter prevents backflow; an incompetent lower esophageal sphincter is believed to be the primary cause of reflux esophagitis. Other causes include a hiatal hernia (see the Hiatal Hernia section), prolonged gastric intubation (i.e., use of a feeding tube), ingestion of corrosive chemicals, certain medications, infections, mucosal alterations, and systemic diseases such as lupus. The syndrome of gastroesophageal reflux is sometimes referred to as gastroesophageal reflux disease (Levy, Stamm, and Meiner, 2002; Williams, 2002).

Esophagitis is simply an inflammation of the esophagus. Most often this results from gastroesophageal reflux caused by either prolonged vomiting or an incompetent lower esophageal sphincter. The amount of mucosal damage is related to the contact time between the esophageal mucosa and the gastric contents, as well as the acidity and quantity of gastric secretions.

Hydrochloric acid from the stomach alters the pH of the esophagus and allows mucosal protein to be denatured. The pepsin in gastric secretions has proteolytic properties that are enhanced when the pH is around 2.0. The combination of pepsin and hydrochloric acid increases the possibility of damage. Reflux has been shown to cause an inflammation that penetrates to the muscularis layer, resulting in motor dysfunction and decreased esophageal clearance. The end results are increased esophageal contact time, more muscle damage, and increased amounts of reflux.

Symptoms include heartburn; retrosternal discomfort; and the regurgitation of sour, bitter material. Symptoms are often precipitated by the ingestion of a large amount of fatty or spicy foods or alcohol. Strictures may develop that make food passage difficult. Dysphagia for both liquids and solids increases when severe obstruction occurs. If regurgitation occurs often, substernal pain may result, occasionally mimicking a heart attack. Reflux may be aggravated by postural changes, such as lying supine when sleeping, but may occur in any position. Pulmonary aspiration as a result of reflux is common when the disease is severe and leads to pneumonia.

Hiatal Hernia. A hiatal hernia is a major cause of reflux and esophagitis and occurs when part of the stomach protrudes through an opening of the diaphragm (Fig. 26-3). The condition may be intermittent or continuous. The continuous type is least common, accounting for only about 10% of cases. Either part or all of the stomach, and even the intestines, may herniate, causing dyspepsia, severe pain, and often a gastric ulceration. The intermittent type, or sliding hernia, occurs with changes in position or with increased peristalsis. The stomach is forced through the opening of the diaphragm when the person is prone and moves back to its normal position when the person stands up. Most hiatal hernias are asymptomatic and require no treatment. Symptoms, when they arise, include heartburn, gastric regurgitation, dysphagia, and indigestion. These symptoms are accentuated (1) when in the supine position after meals, (2) after overeating, (3) after physical exertion, or (4) with a sudden change in posture.

NURSING MANAGEMENT

Assessment

Assessment begins with a history of symptoms and possible aggravating factors. Older clients may use terms such as *indigestion* or *heartburn*, rather than *pain*, and these words need to be clearly defined. Clients also may not understand what

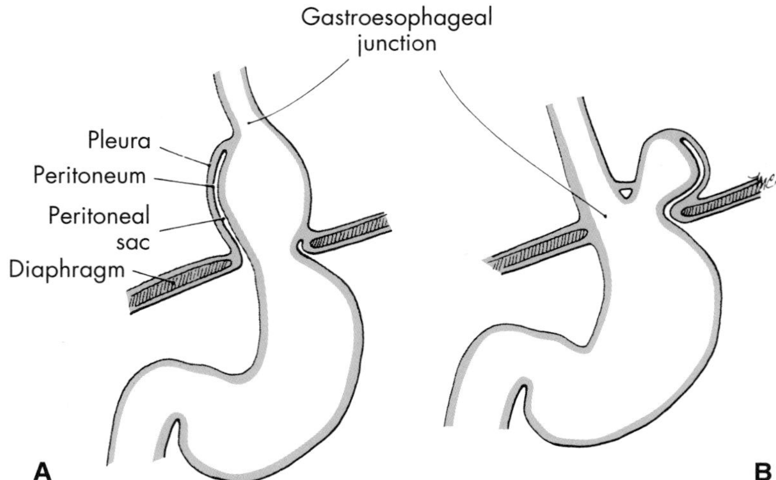

Fig. 26-3 Hiatal hernias. **A,** Sliding. **B,** Rolling. (From Price S, Wilson L: *Pathophysiology: clinical concepts of disease processes,* ed 6, St Louis, 2003, Mosby.)

regurgitation means, especially in relationship to vomiting. The nurse should determine a client's use of tobacco and alcohol; these are contributing factors. Drug and diet history are also important components of the assessment. Physical examination may be unremarkable (Seidel et al, 2003).

Diagnosis

Nursing diagnoses for an older client with gastroesophageal reflux include:

- Risk for aspiration related to regurgitation
- Altered nutrition: less than body requirements related to pain or dysphagia
- Knowledge deficit: disease process and treatment modalities related to lack of exposure

Planning and Expected Outcomes

It is essential to determine whether a client is ready to learn the preventive measures necessary for reducing symptoms. The presence of additional health problems may affect an older client's ability to participate in an educational plan or carry out the interventions.

Expected outcomes for an older client with gastroesophageal reflux include:

1. Client will remain free from aspiration.
2. Client will maintain weight within 10% of ideal body weight.
3. Client will verbalize understanding of the disease process and treatment approaches.

Intervention

Nursing management of older clients with gastroesophageal reflux includes maintenance of adequate nutrition, prevention of aspiration, and instruction to clients and their families about the disease process and treatment approaches (see Client/Family Teaching box). Support from caregivers, spouses, or significant others is a key to success.

Evaluation

Evaluation includes documentation of achievement of expected outcomes, prevention of complications, and appropriate dietary and lifestyle changes. Since most clients improve after 1 month of conservative management with antacids and lifestyle changes, it is important for the nurse to ascertain if symptoms have subsided. If they have not, referral for further medical management is warranted.

Client/Family Teaching

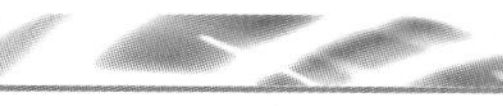

HEARTBURN, HIATAL HERNIA, OR REFLUX

Nutrition and Diet

Eat high-protein, low-fat foods.
Avoid foods containing caffeine and chocolate.
Avoid carminatives (e.g., spearmint, peppermint).
Eat small, frequent meals.
Eat easily digestible foods.
Achieve and maintain ideal body weight.

Habits

Avoid smoking.
Avoid alcohol.

Activity and Rest

Avoid lying down or bending over for 2 hours after meals.
Avoid wearing tight belts or girdles during or after meals.
Sleep with upper body elevated 4 to 6 inches; use blocks, not pillows, under front legs of bed.

From Levy RA, Stamm L, Meiner SE: Conservative management of GERD: a case study, *MEDSURG Nurs* 11(4):169, 2002.

Gastritis

Gastritis refers to inflammation of the gastric mucosa and occurs in acute or chronic forms. Although hydrochloric acid is present in gastritis, the amount of secretion does not have to be excessive.

Acute gastritis causes transient inflammation, hemorrhage, and erosion into the gastric mucosal lining. Although the cause may be undetermined, it is frequently associated with alcoholism; aspirin or nonsteroidal antiinflammatory drug (NSAID) ingestion; smoking; and severely stressful conditions such as burns, trauma, central nervous system damage, chemotherapy, and radiotherapy.

Chronic gastritis is an inflammation of the stomach lining that may occur repeatedly or continue over a period of time. Among its possible causes are ulcers, hiatal hernias, vitamin deficiencies, chronic alcohol use, gastric mucosal atrophy, achlorhydria, and peptic ulceration. The continual loss of gastric mucosa eventually decreases gastric secretion and may lead to pernicious anemia, PUD, or gastric cancer.

The major symptom of gastritis is abdominal pain. Other symptoms include indigestion, distention, decreased appetite, nausea, and vomiting. Many clients with chronic gastritis are asymptomatic.

Pernicious Anemia

Pernicious anemia is a condition most often seen in older adults. Degeneration of the parietal cells in the gastric mucosa causes a decrease in production of the intrinsic factor. This reduces the absorption of vitamin B_{12}, which impairs the production of red blood cells. This results in large, oval, fragile cells that have a short lifetime (Lewis, Heitkemper, and Dirksen, 2004). The resulting condition is known as pernicious anemia and can be treated only with injections of vitamin B_{12}. Oral vitamin B_{12} cannot be absorbed and cannot be substituted for the injections, which must be continued throughout the life span.

NURSING MANAGEMENT

 Assessment

Assessment begins with a history and review of systems, which may include complaints of indigestion, abdominal or epigastric discomfort, nausea, vomiting, or anorexia. Questioning clients about possible GI blood loss (e.g., hematemesis, melena) is also important. With acute gastritis, signs of dehydration may be present.

 Diagnosis

Nursing diagnoses for an older client with gastritis include:

- Acute pain related to epigastric discomfort and/or cramping secondary to acidity
- Deficient fluid volume related to decreased intake and/or vomiting and blood loss
- Knowledge deficit: disease process related to lack of exposure

 Planning and Expected Outcomes

Since most clients receive treatment on an outpatient basis, the nurse must determine an older client's ability to adhere to the recommended treatment strategies. Expected outcomes for an older client with gastritis include:

1. Client will experience relief of epigastric symptoms.
2. Client will maintain adequate fluid and electrolyte balance.
3. Client will verbalize understanding of the disease and factors attributed to the disease.

Intervention

Nursing management of an older client with gastritis includes acid-suppressing medications as ordered; small, frequent, easily digested meals; maintenance of a calm environment to decrease the effects of stress; monitoring of fluid and electrolyte status; and teaching the older client about precipitating and contributory factors. GI bleeding is a possible complication of gastritis, and prevention and early diagnosis are important. An older client must understand the necessity of limiting or eliminating alcohol and tobacco use, avoiding aspirin and other NSAIDs, and seeking prompt medical attention for symptoms of indigestion and epigastric pain.

 Evaluation

Evaluation includes documentation of achievement of expected outcomes, a decrease in symptoms, and lack of evidence of a GI hemorrhage or other complications. The nurse should note an older client's adherence to the necessary lifestyle changes.

Peptic Ulcer Disease

PUD is an ulcerative condition of the GI tract that results from an imbalance between the aggressive forces of gastric acid and pepsin and the defensive forces in the gastric and duodenal mucosa. Although PUD refers to injury anywhere in the GI tract, the most common occurrence is in the stomach and duodenum.

The exact cause of peptic ulcers is unclear, but research indicates conditions that predispose individuals to their development. In some cases there is an increased production of hydrochloric acid in the stomach. This situation is most common with duodenal ulcers (DUs), and it is thought to be due to an increased number of parietal cells. Another factor is a decreased resistance of the gastric mucosa to even normal levels of gastric acid. This occurs most commonly in conjunction with certain medications (NSAIDs, indomethacin [Indocin]) and disorders like chronic gastritis. For years these two factors were believed to be the pathogenesis of ulcer disease, and treatment was focused on maintaining acid levels that were not harmful to the mucosa. However, in 1994 participants in a conference sponsored by the National Institutes of Health concluded that a bacterium, *Helicobacter pylori,* was a causative factor in most cases of PUD (Brozenec, 1996). This organism secretes a urease that generates free ammonia and a protease that breaks down the gastric mucus. It is believed to be present in virtually all clients with DUs and about 70% of those with gastric ulcers. When documented *H. pylori* infection is present, medical treatment can include antacids, H_2 blockers (e.g., ranitidine), or gastric acid pump

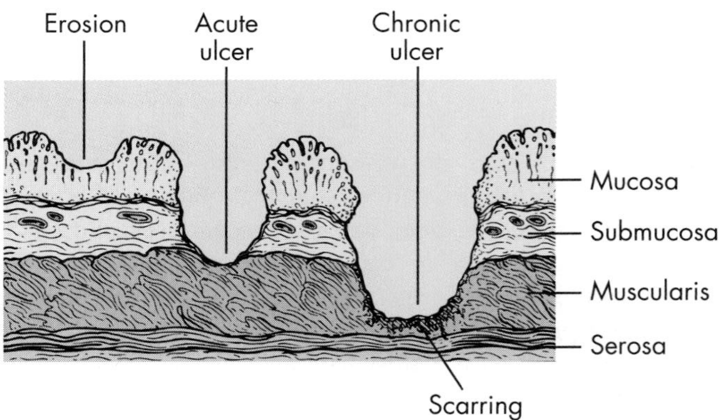

Fig. 26-4 Peptic ulcers, including an erosion, acute ulcer, and chronic ulcer. (Redrawn from Price SA, Wilson LM: Pathophysiology: clinical concepts of disease processes, ed 5, St Louis, 1997, Mosby. In Lewis S, Heitkemper M, and Dirksen S: *Medical-surgical nursing: assessment & management of clinical problems,* ed 6, St Louis, 2004, Mosby.)

inhibitors (e.g., omeprazole) and antimicrobials (Price and Wilson, 2003).

Ulcer disease affects 10% to 15% of the general population. DUs account for approximately 80% of all peptic ulcers, and the pyloric region is the most common site of all peptic ulcers. Although DUs tend to occur in people 20 to 40 years of age, gastric ulcers occur more often in persons over age 40.

Both genetic and environmental factors have been proposed as the cause of peptic ulcers, since both gastric ulcers and DUs tend to occur in families. At present, no direct evidence exists that indicates dietary or occupational factors as causes of ulcer disease. In addition, although psychologic factors such as anxiety or stress play a role in the response of peptic ulcers to treatment, little evidence supports the common belief that a person with the type A personality, striving for perfection, develops ulcers. However, prolonged stress can produce a stress ulcer (see Stress Ulcers).

Gastric Ulcers. In gastric ulcers the level of hydrochloric acid secretion is usually normal or reduced. The problem lies in the increased rate of diffusion of gastric acid back into the tissue. Clients with benign gastric ulcers should be encouraged to receive frequent follow-up monitoring, since these ulcers can become malignant.

The most common symptom with gastric ulcers is epigastric pain, with variable pain relief after eating. Nausea, vomiting, and weight loss are common. Hemorrhage resulting from perforation occurs in 25% of these individuals and is often excessive. Perforation of the ulcer into the peritoneal cavity is less common than with a DU. Healing and recurrences are common. A lack of healing or failure to decrease in size suggests malignancy.

Duodenal Ulcers. In contrast to gastric ulcers, people with DUs have a normal back diffusion of gastric acid but an increased rate of gastric acid secretion. They also have increased emptying rate of acid from the stomach to the duodenum. If the increase in acid is not buffered in the stomach, the acid is propelled into the duodenum, leading to irritation of the duodenal mucosa. It is believed that the bacterium *H. pylori* migrates from the stomach to the duodenum in the presence of dysplastic changes in the duodenal mucosa.

Evidence that the disease has a strong family history and occurs among those with type O blood groups supports a genetic theory. Most of these ulcerations occur in the first part of the duodenum, close to the pylorus.

Typically the symptoms of DU are patterned by periods of exacerbation and remission and follow a pain-food-relief pattern, with the pain beginning 90 minutes to 3 hours after eating. The pain is immediately relieved by food or antacids and is located in the midepigastrium, sometimes radiating to the back. Other GI symptoms include heartburn and regurgitation of sour acidic juice into the back of the throat. Anorexia and weight loss are rare because the client usually seeks food to relieve the pain. A DU may rupture because of erosion through the duodenal wall, and this leads to contamination of the peritoneal cavity (peritonitis). A slowly bleeding ulcer may reveal guaiac positive stools. On physical examination the only abnormality is possibly a tender epigastrium.

Stress Ulcers. Stress ulcers, or erosions, may occur after a major insult to the body, such as burns, sepsis, or head trauma. Although termed an ulcer, these erosions are superficial mucosal defects of the stomach mucosa that usually do not penetrate the muscularis layer. Unlike gastric ulcers or DUs, there are usually several lesions with stress ulcers.

Two mechanisms for producing stress ulcers have been proposed: (1) mucosal ischemia resulting from a lack of blood supply to the gastric mucosa during the after-stress period and (2) increased sensitivity of the gastric mucosa to hydrochloric acid and pepsin.

The major clinical manifestation of stress ulcers is massive, painless, gastric bleeding with an onset of 2 to 15 days after the initial insult. Signs include hematemesis and melena, rarely including pain. Because of the danger of bleeding after acute stress and the difficulty of stopping it once it has started, preventive measures are routinely used to decrease hydrogen ion secretion and neutralize gastric acid. These include administration of antacids and histamine blockers and/or sucralfate.

NURSING MANAGEMENT

Assessment

Assessment begins with evaluation of a client's complaint of abdominal or epigastric pain, the most common symptom of peptic ulcers. The pain should be assessed for presence, location, character, and especially alleviating and precipitating factors. Peptic ulcer pain is usually described as a gnawing, burning, or aching, usually in the epigastric area, and may radiate around to the back. The pain usually begins when the stomach is empty and may disappear with the ingestion of food or an antacid. Because of this, the pain often occurs at night when the stomach is empty, especially with DUs.

A client may also exhibit signs of complications of the peptic ulcer. Hemorrhage may be manifested as either melena or hematemesis. Perforation in an older client may not be manifested by a rigid abdomen, as it so often is with younger individuals. Occasionally, the only sign of perforation in an older adult is abdominal pain, which may have a blunted presentation. An obstruction may be manifested by weight loss or projectile vomiting, but it may produce only subtle findings early in its course in older adults.

Diagnosis

The most frequently used nursing diagnoses for an older client with PUD include:

- Acute pain related to mucosal lesions
- Knowledge deficit: disease process and treatment related to lack of exposure
- Noncompliance with lifestyle changes related to complexity of the regimen.

Planning and Expected Outcomes

Since not all older clients with PUD have the same set of symptoms, the nurse must determine individual client needs with regard to education and other interventions. Expected outcomes for an older client with PUD include:

1. Client will report a decrease in abdominal or epigastric pain.
2. Client will adhere to the prescribed dietary, activity, and medication regimen.
3. Client will acknowledge aggravating factors, such as smoking, alcohol use, stress, or frequent use of aspirin or NSAIDs.

Intervention

Nursing management for an older client with PUD includes education of the client on lifestyle changes, dietary modifications, and medications that may be used in the treatment plan. Lifestyle changes include cessation of smoking, cessation of alcohol consumption, and avoidance of other irritants such as aspirin-containing products and NSAIDs. In addition, stress reduction techniques such as exercise, relaxation training, biofeedback, and other appropriate outlets should be explored and individualized, depending on client needs and wishes. Dietary changes include avoiding foods that are irritating to the mucosa of the stomach, such as caffeine, alcohol, and foods that cause pain.

Medications need to be taken as prescribed. An older client needs to be instructed that the only medications that can immediately decrease the abdominal or epigastric pain are antacids. Other medications should be taken exactly as ordered, but the client should be reminded that these take longer to provide relief. The client should also understand that antacids last only 20 to 30 minutes, while acid suppressants have a long-term effect. Another important point to discuss with the older client is the effect of ulcer medication on other drugs. For example, cimetidine, a histamine-blocking agent, interferes with the metabolism of warfarin, theophylline, and phenytoin.

If surgery is performed, more dietary modifications may be necessary due to a reduction in the size of the stomach. A response known as *dumping syndrome* is common after gastric resection; it is manifested by dizziness, nausea, and diaphoresis after meals. The institution of small, frequent meals that are low in carbohydrates will diminish the incidence of these symptoms. Resting after eating and drinking fluids between (rather than during) meals will also help alleviate these symptoms. Maintaining adequate nutrition and fluid and electrolyte balance is especially important for older clients and can be achieved by these dietary modifications.

Evaluation

Evaluation includes documentation of achievement of the expected outcomes, prevention of complications, elimination of symptoms, and an increased knowledge base regarding PUD. Any complications of the recommended medical treatments should be noted.

Enteritis

Enteritis, or gastroenteritis, is an inflammatory process of the stomach or small intestine. It may be caused by bacteria, viruses, medications, radiation, ingestion of irritating foods, or allergic reactions. Bacterial enteritis is often caused by ingestion of food that is contaminated by bacteria-containing toxins; it is commonly known as food poisoning. Examples of these bacteria include *Staphylococcus aureus*, salmonellae, and *Clostridium botulinum*.

In addition, enteritis may result from parasitic infections such as amebiasis and trichinosis. In amebiasis the cause is a protozoal parasite that primarily invades the large intestine. It is the inactive form, the cyst, that when ingested in fecally contaminated food or water will pass into the intestines. There, the active form is released and enters the intestinal wall, causing ulceration of the intestinal mucosa. Amebiasis is found primarily in tropical countries and where there is poor sanitation. Trichinosis, on the other hand, is transmitted through improperly cooked pork and is caused by the larvae of a roundworm that becomes imbedded into the striated muscles of animals that eat the infected pork. When the infected pork is eaten, the larvae live and develop in the host's intestine. The larvae are released and move toward the host's muscles, where they can remain for many years. Acute enteritis is a result of direct bacterial or viral infection or the effect of the toxins produced by the bacteria. This results in either an increased secretion of water into the intestinal lumen or an increase in motility, causing large amounts of food and fluid to be excreted. In general, enteritis causes inflammatory changes in the intestinal mucosa, which return to normal when the offending agent is removed.

The pathologic process has varying manifestations that result in symptoms of abdominal cramping, profuse diarrhea, and vomiting. With this profuse diarrhea, large amounts of fluid and electrolytes may be lost, leading to dehydration and electrolyte imbalances of hyponatremia and hypokalemia. Older adults are particularly at risk for dehydration, and prompt treatment is required.

NURSING MANAGEMENT

Assessment

Assessment begins with a history of recent food intake; nausea; vomiting; and diarrhea, including amount, duration, frequency, and stool characteristics. Fever and abdominal discomfort may also be present. The nurse should inquire about recent drug use, especially antibiotics, and recent travel. If food poisoning is suspected, the nurse should also question the client regarding possible sources of contamination. Physical examination includes inspection of mucous membranes, assessment of orthostatic blood pressures, and urine-specific gravity, which are helpful in assessing hydration status.

Diagnosis

The most common nursing diagnoses for an older client with enteritis include:

- Deficient fluid volume related to vomiting and diarrhea
- Diarrhea related to intestinal inflammation

Planning and Expected Outcomes

Expected outcomes for an older client with enteritis include:

1. Client will maintain adequate fluid volume and electrolyte balance.
2. Client will have a continual decline in the number of liquid, nonformed stools until baseline is achieved.

Intervention

Nursing management of an older client with enteritis includes maintenance of hydration and monitoring of fluid and electrolyte status. With severe vomiting and diarrhea, intravenous hydration and hospitalization are required. With milder forms of enteritis, clear liquids may be offered at home. In all cases, monitoring for signs and symptoms of dehydration is imperative. In addition, it is important for the nurse to determine if an older client has someone nearby to monitor the status of the condition in case it worsens. Older clients need to be taught signs and symptoms of dehydration, as well as when to seek further medical care. Prevention of bacterial and parasitic enteritis should also be discussed, stressing the need for thorough hand washing, especially before meals and food preparation.

Evaluation

Evaluation includes documentation of achievement of the expected outcomes, prevention of complications, and return to baseline status. The nurse should monitor the older client for a decrease in symptoms as the problem resolves. Careful monitoring of oral intake and tolerance of advancing diet is also noted.

Intestinal Obstruction

Intestinal obstruction occurs whenever there is partial or complete blockage of GI contents in either the small or large intestine. This can be the result of several conditions, which are usually classified as mechanical or nonmechanical obstructions.

Mechanical obstructions are the most common and primarily caused by tumors, adhesions, or hernias (Fig. 26-5). Another mechanical cause of intestinal obstruction is volvulus, or the twisting of a part of the intestine. Although this is a rare cause of obstruction overall, it is more common in older adults because the mesenteric ligaments weaken over time.

Nonmechanical causes of intestinal obstruction involve decreased or absent peristalsis resulting from neurologic or vascular disorders. In these situations movement of intestinal contents is stopped without the presence of an obstructing object.

A common example of intestinal obstruction from neurologic causes is an *ileus*. This is a general term used to describe failure of the bowel contents to move forward because of lack of peristalsis. It may occur in the small or large intestine and may also be called *adynamic* or *paralytic ileus*. An ileus may occur when peristalsis becomes diminished or absent because of a triggering of the inhibitory reflex by a noxious stimuli such as anesthesia, peritoneal injury, interruption of the nerve supply, abdominal injury or surgical manipulation, intestinal ischemia, or electrolyte imbalances. It is a common postoperative problem, especially after abdominal surgery.

Vascular disorders cause intestinal or mesenteric ischemia and the resultant obstruction. Prolonged ischemia results in death of the surface of the villi and epithelial cells, which in turn impairs the absorption of nutrients. In addition, the mucosal layer becomes necrotic and peristalsis diminishes. Although intestinal or mesenteric ischemia is relatively rare, its high mortality rate and predominance in older adults make it important for nurses caring for older adults. Some degree of intestinal ischemia is present in all clients who have a history of other forms of ischemia, thrombosis, or infarction, or in clients who have chronic ischemia, such as those with atherosclerosis. The majority of these clients have a history of cerebrovascular, peripheral vascular, and/or coronary artery disease. Ischemic bowel disease comprises a spectrum of acute and chronic syndromes that usually affect older adults. The major syndromes of ischemic intestinal disease include acute embolic ischemia, acute thrombotic occlusion (ischemia colitis), nonocclusive ischemia, chronic intestinal ischemia (abdominal angina), and venous occlusive disease.

Whatever the cause of intestinal obstruction, after the blockage occurs, the bowel becomes distended by gas and air proximal to the area of blockage. If the process continues, gastric, biliary, and pancreatic secretions, along with water, electrolytes, and serum proteins, begin to accumulate in the area, causing an increase in intraluminal pressure. A third-space shift may occur when the circulating blood volume decreases as a result of the movement of water into the intestinal lumen, which may lead to dehydration, electrolyte imbalances, and hypovolemia.

Clinical findings with an obstruction include the acute onset of severe cramping pain that correlates roughly to the

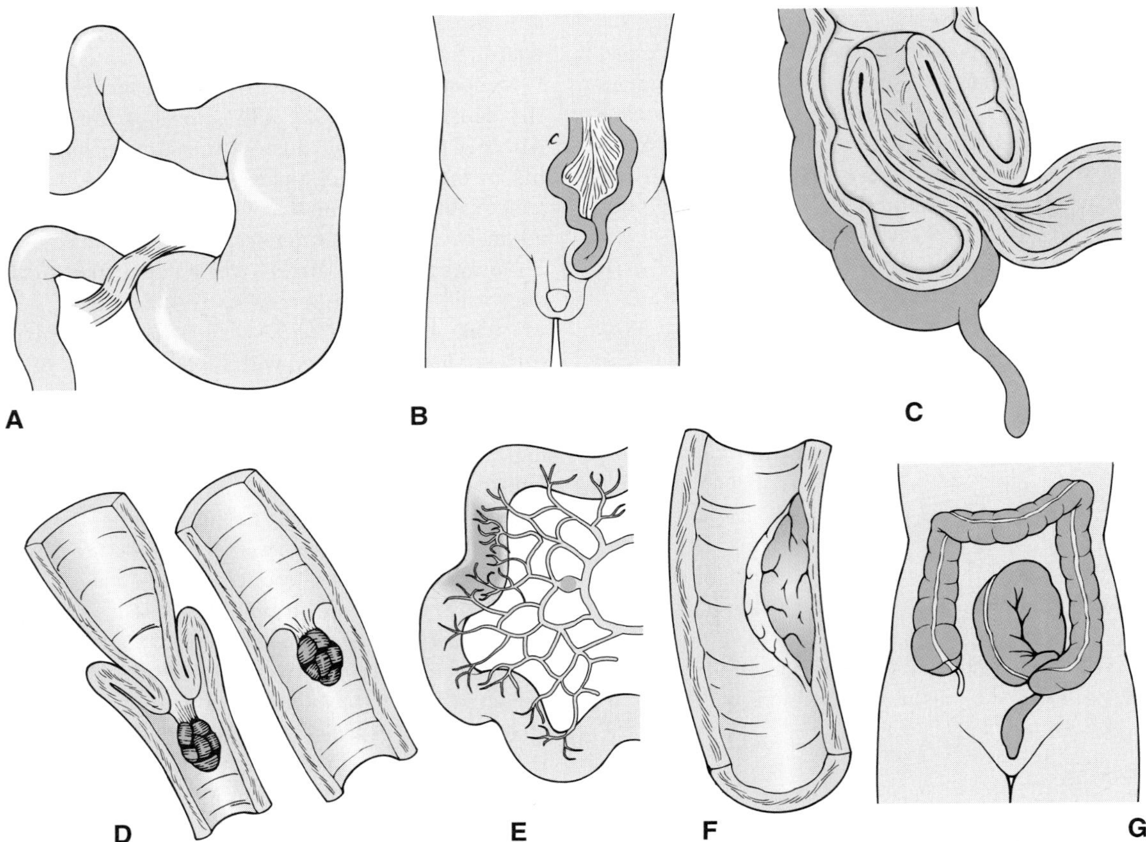

Fig. 26-5 Bowel obstructions. **A,** Adhesions. **B,** Strangulated inguinal hernia. **C,** Ileocecal intussusception. **D,** Intussusception from polyps. **E,** Mesenteric occlusion. **F,** Neoplasm. **G,** Volvulus of the sigmoid colon. (From Lewis S, Heitkemper M, Dirksen S: *Medical-surgical nursing: assessment and management of clinical problems,* ed 6, St Louis, 2004, Mosby.)

area or level of obstruction. The pain may actually decrease in severity as the distention of the bowel increases. In mesenteric ischemia the clinical presentation is initially very nonspecific and can mimic other, more common abdominal problems such as diverticulitis, appendicitis, and cholecystitis. Although the major symptom is abdominal pain, the clue to mesenteric ischemia is that the pain is out of proportion to what is found on physical examination. Atherosclerotic ischemia may create an angina-like cramping abdominal pain that becomes worse after meals and then dissipates. In colonic ischemia the pain is worse in the left lower quadrant. Vasospasm and emboli produce an acute, severe abdominal pain with associated vomiting and diarrhea.

Abdominal distention will be present, especially if the obstruction is in the lower small intestine or colon. Percussion will elicit tympany because of the accumulation of gas and air in the bowel. There will be hyperactive bowel sounds above the site of a mechanical obstruction as the intestine attempts to push the contents downward; the increase in the rate and force of peristalsis may cause borborygmi (loud and high-pitched bowel sounds); these may progress to an absence of bowel sounds as the condition persists. Bowel sounds below the site will be absent, and with an ileus, they will be totally absent. Vomiting is almost always present and may (rarely) be bilious or feculent depending on the level of the obstruction. Diarrhea may occur if the obstruction is not complete, allowing watery contents to pass the obstruction. The client may develop signs of dehydration and shock. Symptoms of perforation occur if the ileus is not treated.

Complications of intestinal obstruction include perforation of the bowel, chemical or bacterial peritonitis, hypovolemic shock, and septic shock. The increased pressure on the mucosa of the affected bowel segment may lead to bowel necrosis, resulting in changes in the permeability of the bowel wall. Normal bacteria of the intestine can then escape into the peritoneal cavity, causing peritonitis that can escalate to bacteremia. Perforation of the thinned intestinal wall results in the loss of fluid into the abdominal space, chemical peritonitis, and possible abscess formation. Infection and loss of fluid and electrolytes are major problems. Hypovolemic shock may result when there is a shift of fluid greater than 10% of body weight. Septic shock may also occur as a result of the contamination of the bloodstream in the peritoneum when the bowel ruptures or becomes gangrenous.

Sepsis and hypovolemic shock are life threatening and must be treated aggressively.

NURSING MANAGEMENT

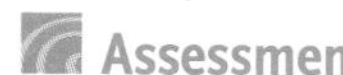

Assessment

Assessment begins with a thorough history of the precipitating event, focusing on the type and frequency of vomiting and diarrhea (e.g., profuse, fecal) and the location and character of pain (e.g., cramping, constant, diffuse). A sudden change in a client's description of abdominal pain from generalized and dull to localized and sharp must be taken seriously; this is a characteristic presentation of peritonitis. Physical examination should focus on the presence and character of bowel sounds (e.g., loud, frequent, absent, weak), presence of abdominal distention, vital signs, and urinary output. Sudden elevation of temperature is another classic sign of peritonitis.

Diagnosis

Nursing diagnoses for an older client with an ileus or bowel obstruction include:

- Deficient fluid volume related to loss of body fluids
- Acute abdominal pain related to increased peristalsis
- Altered nutrition: less than body requirements related to vomiting and obstruction.

Planning and Expected Outcomes

Expected outcomes for an older client with an ileus or intestinal obstruction include:

1. Client will maintain adequate fluid volume and electrolyte balance.
2. Client will verbalize a tolerable level of discomfort.
3. Client will regain and maintain adequate nutrition as evidenced by achievement of preillness body weight.

The older adult client with a bowel obstruction requires careful and close observation, since the classic signs of pain and fluid loss may be blunted.

Intervention

Nursing management of an older client with an ileus or intestinal obstruction includes maintenance of hydration and promotion of comfort. Dehydration can be prevented by providing intravenous fluids and electrolytes as ordered. Monitoring intake and output and urine-specific gravity, as well as monitoring for signs of fluid overload or dehydration, is important. Nasogastric or nasointestinal tubes are usually required for decompression, and maintenance of their patency and placement is imperative. Pain relief measures may require medication; however, narcotics are sometimes not allowed because of their effects on the bowel and their masking of important symptoms. Other comfort measures include repositioning, mouth care, skin care, and music or meditation. If surgery is required, preparation of the client and family concerning what should be expected is also important.

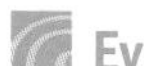

Evaluation

Evaluation includes documentation of achievement of expected outcomes and prevention of complications (see Nursing Care Plan). Vital signs, intake and output, bowel sounds, and bowel elimination patterns should also be recorded. If surgery was performed, monitoring of the incision site and wound healing status is necessary.

Diverticula

Diverticula are saclike protrusions of the mucosa along the GI tract. These small sacs are formed by herniation of the mucous membrane outward through a separation in circular muscle fibers of the intestine. Diverticula are a result of increased intraluminal pressure, and can develop in any part of the digestive tract. They occur most often in the descending and sigmoid colon. Colonic diverticula are usually multiple.

The exact cause of diverticula is unknown. Because of the frequency of diverticula in older adults, it is thought they are related to the blood supply or nutrition of the bowel. Lack of dietary fiber or roughage and decreased fecal bulk have also been correlated with this process. With an increase in food bulk (as with consumption of dietary fiber) the pressure in the colon decreases. In contrast, when there is little waste in the colon, stronger muscle contractions are necessary to excrete it, and the pressure increases. This increase in pressure leads to muscle hypertrophy and the development of diverticula. In this manner diverticula have also been linked to chronic constipation and older adults who are obese. Atrophy of the musculature of the bowel wall may weaken the intestine and be another factor in the development of diverticula in older adults. The presence of multiple diverticula that are not inflamed is termed *diverticulosis.* This is a disease of middle and old age. Diverticulosis increases with age, and in the population over 85 years of age, two thirds have diverticuli (Price and Wilson, 2003). It is the most common disease of the colon in the Western world. Usually diverticulosis is symptom free and is often diagnosed as an incidental finding on x-ray study or sigmoidoscopy. Vague abdominal discomfort may be described.

Diverticulitis is an inflammation of or around a diverticular sac that is usually caused by the retention of undigested food, stool, and bacteria in the sac. This hard mass is termed a *fecalith.* In diverticulitis the stasis in the sac leads to inflammation and/or infection. The mucous membranes may erode or perforate blood vessels, causing bleeding. Obstruction of the large intestine, fistulae, and abscesses may result. Rupture of the infected material into the peritoneal cavity may result in peritonitis. Approximately 15% of those with diverticulosis develop diverticulitis (Clarren, 2004).

Nursing Care Plan

Ileus: Obstruction Resulting from Diverticulitis

Clinical Situation: Mrs. B is a 72-year-old retired seamstress who was recently admitted to the emergency room with abdominal pain. She was brought in by her daughter and son-in-law with whom she lives. Her daughter reported that her mother had been complaining of abdominal pain for the past 24 hours, and since it did not subside, she encouraged her to seek medical attention. Over the past 24 hours, Mrs. B reported left-sided lower abdominal pain; nausea; and, more recently, vomiting. She was unsure whether she had a fever. Her daughter added that her mother had had a lot of constipation recently, for which Mrs. B had taken various types of laxatives.

Her medical history includes hypertension, for which she takes nifedipine extended release (Procardia XL) and hydrochlorothiazide; and hypercholesterolemia, for which she takes lovastatin (Mevacor) on a daily basis. Her daughter also remembers her doctor telling her mother a few years ago that she had diverticulosis, which was diagnosed from an incidental finding on an x-ray study. Her only past surgery was an uncomplicated cholecystectomy about 20 years ago for cholecystitis. Mrs. B stated that she was on no particular diet and has had few weight fluctuations over the past few years.

Physical examination reveals a thin woman, weighing 128 lb, with temperature of 100.9° F (38.3° C) (orally), pulse of 98 beats/min, respiratory rate of 24 breaths/min, and blood pressure of 140/84 mm Hg. She is lying on the stretcher curled in a semifetal position. Her abdomen is not obviously distended, and her only scar is a midline incisional scar from her previous cholecystectomy. She has loud, high-pitched bowel sounds, but no audible bruits. Her abdomen is tender, and a firm mass, possibly feces, is palpable in the lower left quadrant. She has no elicitable rebound tenderness. She has tenderness on rectal examination and is thought to have stool high up in her rectal vault. However, her hemoccult is guaiac negative.

Laboratory tests reveal a white blood cell count of 90,000 µl and normal hemoglobin. Urinalysis is normal, as are serum electrolytes. Serum amylase is 500 units/dl. A plain abdominal x-ray study is ordered and reveals air-fluid levels but no free air on the abdomen. She is given the diagnosis of ileus or obstruction resulting from diverticulitis.

Mrs. B was admitted to a general medical unit and had a surgical consultation. She was placed on intravenous fluids, restricted to NPO status, and had a nasogastric tube placed on high intermittent suction. Intravenous antibiotic therapy was begun and continued for the remainder of her hospitalization. She was monitored closely and managed medically. She was found to have an ileus only and never required surgery for a small bowel obstruction or perforation. She was discharged to home on the eighth day after admission, and was receiving on her previous medications.

Nursing Diagnosis

Fluid volume deficit related to active loss of body fluid secondary to nasogastric tube output

Altered nutrition: less than body requirements related to prolonged NPO status

Constipation related to decreased mobility, daily ingestion of constipating medications, and lack of dietary fiber

Knowledge deficit: diverticular disease related to lack of exposure to knowledge about prevention and complications

Pain (abdominal) related to reluctance to take pain medication

Outcomes

Client will maintain adequate fluid volume and electrolyte balance.

Client will maintain preadmission weight.

Client will establish a regular pattern of bowel movements.

Client and family will be able to verbalize dietary changes and be able to prevent constipation and further complications.

Client will obtain pain relief.

Interventions

Monitor vital signs every 4 hours or as ordered.

Maintain intravenous therapy as ordered.

Monitor intake and output (hourly); skin moisture, color, and (nonarm) turgor; urine-specific gravity (every 4 hours); serum electrolytes; and level of consciousness.

Weigh client every day or as ordered.

Monitor serum albumin and protein.

Administer intravenous total perineal nutrition as ordered.

When client is no longer NPO, encourage high-protein, high-calorie foods.

Administer stool-softening medications, if ordered.

When client is no longer NPO, encourage a daily fluid intake of 2 L and consumption of high-fiber foods. Teach fiber-rich foods to be included in the diet.

When the client is able, encourage her to increase activity level.

Teach about constipating side effects of medications.

Provide client and family with written and verbal information concerning the importance of a high-fiber diet, the need to maintain an adequate fluid intake, and the need for light exercise.

Provide client and family with written and verbal information concerning complications of diverticulosis, such as diverticulitis.

Assess and monitor degree of pain every 4 hours.

Provide client with verbal and written instruction about analgesics.

Provide other measures of pain relief, such as guided imagery, repositioning, and diversional activities.

Provide encouragement by informing client that pain will decrease as the ileus improves.

Clinical manifestations of symptomatic diverticular disease include constipation or diarrhea and left-sided lower abdominal pain. Over half of clients with diverticulitis experience some change in bowel habits; most complain of constipation. Other symptoms include flatulence, nausea, and vomiting. Older adults with diverticulitis may be afebrile, with little abdominal discomfort. Complications include perforation and peritonitis, ureteral obstruction, and significant lower GI bleeding. Surgery may be necessary if an obstruction or perforation is suspected.

NURSING MANAGEMENT

Assessment

Assessment begins with an older client's history of elimination patterns and changes in these patterns, such as frequency of defecation, stool characteristics (e.g., color, size, and consistency), toileting habits, and course (e.g., improving or worsening; recurrent or chronic changes in bowel habits). Exercise patterns, pain, bloating, nausea, vomiting, medical history (e.g., hemorrhoids, bowel surgery), and family history of bowel problems such as polyps or colon cancer are also important. With diverticulitis the client may have fever and chills. Physical examination may be unremarkable, but it may also reveal left lower quadrant tenderness or a guaiac-positive stool.

Diagnosis

The most common nursing diagnoses for an older client with diverticulosis or diverticulitis include:

- Risk for constipation related to decreased fluid and/or bulk in the diet
- Acute pain related to bowel obstruction
- Knowledge deficit: disease process, prevention, and treatment related to lack of exposure

Planning and Expected Outcomes

Expected outcomes for an older client with diverticulosis or diverticulitis include:

1. Client will experience fewer episodes of constipation as evidenced by establishment of a regular pattern of bowel activity.
2. Client will verbalize pain relief and remain free from abdominal pain.
3. Client will verbalize self-care practices to minimize symptoms of diverticulosis and prevent complications of diverticulitis.

Intervention

Nursing management of an older client with diverticulosis or diverticulitis includes the prevention and elimination of constipation and the initiation of dietary changes. This includes teaching the client and family about the development of diverticula and the escalation to diverticulitis. In addition, teaching should include the need to eat high-fiber foods and the importance of achieving and maintaining adequate fluid status. Clients should be encouraged to consume up to 2000 ml of fluids each day, unless contraindicated by cardiac status. High-roughage foods like nuts, popcorn, corn, celery, and other fresh vegetables should be avoided. Methods to relieve or prevent constipation include an increase of fluids and fiber, light exercise on a regular basis, and a toileting program.

An older client with diverticulitis needs pain management (with antispasmodics, analgesics, or other measures such as a heating pad), bowel rest (intravenous fluids if on NPO [nothing by mouth] status), and hospitalization if acutely ill. The nurse should teach self-care practices that promote bowel regularity and should administer stool softeners (such as docusate [Colace]) as necessary. Again, preventing constipation is of the utmost importance.

Evaluation

Evaluation includes documentation of achievement of the expected outcomes, prevention of complications, and maintenance of regular bowel patterns and habits. Asking an older adult to verbalize how he or she has incorporated the self-care practices into daily life is an effective way to ascertain whether the client understands the disease and can work to prevent complications.

Polyps

A polyp is any growth that protrudes from a mucous membrane in the GI tract; it is often found in the large intestine, where it protrudes into the lumen of the bowel. A polyp may be sessile (flat, broad, and attached directly to the intestinal wall) or pedunculated (attached to the wall by a thin stem). Polyps may form as a result of abnormal mucosal maturation or inflammation and are nonmalignant. Those which arise from epithelial proliferation and dysplasia are termed *adenomatous polyps* or *adenomas.* The majority of intestinal polyps occur in the rectosigmoid colon, are multiple, and increase in frequency with age (they are found in more than half of all persons ages 60 or older).

The most common type of nonmalignant polyps is termed *hyperplastic.* These rarely grow large and never cause clinical symptoms. Adenomas are true neoplastic lesions and are closely linked to colorectal adenocarcinoma. The size is the main risk determinant for malignancy. Many clients with polyps are asymptomatic. These growths are often discovered incidentally by sigmoidoscopy or barium enema. Occasionally they may bleed, causing bright red blood in the feces. If the polyp is large enough, it may cause an obstruction.

NURSING MANAGEMENT

 Assessment

Assessment begins with a thorough history of any changes in an older adult's routine pattern of elimination and any symptoms such as blood in the stool or on the toilet paper. A careful family history should be obtained, especially as it pertains to polyps. Physical examination may be unremarkable; however, a guaiac-positive stool may be found on rectal examination.

Diagnosis

The most common nursing diagnoses for an older client with polyps include:

- Knowledge deficit: disease process, importance of treatment, and follow-up related to lack of exposure
- Fear related to knowledge deficit of the disease

Planning and Expected Outcomes

Expected outcomes for an older client with polyps include:

1. Client will verbalize knowledge of disease process and potential outcomes.
2. Client will obtain medical follow-up as suggested by the American Cancer Society or a health care provider.

Intervention

Nursing management of an older client with polyps includes education and reinforcement of the American Cancer Society's suggested guidelines to prevent colorectal cancer. In addition, the client who is to undergo a colonoscopy may need reinforcement of the importance of having the polyps removed. Reminders may need to be given to older clients as to when it is time to have another screening sigmoidoscopy (according to their health care provider or American Cancer Society guidelines). Clients may also need to be reminded that, although polyps are often asymptomatic, they may bleed. The presence of any blood in the stool requires a repeat sigmoidoscopy or colonoscopy.

Evaluation

Evaluation includes documentation of achievement of the expected outcomes and prevention of complications, such as obstruction or invasive colorectal cancer.

Hemorrhoids

Hemorrhoids are dilations of the veins in the mucous membrane inside or outside the rectum. These dilations are common and develop in susceptible people as a result of an increase in pressure in the hemorrhoidal venous plexus. Hemorrhoids are often related to the presence of varicose veins and may be referred to as varicose veins of the rectum. Predisposition may result from constipation, uterine fibroids, pregnancy, liver disease, prolonged standing, prostatic disease, or tumors of the rectum.

Internal hemorrhoids may cause minor bleeding with defecation. The dilated venous sacs may protrude into the anal and rectal canals, where they become exposed, resulting in pain; thrombus, ulcerations, and bleeding then develop. External hemorrhoids produce varying degrees of pain, as well as pressure, itching, irritation, and a palpable mass. Bleeding occurs only if the external hemorrhoid is injured or ulcerated. Usually blood loss is insignificant, but chronic anemia may occur (Hill, 2004).

NURSING MANAGEMENT

 Assessment

Assessment begins with an older client's history of constipation and symptoms of anal and rectal pain or blood in stool or on toilet paper. In addition, a medical and family history of bowel problems such as polyps or colon cancer is also important. Physical examination may be unremarkable except for a painful anus and rectum—painful to the point where thorough examination may be difficult. However, a prolapsed hemorrhoid may be detected and should be assessed for swelling, thrombosis, and ischemia. Guaiac-positive stool may be found.

Diagnosis

The most common nursing diagnoses for an older client with hemorrhoids include:

- Risk for constipation related to pain on defecation
- Acute pain in the anal and rectal area related to swelling and inflammation
- Knowledge deficit: treatment and prevention related to lack of previous exposure

Planning and Expected Outcomes

Expected outcomes for an older client with hemorrhoids include:

1. Client will experience fewer episodes of constipation.
2. Client will establish a regular pattern of bowel elimination.
3. Client will report a decrease in anal and rectal pain.
4. Client will verbalize knowledge of self-care practices to minimize occurrence of hemorrhoids.

Intervention

Nursing management of an older client with hemorrhoids includes the prevention and elimination of constipation. This includes a review of high-fiber, high-roughage foods, including indigestible fiber like whole grains, legumes, and fresh fruits and vegetables. Adequate intake of fluids is also important. Older clients should be encouraged to consume up to 2000 ml of fluids each day unless contraindicated. The nurse should encourage light exercise on a regular basis and review the importance of a regular toileting routine. Over-the-counter anesthetic ointments and creams and sitz baths may be used for pain relief. Clients should be encouraged not to strain when defecating; this may make hemorrhoids worse. The nurse should emphasize that it is important to report any rectal bleeding to rule out the possibility of a more serious disorder.

Evaluation

Evaluation includes documentation of achievement of the expected outcomes, prevention of complications, and maintenance of regular bowel patterns and habits.

DISORDERS OF THE ACCESSORY ORGANS

Cholelithiasis and Cholecystitis

Cholelithiasis is the presence or formation of gallstones in the gallbladder. Gallstones are composed primarily of cholesterol, bile salts, bilirubin, calcium, and proteins. The incidence of gallstones varies among racial groups and countries; however, it is not known whether this is a result of environmental or genetic factors. Risk factors like obesity, female gender, multiparity, sedentary lifestyle, and advancing age increase the incidence of gallstones (Price and Wilson, 2003; Lewis, Heitkemper, and Dirksen, 2004).

The formation of gallstones is primarily metabolic and results from increased cholesterol saturation (because of obesity, estrogen, or resection of the terminal ileum), increased levels of bilirubin (hemolytic anemias), or increased serum cholesterol. In addition, slow emptying of the gallbladder may produce stasis and encourage the aggregation of cholesterol crystals, eventually leading to stone formation. The majority of gallstones in Western cultures are cholesterol stones; other stones are classified as biliary pigment stones.

Gallstones may be present for many years without signs and symptoms. Of clients with gallstones, 20% to 50% are asymptomatic. The classic symptom is a right–upper quadrant pain, ache, or pressure that may radiate to the right scapular area. The pain begins suddenly, often directly after a meal. The pain can last from 15 minutes to 6 hours, and nausea and vomiting may occur. These attacks of pain can occur as infrequently as once every few years or as often as every few days. Often these episodes are precipitated by the ingestion of fatty foods. The symptoms of biliary pain are due to an obstruction of the cystic or common bile duct causing increased pressure and distention of the gallbladder. Often the pain is so severe it is confused with a heart attack. When the stones lodge along the biliary tract, they obstruct the flow of bile. This may result in jaundice because of the blockage of the flow of bilirubin. When the common bile duct becomes blocked, the bile cannot enter the duodenum, so stools are clay colored because they lack the pigment. In addition, obstruction of the common bile duct may cause biliary pain, jaundice, pancreatitis, or cholangitis (inflammation of the bile ducts).

Cholecystitis may be acute or chronic and is usually associated with gallstones or other obstructions of the biliary system. The inflammation in cholecystitis results in a thickening of the wall of the gallbladder, which can lead to ischemia; necrosis; gangrene; and possible perforation of the gallbladder itself, leading to peritonitis. In chronic cholecystitis the walls become thickened and inefficient at emptying. This is a result of chronic chemical or mechanical irritation from stones exerting pressure on the mucosa or from biliary stasis.

NURSING MANAGEMENT

Assessment

Assessment begins with a history of episodes of pain, identifying the location, quality, and duration. Other symptoms include nausea and vomiting. Precipitating factors (e.g., large, fatty meals) and alleviating factors (e.g., pain relievers, changes of position) need to be documented. Physical examination may reveal a tender right upper quadrant and possibly jaundice.

Diagnosis

The most common nursing diagnoses for an older client with cholelithiasis or cholecystitis include:

- Acute pain related to gallbladder inflammation
- Knowledge deficit: condition and treatment options related to lack of previous exposure
- Sleep pattern disturbance related to pruritus and pain

Planning and Expected Outcomes

Expected outcomes for an older client with cholelithiasis or cholecystitis include:

1. Client will experience pain relief.
2. Client will verbalize knowledge of the disease process, prevention of complications, and treatment options available.
3. Client will verbalize a feeling of being rested after nighttime sleeping.

Intervention

Nursing management of an older client with cholelithiasis or cholecystitis includes providing pain relief and instructing the client and family about the disease process, treatment options, and potential complications. Older clients with cholelithiasis need to know that foods high in fat may precipitate an attack of pain. They need to be aware of treatment options, including types of surgery, medical dissolution, and lithotripsy, as well as the advantages and disadvantages of each. The client with cholecystitis may require hospitalization and may receive an intravenous tube and antibiotics. If managed at home, clients need to be on a clear liquid diet until pain is resolved and then slowly advance to a regular diet, avoiding fatty foods. Signs and symptoms of complications need to be reviewed with both clients and their families. Additional nursing care is based on an older client's response to initial treatment.

Evaluation

Evaluation includes documentation of achievement of expected outcomes, prevention of complications, prevention of infection, and assessment of a client's knowledge of the disease process. The nurse also evaluates the client's response to food intake and monitors the client's food selections to ensure dietary compliance.

Pancreatitis

Pancreatitis is an inflammation of the pancreas and often has no known cause. The disorder may be acute or chronic, and the acute phase may become chronic after several acute attacks. In acute pancreatitis the organ returns to normal after treatment. In chronic pancreatitis, permanent and progressive destruction of the pancreas occurs, whereby the normal tissue is replaced by fibrous tissue.

Acute pancreatitis may be alcohol induced or related to biliary tract disease. Pancreatitis related to biliary tract disease is more likely to occur in women in their late 50s and 60s. Approximately 40% of acute pancreatitis is related to biliary disease, and another 40% results from alcoholism. Of the remaining cases, 5% are associated with other conditions, and the cause of the remainder is unknown. In the United States the primary cause of chronic pancreatitis is alcoholism.

Acute pancreatitis is believed to be caused by activation of pancreatic enzymes, which may cause autodigestion of the pancreas. The initiation of activation of the enzymes is thought to result from reflux of bile into the pancreatic duct, obstruction of the pancreatic duct, ischemia, anorexia, trauma, and toxins. The etiology of chronic pancreatitis is not well understood.

Symptoms include severe abdominal pain in the epigastric to the right upper quadrant area, occasionally radiating through to the back. Pain is usually more intense when lying supine, and the client often remains in a flexed position to relieve pain. Nausea, vomiting, abdominal distention, and fever are common. In chronic pancreatitis the pain may be continuous and accompanied by weakness and jaundice. In addition, in chronic pancreatitis the stools often become bulky, fatty, and foul smelling, and weight loss may occur because of malabsorption. Glucose intolerance is a late sign of chronic pancreatitis.

NURSING MANAGEMENT

Assessment

Assessment begins with an older client's history of precipitating factors such as alcohol abuse or the presence of gallstones. Symptoms of abdominal pain, anorexia, nausea, and vomiting need to be assessed in detail. The client may be in tremendous pain and unable to answer, so reliance on a family member may be necessary. Depending on the client's pain, physical examination may be difficult.

Diagnosis

The most common nursing diagnoses for an older client with pancreatitis include:

- Deficient fluid volume related to nausea or vomiting; restricted oral intake
- Acute pain related to obstruction of the pancreatic tract
- Altered nutrition: less than body requirements related to anorexia and vomiting

Planning and Expected Outcomes

Expected outcomes for an older client with pancreatitis include:

1. Client will maintain adequate fluid volume and electrolyte balance.
2. Client will obtain pain relief.
3. Client will stabilize and maintain weight.
4. Client will not experience complications.

Intervention

Nursing management of an older client with pancreatitis includes maintenance of fluid and electrolyte balance, pain relief measures, and prevention of complications. This includes monitoring intravenous therapy, vital signs, intake and output, serum electrolyte values, and weight. Pain management can be extremely difficult, especially for clients with chronic pancreatitis. Often the expertise of a pain consultant is necessary (see Chapter 15).

An important consideration in acute pancreatitis is the prevention of recurrence. When pancreatitis results from alcohol abuse, teaching should center on the dangers of alcoholism and implications for the future. Referral and counseling may be needed. For the client with pancreatitis resulting from biliary tract disease, teaching about high lipid levels is important; providing information and emotional support is important for clients who may need surgery.

Evaluation

Evaluation includes documentation of achievement of expected outcomes, prevention of complications, prevention of recurrence (for acute pancreatitis), and maintenance of adequate nutrition. Older adults who are addicted to alcohol may go through withdrawal, requiring the nurse to carefully monitor and record client responses to treatment of this secondary problem.

Hepatitis

Hepatitis is a general term referring to inflammation of the liver. It may be caused by a variety of factors such as chemicals and alcohol, but the most common cause is viral infection. Although five major viruses can act as the causative agent for hepatitis, the hepatitis A, B, and C viruses are most common in the United States.

Hepatitis A, formerly called infectious hepatitis, is caused by a ribonucleic acid (RNA) virus. The primary mode of transmission of this organism is the fecal-oral route, commonly through ingestion of contaminated food or water. Risk groups for hepatitis A include institutional populations, such as clients in daycare centers, and travelers to endemic areas. The clinical disease tends to be mild and of short duration. There is no residual liver disease following recovery and no indications of a chronic state.

Hepatitis B, formerly called serum hepatitis, is caused by a deoxyribonucleic acid (DNA) virus. This virus is transmitted through blood and body fluids, with risk factors including intravenous drug use and sexual contact. It is considered a sexually transmitted disease by the Centers for Disease Control and Prevention (CDC). Hepatitis B follows a more severe course than hepatitis A, with an increased risk for liver disease (cirrhosis, cancer). There is also a 5% to 10% incidence of a chronic state, defined as continuing to test positive for the viral antigen for 6 months or longer. These individuals may be asymptomatic or have subclinical symptoms; however, they remain contagious as long as the antigen is present.

Hepatitis C is caused by a small RNA virus and represents 85% to 90% of transfusion-related hepatitis cases. The clinical course is usually milder than with hepatitis B, and a client can even be asymptomatic. The major concern with hepatitis C is that a chronic condition develops in more than 50% of individuals.

The pathophysiologic events leading to the liver inflammation seen in hepatitis are similar for all of the viruses. Once the virus is introduced to the individual by its specific mode of transmission, it enters the circulation and seeks out hepatic tissue. The virus enters the cell and uses the host cell's DNA to reproduce itself. This may directly injure or kill the hepatocyte, believed to be the primary cause of cell damage in hepatitis A, or the responding immunologic cells may harm the liver cell in the process of destroying the virus, the probable pathologic cause in hepatitis B and C (Table 26-1).

The clinical picture of hepatitis is essentially the same for all the viruses, with the overall course being shorter for hepatitis A. Typically the illness is divided into three phases. In the *prodromal phase,* clients have generalized symptoms of malaise, fatigue, possible right upper quadrant pain, nausea and vomiting, anorexia, and a low-grade fever. Clients often think they have the flu, or the symptoms are so mild that the individuals do not recall experiencing them. The second phase, when jaundice and dark urine appear, is termed the

TABLE 26-1 Viral Hepatitis

	TYPE A	TYPE B	TYPE C
Transmission	Fecal-oral route (formerly called infectious hepatitis)	Parenteral; close personal contact (formerly called serum hepatitis)	Parenteral; close personal contact; primary cause of transfusion-related hepatitis
Incubation period	15 to 45 days	30 to 180 days	20 to 90 days
Risk groups	Institutional populations, including daycare centers, and travelers to endemic areas	Intravenous drug use and sexual contact; considered by the CDC to be a sexually transmitted disease	Recipients of blood or blood product transfusions
Course of disease	Clinical course tends to be mild and of short duration; no residual liver disease following recovery	Course more severe than with hepatitis A	Milder course
Chronic state	No	5% to 10% of clients asymptomatic or with subclinical symptoms; however, they remain contagious as long as antigen is present	40% to 60%
Liver cancer risk	None	Yes (also other liver disease like cirrhosis)	Yes

icteric phase. Sometimes jaundice does not occur. Clients may actually start to feel better during this phase. Finally, in the *convalescent phase,* jaundice and other symptoms disappear, and clients feel fully recovered. It is important that clients understand that it will take 3 to 6 months for the liver to return to normal functioning status. Care should be taken regarding rest and drug and alcohol consumption during this phase; a relapse can occur.

NURSING MANAGEMENT

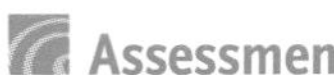

Assessment

Assessment begins by reviewing with the client any possible exposure to a hepatitis virus. The nurse should ask questions about recent travel, food intake, blood transfusions, and close contact with persons who may have had hepatitis in the past. Clinical manifestations include skin color, right upper quadrant tenderness, fatigue, and malaise. The nurse should question the client about changes in functional status, for example, whether the client's activity level and ability to perform activities of daily living (ADLs) have decreased from baseline levels. The nurse should also review nutritional intake and assess for anorexia, as well as question changes in the way clothes fit and ask if family and friends have noticed weight loss in the client. Palpation of the abdomen may reveal an enlarged liver.

Diagnosis

Nursing diagnoses for an older client with hepatitis include:

- Ineffective health maintenance related to knowledge deficit about hepatitis, treatment regimen, and prevention of spread
- Activity intolerance related to generalized weakness
- Altered nutrition: less than body requirements related to anorexia, nausea, and liver dysfunction
- Ineffective therapeutic regimen management related to lack of knowledge

Planning and Expected Outcomes

Expected outcomes for an older client with hepatitis include:

1. Client will verbalize the causes of hepatitis, the treatment plan, and mechanisms to prevent spread to others.
2. Client will participate in ADLs without experiencing fatigue.
3. Client will consume a well-balanced, high-calorie diet as evidenced by food diary.
4. Client will demonstrate self-care activities as much as possible within limitations.

Intervention

The nurse must teach clients and their significant others about the spread of hepatitis and mechanisms of prevention. Depending on the specific mode of transmission of the particular virus, the nurse should also discuss hygienic practices in the home, especially when dealing with feces; proper disposal of needles used for medications; and purchase and preparation of certain foods like shellfish.

The nurse should explain that rest is an important treatment in hepatitis, and activities such as visiting, cooking, and housework need to be curtailed. Frequent rest periods will be necessary; nursing interventions may be needed to allow an older client adequate, uninterrupted rest periods.

A high-carbohydrate, low-fat diet is best tolerated by a client with hepatitis. Several small feedings throughout the day will help alleviate the effect of anorexia. Fluid intake should increase to 2000 to 3000 ml/day unless contraindicated by cardiovascular status.

The cause of jaundice should be explained, and the client should be warned that there may be a change in the color of the urine, skin, and sclera. The client must understand that this is a temporary condition that will completely resolve once the course of the disease is finished.

If pruritus is present from the jaundice, the nurse should discuss the use of nonalcohol lotions, soft clothes and linens, and tepid baths using as little mild soap as possible. The nurse should instruct clients and caregivers about keeping clients' fingernails short to avoid injury from scratching.

Evaluation

Evaluation includes documentation of achievement of the expected outcomes, coupled with the client's successful self-management of the disease. Careful attention to an older adult's food intake, weight trends, and activity tolerance is crucial.

Alcoholic Cirrhosis

Cirrhosis is a general term referring to a chronic disorder of the liver in which there is permanent, irreversible destruction of the hepatocytes and the normal architecture of the organ. Although there are several causes for this disease, about 80% of cases in the United States are due to alcohol abuse.

Alcoholic cirrhosis is also known as Laënnec's cirrhosis, portal cirrhosis, or nutritional cirrhosis. The progressive loss of functioning liver tissue is manifested by the appearance of general signs and symptoms of liver failure; over time, other manifestations of declining liver function will appear (Fig. 26-6). Early signs and symptoms of liver failure from cirrhosis are similar to those of hepatitis. The client experiences fatigue; malaise; anorexia; change in bowel habits (either diarrhea or constipation); nausea and vomiting; and dull, heavy pain in the right upper quadrant. Later symptoms include jaundice and edema in peripheral sites. Ultimately, serious complications like bleeding, portal hypertension, ascites, and encephalopathy develop. Bleeding tendencies are the result of declining clotting and coagulation factors. One

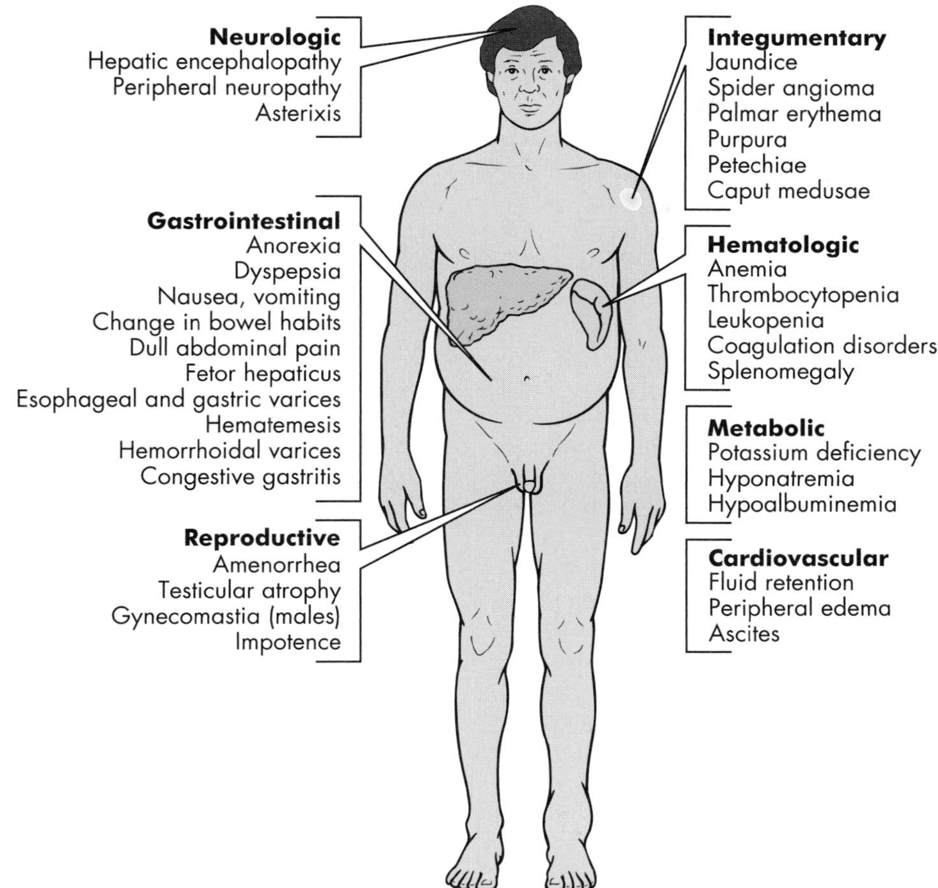

Fig. 26-6 Systemic clinical manifestations of liver cirrhosis. (From Damjanov I, Linder J, editors: *Anderson's pathology*, ed 10, St Louis, 2004, Mosby.)

of the many functions of the liver is the production of clotting factors V, VII, IX, and X, as well as fibrinogen and prothrombin. Decreased amounts of these proteins result in a bleeding diathesis in any client with advanced liver disease from any cause.

Ascites is the accumulation of serous fluid in the abdominal cavity. It is the result of several factors relating to poor liver function, but the most important of these is the decreased production of albumin by the liver. Insufficient amounts of this major plasma protein in the blood cause the escape of plasma fluid into the abdominal space. Another factor is the increased venous pressure from portal hypertension, which forces the fluid out of the vessel. The most serious effect of ascites is respiratory compromise, which occurs when the diaphragm is pushed upward by the increasing abdominal fluid, thus decreasing thoracic space for pulmonary excursion.

Portal hypertension is an increase in pressure in the portal vein and its feeders as a result of liver congestion or obstruction. In addition to contributing to the development of ascites, portal hypertension and the backflow of venous blood cause severe problems with hemorrhoids, splenomegaly, and esophageal varices. The effect of portal hypertension on the esophageal veins is the most dangerous, since these vessels are fragile and susceptible to rupture with any increase in intraabdominal pressure. Clients who bleed from esophageal varices are gravely ill. One third of all deaths from cirrhosis are from esophageal varices. A late-stage event in long-term liver disease is the development of *encephalopathy*, which is due to the diseased liver being unable to carry out its function of detoxification of toxic metabolic byproducts. One of the most critical of these is ammonia, an end product of protein metabolism. Although it is not clear whether the ammonia is directly toxic to the brain or interferes with glucose uptake, decreasing blood ammonia levels is correlated with successful treatment. A client with high ammonia levels will begin to exhibit changes in behavior, irrationality, agitation, combativeness, and muscle tremors (asterixis). If it remains untreated, hepatic coma ensues, which has a mortality rate of 90%.

NURSING MANAGEMENT

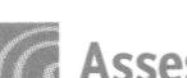

Assessment

Assessment of the client with cirrhosis involves a careful history of the onset and duration of symptoms. The nurse should question the client about changes in the color of the stool, rectal bleeding, and bloody emesis. A thorough physical assessment of all body systems, especially the skin and abdomen, and respiratory and mental status is indicated. Nutritional status is also important.

Diagnosis

Nursing diagnoses for an older client with cirrhosis include:

- Risk for impaired skin integrity related to pruritus, edema, and ascites
- Ineffective breathing pattern related to increased pressure on diaphragm secondary to ascites
- Risk for injury related to decreased clotting factors
- Acute confusion related to increased serum ammonia levels
- Altered nutrition: less than body requirements related to anorexia, nausea, and vomiting
- Risk for situational low self-esteem related to guilt about damage done to self and significant others

Planning and Expected Outcomes

Expected outcomes for an older client with alcoholic cirrhosis include:

1. Client will be free from skin breakdown.
2. Client will demonstrate ability to pace activity and ADLs within current ventilatory function.
3. Client will remain free from injuries and bleeding.
4. Client will demonstrate resolution of cerebral dysfunction as evidenced by no injury to self or others; achieve an appropriate sleep-wake pattern; and communicate meaningfully with others and oriented to time, person, and place.
5. Client will maintain or gain weight to an appropriate level.
6. Client will identify positive aspects about self and express an optimistic outlook regarding relationships.

Intervention

Interventions for an older adult with cirrhosis can be multiple and complex, with a major focus of preventing the common complications. Skin care is a priority. The nurse should inspect the skin daily for signs of breakdown or redness and keep the skin clean and dry, especially after toileting. The nurse should use pressure-relieving devices on a client's bed and chair to provide even weight distribution. He or she must also teach clients and caregivers the importance of changing position every 2 hours; a bed trapeze may be provided to facilitate lifting and position changes.

The nurse should position the client in a semi-Fowler's or high Fowler's position to promote maximum chest expansion and maintain oxygen supplementation as indicated. Lung sounds must be assessed at least daily.

To prevent bleeding, the nurse should limit the number of venipunctures and use the smallest needle possible. A soft toothbrush or oral swabs can be used for mouth care; male clients should use an electric razor to shave. The environment should be kept free of clutter. If the client is confused or combative, the nurse should keep the side rails up and pad them to prevent injury.

A client's orientation and psychomotor function are assessed. The nurse should reorient the client on a consistent basis and limit the number of new people who enter the room. Mouth care should be provided before meals, and the environment should be conducive to eating. Small, bland feedings can be given, especially if the client complains of nausea. The nurse should consider the client's food preferences and remember that a high-carbohydrate, no protein or low-protein, low-fat diet will be ordered; he or she should also remember that fruit juices are often well tolerated by individuals with anorexia.

The nurse should encourage the client to discuss feelings about self-esteem, while maintaining a judgment-free environment at all times. The nurse should also reinforce positive abilities and traits and help the client identify negative automatic behaviors. Resources such as pastoral care can be used as indicated.

Evaluation

Evaluation includes documentation of achievement of the expected outcomes and prevention or early detection of complications. Given the long-term nature of the condition, the nursing care plan should be reviewed and updated on a regular basis.

Drug-Induced Liver Disease

Since one of the major functions of the liver is the metabolism and detoxification of chemicals, including drugs, it is clear that this organ is subject to potential damage from these substances. Hepatic injury may result from direct toxicity, conversion of a drug to an active toxin, or immune mechanisms responding to the presence of a "foreign" invader.

Some agents cause liver cell damage in all individuals at a predictable dose level. A common example of a dose-related toxic drug is acetaminophen, the basic ingredient of Tylenol. With overdosage of these agents, the normal metabolic pathway is exhausted and alternative means are used to clear the drug from the body. These mechanisms yield toxic byproducts. Carbon tetrachloride and chloroform, used in industry, are examples of chemical agents that cause liver disease.

Drugs and chemicals that cause liver damage in an unpredictable manner are said to have *idiosyncratic* toxicity. These reactions are unrelated to dose and occur only in a small percentage of susceptible individuals. Idiosyncratic toxicity is manifested in a variety of ways. There may be massive hepatocellular injury. Drugs like isoniazid, halothane, and methyldopa may cause liver necrosis and possibly hepatic failure. Ingestion of poisonous mushrooms causes massive cell destruction. Substances like vinyl chloride lead to sclerosis of the portal venules and portal hypertension. Another hepatic response to toxic exposure is cholestasis, an arrest or cessation of normal bile flow. This response is caused by drugs like anabolic steroids, oral contraceptives, phenothiazines, and oral antidiabetic drugs. Other manifestations of liver disease from idiosyncratic toxicity are acute or chronic hepatitis, fatty changes in the liver, and mass lesions such as liver cell adenoma and hyperplasia.

The clinical manifestations of toxic liver disease are similar to those of hepatitis. At first, GI and influenza-like symptoms appear. Clients first may be seen with jaundice, especially with the cholestatic presentation. Hepatomegaly and other signs of liver damage may also appear. The onset of symptoms may be immediate or several weeks to months after exposure to the hepatotoxic agent. In some cases the onset of liver failure is abrupt and the clinical course lasts only a few days, with outcomes of resolution, organ transplantation, or death.

NURSING MANAGEMENT

Assessment

In addition to previously discussed assessments related to liver disease, it is essential that information be obtained regarding the exact name of the ingested substance, the dosage and amount taken, and the length of time since ingestion occurred. History of emesis after ingestion is also pertinent.

Diagnosis

The most common nursing diagnoses for an older client with drug-induced liver disease include:

- Knowledge deficit: disease cause, treatment regimen, and outcome related to lack of exposure
- Risk for injury related to end-stage liver failure

Planning and Expected Outcomes

Expected outcomes for an older client with drug-induced liver disease include:

1. Client will verbalize understanding of disease process and interventions.
2. Client will not experience life-threatening complications of liver failure.

Intervention

Nasogastric suction, if required, needs to be approached by the nurse calmly. The nurse needs to make the patient comfortable and lubricate the tube to minimize discomfort. The nurse should also discuss the adverse effect of certain medications with the client and provide written material as reminders to avoid these drugs. The nurse must monitor the client carefully for signs and symptoms of liver failure, percuss liver size, assess the skin and sclera of the eyes, and monitor the level of consciousness.

Interventions for older adults presenting with complications of liver failure are discussed in the section on Alcoholic Cirrhosis.

Evaluation

Evaluation includes documentation of achievement of the expected outcomes and prevention of complications.

GASTROINTESTINAL CANCERS

Cancers of the GI system account for more than 25% of cancer deaths in the United States each year, and they are one of the top three causes of cancer deaths in both men and women. Most tumors of the GI tract are adenocarcinomas, with the exception of the esophagus and anus, where squamous cell malignancies predominate.

Although the GI tract is complex because it is made up of a variety of organs, one problem is universal: the delay in diagnosis of many cancerous states because of vague, nonspecific symptoms that can be somewhat relieved by self-treatment for a time.

In general, incidence of cancers of the GI tract increases with age. The age ranges for several GI cancers should be considered: oral, 40 to 70 years; esophageal, 50 to 70 years; stomach, 50 to 70; liver, 60 to 70; pancreas, 60 to 70; and colon, 55 to 75.

Oral Cancer

Oral cancer commonly includes cancer of the salivary glands, floor of the mouth, tongue, and lips. Although not common (i.e., it represents 3% of all cancers), oral cancer can be devastating for older adults because it can affect appearance, speaking, and eating.

The causative factors have not been well researched. However, risk factors focus on exposure to carcinogenic agents because the mouth is a conduit for air, food, fluids, and tobacco products. These carcinogenic agents include cigarettes, ethyl alcohol, snuff, chewing tobacco, betel nut, and chemicals used in the textile industries and leather manufacturing. Other precipitating factors include pernicious anemia and iron deficiency anemia.

The majority of oral cancers are squamous cell carcinomas. These tumors typically occur in clients between the ages of 40 and 70 years and are more prevalent in men than women. Cancer of the tongue, usually a squamous cell carcinoma, is more prevalent in men than women. This cancer begins as an ulceration, which may be precipitated by chronic irritations from tobacco, food, alcohol, occupational exposures, or malocclusion of the teeth. With growth of the tumor, the cancer metastasizes to the floor of the mouth and lymph nodes of the neck. Unfortunately, metastasis to the neck has already occurred in more than 60% of people when the diagnosis is made. This is partly because of the great vascular and lymph drainage of the tongue and the location of the lesion, which may go unnoticed by a client.

Cancer of the lips usually results from squamous cells, but it may also be caused by basal cell carcinoma. These cancers are usually a result of prolonged exposure to the sun and pipe smoking.

Oral cancers are classified according to four stages. Stages I and II involve a local tumor only with no lymph node spread or metastases. In stage III the tumor is 4 cm, and there may be palpable lymph nodes. In stage IV the tumor is invasive, with metastases to the lungs or liver.

NURSING MANAGEMENT

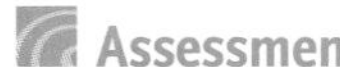

Assessment

Assessment begins with a history of symptoms such as pain of the lips, gums, and floor or roof of mouth or with palpation or visualization of a lump or other abnormality. A history of previous experiences with cancer (either oral or other forms) and an older client's concomitant medical illnesses and medications are necessary. The physical examination includes a complete and thorough oral examination, focusing on palpating and visualizing any abnormalities, especially on the floor and roof of the mouth. Foul breath may be noted.

Diagnosis

Nursing diagnoses for an older client with oral cancer include:

- Impaired oral mucous membrane related to the trauma of surgical incisions
- Altered nutrition: less than body requirements related to pain and difficulty chewing and swallowing
- Body image disturbance related to difficulty accepting postoperative disfigurement secondary to surgical resection
- Anxiety related to diagnosis of cancer

Planning and Expected Outcomes

Expected outcomes for an older client with oral cancer include:

1. Client's lesions and incisions will heal without infection.
2. Client will maintain weight within acceptable range for height and age.
3. Client will accept body image changes imposed by treatment as evidenced by the ability to verbalize fears and concerns related to disfigurement.

Intervention

Nursing management for an older client with oral cancer includes maintenance of adequate nutrition, promotion of oral hygiene, provision of comfort, and facilitation of communication.

When part or all of the tongue is removed, the client may have difficulty swallowing and speaking. Referral to a speech therapist is useful for retraining in swallowing and speaking. Liquid diets and gavage feedings may be used to maintain adequate nutrition. Mouth care and oral hygiene are important to promote healing. Disfigurement and a poor prognosis may lead to coping difficulties that require counseling. The nurse should encourage the client to verbalize feelings and frustrations and attend support groups that may facilitate adjustments.

Evaluation

Evaluation includes documentation of achievement of the expected outcomes, including maintenance of nutrition, prevention of infection, and resumption of activities.

Esophageal Cancer

In the United States esophageal cancer accounts for approximately 23% of all GI cancers (Price and Wilson, 2003). Unfortunately, these malignancies usually remain asymptomatic until they are surgically unresectable because of extension. In addition, many people with esophageal cancer attribute its signs and symptoms to some of the more common disorders that affect older adults. Because of this fact, clients with esophageal cancer have one of the worst prognoses of all malignancies of the GI tract.

Esophageal malignancy usually occurs between ages 50 and 70, but in general develops at a younger age in blacks compared with whites. In addition, incidence is higher among men than women.

Although the cause of esophageal cancer is unknown, a strong correlation exists between esophageal cancer and heavy alcohol intake, cigarette smoking, and chronic gastric reflux (Barrett's esophagus). There is also a relationship between preexisting hiatal hernia and esophageal diverticula.

Morphologically the most common cancer is squamous cell, since it is the major cell type that lines the esophagus. This malignancy may grow around the esophagus at the level of the diaphragm, impinging on the lumen of the tube, or it may cause a bulky, ulcerating tumor mass. Most tumors are found in the middle and lower third of the esophagus. The tumor often spreads by invasion of the surrounding structures and can affect the mediastinum, trachea, lungs, bronchi, and major vessels. In addition, it metastasizes through the lymph system, with flow being either cephalic or caudal. The tumor also metastasizes by hematogenous spread of tumor cells or tumor emboli. Distant metastases to lung, liver, adrenal glands, brain, bone, and kidney are common. There are no adequate screening procedures and no tumor markers to help with diagnosis and response to treatment. The proximity of the tumor to the aorta and the trachea, in addition to the potential for spread to the cervical lymph system, results in a generally poor prognosis. The natural history of the disease includes swallowing difficulties, malnutrition, cachexia, pneumonia, and eventual death.

The earliest complaint is usually a mild dysphagia that becomes progressively worse, starting with problems with solids only and progressing to an inability to swallow liquids. Painful swallowing is present in about 50% of cases. Other symptoms include substernal pressure, fullness, and indigestion. Eventually weight loss is a common complaint, as is general malaise and anorexia. Laryngeal nerve involvement may cause hoarseness and deepening of the voice. Postprandial regurgitation of undigested food may motivate the person to seek medical attention. Hematemesis and guaiac-positive stools are uncommon. Invasion of surrounding structures by the tumor may lead to back pain or respiratory distress. Although symptoms may be present for only weeks or months, the carcinoma can be advanced at diagnosis.

NURSING MANAGEMENT

Assessment

Assessment begins with an accurate history, focusing on risk factors for esophageal cancer. A review of systems may reveal symptoms of dysphagia, eating difficulties, and aspiration. Physical examination will probably reveal few findings definitive of the diagnosis. However, in advanced disease, the nurse may find palpable lymph nodes and perhaps organ enlargement resulting from metastasis. Other findings include significant and recent weight loss (Smith, Cokkinides, and Eyre, 2004).

Diagnosis

Nursing diagnoses for an older client with esophageal cancer include:

- Altered nutrition: less than body requirements related to inadequate intake of nutrients in the diet because of dysphagia
- Risk for aspiration
- Fear related to uncertain prognosis, possible disfigurement, and loss of ability to eat

Planning and Expected Outcomes

Expected outcomes for an older client with esophageal cancer include:

1. Client will initially stabilize weight and then achieve an individually determined weight gain.
2. Client will remain free from aspiration.
3. Client will verbalize fears related to the diagnosis and prognosis.

The medical treatments of radiotherapy, chemotherapy, and surgery will require additional, specific nursing interventions. The nurse should include the older adult and family in planning all aspects of nursing care related to any one or a combination of these modalities.

Intervention

Nursing management of an older client with esophageal cancer includes maintenance of hydration and nutritional status, prevention of aspiration, maintenance of comfort, and provision of emotional support. Optimizing nutritional status and preventing further weight loss can be accomplished with small, frequent feedings; high-protein, high-calorie foods; supplements such as Ensure; and tube feedings if necessary. Nursing care to prevent aspiration focuses on assessment of respiratory status, assessment of difficulty with eating and drinking, and proper positioning during and after eating.

The nurse's role in the prevention and early detection of esophageal cancer may lead to early identification and perhaps improved prognosis for older clients. Persons with risk factors for esophageal cancer should be instructed to reduce or eliminate these factors and be counseled regarding the need for frequent medical follow-up. Counseling on proper nutrition and elimination of smoking and alcohol is important for prevention. Older clients with frequent upper GI complaints should be advised to seek medical attention immediately.

Evaluation

Evaluation includes documentation of achievement of the expected outcomes, prevention of aspiration, and maintenance of adequate nutrition (see Nursing Care Plan).

Gastric Cancer

As with other forms of GI cancer, gastric cancer is insidious. Symptoms may be vague until the cancer has infiltrated and spread throughout the body, when the overt signs of cancer become evident. In addition, stomach cancer mimics other diseases such as ulcers and gastritis, so misdiagnosis and self-medication for chronic "stomach problems" are common and may delay the diagnosis and treatment of stomach cancer.

The incidence of gastric cancer is increasing in certain areas of the world and decreasing in others. For example, the highest incidence is currently in Japan, and the lowest is in the United States. Furthermore, the incidence of gastric cancer has decreased in the United States and occurs more often in lower socioeconomic groups (Price and Wilson, 2003). Gastric cancer usually occurs between the ages of 50 and 70 and strikes men twice as often as women. It occurs

Nursing Care Plan
Esophageal Cancer

Clinical Situation: Mr. E is a 65-year-old retired factory worker and veteran who comes to the Veterans Administration outpatient satellite clinic with the complaint of dysphagia. Within the past 4 months he has had pain and difficulty swallowing solid food; he therefore progressed to eating soft, then liquid foods. But within the past month this has progressed to problems with swallowing even liquids. He reports one episode of nocturnal regurgitation this last week. Other symptoms include a loss of 20 pounds over the past 6 months, fatigue, and a dull backache. Mr. E sheepishly admits that he still smokes, but has cut down from two packs to one pack a day. In addition, he admits to ingestion of beer and hard liquor, although he has cut down in amount and frequency over the past few years, since the death of his wife.

His medical history is unremarkable, except an amputation of two fingers on his right hand while he was in the service. He lives alone but near his daughter, whom he states convinced him to come to the clinic when he did not eat anything at her recent Thanksgiving dinner.

Physical examination reveals a thin but well-developed older man, with a weight of 140 lb, temperature of 98° F (36.6° C), pulse of 80 beats/min, respiratory rate of 18 breaths/min, and blood pressure of 120/82 mm Hg. Inspection of his pharynx reveals no abnormalities except for poor dentition. Examination of his abdomen and rectal area is also unremarkable. Laboratory values reveal iron deficiency anemia, but initial screening is otherwise unremarkable. He is scheduled for an endoscopy the next day. He returns to the clinic 1 week later to get his results, and his diagnosis is esophageal cancer. He is scheduled for radiotherapy and possibly surgery once the tumor has shrunk in size.

Nursing Diagnosis

Imbalanced nutrition: less than body requirements related to inadequate intake of nutrients secondary to dysphagia
Impaired swallowing related to mechanical obstruction secondary to tumor
Fear related to uncertain prognosis, possible disfigurement, and loss of ability to eat
High risk for aspiration related to dysphagia

Outcomes

Client will stabilize weight.
Client will swallow safely without gagging or aspirating.
Client will maintain adequate nutrition and hydration.
Client and family will identify sources of fears and acquire knowledge to deal with the fears.

Interventions

Encourage small, frequent meals. Encourage the use of high-protein, high-calorie foods and the use of supplements such as Ensure. Refer to dietitian if necessary for specific recommendations.
Discuss possibility of the use of tube feedings with client to supplement nutrients or as the sole means of delivering necessary nutrients.
Arrange for a speech therapist consultation to provide instruction regarding swallowing.
Instruct client and family regarding need for upright positioning during and after eating.
Instruct client and family to rotate the client's head toward the affected side to facilitate swallowing.
Provide rest periods before, during, and after feedings.
Provide thick liquids first, adding thin liquids last; begin with cold liquids and progress to hotter ones.
Begin with pureed foods, progressing to soft ones, while taking small bites.
Encourage client and family to verbalize fears.
Provide information to reduce distortions in perceptions.
Encourage client and family to attend cancer support groups.
Instruct client and family about impending treatments such as surgery and radiotherapy.
Assess client's ability to eat and drink.
Assess respiratory status before, during, and after eating.
Monitor for signs of aspiration: dyspnea, cough, wheezing, tachycardia, and elevated temperature.
Observe and record color and character of sputum.
Consult with speech therapist for techniques to improve swallowing.
Instruct client and family to keep head elevated during and after eating or feedings.

twice as often among black men and women compared with whites and seems to have a familial connection. The reasons for these geographic and cultural incidences are unclear.

The cause is unknown, although the incidence is higher when gastric acid is low, as with chronic gastritis and pernicious anemia. Gastric cancer is also associated with environmental and genetic factors, including diet (e.g., poor nutrition, food additives, vitamin A deficiency), low socioeconomic status, and urban residence. It may also be precipitated by polyps or degenerative changes in gastric ulcers, as well as achlorhydria. Finally, there are occupational risks, such as for rubber and coal workers and those working in nickel refineries. There is also a relationship between gastric cancer and infection with *H. pylori*.

Most gastric cancers are adenocarcinomas and occur in either polypoid, ulcerative, or infiltrative forms. The ulcerative form is the most common and produces symptoms similar to those of peptic ulcers. The tumor usually arises in the antrum, the lower third of the stomach. The tumor causes ulceration, obstruction, and hemorrhage. It may metastasize by extension and infiltration along the mucosa into the stomach wall and lymph vessels in three ways: (1) by lymphatic or vascular embolism to regional lymph nodes, (2) by direct extension to adjacent organs, and (3) by bloodborne spread. The tumor may metastasize to the lung, bone, liver, spleen, pancreas, peritoneum, and esophagus.

Because of its elusive nature, gastric cancer is usually well advanced when symptoms begin to appear. When they occur, they are vague and of variable duration. Because of this, people usually delay seeking medical attention for a few months after the initial onset of symptoms. Initially, the client may complain of a vague, uneasy sense of fullness, indigestion, and distention after meals, which may be passed off as stomach upset. As the disease progresses, anorexia, nausea, and vomiting may develop and lead to weight loss. Other symptoms include dysphagia, back pain, weakness, fatigue, hematemesis, and a change in bowel habits. Unfortunately, definitive clinical signs occur mostly with advanced disease and include weight loss, pain, vomiting, anorexia, dysphagia, and a palpable abdominal mass. The prognosis is generally poor (5% to 15% 5-year survival rate).

NURSING MANAGEMENT

Assessment

Assessment begins with a thorough history and review of symptoms pertaining to the GI system, particularly symptoms that an older client may not offer as a complaint unless asked. These include indigestion, discomfort after eating, nausea, anorexia, vomiting, or any chronic "stomach problem." In addition, the nurse should question older adults regarding changes in dietary or bowel patterns and habits, use of prescription and over-the-counter medications, and use of home remedies. Physical examination may reveal no obvious abnormalities except that, when advanced, the tumor may be palpable, especially through the thin skin and musculature of an older client's abdomen. In addition, lymph nodes may be palpable when metastases have occurred.

Diagnosis

The most common nursing diagnoses for an older client with gastric cancer include:

- Anticipatory grieving related to poor prognosis
- Altered nutrition: less than body requirements related to gastric distress
- Acute pain related to gastric distress and discomfort

Planning and Expected Outcomes

Expected outcomes for an older client with gastric cancer include:

1. Client will discuss thoughts and feelings related to the diagnosis with appropriate people.
2. Client will use appropriate resources for support counseling.
3. Client will maintain adequate nutrition as evidenced by stabilization and maintenance of weight and consumption of a well-balanced, high-calorie diet.
4. Client will effectively manage pain as evidenced by verbalization of comfort and pain relief after analgesic use.

Intervention

Nursing management of an older client with gastric cancer includes maintenance of hydration, nutrition, and fluid and electrolyte balance, and provision of emotional support to the individual and family. Many clients and their families feel guilty and negligent about the delay in seeking medical attention for the vague symptoms of gastric cancer. The nurse can support clients and families by dispelling misconceptions and offering a realistic sense of hope.

Nursing care should also focus on the prevention and early diagnosis of gastric cancer, including encouragement for all older clients with GI symptoms, however trivial, to seek medical attention. In addition, identifying those at risk and encouraging them to seek medical care for evaluation on a regular basis is also important.

Evaluation

Evaluation includes documentation of achievement of the expected outcomes, prevention of malnutrition, maintenance of comfort, and continued family support. As the disease advances and the older client becomes more debilitated, the focus of care will change, requiring the nurse to collaborate and coordinate with other health care team members regarding alternative care arrangements.

Colorectal Carcinoma

Colorectal carcinoma is one of the most common cancers for both men and women in the United States. Cancer of the large intestine is the third most common cause of death from a malignancy for both men and women. Colorectal cancer affects both genders equally, and the probability of developing it increases with age. Therefore age is a significant risk factor for colorectal cancer; risk increases rapidly above age 55 and doubles with each successive decade, reaching a peak at age 75.

Although the cause of colorectal cancer is unknown, research has indicated that diet, environment, and genetics all play important parts in the development of the disease. Colon cancer is more prevalent in the United States, probably because the American diet is much lower in fiber than (for example) the African diet. A diet high in fat and refined carbohydrates and low in roughage is considered a risk factor for colorectal cancer. Citizens of developing countries with a lower incidence of colorectal cancer generally eat diets high in fiber. In more Westernized civilizations, fiber intake decreases, since the diet is composed of more refined foods. Since a high-fiber diet reduces transit time, it appears to limit the time the colon is exposed to cancer promoters (Rex et al, 2000).

Genetic studies also suggest an inheritable susceptibility to colorectal cancer. Individuals with first-degree relatives diagnosed with colorectal cancer have double the risk for the development of adenomatous polyps, which are considered to be precursors of carcinoma.

Adenocarcinoma accounts for 95% of the carcinomas of the colon. The tumors tend to grow slowly and may remain asymptomatic for a long time. Cancer of the rectum is manifested as bright red bleeding through the rectum, along with changes in the characteristics of the stool. Carcinomas in the sigmoid and descending colon tend to grow around the bowel, encircling it and leading to an obstruction. For these clients, a change in bowel habits is a common symptom. On the right side, few symptoms are seen. If present, crampy abdominal pain may be difficult to pinpoint. Anemia may also be present. Tumor growth is by direct invasion and local extension; however, once it has invaded the lymph and vascular channels, metastases are likely. Metastases to the liver and lymphatic system are common, although other sites include brain, lung, bones, and adrenal glands. Clinical manifestations depend on the location and extent of the tumor. Left-sided lesions often cause melena, diarrhea, constipation, and a feeling that there is retained stool. Right-sided tumors often cause weakness, malaise, and weight loss. Abdominal pain is rare with either type and may result from obstructions or nerve involvement. An obstruction is often the first sign of the disease. Often, if a mass is palpated on physical examination or a routine rectal examination, the stool is guaiac positive. Although the duration of symptoms is not effective in predicting the degree of tumor advancement, the early diagnosis of cancer in asymptomatic persons has been shown to be related to improved survival.

Colon cancers produce a wide variety of tumor antigens; the carcinoembryonic antigen (CEA) is the most well-known. CEA levels are used to gauge the effectiveness of therapy and may be useful at the time of diagnosis for prognostic value. In addition, it is used to monitor for recurrence. The CEA's current use in mass screening and detection is limited.

NURSING MANAGEMENT

Assessment

Assessment begins with an older client's history of symptoms, such as diarrhea, constipation, abdominal pain, blood in stool, or melena. Generalized symptoms may have been overlooked by an older client; these include malaise, weight loss, weakness, and fatigue. Eliciting a family history of colorectal cancer, polyps, and any previous bowel surgeries is also important. Because of the potential for multiple losses with colorectal cancer, the nurse must also assess an older client's coping skills and abilities. Physical examination may reveal a mass in the abdomen or a guaiac-positive stool, or it may be unremarkable.

Diagnosis

The most common nursing diagnoses for an older client with colorectal cancer include:

- Altered nutrition: less than body requirements related to anorexia
- Acute pain related to GI distress
- Body image disturbance related to a colostomy

Planning and Expected Outcomes

Expected outcomes for an older client with colorectal cancer include:

1. Client will maintain weight and adequate nutrition.
2. Client will verbalize comfort after taking an analgesic.
3. Client will verbalize acceptance of permanent or temporary body changes resulting from a colostomy.

Intervention

Nursing management of an older client with colorectal cancer depends on the stage of the disease and the treatment modalities necessary. In general, older clients are at risk for weight loss and malnutrition as a result of the cancer and symptoms of vomiting or diarrhea. Eating small, frequent, high-calorie, high-protein meals should be encouraged. Allowing clients to eat some of their favorite foods on a regular basis may help maintain weight. The use of supplements such as Ensure or nighttime tube feedings may be necessary to maintain adequate nutrition. Not every client with colorectal cancer complains of pain, but if present, pain can be managed with both pharmacologic and nonpharmacologic relief measures (see Chapter 22). If an older client requires a colostomy either for treatment or as a palliative measure, the client should be encouraged to verbalize and express feelings on a regular basis. Referral to a support group or counseling may be necessary. Having an older client speak with or visit someone with a colostomy may help reduce anxiety, concerns, and fears associated with it. If the colorectal cancer is completely resected, reminding and encouraging the older client to have follow-up examinations and procedures to check for recurrence is of the utmost importance.

Evaluation

Evaluation includes documentation of achievement of the expected outcomes and prevention of complications. In addition, documentation of the client's methods of coping with the lifestyle changes imposed by the various treatment modalities is essential.

Pancreatic Cancer

Pancreatic cancer is the fourth leading cause of death in the United States. Fewer than 20% of affected individuals survive

1 year after diagnosis, and there is only a 10% 5-year survival rate. The disease usually affects older adults ages 60 to 70, and it affects men more than women. It is believed that race and ethnicity may be factors in the development of pancreatic cancer.

An increased risk attributable to environmental factors has been suggested, since the incidence is higher in those who are exposed to industrial pollutants or who live in urban areas. In addition, pancreatic cancer has been correlated with alcohol abuse, high-fat diets, tobacco use, chronic pancreatitis, and low socioeconomic status. Pancreatic cancer occurs twice as often in heavy smokers as in nonsmokers (Lewis, Heitkemper, and Dirksen, 2004).

Cancer of the pancreas is primarily an adenocarcinoma. Although the head, body, or tail of the pancreas may be involved, it is primarily a disease of the exocrine portion of the gland. It arises in the head of the organ in 60% to 70% of cases.

As tumor growth advances within the pancreas or on lymph nodes along the biliary tree, obstruction and compression of the common bile duct can result. Eventually the carcinoma may infiltrate the duodenum, stomach, transverse colon, spleen, kidney, and surrounding blood vessels. Invasion by the celiac nerve plexus accounts for the severe pain associated with cancer of the body or tail of the pancreas. Cancer of the pancreas grows rapidly, so at the time of diagnosis, the cancer has invaded locally or metastasized in 90% of individuals. Metastasis occurs through the bloodstream and by peritoneal seeding, causing frequent cancers in the lung and bone.

Symptoms generally occur late in the course of the disease and are vague and insidious in onset. Although manifestations of the disease differ according to the location of the tumor within the pancreas, the symptoms generally include anorexia, weight loss, nausea, and pain. Jaundice is a late sign.

NURSING MANAGEMENT

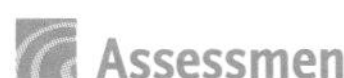

Assessment

Assessment begins with a history of symptoms and a review of possible precipitating causes of pancreatic cancer (e.g., environmental exposure to toxins, tobacco use, chronic alcohol ingestion and abuse). An accurate assessment of the pain pattern is also important. The nurse should obtain a symptom analysis for any of the usual symptoms of nausea, vomiting, weight loss, weakness, and stool changes. Physical examination may be unremarkable.

Diagnosis

Nursing diagnoses for an older client with pancreatic cancer include:

- Acute pain related to abdominal discomfort
- Ineffective coping related to terminal diagnosis
- Compromised family coping related to terminal diagnosis

Planning and Expected Outcomes

Expected outcomes for an older client with pancreatic cancer include:

1. Client will remain free from pain.
2. Client and family will verbalize concerns and feelings related to the diagnosis and prognosis.
3. Client and family will demonstrate improved coping strategies as evidenced by incorporation of alternative coping behaviors and techniques in their interactions.

Intervention

Nursing management for an older client with pancreatic cancer focuses on provision of pain relief and encouragement to verbalize feelings. Pain relief may require narcotics, and the client and family may require teaching concerning their prolonged use. Other nonpharmacologic measures of pain relief (e.g., diversional activities, repositioning, meditation, massage) need to be offered. The client and family may benefit from attending a support group for cancer clients. However, because of the poor prognosis, encouraging families to spend time with the older client is also important. Assisting the client and family in dealing with an imminent death may also be necessary.

Evaluation

Evaluation includes documentation of achievement of expected outcomes, prevention of complications, and provision of a comfortable environment.

Metastatic Liver Disease

Although primary cancers of the liver are associated with hepatitis B and C and cirrhosis, it is 20 times more likely that liver cancer is metastatic. In the case of metastatic disease the common original sites are the lung, breast, kidney, and other organs in the GI tract. Most often there are multiple masses in the liver, with spread throughout the organ via its massive vascular system. The diagnosis of liver metastasis is usually an indicator that the primary cancer is incurable. Signs and symptoms of liver involvement are the late signs of organ failure (e.g., ascites, portal hypertension), so by the time of diagnosis of the spread, the overall prognosis is poor. The 5-year survival rate is 5%; if untreated, death will occur 6 to 8 weeks following diagnosis. The cause of death is commonly pneumonia, malnutrition, emboli, hepatic failure, or hemorrhage.

Nursing management of older clients with metastatic liver disease is similar to that for clients with alcoholic cirrhosis, so the reader is referred to that section in this chapter.

Home Care

1. Regularly monitor and assess the diagnosed GI disease or disorder for signs and symptoms indicating exacerbation or instability.
2. Weigh at regular intervals to monitor weight loss or gain; encourage homebound older adults to use nutritional supplements if indicated.
3. Teach caregivers and homebound older adults appropriate dental hygiene practices.
4. Instruct caregivers and homebound older adults on reportable signs and symptoms related to any GI problem or disorder and when to report these symptoms to the home care nurse or health care provider.
5. Instruct caregivers and homebound older adults on the name, dose, frequency, side effects, and indications of both prescribed and over-the-counter medications being used to treat the identified GI problem.
6. Instruct caregivers and homebound older adults about laboratory indices used to evaluate GI disturbances. Inform them of the results of any tests after the health care provider has been notified.
7. Assess and instruct older adults on the importance of maintaining hydration in the presence of GI disturbance.
8. Instruct caregivers and homebound older adults on all aspects of any treatments used to provide nutritional support in the absence of a functioning GI system (e.g., enteral nutrition, total parenteral nutrition, formula supplements).

SUMMARY

Many of an older adult's health concerns are related to the GI system. Since these problems are often amenable to appropriate self-care practices, the nurse is responsible for teaching prevention and self-management strategies to these clients (see Chapter 8, Health Promotion and Illness/Disability Prevention). However, the nurse must also teach older adults that GI-related symptoms should not be dismissed as part of the normal aging process; they should be reported so that an accurate determination can be made and timely interventions instituted.

Key Points

- A decline in normal function of the GI tract may occur with aging without an effect on physiologic processes.
- A significant decrease of liver function is not an inevitable outcome of aging, but because the incidence of chronic disease increases with advancing age, liver disorders are more common in older adults.
- Any weight loss or complaint of dysphagia, indigestion, heartburn, vomiting, change in appetite, or change in stool in an older client warrants prompt evaluation by the health care provider.
- Primary and secondary prevention of problems in the GI tract should be part of the care for all older clients.
- Smoking, alcohol, and dietary factors are important risk factors for the development of GI cancers in older clients.
- Gastric ulcers have a higher incidence of becoming malignant than do DUs.
- Intestinal ischemia should be included in the differential diagnosis of an older client with a history of cardiovascular disease who complains of abdominal pain.
- A guaiac-positive stool in an older adult should be considered pathologic until proven otherwise.
- Intestinal polyps and a positive family history of polyps are the largest risk factors for the development of colorectal cancer.
- Although 60% of polyps and cancers are visualized with flexible sigmoidoscopy, a colonoscopy is necessary to detect any suspected cancers in the right colon.
- Although treatment of asymptomatic gallstones is not currently recommended, the rise in new therapeutic treatment options for cholecystitis should lead to a decline in morbidity and mortality previously associated with cholecystectomies in older adults.
- GI cancers present a common concern in that the symptoms are often overlooked or self-treated until the disease has become well established.
- Although the incidence of pancreatic cancer is increasing in the United States, treatment remains palliative.
- The high correlation between polypharmacy, increased drug consumption, and age makes the older person more prone to drug-induced liver disorders.

Critical Thinking Exercises

1. Your client, a 67-year-old man, has smoked at least a pack of cigarettes a day for the past 49 years. At present he is being treated for gastric ulcers. What relationship, if any, exists between his age, smoking history, and GI disorder?
2. Your 85-year-old grandfather confides in you that he has recently had bright red blood in his stools but thinks it is because of hemorrhoids. He is reluctant to see his doctor because he does not want to go into the hospital. What advice should you give him? Why are bloody stools of particular importance in older adults?
3. A 62-year-old man is admitted to the hospital with a diagnosis of cirrhosis of the liver. During the shift report his primary care nurse states that he has been agitated and anxious but has not exhibited any manifestations of alcohol withdrawal. What assumptions did the nurse make? Are these assumptions valid? Explain.
4. Discuss the nursing care measures that would be similar for an older adult client with cirrhosis and one with hepatitis.

REFERENCES

Bottomley J, Lewis C: *Geriatric rehabilitation: a clinical approach,* ed 2, Philadelphia, 2003, Prentice Hall.

Brozenec S: Ulcer therapy update, *RN* 59(9):48, 1996.

Clarren DS: Diverticular disease. In Meiner S, editor: *Care of gastrointestinal problems in the older adult,* New York, 2004, Springer.

Coleman P: Improving oral health care for the frail elderly: a review of widespread problems and best practices, *Geriatr Nurs* 23(4):189, 2002.

Ghezzi E et al: Longitudinal influence of age, menopause, hormone replacement therapy, and other medications on parotid flow rates in healthy women, *J Gerontol Med Sci* 55A:34, 2000.

Hill C: Hemorrhoids and problems of the anus and rectum. In Meiner S, editor: *Care of gastrointestinal problems in the older adult,* New York, 2004, Springer.

Levy RA, Stamm L, Meiner SE: Conservative management of GERD: a case study, *MEDSURG Nurs* 11(4):169, 2002.

Lewis S, Heitkemper M, Dirksen S: *Medical-surgical nursing: assessment and management of clinical problems,* ed 6, St Louis, 2004, Mosby.

Lyder C, Molony S: Topics in gastrointestinal care. In Molony SL, Waszynski CM, Lyder CH, editors: *Gerontological nursing: an advanced practice approach,* Stamford, Conn, 2003, Appleton & Lange.

Miller C: *Nursing for wellness in older adults: theory and practice,* ed 4, Philadelphia, 2004, Lippincott Williams & Wilkins.

Morley J: Pathophysiology of anorexia, *Clin Geriatr Med* 18:661, 2002.

Price S, Wilson L: *Pathophysiology: clinical concepts of disease processes,* ed 6, St Louis, 2003, Mosby.

Rao S: Constipation: evaluation and treatment, *Gastroenterol Clin North Am* 32:659, 2003.

Rex DK et al: ACG recommendations on colorectal cancer screening for average and higher risk patients, *Clin Pract* April 2000. Accessed on website: www.acg.gi.org/patientinfo/cork/CRC2000.pdf

Seidel HM et al: *Mosby's guide to physical examination,* ed 5, St Louis, 2003, Mosby.

Ship J, Pillemer S, Baum B: Xerostomia and the geriatric patient, *J Am Geriatr Soc* 50:535, 2002.

Smeltzer S, Bare B: *Medical-surgical nursing,* ed 10, Philadelphia, 2004, Lippincott Williams & Wilkins.

Smith R, Cokkinides V, Eyre H: American Cancer Society Guidelines for the early detection of cancer, *Cancer J Clin* 54:41, 2004.

US Department of Health and Human Services: *Healthy People 2010,* McLean, Va, 2000, International Medical Publishing.

Williams J: Gastroesophageal reflux disease, *Geriatr Nurs* 26(5):195, 2002.

27 Musculoskeletal Function

SUE E. MEINER, EdD, APRN, BC, GNP

Learning Objectives

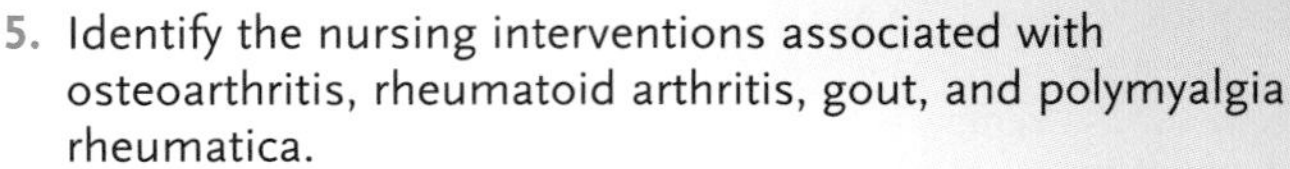

On completion of this chapter, the reader will be able to:

1. Describe the normal structure and function of the musculoskeletal system.
2. Discuss the age-related changes in the musculoskeletal system.
3. Discuss the nursing management of clients with fractures of the hip, wrist, clavicle, and vertebrae.
4. Distinguish differences among osteoarthritis, rheumatoid arthritis, gout, and polymyalgia rheumatica.
5. Identify the nursing interventions associated with osteoarthritis, rheumatoid arthritis, gout, and polymyalgia rheumatica.
6. Discuss the pathophysiology, treatment, and nursing management of osteoporosis.
7. Describe the indications and nursing management for clients with amputations.
8. Discuss the causes and management of common foot problems in older adults.

Musculoskeletal problems are common among older adults. AARP (1997) found that 40% of older adults living in the community are diagnosed with arthritis, and 17% report having other chronic problems of the musculoskeletal system. Complaints in the musculoskeletal system are common, since normal aging predisposes people to the development of diseases such as osteoarthritis and osteoporosis. Diseases of the musculoskeletal system are generally not fatal but can cause chronic pain and disability. Chronic conditions of the musculoskeletal system may contribute to impaired function and disability in older adults in the areas of self-care and mobility. They may suffer impairments in the ability to perform activities of daily living (ADLs), such as bathing, dressing, and eating, and instrumental activities of daily living (IADLs), such as managing finances, preparing food, managing transportation, and keeping house. Functional impairment of ADLs and IADLs can be devastating to older adults who desire to maintain independence. When dependence occurs, it can result in loss of self-esteem, the perception of decreased quality of life, and depression (see Cultural Awareness box).

AGE-RELATED CHANGES IN STRUCTURE AND FUNCTION

The musculoskeletal system is affected in numerous ways by the aging process. A pronounced decrease in muscle mass and muscle strength occurs gradually over time. The actual number of muscle cells decreases, and they are replaced by fibrous connective tissue. As a result, muscle mass, tone, and strength decrease. The elasticity of ligaments, tendons, and cartilage decreases, as does bone mass, which results in weaker bones. The intervertebral disks lose water, causing a narrowing of the vertebral space. This shrinkage may result in a loss of 1.5 to 3 inches of height. The lordotic or convex curve of the back flattens, and both flexion and extension of the lower back are decreased. Posture and gait change. Posture, as a result of the changes in the spine, assumes a position of flexion. Changes in posture result in a shift in the center of gravity. In men, the gait becomes small stepped with a wider-based stance. Women become bow-legged, with a narrow standing base, and walk with a waddling gait. The articular cartilage erodes in older adults. This has not been proven to be either a direct result of the aging process or the result of wear and tear on the joint.

All the changes mentioned may cause pain, impaired mobility, self-care deficit, and increased risk of falls for older adults. Approximately one third of those ages 65 and older have falls each year. About 2% of this group is hospitalized as a result of injuries incurred during the fall (King and Tinetti, 1996).

It has been estimated that half the residents in nursing facilities have falls each year. Falls are the most common cause of accidental death in older adults (see Chapter 12). When falls result in injury and hospitalization, the risk of iatrogenic illness and immobility can lead to a downward trajectory, which can ultimately result in death. Falls may also

NOTE: A special thanks for the work done by Karen Van Dyke Lamb and Marilyn Cummings on the previous edition of this chapter.

Cultural Awareness

BIOCULTURAL VARIATIONS IN THE MUSCULOSKELETAL SYSTEM

BONE	REMARKS
Frontal	Thicker in black men than white men
Parietal/occipital	Thicker in white men than in black men; occipital protuberance palpable in Eskimos
Palate	Tori (protuberances) along suture line of hard palate, which is problematic for denture wearers Incidence: Blacks: 0% Whites: 24% Asian-Americans: up to 50% Native Americans: up to 50%
Mandible	Tori (protuberances) on lingual surface of mandible near canine and premolar teeth, which is problematic for denture wearers Most common in Asian-Americans and Native Americans; exceeds 50% in some Eskimo groups
Humerus	Torsion or rotation of proximal end with muscle pull Larger in whites than in blacks Torsion in blacks is symmetric; torsion in whites usually greater on right side than on left
Radius/ulna	Length at wrist variable Ulna or radius may be longer Equal length: Swedish: 61% Chinese: 16% Ulna longer than radius: Swedish: 16% Chinese: 48% Radius longer than ulna: Swedish: 23% Chinese: 10%
Vertebrae	24 vertebrae found in 85% to 93% of all people; racial and gender differences reveal 23 or 25 vertebrae in select groups (23 vertebrae in 11% of black women; 25 vertebrae in 12% of Eskimo and Native American men) Related to lower back pain and lordosis
Femur	Convex anterior: Native Americans Straight: blacks Intermediate: whites
Pelvis	Hip width 1.6 cm (0.6 in) smaller in black women than in white women; Asian-American women have significantly smaller pelvises
Second tarsal	Second toe longer than great toe Incidence: Whites: 8% to 34% Blacks: 8% to 12% Vietnamese: 31% Melanesians: 21% to 57%
Height	Clinical significance for joggers and athletes White men 1.27 cm (0.5 in) taller than black men and 7.6 cm (2.9 in) taller than Asian-American men White women equal to black women Asian-American women 4.14 cm (1.6 in) shorter than white or black women
Composition of long bones	Longer, narrower, and denser in blacks than in whites; bone density in whites greater than in Chinese, Japanese, and Eskimos Osteoporosis lowest in black men; highest in white women

Continued

Cultural Awareness *cont'd*

BIOCULTURAL VARIATIONS IN THE MUSCULOSKELETAL SYSTEM—cont'd

MUSCLE	REMARKS
Peroneus tertius	Responsible for dorsiflexion of foot Muscle absent: Asian-Americans, Native Americans, and white: 3% to 10% Blacks and Berbers: 10% to 15% (Sahara desert): 24% No clinical significance because tibialis anterior also dorsiflexes the foot
Palmaris longus	Responsible for wrist flexion Muscle absent: Whites: 12% to 20% Native Americans: 2% to 12% Blacks: 5% Asian-Americans: 3% No clinical significance because three other muscles are also responsible for flexion

Data from Overfield T: *Biologic variation in health and illness: race, age, and sex differences*, ed 2, Boca Raton, Fla, 1995, CRC Press.

cause a cycle of disuse. This pattern of disuse usually occurs after the individual has experienced repeated falls. The fall experience causes a fear of falling. To avoid falls, the individual decreases mobility; with decreased mobility, muscle strength decreases, joints become stiff, and pain develops, resulting in disability, loss of independence, and frailty.

Current research has documented that some of the diseases and decline in the musculoskeletal system can be decreased or prevented through the use of regular programs of active exercise and resistive muscle strengthening.

COMMON PROBLEMS AND CONDITIONS OF THE MUSCULOSKELETAL SYSTEM

Fractures are common problems for older adults that often result in some loss of functional ability. A *fracture* is a break or disruption in the continuity of the bone. Fractures may occur because of trauma to a bone or joint, or they may be the result of pathologic processes such as osteoporosis or neoplasms. When bones are subjected to more stress than can be withstood, a fracture occurs. Stresses on bones may be from major trauma such as automobile accidents or falls. Falls are the most common cause of fractures in older adults. The most frequently occurring fractures among older adults are hip fractures, fractures of the proximal femur, Colles' (wrist) fractures, vertebral fractures, and clavicular fractures. Fractures are classified as open or closed by the location and type of fracture (Fig. 27-1).

The completed process of bone healing is termed *union*. After fractures occur, regenerative cells (fibroblasts and osteoblasts) move to the fracture site and lay down a fibrous matrix of collagen—the *callus*. This process usually occurs within 7 days of the injury. As the healing process takes place, the callus bridges the fracture site and the distance between the bone fragments decreases. In the final stage of bone healing, remodeling (absorption of excess cells and calcification), occurs.

The history given by a client with a fracture includes trauma followed by immediate local pain. Tenderness, swelling, muscle spasm, deformity, bleeding, and loss of function are also seen with fractures (see Emergency Treatment box).

Hip Fracture

Hip fractures are the most disabling type of fracture for older adults. They usually are caused by falls with direct trauma to the hip. Approximately 24% of clients with hip fracture die within 1 year after the injury (Wolinsky, Fitzgerald, and Stump, 1997). The complications of hip fracture are generally related to immobility. They include pneumonia, sepsis from urinary tract infections, and pressure ulcers. With the growing number of older adults, especially those over age 75, it is expected that the incidence of hip fractures will increase.

Hip fractures are classified by their locations. *Intracapsular* fractures, or subcapital fractures, occur within the hip capsule. *Extracapsular* fractures occur outside or below the capsule and are referred to as intertrochanteric and subtrochanteric locations (Fig. 27-2).

After the fall or injury that results in the fractured hip, the client has an affected extremity that is usually externally rotated and shortened. Tenderness and severe pain at the fracture site may be present. Immediately after the injury, the joint should be immobilized. Buck's or Russell traction (Fig. 27-3) is used until the client is stabilized. After the client is stabilized, surgical repair, the preferred treatment, is performed. The type of surgical repair depends on the location and type of fracture and can include internal fixation with pins, plates, and screws, or prosthetic replacement of the femoral head (Fig. 27-4).

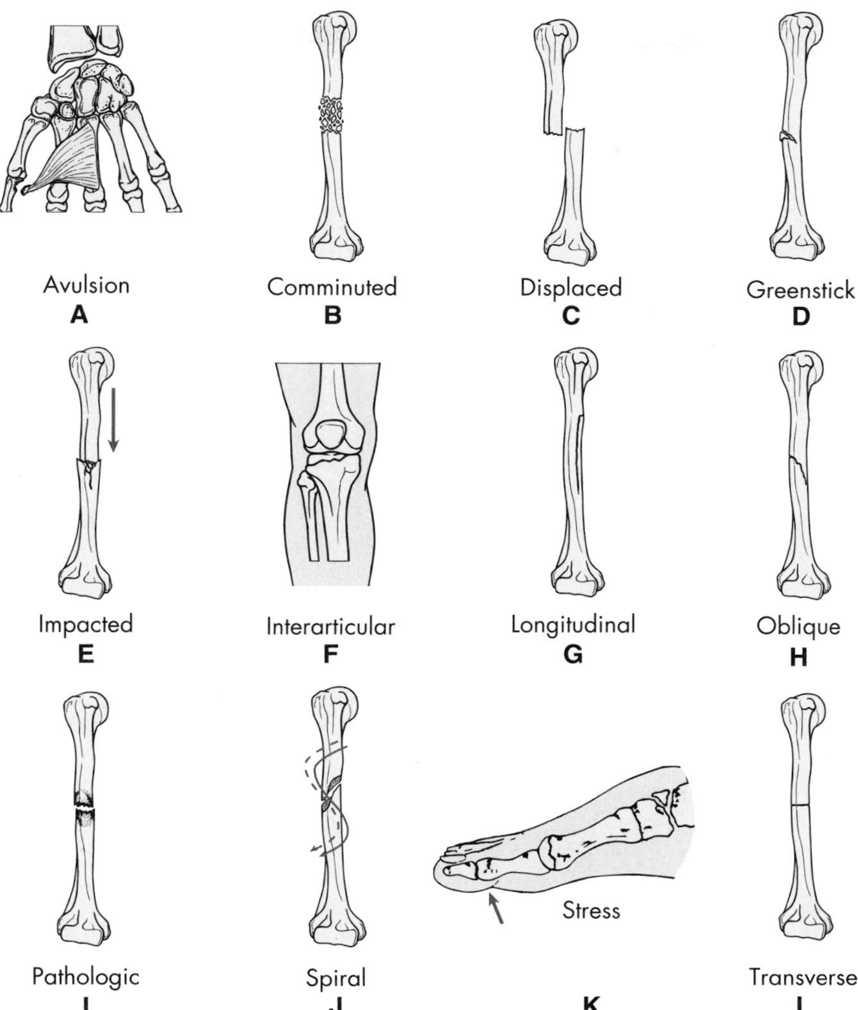

Fig. **27-1** Types of fractures. **A,** An avulsion is a fracture of bone resulting from strong pulling effect of tendons or ligaments at bone attachment. **B,** A comminuted fracture is a fracture with more than two fragments. The smaller fragments appear to be floating. **C,** A displaced (overriding) fracture involves a displaced fracture fragment that is overriding the other bone fragment. The periosteum is disrupted on both sides. **D,** A greenstick fracture is an incomplete fracture with one side splintered and the other side bent. The periosteum is not torn away from the bone. **E,** An impacted fracture is a comminuted fracture in which more than two fragments are driven into each other. **F,** An interarticular fracture is a fracture extending to the articular surface of the bone. **G,** A longitudinal fracture is an incomplete fracture in which the fracture line runs along the axis of the bone. The periosteum is not torn away from the bone. **H,** An oblique fracture is a fracture in which the line of the fracture extends in an oblique direction. **I,** A pathologic fracture is a spontaneous fracture at the site of a bone disease. **J,** A spiral fracture is a fracture in which the line of the fracture extends in a spiral direction along the shaft of the bone. **K,** A stress fracture is a fracture occurring at the site of a muscle attachment. It is caused by a sudden, violent force or repeated, prolonged stress. **L,** A transverse fracture is a fracture in which the line of the fracture extends across the bone shaft at a right angle to the longitudinal axis. (From Lewis S, Heitkemper M, Dirksen S: *Medical-surgical nursing: assessment and management of clinical problems,* ed 5, St Louis, 2000, Mosby.)

EMERGENCY TREATMENT

FRACTURES

If a fracture is suspected, assess injured area for:

- Movement
- Pain
- Color
- Temperature
- Pulse
- Sensation

If fracture is open and bleeding is present:

- Apply pressure.
- Apply sterile dressing.
- Immobilize the fracture site.

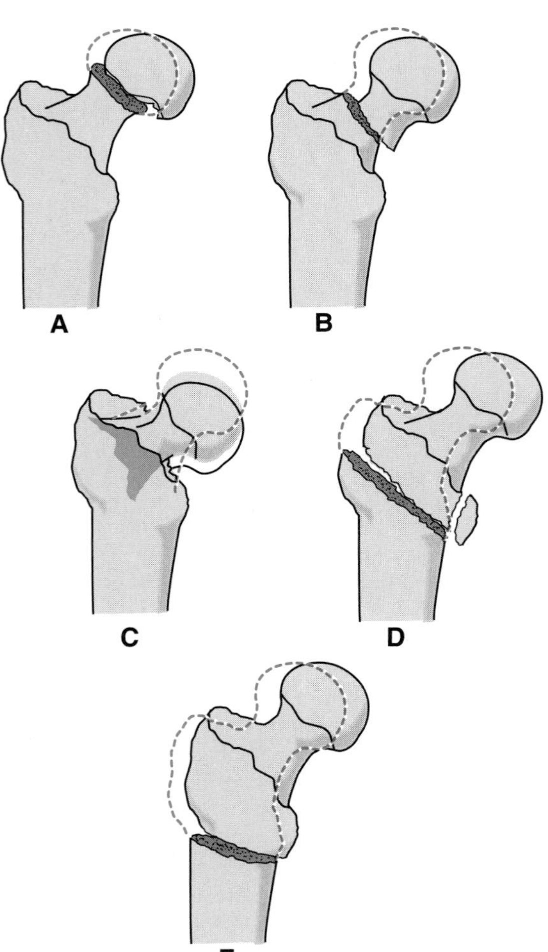

Fig. 27-2 Fractures of the hip. **A,** Subcapital fracture. **B,** Transcervical fracture. **C,** Impacted fracture of base of neck. **D,** Intertrochanteric fracture. **E,** Subtrochanteric fracture. (From Phipps W, Sands J, Marek J: *Medical-surgical nursing: concepts and clinical practice,* ed 6, St Louis, 1999, Mosby.)

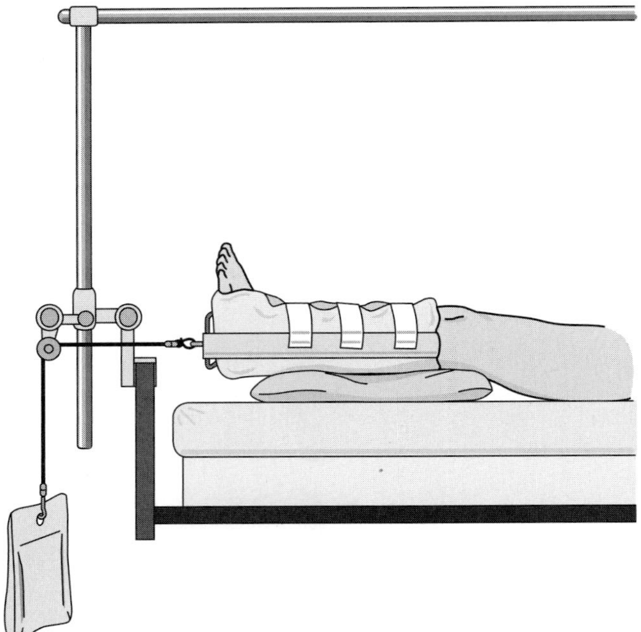

Fig. 27-3 Buck's extension. Heel is supported off bed to prevent pressure on heel, weight hangs free of bed, and foot is well away from footboard of bed. The limb should lie parallel to the bed unless prevented, as in this case, by a slight knee flexion contracture. (From Phipps W, Sands J, Marek J: *Medical-surgical nursing: concepts and clinical practice,* ed 6, St Louis, 1999, Mosby.)

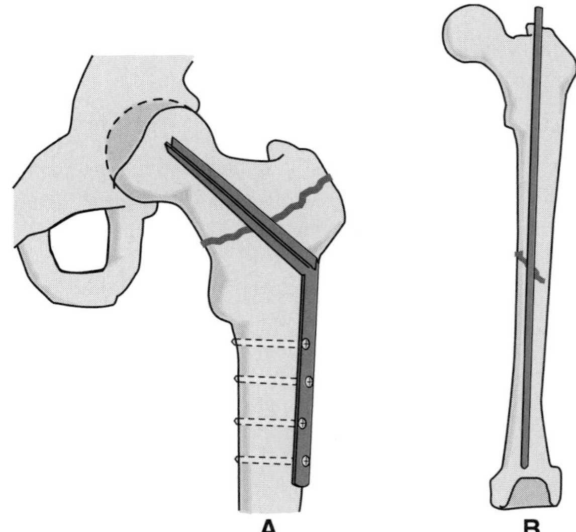

Fig. 27-4 **A,** Neufeld nail and screws, used in the repair of intertrochanteric fracture. **B,** Küntscher nail (intramedullary rod) used in repair of midshaft femoral fracture. (From Phipps W, Sands J, Marek J: *Medical-surgical nursing: concepts and clinical practice,* ed 6, St Louis, 1999, Mosby.)

NURSING MANAGEMENT

Assessment

Hip fractures are most often related to falls. After any fall or other injury that may cause hip trauma, the nurse assesses the hips and lower extremities for evidence of fracture. This includes inspecting the site for direct evidence of fracture, shortening of the extremity, and abnormal rotation. Also assessed is the presence of pain or tenderness at the site of the injury.

Diagnosis

Nursing diagnoses for a client with hip fracture include:

- Pain related to discomfort from the muscle and bone trauma
- Impaired physical mobility related to immobilization of fracture and healing process
- Risk for impaired skin integrity related to the immobilization required for healing
- Risk for infection related to possible impaired wound healing, compromised nutrition, and effects of immobility
- Self-care deficit (bathing and hygiene, grooming, dressing, and toileting) related to discomfort and impaired mobility
- Impaired home maintenance management related to decreased independence and recovery period needed for fracture healing

Planning and Expected Outcomes

Nursing care of a client with a hip fracture involves the perioperative, postoperative, and rehabilitation periods. Each of these stages of treatment and recovery requires specific nursing interventions and includes the following expected outcomes:

1. Client will report minimum discomfort and adequate level of pain control.
2. Client will remain free from postoperative complications, such as altered skin integrity and wound infection.
3. Client will adhere to the prescribed physical therapy regimen to regain function of the affected joint.
4. Client will be able to participate in physical and occupational therapies.
5. Client will be able to safely demonstrate use of assistive devices for mobility and ADLs.
6. Client will be able to return to the preinjury level of independence with appropriate support and assistive devices.

Intervention

On arrival in the acute care setting, the client has his or her medical condition and hip fracture assessed and stabilized. Surgical intervention is usually recommended but is considered elective and therefore requires stability of major health conditions. During this preoperative period the nurse's main focus is on keeping the client comfortable and hydrated and preventing complications of immobility. Preoperatively, hip fractures can produce severe muscle spasms causing intense pain. Pain medications, traction or immobilization (Fig. 27-5), and proper positioning are used to manage the pain. Preoperative education should include information regarding the surgical procedure, postoperative treatments, potential complications, and expected outcomes for rehabilitation and recovery.

The immediate postoperative period requires monitoring of vital signs and intake and output. Turning, deep breathing, and coughing are used to prevent respiratory complications. The operative site is monitored for signs of infection and bleeding. Movement, circulation, and sensation of the extremity are assessed to determine impaired circulation. Mental status should be assessed and any changes noted. Postoperative delirium may occur in older clients following hip fracture; the effects of surgery, anesthesia, analgesic medications, loss of familiar surroundings, pain, and immobility

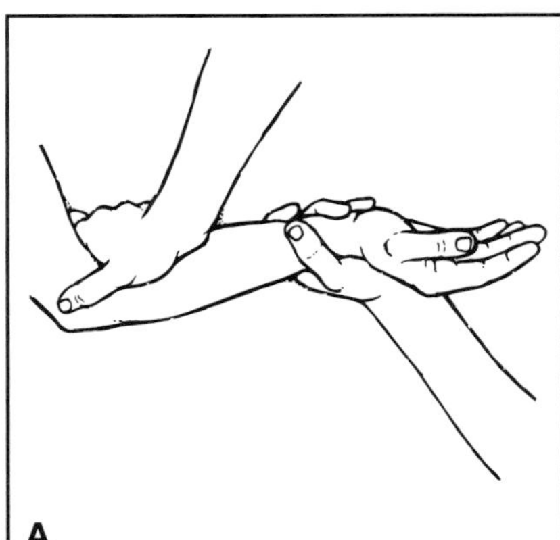

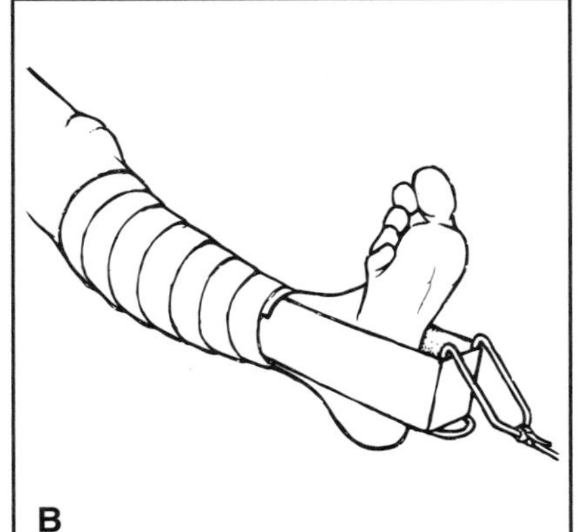

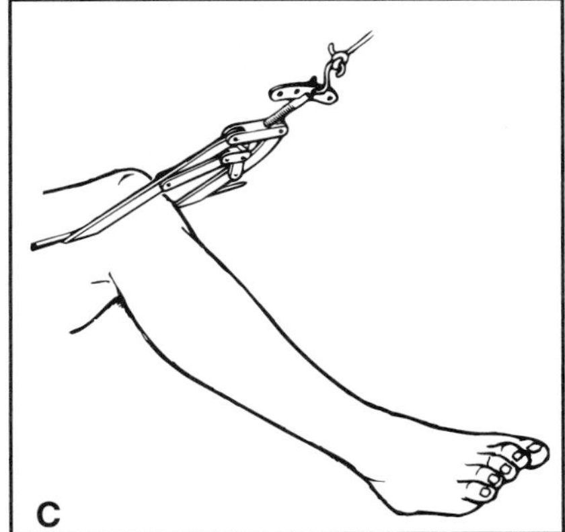

Fig. 27-5 Traction techniques, including **A,** manual; **B,** skin; and **C,** skeletal. (Illustration from the Traction Handbook ©2005 Zimmer Orthopaedic Surgical Products, Inc.)

may increase the potential for delirium. Care planning should include familiarizing the client with his or her surroundings, providing for safety, instituting comfort measures, decreasing anxiety, and assisting with maintaining a sense of independence and identity (see Chapter 29) (see Research box).

Pain is managed through careful administration of pain medication. Because of the normal physiologic aging changes that affect pharmacokinetics and pharmacodynamics, older adults are at risk for developing changes in mental status, respiratory depression, and sedative effects with the use of narcotic analgesics (see Chapter 22). To prevent these problems, lower initial doses of narcotics than those used with younger adults may be used. The individual's response to the pain medication and the pain are closely monitored. If low doses are tolerated, the dose may be carefully increased. Keeping the affected extremity in alignment during turning also decreases pain. This is done using pillows between the knees or an abduction splint.

Clients who have their fractures repaired with hemiarthroplasty are at risk for dislocation. The nurse should give the client and family instructions on preventing dislocation. Dislocation may occur when the joint is adducted and internally rotated. Activities to avoid include crossing the legs and feet while seated, sitting on low seats, and adducting the legs when lying on the nonoperated side. The client is instructed not to put on socks or shoes without the aid of assistive devices, not to cross legs, not to lie on the affected side, to use a raised toilet seat and a shower chair, and to use a pillow between the legs while in bed. Activities that can cause dislocation should be avoided for 6 weeks until muscles surrounding the joint are healed and the joint is stabilized. Symptoms of dislocation are sudden severe pain and external rotation of the leg.

Following the devastating events of hip fracture and surgery, comprehensive multidisciplinary rehabilitation focuses on returning the client to the prior level of function and preventing disability. Specific areas of treatment are gait and transfer training, muscle strengthening through active assistive exercises, teaching the use of adaptive techniques for dressing, and teaching the correct use of assistive devices. Walkers and canes will be used by the client (Fig. 27-6), and the nurse must ensure that the client uses safe technique with either device (see Client/Family Teaching box).

Research

SAMPLE/SETTING

The sample consisted of 26 older adult clients with hip fractures who were admitted through the emergency department of an academic medical center.

METHODS

The subjects' cognitive and ADL status was monitored from admission to 5 days after surgery.

FINDINGS

Approximately 73% showed cognitive impairment sometime before or after surgery, or at both times. Cognitive function seemed most vulnerable to becoming impaired after surgery. A relationship between cognitive and functional status was found. Clients with impaired cognitive status were more dependent in ADLs.

IMPLICATIONS

It is crucial to assess the baseline mental status of clients with hip fractures accurately and to monitor changes throughout the course of hospitalization. Assessment of mental status should be linked to functional ability to enhance postoperative outcomes.

Milisen K, Abraham IL, Broos PL: Postoperative variation in neurocognitive and functional status in elderly hip fracture patients, *J Adv Nurs* 27(1):59, 1998.

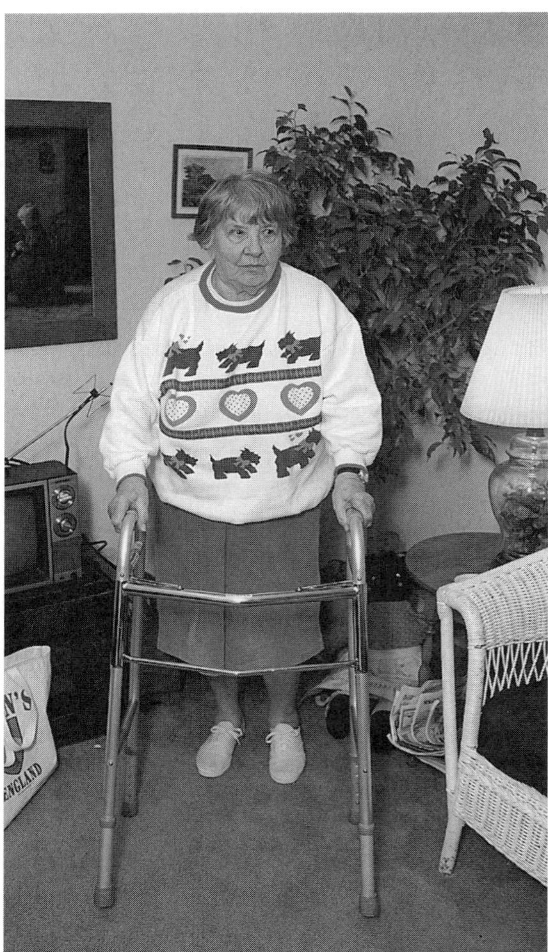

Fig. 27-6 Walking with a walker. The walker is moved about 6 inches in front of the resident. Both feet are moved up to the walker. (From Potter PA, Perry AG: *Fundamentals of nursing: concepts, process, and practice,* ed 2, St Louis, 1985, Mosby.)

Client/Family Teaching

CORRECT USE OF WALKERS

A walker should always rest on all four legs, never two.
Correct body position should be maintained:

- Posture erect
- Elbows slightly bent
- Wrists extended
- Shoulders relaxed

Sturdy, comfortable, hard-soled shoes should be worn.
Walker and affected leg should be moved together.
Be alert for hazards such as uneven surfaces or wet floors.

The loss of independence and decreased functional ability should also be addressed during rehabilitation. These losses can lead to depression (see Chapter 14). The nurse's role is to identify the client's strengths, give positive feedback, and reinforce the progress made in achieving goals. Discharge planning focuses on using family and social support networks and ongoing therapy programs.

Evaluation

Successful achievement of the expected outcomes after hip fracture will allow the client to return to a preinjury level of function. Those living independently should be successful in meeting goals of therapy and regain their self-care abilities, allowing for return home. Home health agencies may also be useful in successfully returning the client to the community.

Clients who were living in other types of health care facilities before the injury should be expected to return to their previous level of activity. Complications will prolong the recovery period and may lead to long-term changes in level of independence. Clients should report minimum pain at the fracture or surgical site and intact skin integrity. Muscle strength, joint movement, level of mobility, and degree of safety while performing ADLs will be continually evaluated throughout the recovery period. Continued physical and occupational therapies may be required to achieve goals and expected outcomes (see Nursing Care Plan).

Nursing Care Plan
Fractured Hip

Clinical Situation: Ms. W is an 88-year-old executive secretary who is admitted to the skilled nursing unit of the local hospital for restorative care after surgical repair of a fractured left hip. The hip was repaired with femoral head prosthesis. Ms. W fell when getting on the city bus. Before this incident, Ms. W worked 3 days a week. Her general health status is good. She lives alone on the second floor of a two-story building. Her only family is a niece who lives 60 miles away.

On admission, Ms. W is a slender woman who looks younger than her stated age. She is in no acute pain. The left hip incision is clean and dry with the staples intact. Ms. W transfers with the moderate assistance of two people. During the transfer she becomes tense and tells the nurses that she is afraid of falling and that she has to get on her feet so that she can get back to work. Because the surgical procedure has caused decreased range of motion and weakness in her left leg, Ms. W requires assistance with bathing and dressing her lower extremities.

Nursing Diagnoses

Impaired physical mobility related to alteration in musculoskeletal function as a result of fracture and surgical repair
Self-care deficit of bathing and dressing lower extremities related to alteration in musculoskeletal function secondary to fracture and surgical repair
Knowledge deficit: home care programs related to limited exposure

Outcomes

Client will walk 50 feet with a pickup walker.
Client will bathe and dress lower extremities with the use of assistive devices.
Client will verbalize knowledge of home care program.
Client will verbalize satisfaction with discharge plans.

Interventions

Consult with physical therapist for a program of muscle strengthening, transfer training, and gait training.
Reinforce physical therapy training.
Give positive feedback for gains made.
Instruct client to take deep breaths and relax before transfers.
Assist with transfers.
Give specific instructions before transfers. Instruct on hip precautions.
Teach use of a walker.
Give pain medication 30 to 60 minutes before physical therapy.
Consult with occupational therapist for specific assistive devices.
Teach use of assistive devices. Allow adequate time for bathing and dressing.
Give positive feedback for gains made.
Assess support systems and need for home services.
Instruct on wound care, home safety, and home exercise program.
Plan for discharge with client and team members.
Use community services, visiting nurse, physical therapy, and niece for assistance.

Colles' Fracture

Colles' fracture is a fracture of the distal radius that is usually a result of reaching out with an open hand to break a fall. This fracture is seen most often in older women with osteoporosis. Clients with a Colles' fracture have pain at the site of the fracture that begins immediately after the traumatic episode; local edema, swelling, and a visible deformity from the displacement of the distal bone fragment are also present. Treatment of a Colles' fracture is usually closed reduction and immobilization with a forearm splint or cast. Nursing measures include elevating the extremity to decrease edema and neurovascular assessment to monitor for complications. The client is instructed to actively move the thumb and fingers to improve venous return and decrease edema. Range-of-motion exercises for the elbow and shoulder prevent stiffness of the extremity.

Clavicle Fracture

Clavicle fractures, like Colles' fractures, can occur after a fall on an outstretched hand or on a fall to the shoulder. The majority of these fractures occur in the middle third of the clavicle. Clients with a fractured clavicle have point tenderness, local edema, and crepitus. The shoulder is noticeably deformed, dropping downward, forward, and inward. Treatment of a clavicle fracture includes reduction of the fracture and immobilization with a sling or cast. Nursing measures include monitoring for neurovascular complications such as compartment syndrome, elevating the extremity, and actively moving the hand and fingers.

Casts and Cast Care. Casts are one type of device used to immobilize an injured body part. They maintain proper positioning of the injured area, prevent further deformity, protect realigned bones, and promote healing. Used on the lower extremities, they may also allow for earlier weight bearing.

Casting materials include plaster of Paris or synthetic materials such as fiberglass. After application, plaster of Paris casts should be left uncovered to air dry. Drying time depends on the size and thickness of the cast and may take up to 48 hours. The nurse should support this type of cast with the palms of the hands rather than with the fingers to prevent indentations in the cast during the drying time. Synthetic cast materials harden quickly during and after application. The surface of this type of cast may be rough and can be covered with a stockinet.

Clients are instructed to keep both types of casts dry; plastic or purchased cast protectors may be used during showering or bathing. Synthetic casts are immersed in water only with physician approval and should be dried thoroughly afterward. A hair dryer set at a low temperature may be used for this purpose.

Clients are instructed to keep the extremity elevated to the level of the heart to decrease edema. The client should also be instructed to maintain movement of the extremity to prevent muscle atrophy and joint stiffness above or below the cast (see Client/Family Teaching box). Nursing care includes assessment for potential areas of skin irritation or breakdown. The client should be instructed to report any redness or discomfort along the edges of the cast and any signs of drainage or odor coming from the cast.

Neurovascular assessment of the extremity is done to determine that the cast is not constrictive. Excessive constriction caused by the cast could result in compartment syndrome, leading to ischemia and tissue destruction of the extremity. Any change in capillary refill, skin color, skin temperature, or excessive pain not controlled with medication should be immediately reported to the physician.

Casts are generally used to immobilize fractures for 6 to 8 weeks. A variety of assistive devices may be used for clients with lower extremity casts (Fig. 27-7). The nurse prepares the client for self-care and prevention of complications during this treatment period.

Osteoarthritis

Osteoarthritis, also known as degenerative joint disease, is a noninflammatory disease of joints that is characterized by progressive articular cartilage deterioration with the formation of new bone in the joint space. This is the most common type of arthritis seen in older adults.

The exact cause of osteoarthritis is not well understood. The degeneration of the joint is not caused by aging alone. Age, trauma, lifestyle, obesity, and genetics have been cited as predisposing factors in the development of osteoarthritis.

In osteoarthritis the articular cartilage thins and is lost, particularly in areas of increased stress. As the cartilage deteriorates, there is a proliferation of bone at the margins of the joints. When the joint cartilage is lost, the two bone surfaces come into contact with each other. This results in joint pain. The distal interphalangeals, proximal interphalangeals, knees, hips, and spine are the joints most commonly affected by osteoarthritis.

The most common symptom is a gradual onset of aching joint pain. The pain occurs with activity and is relieved with rest. Stiffness after periods of inactivity that resolves with activity is also seen in osteoarthritis. Crepitus, a grating

Client/Family Teaching

CAST CARE

Keep casted extremity elevated for the first 24 hours.
When cast is wet, lift with palms of hands.
Observe the extremity for swelling, color changes, movement, and sensation.
If any changes occur, contact health care provider.
Do not put anything inside the cast.
Do not get plaster cast wet; cover with plastic for bathing.

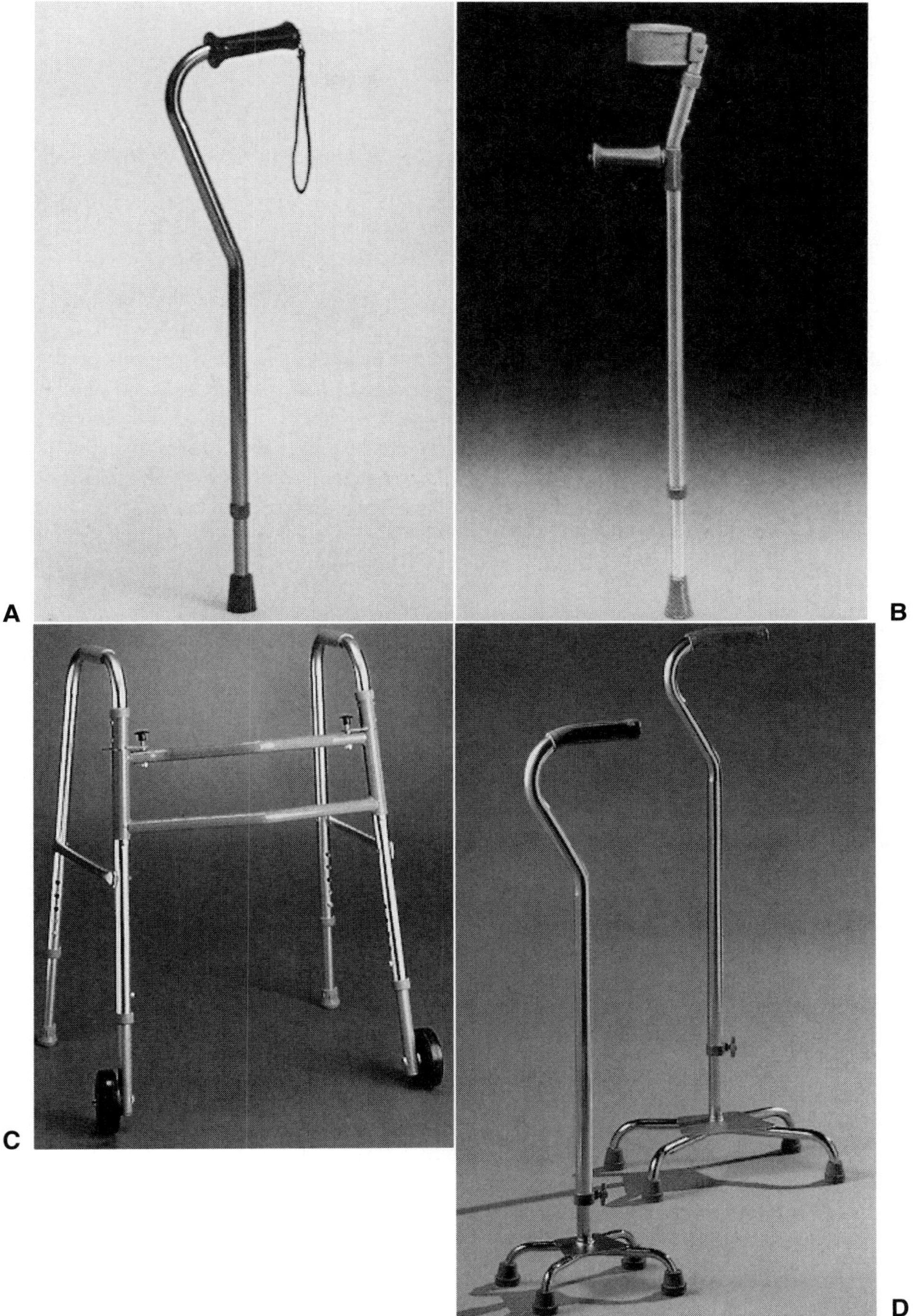

Fig. 27-7 Assistive devices. **A,** Ortho cane with wrist strap. **B,** Forearm crutch stabilizes elbow during walking. **C,** Walker with front wheels allows constant contact with the ground. **D,** Quad cane offers more support than a single-stem walker. (**A** and **B**, Courtesy Graham-Field Inc., Bay Shore, NY. **C** and **D**, Courtesy Sammons Preston, Inc., an AbilityOne Company, Bolingbrook, Ill.)

sound and sensation, may be heard and felt with range of motion in affected joints. Affected joints also have a decreased range of motion. The degeneration of the joint structure may result in muscle spasm, gait changes, and disuse of the joint. Bony enlargements, called Heberden's nodes (Fig. 27-8), may be seen on the distal interphalangeals.

NURSING MANAGEMENT

Assessment

Nursing assessment of a client with osteoarthritis begins with a thorough history of the problem. Data gathered include information about the onset, location, quality, and duration of the joint pain. Questions about precipitating factors, medications used, and impact on functional abilities should be asked. Affected joints should be inspected for pain, tenderness, swelling, redness, crepitation, and range of motion.

Diagnosis

Nursing diagnoses for the older adult client with osteoarthritis include:

- Pain related to inflammation and deterioration of the joint cartilage
- Impaired physical mobility related to lower extremity joint stiffness
- Self-care deficit (specify) related to limitations in joint movement and strength

Planning and Expected Outcomes

The focus of the nursing care plan is to protect and preserve joint motion and function. Expected outcomes for this client are individualized and specific to the joints affected. Outcomes include:

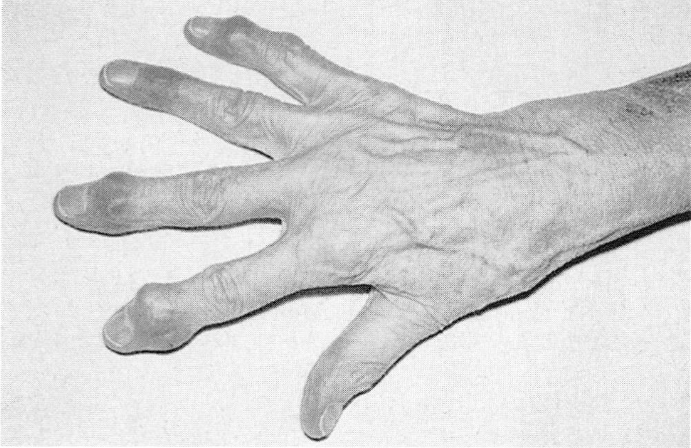

Fig. 27-8 Right hand of a 71-year-old woman with osteoarthritis and Heberden's nodes. (From Kamal A, Brockelhurst JC: *Color atlas of geriatric medicine*, ed 2, St Louis, 1991, Mosby.)

1. Client will verbalize improved level of comfort with activities.
2. Client will be able to successfully use various adaptive devices in maintaining independence in ADLs and IADLs.
3. Client will demonstrate safe use of assistive devices for ambulation.

Intervention

Instructions on joint protection and energy conservation are given. For clients with mild pain, a gentle exercise program that improves muscle tone and prevents joint stiffness may be used. Rest periods between activities are recommended. Heat or cold therapy to the joints may also be used to decrease joint pain. Simple measures such as a warm bath or shower in the morning may help reduce the early morning stiffness that may accompany the pain. Other pain relief interventions may be incorporated into the treatment plan (see Chapter 15).

The physician may also prescribe various nonsteroidal antiinflammatory drugs (NSAIDs) and nonopioid analgesics to help control the pain. Clients may initially be given over-the-counter medications and then gradually be advanced to a prescription antiinflammatory agent. Other medical treatment options for more severe pain may include directly injecting the painful joint with steroids. This can be done 2 or 3 times yearly for chronic pain. More recent developments in arthritis treatment include the injection of hyaluronic acid into a painful knee joint that has not responded to more conservative measures. The nurse should educate the client about these conservative measures for treating the symptoms of arthritis. Information regarding correct dosing of oral medications, contraindications, side effects, and adverse effects should be provided.

When conservative measures for treating chronic arthritis pain fail and the client becomes more disabled, surgical procedures may be considered. The main indications for surgery are severe pain and increasing disability. The surgical procedure most often used is arthroplasty, a surgical replacement of the involved joint. Joint replacement surgery is currently successful for many joints that may be involved with arthritis, including the shoulders, elbows, fingers, hips, and knees.

Other surgical options include arthroscopic procedures and joint fusion surgery. These procedures do not replace the joint but may result in improved function and reduced pain.

For clients undergoing joint replacement surgery for the hip or knee, the preoperative period focuses on education about the surgical procedure, its risks, any potential complications, and the postoperative course. After surgery the goals of nursing care are to prevent complications, relieve surgical pain, and assist the client in achieving a higher level of function and activity.

Major complications after joint replacement surgery may include thromboembolism, joint or wound infection, blood loss, nerve injury, joint dislocation, and surgical pain. Use of critical pathways or care paths in most institutions has resulted in shortened hospital stays, fewer incidents of complications, and improved outcomes (Theis, 1998).

Nursing interventions in the postoperative period include measures to prevent infection, control pain, and assist with daily activities. Aseptic precautions should be taken with surgical wound dressings, urinary catheters, and surgical drains to prevent infection. The client may be given prophylactic antibiotics for a short time (24 hours) after surgery.

Infections of the joint replacement are a serious complication. The incidence of deep infection of joint replacements is 0.5% to 1%. The infection may be a result of contamination during surgery, hematoma formation, or delayed wound healing, or it may be hematogenous from a distant site, such as a urinary tract infection. The most common contaminants are staphylococci and gram-positive aerobic streptococci. Because the new joint is a foreign body, pathogens may be introduced that will persist on the metal or plastic surfaces of the prosthesis, leading to chronic deep infection of the joint.

Clients with rheumatoid arthritis, diabetes mellitus, or poor nutritional status and those receiving long-term corticosteroid therapy are at increased risk for developing joint infections. If infection occurs in a joint replacement, long-term intravenous antibiotic therapy is instituted for at least 6 weeks. In some cases the infected joint may be replaced. Joint infections may lead to increased disability and prolonged rehabilitation. Various prophylactic measures may be used to prevent deep venous thrombosis. These may include various lower extremity compression devices, oral or injectable anticoagulants, and physical therapy to mobilize the client.

Pain control during the first 24 to 48 hours may be accomplished with intravenous or epidural administration of narcotic analgesics. Patient-controlled analgesia is frequently used to provide adequate pain control. As the client's pain decreases, oral analgesics will be ordered. Mild analgesics may be required for up to 6 weeks postoperatively as the surgical site heals.

Clients who have total hip replacement surgery are at risk for hip dislocation. The hip should be maintained in a position of abduction and neutral alignment. Some physicians may require the use of pillows or abduction splints while the client is in bed. Nurses should reinforce hip precautions as described in the Client/Family Teaching box.

The goal of total knee replacement surgery is to restore at least 90 degrees of knee flexion. To achieve this, active and passive physical therapy is instituted. In addition, the physician may order a continuous passive motion device, which continuously moves the knee through a preset range of flexion and extension. Rehabilitation for a client with a joint replacement begins within 24 to 48 hours of the surgical procedure and includes muscle strengthening and range-of-motion exercises. The client is instructed on the use of a cane, walker, or crutches. Occupational therapy provides the client with instructions for independence in daily activities. A short stay in a rehabilitation facility may follow the acute hospital stay. However, many clients are able to quickly return to their own home with continued home therapy services.

Client/Family Teaching

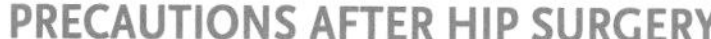

PRECAUTIONS AFTER HIP SURGERY

Sit with your hips at a 90-degree or greater angle.
Do *not* bend forward more than 90 degrees.
Do *not* lift the knee on the operated side higher than your hip.
Do *not* cross legs at knees or ankles.
Keep pillows between your legs when lying on your side or your back.
Do *not* bend to put on shoes; use a long shoehorn.
Do *not* bend down to reach items on the floor.
Do *not* sit in low chairs.

Evaluation

The goals in caring for a client with osteoarthritis are to relieve pain and restore function. Clients should report minimum pain and improved ability to perform ADLs. Conservative measures (as outlined earlier) will improve mobility and increase comfort for many older clients. If surgical intervention is used, the client needs to understand the expected outcomes, as well as the risks associated with the procedure. Clients with osteoarthritis may benefit from support groups and group exercise programs especially designed for clients with arthritis. The client's self-care practices should include regular exercise, the use of adaptive devices if necessary, and adherence to prescribed medication regimens. Understanding the disease process and treatment measures will assist an older adult in maintaining function and independence (see Research box).

Spinal Stenosis

Symptomatic osteoarthritic changes of the spine leading to functional limitation and pain in older adults are becoming more common. Lumbar spinal stenosis is one of the most frequently encountered, clinically important degenerative spinal disorders in the aging population (Spivak, 1998). Degenerative spinal stenosis is a bony overgrowth of the facet joints of the vertebrae, which leads to narrowing of the spinal canal and possible compression of the nerve roots. Although spinal stenosis can occur at any level of the spine, it is most frequently seen in the lumbar region at levels L3 and L4 (Fig. 27-9). Degeneration of the vertebral joints and disks of the spine, along with nerve compression, leads to progressive back pain and possible weakness of lower extremities. Clients with spinal stenosis may develop claudication-like symptoms of burning and numbness in their lower extremities.

Research

SAMPLE/SETTING

Subjects included 22 men and 23 women who suffered from hip dysfunction with arthritic pain and impaired mobility.

METHODS

To determine health status following total hip replacement, subjects were tested before surgery and 3½ months later with the Arthritic Impact Measurement Scale.

FINDINGS

There were significant improvements in pain levels and physical activity following total hip replacement.

IMPLICATIONS

Nurses can provide clients who are contemplating arthroplastic surgery with information about the advantages and disadvantages of the procedure so they can make informed choices about surgery and managing their health problems.

Brodie L, Sloman R: Changes in health status of elderly patients following hip replacement surgery, *J Gerontol Nurs* 24(3):5, 1998.

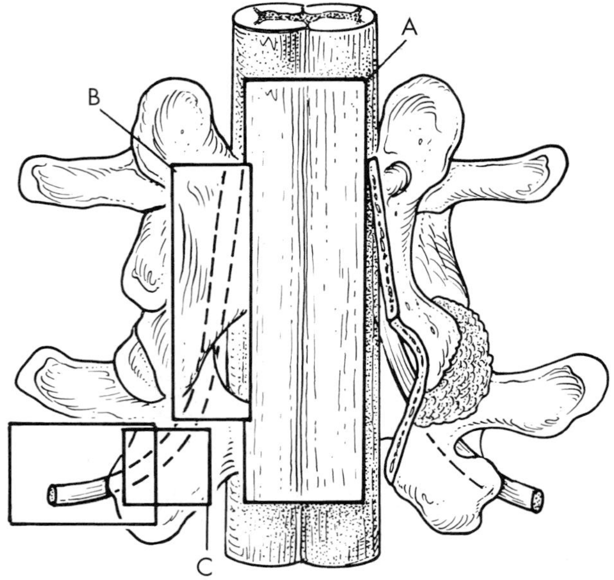

Fig. 27-9 Three-dimensional illustration of segmental stenoses. *A*, Anatomic; *B*, segmental; *C*, pathologic. (Redrawn from Ciric I et al: The lateral recess syndrome: a variant of spinal stenosis, *J Neurosurg* 53:433-443, 1980.)

NURSING MANAGEMENT

Assessment

Goals of nursing assessment focus on the client's symptoms. Exact location of pain or numbness, duration of the symptoms, and successful pain relief measures should be identified. Pain caused by degenerative spinal stenosis tends to occur primarily in the back and buttocks, but it may also radiate into the thighs, calves, and feet. The pain may be unilateral or bilateral and generally worsens with prolonged standing or activity. Symptoms are generally relieved with flexion of the spine. Clients can usually report specific positions or activities that aggravate or reduce their symptoms. They may report that activities such as leaning over a grocery cart lessen their pain. Comfort levels during routine ADLs should always be assessed.

Diagnosis

Nursing diagnoses for a client with spinal stenosis include:

- Chronic pain related to spinal nerve root narrowing
- Impaired physical mobility related to discomfort with walking and movement
- Risk for activity intolerance related to chronic pain
- Risk for injury related to pain and difficulty with ambulation

Planning and Expected Outcomes

The focus of the nursing care plan for a client with spinal stenosis is to manage chronic pain, maintain strength and mobility, and promote independence with daily activities. Severity of symptoms and assessment of current limitations of activity will determine the individual needs of clients with degenerative spinal stenosis. Expected outcomes include:

1. Client will report minimum or tolerable level of pain.
2. Client will demonstrate improved mobility and tolerance of activity.
3. Client will be able to incorporate a plan for lifestyle modifications that includes activity and rest.
4. Client will demonstrate safe use of assistive devices and make necessary environmental changes to promote safety.

Intervention

Nursing care for a client with spinal stenosis depends on the severity of spinal cord narrowing, the client's state of health, and the degree of pain and immobility. For the client being treated conservatively, the nurse should instruct the client to allow sufficient periods of rest, with limitations of activities that produce pain. Physical therapy for range of motion and muscle strengthening may be ordered by the physician. Pain relief measures should be initiated and then evaluated for their effectiveness. The physician may order NSAIDs and possibly analgesics for more severe pain. Use of pain assessment scales will help determine pain patterns, severity of pain, and the effectiveness of pain relief measures.

Other nursing measures to relieve pain include the use of heat or cold applications to the back, massage therapy, relaxation techniques, and position changes for the client while in bed. Clients with unrelieved chronic pain may be considered for pain team consultation and multidisciplinary treatment efforts.

In many clients with chronic pain, depression may accompany and increase the intensity of the pain symptoms. A physician consultant may recommend the use of mild antidepressant medication in addition to the other pain relief measures.

Evaluation

The client's ability to perform ADLs independently with minimum discomfort should be evaluated by self-report and observation. The effectiveness of pain relief measures should be discussed with the client, and changes made when medications have lost their effectiveness. For clients undergoing epidural injections or surgical procedures, the nurse should reinforce instructions about precautions and activities. The client should be able to verbalize potential complications and expected outcomes of treatment. Documentation of client interactions should include use of an appropriate pain scale and information about current activity level and restrictions.

Rheumatoid Arthritis

Rheumatoid arthritis is a chronic, systemic, inflammatory disease that causes joint destruction and deformity and results in disability. The onset of the disease most commonly occurs in the third or fourth decade. However, rheumatoid arthritis can also develop in older adults. When present in older adults, the disease is usually a chronic problem.

The cause of rheumatoid arthritis is not known. The most widely accepted theory is that it is an autoimmune disease that causes inflammation, most often in the joints but sometimes also in connective tissue. Joint involvement most often starts with the proximal interphalangeals, metacarpophalangeals, and wrists; in the later stages of the disease, knees and hips are affected.

In the initial phase of rheumatoid arthritis the synovial membrane becomes inflamed and thickens, with an increased production of synovial fluid. The change is called *pannus*. As the pannus tissue develops, it causes erosion and destruction of the joint capsule and subchondral bone. These processes result in decreased joint motion; deformity; and finally ankylosis, or joint immobilization.

The course of rheumatoid arthritis is variable. Generally the onset is gradual and the course is one of remissions and exacerbations. The symptoms are painful, stiff joints; decreased range of motion in the joints; joint swelling; and deformity (Fig. 27-10). The joint stiffness is present in the morning and lasts from 30 minutes to 6 hours. On examination, the affected joints are warm and swollen. Deformities of the joints include ulnar deviation of the wrists, boutonnière deformity caused by contractures of the distal and proximal interphalangeal joints, and swan-neck deformity caused by contractures of the distal interphalangeal joint (Fig. 27-11).

Systemic symptoms may include fatigue, anorexia, weight loss, and anemia. Rheumatoid arthritis in older adults may appear atypically; that is, large joints are affected more often and onset may be more sudden than in younger adults. Fatigue, weakness, and fever may be present (Table 27-1).

NURSING MANAGEMENT

Assessment

A careful nursing history is taken. Questions are asked about family history and constitutional symptoms, including fever, anorexia, weight loss, fatigue, and duration of the joint stiffness. On physical examination, the affected joints are inspected for symmetric involvement, pain, tenderness, swelling, heat, erythema, and deformity.

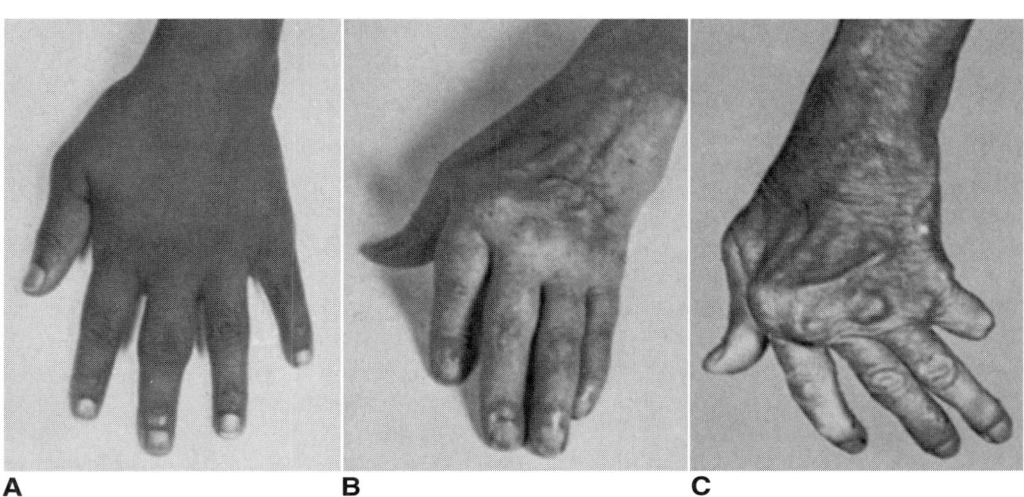

Fig. 27-10 Rheumatoid arthritis of the hand. **A,** Early stage. **B,** Moderate involvement. **C,** Advanced stage. (From Brashear H, Raney R: *Handbook of orthopaedic surgery*, ed 10, St Louis, 1986, Mosby.)

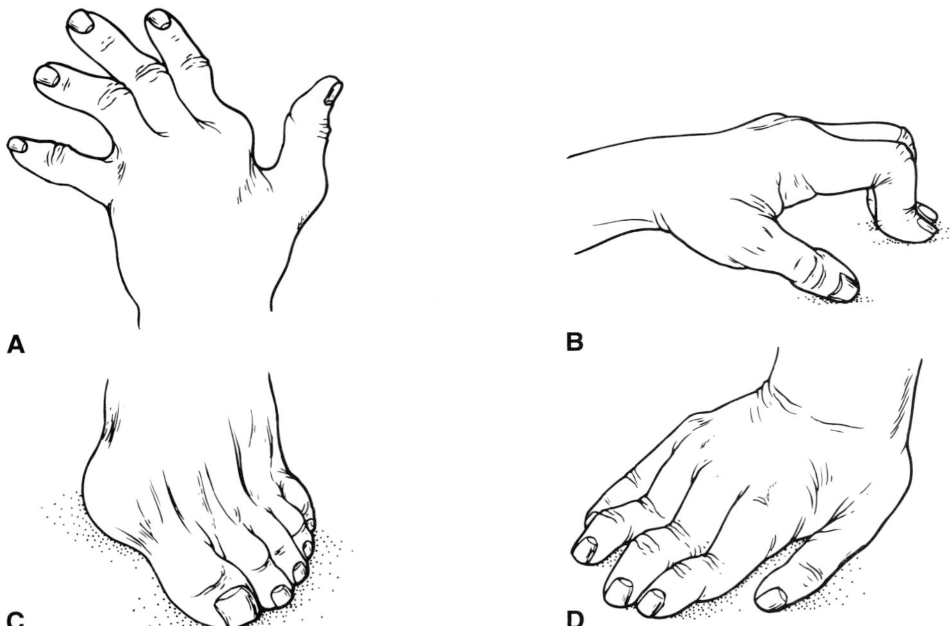

Fig. 27-11 Typical deformities of rheumatoid arthritis. **A,** Ulnar drift. **B,** Boutonnière. **C,** Hallux valgus. **D,** Swan-neck deformity. (From Lewis SM, Heitkemper M, Dirksen S: *Medical-surgical nursing: assessment and management of clinical problems*, ed 6, St Louis, 2004, Mosby.)

TABLE 27-1 Differentiating Rheumatoid Arthritis from Osteoarthritis

	RHEUMATOID ARTHRITIS	OSTEOARTHRITIS
Age at onset	3rd and 4th decades	5th and 6th decades
Onset	Gradual	Gradual
Disease course	Exacerbations and remissions	Variable, progressive
Duration of stiffness	1 to 24 hr	30 min or less
Joint pain	Worse in morning	Worse after activity
Joints involved	Proximal interphalangeal Metacarpophalangeal Metatarsophalangeal Knees, hips, wrists	Distal interphalangeal Knees, hips Lumbar, cervical Spine
Symmetric pattern	Almost always	Occasionally
Constitutional manifestations	Present	Absent
Synovial fluid	Increased cells Decreased viscosity	Few cells Normal viscosity
X-ray findings	Abnormalities present	Abnormalities present
Erythrocyte sedimentation rate	Almost always elevated	Occasionally elevated
Positive rheumatoid factor	Almost always	Never

Diagnosis

Nursing diagnoses for a client with rheumatoid arthritis include:

- Pain related to swollen, inflamed joint tissue
- Impaired physical mobility related to the joint deformities and inflammation
- Fatigue related to systemic disease process
- Potential for altered nutrition: less than body requirements related to loss of appetite
- Self-care deficits in ADLs related to the loss of motion and strength in painful, swollen joints
- Body image disturbance related to the gradual onset of joint deformities.

Planning and Expected Outcomes

Prevention of joint deformities, control of symptoms, and maintenance of the client's abilities to have an active lifestyle are the focus of intervention for a client with rheumatoid arthritis. Outcomes for the client include:

1. Client will maintain normal joint motion in affected joints, with minimum deformities.
2. Client's pain related to inflammation will be well controlled.
3. Client will be able to maintain optimum functional status.

Intervention

Clients with rheumatoid arthritis and their families require extensive education to cope effectively with the chronic nature of this disease. The nurse needs to discuss with them pain management, drug therapies, maintenance of self-care activities, promotion of safe mobility, methods of joint protection and precautions, and management of overall health.

Education on pain management includes information on appropriate medications that have been prescribed and over-the-counter remedies that a client may be using. The client should be informed that stress and anxiety can cause muscle tension and worsen joint pain. Progressive relaxation and guided imagery are taught to decrease anxiety and stress. Application of heat and cold to the affected joints decreases cutaneous nerve stimulation. Ice packs are applied to joints during periods of acute inflammation. Moist heat is useful in relaxing muscles and increasing joint mobility.

The role of the nurse in medication management is to teach the client about the action, side effects, and special precautions related to the specific medications (Table 27-2). In addition to the medications listed in Table 27-2, newer pharmacologic and biologic agents are being researched and developed for use in clients with rheumatoid arthritis. Recently the Cox-II inhibitors were found to be a risk for cardiac problems such as myocardial infarction and stroke. The information was

TABLE 27-2 Drug Use, Side Effects, and Nursing Implications

DRUG	RATIONALE FOR USE	SIDE EFFECTS	NURSING IMPLICATIONS
Salicylates: Aspirin	Used in early disease phase; analgesic, antipyretic, and antiinflammatory	Gastrointestinal irritation; slight elevation of liver enzymes; tinnitus (reversible)	Administer with milk or food. Teach use of enteric-coated tablets. Evaluate for gastrointestinal pain or bleeding, as well as tinnitus.
NSAIDs			
Long term: Diclofenac Fenoprofen Flurbiprofen Ibuprofen Indomethacin Ketoprofen Meclofenamate Mefenamic acid Nabumetone Naproxen Oxaprozin Piroxicam Salsalate Sulindac Tolmetin	Used when salicylates are ineffective; analgesic, antipyretic, and antiinflammatory actions; generally inhibit prostaglandin synthesis	Gastrointestinal irritation; diarrhea; fluid retention, edema; interstitial nephritis; nephrotic syndrome; dizziness, tachycardia, blurred vision, headaches; cholestatic hepatitis; bone marrow depression	Must be administered for 1 to 2 weeks before a therapeutic response is seen. Administer with food or antacids. Assess for gastrointestinal pain and occult bleeding. Teach client to avoid alcohol. Evaluate renal and hepatic function regularly.
Short term: Phenylbutazone	Specific for adjunctive use	Same as above	Same as above; 1-week trial is suggested. Evaluate CBC. Use with caution in older adults.
Oxyphenbutazone	Effective for articular symptoms in some clients	Same as above	Same as above; use under close medical supervision.
Antimalarials: Hydroxychloroquine sulfate Hydroxychloroquine phosphate	Used for severe destructive disease; 3 to 6 months needed to reach therapeutic levels	Gastrointestinal irritation; skin rash and changes; retinal changes; bone marrow depression	Advise ophthalmologic examination every 4 to 6 weeks. Allow 6 to 8 weeks for therapeutic effects to begin.

Continued

TABLE 27-2 **Drug Use, Side Effects, and Nursing Implications—cont'd**

DRUG	RATIONALE FOR USE	SIDE EFFECTS	NURSING IMPLICATIONS
			Evaluate CBC regularly. Assess for gastrointestinal effects, headaches, dizziness, hearing effects, and hepatotoxicity. Evaluate for water and sodium retention.
Auranofin	Effects cumulative, slow onset of effects (8 to 14 weeks); dosage may be gradually decreased after remission	Proteinuria; interstitial fibrosis; metallic taste	Teach skin care. Evaluate gastrointestinal discomfort. Check urine for blood and protein.
Penicillamine	As effective as gold but more toxic; unknown mechanism of action; effects seen in 2 months	Gastrointestinal irritation; taste alterations; blood dyscrasias; skin rash; stomatitis; nephrotic syndrome, glomerulonephritis; autoimmune syndrome; proteinuria	Evaluate CBC, liver, and renal function weekly for 2 months, then monthly. Teach client to report sore throat or fever. Take between meals because food decreases absorption.
Antirheumatics: Gold sodium thiomalate Aurothioglucose	Used when salicylates and NSAIDs fail; remission-inducing action suppresses inflammation	Skin rashes, pruritus; stomatitis; diarrhea; blood dyscrasias; hepatitis	Give with NSAIDs until efficacy is reached. Assess CBC and renal and liver function often.
Steroids: Systemic Prednisone Prednisolone Hydrocortisone	For use with incapacitating disease; used cautiously and preferably short term	Multiple toxic effects, including osteoporosis, gastric ulcers, risk of infection susceptibility, hirsutism, acne, emotional lability, menstrual irregularities, edema, moon facies, hypokalemia, cataracts, glaucoma	Teach client not to stop medication abruptly. Administer for short periods and taper dose slowly. Monitor for side effects, including hypertension and hyperglycemia.
Intraarticular	Used when only 1 or 2 joints are involved; used for pain relief, to increase function; benefits last 2 weeks to several months; joints most amenable are ankles, knees, hips, shoulders, and hands	Same as above	Teach client that effects may be short lived. Advise that administration is limited to 2 to 4 infections per year per joint.
Immunosuppressives: Azathioprine Methotrexate Cyclophosphamide	Used with advanced disease; affect immune system to decrease inflammation; teratogenic potential	Hepatitis, cirrhosis; gastrointestinal ulcers; susceptibility to infection; bone marrow suppression; alopecia; skin rash	Evaluate CBC, liver function, and renal function weekly. Assess older adults closely for signs of toxicity.

Modified from Moore KA: Arthritic disorders. In Salmond SW, Mooney NE, Verdisco LA, editors: *Core curriculum for orthopaedic nursing*, ed 3, Pitman, NJ, 1996, National Association of Orthopaedic Nurses.

identified after two of the three main drugs were already being prescribed for thousands of individuals across the United States. The two durgs that were taken off of the market (as of April 2005) were valdicoxib (Bextra) and rofecoxib (Vioxx). Celecoxib (Celebrex) is still available by prescription for the treatment of osteoarthritis, rheumatoid arthritis in adults, and management of acute pain. The Federal Drug Administration is continuing to investigate celecoxib to determine if it continues to be a safe drug. For the latest information, access http://www.fda.gov/bbs/topics/ANSWERS/2004/ANS01336.html. Other disease-modifying drugs such as leflunomide (Arava) and etanercept (Enbrel) are entering the field of treatment for rheumatoid arthritis to reduce signs and symptoms and to retard structural damage and improve physical functioning (Keystone et al, 2004; Savage, 2005; Wolfe, Zhao, and Pettitt, 2004).

Fatigue and decreased mobility of the joints of the upper extremities contribute to self-care deficits. Occupational therapists work with clients to improve joint function and prevent disability. The modalities used include exercises, splints, methods to protect joints, and assistive devices. Splints may be used to protect joints, maintain joint function, and decrease pain. The nurse reinforces the use of these devices and monitors correct usage.

Limitations of mobility because of pain and joint stiffness can lead to disuse and greater disability. To prevent excessive disability, the client is taught body mechanics and proper body alignment and is given recommendations for an exercise program. Using good body mechanics and keeping the body in a position of optimum alignment decrease joint stress and fatigue. Physical therapists prescribe individualized therapeutic exercise programs, which include strengthening and stretching exercises, range-of-motion exercises, and endurance training.

Fatigue is a common constitutional symptom of rheumatoid arthritis. Fatigue can interfere with the older adult's achievement of optimum functional independence. Methods used to decrease fatigue include balancing rest with activity, scheduling short rest periods (1 to 2 hours), practicing relaxation techniques, and adapting the environment to simplify work. Coping with chronic illness, pain, deformity, and alterations in body image can predispose a client to depression. If clinical depression occurs, medical evaluation and treatment are indicated.

The joint deformities and alteration in body image can lead to alteration in sexual function. The nurse should be aware of this and openly discuss issues of sexuality and methods of maintaining physical intimacy. Suggestions may include using analgesics before sexual activity, planning rest periods before sexual activity, assuming alternative positions, and encouraging alternative methods of maintaining physical intimacy (see Chapter 13).

Adults with rheumatoid arthritis require many supports to cope with this chronic, disabling disease. The nurse's role is to provide the older adult with information about resources that are available so that optimum levels of functioning can be reached. A good resource is the Arthritis Foundation (1314 Spring Street, NW, Atlanta, GA 20309; [800] 283-7800; www.arthritis.org), which publishes educational materials that address exercise programs, work simplification, and the disease process. Support groups and self-help classes taught in 6-week sessions are conducted by local chapters. The content of the classes includes self-efficacy, exercise, pain management, depression, stress management, and nontraditional therapies.

Evaluation

The older adult with rheumatoid arthritis will experience minimum discomfort and be able to maintain an acceptable level of function and mobility. With advances in drug therapy and active participation by the client in activities to prevent joint deformities, the client will experience less deformity, increased comfort levels, and understanding of the disease process.

Gouty Arthritis

Gout is a disease in which acute attacks of arthritis pain occur as a result of elevated levels of serum uric acid. During acute gout attacks, joint inflammation is caused by sodium urate crystals in the joint. Gout is classified as *primary* or *acquired*. Primary gout is an inborn disease of purine metabolism. Acquired gout is caused by medications that affect excretion of uric acid. These medications include thiazide diuretics, such as hydrochlorothiazide. Gout usually occurs in the middle years but also affects older adults; it is more prevalent in men than women.

In gout there may be an excessive production or a decreased urinary excretion of uric acid. The excess monosodium urate salts are deposited in joints and surrounding connective tissue. The deposits of the uric acid crystals are called *tophi* (Fig. 27-12).

Gout can manifest as an acute or a chronic condition. The onset of gout is sudden and is manifested by an acute attack of pain in one or more joints. The most commonly affected area is the great toe. Other joints affected by gout include the ankle, knee, wrist, and elbow. The affected joint becomes hot, reddened, and tender. The pain can be severe and interfere with mobility, self-care, and functional abilities. Chills and fever may also be present. Acute attacks of gout usually subside in 7 days regardless of treatment. In chronic gout the uric acid crystals cause bone destruction and deformity. Uric acid crystals can also be deposited in the kidney and cause nephrolithiasis.

NURSING MANAGEMENT

Assessment

The onset of an acute gout attack is identified by the presence of warmth, swelling, cutaneous erythema, and severe pain in

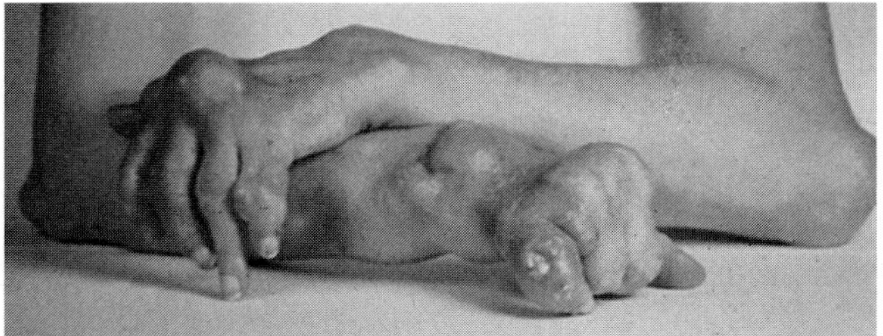

Fig. 27-12 Tophaceous gout. (Reprinted from the Clinical Slide Collection on the Rheumatic Diseases, ©1991, 1995, 1997. Used by permission of the American College of Rheumatology. In Seidel HM et al: *Mosby's guide to physical examination*, ed 4, St Louis, 1999, Mosby.)

the affected joint. The initial attack is usually in one joint, and in 50% of clients it will involve the first metatarsophalangeal joint (Edwards, 1997). The pain is intense, and the joint is sensitive to even the slightest touch. Other symptoms may include fever, chills, and malaise. Intervals between initial attacks and subsequent acute episodes will vary, but the attacks usually become more frequent and involve more joints.

Clients with chronic gouty arthritis usually report 10 or more years of previous acute gout attacks. The involved joints are chronically uncomfortable and swollen, although the intensity of the pain is less than in the acute episodes. Tophi may or may not be detected on physical examination.

Nursing assessment should identify other risk factors or conditions that may predispose the client to development of gout. These factors include obesity, hypertension, alcohol ingestion, use of diuretics, recent trauma, and hyperlipidemia.

Diagnosis

Nursing diagnoses for a client with gouty arthritis include:

- Pain, acute or chronic, related to joint inflammation and swelling
- Impaired physical mobility related to joint deformity and discomfort secondary to disease process
- Risk for activity intolerance related to pain

Planning and Expected Outcomes

The overall management plan for an older adult with gouty arthritis, either acute or chronic, is to decrease the pain and other associated symptoms. Expected outcomes for a client with gout include:

1. Client will verbalize increased comfort and pain relief with the use of appropriate analgesics and NSAIDs.
2. Client will be able to verbalize understanding of the disease process.
3. Client will incorporate appropriate diet modifications and lifestyle changes, such as weight loss and avoidance of alcohol.
4. Client will modify his or her activity and rest pattern based on limitations imposed by pain.
5. Client will incorporate health practices to minimize recurrent attacks.

Intervention

In the acute phase the goal of nursing management is to relieve pain. During an acute attack of gout the pain may be so severe that the client is unable to bear weight or to tolerate clothing or blankets on the affected joint. Colchicine is an effective medicine for the treatment of pain and inflammation of acute gout; severe pain subsides within 48 hours. The use of NSAIDs, especially indomethacin, provides comparable relief to colchicine. Other pain relief measures include analgesics, elevation of the affected extremity, immobilization of the joint, and heat or ice packs to the area.

Nursing interventions for chronic gout also focus on pain relief measures and prevention of recurrent attacks of gout. This is accomplished through client education. Because obesity and diets high in protein have been linked to gout, information about the role of dietary habits is provided. Foods that are high in purines, such as shellfish and organ meats, should be avoided. Alcoholic beverages should also be avoided. Obese clients should have weight reduction diets or programs recommended. A consultation with a dietitian for diet modifications may be helpful.

Allopurinol is the medication of choice for clients with chronic gout symptoms. Probenecid, a uricosuric agent, is another medication that may be used. Clients must be closely monitored for renal function during drug therapy. To discourage the formation of renal stones, the client should be encouraged to have a daily intake of 2 to 3 L of fluid unless contraindicated. The client should also be instructed to avoid salicylates, which could inhibit drug effects.

Evaluation

Clients with acute or chronic gout should be able to maintain a healthy lifestyle, incorporating the changes suggested during treatment. The client must understand the drug therapy for acute attacks and chronic treatments. Pain management should allow a client to participate fully in ADLs and allow for full mobility.

Osteoporosis

Osteoporosis is considered the most common metabolic bone disorder, affecting 25 million men and women in the United States. It is estimated that there are 1.5 million bone fractures every year secondary to osteoporosis (Ybarra et al, 1996). The disease primarily affects women but also occurs in one out of six men. Osteoporosis is commonly referred to as porous bone or brittle bone disease and is distinguished by a reduction in the bone mass and a loss of bone strength.

Bone is constantly remodeling itself throughout life, and the process of maintaining bone is constant. Old bone cells are removed (resorbed) by osteoclasts, and new bone cells are formed by osteoblasts. The complete process of bone remodeling takes 4 to 8 months. Bone mass is accumulated in the early part of life, with bone mineral density (BMD) increasing until approximately age 30, when peak bone mass is attained. Anything that interferes with the normal process of bone remodeling can possibly lead to the development of osteoporosis. Conditions that contribute to this process include renal or hepatic failure and endocrine disorders such as hyperthyroidism or hyperparathyroidism. Other risk factors include heredity and genetic predisposition, lifestyle factors, and age. With osteoporosis, an alteration in the bone remodeling process occurs and the rate of bone resorption exceeds the rate of bone formation, leading to decreased bone mass.

Osteoporosis is classified as primary and secondary osteoporosis. Although the cause of primary osteoporosis is not clearly understood, it is further classified into postmenopausal (type I) and age associated (type II). Type I osteoporosis is related to menopausal estrogen deficiency and is seen in women between the ages of 51 and 75. In type I the trabecular bone in the vertebral column, hips, and wrists is weakened. Because type I osteoporosis is related to estrogen deficiency, it is seen 6 times more often in women than in men. Type II osteoporosis occurs in both men and women over age 70 and produces a gradual loss of cortical bone. Because this cortical bone provides support in the body, weakening of the bone is a predisposing factor to hip fractures. Age-related changes in vitamin D synthesis that result in decreased calcium absorption are thought to be the cause of type II osteoporosis.

Secondary osteoporosis, seen in 15% of the cases, is the result of diseases such as hyperthyroidism, hyperparathyroidism, gastrointestinal disorders, neoplasms, and alcoholism. In women, early oophorectomy is a cause of secondary osteoporosis. Long-term use of corticosteroids, methotrexate, aluminum-containing antacids, phenytoin, and heparin can result in secondary osteoporosis. Prolonged immobility, which causes calcium excretion, is also a cause of secondary osteoporosis.

Certain risk factors for the development of osteoporosis have been identified (Box 27-1). Risk factors that can be modified with lifestyle changes involve calcium intake, exercise, cigarette smoking, and consumption of alcoholic beverages. Age, race, gender, and body frame are risk factors that cannot be changed. The nurse can educate the client about these risk factors, making suggestions to modify lifestyle and nutrition. Three key essentials to preventing osteoporosis throughout life are appropriate diet, exercise, and lifestyle changes (Drugay, 1997).

Osteoporosis is called a "silent killer" because frequently no clinical symptoms appear until fractures occur. The initial complaint may be back pain or fatigue. The fatigue results from the increased demand on muscles to keep the body in an upright position with a decreased bone mass. Osteoporotic fractures are most commonly seen in the vertebrae of the thoracic spine, the femoral neck, and the wrist. Fractures may occur with routine activities such as bending, lifting, coughing, and straining at stool. Osteoporosis of the spinal vertebrae causes a loss of height of 1 to 2.5 inches. Also seen is the "dowager's hump," or kyphosis, which results from the vertebrae sliding on top of each other (Fig. 27-13).

Conventional x-ray studies can detect evidence of osteoporosis, although this is often done retrospectively after a fracture. Unfortunately, at least 30% of bone mass must be lost before the disease is apparent on standard x-ray studies. To evaluate bone mass in individuals suspected of having osteoporosis or those considered at risk for development of the disease, determination of BMD appears irrefutable. Bone densitometry is commonly done with dual-energy x-ray absorptiometry (DEXA). This procedure is simple, is noninvasive, uses a low radiation dose, and is completed in less than 30 minutes. Many physician offices are now equipped with a DEXA machine for quick and simple screening of clients. Measurement sites include the hip or lumbar spine and peripheral sites such as the wrist. Scores computed from the testing compare the subject's score with those of normal young adults for peak bone mass and with sex- and age-matched controls. Criteria for diagnosis of osteoporosis have been established by the World Health Organization and are based on standard deviations from the norm. Laboratory blood studies are obtained to differentiate osteoporosis from other diseases that can cause bone loss. Complete blood count (CBC), serum calcium, serum phosphorus, alkaline phosphatase, and urinary calcium are all normal in osteoporosis.

BOX 27-1 Risk Factors for Development of Osteoporosis

- Female gender
- Increasing age
- White race
- Thin body frame
- History of bilateral oophorectomy
- Alcoholism
- Cigarette smoking
- Calcium intake below daily requirements

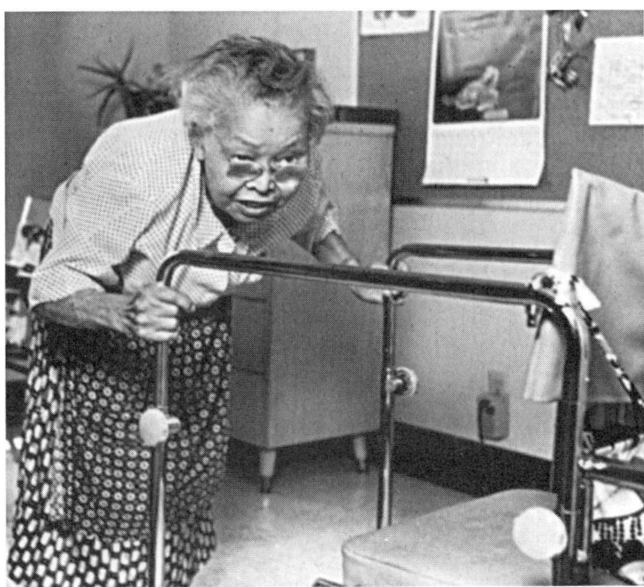

Fig. 27-13 Kyphosis has caused this elderly woman to stoop very low. This reduction of chest cavity size makes oxygen exchange difficult. (Courtesy Ken Yamaguchi. In Castillo HM: *The nurse assistant in long-term care: a rehabilitative approach*, St Louis, 1992, Mosby.)

Measures to address osteoporosis should be directed at minimizing bone loss in older adults and preserving the current level of bone mass. Client education and developing awareness of the disease are critical for prevention and risk reduction. Changing lifestyle risk factors, nutritional counseling, and pharmacologic management are strategies used to prevent osteoporosis.

Adequate nutritional intake of calcium should be instituted in early childhood and continued throughout the life span. The current recommendation for daily calcium intake is 1000 mg for men and premenopausal women ages 25 through 49, 1500 mg for postmenopausal women who are not taking estrogen, 1000 mg for postmenopausal women taking estrogen, and 1500 mg for men and women above age 65 years. Milk, either low-fat or nonfat, is a good source of calcium and vitamin D. Table 27-3 identifies dietary sources of calcium. Many of these food items are also good sources of vitamin D, which is essential for the synthesis of calcium.

TABLE 27-3 Dietary Sources of Calcium

FOOD	SERVING	CALCIUM CONTENT (IN mg)
Milk		
Skim	8 oz	302
2% fat	8 oz	297
Whole	8 oz	291
Cheeses		
Swiss	1 oz	272
Processed American	1 oz	174
Mozzarella	1 oz	207
Cottage cheese	1 oz	135
Other dairy products		
Yogurt, lowfat	8 oz	415
Ice cream, vanilla	1 cup	176
Ice milk, vanilla	1 cup	274
Seafood		
Oysters	1 cup	226
Pink salmon, canned with bones	3 oz	167
Vegetables		
Collards, frozen or fresh	1 cup	357
Broccoli, fresh	1 cup	177
Broccoli, frozen	1 cup	94
Mustard greens	1 cup	104
Dried beans (cooked and drained)		
Navy beans	1 cup	90
Pinto beans	1 cup	86
Red kidney beans, canned	1 cup	74
Other foods		
Blackstrap molasses	2 tbsp	274
Tofu	4 oz	108

Modified from US Department of Agriculture: Human nutrition information servings, *Home Garden Bullet* 72, 1985.

For individuals unable to consume adequate calcium, supplements are recommended. Various forms of calcium supplements are available. Calcium carbonate is thought to be the best supplement because it contains 40% elemental calcium, is the least expensive, and requires taking the least number of tablets. Calcium supplements should be taken with meals and followed by at least 10 oz of water to promote absorption.

Exercise programs that include weight bearing and resistance have been shown to prevent bone loss. Beneficial exercises for older adults include walking, low-impact aerobics, vigorous water exercises, and racquet sports. Exercises should be done 3 times a week for 30 to 60 minutes for best effect. Postural exercises to prevent or minimize kyphotic deformity are also of benefit to older adults. Moderation in any exercise program is always recommended.

Postmenopausal estrogen replacement therapy (ERT) will prevent or stabilize the process of osteoporosis. Estrogen has a direct role in regulating bone metabolism, attaching to receptor sites on the osteoblasts and decreasing bone resorption. It also has a positive effect on calcium absorption, promoting the synthesis of calcitonin and increasing vitamin D receptors in the osteoblasts. The controversy with ERT is that it may contribute to an increased incidence of endometrial cancer and possibly an increased risk for breast cancer. The addition of progestin in hormone replacement may reduce the potential risk of endometrial cancer. ERT and its impact on prevention or treatment of osteoporosis are still undergoing much study. ERT is generally started as early as possible in the postmenopausal period if indicated. The benefits of ERT in decreasing the incidence of hip fracture may outweigh the risks. ERT is contraindicated for those who have a history of breast cancer or thromboembolic disease. Low-dose estrogen (0.625 mg of conjugated estrogen) is prescribed in ERT. Individuals receiving ERT should perform breast self-examination monthly and undergo mammography annually. If abnormal vaginal bleeding occurs, medical evaluation is indicated.

Other pharmacologic agents that are being used to retard the progression of osteoporosis and maintain bone mineral content have been approved. These so-called antiresorptive agents act by inhibiting the osteoclasts, thereby preventing bone resorption. Alendronate sodium (Fosamax) has been found to produce a significant reduction in bone resorption, and treatment with the drug has shown significantly increased bone mass at the lumbar spine, hip, and total body (Pitocco et al, 2005). Fosamax has been approved for treatment of postmenopausal osteoporosis and approved for prevention of osteoporosis in clients at risk. It can be used in both men and women because it is a nonhormonal compound. The drug requires client education because it is poorly absorbed from the gastrointestinal tract if not taken correctly. Special instructions include taking it daily, 1 hour before any food or medications. It is taken with 6 to 8 oz of water, and the client must remain upright for at least

30 minutes after taking the drug. Fosamax should be taken cautiously by clients with active upper gastric disease, and side effects for all clients may include abdominal pain or gastric distress. Ability to comply in the administration of this drug should be considered in the older adult population (Christensen et al, 2005).

Another antiresorptive drug used to treat osteoporosis is calcitonin in either a parenteral or nasal spray preparation. Oral administration is not appropriate because the drug is a polypeptide hormone and is destroyed in the gastrointestinal tract. The nasal spray preparation is a formulation of synthetic salmon calcitonin, and it has been approved for use for the treatment of osteoporosis in women who are at least 5 years postmenopausal, have low bone density, and are not candidates for ERT. Marketed under the brand name Miacalcin, calcitonin is generally administered daily in one puff, alternating nares. Because the drug may elicit a systemic allergic reaction in certain individuals, intradermal skin testing may precede the initial dosage. Systemic adverse effects of the nasal route are reported as being minimum but may include nasal discomfort, occasional rhinitis, and itching of the nasal mucosa.

The newest drug approved for prevention of osteoporosis is raloxifene hydrochloride (Evista). This drug is a selective estrogen receptor modulator (SERM) and has an estrogen-like effect on bone metabolism. The benefit of SERMs is still being investigated, but it appears that they do not have the same estrogen effect on uterine and breast tissue, thereby decreasing the risk of cancer. They may also have beneficial effects on heart disease risk factors. Other agents that are beneficial include sodium fluoride to stimulate osteoblasts and parathyroid hormone to stimulate bone formation (Gibney et al, 2005).

NURSING MANAGEMENT

Assessment

Nursing assessment of older clients should include a thorough health history on the client's family history, presence of risk factors, level of exercise, alcohol and caffeine intake, and smoking. Women should be assessed for age of onset of menopause, use of ERT, date of last mammogram, and history of breast or uterine cancer. All clients should be asked about their lifelong intake of calcium, history of fractures, presence of pain, and history of falls. Physical examination includes inspection to determine the presence of kyphosis, gait impairments, muscle weakness, and cognitive impairments.

Diagnosis

Nursing diagnoses for an older client with osteoporosis include:

- Altered nutrition: less than body requirements related to decreased intake of calcium and vitamin D
- Risk for injury related to weakening of the bones
- Pain related to inadequate pain relief secondary to bone fractures
- Body image disturbance related to spinal deformities and loss of height
- Knowledge deficit: disease process, risk factors, and measures of prevention related to lack of previous exposure

Planning and Expected Outcomes

Awareness of the risk factors and education about the lifetime prevention of osteoporosis and its complications, such as falls and fractures, are the most important aspects of planning the care of older adults with osteoporosis. Expected outcomes for a client with osteoporosis include:

1. Client will demonstrate taking precautions at home and in the community to prevent falls and activities that may result in fractures.
2. Client will report adequate level of pain control in presence of bone fractures.
3. Client will consume nutritional supplements, food products, and medications recommended or prescribed for meeting dietary needs, as evidenced by diet log.
4. Client will verbalize acceptance of changes brought about by the disease and understanding of the treatment and prevention of further deformities (see Research box and Health Promotion box).

Research

SAMPLE/SETTING

The subjects were 247 women recruited from worksites, primary health care providers, and a health fair.

METHODS

The Facts on Osteoporosis quiz, a 25-item true-false test related to self-care, risk factors, and prevention of osteoporosis, was used to assess participants' knowledge of osteoporosis.

FINDINGS

The average score was 16. Participants had the lowest number of correct responses to questions about the risk factors of alcohol abuse and high caffeine intake and about the availability of treatment.

IMPLICATIONS

There is a need for nurses to educate women concerning the risk factors, prevention strategies, and treatment of osteoporosis.

Alinger RL, Emerson J: Women's knowledge of osteoporosis, *Appl Nurs Res* 11(3):111, 1998.

Health Promotion/Illness Prevention

Musculoskeletal Function: Osteoporosis

HEALTH PROMOTION

- Routine weight-bearing exercises that do not stress the joints, such as walking
- Achievement of ideal body weight
- Initiation of a weight-training program
- Smoking cessation
- Decreased intake of alcohol and caffeine

DISEASE PREVENTION

- Participation in regular program of weight-bearing exercises
- Avoidance of injury and falls
- Maintenance of adequate dietary intake of calcium and supplementation with oral calcium supplements as indicated
- Consideration of hormone replacement therapy
- Little to no intake of alcohol and caffeine
- Avoidance of smoking

Intervention

The nurse's role focuses on client education about the disease process, strategies to prevent further injury or deformity, and measures to promote decreased loss of bone. Education should emphasize the identification and minimization of controllable risk factors. These include cigarette smoking, excessive use of alcohol, and caffeine intake. Exercise programs are recommended that will place some stress on the bones, such as walking and lifting light weights, to strengthen them. Additional information for osteoporosis education and programs can be found through the National Osteoporosis Foundation (1232 22nd Street, NW, Washington, DC 20037; [202] 223-2226; www.nof.org).

Compression fractures of the vertebrae can cause pain, loss of function, and disturbance in body image brought about by the gradual loss of height that can occur with multiple fractures. Control of pain is achieved through the use of analgesics, NSAIDs, positioning, and relaxation techniques. Other pain management modalities include transcutaneous electrical nerve stimulation, various back supports or braces, and formal pain management consultation. Body image can be supported by discussions of acceptance of changes that have occurred, but with a focus on prevention of further injury and deformity.

Nursing care of the older adult with a hip fracture or other fracture secondary to osteoporosis includes the interventions previously noted in this chapter.

Evaluation

A client with osteoporosis should be able to describe measures that can be taken to decrease the potential for development of the disease and maintain a safe living environment to reduce the risk of injury resulting from falls. The client will be able to describe the benefits of appropriate diet, lifestyle modifications, and diet supplements or medications if needed. The older adult will also be able to participate in regular exercise programs and to identify resources available for prevention of disease (see Nursing Care Plan).

Nursing Care Plan

Osteoporosis with Fractured Thoracic Vertebrae

Clinical Situation: Mrs. R is a 79-year-old widow who has severe osteoporosis and who recently fractured her T4 and T5 vertebrae. After the fracture she complained of severe pain, which limited her daily activity and caused her to spend most of the day in bed. The period of bed rest has left her weak. Before the fracture she was independent in mobility and self-care. She drove and participated in activities with her friends on a regular basis. She is referred to the home care agency for pain management and physical therapy to upgrade her ADL skills and endurance.

Mrs. R has no other health problems. She lives alone in a two-story house. The bathroom is on the second floor. Since the fracture, Mrs. R has stayed on the second floor all day except for one trip a day to the kitchen on the first floor to fix a meal. Mrs. R's major support is her daughter, who lives in another state. She has several close friends, but they are unable to help her because of their health problems.

On the admission visit, the nurse finds Mrs. R's house to be in an unsafe condition. The rooms and stairs are cluttered with papers, boxes, and other objects. Mrs. R tells the nurse that her pain is somewhat improved, but it still limits her ability to take care of herself and her home. She also tells the nurse, "I don't understand this osteoporosis; how did that cause my fractures?"

Nursing Diagnoses

High risk for injury related to unsafe environment
Knowledge deficit: osteoporosis related to lack of exposure
Impaired physical mobility related to pain and musculoskeletal impairment
Pain related to inadequate knowledge of pain management
Self-care deficit: bathing and dressing lower extremities related to pain and prolonged immobility

Outcomes

Client will remain free from fracture or other injuries and will verbalize unsafe features of home and a plan to correct.

Continued

Nursing Care Plan
Osteoporosis with Fractured Thoracic Vertebrae—cont'd

Client will verbalize basic information about the disease process, outcomes, and treatment.
Client will safely walk 100 feet using pickup walker and will participate in a daily exercise program.
Client will verbalize that pain is tolerable. Pain will not interfere with ability to participate in daily activities.
Client will bathe and dress lower extremities with the use of assistive devices.

Interventions

Discuss outcomes of unsafe environment: risks of falling and fracture as a result of cluttered environment.
Use homemaker and friends to reduce clutter and encourage use of safety aids.
Teach safe transfer and ambulation techniques, wearing of sturdy supportive footwear, avoidance of lifting heavy objects, and how to bend from the knees when lifting.
Provide information and instruction on osteoporosis, including the pathophysiology of the disease; treatment regimen; and medication schedule, doses, and side effects.
Stress the importance of dietary intake of calcium and provide information on foods that are high in calcium.
Consult with physical therapy for a program of muscle strengthening, endurance development, stair training, and regular exercise.
Reinforce physical therapy training.
Give positive feedback for gains made.
Instruct client to make limited trips up and down stairs until strength is improved.
Instruct client on taking pain medication before the exercise program and the need for regular rest periods throughout the day.
Assess pain and effectiveness of prescribed medication.
Instruct client to take pain medication before activities and on a regular basis until pain diminishes.
Instruct client on the use of diversional activities and relaxation techniques.
Assist client in setting short-term, realistic goals.
Consult with occupational therapist for specific assistive devices.
Instruct client on use of assistive devices.
Provide assistance, supervision, and teaching as needed to promote self-care.
Give positive feedback for gains made.

Paget's Disease

Paget's disease (osteitis deformans) is an inflammatory disease of the bone in which both osteoclasts and osteoblasts proliferate. The processes of bone formation and bone resorption do not always proceed at the same rate. The cause of Paget's disease is not known. Recent evidence supports the theory that a viral infection of the osteoclasts causes the disease. There is also a possible familial predisposition to Paget's disease, which occurs most often in men over age 40, with a higher incidence in individuals older than 80 years of age.

Increased activity of osteoclasts leads to increased bone resorption. Bone formation is increased to compensate. This abnormal remodeling causes deformed and enlarged bones. Vascularity in the abnormal bones is increased, which results in excessive warmth over the bones involved. Bones affected by the disease are structurally weak and prone to pathologic fractures.

The onset of Paget's disease is insidious. Bones most often involved are the pelvis, femur, skull, tibia, and spine. The first symptom is bone pain, which is not relieved with rest and movement. The intensity of the pain varies from mild to severe; quality can be stabbing or dull. If bones of the skull are involved, headache and conductive hearing loss may occur. Barreling of the chest, kyphosis, skull enlargement, and bowing of the tibia and femur are commonly seen bone deformities. The bowing of legs and kyphosis lead to reduction in height.

The prognosis for clients with Paget's disease is not favorable because of the complications that may develop. These include pathologic fracture and loss of hearing related to changes in the temporal bone. The overgrowth of the spinal vertebrae can cause cord compression and paralysis.

NURSING MANAGEMENT

 Assessment

Nursing assessment should include a thorough health history, including information about known family history of the disease. The nurse should assess for warmth, deformity, pain, and erythema over long bones; assess range of motion in joints; and evaluate the presence of any weakness, ataxia, or hearing loss.

Diagnosis

Nursing diagnoses for a client with Paget's disease include:

- Pain related to bone deformity and possible joint involvement
- Impaired mobility related to bone deformity, fracture, or pain
- Risk of injury related to limitations of mobility and altered bone metabolism
- Altered body image related to bone deformities and disturbance in function

Planning and Expected Outcomes

Nursing care of the client should focus primarily on pain management, if necessary, and the issues of chronic disease. Addressing the alterations in body image and impaired mobility are also critical. Expected outcomes include:

1. Client will achieve satisfactory comfort level with pain management techniques and medications.
2. Client will modify home environment and take precautions in the community to prevent injuries.
3. Client will verbalize understanding of the chronic nature of the disease and appropriate therapies.
4. Client will make positive coping statements related to potential altered body image.

Intervention

Nursing care of a client with Paget's disease includes education regarding the disease and treatment. Pain management should be addressed; pain is usually the presenting symptom. The pain is usually a deep, aching type of bone pain that may worsen with activity, especially with weight-bearing activities in clients with spinal or lower extremity deformities. Various methods of pain relief may be attempted, including use of NSAIDs and analgesics. Other nursing interventions include instructing a client on use of heat or cold, rest periods, and other pain relief measures (see Chapter 15).

The client's safety and mobility issues should be assessed. Instruction on simple exercises and the use of assistive devices or consultation with physical or occupational therapists may be of benefit. Occasionally, the client's disease may involve the hip or knee joint, resulting in chronic, severe pain and deformity. Arthroplasty may be recommended to correct the deformity and relieve pain.

Helping the client maintain mobility and independence with daily activities may also positively affect the client's body image and attitude toward the chronic disease. Discussions of long-term prognosis and treatment may offer encouragement.

Evaluation

Nursing evaluation of a client with Paget's disease includes documentation of the client's ability to perform ADLs and understanding of the importance of therapy for prevention of pain, deformity, and loss of function.

Osteomyelitis

Osteomyelitis is an infection of the bone that can be either acute or chronic. Acute osteomyelitis resolves in 4 weeks when treated with antibiotics. Chronic osteomyelitis lasts longer than 4 weeks and does not respond to initial treatment with antibiotics.

Invasion of the bone by microorganisms is the cause of osteomyelitis. Microorganisms enter the body directly through an open fracture or stage IV pressure ulcer. Bloodborne bacteria from distant sources such as urinary tract infections can indirectly inoculate the bone. *Staphylococcus aureus* is the most common bacteria seen in osteomyelitis. Other causative agents are gram-negative bacteria such as *Escherichia coli* and *Pseudomonas aeruginosa*. Osteomyelitis is seen most often in older adults as a complication of a stage IV pressure ulcer.

Bacteria enter the bone through the blood supply and lodge in an area of the bone where sluggish circulation occurs. The bacteria multiply, resulting in an inflammatory response. Pus and vascular congestion develop, causing increased pressure in the bone, which leads to ischemia and vascular compromise. The necrotic bone separates from living bone. The devitalized areas are called *sequesta*.

In an older adult with osteomyelitis related to a bone injury the presenting signs are localized pain, tenderness on palpation, erythema, warmth to touch, and edema. In osteomyelitis related to infected pressure ulcers the symptoms may be subtle changes in mental status, low-grade fever, and increased purulent wound drainage. These signs and symptoms may go unnoticed until sepsis occurs.

If treated early, osteomyelitis has a good prognosis. The older adult may not have the classic signs of infection. Often, the first sign of osteomyelitis may be sepsis; in these cases, the prognosis is poor.

NURSING MANAGEMENT

Assessment

The nurse caring for an older adult with osteomyelitis or at risk for developing osteomyelitis must be aware of the subtlety of the presenting signs and symptoms of infection. Presenting symptoms vary in older adults and range from severe, acute onset to a clinical picture of chronic, subacute illness with minimum pain. Nursing assessment should focus on identification of risk factors predisposing a client to osteomyelitis, careful examination of any preexisting wounds or infections, and monitoring vital signs and diagnostic test results.

Diagnosis

Nursing diagnoses for a client with osteomyelitis include:

- Pain related to swelling and tenderness
- Impaired skin integrity related to infected wounds
- Risk for impaired physical mobility related to lower extremity pain

Planning and Expected Outcomes

Planning care for a client with osteomyelitis should include a multidisciplinary approach. Treatment for this condition may be prolonged and therefore may require additional emotional and physical support. The long-term treatment for this problem requires family and significant others to be involved in the planning process. Expected outcomes include:

1. Client will report minimum discomfort and adequate pain control.
2. Client will verbalize understanding of the need for long-term therapy to eliminate infection.
3. Client will demonstrate safe and independent mobility.
4. Client will exhibit intact skin surfaces and no evidence of further infection.

Intervention

Prevention of osteomyelitis includes using sterile technique during dressing changes and following strict wound precautions. A client with infected pressure ulcers will most likely be functionally impaired and return to a long-term care setting for completion of intravenous antibiotic treatment. Clients with osteomyelitis as a result of other causes will be discharged while receiving oral antibiotics. Discharge planning involves teaching about the importance of completing the course of oral antibiotics, methods to prevent infection, and specific techniques of wound management. An alternative treatment is a medication pump that is surgically implanted to deliver continuous antibiotic to the infection site.

The long-term treatment of chronic osteomyelitis creates psychologic coping issues. Lengthy hospitalizations, immobility, and dependence can lead to feelings of anger and decreased self-worth. To help clients cope more effectively, the nurse should allow them to make informed decisions about care and should consult with therapeutic recreation specialists for diversional activities. The prolonged immobility can lead to the complications of immobility and self-care deficits. To prevent these problems, physical and occupational therapists are consulted to provide individualized exercise programs that promote optimum function and prevent disability.

Evaluation

Clients with osteomyelitis should participate fully in all aspects of care. Any wounds or other potential sources of infection should show progressive healing. The client should be able to verbalize understanding of the chronic nature of treatment, and documentation should include the client's involvement in wound care or antibiotic therapy. Older clients may have difficulty adjusting to the extended hospitalizations required for therapy, and the nurse can facilitate appropriate consultations.

Amputation

Amputation of the lower extremity is a common surgical procedure in older clients. The level of amputation depends on the extent of the disease process. Peripheral vascular disease (PVD), infection, neoplasm, and traumatic injury may all lead to lower extremity amputation, with PVD being the most common cause in older adults. In PVD caused by atherosclerosis and diabetes, circulation is inadequate to maintain cellular function.

Atherosclerosis and diabetes are predisposing factors in the development of foot or extremity ulcers. The ulcers can be chronically infected. Osteomyelitis with bone destruction results in amputation of the extremity.

In PVD, chronic obstruction of the arteries results in inadequate circulation that causes tissue hypoxia. When the tissues are inadequately perfused for prolonged periods, atrophy of the underlying tissue occurs. This decreased circulation leads to delayed healing of injured feet or lower extremities. When ischemic ulcers do not heal, infection and necrosis or gangrene develop.

Gangrene manifests as a blackened area. The temperature in the affected area is lower than that of the unaffected area, and pain may be present. With the chronically infected extremity ulcer, the ulcer persists despite treatment with antibiotics.

NURSING MANAGEMENT

Assessment

Before the surgical procedure, a complete nursing assessment is done to determine the presence of other diseases and their effect on function. The focus of this assessment is on mobility and self-care ability. How do clients walk? Are assistive devices required? What is the extent of self-care abilities? Assessment of the affected limb includes peripheral pulses, temperature, sensation, and movement. The specific characteristics of the ulcer or gangrenous area are noted, including location, size, and color. The individuals' perception of the surgery is ascertained. Clients are asked how they feel about the impending surgical procedure and how they see the amputation affecting their health and lifestyle.

Diagnosis

Nursing diagnoses for an older client undergoing amputation include:

- Pain secondary to surgical procedure and phantom limb sensation
- Body image disturbance related to amputation, impaired mobility, and prolonged immobilization
- Potential for alteration in skin integrity related to disease process, surgical procedure, and immobility
- Impaired physical mobility related to loss of extremity
- Activity intolerance related to immobility
- Ineffective individual coping related to loss

Planning and Expected Outcomes

Nursing care of the client undergoing amputation includes planning for the client's preoperative, postoperative, and rehabilitative periods. Multidisciplinary planning is critical for the client's recovery and long-term prognosis. Expected outcomes include:

1. Client will report pain relief with the administration of analgesics.
2. Client will demonstrate acceptance of body image change, as evidenced by positive statements regarding body and active involvement in treatment of the stump.
3. Client's incisional area will remain clean without evidence of infection.
4. Client will safely perform self-care activities within his or her activity and energy expenditure limitations.

Intervention

Client education is an important nursing role in preventing amputation. Because the majority of amputations are a result of PVD, clients need knowledge of how to control the factors that can lead to amputation. Clients with diabetes and PVD are taught how to inspect and care for their feet and lower extremities. Instructions include information on promptly notifying a health care provider if there are changes in temperature, sensation, and color. If a sore develops, prompt treatment must be sought. Methods to protect the lower extremity from injury are included in the teaching plan.

Preoperative Care. Amputation is a major threat to an individual's body image and has the potential to lead to ineffective coping. To assist with adjustment in the postoperative phase, the nurse provides extensive information about the surgical procedure, including the purpose of the amputation, the potential use of a prosthesis, and the rehabilitation program. To assist in the rehabilitation phase, the nurse teaches exercises to strengthen upper extremities. Postoperative care, including information about positioning, turning, compression bandaging, and pain control, is discussed. Clients also require information about phantom sensations and phantom limb pain. Phantom limb sensation is the feeling of tingling, itching, or aching in the limb; phantom limb pain is a painful sensation that occurs after the amputation; both may become chronic.

Postoperative Care. Routine postoperative care is provided in the immediate postoperative period. Clients are monitored carefully for complications that may be a result of preoperative health problems. Complications include hemorrhage and infection. The postoperative dressing depends on the type of prosthesis that will be used. The client has either an immediate prosthetic fitting or a delayed prosthetic fitting. Because older adults may be debilitated from multiple chronic illnesses and the chronic condition that caused the amputation, they will probably have a delayed prosthetic fitting. Dressings are either rigid or soft in delayed prosthetic fittings. The rigid dressing may be made from either plastic or plaster of Paris. The advantage of this type of dressing is that it decreases edema. Soft dressings consist of Kerlix gauze covered with an elastic wrap that acts as a compression dressing. The compression dressing is used to support the tissues, to decrease pain and edema, and to promote shrinking of the stump. The soft dressing is changed daily using sterile technique. The wound is assessed for signs and symptoms of infection. A dry dressing is applied directly to the suture site.

In the immediate postoperative period (48 to 72 hours), pain medication is given on a regular schedule. Because of age-related changes in pharmacokinetics and pharmacodynamics, clients receiving narcotic analgesics should be monitored closely for response and side effects (see Chapter 22). The effect of narcotics may last longer and may also result in excessive sedation, confusion, or respiratory depression. Initial doses may be lower than those used for younger adults. However, based on the individual's pain relief and tolerance, doses may be increased. Morphine sulfate is the medication used most often in this phase of care. Box 27-2 provides guidelines for pain management.

Rehabilitative Care. The rehabilitative phase starts immediately after surgery with the application of the dressing. The dressing is important for prosthesis fitting because it shapes the stump for the prosthesis. The compression dressing is worn continuously and removed at least 2 times a day. Care is taken to properly apply the dressing. It should be wrapped snugly and securely, but not so tightly that it impairs circulation. A stump shrinker, a continuous tube of elasticized fabric closed at one end, may be used instead of the wrap.

When the client's condition is stable, physical therapy begins. Nursing goals for this phase include preventing complications and assisting the client in reaching an optimum level of function. The physical therapy program includes active range of motion, upper extremity strengthening, and gait training. For ambulation, walkers are used with older adults rather than crutches, since crutches require greater upper extremity strength and endurance. The nurse reinforces the exercise program and assists the client in practicing safe transfer techniques.

Prosthetic Fitting and Adaptation. Not all older adults are candidates for prostheses. Multiple chronic illnesses may result in a state of debilitation in which the client will not have the strength and reserve to complete a program of intense prosthetic training. These clients are taught transfer techniques and wheelchair mobility.

BOX 27-2 Guidelines for Postoperative Pain Management

- Give the lowest possible effective dose.
- Increase intervals between doses.
- Combine narcotics with nonnarcotic analgesics.
- Closely monitor effectiveness and response.

Delayed prosthetic fitting takes place when the stump is healed and well molded. The fitting is done by a prosthetist, who makes a mold of the stump. As the stump shrinks, adjustments in the prosthesis are made. The client is instructed to assess the stump daily for signs of irritation from an ill-fitting prosthesis.

The physical therapist and prosthetist instruct the client in the use of the prosthesis. The physical therapist also works on gait training. The nurse reinforces the teaching and provides the amputee with reinforcement on performance. Fig. 27-14 shows different types of prostheses.

The individual who has had an amputation experiences a loss and a major threat to body image. The normal response to loss is grief. The grieving process and adjustment to the loss are an individualized response characterized by vacillations in the recognized stages of grief: denial, isolation, anger, bargaining, depression, and acceptance.

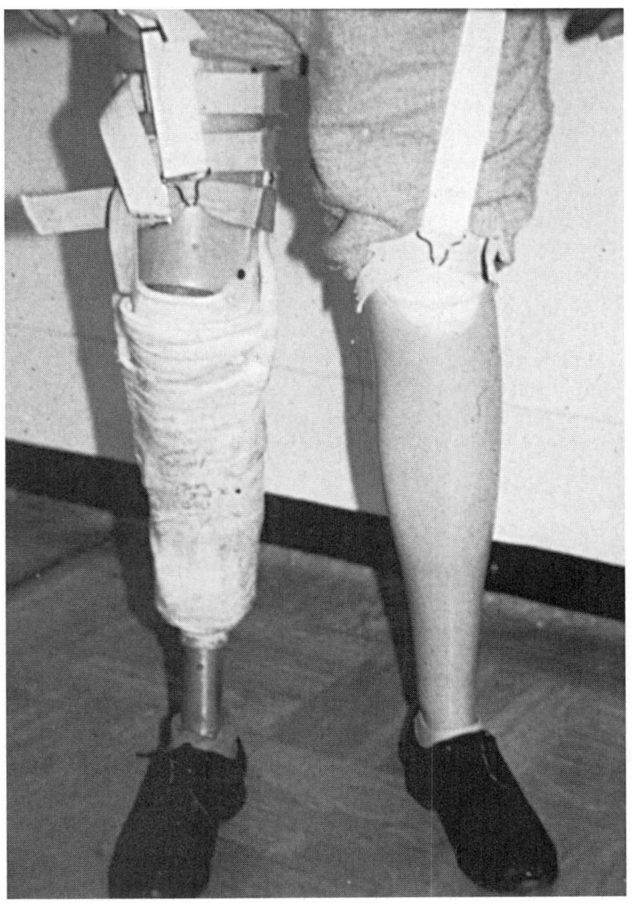

Fig. 27-14 Two types of prosthesis. Patellar tendon-bearing type, below-the-knee prosthesis with cuff suspension *(left)*. Early fitting below-the-knee rigid plaster dressing with pylon *(right)*. (From Lewis S, Heitkemper M, Dirksen S: *Medical-Surgical nursing: assessment & management of clinical problems*, ed 3, St Louis, 1992, Mosby.)

Body image is an individual's subjective perception of the body. Gradual changes in body image are easier to adapt to than those which have an abrupt onset, such as the change experienced by an amputee. The adaptation to the change in body image does not always reflect the extent of the injury, but it is related to that individual's feelings toward himself or herself as a total person. The role of the nurse is to help amputees discover a new self. Traumatic changes in body image may be characterized by revulsion in viewing the amputation. Viewing the amputation and looking in the mirror at the total self-picture may be difficult. Accepting the body changes is a gradual process. The nurse must allow the client time to work through this process. The nurse can ask broad, open-ended questions about the body changes, such as, "How do you see yourself?" and "How do you think others see you?" (Ebersole, Hess, and Luggen, 2004). Talking with other amputees one-on-one and in support groups is helpful for clients in adapting to changes in body image. The nurse should give positive and realistic feedback about the individual's progress in functional abilities (see Nursing Care Plan).

Evaluation

Evaluation is based on achievement of expected outcomes as evidenced by the client exhibiting a positive outlook about the body changes; performing self-care and other activities safely and adequately; and experiencing pain relief over time, until eventually analgesic pain medication is not needed. Documentation of these activities is critical for the multidisciplinary evaluation of the client's progress and is used as the basis for further care planning.

Polymyalgia Rheumatica

Polymyalgia rheumatica is a chronic inflammatory condition characterized by sudden onset of muscle stiffness and aching (myalgia) in the neck, shoulders, and hip girdle. The disease occurs after the age of 50 years, most often in those 65 years and over. Women are affected more than men. The cause of polymyalgia rheumatica is not known. Infection and an altered immune response have been suggested but not proven as the cause. Likewise, a genetic predisposition is suggested, but not confirmed. The pathophysiology of polymyalgia rheumatica is not clearly understood.

The clinical presentation of polymyalgia rheumatica is similar to that of rheumatoid arthritis and osteoarthritis. Symptoms include muscle stiffness and aching in the neck, shoulders, and hip girdle. The muscle stiffness is present in the morning and lasts more than 1 hour. Constitutional symptoms such as fever, malaise, anorexia, and weight loss may be present. Initially the pain may be limited to one area, but it generally develops in a symmetric fashion. Objective signs of muscle weakness are not present on physical examination. Joint swelling is usually absent, and there are no

Nursing Care Plan
Amputation

Clinical Situation: Mr. C is a 75-year-old retired truck driver with a medical history of type 2 diabetes, PVD, and a chronic right foot ulcer. Because the foot ulcer did not respond to conservative treatment, he underwent a right below-the-knee amputation. Before this surgical procedure, Mr. C had been hospitalized for 3 weeks for treatment of the foot ulcer. During the hospitalization he became weak and deconditioned. He now requires assistance with eating and ADLs and maximum assistance for transfers. Mr. C complains of phantom limb pain and requires pain medication every 4 to 6 hours.

The prolonged illness, hospitalization, and amputation have caused Mr. C to feel hopeless. He has told the nurses he is tired of being in the hospital, sick, and in pain. Mr. C has also verbalized feelings about not being the man he once was. He does not initiate any self-care and needs encouragement to complete self-care. Mr. C has a supportive wife and family. His wife has rheumatoid arthritis and thinks it will be difficult for her to care for her husband unless he participates in his care and is rehabilitated with a prosthesis. Mr. C is stable 2 days postoperatively and is beginning physical therapy for preprosthetic training.

Nursing Diagnoses

Body image disturbance related to amputation, impaired mobility, and prolonged hospitalization
Pain related to surgical procedure and phantom limb sensation
Potential for alteration in skin integrity related to disease process, surgical procedure, age-related changes, and immobility
Impaired physical mobility related to below-the-knee amputation and prolonged immobility
Activity intolerance related to prolonged immobility, deconditioning, and disease processes
Ineffective individual coping related to amputation
Potential for ineffective family coping related to spouse's chronic illness and disability

Outcomes

Client will verbalize feelings of acceptance of change in body image.
Client will verbalize that pain is tolerable.
Pain will not interfere with ability to participate in ADLs.
Incision will heal without signs or symptoms of infection.
Skin will remain free from pressure ulcers.
Client will transfer independently and walk 10 feet with a pickup walker.
Range of motion will remain within normal limits.
Flexion contracture will not develop.
Client will attend and participate in a daily therapy program with normal physiologic response.
Client will use effective coping strategies and participate in a rehabilitation program.
Family will use effective coping strategies and support client's participation in the rehabilitation process.

Interventions

Allow verbalization of feelings; actively listen to feelings.
Give positive feedback for progress made in self-care and mobility and for aspects of general appearance.
Encourage normal activities such as dressing in street clothes.
Encourage participation in support groups.
Assess pain and effectiveness of medications.
Administer pain medications as ordered.
Provide diversional activities and alternative treatments such as relaxation techniques.
Assess incision and pressure areas (use a risk assessment scale) daily for signs of infection or pressure ulcers.
Change surgical dressing with aseptic technique.
Reposition every 2 hours; position to keep pressure off bony prominences.
Teach client how to change positions.
Provide adequate caloric, protein, and fluid intake.
Wrap stump with compression dressing or stump shrinker.
Consult with physical therapy for a program of muscle strengthening, transfer training, and gait training.
Reinforce physical therapy training.
Give positive feedback for gains made.
Teach transfer techniques; assist with transfers.
Teach safe use of walker.
Give pain medications 30 to 60 minutes before therapy.
Do not elevate stump on pillows.
Keep stump in good alignment; prevent flexion contractures.
Reinforce use of active range-of-motion exercises.
Encourage lying on the abdomen for 30 minutes 2 times a day.
Encourage participation in therapy program.
Gradually increase activity.
Allow at least 60 minutes of rest after therapy.
Monitor vital signs before, during, and after therapy.
Assist client in identifying previously successful coping skills.
Suggest and describe effective coping skills.
Encourage activities that enhance self-esteem.
Encourage use of support systems.
Encourage participation in amputation support group; include family, especially spouse, in support group.
Encourage spouse's verbalization of feelings when client is not present.
Suggest and describe effective coping skills.
Suggest taking time to care for self.

limitations in range of motion. The symptoms last at least 4 weeks without treatment.

Polymyalgia rheumatica is treated with NSAIDs and steroids, and generally shows a significant improvement in symptoms 1 to 2 days after the beginning of treatment. This marked improvement so soon after initiation of treatment is not seen in rheumatoid arthritis or osteoarthritis.

NURSING MANAGEMENT

Assessment

A thorough history of the client's symptoms, a physical examination, and a functional assessment are important in determining the effect of the disease on functional abilities.

Diagnosis

Nursing diagnoses for a client with polymyalgia rheumatica include:

- Pain related to muscle stiffness and aching
- Altered mobility related to pain and muscle stiffness
- Fatigue related to systemic symptoms
- Self-care deficit related to muscle stiffness
- Potential for ineffective coping related to chronic nature of disease

Planning and Expected Outcomes

Expected outcomes for an older client with polymyalgia rheumatica include:

1. Client will report pain relief with initiation of treatment.
2. Client will correctly describe pharmacologic therapy, including purpose, action, and side effects of prescribed drugs.
3. Client will establish an activity and rest pattern based on limitations imposed by the disease.
4. Client will incorporate effective coping strategies in disease management.
5. Client will correctly state the treatment rationale and prognosis.

Intervention

The medical diagnosis of polymyalgia rheumatica is difficult to make; because symptoms are similar to those of rheumatoid arthritis and osteoarthritis, it is often misdiagnosed. The client who has been to many physicians in an attempt to receive the correct diagnosis and proper treatment may be frustrated, angry, and worn out. The nurse should listen to the client's concerns and give information about the disease and treatment plan. This includes information about treatment with and side effects of corticosteroids. The nurse monitors for the development of side effects. The client is reassured that the dose of medication will be tapered and eventually the symptoms will subside.

Evaluation

Clients with polymyalgia rheumatica need to understand the chronic nature of the disease and be able to maintain functional abilities. Pain management is necessary for the older client to perform ADLs, so the client will need to be familiar with the medications and their side effects. Providing appropriate education about the disease and symptom management will assist in acceptance. Documentation of education, pain assessment, and functional abilities is important for ongoing planning and care of the client.

FOOT PROBLEMS

The foot is often overlooked in assessment and care of older adults. Foot problems, especially pain, are common in older adults. The incidence and severity of foot problems increases with age. After age 65, 75% of the population complains of foot problems. More than 80% of those over age 55 demonstrate arthritic changes on x-ray examination. Foot problems may cause an unsteady gait and result in falls (Karpman, 1995).

The foot is a complex structure composed of 26 bones; 33 joints; and numerous ligaments, tendons, and muscles. The foot is necessary for ambulation. During standing and ambulation, the foot provides body support and absorbs shock. Painful feet can be the result of congenital deformities; weak structure; injuries; and diseases such as diabetes, rheumatoid arthritis, and osteoarthritis. Ill-fitting shoes result in foot pain by crowding the toes and impeding normal movement. As people age, the feet show signs of wear and tear. The cushioning layer of fat on the soles of the feet becomes thin. Years of walking cause the metatarsal bones to spread and the ligaments to stretch, which results in wider feet.

Corns

Corns are thickened and hardened dead or hyperkeratotic tissue that develops over bony protuberances. Corns often cause localized pain. Corns are caused by ill-fitting or loose shoes that constantly place pressure on bony prominences. Soft corns are produced by the bony prominence of one toe rubbing against the adjacent toe in the web space between the toes. Soft corns are macerated because of moisture in the web space (Fig. 27-15).

Warm water soaks are used to soften corns before gentle rubbing with a pumice stone or callus file. Another treatment is gentle débridement by a podiatrist. To relieve pain and prevent the development of corns, moleskin or cotton pads are placed over areas of rubbing and pressure. Wider and softer shoes are recommended. Topical applications of salicylic acid should be avoided in older adults because they may cause irritation, burns, or infection, especially in those with diabetes and impaired circulation.

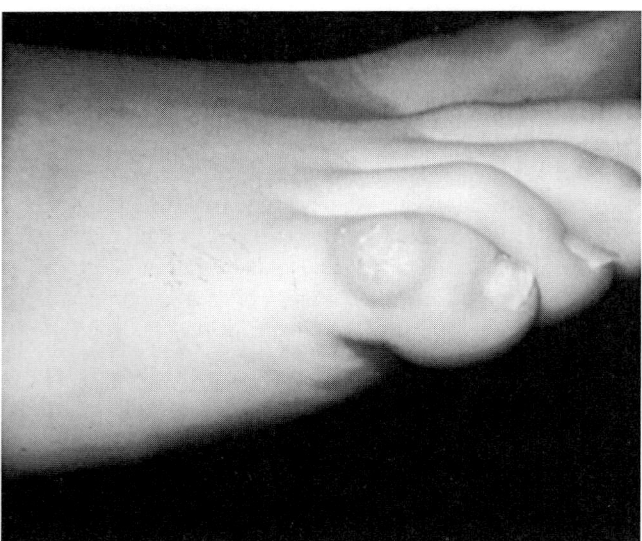

Fig. 27-15 Hard corn on lateral aspect of fifth toe over prominent condyles of proximal phalanx. (Reprinted with permission from Coughlin MJ: *Postgrad Med* 75:191, 1984.)

Calluses

Calluses, or plantar keratoses, are dead tissue found on the plantar surfaces of the feet. They form under the metatarsal heads, most commonly the second and third heads. About half of people over 65 years of age have some degree of plantar calluses. The aging changes of decreased toe function and decreased fat padding contribute to their development. Soft-soled shoes with the addition of insoles are recommended. Treatment is the same as for corns.

Bunions

Bunions, or hallux valgus, have the greatest prevalence in those over 50 years of age, with women experiencing them 4 times more often than men, since women tend to wear narrow, pointed, high-heeled shoes. Arthritis and other age-related changes such as ligament and tendon atrophy predispose older adults to bunions.

Bunions appear as bony protuberances on the side of the great toe (Fig. 27-16). In bunions the large toe angles laterally toward the second toe. As the great toe rubs against the shoe, the bursa becomes inflamed, resulting in bursitis and pain. Initial treatment of bunions is with soft leather shoes that are flat, wide, and lace-up. Walking or running shoes with a wide toe box prevent rubbing on the bunion. Moleskin bunion pads can be used to protect the bony protrusion. NSAIDs may be prescribed to reduce inflammation and pain. Surgical interventions are used after conservative treatment has failed. The surgical procedure includes removal of the bursa sac and correction of the bony deformity.

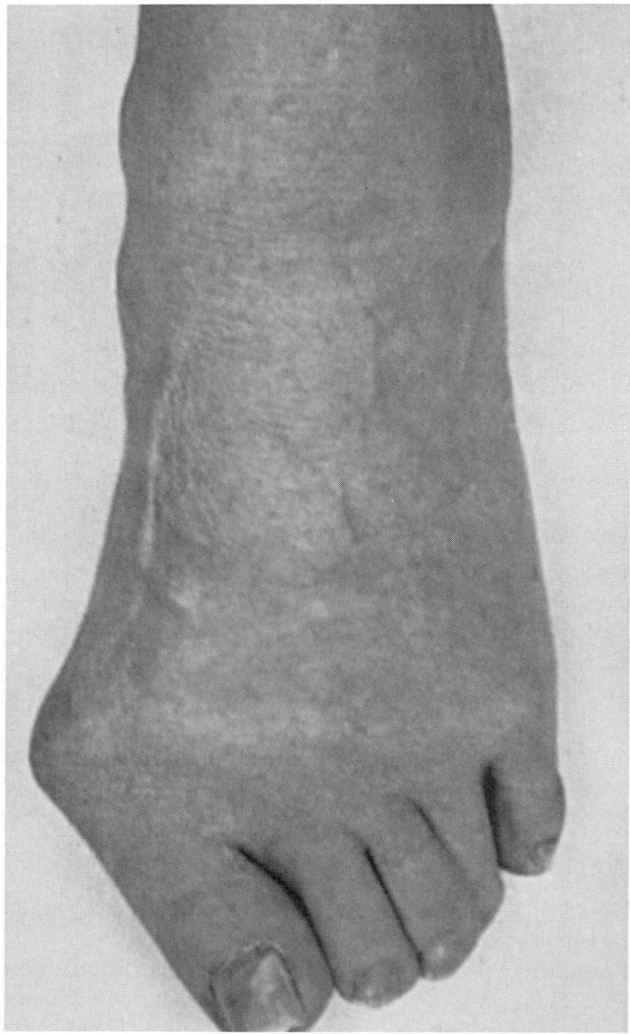

Fig. 27-16 Hallux valgus angulation of first three toes; overlapping of middle toe on fourth toe; and wide, flat metatarsus. (From Mann RA, Coughlin MJ: *Surgery of the foot and ankle,* vol 1, ed 6, St Louis, 1993, Mosby.)

Hammertoe

Hammertoe is a deformity of the second toe. In this deformity the metatarsophalangeal joint is dorsiflexed, the proximal interphalangeal joint is plantar flexed, and there is callus formation on the dorsum of the proximal interphalangeal joint and the end of the affected toe. The result is a toe that is in a clawlike position (Fig. 27-17). Improperly fitted shoes, muscle weakness, and arthritis are causes for hammertoe. Symptoms include pain and burning on the bottom of the foot and problems walking in shoes. Initially, pain may be relieved with a moleskin toe pad. Other treatments for hammertoe include metatarsal arch support, orthotics, splints, and passive manual stretching of the proximal interphalangeal joint. Surgical correction is done if the conservative treatment is ineffective.

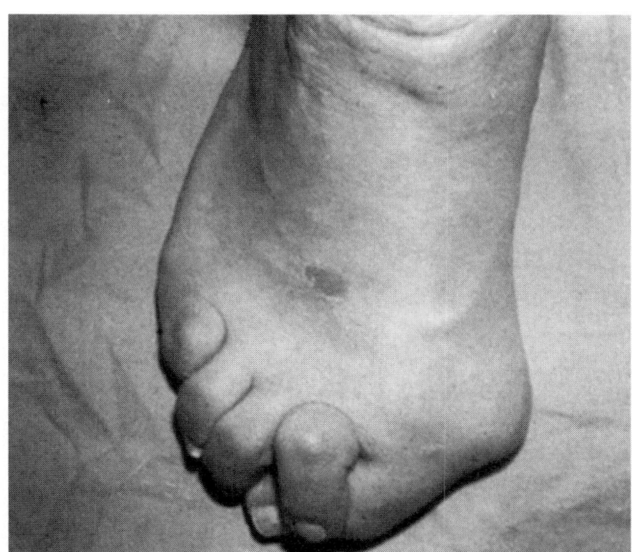

Fig. 27-17 Hammertoe associated with hallux valgus. (From Crenshaw AH, editor: *Campbell's operative orthopaedics*, vol 4, ed 8, St Louis, 1992, Mosby.)

Nail Disorders

Toenail problems are common in older adults. Older adults with problems of the nails should be referred to a podiatrist.

Onychauxis is hypertrophic nails with the nail borders curving into the soft tissue of the toes. This disorder can cause nail bed ulcers, infection, and pain.

Onychomycosis is a localized fungal infection of the toenail that is seen most frequently in older adults. Degeneration of the nail plate causes changes in the growth and appearance of the nail. Onychomycotic nails may have simple scaling or may be totally destroyed by the fungus. Initially the nail becomes brittle and hypertrophic. The nails can be white, yellow, or brown. Ridges and pitting of the nail are common. Generally the infection spreads between the nails. Predisposing factors for onychomycosis are moisture, poor footwear, recurrent trauma, and diabetes.

Treatment of onychomycosis is difficult because of the composition of the nail and the involvement of the nail matrix. Topical antifungals such as clotrimazole are generally used for several months. The oral antifungal agents such as terbinafine and itraconazole are generally not used with older adults because many have a decreased pedal blood supply. Clients with onychomycosis that does not respond to topical antifungal agents should be referred to the podiatrist. The podiatrist will débride the nail at periodic intervals.

Client Education

The nurse should educate the older adult about the predisposing factors, prevention, and treatment of onychomycosis and the need for ongoing foot care, including inspection of feet for signs of infection and application of the medication.

The nurse has an important role in educating clients about proper foot care and footwear. Well-fitted shoes are essential to the prevention of foot problems. The shoe should not crowd the toes and should be of the correct length and width. Shoes that are too short or narrow can force the great toe into a position of hallux valgus. Shoes should be wide enough to allow bending of the toes and movement of the foot muscles. Adequate arch support should be provided. Women should not wear high heels.

Clients should be taught foot care that includes daily hygiene and changing of socks. Socks or stocking should be loose enough to avoid the development of pressure ulcers. Toenails should be trimmed with nail clippers; clients with impaired vision, impaired mobility, or self-care deficits may require assistance to perform this task safely. To prevent the development of ingrown toenails and infections, the nails should be trimmed straight across. If persistent foot problems develop, a podiatrist should be consulted.

MUSCLE CRAMPS

Idiopathic muscle cramps without muscle weakness are common in older adults. The cramps can start during rest or after minor exercise. Muscle cramps generally affect the calf or foot muscles, producing plantar flexion of the foot or toes. They occur most frequently at night during sleep.

Prevention of muscle cramps can be achieved by stretching the affected muscles for several minutes at bedtime. After the cramping occurs, stretching will generally relieve the discomfort. The calf muscles should be stretched for two or three 1-minute intervals with 1-minute rest periods between stretches. Stretching exercises improve muscle flexibility and reduce the motor activity in the affected muscles.

Quinine sulfate is sometimes prescribed for muscle cramps; however, its effectiveness has been questioned. The side effects of quinine therapy for muscle cramps can increase concentration of digoxin, and overdose can cause confusion.

SUMMARY

Problems of the musculoskeletal system can have a great effect on the day-to-day life of older adults. Conditions such as osteoarthritis, rheumatoid arthritis, osteoporosis, and fractures can result in functional disability, chronic pain, and decreased quality of life. The role of the nurse working with clients with musculoskeletal disorders is to promote safe, optimum function in mobility and self-care. Interventions to promote comfort and to relieve pain are critical in the maintenance of function. To prevent serious disability, it is essential that clients resume activity as soon as possible after

Home Care

1. Assessment of the musculoskeletal system includes examination of bones, muscles, and joints in homebound older adults.
2. Instruct caregivers and homebound older adults about reportable signs and symptoms related to the musculoskeletal system disease or disorder being treated and when to report these changes to the home care nurse or physician.
3. Instruct caregivers and homebound older adults on the name, dose, frequency, side effects, and indications of both the prescribed and over-the-counter medications being used to treat the identified musculoskeletal problem.
4. Musculoskeletal problems increase safety hazards (e.g., falls) in homebound older adults.
5. Assess for functional impairments, such as inability to provide self-care and perform IADLs. If necessary, have social worker identify community resources for additional assistance with identified impairments, such as transportation and food preparation.
6. Assess the activity tolerance level, which may be affected by musculoskeletal problems.
7. Instruct caregivers and homebound older adults about the diagnosed musculoskeletal disease or disorder, focusing on self-care measures that maintain or promote independence.
8. Have the physical therapist and occupational therapist evaluate and teach caregivers and homebound older adults how to adapt the environment based on the specific musculoskeletal problem (e.g., gait training, use of handheld devices to assist with eating, splints, prostheses).
9. Encourage ambulation in a safe manner. Stretching exercises that improve posture should be part of the nursing interventions.
10. An exercise program may be suggested after consulting with the physician.
11. Instruct caregivers and homebound older adults on the necessity of calcium supplements and exercise to maintain proper skeletal function and prevent bone loss.

episodes of acute illness. A key nursing role is to educate clients about the importance of musculoskeletal activity in maintaining function.

Key Points

- A high incidence of musculoskeletal disorders exists in older adults.
- Musculoskeletal disorders are a major cause of functional impairments in older adults.
- Age-related changes in the musculoskeletal system can predispose older adults to falls.
- The most common sites of fractures in older adults are hip, wrist (Colles' fracture), and vertebrae.
- Demographic factors associated with osteoporosis include female gender, age, and white race.
- Lower extremity amputations in older adults are most often the result of PVD or diabetes.
- Symptoms of osteoarthritis, rheumatoid arthritis, gouty arthritis, and polymyalgia rheumatica are similar, yet treatments differ.
- Physical activity and exercise are key to preventing disability from musculoskeletal disorders in older adults.

Critical Thinking Exercises

1. An 80-year-old woman has suffered a musculoskeletal injury that requires a period of bed rest and limited mobility. How will age affect her ability to tolerate a period of decreased mobility? Explain.
2. You are caring for two clients: a 72-year-old man with gouty arthritis and a 68-year-old woman with rheumatoid arthritis. What aspects of their care will be similar? What aspects will be different?
3. A 73-year-old man has lived a fairly sedentary lifestyle as an accountant. Now that he is retired, he recognizes the need to be active to maintain his health as long as possible. He is concerned, however, that it is too late for him to start exercising because he has never engaged in such activities. What encouragement, if any, can you give to him, and what suggestions can you make for an exercise program?

References

AARP: *A profile of older Americans: 1997,* Washington, DC, 1997, US Department of Health and Human Services.

Christensen PM et al: Cost effectiveness of alendronate in the prevention of osteoporotic fractures in Danish women, *Basic Clin Pharmacol Toxicol* 96(5)387-396, 2005.

Drugay M: Breaking the silence: a health promotion approach to osteoporosis, *J Gerontol Nurs* 23(6):36, 1997.

Ebersole P, Hess P, Luggen AS: *Towards healthy aging: human needs and nursing response,* ed 6, St Louis, 2004, Mosby.

Edwards NL: Gout: clinical and laboratory findings. In Klippel JH, editor: *Primer on rheumatic diseases,* Atlanta, 1997, Arthritis Foundation.

Gibney J et al: Metabolic effect of Raloxifene and oral estrogen in postmenoausal and growth hormone–deficient women, *J Clin Endocrinol Metabol* 26(5):173-181, 2005.

Karpman R: Foot problems in the geriatric patient, *Clin Orthoped Relat Res* 316:59, 1995.

Keystone EC et al: Once-weekly administration of 50-mg etanercept in patients with active rheumatoid arthritis: results of a multicenter, randomized, double-blind, placebo-controlled trial, *Arthritis Rheumatol* 50(2):353-363, 2004.

King MB, Tinetti ME: A multifactorial approach to reduce injurious falls, *Clin Geriatr Med* 12(4):745, 1996.

Pitocco D et al: Six-month treatment with alendronate in acute charot neuroarthropathy: a randomized controlled trial, *Diabetes Care* 28(5):1214-1215, 2005.

Savage R: Cyclo-oxygenase-2 inhibitors: when should they be used in the elderly? *Drugs Aging* 22(3):185-200, 2005.

Spivak JM: Current concepts review—degenerative lumbar spinal stenosis, *J Bone Joint Dis* 80-A(7):1053, 1998.

Theis LM: Cost containment and quality coexisting in total joint care, *Orthoped Nurs* 17(6):70, 1998.

Wolfe F, Zhao S, Pettitt D: Blood pressure destabilization and edema among 8538 users of celecoxib, rofecoxib, and nonselective non-steroidal anti-inflammatory drugs (NSAIDs) and nonusers of NSAIDs receiving ordinary clinical care, *J Rheumatol* 31(6):1143-1151, 2004.

Wolinsky FD, Fitzgerald JF, Stump TE: The effect of hip fracture on mortality, hospitalization, and functional status: a prospective study, *Am J Pub Health* 87(3):398, 1997.

Ybarra J et al: Osteoporosis in men: a review, *Nurs Clin North Am* 31(4):805, 1996.

28 Urinary Function

SABRINA FRIEDMAN, MSN, PhD, EdD, FNP

Learning Objectives

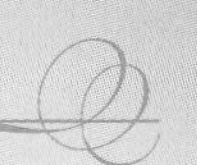

On completion of this chapter, the reader will be able to:

1. Describe how aging affects normal bladder function.
2. List four possible causes of acute incontinence.
3. List the types of persistent incontinence and their clinical characteristics.
4. List the components of a continence history.
5. Discuss the role of functional and environmental assessment in the evaluation of urinary incontinence.
6. Discuss how the nurse can use tests of provocation in making a nursing diagnosis of clients with urinary incontinence.
7. Describe the behavioral interventions used to treat urinary incontinence in cognitively intact clients.
8. Develop a client teaching plan for a client with urge incontinence.
9. Develop a caregiver teaching plan for a client with functional urinary incontinence resulting from dementia.
10. Describe the effects of normal aging on renal function.
11. Identify the possible causes of acute and chronic renal failure.
12. Identify the treatment options for clients with bladder cancer.
13. List supportive services for the individual who has undergone a cystectomy.
14. Differentiate between benign prostatic hypertrophy and prostate cancer.
15. Identify the treatment options for clients with prostate cancer.
16. Apply the nursing process in the care of older adults with select urinary system conditions.

Urinary incontinence (UI) is one of the most common health problems affecting older adults. The Agency for Health Care Policy and Research (AHCPR, 1996) defines urinary incontinence as an involuntary loss of urine that is sufficient to be a problem. It is a major clinical problem and a significant cause of disability and dependency. Physical health, psychologic well-being, social functioning, and health care costs can be adversely affected by incontinence. Individuals with UI are at increased risk for urinary tract infection (UTI), skin problems (e.g., rash, infections, breakdown), and falls. Incontinence can cause psychologic distress and social isolation. It is a cause of caregiver burden and may be a factor in the decision to place older individuals in long-term care facilities. The cost of medical managing of UI is staggering.

AGE-RELATED CHANGES IN STRUCTURE AND FUNCTION

Contrary to the belief of many older adults and (unfortunately) some health care providers, aging is not the sole cause of UI. However, aging does affect the lower urinary tract (Fig. 28-1). These age-related changes increase an older adult's susceptibility to other insults to the lower urinary tract. As a result, these insults (e.g., drug side effects, UTIs, conditions impairing mobility) are more likely to produce incontinence in older clients than in younger ones.

With age, bladder capacity decreases, the prevalence of involuntary bladder contractions increases, and more urine is produced at night. The reduction in bladder capacity and increased involuntary bladder contractions can lead to urgency and frequency. Many older adults find that they have to empty their bladders more often than they did when they were younger. Increased urine formation at night leads to nocturia. Nocturia is very common; close to 70% of community-dwelling older adults get up once a night to empty their bladders, and 25% get up twice (Ouslander, 2003).

Changes occur in the urethra because of the aging process and the decreased levels of estrogen after menopause. Thinning and increased friability of the urethral mucosa can contribute to urgency and frequency. A decrease in muscle tone and bulk can decrease urethral resistance. In addition to the changes in the urethra, declining estrogen levels affect pelvic floor muscle tone and function.

Although it is not considered a normal change associated with aging, as men get older the prevalence of prostatic hypertrophy increases. Enlargement of the prostate can interfere with bladder emptying and can also precipitate involuntary bladder contractions.

PREVALENCE OF URINARY INCONTINENCE

As many as one in three older adults living in the community have some degree of UI. Of these, one in four has frequent

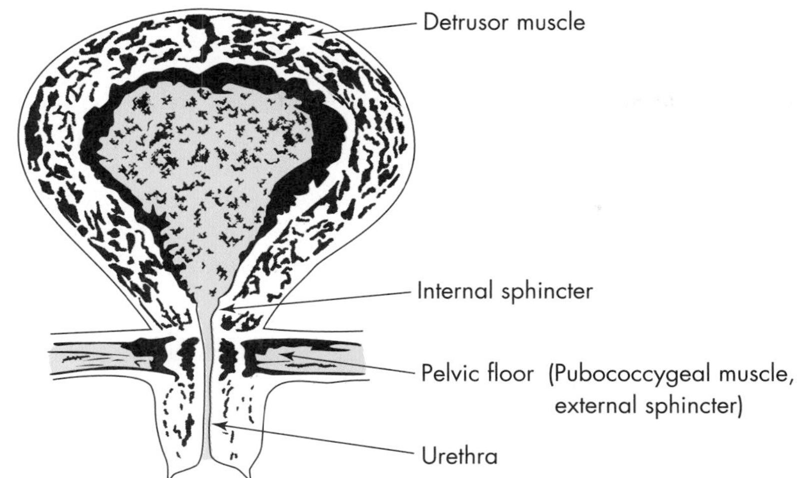

Fig. 28-1 The urinary bladder. (From Burke M, Walsh M: *Gerontologic nursing care of the frail elderly*, St Louis, 1992, Mosby.)

incontinent episodes (AHCPR, 1996). UI is twice as prevalent among women as men. Among homebound individuals, prevalence rates as high as 53% have been reported (Ouslander, 1999). UI is even more common among nursing facility residents. At least half of the 1.5 million Americans in nursing facilities suffer from UI (AHCPR, 1996). It is estimated that 20% to 35% of older adults in acute care settings are incontinent (Ouslander, 2003).

Myths and Attitudes

Despite the significant number of older adults with UI, most do not report the condition or seek medical treatment. This may be because they are embarrassed, believe it is not important enough to mention, or believe it cannot be treated. Research studies have indicated that common beliefs about UI may lead older clients, particularly older women, to think that incontinence is normal and not worth reporting to health care providers.

Although little systematic information exists about health care professionals' knowledge and attitudes about UI, some evidence suggests that many do not see incontinence as a treatable problem (AHCPR, 1996). Many health care providers do not ask clients about incontinence. Even when clients inform them about incontinence, many providers ignore the problem and do not provide adequate diagnosis and treatment.

COMMON PROBLEMS AND CONDITIONS

Acute Incontinence

UI is generally classified as either acute (transient) or chronic (persistent). Acute incontinence has a sudden onset, is generally associated with some medical or surgical condition, and generally resolves when the underlying cause is corrected (Ouslander, 2003) (Box 28-1). Medication is a common cause and should always be suspected as a potential cause of new incontinence. Although the exact prevalence of acute incontinence is not known, any new onset of incontinence should be considered acute, and possible precipitating causes should be ruled out. Addressing the cause has the potential to resolve the incontinence.

Chronic Incontinence

Persistent incontinence is not related to an acute illness. It continues over time, often becoming worse. Major types of

BOX 28-1 Causes of Acute Urinary Incontinence

Restricted mobility
Fecal impaction
Delirium
UTIs
Endocrine disorders
- Poorly controlled diabetes mellitus
- Hypercalcemia

Alcohol
Medications
- Anticholinergics
- Beta-adrenergic medications
- Alpha-adrenergic blockers
- Alpha-adrenergic agonists
- Calcium channel blockers
- Diuretics
- Psychotropics
- Narcotics

persistent incontinence include stress, urge, overflow, and functional incontinence (AHCPR, 1996). These types of incontinence can occur in combination, causing mixed incontinence. This is quite common in the older adult population (Ouslander, 2003).

Stress Incontinence. Stress incontinence is commonly seen in older women, who involuntarily lose urine as the result of a sudden increase in intraabdominal pressure. Stress incontinence occurs as pressure in the bladder (intravesical pressure) exceeds urethral resistance when intraabdominal pressure increases in the absence of a detrusor (bladder) contraction. This can occur because of loss of normal support of the bladder neck and proximal urethra or because the proximal urethra no longer functions as a sphincter (Haab, Zimmern, and Leach, 1996). This damage can be the result of pregnancy, vaginal delivery, trauma during gynecologic or urologic surgery, obesity, or chronic coughing (Ouslander, 1999). Individuals with stress incontinence often leak urine with physical exertion such as coughing, sneezing, laughing, lifting, and exercise. Older women may report leakage when they change position (e.g., get out of a chair) or lift a small child. These activities increase intraabdominal pressure, which increases bladder pressure. If the urethra, supporting tissues, and bladder neck are abnormal, urethral resistance may be too low to withstand the increased pressure on the bladder, which results in involuntary urine loss. Typically, a small to moderate amount of urine is lost (Gibbons and Choe, 2004). Stress incontinence is uncommon in men, but it can occur as a result of injury to the sphincter during prostate surgery or radiation therapy (Ouslander, 2003).

Urge Incontinence. Urge incontinence is also common in the older adult population. Urge incontinence is usually, although not always, associated with abnormal detrusor contractions (AHCPR, 1996). Common causes of urge incontinence include local genitourinary conditions such as cystitis, urethritis, tumors, stones, and diverticula, as well as central nervous system disorders such as stroke, dementia, and Parkinson's disease (Ouslander, 2003). Individuals with urge incontinence typically give a history of involuntary urine loss after a sudden urge to void. Urgency and involuntary urine loss can be precipitated by the sound of running water, cold weather, or the sight of a toilet. Urinary accidents are sometimes large. Urge incontinence is often accompanied by nocturia and complaints of frequency. Urge incontinence can be classified as one of the following types, based on etiology and the bladder abnormality (AHCPR, 1996):

1. Detrusor hyperreflexia (DH), when the uninhibited bladder (detrusor) contractions are caused by a neurologic problem (e.g., stroke).
2. Detrusor instability (DI), when there is no underlying neurologic problem.
3. Detrusor sphincter dyssynergia (DSD), when the uninhibited bladder contraction is accompanied by contraction of the external sphincter. This results in urinary retention and may be seen in clients with suprasacral spinal cord lesions and multiple sclerosis.
4. Detrusor hyperactivity with impaired bladder contractility (DHIC), when uninhibited bladder contractions are accompanied by impaired contractility during voluntary voiding. As a result, the client must strain to empty his or her bladder either completely or incompletely. This type of urge incontinence may be seen in frail older adults.

Overflow Incontinence. Overflow incontinence occurs when a chronically full bladder increases bladder pressure to a level higher than urethral resistance, causing the involuntary loss of urine. Based on the history alone, overflow incontinence may be difficult to differentiate from stress or urge incontinence. It accounts for only a small number of incontinence cases in older adults. Typically, individuals with overflow incontinence complain of frequent loss of small volumes of urine. They may have both daytime and nighttime accidents. Additional complaints may include always being wet, frequency of urges, a weak urine stream, hesitancy (difficulty starting to pass urine), interrupted voiding, or feeling of incomplete emptying (McDowell et al, 1996). Overflow incontinence can occur as a result of an atonic bladder that does not contract adequately (e.g., from diabetic neuropathy, anticholinergic medications, or spinal cord injury); a mechanical obstruction to bladder emptying (e.g., prostatic hypertrophy, a large cystocele, or uterine prolapse); or dyssynergia, a condition in which the urethral sphincter contracts during bladder contraction, preventing the bladder from emptying (e.g., from multiple sclerosis) (AHCPR, 1996).

Functional Incontinence. In functional incontinence, involuntary urine loss occurs as a result of inability or unwillingness to toilet appropriately and from physical, mental, psychologic, or environmental factors. Clients with physical disabilities affecting gait may have difficulty reaching the bathroom in a timely manner. Clients with cognitive impairment may not recognize their need to void or may have difficulty finding the toilet and preparing to void. Those with psychologic problems such as severe depression may lack the motivation to toilet appropriately. Environmental factors may play a role in causing incontinence, especially in acute and long-term care settings. Clients who are confined to beds or are restrained are dependent on caregiver assistance to the toilet. If that assistance is not available in a timely manner, the client is often incontinent. This is especially true if the client also has urgency. Functional incontinence should be a diagnosis of exclusion.

Mixed Incontinence. Mixed incontinence is described as a combination of two or more other types: stress, urge, overflow, or functional incontinence. Among community-dwelling older adults, mixed urge and stress incontinence is common. In clients with dementia or severe mobility problems, mixed urge and functional incontinence is common. This condition should be thoroughly evaluated to delineate which symptoms are most bothersome to the patient so appropriate treatment may be assigned (Gibbons and Choe, 2004).

Diagnosis of Urinary Incontinence

The purpose of the diagnostic evaluation for UI is threefold (Ouslander, 2003):

1. To identify potentially reversible factors that may be contributing to the incontinence
2. To identify clients who need more than a basic evaluation
3. To determine the type of incontinence so appropriate treatment can be initiated

The basic evaluation for UI includes a history, physical examination, postvoid residual (PVR), and urinalysis. This evaluation is indicated for all clients with incontinence and is often sufficient to diagnose the type of incontinence and guide therapy (AHCPR, 1996). A PVR over 100 ml may indicate inadequate bladder emptying. A clean urine specimen should be collected for urinalysis. If there is a delay in processing a urine specimen, it should be refrigerated.

The majority of cases of incontinence can be cured or significantly improved with careful evaluation to identify treatable factors contributing to the incontinence, followed by implementation of appropriate medical and nursing interventions. Evaluation of the success of any efforts to restore urinary incontinence should be based on an older person's satisfaction and tolerance of the interventions and strategies to achieve the outcome.

NURSING MANAGEMENT

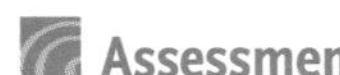

Assessment

The purpose of the nursing assessment for UI is to determine the type of incontinence and the factors contributing to it so that appropriate nursing interventions can be planned and implemented. In addition, the nursing assessment allows the nurse to identify those clients who need to be referred to a physician or nurse practitioner for more complete evaluation. The assessment consists of a history assessment, functional assessment, environmental assessment, psychosocial assessment, physical examination, tests of provocation, and evaluation of bladder habits.

History. During the history assessment, information is collected about the client's incontinence symptoms and bladder habits; general health and functional status; medical problems; current medications; and past medical, surgical, and obstetric history. If clients are able to provide the history, they are the most accurate source of data. In situations in which a client has cognitive impairment, however, the nurse may have to rely on secondary sources such as family caregivers or medical records.

During the incontinence history assessment, the following information should be collected:

- The onset of the incontinence
- The frequency and volume of accidents
- The circumstances that cause urine loss, including (1) any leaking of urine when the client coughs, sneezes, laughs, changes positions, climbs steps, exercises, has an urge to void, hears running water, is cold, or is sleeping; (2) any involuntary urine loss caused by caffeine, alcohol, or any medication; and (3) whether the client leaks urine without being aware that it occurred, has any postvoid dribbling, or leaks continuously
- Bladder habits, including the frequency and volume of daytime and nighttime urination
- Daily fluid intake, including caffeine intake
- Self-management techniques the client uses to manage the incontinence (e.g., frequent voiding, restricting the volume or type of fluid, incontinence products, urine collection devices)
- Previous evaluation and treatment of the incontinence, including the client's perception of the effectiveness of previous treatment measures
- Any other urinary tract symptoms, including urgency, burning, pain, hematuria, weakness of the urinary stream, intermittent stream, and difficulty emptying the bladder completely
- Bowel habits, including constipation, laxative use, and fecal incontinence

In addition to the incontinence history, the nurse should also obtain a general health history. The nurse should inquire about current medical problems and specifically ask about problems that can affect bladder function (e.g., diabetes mellitus, congestive heart failure, bladder and kidney infections, strokes, Parkinson's disease, depression, memory problems, mobility problems, problems with coordination, and other neurologic problems or injuries); ask about current medication and treatment, including the use of over-the-counter medication; inquire about previous surgeries, including past urologic or gynecologic surgery; for men, ask specifically about prostate surgery and radiation; for women, obtain an obstetric history, including information about the number of pregnancies, type of deliveries, any complications during delivery, and birth weights of the infants; and for postmenopausal women, inquire about estrogen replacement therapy.

Functional Assessment. Because function problems often contribute to UI, functional assessment is one of the most important parts of the evaluation. Information should be collected about the client's ability to perform normal activities of daily living (ADLs), including grooming, dressing, getting in and out of bed, and walking. Clients who have difficulty performing these ADLs often have difficulty toileting.

Functional status can be assessed by unstructured questioning or by using a structured questionnaire such as the Older Americans Research and Service Center Instrument (OARS) (Duke University Center for the Study of Aging and Human Development, 1978) or the Katz Index of ADLs (Katz et al, 1963) (see Chapter 4).

Direct observation provides the most valuable information about the client's mobility and toileting ability. The following observational guide can be used in practice (Burgio and Goode, 1997):

1. Place the client 15 feet from the toilet.
2. Ask the client to approach the toilet, either on foot or in a wheelchair, and to prepare and position for voiding.
3. Note the time it takes the client to reach the toilet and any difficulty in getting undressed or positioning for voiding.
4. If the client is unable to toilet independently and a caregiver normally assists the client, observe the toileting procedure with caregiver assistance.

Mental status should be assessed during the functional assessment. Cognitive ability can affect the client's ability to recognize the need to urinate, locate the toilet, and undress for toileting. In addition, knowledge of a client's cognitive status is essential for planning nursing interventions for incontinence. The most efficient way to assess cognitive status is to use a standardized instrument such as the Folstein MiniMental State Examination (Folstein, Folstein, and McHugh, 1975) (see Chapter 4).

Environmental Assessment. Environmental barriers can contribute to UI. For example, the bathroom may be too far away or inaccessible to the client, or the toilet may be too low or difficult for the client to get on and off. The client may need assistance in toileting, which may not be readily available. For these reasons, environmental assessment is an important component of the evaluation of UI. It is necessary to note:

- Proximity of the toilet
- Any barriers between the client's usual location and the toilet, such as poor lighting, steps, furniture, or other objects
- The size of the bathroom: Is it large enough to accommodate the client and any assistive devices (wheelchair or walker) that must be used?
- Toilet height: Is it adequate or too high or low?
- Presence of grab bars, if needed
- Availability of caregiver or nursing staff assistance if needed
- Availability of a call bell if needed

Psychosocial Assessment. Psychosocial assessment focuses on the effect of incontinence on the client's life and on the availability and quality of caregiver assistance. The nurse should ask the client how incontinence has affected social activities (e.g., visiting family and friends, attending social functions and church), self-esteem, mood, sexual activity, and family relationships; the nurse should also assess the client's desire and willingness to participate in a treatment program for incontinence. Effective nursing interventions for UI require active client involvement, so motivation is an essential component to success. If a client does not want treatment for incontinence, the reasons should be explored. Is the reason, for example, a lack of knowledge; depression; or an overwhelming physical, social, or psychologic problem?

If the client depends on another person's assistance in toileting, caregiver assessment is an essential component of the psychosocial assessment. Is the caregiver (1) physically able to assist the client, (2) available on a consistent basis, and (3) willing to assist the client? What is the caregiver's attitude toward the client and toward incontinence? Does the caregiver have an adequate understanding of the problem and its management?

Physical Examination. The physical examination should include:

- Inspection of gait and balance
- Neurologic assessment of any weakness, paralysis, or sensory deficit in the lower extremities, which can affect a client's ability to toilet
- Abdominal examination for bladder distention, suprapubic tenderness (occurs in bladder infections), and costovertebral angle tenderness (occurs in kidney infections)
- Rectal examination for fecal impaction; rectal sensation and tone; and, for men, the size, shape, and consistency of the prostate gland
- Measurements of sitting and standing blood pressure to detect orthostatic hypotension and dizziness
- Pelvic examination, including inspection of the vagina for atrophic changes, vaginitis, cystocele, rectocele, or uterine prolapse, any of which can contribute to UI

Tests of Provocation. Additional useful information can often be gathered by performing simple tests of provocation while the client has a full bladder. The physician or advanced practice nurse generally performs these during urodynamic testing. They can, however, also be performed if the client has a full bladder from drinking fluids. A number of useful tests are listed in this section. During each maneuver, the nurse should note any involuntary urine loss either by direct observation or by checking a previously applied dry absorbent pad. If the client leaks urine during any of the maneuvers, ask the client to try to stop the flow of urine. This allows the nurse to evaluate pelvic floor muscle strength:

1. Ask the client to cough 3 or 4 times while in a supine position.
2. Ask the client to stand; note any involuntary urine loss during the position change.
3. Ask the client to cough 3 or 4 times while standing.
4. If the client's physical condition permits, ask him or her to bounce on the heels 3 or 4 times.

5. Have the client listen to running water.
6. Ask the client to walk to the bathroom.
7. Have the client wash his or her hands.

The first four of these are stress provocations, whereas the fifth and seventh are urge provocations. Leaking when walking to the bathroom can be due to urge incontinence (i.e., the client experiences an urge to void) or stress incontinence (i.e., the physical activity of walking can result in leaking in some clients with severe stress incontinence).

Bladder Habits. One of the most effective ways to assess bladder habits is to ask the client or caregiver to keep a diary of the frequency of urination and any incontinent episodes, their relative volume, and the circumstances that precipitated their occurrence (e.g., coughing, sneezing, urgency, changing position). Fig. 28-2 shows a sample bladder diary. Bladder diaries can be used in the home, hospital, or nursing facility and can be kept by the client or caregiver. They provide a more objective and accurate measure of a client's bladder habits than can be obtained by recall alone. They can be especially useful for a client who has short-term memory problems. If they are to be accurate, however, clients and caregivers need careful instructions on their maintenance.

Collecting bladder diaries during assessment helps establish the type of UI and aids in planning nursing interventions. During treatment, diaries allow the nurse to assess progress and evaluate the effectiveness of interventions (Burgio, 2004).

Diagnosis

The data collected during assessment and the nurse's knowledge of UI often permit diagnosis of the client's type of incontinence. Sometimes, however, a more complex evaluation is needed to determine the cause of and most appropriate treatment for UI. In any new case of incontinence the nurse should consider acute and potentially reversible causes. If acute incontinence is ruled out or treated and involuntary urine loss continues, a diagnosis of persistent or chronic incontinence must be considered.

The following nursing diagnoses are appropriate in clients with persistent incontinence: stress incontinence, urge incontinence, overflow incontinence, functional incontinence, and mixed incontinence.

Stress Incontinence.

History—Client reports leaking urine with activities that increase intraabdominal pressure (e.g., coughing, sneezing, laughing, lifting, position changes, walking, climbing steps, exercise).

Objective observations—Leaking urine with stress provocation; signs of pelvic floor relaxation (e.g., cystocele, rectocele, uterine prolapse) observed on pelvic examination

Bladder records—Documentation of urine loss during physical activities that increase intraabdominal pressure

Urge Incontinence.

History—Client reports a sudden urge to void, followed by involuntary urine loss; may also report that running water or cold weather precipitates involuntary urine loss.

Objective observations—Leaking urine with urge provocation

Bladder records—Documentation of urine loss associated with urgency; frequent urination and nocturia also frequently recorded

Overflow Incontinence.

History—Client histories vary, but they often show frequent involuntary urine loss of small amounts. Urine loss may be associated with physical exertion. Complaints may include decreased force of the urine stream, hesitancy, a feeling of incomplete bladder emptying, and frequent urination of small amounts of urine. Clients may also have risk factors for urinary retention, such as diabetes or the use of anticholinergic medications.

Objective observations—An elevated PVR (greater than 100 ml) is the hallmark of overflow incontinence. This should be part of the initial evaluation of clients with UI. On abdominal examination a distended bladder may be detected on percussion or palpation. In cases where overflow incontinence is related to prostatic hypertrophy, an enlarged prostate can be detected by rectal examination. In women a large cystocele observed during pelvic examination may suggest the cause of overflow incontinence.

Bladder records—Documentation of frequent small-volume urinary accidents

Functional Incontinence.

History—Client or caregiver reports large-volume urine loss in places other than the toilet, commode, bedpan, or urinal in the absence of symptoms of stress, urge, or overflow incontinence. The client may be unaware of the need to void or have significant mobility impairment.

Objective observations—In pure functional incontinence, there is no leaking with stress or urge provocation and normal PVR. Mental status examination may reveal cognitive impairment. Functional assessment may reveal impaired mobility and toileting skills.

Bladder records—Documentation of involuntary urine loss (often large accidents) without symptoms of urge or stress incontinence

Planning and Expected Outcomes

For all types of UI the nurse must determine the client's and caregiver's motivation and willingness to carry out the recommended self-care practices and interventions.

Stress Incontinence. The long-term goal is that the client will reduce or eliminate the number of stress accidents. Short-term goals include:

NAME: ______________________ DATE: ______________________

Instructions:

1. In the 1st column, mark the time every time you void.
2. In the 2nd or 3rd column, mark every time you accidently leaked urine.
3. In the 4th column, enter the event that caused the accident, or the circumstances of the accident.

URINATED IN TOILET	SMALL ACCIDENT	LARGE ACCIDENT	REASON FOR ACCIDENT

No. of Pads Used Today: __________ No. of Accidents: __________

Comments: ____

____

Fig. **28-2** Bladder diary. (Courtesy of Benedum Geriatric Continence Program, University of Pittsburgh, Pittsburgh, Pa.)

1. Client will master behavioral interventions (e.g., pelvic floor muscle exercises, stress strategies) designed to decrease the number of stress accidents.
2. Client will recognize factors that precipitate stress accidents and use interventions to prevent accidents.

Urge Incontinence. The long-term goal is that the client will reduce or eliminate urge accidents. Short-term goals include:

1. Client will master behavioral interventions (e.g., pelvic floor muscle exercises, urge strategies, bladder retraining) designed to decrease urge accidents.
2. Client will recognize factors that precipitate urge accidents and use interventions to prevent accidents.

Overflow Incontinence. The long-term goal is that the client reduces or eliminates incontinence caused by urinary retention and overflow. Short-term goals for the client vary depending on the underlying mechanism responsible for the incontinence, but they might include:

1. Client will seek urologic evaluation of incontinence.
2. If client has an acontractile bladder, client will master in-and-out self-catheterization.

Functional Incontinence. The long-term goal is that, with caregiver assistance, the client will reduce or eliminate urinary accidents. Short-term goals for the caregiver include:

1. Caregiver will master behavioral interventions designed to decrease urinary accidents.
2. Caregiver will remove environmental barriers to proper toileting.

Intervention

Nursing interventions for UI focus on behavioral therapies. The effectiveness of these interventions has been demonstrated in a number of research studies (Burgio et al, 1998; Burgio et al, 1988; McDowell et al, 1996; Wyman et al, 1998). In 1988 the National Institutes of Health (NIH) held a consensus conference to review the status of knowledge on UI. The conference stated: "As a general rule, the least invasive or least dangerous procedures should be tried first. For many forms of incontinence, behavioral techniques meet this criterion" (NIH Consensus Development Conference, 1990). Despite the effectiveness of these techniques, many nurses are not skilled in their implementation. The most appropriate behavioral intervention depends on the type of incontinence and a client's cognitive status (Du Moulin et al, 2005).

Cognitively Intact Clients. Two behavioral interventions useful in cognitively intact individuals are bladder retraining and pelvic floor muscle exercises. These interventions may be used alone or in combination, depending on the type of incontinence.

Bladder Retraining. The client is encouraged to adopt a gradually expanding voiding schedule. Retraining is useful for correcting the habit of frequent toileting and for diminishing urgency. A schedule is established for voiding times, and voiding because of urgency is discouraged. This procedure is most useful for clients with urge incontinence and frequent urination.

Pelvic Floor Muscle Exercises. Pelvic floor muscle exercises were first reported as a treatment for UI by Kegel (1948). These exercises consist of alternating contraction and relaxation of the levator ani muscles, which are the muscles of the pelvic floor. These muscles, including the pubococcygeal muscle surrounding the midportion of the urethra, contract as a unit. In older adults these muscles are often weak from disuse atrophy. Performed correctly, pelvic floor muscle exercises strengthen the muscles, increase urethral resistance, and allow the client to use the muscles voluntarily to prevent urinary accidents.

Clinicians often use verbal feedback during digital examination of the rectum or vagina to help clients identify their pelvic floor muscles. The nurse inserts two fingers into the vagina or one into the rectum and asks the client to contract the pelvic floor muscles. Approximately one third of clients are correctly able to identify and contract their pelvic floor muscles on digital examination and can use this exercise as a successful intervention for UI. The majority of older clients, however, need additional help in identifying and learning to use their pelvic floor muscles. These clients often benefit from pelvic floor muscle biofeedback. Biofeedback is not a treatment in itself, but if appropriately used, it can facilitate acquisition of the ability to contract and to use the pelvic floor muscles to prevent involuntary urine loss (Burgio and Goode, 1997). During biofeedback, the client is given immediate auditory and/or visual feedback of pelvic floor muscle contractions.

A variety of techniques, including vaginal probes, rectal probes, and surface electromyography, have been used to provide biofeedback. Simultaneous feedback of pelvic floor and abdominal activity can assist the client in learning to contract the pelvic floor muscles while keeping the abdominal muscles relaxed (Burgio and Goode, 1997). This therapy is more effective when used in conjunction with Kegel exercises.

After training with biofeedback or verbal feedback, the client must practice pelvic floor muscle exercises at home. The client should be instructed to practice contracting and relaxing the pelvic floor muscles at least 45 times a day, in three or four practice sessions. The client should exercise lying down, sitting, and standing. This facilitates the client's ability to identify and use the muscles in any position. The nurse should remind the client to relax the abdominal muscles when exercising as this is essential to successful performance of exercises. The nurse can ask clients to try occasionally to slow or stop their urine stream while voiding. This allows them to monitor their progress in using and strengthening the correct muscles (Box 28-2).

BOX 28-2 Pelvic Floor Muscle Exercise Instructions

1. Do 45 pelvic floor muscle exercises every day.
2. Do the exercises in three sets, 15 exercises at a time, 3 times a day.
   - Do 15 lying down in the morning.
   - Do 15 standing up in the afternoon.
   - Do 15 sitting in the evening.
3. For each exercise:
   - Squeeze for ______ seconds.
   - Relax for ______ seconds.
4. Remember to relax all the muscles in the abdomen and continue to breathe normally when doing these exercises.

Once clients master the exercises, they should be taught strategies to prevent involuntary urine loss (stress and urge strategies). Clients with stress accidents should be instructed to contract their pelvic floor muscles before and during activities that precipitate leaking such as coughing, sneezing, lifting, or changing position. Those with urge incontinence can be taught to contract their pelvic floor muscles to inhibit involuntary bladder contractions. A client should respond to an urge to void by relaxing and contracting the pelvic floor muscles 3 or 4 times quickly. When the urgency subsides, the client should walk to the toilet at a normal pace (Box 28-3).

Cognitively Impaired Clients. The techniques already described (bladder retraining, pelvic floor muscle exercises, and biofeedback) require active client involvement. Treating UI in individuals with cognitive impairment requires the use of other behavioral techniques that depend on the caregiver rather than the client. These include scheduled toileting, habit training, and prompted voiding. The success of these techniques in large part depends on the availability and motivation of the caregiver and the dedication of the nursing staff.

Scheduled Toileting. The client is assisted in voiding on a regular, preset schedule. Family or professional caregivers simply take the client to the toilet at the scheduled times, often every 2 hours.

Habit Training. Patterned urge response training (PURT) is an example of habit training. Initially a client's baseline voiding pattern is assessed. Once the client's normal voiding pattern is established, the client is assisted in voiding at the established times. In her research on PURT, Colling used continuous electronic monitoring of voiding frequency to establish the precise voiding pattern of each subject (Colling et al, 1992a).

Prompted Voiding. Prompted voiding is most successful with clients who can recognize the need to void. It depends on active caregiver and client involvement. The goal is to increase a client's awareness of the need to void and, it is hoped, increase the frequency of self-initiated toileting. Clients are approached on a regular schedule, asked if they are wet or dry, and then prompted to toilet (Box 28-4). A client should never be forced to toilet or reprimanded for failing to toilet appropriately. Self-initiated toileting should not be discouraged.

It is not clear whether the benefits of toileting cognitively impaired individuals regularly during the night outweigh the disruption it causes to their sleep (Ouslander, 1999). To relieve the stress that can occur due to sleep disruption for both caregiver and client, toileting protocols can be modified during the nighttime hours.

Other Nursing Interventions. Individuals with UI may decrease fluid intake as a way of trying to prevent accidents. This is not an effective primary method of managing incontinence. Adequate fluid intake is important, especially for older adults who already have a decrease in total body water and are at risk for dehydration. In addition, inadequate fluid intake contributes to constipation, another problem commonly seen in the older adult population. The clients and caregivers should be cautioned not to decrease fluid intake to less than 6 glasses a day.

Individuals with incontinence, particularly those with urge accidents, should be advised to eliminate or restrict their caffeine intake. This includes coffee, tea, caffeinated colas, and chocolate. Caffeine has been shown to increase the occurrence of abnormal detrusor contractions, which are the cause of urge incontinence.

Some older adults, even those who are continent, complain of frequent nocturia that disrupts their sleep. Getting up once at night is probably a normal effect of aging. For

BOX 28-3 Urge Strategies

When a client has an urge to void, the nurse should instruct the client to:

1. Stop and relax.
2. Squeeze the pelvic floor muscles 3 or 4 times quickly; the client should not hold.
3. Wait for the urge to pass, and then walk slowly to the bathroom during the calm period.

BOX 28-4 Prompted Voiding Instructions

1. Approach the client at the scheduled times and ask if he or she is feeling wet or dry.
2. Check to see if the client is wet or dry.
3. If the client correctly identified present continent status, give positive feedback.
4. Ask the client if it is preferable to use the toilet. If the response is yes, toilet the client; if it is no, encourage the client. *Never* force the client to toilet.
5. Give positive feedback for appropriate toileting. Do not give any negative feedback.

clients who get up more often and think that the quality of their sleep is disrupted, some measures may be helpful, such as restricting fluid intake in the evening. Although it is important for clients to have adequate fluid intake, individuals with frequent nocturia should drink the bulk of this fluid before dinner. These individuals should be advised to eliminate caffeine in the evening. Going to bed with swollen ankles and feet increases nocturia. Clients with such swelling should be advised to elevate their legs for several hours during the afternoon to limit the amount of edema present at bedtime (Box 28-5).

Frail older adults are at increased risk for constipation and fecal impaction, which can cause acute incontinence and exacerbate persistent incontinence. Nurses should assess bowel habits regularly and institute preventive measures such as increased fiber intake, adequate fluids, and increased activity levels.

UI increases the risk of skin rashes, infections, and breakdown. Frequent changes of incontinence pads and scrupulous skin care provide the best protection against these complications. For short-term use in conjunction with other treatment measures, incontinence pads or garments provide convenience and comfort. However, they are expensive for long-term use and can be associated with skin rashes and breakdown if not changed often. They should not be used as a substitute for the evaluation and treatment of incontinence.

For men, external collection devices may be less expensive and less time consuming than incontinence pads or garments. They are, however, associated with a number of complications including UTI, skin breakdown, and ischemic disease resulting from penile constriction (AHCPR, 1996). Practical external collection devices are not available for women.

The use of external collection devices requires proper preparation of the penile surface before application. The penis should be thoroughly washed and dried. It may be necessary to trim excessive hair from around the penile shaft. An adhesive-enhancing skin preparation should be applied to the penile shaft and allowed to dry before condom application. Self-adhesive condom catheters, although more expensive than regular condom catheters, eliminate the need for adhesive tape. The penis should be gently squeezed with the condom in place until the condom adheres securely to the penis. If a regular condom catheter is used, two-sided tape should be applied around the shaft of the penis in a spiral fashion. The client or caregiver should slowly unroll the condom catheter over the tape and squeeze the penis gently until the condom adheres to the tape. For a more secure fit, a second strip of tape should be applied (again in a spiral fashion) on top of the condom. Stretchable adhesive tape should always be used; plain adhesive, silk, or paper tape should never be used. The use of nonstretchable tape can result in tissue ischemia. The condom catheter should be removed daily, and the penis should be inspected for irritation or skin breakdown (AHCPR, 1996). The skin should be washed and dried before reapplication. If there is any evidence of trauma or infection, the condom should not be reapplied.

Individuals with overflow incontinence should be referred to a urologist to correct treatable causes. If the cause of incomplete bladder emptying is not correctable, measures such as Credé's method may help empty the bladder. Credé's method is performed by applying pressure over the suprapubic area to aid in the elimination of residual urine during a voiding session. If this is ineffective in emptying the bladder, the treatment of choice is often intermittent in-and-out catheterization using sterile technique. Because of the high risk of associated bladder infections and urinary sepsis, indwelling catheters should be used to treat incontinence only in select circumstances (Ouslander, 2003) (Box 28-6).

Evaluation

Evaluation is an integral, ongoing component of the management of UI. Client goals are the focal point of evaluation. A client's perception of the effectiveness of and satisfaction with his or her treatment should be assessed and documented. A number of older adults with incontinence may require more than one treatment modality to achieve a satisfactory reduction in incontinence episodes. As a result, the care plan often evolves over time (see Nursing Care Plans).

AGE-RELATED RENAL CHANGES

The process of aging results in anatomic and functional changes in several body systems. These changes include the cardiovascular, respiratory, gastrointestinal, and neurologic

BOX 28-5 Management Suggestions for Nocturia

- Restrict fluids after dinner. It is important to drink enough fluids (usually six to eight glasses a day), but the bulk of fluids should be drunk during the day.
- Eliminate caffeine in the evening (e.g., caffeinated cola, tea, chocolate).
- Elevate the legs in the afternoon so the feet and ankles are not swollen when going to bed.

BOX 28-6 Indications for Use of Indwelling Catheters

- Urinary retention that cannot be corrected medically or surgically; cannot be managed practically by intermittent catheterization; *and* is causing persistent overflow incontinence, symptomatic UTIs, and/or renal dysfunction
- Pressure sores or skin lesions that are being contaminated by incontinent urine
- Provision of comfort for terminally ill or severely impaired clients

Nursing Care Plan
Mixed Incontinence

Clinical Situation: Ms. N is a 71-year-old retired retailer who was discharged from the hospital after treatment for a diabetic foot ulcer. The nurse sees her 2 times a week to change the dressing and assess wound healing. Ms. N's medical problems include having type 2 diabetes mellitus for 20 years, complicated by peripheral neuropathy. She also has coronary artery disease with two myocardial infarctions in the past, hypertension, hiatal hernia, diverticulitis, and osteoarthritis. She has had both hips replaced. She walks with a cane, and her gait is slow and sometimes unsteady. Her current medications include NPH insulin, ibuprofen, diltiazem extended release (Cardizem CD), triamterene and hydrochlorothiazide (Dyazide), nitroglycerine, and oxybutynin. Her over-the-counter medications include vitamins A, D, and E; Metamucil; and Tums. She needs assistance with personal grooming and bathing.

She has had problems with constipation but finds that daily Metamucil keeps her regular. Ms. N has been incontinent for 5 years. She describes both stress and urge accidents and states that she has about 14 accidents per week. She denies nocturia. She drinks three or four cups of regular coffee or tea a day and drinks a considerable amount of iced tea in the summer. She has seen a urologist who put her on oxybutynin, which she has been taking for 2 years. Although it somewhat decreased her accidents, she does not think it is very effective. She finds the incontinence disturbing and wishes there was something more she could do to treat it.

Nursing Diagnoses
Mixed urinary incontinence

Outcomes
Client will master pelvic floor muscle exercises.

Client will experience a decrease in the number of urinary accidents.

Interventions
Ask client to keep baseline bladder diaries before treatment.

Teach client pelvic floor muscle exercises using verbal feedback of pelvic floor muscle contractions during rectal examination.

Provide written instructions for practicing the exercises.

Ask client to continue to keep bladder diaries during treatment.

Review the diaries and assess client's progress during weekly visits.

Once client has mastered the exercises, teach urge and then stress strategies if indicated by the diaries.

If client is unable to identify her pelvic floor muscles using verbal feedback or is not making adequate progress, refer her to the continence nurse specialist for biofeedback.

Advise client to substitute decaffeinated coffee and tea for the regular coffee and tea she now drinks.

Nursing Care Plan
Functional Incontinence

Clinical Situation: Mrs. P is an 80-year-old retired school teacher who receives visits from a nursing agency for congestive heart failure. Mrs. P was diagnosed with dementia 4 years ago. She lives with her daughter, who is also her caregiver. In addition to dementia, Mrs. P has macular degeneration. She is blind in her left eye and has significantly impaired vision in her right. She fell and fractured her left hip 1 year ago. She walks with the assistance of a walker. She has a moderate amount of ankle and foot edema bilaterally. She also suffers from frequent constipation. Her current medications include hydrochlorothiazide, a calcium channel blocker, and a stool softener. Mrs. P is able to get in and out of bed by herself but requires assistance with all other ADLs. She has been incontinent of urine for 2 years. Mrs. P generally knows when she needs to void but leaks urine before she gets to the bathroom. Mrs. P wears incontinence undergarments. She also has enuresis and is usually wet in the morning.

Nursing Diagnoses
Functional incontinence

Outcomes
Client's caregiver will master a prompted voiding/toileting program with client.

Client will experience a decrease in the number of incontinent episodes.

Interventions
Collect baseline bladder diaries to establish the frequency of urinary accidents and what precipitates them.

Assess caregiver's willingness to participate in a behavioral program to treat client's incontinence.

Teach caregiver how to implement a prompted voiding program.

Assess client's understanding by having her conduct a return demonstration of the technique.

Visit weekly to assess implementation and success of the program.

Have caregiver keep bladder diaries during treatment.

Assess client's daily fluid intake.

If daily fluid intake is less than six to eight glasses of fluid per day, instruct caregiver to increase client's fluid intake.

Instruct caregiver to restrict client's fluids in the evening, providing the bulk of her fluids during the day.

Instruct caregiver to restrict client's caffeine intake, with no caffeine in the evening.

Instruct caregiver to have client elevate her legs in the afternoon to reduce the amount of edema.

systems. Understanding changes in the renal system requires understanding the effects of aging on the kidney. Kidneys of older adults are smaller than those of younger persons and have a decreased blood flow and glomerular filtration rate (GFR). Whether these changes can be attributed to the aging process alone or are associated with disease remains controversial. Despite the anatomic and functional changes associated with age, the kidneys remain capable of performing their functions well into the ninth decade of life unless acute illness or comorbidities result in renal dysfunction.

Anatomic changes that occur with age relate to the kidney's size and weight. Kidney length decreases by about 0.5 cm for each decade after the age of 50. Kidney weight also diminishes gradually. A normal adult kidney weighs 150 to 200 g by age 30. By age 90 the average weight of a kidney is 110 to 150 g. Reduction in mass occurs mostly in the renal cortex, whereas the medulla is typically spared. Glomeruli are also affected by the aging process; there is an increase in the number of sclerotic glomeruli, which are presumed to be nonfunctional.

Renal blood flow in an adult is approximately 600 ml/min. With aging, this blood flow decreases by 10% for every decade beyond the age of 40. With decreases in renal mass, functioning glomeruli, and blood flow, GFR will be affected. GFR remains stable until age 30 to 35, and then falls at a rate of 8 to 10 ml/min per 1.73 m^2 per decade.

The effect of aging on the renal system has strong implications for clinical management. Dosages of medications that are excreted by the kidneys should be adjusted. One should be aware that older adults lack adaptive mechanisms; therefore fluid and electrolyte alterations should be expected in the presence of acute illness. It is also important to recognize comorbidities that are likely to affect renal function in the older adult population, such as cardiovascular disease and diabetes.

COMMON PROBLEMS AND CONDITIONS

Acute Renal Failure

Acute renal failure (ARF) is the sudden loss of renal function. It is typically accompanied by retention of metabolic waste products, fluid and electrolyte alterations, and an acid-base disturbance. It may or may not be associated with oliguria. ARF can be classified as either prerenal, intrarenal, or postrenal depending on the causative factor (Box 28-7).

Prerenal failure occurs as a result of inadequate perfusion. There is no parenchymal damage; therefore, if hypoperfusion has not been prolonged, restoring perfusion should restore renal function. Intrarenal failure occurs as a result of intrinsic abnormalities within the kidney and may be due to nephrotoxic medications, prolonged ischemia, transfusion reactions, or crushing injuries. Acute tubular necrosis (ATN) is the most common cause of intrarenal failure. There are three stages of ATN:

1. The *oliguric stage* lasts from 7 to 21 days and is the period where urine output is less than 400 ml/day. Blood urea nitrogen (BUN) and creatinine rise continuously during this stage.
2. The *diuretic stage* lasts from 7 to 14 days. Clients can lose a large volume of fluid during this time while the BUN plateaus.
3. The *convalescent stage* can last for 12 months and begins from the time the BUN and creatinine are stable until the client is able to return to normal activity and urine output is normal.

Intrarenal failure involves parenchymal damage, so clients may occasionally require temporary dialysis treatments until the kidneys can resume control of fluid and electrolytes and maintain homeostasis. Postrenal failure is due to an obstructive or mechanical process in the urinary tract that will not permit the outflow of urine. Removal of the obstructive process should restore renal function.

BOX 28-7 Causes of Acute Renal Failure

PRERENAL

Hypovolemia
- Dehydration
- Hemorrhage
- Burns
- Gastrointestinal loss (e.g., vomiting, diarrhea)
- Shock

Cardiovascular failure
- Myocardial infarction
- Arrhythmias
- Cardiogenic shock
- Congestive heart failure

Renal artery stenosis or thrombosis

Altered peripheral vascular resistance
- Neurogenic shock
- Septic shock
- Anaphylactic shock

Antihypertensive medications

INTRARENAL

Acute glomerulonephritis
Acute tubular necrosis
Nephrotoxic medications
Radiocontrast dye
Renal ischemia
Vasopressors

POSTRENAL

Mechanical
- Renal calculi
- Strictures
- Prostatic disease
- Tumors

Functional
- Neurogenic bladder

Adapted from Copstead L: *Perspectives on pathophysiology*, Philadelphia, 1995, WB Saunders.

For older adult clients who experience ARF, evaluation should begin with an attempt to determine the causative factor. Once that factor is removed, renal function typically resumes. Clinical manifestations of ARF may include electrolyte disturbances, metabolic acidosis, and uremic symptoms (e.g., anorexia, nausea, anemia, fatigue, resistance to infection, edema, and crackles). The client may also have a history of exposure to nephrotoxic substances, recent blood transfusion, or recent UTI. Mortality can be as high as 60%.

The diagnosis of ARF is made based on the development of decreased urinary output (usually less than 400 ml/day), an elevation in BUN, an elevation in serum creatinine, and a decrease in creatinine clearance. In older adults, interventions consist of modifying diet, ensuring adequate hydration, and maximizing cardiac output, thereby increasing renal blood flow. The death rate for ARF in older debilitated adults is higher than in younger clients.

Chronic Renal Failure

Chronic renal failure (CRF) is a progressive, irreversible loss of renal function that develops over time (Box 28-8). The symptoms manifested depend on the extent of the disease. There are three types of CRF:

1. Decreased renal reserve, in which only 40% to 75% of the nephrons are functional. This type of CRF can be managed successfully with diet modifications; the client is generally asymptomatic.
2. Renal insufficiency, in which only 20% to 40% of the nephrons are functional. Clients experience mild azotemia and have a mildly elevated BUN and creatinine. This type of CRF can be managed successfully with diet and medications.
3. End-stage renal disease (ESRD), in which only 15% of the nephrons are functional. These clients have an elevated BUN and creatinine and require dialysis treatments for life or until a successful renal transplant can be performed. ESRD is accompanied by azotemia, fluid and electrolyte imbalances, and acid-base disturbances. Alterations in the neuromuscular, cardiovascular, and gastrointestinal systems are not uncommon. Older clients who have renal insufficiency are at risk for development of ESRD when an acute illness occurs, especially if comorbidities exist (see Client/Family Teaching box).

BOX 28-8 Causes of Chronic Renal Failure

Congenital disorders
Cystic disorders
Tubular disorders
Infections
Systemic disorders
- Diabetes
- Hypertension
- Scleroderma
- Systemic lupus erythematosus
- Amyloidosis

Modified from Copstead L: *Perspectives on pathophysiology,* Philadelphia, 1995, WB Saunders.

Client/Family Teaching

CHRONIC RENAL FAILURE

Your kidneys perform crucial functions that affect all parts of your body. Your kidneys, in fact, keep the rest of your body in balance and working properly. When chronic renal (kidney) disease causes the kidneys to fail, your whole body stops functioning correctly and you can become extremely ill unless the condition is treated.

How Do the Kidneys Function?

The kidneys are located at the bottom of the rib cage, one on each side of the spine. Each is about the size of a fist and contains about 1 million functioning units, called nephrons. The nephrons' job is to cleanse the blood of toxic wastes and excess fluid and to add needed chemicals such as hormones and vitamins. The cleansed blood is then returned to the bloodstream. About 200 qt of fluid are filtered through the kidneys every 24 hours. Of this fluid, 2 qt are eliminated as urine and the rest is retained in the body.

The kidneys are responsible for regulating the body's salt, potassium, and acid content. They also control the production of red blood cells and regulate blood pressure.

What Causes Chronic Renal Disease?

There are several different types and causes of chronic renal disease. *Glomerulonephritis,* which can arise from a number of immune disorders, is an inflammation of the kidney and can damage the nephrons. *High blood pressure,* whether a result of a kidney disorder or a cause of kidney disease, can hasten kidney failure. *Diabetes mellitus* may cause kidney disease. *Polycystic kidney disease* is an inherited disorder in which cysts form on kidney tissue and eventually destroy the healthy kidney tissue. *Congenital anomalies* can cause obstructions, which can lead to infection and destruction of kidney tissue. *Interstitial nephritis,* usually caused by drug use, is an inflammation of kidney tissue and leads to eventual destruction of the kidney. *Nephrotic syndrome* can occur with a variety of kidney problems, including glomerulonephritis, diabetes, and infections.

What Are the Signs of Renal Failure?

Because kidney failure sometimes gives no warning signs, it can go undiagnosed until it is well advanced. However, there are six warning signs of kidney disease that you should be aware of:

Client/Family Teaching—cont'd

1. High blood pressure
2. Puffiness around the eyes and swelling in the hands and feet (edema)
3. Pain in the kidney area (the small of the back just below the ribs)
4. Difficulty urinating or burning during urination
5. More frequent urination and urinating during the night
6. Passage of bloody or cola-colored urine

How Is Renal Failure Treated?

When kidney failure is in its early stage, it may be slowed by special diets, medication, or both. However, as the disease progresses and the kidneys no longer perform their duties of removing bodily wastes, other treatments must be used. The blood must be cleansed by using an artificial kidney (hemodialysis) or by introducing a cleansing solution into the abdomen (peritoneal dialysis). A kidney transplant, in which a healthy, donated kidney replaces the failed kidneys, can restore normal kidney function.

Outlook

There is no cure for chronic renal disease. Following the program your health care provider prescribes for you is vitally important to help you live with kidney failure. Thousands of people who have the disease are living active, productive lives.

From Brundage DJ: *Renal disorders,* St. Louis, 1992, Mosby.

The diagnosis of CRF is usually made based on a decrease in creatinine clearance, an elevation of BUN level, and a decrease in red blood cells. The remainder of the evaluation is identical to that for a client with ARF. Treatment of renal failure in an older adult is initially conservative. Older adult clients with ESRD generally have concomitant illness, such as diabetes, cardiac disease, or cancer.

NURSING MANAGEMENT

Assessment

Assessment of an older adult with kidney disease should include a thorough health history and physical examination; special attention should be paid to the medication history. Box 28-9 summarizes the nursing history and physical assessment data to be obtained.

BOX 28-9 Nursing Assessment of Renal System

HISTORY

Personal or family history of renal disease
Recent surgeries or illnesses (predisposing to renal dysfunction)
Symptoms
- Urine (e.g., frequency, color, amount, appearance)
- Nausea and vomiting
- Anorexia
- Weight loss
- Confusion
- Fatigue
- Pruritus
- Edema

Medications (e.g., antibiotics, antineoplastics, and nonsteroidal antiinflammatory drugs)
Diet
Current support systems

PHYSICAL ASSESSMENT

Neurologic status: altered mental status and presence of asterixis
Cardiopulmonary status: rales and pericardial rub
Gastrointestinal status: nausea and vomiting, abdominal discomfort, and toleration of diet
Musculoskeletal status
Ophthalmoscopic examination and visual inspection

Diagnosis

Appropriate nursing diagnoses for a client with renal failure include:

- Fluid volume excess related to compromised urinary regulatory mechanisms
- Altered nutrition: less than body requirements related to anorexia
- Risk for infection related to a compromised immune system
- Knowledge deficit: disease process, treatment regimen, and follow-up care related to lack of exposure
- Ineffective coping related to uncertain outcome of illness
- Activity intolerance related to fatigue secondary to renal failure
- Self-care deficit related to weakness and fatigue
- Risk for impaired skin integrity related to pruritus and immobility

Planning and Expected Outcomes

The development of a care plan for an older adult with renal failure must include the client and family or significant others because of the potential for self-care deficits. Expected outcomes include:

1. Client will achieve a normal level of fluid volume use as evidenced by reestablishment of baseline "dry" weight.

2. Client will consume a well-balanced, appropriately restricted diet on a regular basis.
3. Client will remain free from infection as evidenced by an afebrile state during hospitalization.
4. Client will demonstrate knowledge of the disease process and therapeutic regimen as evidenced by adherence to prescribed self-care and other treatment measures.
5. Client will demonstrate the use of effective coping strategies as evidenced by verbalization of feelings and seeking of support.
6. Client will demonstrate the ability to carry out ADLs without undue stress or fatigue.
7. Client will maintain skin integrity as evidenced by no reddened areas or broken skin.

Intervention

Interventions for an older adult with renal failure should focus on maintaining fluid and electrolyte balance; monitoring nephrotic symptoms; educating about treatment regimens, diet management, and medication usage; and managing fatigue and low energy levels. Clients and significant others must be educated on the prescribed diet and fluid intake. The typically prescribed diet is a low-protein, low-sodium, and low-potassium diet. At times the diet is less than palatable, so with the normal age-related changes in the sense of taste and smell, adherence to a renal diet presents a challenge. The use of spices and seasonings to enhance taste may be helpful. For those individuals with renal failure who experience nausea resulting from uremic symptoms, it might be beneficial to administer a prescribed antiemetic before meals (Boxes 28-10 to 28-12 and Client/Family Teaching box).

With the varied treatment options available to the individual with renal failure, it is important to educate clients and significant others about prescribed modalities. The American Kidney Foundation can provide educational information and assist with transportation to dialysis centers in some areas.

Evaluation

Evaluation is an important component in the care of older adults with CRF. Subjective data include the client's reported symptoms and quality of life. Objective data include improved or stable renal function as evidenced by stable BUN and creatinine, hematocrit, and fluid and electrolytes.

Urinary Tract Infection

UTI and asymptomatic bacteriuria are common in the older adult population. The prevalence of bacteriuria increases dramatically in women and men over the age of 80. The incidence of bacteriuria is higher in women than men partly because of the close proximity of the urethra to the rectum meatus. The incidence is also higher for residents of extended care or nursing facilities compared with those living

BOX 28-10 Renal Diet

Managing the diet of a client with renal failure is a challenge. One must be able to provide a balance between sufficient calories and protein. Clients in renal failure typically have a high metabolic demand that requires a high caloric intake. Sufficient amounts of protein and calories must be provided to prevent catabolism while preserving renal function. A renal diet is typically restricted in fluid, sodium, potassium, and protein. How restricted the diet is depends on the degree of renal dysfunction. A dietitian should be involved to assist with diet modification. Following the diet prescribed by the physician will prevent further complications of renal dysfunction.

CALORIES

Calories are important for maintaining energy and preventing weight loss. Much of the caloric intake can come from carbohydrates and unsaturated fat. If there is a need to increase caloric intake, margarine and oils that are low in cholesterol may be considered. Jams, jellies, sugar, and honey may also be added to the diet.

POTASSIUM

Alterations in potassium can cause significant illness and even life-threatening arrhythmias of the heart. It is important to maintain a low-potassium diet because, in renal failure, the kidneys are unable to rid the body of potassium in normal quantities. Foods high in potassium include dried beans, nuts, fruits, vegetables, chocolate, mushrooms, potatoes, and prune juice.

SODIUM

An elevation in sodium will cause fluid retention. This can lead to congestive heart failure and edema. It is very important to control the intake of sodium. Teaching clients to get into the habit of reading labels on food packages is essential.

FLUID

Fluid intake consists of anything that becomes a liquid at room temperature. Too much fluid can lead to weight gain, congestive heart failure, edema, shortness of breath, and high blood pressure. The amount of fluid intake dependent on the degree of renal dysfunction.

VITAMINS AND MINERALS

Vitamin supplementation is often necessary in clients with renal failure. Typically supplements of folic acid, pyridoxine, and water-soluble vitamins are necessary.

Adapted from Copstead, L: *Perspectives on pathophysiology*, Philadelphia, 1995, WB Saunders.

BOX 28-11 What is Peritoneal Dialysis?

Peritoneal dialysis is a type of dialysis that is performed when the renal system fails and can no longer adequately control the removal of waste products. It is indicated when medications and changes in diet and fluid intake can no longer control renal dysfunction.

A membrane in the abdomen called the peritoneum lines the abdominal organs and the abdominal wall. This membrane is porous and has a rich supply of blood. Before peritoneal dialysis can begin, a catheter is inserted into the peritoneal cavity; this permits the fluid to run in. A prescribed dialysate solution is run into the peritoneum and permitted to dwell for a period of time. During the dwell period, waste products are removed from the blood through the peritoneal wall into the dialysate solution.

The physician chooses one of three types of peritoneal dialysis, based on the client's need.

Continuous ambulatory peritoneal dialysis (CAPD) was first described in 1976 but not widely used until 1978. CAPD is done continuously, 7 days a week. It involves the use of an indwelling catheter, connective tubing, and dialysate. If the client needs certain electrolytes, they can be added to the dialysate solution. During the dwell period, these substances move through the porous membrane and into the client's blood supply in an effort to restore normal electrolyte concentrations. Dialysate dwells in the peritoneal cavity for a 4- to 8-hour period while "dialysis" occurs. The tubing is clamped and the bag rolled up under the client's clothing. Normal daily activities can be accomplished during the dwell time. Once the dwell period ends, the dialysate is drained and the peritoneum filled with a new bag of dialysate. CAPD is used primarily for clients with ESRD. Clients and their families are educated on the process, and it is performed in the home.

Intermittent peritoneal dialysis (IPD) is not performed as often as it once was, but when indicated, it is done in an acute care setting 3 to 5 times a week. IPD involves an indwelling catheter, dialysate, and a machine. The treatment is carried out while the client is asleep, and it takes 8 to 12 hours to complete. During the day the client has no fluid in the abdomen and remains "dry."

Continuous cyclic peritoneal dialysis (CCPD) uses an indwelling catheter, dialysate, and a cycling machine. Before going to sleep, the individual must connect to the machine, which will cycle dialysate solution in and out of the peritoneum 3 to 5 times a night, allowing for a prescribed dwell period. In the morning the last cycle runs in and is permitted to dwell for the entire day. At the end of the day, the solution is drained, the client connects to the cycler, and the process is restarted. Occasionally, CCPD clients require a manual exchange of dialysate during the day to allow for better clearance of waste products. In this instance, CCPD becomes a combination of IPD and CAPD. CCPD may be accomplished in the home once the client and family have been educated on the procedure; it is performed continuously 7 days a week.

COMPLICATIONS

Complications associated with peritoneal dialysis include peritonitis, an infection of the peritoneal wall. Infections involving the catheter tunnel and the exit site of the catheter can also occur. It is important for the client to recognize and immediately report signs of infection (e.g., abdominal pain, fever, dialysate solution that is cloudy once drained from the abdomen).

OUTLOOK

Peritoneal dialysis is an alternative for a failed renal system, but it does not cure the disease. Clients with chronic renal failure need to undergo some form of dialysis for the remainder of their lives as a bridge to successful transplantation. Many clients lead nearly normal lives despite peritoneal dialysis and modifications in diet and fluid intake.

Data from Hazzard W et al: *Principles of geriatric medicine and gerontology,* ed 5, Philadelphia, 2003, McGraw-Hill

at home. Higher rates of bacteriuria in nursing facilities are likely caused by the increased incidence of soiling, incomplete bladder emptying, and bladder catheterization. Risk factors for development of UTI in nursing facility residents include cardiovascular accident, cognitive impairment, decreased functional status, bladder catheterization, and antibiotic use (Hazzard et al, 2003). *Escherichia coli* continue to be the most common infectious organism. Other common organisms are *Proteus, Klebsiella, Enterobacter, Serratia,* and *Pseudomonas* organisms.

Clinical presentation of UTI in older adults will likely include dysuria, urgency, frequency, and hematuria secondary to damaged superficial blood vessels in the mucosa of the bladder. These symptoms are typical for lower UTIs. If the infection is in the upper urinary tract, older clients may manifest fever, chills, and flank tenderness in addition to mental status changes. If an older client is experiencing bacteremia as well, signs and symptoms of septic shock may be seen. However, the nurse is cautioned to remember the often atypical presentation of acute illness in older adults (see Chapter 4).

NURSING MANAGEMENT

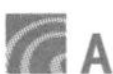 Assessment

A subjective assessment of urinary elimination patterns should be completed. This assessment should include normal voiding patterns and alterations in those patterns. The characteristics of the urine should also be noted. In addition, a mental status examination may be indicated; an older adult with infection may be delirious.

BOX 28-12 What Is Hemodialysis?

Hemodialysis is a type of dialysis that is performed when the renal system can no longer clear wastes effectively. It is indicated when medications and alterations in diet and fluid intake are no longer effective in the management of renal disease. Hemodialysis involves the use of an artificial kidney and a dialysis machine. Each hemodialysis treatment lasts 3 to 4 hours and typically is performed 3 times a week. Hemodialysis differs from peritoneal dialysis in that the clearance of waste products occurs outside the body and the treatments cannot be done at home but rather at an outpatient dialysis center.

For hemodialysis to occur, one must have access to the bloodstream. This access could be a large intravenous tube placed in a vein of the neck or chest. If the client has chronic renal failure, a permanent access, termed a *fistula* or a *graft*, is surgically placed. During the hemodialysis treatment the client's blood and a prescribed dialysate solution circulate continuously through the artificial kidney. Clearance of waste products and stabilization of electrolytes occur at this time. When the treatment is complete, the nurse returns the dialysized blood to the client and removes the needle access to the fistula or graft. The first few hemodialysis treatments are slow and short to avoid any complications.

COMPLICATIONS

Complications that may occur during or after hemodialysis treatment consist of low blood pressure, rapid heart rate, and dry mouth, which could indicate that too much fluid has been removed. The client could also experience high blood pressure, fast heart rate, and shortness of breath, which could indicate that not enough fluid has been removed from the body. If these symptoms occur during a treatment, the client should be instructed to notify the nurse immediately. If they occur after a treatment and the client is at home, it is important to immediately notify the physician.

Client/Family Teaching

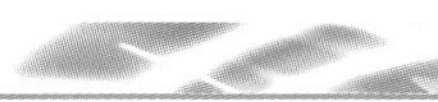

MANAGEMENT OF RENAL FAILURE

Client education should include the following factors:

- Cause of the renal failure
- Prescribed diet and fluid regimen
- Self-observation skills (e.g., measuring temperature, pulse, respiration, blood pressure, intake and output, daily weight)
- Personal hygiene
- Exercise and rest programs
- Medication regimen (e.g., name, purpose, dosage, dosing schedule, adverse reactions)
- Schedule of medical follow-up

Modified from Brundage DJ: *Renal disorders*, St Louis, 1992, Mosby.

Diagnosis

Nursing diagnoses for an older adult client experiencing a UTI include:

- Pain related to altered urinary elimination
- Altered urinary elimination related to the infectious process

Planning and Expected Outcomes

Expected outcomes for an older client with a UTI include:

1. Client will be free from pain as evidenced by reports of no further dysuria or burning with urination.
2. Client will resume normal voiding pattern, free from frequency, urgency, and dysuria.

Intervention

Nursing management should focus on education of older adults, including appropriate perihygiene measures such as front-to-back wiping techniques, adequate daily fluid intake, adherence to prescribed medication regimen, and reportable signs and symptoms of a recurrent infection. Sterile technique should be used with urinary catheterization.

Evaluation

Evaluation includes documentation of achievement of the expected outcomes and prevention of symptomatic UTI. Other key areas to document include the urine characteristics, intake and output, and any education provided.

Bladder Cancer

Bladder cancer is the most common form of cancer originating in the urinary system and is most often found in persons 50 to 70 years of age. Approximately 90% of all bladder cancers originate in the epithelial lining of the urinary tract. The other 10% are typically adenocarcinoma, squamous cell carcinoma, or sarcoma. Most bladder tumors are easily resected but may metastasize to the bladder wall, pelvis, liver, lungs, or bone. The causes of bladder cancer have not been clearly identified, but it is believed that 20% to 30% of them may be occupation related. Individuals with a history of industrial exposure to dyes, rubber, chemicals used in processing leather, and paint are at high risk for developing bladder cancer. Sewage workers and laboratory technicians are at risk for bladder cancer as well. Cigarette smoking also predisposes one to bladder cancer. Bladder cancer occurs more often in men than women.

Signs and symptoms of bladder cancer include painless hematuria, dysuria, urgency, burning with urination, frequency, and nocturia. If the tumor is large, late signs include suprapubic pain. A large tumor may also cause urinary obstruction, which in turn could cause low back and pelvic pain and predispose a client to postrenal failure.

NURSING MANAGEMENT

Assessment

Nursing assessment should include a thorough history with attention to changes in urinary elimination patterns. Subjective assessment should focus on the presence of pain, hematuria, dysuria, urgency, frequency, and voiding of small volumes. Objective assessment findings include gross or microscopic hematuria.

Diagnosis

Nursing diagnoses appropriate for an older client with bladder cancer include:

- Anxiety related to uncertain prognosis
- Altered urinary elimination related to surgical diversion
- Risk for body image disturbance related to surgical diversion
- Ineffective coping related to uncertain outcome of treatment
- Risk for sexual dysfunction related to anatomic alterations

Planning and Expected Outcomes

Developing a care plan for a client with bladder cancer involves the client, family, and significant others. Expected outcomes include:

1. Client will experience reduced anxiety as evidenced by a decrease in symptoms.
2. Client will develop a routine for managing urinary diversion.
3. Client will verbalize acceptance of urinary diversion and associated changes.
4. Client will demonstrate the use of effective coping strategies as evidenced by verbalization of feelings and seeking of support.
5. Client will verbalize sexual concerns.
6. Client will express satisfaction with alternative positions for intercourse.

Intervention

Nursing interventions for clients with bladder cancer focus on client education, psychosocial support, management of pain, and maintenance of adequate fluid and nutritional intake. The majority of clients with bladder cancer undergo a cystectomy and require education regarding the management of urinary diversion devices. To compound the fears and concerns a client has regarding a diagnosis of cancer, there is also a social stigma associated with the excretion of body fluids from an external device. Since clients may have difficulty coping, it is important to encourage them to verbalize fears and concerns and to refer them to the appropriate supportive services if necessary.

If a client requires chemotherapy, nursing interventions include monitoring for UTI, irritative voiding symptoms, allergic reactions, and bone marrow suppression. Client education should include instructions for follow-up care and the importance of cystoscopy every 3 months for 1 year, then every 6 months to 1 year thereafter. The client should be counseled to stop smoking as well.

Evaluation

Evaluation of nursing interventions is based on resolution of hematuria and a return of patterns of urinary elimination to premorbid conditions or the establishment of a new pattern of regular, complete bladder evacuation. Documentation of achievement of the expected outcomes is key.

Benign Prostatic Hypertrophy

Benign prostatic hypertrophy (BPH) is an age-related enlargement of the prostate gland that constricts the urethra and obstructs the outflow of urine. Approximately 90% of men may be diagnosed with BPH by the age of 80. The exact cause of BPH is unknown, but it is associated with aging and age-associated changes in hormones (Hazzard et al, 2003).

In early prostatic enlargement the client may be asymptomatic because the muscles may initially compensate for increased urethral resistance. As the prostate gland enlarges, the client begins to manifest symptoms of an obstructive process. The symptoms may include hesitancy, decrease in the force of urinary stream, terminal dribbling, sensation of full bladder after voiding, and urinary retention. Urethral obstruction may cause urinary stasis, UTI, hydronephrosis, and renal calculi.

The purpose of the diagnostic evaluation of BPH is to evaluate the extent of the obstruction and rule out a metastatic process. Diagnostic evaluation includes a history and physical examination, digital rectal examination (DRE), and measurement of BUN and serum creatinine. The most valuable tool for assessing urinary obstruction is the measurement of urinary flow rate. An abdominal ultrasound and cystourethroscopy are also used to screen for prostate obstruction.

NURSING MANAGEMENT

Assessment

The purpose of the nursing assessment for an individual with BPH is to determine the extent of prostate enlargement and its effect on function so that appropriate nursing interventions can be planned and implemented. The assessment consists of a history, physical examination, and evaluation of voiding patterns (Box 28-13).

Diagnosis

Nursing diagnoses appropriate for the client experiencing BPH include:

- Altered urinary elimination related to bladder outlet obstruction
- Urinary retention related to blockage secondary to BPH
- Risk for infection related to stasis
- Potential for sexual dysfunction related to erectile dysfunction

Planning and Expected Outcomes

Expected outcomes for a client with BPH include:

1. Client will maintain a regular schedule of complete bladder emptying.
2. Client will effectively use Credé's method to facilitate bladder emptying.
3. Client will remain free from UTI as evidenced by use of measures to prevent infection.
4. Client will verbalize sexual concerns and describe measures to cope.

If surgery is indicated, expected outcomes might include:

1. Client will have minimum postoperative pain as evidenced by statements indicating such.
2. Client will regain urinary control as in the premorbid state.

BOX 28-13 Nursing Assessment for Benign Prostatic Hypertrophy

HISTORY

General health
Functional status
Medical and surgical history
Current medications
Voiding habits and patterns

- The initiation and caliber of the urinary stream
- The presence of obstructive symptoms
  - Diurnal frequency
  - Nocturia
  - Hesitancy
  - Urgency
  - Urge incontinence
  - Incomplete bladder emptying
  - Postvoid dribbling
  - Signs and symptoms of urinary tract infection
- Dysuria
- Frequency

PHYSICAL EXAMINATION

The physical examination is usually conducted by the physician or an advanced practice nurse and includes:
DRE of the prostate gland to evaluate the size, shape, and consistency of the prostate
Abdominal examination to determine the presence of bladder distention, suprapubic tenderness, and costovertebral angle tenderness

Intervention

Nursing interventions for BPH focus on client education regarding the diagnosis and management of the disease. Education regarding the management of alterations in urinary elimination should include establishment of a frequent voiding schedule and, if prescribed, self-catheterization techniques. The educational plan should also include teaching clients about the sympathomimetic actions of decongestant medications and diet pills.

Nursing interventions must also take into account the treatment regimen. For clients treated with nonsurgical methods, interventions should focus on education about signs and symptoms of progressive BPH. These include urgency, frequency, inadequate bladder emptying, reduced urinary stream, the prescribed medication regimen, and potential adverse reactions. For clients undergoing surgery, nursing interventions should initially focus on immediate postoperative care. Most surgical procedures require general anesthesia and a few days of hospitalization. Interventions should focus on maintaining clients' levels of function and preventing iatrogenic effects associated with hospitalization, such as immobility, sensory deprivation, and social isolation. After hospitalization clients require education related to prescribed temporary activity restrictions, signs and symptoms of urinary obstruction, and possible temporary incontinence. Surgical interventions may result in a temporary sexual dysfunction; clients should be given the opportunity to verbalize concerns and to be referred to appropriate supportive services, such as a urologist or a certified sex therapist (see Client/Family Teaching box).

Client/Family Teaching

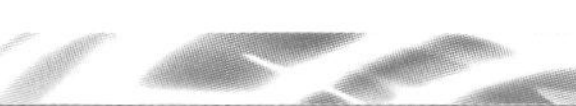

BENIGN PROSTATIC HYPERTROPHY

BPH can alter the flow of urine. Any of the following symptoms could indicate BPH and should be reported to the physician immediately:

- Hesitancy or difficulty beginning to urinate
- Frequent need to urinate during the day as well as at night
- Leakage of urine
- Sensation of a full bladder after having just gone to the bathroom
- Weaker-than-normal flow of urine

Evaluation

Evaluation of interventions is based on the return of urinary function to the premorbid state, relief of urinary symptoms, avoidance or prompt management of UTIs, and return to satisfactory sexual activity. Documenting care of a client with BPH includes noting the effectiveness of the nursing interventions, including validation of the client's understanding of the disease process and treatment regimen. The nurse also records the client's urinary elimination patterns.

Prostate Cancer

Prostate cancer is rarely seen before the age of 50, and is considered a disease of aging. It is the second leading cause of cancer-related death among men in the United States (Holden and Emery, 2004). Death from prostate cancer is more common in black men than in white men. Black men have a 60% higher incidence rate and a twofold higher mortality rate (Holden and Emery, 2004). The cause of prostate cancer is unknown, but there is an increased risk for those who have a family history of the disease. Prostate cancer can spread through the lymphatic system or the bloodstream.

Most prostatic cancers are adenocarcinomas, but they may be transitional cell carcinomas, squamous cell carcinomas, or sarcomas. The pelvic lymph nodes and the skeleton are the most frequent sites for metastasis. The body organs most frequently involved in metastasis include the liver, lungs, and adrenal glands.

Early prostate cancer is typically asymptomatic. As the disease spreads to the urethra, it may cause symptoms of urinary obstruction. If obstruction of the urethra occurs, the client may manifest symptoms of postrenal failure. Other symptoms may include perineal and rectal discomfort, weakness, nausea, hematuria, and lower extremity edema (with metastasis to pelvic nodes). Skeletal pain and pathologic fractures may indicate advanced disease with metastases.

It is extremely important for men to follow the recommendations of the American Cancer Society regarding screening for prostate cancer so that early detection can occur and treatment, if indicated, can begin early in the course of the disease.

NURSING MANAGEMENT

Assessment

Assessment of a client with prostate cancer is essentially the same as that for a client with BPH. The nurse should assess the client's health beliefs and fears related to a malignant process.

Diagnosis

Appropriate nursing diagnoses for a client with prostate cancer include:

- Altered urinary elimination related to bladder outlet obstruction
- Anxiety related to uncertain prognosis
- Sexual dysfunction related to treatment measures
- Knowledge deficit: treatment modalities and prognosis related to lack of previous exposure

Planning and Expected Outcomes

Expected outcomes for a client with prostate cancer include:

1. Client's urinary elimination patterns will return to premorbid parameters.
2. Client's expressions of anxiety about diagnosis, treatment, and prognosis will be replaced with understanding of the prognosis.
3. Client and partner will have a mutually satisfying sexual relationship.
4. Client will demonstrate knowledge of treatment methods and prognostic indicators.

Intervention

Nursing interventions for a client with prostate cancer include educating the client on diagnostic tests and treatment options. If surgery is indicated, nursing interventions should include:

1. Administration of analgesics for pain control
2. Suggestion of options for sexual counseling if the client indicates a need
3. Education of the client on the importance of a follow-up check of prostate-specific antigen (PSA) levels and evaluation for disease progression

If hormonal therapy is indicated, the nurse should educate the client on the administration of intramuscular or subcutaneous injections. If bone metastasis has occurred, the nurse should encourage safety measures around the home to decrease the incidence of pathologic fractures. The client should be educated on when to report symptoms of worsening urethral obstruction, such as increased frequency, urgency, hesitancy, and urinary retention (see Nursing Care Plan).

Evaluation

Evaluation of interventions is based on a client's relief of symptoms from the obstruction and his return to the premorbid urinary elimination pattern. The client will verbalize an understanding of the disease process, the staging of the tumor, and the recommended treatment. The client and his partner will regain satisfactory sexual relations (see Health Promotion Box).

SUMMARY

The changes that occur in renal function with aging can be challenging for the caregiver and the nurse. Altered urinary elimination can cause problems that have a significant effect

Nursing Care Plan
Prostate Cancer

Clinical Situation: Mr. B is a 71-year-old retired accountant. He has no major health problems at this time. At an annual physical examination he was found to have prostatic enlargement; serum PSA showed a level of 35 ng/ml. He then underwent magnetic resonance imaging and was found to have a grossly enlarged prostate. A needle-guided biopsy was performed, which showed adenocarcinoma of the prostate gland. Because of the large size of the prostate mass, a metastatic evaluation consisting of a bone scan and chest x-ray examination was performed. The metastatic evaluation failed to show any metastatic disease.

Mr. B promptly scheduled a consultation with a urologist at a major medical center for the treatment of the prostate tumor. On evaluation, he was found to have stage C prostate cancer. The decision was made to treat the prostate tumor with a radical prostatectomy.

Mr. B and his children are experiencing anxiety, fear, and anticipatory grief related to the diagnosis. Mr. B lost his wife 5 years ago to ovarian cancer and has many bad memories of the effects of cancer.

Nursing Diagnoses
Anxiety related to diagnosis of cancer

Knowledge deficit: current treatment modalities and prognosis related to lack of previous exposure

Outcomes
Expressions of anxiety about diagnosis and prognosis will be replaced by a realistic understanding of the disease and the likely prognosis as evidenced by satisfactory engagement in activities.

Client and family will verbalize understanding of treatment regimen.

Client and family will seek supportive services.

Interventions
Reassure the client and family that prostate cancers are typically slow growing and treatable.

Reiterate explanation of diagnosis and treatment.

Include family in teaching whenever possible.

Refer client and family to cancer support group services.

Emphasize the importance of continuing present activities.

Assist client in gaining awareness of anxiety.

Teach client relaxation techniques.

Provide written information regarding prostate disease and treatment regimens.

Encourage client and family members to attend educational and supportive services provided by the American Cancer Society.

Health Promotion/Illness Prevention

Urinary Function

HEALTH PROMOTION
- Adherence to prescribed bladder training program, exercises, and techniques for urinary incontinence
- Adherence to a regularly scheduled program of monitoring conditions as appropriate (e.g., PSA, blood pressure, urinalysis, laboratory tests)
- Prompt treatment of urinary tract symptoms

DISEASE PREVENTION
- Participation in a prostate cancer screening program, based on risk established by the health care provider
- Drinking at least eight glasses of water daily, unless contraindicated by other chronic conditions
- Establishment of a routine pattern of urinary elimination
- Use of appropriate hygiene measures to avoid urinary tract contamination

on day-to-day activities and may be embarrassing and disabling. The nurse's role includes assessing, advocating treatment, providing emotional support, and making counseling available when indicated. Individualized care plans should be developed, focusing on promotion of self-care and functional ability (see Health Promotion box).

Key Points

- UI is one of the most common health problems of older adults.
- Although the aging process does affect lower urinary tract function, aging alone does not cause UI.
- Medications, including a number of over-the-counter drugs, can cause acute UI.
- Functional and environmental assessments are important components of the evaluation of UI.
- Bladder diaries provide a more objective measure of the severity and type of incontinence than recall alone and should be part of the evaluation of UI.

Home Care

1. Regularly monitor and assess homebound older adults for signs and symptoms of exacerbation of the diagnosed renal or urinary disease or disorder.
2. Instruct caregivers and homebound older adults on reportable signs and symptoms related to the diagnosed renal or urinary system disorder and when to report these symptoms to the home care nurse or health care provider.
3. Instruct caregivers and homebound older adults on the name, dose, frequency, and side effects of medications prescribed to treat the diagnosed renal or urinary system disease or disorder.
4. Assess functional and environmental factors that contribute to UI in homebound older adults.
5. Instruct caregivers and homebound older adults to keep a voiding diary to help the home care nurse establish the type of UI and plan nursing interventions.
6. Instruct caregivers and homebound older adults on behavioral interventions (e.g., bladder retraining, pelvic floor exercises) to treat UI.
7. If a homebound older adult is cognitively impaired, the success of behavioral techniques (e.g., habit training, PURT, prompted voiding) used to treat UI will depend on the caregiver's availability and motivation.
8. Instruct caregivers and homebound older adults on measures to reduce urinary incontinence and maintain comfort.
9. Use indwelling catheters as a last resort to treat UI.

- Behavioral interventions are the initial treatment of choice for many clients with UI.
- Cognitively intact clients with urge or stress incontinence often respond well to properly taught pelvic floor muscle exercises.
- Once a client masters pelvic floor muscle exercises, the nurse can teach urge or stress strategies to prevent involuntary urine loss.
- Prompted voiding, habit training, and PURT can effectively reduce incontinence in clients with cognitive impairment, but the success of these methods depends on caregiver compliance.
- Aging affects renal function; however, impaired renal function is not a normal consequence of aging. Older adult clients must be assessed and attention directed to adequate hydration, adjusted medication dosages, and the existence of comorbidities that can lead to renal dysfunction.
- There are three types of ARF, and it is a reversible process. The nurse must focus on education regarding proper diet and medications used to treat renal failure to halt the progression of ARF.
- CRF is not reversible but can be managed with medications and diet modification unless it has progressed to ESRD; in this case, dialysis treatments are typically required as a bridge to successful transplantation.
- Alterations in urinary elimination are common in men with BPH. The nurse must be prepared to educate clients regarding medications and Kegel exercises after surgery.
- The importance of PSA screening in black men over the age of 40 and all other men over the age of 50 cannot be stressed enough. Disease progression with prostate cancer can be very quick or very slow, and early detection is extremely important so that optimum treatment can be offered.

Critical Thinking Exercises

1. Your 75-year-old female client complains that she has leakage of urine during the day. What additional information do you need to assess her urinary function?
2. A 78-year-old man is admitted to the emergency department with complaints of nausea, fatigue, and poor appetite. The physician orders a urinalysis, BUN, and creatinine. Why does the physician suspect a urinary problem?

References

Agency for Health Care Policy and Research: *Urinary incontinence in adults: acute and chronic and management,* AHCPR Pub No 96-0682, Washington, DC, 1996, US Department of Health Care Policy and Research.

Burgio KL: Current perspectives on management of urgency using bladder and behavioral training, *J Am Acad Nurse Pract* 16(10suppl):4-7, 2004.

Burgio KL, Goode PS: Behavioral interventions for incontinence in ambulatory geriatric patients, *Am J Med Sci* 314:257, 1997.

Burgio KL et al: Behavioral treatment for urinary incontineyce in elderly patients: initial attempts to modify prompted voiding and toileting procedures, *Behav Ther* 19:345-357, 1988.

Burgio KL et al: Toileting skills and habits in clients of an adult day care center, *J Gerontol Nurs* 17(12):32-35, 1991.

Burgio KL et al: Treatment seeking for urinary incontinence in older adults, *J Am Geriatr Soc* 42:208-212, 1994.

Burgio KL et al: Behavioral versus drug treatment for urge urinary incontinence in older women: a randomized controlled trial, *J Am Med Assn* 1995:2000, 1998.

Colling J et al: The effect of patterned urge-response toileting (PURT) on urinary incontinence among nursing home residents, *J Am Geriatr Soc* 40:135, 1992a.

Colling J et al: Patterned urge response toileting for urinary incontinence: a clinical trial. In Tornquist E et al, editors: *Key aspect of elder care: managing falls, incontinence, and cognitive impairment,* New York, 1992b, Springer.

Duke University Center for the Study of Aging and Human Development: *Multidimensional functional assessment: the OARS methodology,* Durham, NC, 1978, Duke University.

Du Moulin MF et al: The role of the nurse in community continence care: a systematic review, *Int J Nurs Studies* 42(4)479-492, 2005.

Folstein MF, Folstein SE, McHugh PR: "Mini-Mental State": a practical method for grading cognitive state of patients for the clinician, *J Psychiatr Res* 12:189 1975.

Gibbons L, Choe JM: Helping women quell urinary incontinence, *Clin Adv* 7(5):21, 2004.

Haab F, Zimmern PE, Leach GE: Female stress urinary incontinence due to intrinsic sphincteric deficiency: recognition and management, *J Urol* 156:3, 1996.

Hazzard W et al: *Principles of geriatric medicine and gerontology*, ed 5, Philadelphia, 2003, McGraw-Hill.

Holden J, Emery CB: Prostate cancer: primary care providers play critical role, *Adv Nurse Pract* 12(4):28, 2004.

Katz S et al: Studies of illness in the aged—the index of ADL: a standardized measure of biological and psychosocial function, *JAMA* 185:94ff, 1963.

Kegel AH: Progressive resistance exercise in the functional restoration of the perineal muscles, *Am J Obstet Gynecol* 52:242, 1948.

McDowell BJ et al: Characteristics of urinary incontinence in homebound older adults, *J Am Geriatr Soc* 44:963, 1996.

National Institutes of Health Consensus Development Conference: Urinary incontinence in adults, *J Am Geriatr Soc* 38:265, 1990.

Ouslander JG: Urinary incontinence. In Hazzard WR et al, editors: *Principles of geriatric medicine and gerontology*, ed 5, Philadelphia, 2003, McGraw-Hill.

Rose MA et al: Behavioral management of urinary incontinence in homebound older adults, *Home Health Care Nurse* 8(5):10, 1990.

Schnelle JF: Treatment of urinary incontinence in nursing home patients by prompted voiding, *J Am Geriatr Soc* 38:356, 1990.

Shaker HS, Hassouna M: Sacral nerve root neuromodulation: an effective treatment for refractory urge incontinence, *J Urol* 159:1516, 1998.

Wyman JF et al: Comparative efficacy of behavioral interventions in the management of female urinary incontinence, *Am J Obstet Gynecol* 179:999-1007, 1998.

29 Cognitive and Neurologic Function

KRISTAL IMPERIO, PhD, RN, CS, ANP, GNP, and
ELEANOR PUSEY-REID, MS, MEd, RN, CCRN

Learning Objectives

On completion of this chapter, the reader will be able to:

1. Compare and contrast structural changes in the brain and nerve function associated with aging.
2. Describe functional changes in the neurologic system during the aging process.
3. Compare normal, age-related changes of the neurologic system with those associated with cognitive disorders.
4. Differentiate the symptoms of depression, delirium, dementia, and other cognitive disorders.
5. Describe the symptoms and diagnostic tests and interventions of common neurologic disorders in older adults.
6. Use the nursing process in the development of a care plan for clients with common neurologic disorders.
7. Analyze evidence-based practice that enhances management of clients with neurologic disorders.

The number of Americans 65 years old and older is growing rapidly. It is estimated that by the year 2030, every fifth American will be over age 65. People over the age of 65 years represented 12.4% of the population in the year 2000 (Administration on Aging, 2003). In light of these statistics, it is imperative that nurses keep abreast of the most recent findings regarding the development, manifestations, and treatment of cognitive and neurologic problems among older adults. This knowledge will assist nurses in providing safe, effective, and evidence-based nursing interventions.

The brain is a complex web of tissue and structures that allows for a series of intricate functions that continues to astonish the most advanced neuroscientists. Understanding the brain and its function has long been an interest for health care providers. For nurses caring for older persons, the understanding of basic neurologic changes and common disorders is crucial.

STRUCTURAL AGE-RELATED CHANGES OF THE NEUROLOGIC SYSTEM

The nervous system is a network of complex structures that undergo many neurophysiologic changes as an individual ages. Some changes that occur in the brain do not affect all elderly individuals equally, and the individual presentation of neurologic changes varies from person to person. An individual's lifestyle, nutritional intake, genetic makeup, and tissue perfusion are some of the many factors that affect the neurologic system. To appreciate the significant changes that take place with aging, a brief review of the neurologic system is required.

The central nervous system (CNS) is divided into three major functional components: higher level brain or cerebral cortex, lower level brain (basal ganglia, thalamus, hypothalamus, brainstem, and cerebellum), and spinal cord. The brain is divided into three major areas, which include the cerebrum, brainstem, and cerebellum. The cerebrum consist of two hemispheres (right and left); each hemisphere is divided into lobes (frontal, temporal, parietal, and occipital) (Fig. 29-1). Specialized neurons located within the lobes include the hippocampus and the basal ganglia. These are the neurons that undergo structural and physiologic changes during the aging process. Another area of the CNS that undergoes significant changes in the normal aging process is the brainstem (midbrain, pons, and medulla oblongata). The reticular formation (RF) is a complex network of gray matter located primarily in the brainstem area of the CNS. The RF assists and controls many functions, including skeletal muscle movement and sleep-wake cycle, another aspect that is altered in aging (Black, Hawks, and Hogan, 2005).

Cellular and Structural Changes

Neuron. The neuron is the basic unit of the CNS and functions to transmit impulses. Some neurons are motor,

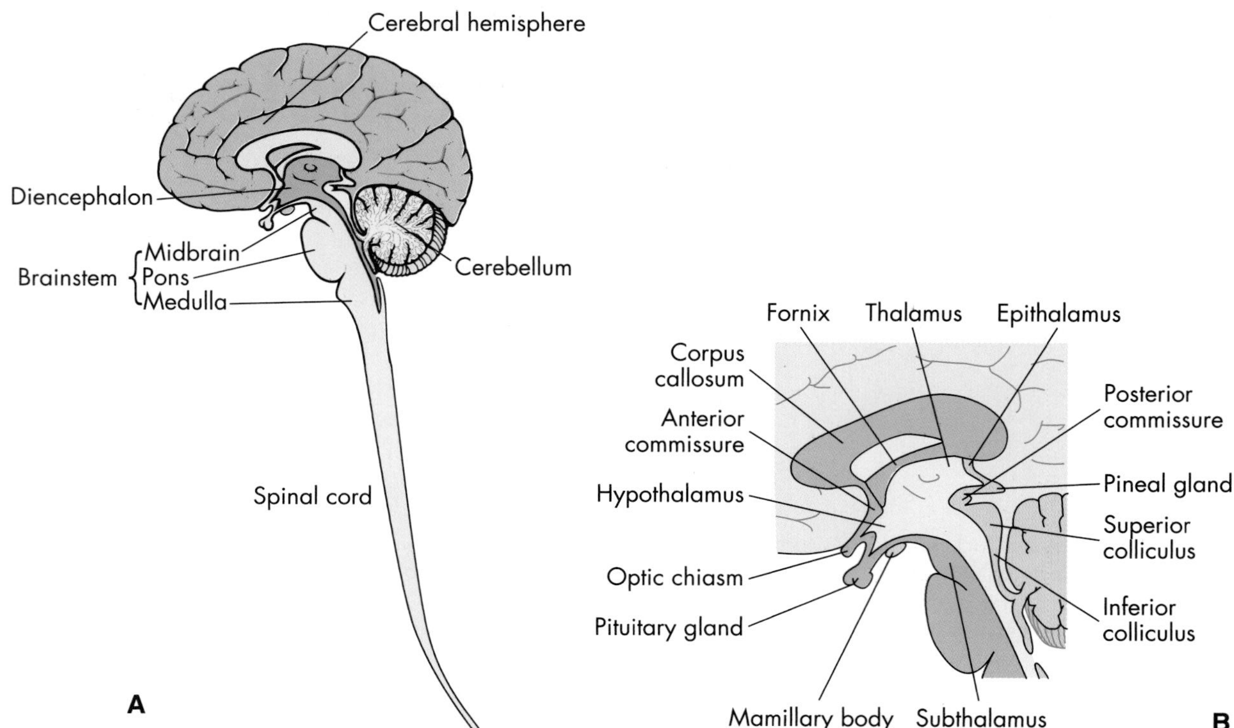

Fig. 29-1 **A**, Major divisions of the CNS. **B,** Diencephalon (thalamus and hypothalamus). (From Lewis SM, Heitkemper MM, Dirksen SR: *Medical surgical nursing: assessment and management of clinical problems*, ed 6, St Louis, 2004, Mosby.)

and some are sensory. Each neuron has a cell body (soma), dendrites, and a single axon (Fig. 29-2). Synapses are structural and functional junctions between two neurons. These are the points at which the nerve impulse is transmitted from one neuron to another or from neuron to efferent organ. The two types of synapses are electrical and chemical.

Neurotransmitters. Neurotransmitters are chemical substances that enhance or inhibit nerve impulses. These substances are necessary in the synaptic transmission of information from one neuron to another. In aging the function of these substances is altered due to the decrease of neurons. With aging there is also a decreased number of neurons

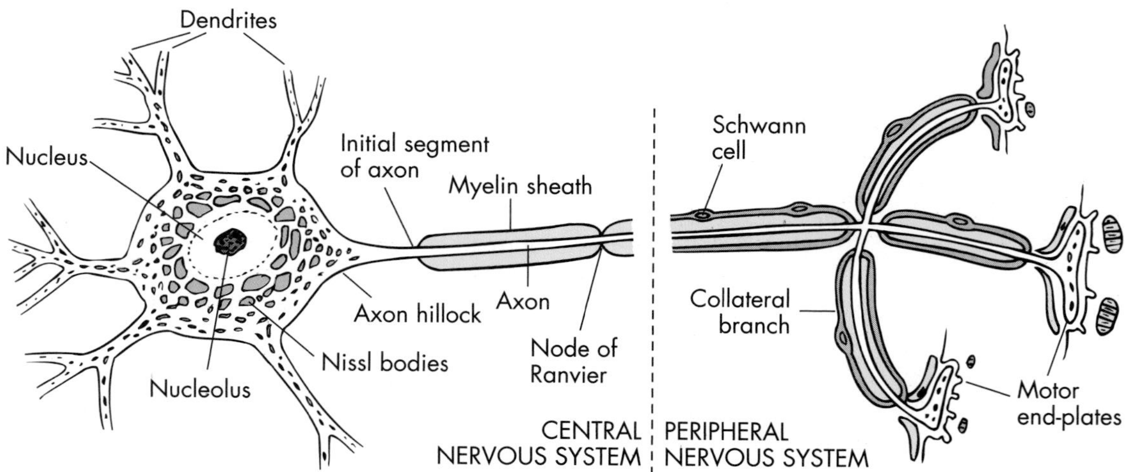

Fig. 29-2 Neuron with composite parts. (From Urden LD, Stacey KM, Lough ME: *Thelan's critical care nursing: diagnosis and management,* ed 3, St Louis, 2002, Mosby.)

in various areas of the brain and deposits of abnormal substances on neuronal cellular structure (dendrites) (McCance and Huether, 2002). The loss of neurons is not as extensive in the process of aging as previously believed. In actuality, large neurons appear to shrink and few are lost. The changes in neuron function are associated with accumulation of lipofuscin (dark fluorescent pigment) granules and neuritic plaques in the cell body of some neurons and some cellular debris in neuroglia cells (Albert, 2002) (Table 29-1).

Neuroglia and Schwann Cells. Neuroglia and Schwann cells are the supportive cells of the CNS, making up approximately half of the brain and spinal cord tissue. Their role is to protect the neurons. As individuals age, the number of these protective cells increases. Each of these cells serves a different function.

Neuroglia cells vary in size and shape and are divided into two main classes: the microglia and macroglia (Fig. 29-3). The microglias are phagocytic scavenger cells related to macrophages that respond to infection or trauma to the CNS. The macroglia cells include astrocytes, oligodendrocytes, and ependymal cells. Astrocytes (astroglia) are star-shaped cells that provide the physical support for the neurons. They also regulate the chemical environment and nourish the neurons. These cells respond to brain trauma by forming scar tissue.

Oligodendrocytes and Schwann cells produce myelin within the CNS and peripheral neurons, respectively. Ependymal cells form the lining of the ventricles, choroid plexuses, and central canal of the spinal cord. These cells help in the regulation of the cerebrospinal fluid (CSF) and blood-brain barrier.

Cerebrospinal Fluid and Ventricular System

CSF is a clear, colorless fluid. Approximately 135 ml of CSF circulates through the ventricles—a system of cavities within the brain—and within the subarachnoid space (80 ml in ventricles and 55 ml in subarachnoid space). The brain and spinal cord float in the CSF, which absorbs shocks; cushions the CNS; and prevents the brain from tugging on meninges, nerve roots, and blood vessels. The choroid plexus (CP) is a group of blood vessels (capillaries) covered with a thin layer of epidermal cell. The CP is responsible for producing approximately 500 ml of CSF per day (Figs. 29-4 and 29-5).

Several physiologic changes are known to occur in the CNS of aging individuals. These changes may include sensory motor changes such as difficulty retrieving explicit memories; altered vision, hearing, taste, and smell; vibratory sensations; and position sense. As a result of neurotransmitters and hypothalamic changes in the aging process, the reticular activating system (RAS) that controls arousal and conscious-

TABLE 29-1 Significant Changes in Aging Nervous System

NEUROLOGIC COMPONENTS	CHANGES
CENTRAL NERVOUS SYSTEM	
Neurons	Shrinkage in neuron size and gradual decrease in neuron numbers Structural changes in dendrites Deposit of lipofuscins granules, neuritic plaque, and neurofibrillary bodies within cytoplasm and neuron Loss of myelin and decreased conduction in some nerves, especially peripheral nerves
Neurotransmitters	Changes in precursors necessary for neurotransmitter synthesis Change in receptor sites Alteration in enzymes that synthesize and degrade neurotransmitters Significant decreases in neurotransmitters, including ACh, glutamate, serotonin, dopamine, and gamma-aminobutyric acid
PERIPHERAL NERVOUS SYSTEM	
Motor	Muscular atrophy—decrease in muscle bulk Decrease in electrical conduction system
Sensory	Decrease in electrical conduction Atrophy of taste buds Alteration in olfactory nerve fibers Alteration in nerve cells of vestibular system of inner ear, cerebellum, and proprioception
Reflexes	Altered electrical conduction of the nerve due to myelin loss Altered reflex responses (ankle, superficial reflexes)
Reticular formation	Physiologic changes in the RAS results in decrease in stages 3 and 4 of the sleep cycle
AUTONOMIC NERVOUS SYSTEM	
Basal ganglia	Slowing of autonomic nervous system response as a result of structural changes in basal ganglia

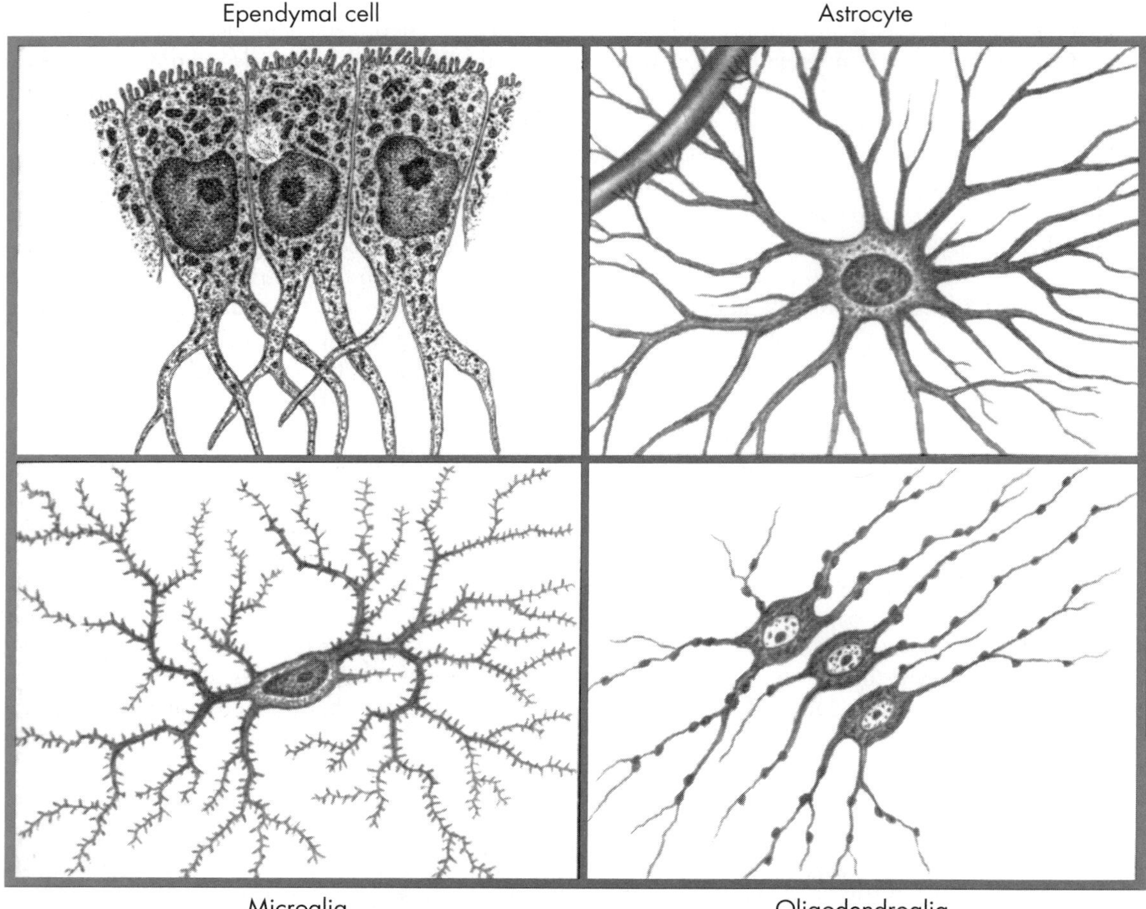

Fig. 29-3 Types of neuroglial cells. (From Thompson JM et al: *Mosby's clinical nursing*, ed 4, St Louis, 1997, Mosby.)

ness from the brainstem to the cerebral cortex is also altered. The neuroendocrine system plays a vital role in the function of the hippocampus. When there is an alteration in this system, gradual changes in memory may be seen.

Hippocampus and the Hypothalamic-Pituitary-Adrenal Axis. The hippocampus is a part of the temporal lobe that plays an important role in memory and learning. Normal aging is associated with changes in the ability to consciously learn and retain new information easily. This occurs as a result of structural changes, synapse loss in the neurons, decreased microvascular integrity, reduction in glucose metabolism, and alterations in the neuroglia cells with aging. As a result of changes in the secretory pattern of the hypothalamic-pituitary-adrenal (HPA) axis, additional alterations occur in the hippocampal area of the brain. The hippocampal area is strongly influenced by HPA hormones (Fig. 29-6). The specific aspects altered by the aging process are the explicit memory (e.g., delayed recall), the ability to learn new information quickly, memory storage, and memory retrieval (Albert, 2002; Miller and O'Callaghan, 2003).

Cerebrospinal Fluid. A reduction in the turnover of CSF with age decreases the distribution and efficiency by which the necessary substances are delivered from the CP to the brain target sites. These substances include the hormones necessary for metabolism and appetite, and the nutrients (e.g., transferrin, glucose, amino acids, and vitamins) necessary for nerve function. A reduction in the turnover of CSF can affect the removal of waste products, toxins (e.g., amyloid peptides, lactate), and drugs. The accumulation of these substances resulting from age-related changes may contribute to diseases causing cognitive decline. One significant factor that reduces the turnover secretion rate of CSF is the age-related increase in resistance from the vascular (sagittal venous sinus) system in the arachnoid (Preston, 2001). These changes occur in various degrees among aging individuals.

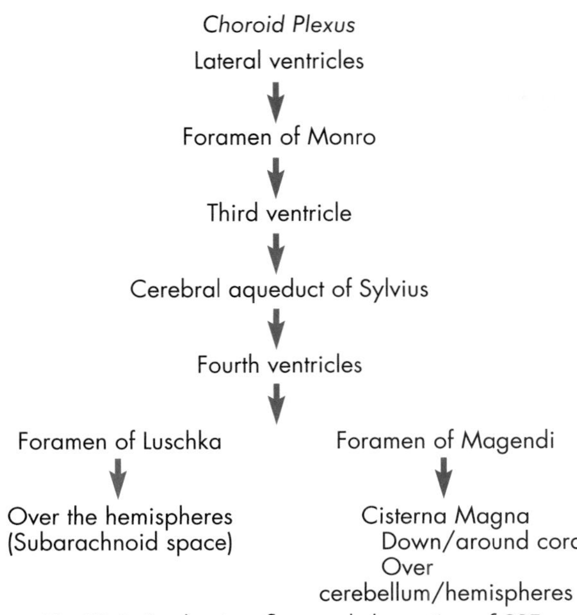

Fig. 29-4 Production, flow, and absorption of CSF.

Balance and Motor Function. The age-related neurodegenerative and neurochemical changes in the cerebellum are believed to be the underlying cause of decline in motor and cognitive function. The neurodegenerative and neurochemical changes, combined with inner ear and vestibular changes, cause many elderly to experience changes in their balance. These changes can further contribute to postural hypotension because of an inability to quickly respond to changes in position. The symptoms of postural hypotension are dizziness or lightheadedness when changing positions rapidly. However, compensatory processes in the cortex and subcortical areas of the brain help aging individuals maintain relatively normal motor performance (Ward and Frackowiak, 2003).

Reticular Formation and Sleep Patterns. The RF is a set of neurons that extends from the upper level of the spinal cord through the brainstem up to the cerebral cortex. The RF contains both motor and sensory tracts that are closely connected with the thalamus, basal ganglia, cerebellum, and cerebral cortex. This group of neural fibers has both excitatory and inhibitory capability. The RF contains a physiologic element, the RAS, which regulates sensory impulses that are transmitted to the cerebral cortex. The lower portion of

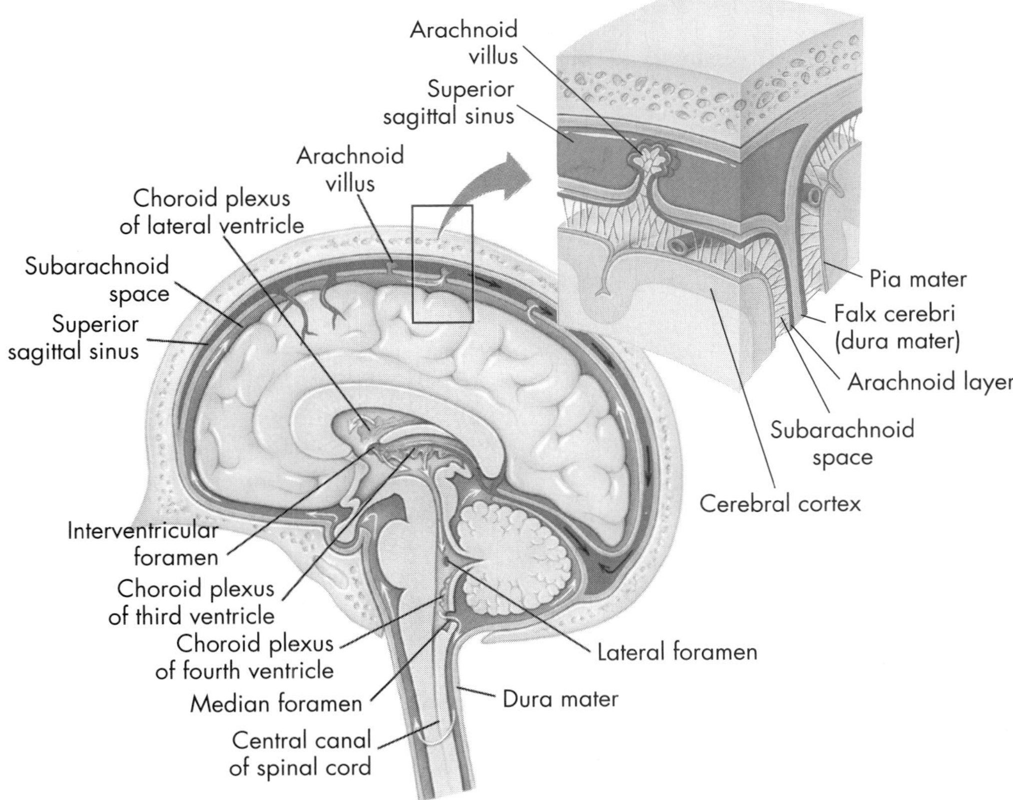

Fig. 29-5 Flow of CSF. (From Thibodeau GA, Patton KT: *Anatomy and physiology*, ed 4, St Louis, 1999, Mosby.)

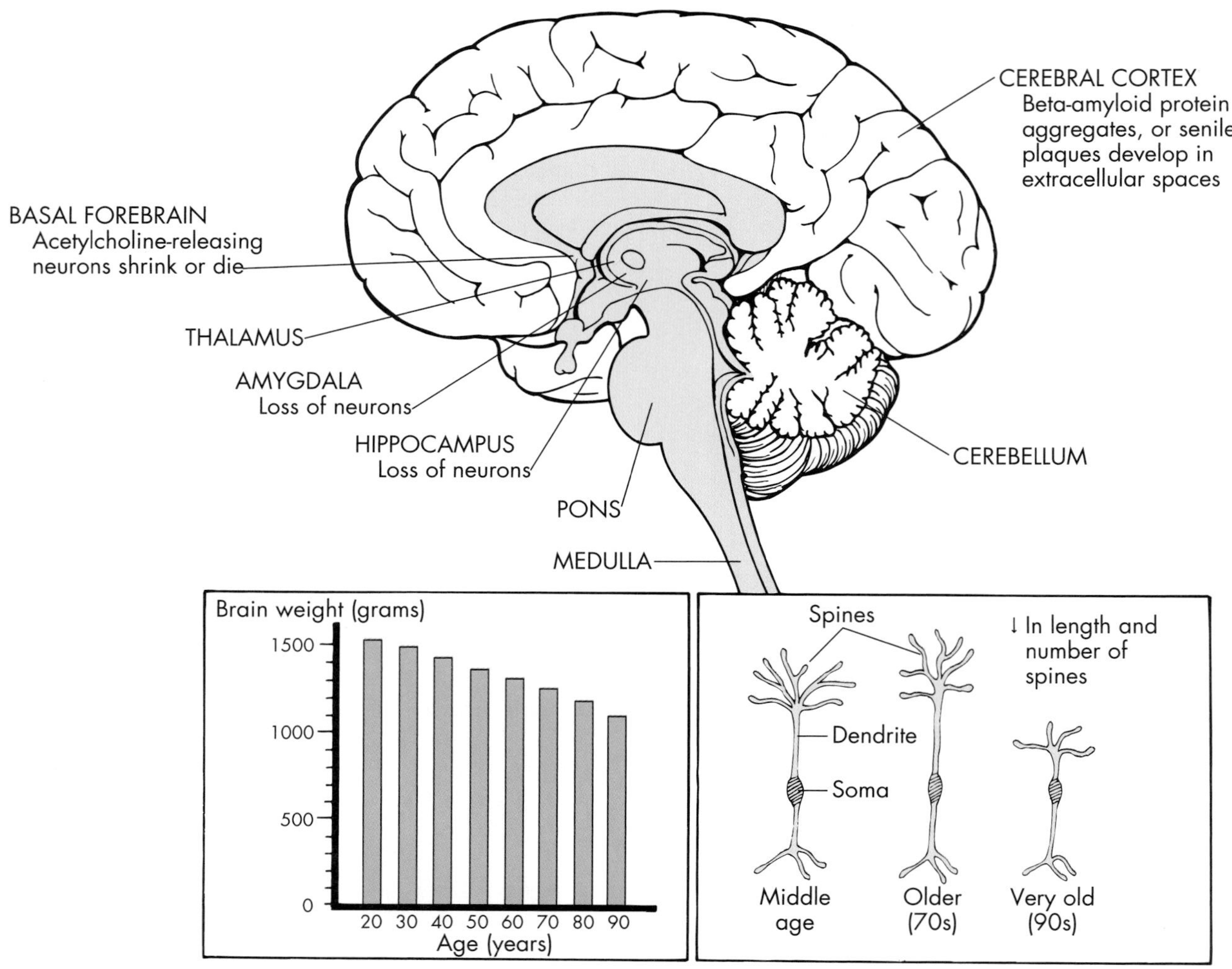

Fig. 29-6 Changes in the brain with aging. (*Bottom left and right* adapted from Selkoe DJ: Aging brain, aging mind, *Sci Am* 267(3):133-142, 1992. Copyright© 1992 by Scientific American, Inc. All rights reserved. *Top* courtesy Carole Donner, Tuscon, AZ.)

the RAS in the brainstem assists in the regulation of the wake-sleep cycle and consciousness (Urden, Stacey, and Lough, 2002).

Sleep disorders are common in aging individuals. Risk factors for sleep disturbances include physical illness; medications; changes in social patterns, retirement, and death of a spouse or loved one; and changes in circadian rhythm. Some sleep disturbances may also be part of the normal aging process resulting from neural changes in the RAS.

Normal sleep is organized into different stages that cycle throughout the night. The sleep stages are classified into the following categories (Vij and Gentili, 2002):

- Rapid eye movement (REM) sleep. This is the stage of sleep during which muscle tone decreases significantly. In advanced aging REM sleep is maintained with minimum show of decline.
- Non-REM sleep. This is subdivided into 4 stages. Stages 1 and 2 constitute light sleep, and stages 3 and 4 are deep sleep or slow-wave sleep. In aging there is an increase in the duration of stage 1 sleep and an increase in the number of shifts into stage 1 sleep. Stages 3 and 4 decrease significantly with age. Among the oldest old people (over 90 years), stages 3 and 4 may disappear completely. Some older women have normal or even increased stage 3 sleep, whereas men have normal or reduced stage 3 sleep.

As individuals age, they spend more time in bed to get the same amount of sleep they obtained when younger; however, the total sleep time is only slightly decreased, with an increase in nocturnal awakenings and daytime napping. Hence older persons often report having earlier bedtimes and an increased sleep latency (time to fall asleep).

Excessive daytime somnolence is not part of normal aging. Somnolence indicates the presence of a pathologic condition. In the aging process there is a decrease in the hypothalamic function; as a result, older clients have been observed to be more easily aroused from sleep by auditory stimuli, suggesting increased sensitivity to environmental stimuli and altered neuroendocrine function (Vij and Gentili, 2002).

Sensorimotor Function. The nervous system depends on specialized sensory receptors to gather information about the internal and external environment. These receptors include those needed for vision, hearing, smell, touch, equilibrium, and pain sensation. Gradual changes occur in these sensory receptor sites as the aging process take place.

Vision changes that occur with aging are significant. The lens of the eye thickens, becoming yellow, cloudy, and less elastic. The thickening of the lens reduces the amount of light passing through the lens. As the lens becomes less elastic, it loses its ability to focus on close objects. The change in elasticity also narrows the visual field and diminishes depth perception. The yellowing of the lens and changes in size and thickening of the cornea make it difficult to see at night. In aging the fluid of the eye also becomes cloudy, reducing light sensitivity. These changes in the eyes lead to gradual decrease in color perception, potentially affecting the ability of older individuals to distinguish between blues, greens, and violets.

The ear consists of the outer ear, middle ear, and inner ear. Presbycusis is the hearing loss associated with the aging process. With presbycusis older persons are unable to hear high frequencies and are unable to clearly hear consonant sounds such as f, g, s, z, t, sh, and ch. Other age-related auditory changes involve the collapse and narrowing of the auditory canal and thickening of earwax, which increase hearing difficulty.

With aging, there is a decrease in the number of taste and smell receptors and slower nerve transmissions, although these losses are highly variable. The loss of taste and smell receptors means that food is not as appetizing to the older adult. Aging adults are also less likely to detect the bad taste or smell of spoiled food. Their reduced ability to smell also may make them unable to rapidly detect smoke, gas leaks, or other toxic fumes.

The somatic receptors respond to touch, pressure, cold, pain, and body position. These receptors also become less sensitive as aging occur. Older individuals therefore experience decreased ability to feel pain and cope with temperature changes. These and additional age-related changes are presented in Table 29-1.

ASSESSMENT OF COGNITIVE FUNCTION

The assessment of neurocognitive function is an essential part of a comprehensive assessment in older adults. Neurocognitive function assessment includes several components and can be easily incorporated into the general assessment of older adults through history, physical examination, and the use of selected screening instruments. A complete mental status assessment should include attention, memory, orientation, perceptions, thought processes, thought content, insight, judgment, affect, mood, language, and higher cognitive functions (see Chapter 14 for the components of cognitive or mental status assessment). Neurologic assessment includes the evaluation of cranial nerves, gait, balance, distal deep tendon reflexes, plantar responses, primary sensory modalities in the lower extremities, and cerebrovascular integrity. Complete neurocognitive examinations should be performed on all older adults to establish baseline function and to detect potentially reversible conditions causing mental and behavioral disturbances.

Few older adults recognize the symptoms of cognitive decline in themselves. It is often a friend or family member who reports these symptoms to the nurse or physician caring for the client. An interview with the friend or family member, physical assessment, and the use of structured mental status assessments assist the nurse in identifying cognitive decline in older adults (Cotter, Clark, and Karlawish, 2003).

One of the early manifestations of cognitive decline may be observed in the functioning of older adults. It is important to include functional assessment as part of the assessment of older adults. Simple questions that may be asked in the history include their ability to perform activities of daily living (ADLs), such as bathing, dressing, toileting, and eating. Instrumental activities of daily living should also be addressed. These activities include ability to clean house, shop, pay bills, and perform other functions that would allow clients to remain independent within their homes.

Selected Cognitive Function Screening Instruments

Functional Assessment. One screening tool that has been used to identify the presence and severity of dementia symptoms based on level of function and cognition in older adults is the Dementia Severity Rating Scale (DSRS) (Clark and Ewbank, 1996). The DSRC is an 11-item instrument that can be easily and quickly administered and covers the areas of memory, orientation, judgment, community affairs, home activities, personal care, speech and language recognition, feeding, incontinence, and mobility or walking. A normal score on this instrument is 4 or less; the score increases as the older person's cognition decreases.

Mental Status Examination. The MiniMental State Examination (MMSE) is one of the most widely used instruments in all settings and is useful for the assessment of orientation, immediate and recent memory, attention, calculation, and language and motor skills (Folstein, Folstein, and McHugh, 1975). Cognitive impairment is identified in individuals with scores of less than 24; however, educational level and age may have an impact on the results and must be taken into consideration when interpreting the results. The Mental State Questionnaire (MSQ) is a 10-item list, one of the shortest instruments used to assess cognitive function. This test is reliable in identifying clients with moderate to severe cognitive impairment. The MSQ is not beneficial for all client evaluations (Alexopoulos and Mattis, 1991). The Blessed Dementia Scale or Short Blessed Test (SBT) is another frequently used screening tool for the assessment of dementia; however, both aging and depression have an effect on BOMC performance (Jorm and Jacob, 1989). The Blessed Orientation-Memory-Concentration Test is a reduced version of the SBT and consists of six questions. This shortened version of the SBT is used by many disciplines.

Depression Assessment. The Geriatric Depression Scale is widely used to identify depression in older adults (Yesavage et al, 1983). Patients answer 30 statements on this screening tool with either "yes" or "no." A score of 11 or greater indicates possible depression and the need for more in-depth evaluation. See Chapter 14 for an in-depth discussion on the evaluation of depression in older adults.

Cognitive Function and Memory in Typical Aging

Forgetfulness as an inevitable consequence of aging is a myth that has had significant influence on society's views of aging. Forgetfulness may affect both the young and old, but should not be confused with true cognitive impairment. In reality, memory and delayed recall are not substantially decreased in older persons. If allowed time to learn new material, older persons experience no more memory loss than younger persons. Cognitive impairment involves mental status changes in addition to higher level cognitive functional changes such as failure to correctly spell common words, compute simple sums, balance a checkbook, drive a car safely, plan a meal, or follow grammatical conventions. Decline in cognitive function is an effect of disease, not an effect of the normal aging process.

COGNITIVE DISORDERS ASSOCIATED WITH ALTERED THOUGHT PROCESSES

Several cognitive disorders are associated with altered thought processes in older adults. These include the three Ds of depression, delirium, and dementia, as well as cranial tumors, subdural hematoma, and normal pressure hydrocephalus. It is often difficult to accurately diagnose the underlying cause of altered thought processes in older adults because of the similarity in their presentations. Nevertheless, accurate assessment and diagnosis are essential to ensure appropriate treatment to improve or potentially reverse the underlying pathophysiologic condition contributing to the individual's impaired cognition.

Depression

Approximately 15% of individuals over the age of 65 have significant depressive symptoms, and about 3% suffer from major depression (*Depression in old age*, 2003). Between the ages of 80 and 84, 17% of men and 22% of women have severe depression, but by age 85, the percentage of older persons with depressive symptoms equalizes (Federal Interagency Forum on Aging-Related Statistics, 2000). In older age, depression is associated with higher suicide rates than in the younger depressed population. Although older Americans make up 13% of the U.S. population, they account for 18% of all suicide deaths. White men over 50 years of age make up 30% of attempted suicides in the United States. A psychologic autopsy of 80 people who committed suicide at an average age of 68 found that 50% of them had a known history of major depression (Arias et al, 2001).

Clinical Manifestations. Depression may manifest itself through signs such as fatigue; constipation; psychomotor retardation; depressed mood; loss of interest, energy, libido, or pleasure; changes in appetite, weight, and sleep patterns; and agitation, anxiety, or crying (American Psychiatric Association [APA], 2000). Depression often is first seen in older adults as cognitive impairment, particularly in the areas of attention and concentration. Depressed older adults may neglect eating or caring for a chronic medical condition, predisposing them to the development of delirium.

Depression is also a common response to serious illness of any kind, particularly multiple sclerosis, hypothyroidism, lupus, hepatitis, acquired immunodeficiency syndrome (AIDS), vitamin deficiencies, and anemia. These conditions may produce depression in a more direct biologic sense. Drugs can also contribute to depressive symptoms (Box 29-1). Older adults require a careful medical history and physical examination before the diagnosis of depression can be made.

Late-life depression is often similar in presentation or may be concomitant to cognitive impairment and dementia caused by neurochemical changes and awareness of the loss of physical or intellectual functioning. Symptoms common to both depression and dementia include irritability, inability to concentrate or feel pleasure, loss of interest in life, and lack of energy and initiative. The term *pseudodementia* has been

BOX 29-1 Medications That May Contribute to Depression

- Amphetamines
- Analgesics, narcotics
- Antihypertensives
- Antimicrobials
- Antineoplastic agents
- Antiparkinsonian agents
- Barbiturates
- Benzodiazepines
- Digoxin
- Hypoglycemic agents (by causing hypoglycemia)
- Phenothiazides
- Steroids
- Sulfonamides

used to describe depression masquerading as dementia. *Pseudodelirium* is the term used when an older adult is seen with an acute confusion found to be due to depression. With a careful assessment, it is possible to make the appropriate diagnosis. Individuals suffering from dementia are more likely to show signs of disorientation and loss of short-term memory and are less likely to feel sadness or guilt or to complain about pain, insomnia, and poor appetite. Table 29-2 offers a comparison of selective features associated with dementia, delirium, and depression. The reader is referred to Chapter 14 for a comprehensive discussion of depression among older persons.

Delirium

Delirium is described in the *Diagnostic and Statistical Manual of Mental Disorders* (DSM-IV-TR) (APA, 2000) as a transient, organic mental syndrome characterized by reduced level of consciousness, reduced ability to maintain attention, perceptual disturbances, and memory impairment. The onset of delirium is short, generally ranging from hours to days. Delirium occurs in all settings, including homes, assisted living facilities, nursing facilities, and hospitals. Frequently, when an older adult becomes delirious in a community setting, it precipitates a hospital admission, in part because of the underlying illness causing the delirium. Delirium occurs in 10% to 65% of older hospitalized clients, with associated morbidity rates as high as 65% within this group (Inouye and Charpentier, 1996).

Risk Factors. The risk factors for delirium include advanced age, CNS diseases, infection, polypharmacy, hypoalbuminemia, electrolyte imbalances, trauma history, gastrointestinal or genitourinary disorders, cardiopulmonary disorders, and sensory changes. These factors can lead to physiologic imbalances increasing the risk for confusion (Balir, 2000). Specific laboratory testing should be guided by clues in the history and physical examination in order to identify the physiologic causes of delirium.

Clinical Manifestations. Symptoms of delirium fluctuate and may include difficulty maintaining concentration or attention to external stimuli and a language disturbance, including slurred, forced, or rambling speech. Disorganized thinking demonstrated by tangential reasoning and conversation is often the presenting symptom. Other common symptoms of delirium include:

- Clouding of consciousness or fluctuation of awareness
- Misperceptions, illusions, or hallucinations
- Disorientation to persons, place, and time
- Memory problems
- Increased or decreased physical activity
- Impaired judgment

Management. Early delirium research focused on the early identification of delirium in hospitalized older adults. Current research focuses on the identification of risk factors and prevention strategies. Multiple instruments have been developed to assess for delirium. The nursing acute confusion assessment

TABLE 29-2 Clinical Features of Depression, Delirium, and Dementia

CLINICAL FEATURE	DEPRESSION	DELIRIUM	DEMENTIA
Onset	Can be abrupt or associated with life events	Sudden onset	Months to years
Duration	Weeks to months	Hours to days	Long term or lifetime
Mood	Consistent; sadness, anxiety, irritability	Labile; suspicious, mood swings	Fluctuating; depressed, apathetic, uninterested
Behavior	Variable; may have psychomotor retardation or agitation	Variable; hypokinetic or hyperkinetic	Variable with psychomotor retardation or agitation
Cognition			
Orientation	Selected disorientation	Impaired with variable severity	Slow decline over time
Alertness	Normal	Lethargic or hypervigilant	Generally normal
Memory	Selective impairment	Impairment of recent memory and attentiveness	Early recent and later remote memory impairment
Thought processes	Intact with themes of hopelessness, helplessness, and self-depreciation	Difficulty maintaining concentration; disorganized; fragmented	Impoverished; impaired abstract thinking; word-finding difficulties; impaired judgment
Perception	Normal	Possible visual, auditory, and tactile hallucinations or delusions	Misperceptions not generally present
Speech and language	Normal to slowed	Slurred, forced, or rambling	Disordered; word-finding difficulties
MiniMental State Examination	Performance fluctuates over time	Acute fluctuations	Moderately stable with decreasing scores over time

instruments include the Clinical Assessment of Confusion–A &B (Vermeersch, 1986; 1992), the VAS-AC (Nagley, 1986), and the NEECHAM Confusion Scale (Neelon et al, 1996). There are also several medical model delirium assessment scales, including the Delirium Rating Scale (Trzepacz, Baker, and Greenhouse, 1988), Delirium Symptom Interview (Levkoff, Besdine, and Wetle, 1986), and Confusion Assessment Method (Inouye et al, 1990). All these instruments have demonstrated sensitivity and specificity for use with hospitalized older adults.

In one study a program was developed for the early detection and treatment of older persons who developed symptoms of delirium during hospitalization (Inouye, 1999). The predictive model used in this study included four risk factors for delirium: visual impairment, severe illness, cognitive impairment, and a high ratio of blood urea nitrogen to creatinine. Intermediate risk for the development of delirium was defined as the presence of one or two risk factors at baseline, and high risk was defined as the presence of three or four risk factors at baseline. Individuals 70 years and older were matched and assigned to either an intervention group or a usual care group. Table 29-3 outlines the assessment and intervention protocols used in this study. The intervention group showed decreased incidence of delirium, but once delirium developed, the intervention group fared no better than the usual treatment group. This study emphasizes the importance of assessment, primary prevention, and early detection of delirium among hospitalized older persons.

Cole, Pimeau, and McCusker (1996) reviewed the literature evaluating the effectiveness of interventions to prevent delirium in hospitalized clients. These researchers identified a broad spectrum of preventive interventions that may be modestly effective, including psychiatric or medical assessment, support, education, and reorientation. They also found that interventions by nurses alone were as effective as interventions by physicians. Delirium management includes rapid diagnosis and treatment of the underlying cause, management of disruptive behaviors, and supportive care. As discussed in the Inouye (1999) study, assessment of changes in older persons' cognition is paramount. A thorough history and physical examination are essential for the identification of the onset, cause, direct physiologic manifestation of a general medical condition, or intoxication with or withdrawal from substances that may be contributing to the onset of delirium (APA, 2000).

The treatment of delirium entails the identification and treatment of the underlying cause. These treatment interventions may be categorized as pharmacologic and nonpharmacologic. Nonpharmacologic approaches include removing bladder catheters, improving nutritional intake, providing reality orientation, decreasing sensory overstimulation or deprivation, and reassuring the older adult and his or her

TABLE 29-3 Risk Factors for Delirium and Intervention Protocols

TARGETED RISK FACTOR AND ELIGIBLE PATIENTS	STANDARDIZED INTERVENTION PROTOCOLS	TARGETED OUTCOME FOR REASSESSMENT
Cognitive impairment*		
All patients, protocol once daily; patients with baseline MMSE score of <20 or orientation score of <8, protocol 3 times daily	Orientation protocol: board with names of care team members and day's schedule; communication to reorient to surroundings Therapeutic-activities protocol: cognitively stimulating activities 3 times daily (e.g., discussion of current events, structured reminiscence, or word games)	Change in orientation score
Sleep deprivation		
All patients: need for protocol assessed once daily	Nonpharmacologic sleep protocol: at bedtime, warm drink (milk or herbal tea), relaxation tapes or music, and back massage Sleep-enhancement protocol: unit-wide noise-reduction strategies (e.g., silent pill crushers, vibrating beepers, and quiet hallways) and schedule adjustments to allow sleep (e.g., rescheduling of medications and procedures)	Change in rate of use of sedative drug for sleep†
Immobility		
All patients: ambulation whenever possible, and range-of-motion exercises when patients chronically nonambulatory, bed or wheelchair bound, immobilized (e.g., because of extremity fracture or deep venous thrombosis), or prescribed bedrest	Early-mobilization protocol: ambulation or active range-of-motion exercises 3 times daily; minimum use of immobilizing equipment (e.g., bladder catheters or physical restraints)	Change in ADL score

Continued

TABLE 29-3 Risk Factors for Delirium and Intervention Protocols—cont'd

TARGETED RISK FACTOR AND ELIGIBLE PATIENTS	STANDARDIZED INTERVENTION PROTOCOLS	TARGETED OUTCOME FOR REASSESSMENT
Visual impairment		
Patients with <20/70 visual acuity on binocular near-vision testing	Vision protocol: visual aids (e.g., glasses or magnifying lenses) and adaptive equipment (e.g., large illuminated telephone keypads, large-print books, and fluorescent tape on call bell), with daily reinforcement of their use	Early correction of vision, ≤48 hr after admission
Hearing impairment		
Patients hearing ≤6 of 12 whispers on Whisper Test	Hearing protocol: portable amplifying devices, earwax disimpaction, and special communication techniques, with daily reinforcement of these adaptations	Change in Whisper Test score
Dehydration		
Patients with ratio of blood urea nitrogen to creatinine ≥18, screened for protocol by geriatric nurse-specialist	Dehydration protocol: early recognition of dehydration and volume repletion (i.e., encouragement of oral intake of fluids)	Change in ratio of blood urea nitrogen to creatinine

From Inouye SK: Risk factors for delirium and intervention protocols, *N Engl J Med* 340(9):669, 1999.
*Orientation score consisted of results on first 10 items on the MiniMental State Examination (MMSE).
†Sedative drugs included standard hypnotic agents, benzodiazepines, and antihistamines, used as needed for sleep.

family members (Insel and Badger, 2002). Pharmacologic approaches may include antibiotics to treat underlying infections and the removal of potentially contributory medications. It may be necessary to use medications for the management of agitation and hallucinations (haloperidol) or alcohol withdrawal symptoms (benzodiazepines). The former must be used judiciously to treat agitation and hallucinations while being cautious to avoid polypharmacy (see Research box).

Dementia

Approximately 6.8 million individuals in the United States have dementia, translating into a prevalence rate of 35.8% among individuals over 85 years of age (Federal Interagency Forum on Aging-Related Statistics, 2000). Not included in these statistics is the phenomenon of potentially reversible dementia. The primary types of dementia include Alzheimer's

Research

OBJECTIVE

To determine whether delirium is a predictor of mortality in older patients seen in emergency departments and discharged home without hospital admission.

SAMPLE/ SETTING

The subjects were 30 delirious and 77 nondelirious patients, ages 66 and older, from two emergency departments in Montreal, who were discharged home without being admitted to the hospital. They were identified and monitored for 18 months after emergency department discharge.

METHODS

Detailed interviews with patients and their proxies and review of medical charts were performed at enrollment. Trained lay interviewers determined delirium status using the Confusion Assessment Method. Subjects were followed up at 6-month intervals for a total of 18 months. Survival analysis was performed using the Cox proportional hazards modeling adjusting for potential confounding variables.

FINDINGS

The analysis revealed a significant association between delirium and mortality after adjustments for age, sex, functional level, cognitive status, comorbidity, and number of medications for the first 6 months of follow-up. The subjects whose delirium was not detected by the emergency department physician or nurse had the highest death rate over 6 months.

IMPLICATIONS

The lack of detection of delirium in the emergency department may be associated with increased mortality within 6 months after discharge. It is important for medical care providers to recognize and treat the symptoms of delirium.

Kakuma R et al: Delirium in older emergency department patients discharged home: effect on survival, *J Am Geriatr Soc* 51(4):443, 2003.

disease (AD), vascular dementia (VaD), Lewy body dementia, and frontotemporal dementia (FTD).

Dementia is a syndrome of gradual and progressive cognitive decline. It has been defined as an alteration in memory in addition to acquired persistent alteration in intellectual function (e.g., orientation, calculation, attention, motor skills) compromising multiple cognitive domains. In dementia, individuals are unable to do the things they used to do because of the mental changes associated with this disease process. Dementia may involve language deficits, apraxia (difficulty with the manipulation of objects), agnosia (inability to recognize familiar objects), agraphia (difficulty drawing objects), and impaired executive function (Knopman, Boeve, and Petersen, 2003).

Although dementia is more common in older persons than in younger persons, it is not part of the normal aging process. Dementia is usually a condition occurring in later life because of changes in neurologic function caused by a disease process. Dementia has been linked to a variety of conditions. Research of the problem has been difficult because of the lack of a standard definition of mild dementia and difficulty in detecting symptoms of early dementia.

Reversible Dementia. Reversible dementia is a phenomenon that occurs when other pathologic conditions masquerade as dementia. Causes of potentially reversible dementia are presented in Box 29-2. It is important to identify and treat the underlying causes of dementia symptoms. Nevertheless, it is important to understand that even if these disorders are identified and treated, not all individuals with dementia symptoms will improve (Larson et al, 2004).

Alzheimer's Disease

AD is the most common form of dementia in older persons and accounts for 60% to 80% of individuals participating in research on dementia (Knopman, 1998). AD is a progressive, neurodegenerative disease characterized by the presence of neurofibrillary tangles composed of misplaced proteins within the brain, cortical amyloid plaques, and granulovascular degeneration of neurons in the pyramidal cell layer of the hippocampus. An estimated 4.5 million Americans have AD, and it is predicted that by 2050 the number of individuals with AD could range from 11.3 million to 16 million (Federal Interagency Forum on Aging-Related Statistics, 2000; Hebert et al, 2003). From the time of diagnosis, individuals with AD survive about half as long as those of similar age without dementia (Larson et al, 2004). The personal and public price of AD is high. Medicare costs for beneficiaries with AD are expected to increase from $31.9 billion in 2000 to $49.3 billion in 2010 (Lewin Group, 2001).

BOX 29-2 Causes of Potentially Reversible Dementia

- Medications
- Ethyl alcohol (ETOH) intoxication or withdrawal
- Metabolic disorders
  - Thyroid disease
  - Vitamin B_{12} deficiency
  - Hyponatremia
  - Hypercalcemia
  - Hepatic dysfunction
  - Renal dysfunction
- Depression
- Delirium
- CNS neoplasm
- Chronic subdural hematoma
- Normal pressure hydrocephalus

Risk Factors. Research has focused on genetic, nutritional, viral, environmental, and other causes of AD. Age is the single most important risk factor for the development of AD, as the number of people with the disease doubles every 5 years beyond age 65.

Genetic Factors. Another risk factor for the development of AD is genetics, particularly in cases of presenile dementia, or dementia seen in individuals under the age of 65. Other genetic mutations cause excessive accumulations of amyloid protein are also associated with age-related (sporadic) AD (Green et al, 2002). AD may be autosomal-dominantly inherited in families with presenile dementia. Chromosome 14 has been linked to early-onset familial AD in over 70% of the cases, and chromosome 19, closely associated with the gene responsible for the encoding of apolipoprotein E, has been linked to late-onset familial AD (Geller et al, 1995). Mutations in chromosome 21, the gene associated with Down syndrome (trisomy 21), have also been linked with development of the disease. All persons with Down syndrome who survive to the third or fourth decade develop the pathologic condition of AD (Geller et al, 1995). In spite of these data, AD is not an exclusively inherited disease.

Viral Factors. Viral illness such as herpes zoster, herpes simplex, or viral encephalitis is believed to be a possible risk factor for AD. Viral infection of the brain has become an important topic of study because of the association of dementia and AIDS. Researchers are studying the origin of the amyloid deposited in the senile plaques of brain cells of clients with AD. The amyloid precursor protein may have an important role in myeloid deposition in AD. Amyloid fibers become entangled around the cerebral blood vessels, and amyloid-laden neuritic plaques replace the degenerating nerve endings.

Environmental Factors. Environmental factors that are potentially associated with cognitive dysfunction include exposure to toxic substances or chemicals. The role of environmental factors in the expression of AD is supported by studies that reveal only a 40% concordance rate for AD in monozygotic twins, as well as by variations in age at the onset of dementia in monozygotic twin pairs. These findings suggest that nongenetic and potentially environmental factors may influence the development of AD. Many of these environmental risk factors require confirmation (Carr et al, 1997). Head trauma occurring early in life with associated loss of consciousness has been associated with the development of AD in later years (Plassman et al, 2000).

Nutritional Factors. Reports suggest an association between AD and vitamin B_{12} deficiency, since low serum vitamin B_{12} concentrations are found in more than 10% of older people and the prevalence of low serum vitamin B_{12} levels has been reported among people with AD. Hyperhomocysteinemia (plasma homocysteine of greater than 14 μmol/L) increased the risks for dementia and AD in an elderly cohort participating in the Framingham study (Seshadri et al, 2002).

Clinical Manifestations. Symptoms of AD that may be identified by family members and nurses include the individual's repeated questions and statements, forgetting to pay bills or take medications, increasing problems with orientation, and geographic disorientation. Other symptoms of AD include pervasive forgetfulness and memory loss, language deterioration, impaired ability to mentally manipulate visual information, poor judgment, confusion, restlessness, and mood swings. Personality changes may include apathy or loss of interest in previously enjoyed activities. Eventually AD destroys cognition, personality, and the ability to function.

Diagnostic Studies. Currently no validated test is available for the diagnosis of AD. Although autopsy remains the gold standard for the diagnosis of AD, clinical diagnosis has become increasingly accurate over the past several years (Knopman et al, 2003). Magnetic resonance imaging (MRI) and positron emission tomography (PET) scans have been used to identify the hippocampal atrophy associated with the diagnosis AD. Because the costs are prohibitive and the findings similar to those of clinical examination for the diagnosis of AD, these tests are not routinely recommended (Knopman et al, 2003).

Treatment. At this time there is no cure for AD. Several pharmacologic options have been introduced to slow the progression of the disease in its early stages. These new medications have transformed the care of AD clients. Tacrine (Cognex) was the first of the cholinesterase inhibitors, but because of the need to frequently monitor a client's liver function, its use is limited. Donepezil (Aricept), rivastigmine (Exelon), and galantamine (Reminyl), all cholinesterase inhibitors, have been found to have fewer side effects and demonstrated greater cognitive and global functional improvement in early and mid-stage AD. These medications may keep some symptoms from becoming worse for a limited time. A fifth drug, memantine (Namenda), was approved for use in the United States. Combining memantine with other AD drugs promises to be more effective than any single therapy. Although cholinesterase inhibitors have been useful for older adults with AD, they have not been shown to have the same effects in older adults with other types of progressive dementia.

Ginkgo biloba, an herbal plant extract, has shown promise in stabilizing and occasionally improving cognitive performance and function in demented older adults for 6 months to a year (Birks et al, 2003). It has been used as a standardized form in Europe for many years, but is sold in the United States as a nutritional supplement. Vitamin supplementation has been attempted and studied, but there is no consensus on the efficacy of this intervention. In a research review by Malouf and Areosa Sastre (2004), there was insufficient evidence to support the efficacy of vitamin B_{12} in improving the cognitive function of people with dementia and low serum B_{12} levels. In another review, Malouf, Grimley Evans, and Areosa Sastre (2004) found no benefit from folic acid with or without vitamin B_{12} in comparison with placebo on any measures of cognition or mood in the clinical trials they reviewed. The results of a 2004 meta-analysis of the role of vitamin E in the treatment of AD were inconclusive (Tabet et al, 2004).

Although nonsteroidal antiinflammatory medications (NSAIDs) have been suggested in the treatment of AD, no evidence exists from randomized double-blind and placebo-controlled trials demonstrating its benefit (Tabet et al, 2004). Because ibuprofen and other NSAIDs have a significant side effect profile, including gastrointestinal bleeding, it needs to be demonstrated that the benefits of such a treatment outweigh the risk of side effects before ibuprofen can be recommended for AD treatment.

Nursing Management. Previously the management of clients with dementia consisted of helping victims and their families through progression of the disorder while allowing them as much dignity and independence as possible. This is clearly still true. However, the focus is now on maintaining cognitive and global function early in the disease process to postpone the need for institutional care.

Vascular Dementia

VaD is the second most frequently occurring type of dementia among older persons (Roman, 2003). It has been estimated that 20% of all dementias have a vascular component (Knopman et al, 2003). Often referred to as multiinfarct dementia, VaD is defined as a loss of cognitive function resulting from ischemic, hypoperfusive, or hemorrhagic brain lesions resulting from cerebrovascular disease or cardiovascular pathologic conditions. VaD is associated with the progressive loss of brain tissue as a result of a series of small brain attacks (infarcts) caused by occlusions and blockages within the arteries to the brain. Individuals who have experienced a cerebrovascular accident (CVA) have an even greater risk of VaD.

Pathophysiologically, asymmetric regions of cerebral softening and hemorrhage are diffuse and irregular. If there is a series of brain attacks, the rate of decline in function increase. Some recovery of function may occur over time, but there is never full recovery. As the damage from the infarcts progresses and accumulates, more widespread evidence of diminished mental ability exists.

Risk Factors. Several medical problems place individuals at risk for the development of VaD. These include arteriosclerosis, blood dyscrasias, cardiac decompensation, hypertension, atrial fibrillation, cardiac valve replacements, systemic emboli for other reasons, diabetes mellitus, peripheral vascular disease, obesity, smoking, and vasospasms in segments of the brain (also referred to as transient ischemic attacks [TIAs]).

Clinical Manifestations. The onset of VaD may be gradual or abrupt. Gradual onset VaD occurs as a result of small lacunar infarcts that affect a very small area of the brain, causing memory, motor, or sensory perceptual function deficits. This phenomenon may not be obvious until several small infarcts have occurred. Abrupt onset VaD presents with immediate neurologic symptoms, such as one-sided weakness, gait abnormalities, or focal neurologic signs. Destruction of the brain tissue resulting from small emboli or brain attacks may be localized or diffuse. The usual progression of VaD follows a stepwise decline rather than the slow, steady decline associated with AD. Patients with VaD have an infarct, decline in function, and then experience a functional plateau before experiencing another insult and subsequent decline.

Symptoms of VaD depend on the location of the infarct and may include:

- Impaired learning and impaired retention of new information
- Impaired handling of new tasks
- Impaired reasoning ability
- Impaired spatial ability and orientation
- Impaired language

These impairments generally interfere with work and social functioning. Other symptoms may include wandering; getting lost in familiar places; moving with rapid, shuffling steps; losing bladder or bowel control; inappropriately displaying emotions; and having difficulty following instructions. Not all brain attacks result in intellectual impairment; some affect movement, vision, or other functions.

Diagnostic Studies. Neuroimaging with either computed tomography (CT) or MRI usually reveals one or more areas of cerebral infarction. VaD is most often associated with diffuse or bilateral cortical or subcortical areas of infarction or microinfarction. Other than neuroimaging and clinical examination, no other diagnostic tests or biomarkers exist for the diagnosis of VaD.

Treatment. Research on the use of donepezil for improving cognitive function, clinical global impression, and ability to perform ADLs in patients with mild to moderate VaD has been promising (Malouf and Birks, 2004). Nimodipine (Nimotop), a calcium channel blocker, has also demonstrated short-term benefit in the treatment of VaD; however, little evidence supports its efficacy with long-term use in VaD (Lopez-Arrieta and Birks, 2004). Cognitive training interventions for individuals with VaD showed no efficacy in a 2004 review of clinical trials using this treatment modality (Clare et al, 2004).

Lewy Body Dementia

Lewy body dementia is a progressive, degenerative brain disorder named after an intracytoplasmic neuronal inclusion, which may be found in the brainstem, diencephalon, basal ganglia, and cerebral cortex (Kalra, Bergeron, and Lang, 1996). The pathologic changes of Lewy body dementia are present in 10% to 20% of autopsies, primarily in the limbic and neocortical regions of the brain (Knopman, 2003). Individuals with Parkinson's disease (PD) have a sixfold increased risk for the development of Lewy body dementia compared with the general population (Aarsland et al, 2001).

Risk Factors. Risk factors associated with the development of Lewy body dementia include advanced age, depression, confusion or psychosis while taking levodopa, and facial masking in individuals with diagnosed PD (Larson et al, 2004).

Clinical Manifestations. The clinical manifestations of Lewy body dementia are similar to those of AD; however, Lewy body dementia is often marked by prominent fluctuations in attention and ability to communicate and by the severity of psychiatric symptoms, particularly visual hallucinations. Lewy body dementia, compared with AD, tends to have more visual-spatial processing impairments and features of subcortical dementia. These include decreased attention and deficits in verbal fluency. Extrapyramidal features are also found in Lewy body dementia, including rigidity, bradykinesia, flexed posture, and shuffling gait. Other symptoms may include:

- Excessive daytime sleepiness and altered arousal
- Periods of reduced attention and concentration
- REM sleep disorder

Diagnostic Studies. No laboratory tests are available for the diagnosis of Lewy body dementia. MRI shows less hippocampal activity than is seen in AD, but these are too minimal to be of diagnostic value (Knopman, 2003).

Management. Management of patients with Lewy body dementia focuses on symptomatic relief when psychiatric and behavioral symptoms become distressing. Treatment for PD is essential in the event of gait and balance alterations.

The use of cholinesterase inhibitors has also been supported in Lewy body dementia (McKeith et al, 2000). Caregiver education and support are important aspects of disease management because of the unique pattern of psychiatric symptoms and motor and cognitive deficits that these patients display (Lantz and Buchalter, 2002).

Frontotemporal Dementia

FTD is a clinical syndrome of exclusion associated with non-AD pathologic conditions and is relatively rare in the clinical setting. This syndrome includes the spectrum of non-AD dementias and is characterized by focal atrophy of the frontal and anterior temporal regions. Pathologically, FTD is variable; some cases may show tau-positive disease (with or without classic Pick bodies), whereas others show ubiquitin-positive inclusions, and still others may lack distinctive histologic features (McKhann et al, 2001).

Risk Factors. The risk factors for FTD are poorly understood.

Clinical Manifestations. Two major clinical presentations of FTD include frontal or aphasic variants. Frontal behavioral variant FTD is associated with progressive changes in personality and social cognition, disinhibition, loss of empathy, changes in eating patterns, ritualized or stereotypic behaviors, and apathy. Aphasic variants of FTD include progressive fluent or nonfluent aphasia (loss of ability to use language), depending on the frontal or temporal focus (Grossman, 2002). Either of these main variants may be associated with motor neuron disease, although the behavioral features typically precede motor symptoms (Bak, 2001).

Pick's Disease. One example of an FTD that is more common in Europe than in the United States is Pick's disease. Pick's disease is an uncommon type of progressive dementia with clinical features similar to those of AD. Often occurring between the ages of 40 and 60, Pick's disease involves atrophy of the frontal and temporal lobes of the cerebral cortex. This atrophy occurs due to neuronal loss, gliosis, and the inclusion of the distinctive Pick's bodies. Individuals with Pick's disease often have more frontal lobe symptoms, particularly behavioral problems.

Diagnostic Studies. Neuroimaging with CT or MRI may be useful in the diagnosis of FTD. Focal atrophy of the prefrontal or temporal regions confirms FTD; however, this finding is not always present. PET scanning may also assist in the confirmation of the clinical diagnosis (Knopman, 2003).

Management. The prognosis of FTD between onset of symptoms and severe dementia ranges from 3 to 10 years. Currently there are no treatments for FTD (Knopman, 2003).

Other Dementia-Related Diseases

Normal Pressure Hydrocephalus. Normal pressure hydrocephalus (NPH) is a rare but potentially reversible condition; if left untreated, it leads to permanent cognitive impairment. In NPH the CSF does circulate to the cerebral subarachnoid space, enlarging the ventricles, but causing no rise in the CSF pressure. It is believed that the majority of cases of NPH are related to prior cerebral insult such as traumatic injury, viral insult, or previous surgery. NPH has a triad of symptoms that present together: gait disturbance (e.g., ataxic, magnetic gait), urinary incontinence, and cognitive dysfunction (Larson et al, 2004). Clients who develop dementia before the gait disturbance have poorer outcomes. Treatment involves placing a shunt to drain the CSF; however, a recent review of research revealed no consistent evidence that the placement of a shunt is effective in the management of NPH (Esmonde and Cooke, 2004).

Dementia may also result from other diseases, including Huntington's disease (formerly called Huntington's chorea), Creutzfeldt-Jakob disease, and infection with human immunodeficiency virus (HIV). These diseases are less common among the older adult population.

Subdural Hematomas. A subdural hematoma is a bleed between the cranium and the cerebral cortex. The pressure created by this bleeding can cause cognitive impairment and neurologic deficits. Older adults are at risk for the development of subdural hematomas caused by brain atrophy and corresponding vascular changes that occur with normal aging and risk for falls and subsequent head injury.

There are two types of subdural hematomas: acute and chronic. Symptoms of acute subdural hematomas develop within 48 to 72 hours after a head injury but are not seen with the typical signs of increased intracranial pressure. Instead, the presentation includes insidious changes in mentation and focal neurologic signs. Chronic subdural hematomas may be due to trauma, but often are not noticed until 3 or more weeks after the initial injury because of slow bleeding into the intracranial space.

Treatments for both acute and chronic subdural hematomas include the evacuation of the hematoma, usually using burr holes with a closed drainage system. Unfortunately, recurrence is not uncommon.

Intracranial Tumors. Intracranial tumors occur more frequently in older adults than in younger adults and can be either benign (meningiomas) or malignant (gliomas). Intracranial tumors in older adults rarely are seen with the typical signs of increased intracranial pressure (e.g., headaches, vomiting, papilledema), but with subtly progressive changes such as withdrawal, isolation, personality changes, and slowly progressive hemiparesis. Because the symptoms are insidious and include cognitive dysfunction and withdrawal, older adults with intracranial tumors are often misdiagnosed with depression or dementia. Later, when focal neurologic signs appear, brain tumors are considered.

The diagnosis of an intracranial tumor is made following a head CT or MRI. The pathologic condition is determined through biopsy, either by tumor extraction or stereotactic needle biopsy under CT or MRI control. Treatment is based on the results of the biopsy and may include surgical extraction followed by radiation if the tumor recurs (meningioma), or surgical extraction followed by radiation and concomitant chemotherapy (malignant glioma). Prognosis is generally poor, with a 23% 1-year survival rate with malignant gliomas.

The decision of whether and how to treat intracranial tumors in older adults is complex, in part because of preexisting illnesses that may complicate neurosurgery, as well as potential complications or side effects following surgery, chemotherapy, and radiation. Treatment in older clients may lead to deficits as serious as if no treatment or limited treatment were given. All treatment decisions should be made in conjunction with individuals and their families.

Amnesic Disorders. Amnesic disorders are characterized by memory impairment that is the result of a general medical condition or the persisting effects of a drug, medication, or toxin. Duration of the disturbance is a qualifier for the diagnosis. Transient disorders are those lasting less than 1 month; chronic disorders last more than 1 month.

Cognitive Disorders Not Otherwise Specified. This category of diagnosis describes those disorders characterized by cognitive dysfunction presumed to be a result of the physiologic effect of a medical condition but that do not meet other criteria.

DIAGNOSTIC ASSESSMENT OF ALTERED THOUGHT PROCESSES

Examination

History, physical examination, behavioral observation, and functional and mental status examinations form the basis for a diagnosis of depression, delirium, and dementia. Medical screening alone is not sufficient for the evaluation of intellectual decline in older adults, but it does provide valuable information to rule out treatable disorders. The only positive diagnosis for dementia-related disorders is brain tissue biopsy or autopsy of the brain. Screening for treatable, reversible causes is essential to identify and implement appropriate treatment for the underlying cause of cognitive dysfunction associated with altered thought processes.

Diagnostic Studies. Laboratory tests are used to assess the nervous system or rule out medical problems causing the disorder. CT scan, MRI, and electroencephalogram (EEG) have been used for diagnosis of delirium or dementia. Pathologically, a CT scan is useful in detecting space-occupying lesions (e.g., intracranial tumors, subdural hematoma, and hydrocephalus) that may lead to dementias. The pathologic changes seen in dementia, including ventricular enlargement, narrowing of the gyri, widening of the sulci, and brain atrophy, may be identified in a CT. Images obtained by MRI have a high resolution and may be useful in detecting multiple subcortical brain attacks and white matter disease. MRI is useful in diagnosis of VaD. The disadvantage of MRI testing is that the test requires the older person to lie motionless for a long time. This may be impossible for older persons with cognitive disorders. Results of EEG may provide important information about mental status. Background frequency of the waking EEG can be correlated with a client's mental state. If the client is severely impaired and the EEG results are normal, this supports the diagnosis of pseudodementia. In early dementia the EEG results may be abnormally slow, indicating a treatable diagnosis. PET is a noninvasive technique that allows assessment of regional glucose use, oxygen consumption, and regional cerebral blood flow. This technique may be useful in differential diagnosis of the hippocampal atrophy seen in AD and the changes associated with FTD.

Laboratory Studies. CSF studies are useful for the identifying reversible causes of dementia. Laboratory screening tests to rule out treatable medical diagnoses may include complete blood count (CBC); electrolytes; chest x-ray examination; urinalysis; liver, kidney, and thyroid function tests; serum B_{12} levels; folate; syphilis serology (if syphilis highly suspected); and drug studies. Genetic testing remains controversial; however, testing for apolipoprotein E epsilon 4 allele has been considered in AD. Routine use of this test may, however, lead to the overdiagnosis of AD.

Postmortem biopsy is considered the only definitive diagnosis to differentiate the type of dementia causing the symptoms. The clinical profile, including history, physical examination, mental status examination, laboratory tests, and behavioral observations, has improved the classification of dementia.

DSM-IV-TR Criteria

The DSM-IV-TR (APA, 2000) is the most widely accepted system of classifying abnormal behaviors and is consistent in most respects with the systems used by the World Health Organization and the International Classification of Diseases. The DSM-IV-TR classification categorizes each disorder as a clinically significant behavioral or psychologic syndrome or pattern that can occur in a person and is associated with present distress and disability; an important loss of freedom; or an increased risk of suffering death, pain, or disability. There is no assumption that each mental disorder is a discrete entity with sharp boundaries between it and other disorders. The disorders are classified for all age groups and are not specific to older adults.

The DSM-IV-TR disorders have been grouped into delirium, dementia, and other cognitive disorders (Box 29-3). These disorders are further subdivided by cause:

Delirium

- Delirium resulting from a general medical condition
- Substance-induced delirium (as a result of a drug or medication or of toxin exposure)
- Delirium resulting from multiple causes
- Delirium not otherwise specified (if the cause is indeterminate)

Dementia

- AD
- VaD
- Dementia resulting from other general medical conditions (e.g., HIV, head trauma, PD, Huntington's disease)
- Substance-induced persisting dementia (resulting from drug abuse, medications, or toxin exposure)
- Dementia resulting from multiple causes
- Dementia not otherwise specified (if the cause is indeterminate)

Cognitive disorder not otherwise specified

- Does not meet criteria for other disorders

BOX 29-3 DSM-IV-TR Criteria for Dementia

1. Memory impairment.
2. At least one of the following:
   a. Aphasia
   b. Apraxia
   c. Agnosia
   d. Disturbance in executive function
3. The disturbances in memory and in those listed in 2 interfere with work, social relationships, or activities.
4. These disturbances do not exclusively occur during an episode of delirium.

TYPES OF DEMENTIA

Dementia of the Alzheimer's type (AD)
- Gradual onset
- Continuing cognitive decline not caused by medical, psychiatric, or neurologic condition

Vascular dementia (VD)
- Focal neurologic signs
- Diagnostic or laboratory evidence of cerebral vascular condition

Dementia not otherwise defined
- Evidence from history, physical examination, laboratory, or diagnostic findings of a specific medical condition contributing to dementia:
  —HIV dementia
  —Head trauma
  —PD
  —Huntington's chorea
  —Pick's disease
  —Creutzfeld-Jacob

Adapted from American Psychiatric Association: *Diagnostic and statistical manual of mental disorders*, ed 4, text revision, Washington, DC, 2004, The Association.

TREATMENT OF ALTERED THOUGHT PROCESSES

Pharmacotherapy

Disease Management. Medication management of each of the disorders described has been presented previously. In summary, medication management of depression requires the use of antidepressant medications. These are described in greater detail in Chapter 22. Medication management for the treatment of delirium may include the discontinuation of medications contributing to the older person's recent mental status changes, or the addition of medications to treat underlying conditions. The advent of cholinesterase inhibitors has revolutionized the treatment of early AD and shown some promise in the treatment of both VaD and Lewy body dementia. These medications work to slow disease progression and decrease agitated behaviors. Pharmacotherapy for altered thought processes in older adults is summarized in Table 29-4.

Behavior Management. Several classes of medications are available to aid in the behavior management of older persons with dementia. These medications include antipsychotics, antidepressants, benzodiazepines, buspirone (BuSpar), and antiepileptics.

Antipsychotics are useful for the treatment of the behavioral response to psychotic symptoms such as a delusions or hallucinations. They are also used to decrease aggression in older adults who may be endangering themselves or others. This is particularly helpful when acute confusion or delirium is thought to be the cause and when the agitation does not allow the nurse or primary caregiver to assess the client. Haloperidol in daily doses of 0.25 to 2 mg orally or intramuscularly is a good choice for acute control of agitation symptoms (Grossberg, 1998). In one meta-analysis, Lonergan, Luxenberg, and Colford (2001) reported that in patients with dementia, haloperidol reduces aggression but does not reduce agitation and increases other adverse events. There is concern over the long-term side effects of major tranquilizers (Box 29-4). Newer agents such as olanzapine (Zyprexa) and risperidone (Risperdal) have been developed to combat or limit these troubling effects, particularly those of orthostatic hypotension and extrapyramidal side effects.

Depression Management. Antidepressants may be helpful in the management of troubling behaviors and for the treatment of depression with dementia. Trazodone, a sedating antidepressant, can be useful in managing wandering at night or reversing the sleep-wake cycle. Trazodone is often used as a first-line medication when an older adult has mild to moderate agitation during the day as well. Small doses of 25 to 50 mg a few times during the day, then a larger dose at

TABLE 29-4 **Pharmacotherapy for Altered Thought Processes in Older Adults**

AGENT	INITIAL DOSE (IN mg)	COMMON ADVERSE EFFECTS
NEUROLEPTICS		
Haloperidol	0.25-0.5 bid	Sedation, extrapyramidal symptoms, akathisia
Olanzapine	5 qhs	Sedation, weight gain
Risperidone	0.25-0.5 bid	Sedation
ANTICONVULSANTS		
Carbamazepine	50-100 bid	Sedation, GI distress, altered drug metabolism
Valproic acid	125-250 qhs	Sedation, GI distress, altered drug metabolism
ANXIOLYTICS		
Lorazepam	0.25-0.5 bid	Sedation, disinhibition, delirium
Buspirone	10-15 bid	Dizziness, nausea
ANTIDEPRESSANTS		
Trazodone	12.5-25 bid	Sedation, orthostasis, ECG changes

From Sutor B, Rummans TA, Smith GE: Assessment and management of behavioral disturbances in nursing home patients with dementia, *Mayo Clin Proc* 76(5):540, 2001.
bid, Twice daily; *ECG,* electrocardiographic; *GI,* gastrointestinal; *qhs,* at bedtime.

BOX 29-4 **Side Effects Associated With Major Tranquilizers**

- Hypotension
- Extrapyramidal reactions
- Delirium or reversible dementia
- Increased sensitivity to heat and cold
- Anticholinergic effects
- Dry mouth
- Blurred vision
- Dilated pupils
- Constipation
- Urinary retention
- Increased heart rate
- Confusion

BOX 29-5 **Side Effects Associated With Antidepressants**

- Drowsiness
- Dry mouth
- Urinary retention
- Nasal congestion
- Delirium
- Increased appetite for sweets
- Increased heart rate
- Blurred vision
- Dizziness or fainting
- Constipation
- Hypotension
- Arrhythmias
- Weight gain

bedtime, are often useful. Clients should be monitored for orthostatic hypotension while taking this medication. Sedation may limit the use of this medication in some older adults. When depression is a concern in a client who is agitated, selective serotonin reuptake inhibitors (SSRIs) such as paroxetine (Paxil), sertraline (Zoloft), and fluoxetine (Prozac) have been helpful in managing agitation. Unfortunately, SSRIs tend to cause transient appetite suppression, especially on initiation of therapy. Fluoxetine, the first SSRI, is often avoided in older adults because of its long half-life (Box 29-5).

Benzodiazepines. Benzodiazepines should be reserved for acute situations and not used for the long-term management of troubling behaviors. The Omnibus Budget Reconciliation Act of 1987 (OBRA) discouraged the overuse of benzodiazepines in long-term care settings. Significant risk factors are associated with the use of benzodiazepines among older adults. These include increased risk for falls, impaired cognition, and addiction with acute withdrawal symptoms between doses or on abrupt cessation of the medication. For short-term use or one-time dosing for acute agitation or combativeness, lorazepam (Ativan), 0.25 to 1 mg orally or intramuscularly, or oxazepam (Serax), 5 to 10 mg orally, may be helpful (Grossberg, 1998).

Buspirone. Buspirone has been found to be useful in the treatment of anxiety-triggered agitation. It is important to educate caregivers that it may take 2 to 6 weeks before the results of this medication are appreciated; therefore it is not useful for acute episodes of agitation. Buspirone is also useful in older adults who have mild to moderate levels of agitation. It has a low side effect profile and a low risk for drug-drug interactions. Buspirone is the only anxiolytic currently exempt from the regulations of OBRA (Grossberg, 1998).

Antiepileptic or Anticonvulsant Medications. Antiepileptic medications are useful when frequent mood fluctuations or sudden outbursts of agitation are problematic. Two medications used most frequently as mood stabilizers are carbamazepine (Tegretol) and divalproex (valproic acid). Both these medications are indicated for moderate to severe agitation with aggressive outbursts in older adults who require long-term management. The advantages of both medications include the ability to monitor serum levels. Carbamazepine has an antikindling effect on CNS electrical activity at serum levels between 4 to 8 mcg/ml (Grossberg, 1998). Unfortunately, multiple drug interactions and potentially serious side effects such as agranulocytosis, ataxia, and hyponatremia limit the use of carbamazepine. Divalproex has fewer side effects and drug interactions, making it more likely to be the first-line agent for treatment of moderate to severe agitation and combativeness among older adults. Titration of the dose to serum levels of 40 to 100 g/ml is considered a therapeutic level.

Individualized Care. When initially considering the use of medications in the treatment of altered thought processes, health care providers must remember that individual responses to medications vary considerably. All medications require close monitoring by health care workers and family members for action and side effects. The recommendation for pharmacotherapy in the older adult is to is "start low, go slow, and titrate upward until benefits or side effects are seen" (Grossberg, 1998). Client and family education is essential when starting a new medication. Education helps create realistic expectations of the medication's benefits and the potential side effects. Every client may respond differently to medication management; therefore individualized care is essential.

NURSING MANAGEMENT

Nurses caring for older adults who have symptoms of an acute cognitive disorder need to support existing sensory perception until the cognitive state returns to the previous level of function. The goal of caring for older persons with dementing disorders should be the maintenance of good health, gross and fine motor skills, and functional behaviors to maximize self-care abilities. The care provided to older adults with dementia is similar in the beginning stages, but it becomes complex and individually focused as the disease progresses. Philosophies about the care of older adults with cognitive and behavioral impairment have changed over the years. Public policy has shifted to encourage family members to care for older adults in their homes, thus decreasing health care costs and individualizing care to meet client needs. Nursing focus has shifted from the caregiver to care coordinator, teaching and assisting the family members with home care, providing supportive care, and serving as a client advocate.

Assessment

Performing a complete baseline physical examination, along with a neurologic examination and mental status assessment, is essential to rule out an atypical presentation of a medical illness in an older adult. Deficits and impairments may be inaccurately attributed to age or disease if accurate and complete baseline information is not available. Verbal and nonverbal responses from the client, family members, and significant others should be used to validate assessment data. The assessment process is ongoing to ensure the accurate collection of information. The purpose of a comprehensive assessment is to determine problem areas, as well as areas of strength on which to base a care plan, including education of families and caregivers.

Assessment data gathered at the time of an acute crisis, such as in a hospital setting, is critical for initial treatment. The special needs of an older adult with a cognitive disorder may require completing the assessment after treatment of the crisis to ensure discrete symptoms are not overlooked and treatment is appropriate for the disorder.

Level of Consciousness. Level of consciousness provides an indication of pathologic processes. Consciousness can be defined as the state of awareness of the self and the environment. The most widely used and accepted tool for measuring consciousness is the Glasgow Coma Scale. The scale measures eye opening, verbal response, and motor response. This may be the appropriate tool to use for assessment of an older person in a critical state whose neurologic status is undetermined or rapidly changing.

Mental Status Examination. Mental status examinations for assessment of mental and cognitive function are necessary to identify impairments that may have significant and permanent effects. The choice of cognitive assessment tool varies depending on the setting and results of the physical examination. An objective assessment may require more than obtaining orientation to person, place, and time and should be considered before labeling a person "disoriented." It is important to thoroughly assess visual and hearing deficits and alter the environment to enhance the validity of the client's response.

Pupil Assessment. Pupil assessment provides neurologic information and assists in the identification of the cause, responses, and location of pathologic condition. Evaluation of an older adult's pupil size and reaction to light may be difficult, since his or her pupils may appear smaller than normal, and light reflex may be sluggish. Pupil response may also be altered by the presence of cataracts, retinal detachment, glaucoma, and sclerotic changes in the iris.

Neurologic Assessment. Neurologic disorders can cause a wide range of motor abnormalities. The extremities should be assessed for muscle strength and tone and compared for symmetry. Many older persons have normal age-related symmetric weakness and muscular fatigue. Decreased vibratory sense in the feet, decreased Achilles tendon reflex, and decreased sensory perception may be caused by the normal loss of neurotransmitters or sensory receptors.

In the event of traumatic injury resulting in increased intracranial pressure, the classic symptoms of headache, vomiting, and papilledema may not appear in older persons or may be more subtle because of normal, age-related changes caused by cerebral atrophy. These changes, including alterations in consciousness, cranial nerve deficits, and motor changes, may mimic cognitive disorders.

Behavioral Assessment. Persons with cognitive disorders commonly demonstrate problematic behaviors. These new behaviors should not be overlooked but should be viewed as symptoms requiring assessment. The type and intensity of the behavior vary depending on the stage of disease, but each behavior exhibited requires a comprehensive, individualized assessment. Identifying the behavior and extenuating circumstances assists in ruling out treatment causes and determining the personal meaning associated with the behavior.

Diagnosis

The selection of nursing diagnoses should be based on the assessment findings. The most commonly used nursing diagnoses for an older adult with cognitive impairment include:

- Activity intolerance related to physical illness
- Altered family processes related to cognitive impairment
- Altered nutrition: less than body requirements related to poor oral intake
- Altered role performance related to cognitive impairment
- Altered thought processes related to cognitive impairment
- Anxiety related to misinterpretation of environmental cues
- Bathing and hygiene self-care deficit related to cognitive impairment
- Bowel incontinence related to cognitive decline and misinterpretation of physiologic needs
- Caregiver role strain related to older adult's cognitive decline and behavioral problems
- Confusion (acute or chronic) related to physiologic, emotional, or environmental processes
- Dressing and grooming self-care deficit related to cognitive impairment
- Fatigue related to increased physical, emotional, and environmental demands
- Fear related to cognitive impairment
- Feeding self-care deficit related to increased cognitive impairment
- Functional incontinence related to inability to interpret physiologic and environmental cues
- High risk for injury related to altered ability to interpret the environment
- Impaired physical mobility related to neurologic deficits
- Impaired social interaction related to cognitive impairment
- Ineffective family coping: compromised due to needs of older adult with cognitive impairment
- Ineffective family coping: disabling related to lack of social supports
- Knowledge deficit: disease process related to lack of previous exposure
- Self-esteem disturbance related to awareness of cognitive deficits
- Spiritual distress related to the impact of cognitive impairment on individual and family

Planning and Expected Outcomes

Expected outcomes for older adults with cognitive changes are adapted for each diagnosis. Expected outcomes include:

1. Client will exhibit no episodes of acute confusion as evidenced by adequate hydration, nutrition, and socialization.
2. Client will maintain continence through the use of visual and verbal cues and a regular bowel and bladder routine.
3. Client and family will demonstrate ability to cope by accessing community agencies for support groups, Internet pages, and home health agencies for respite and support services.
4. Client will exhibit reduced fear and anxiety by establishing routine, keeping familiar objects, and participating individually in activities for calming down (e.g., listening to favorite music, sitting in the sun, retreating to his or her room).
5. Client will demonstrate fewer inappropriate behaviors such as agitation, combative behavior, and mood changes as evidenced by identifying the triggers that cause them and decreasing or eliminating these triggers.
6. Client will demonstrate increased socialization by voluntarily participating in activities.
7. Client will maintain physical health.
8. Family members will participate in activities and care.
9. Spiritual health of the older adult and his or her family will be maintained as evidenced by participation in religious services, communication with their religious organization, and participation in formal and informal spiritual practices.

Intervention

Each older adult will have a different presentation, triggers, and responses to illness; therefore the most effective interventions are based on the assessment and are individualized for each client. When planning interventions, it is important to consider environmental and cultural influences that affect the person's response patterns. Remaining attentive to needs as they are communicated, as well as to changes and responses in behavior, and using creativity in each situation can accomplish this. The best interventions are learned through trial and error, requiring commitment and communication with the family and caregiver.

The efforts of health care personnel and caregivers will result in implementation of the best strategies for managing care of the client with dementia. Identifying the stage of disease provides a baseline for management of care, but because each person's behavioral responses are based on an individual personal history and experiences, it requires persistence to determine approaches that result in desired responses. Positive responses to selected interventions may continue for a time but decline as the disease progresses, resulting in the need to reevaluate strategies. General principles of care should be individualized when caring for people with dementia (Box 29-6).

Communication. Relaying trust, security, care, and support through simple and direct therapeutic verbal and nonverbal communication is essential when caring for older persons with dementia. In some situations older persons are more inclined to respond to the nonverbal messages. The tone of communication should be calm and relaxed. Using eye contact and therapeutic touch when delivering a message helps the client focus on meaning. It is important to use simple words and short sentences along with simple gestures to demonstrate meaning. At times distraction as a form of communication may be necessary to dissuade a person with memory impairments from engaging in undesirable activities. Verbal communication may become less meaningful for the older person with altered thought processes resulting from memory loss, aphasia, apraxia, agnosia, and disorientation. Nevertheless, verbal communication on the part of the caregiver remains essential. Sounds and voices may elicit a response and provide a calming effect and an orientation to reality in these individuals.

Physical Interventions. Assessing the physical health and the ability of individuals with altered thought processes to meet their basic needs is the foundation of nursing care. Independence should be encouraged and self-esteem promoted by maintaining daily hygiene and grooming. Because a limited ability to verbally communicate may prevent an older adult from relaying a problem or symptom, nonverbal cues should be observed and considered indicative of a potential symptom requiring attention.

BOX 29-6 Principles for Implementation of Care for Cognitively Impaired Older Adults

- Monitor and maintain physical health.
- Recognize the meaning of behaviors.
- Adapt the environment (e.g., routines, setting).
- Communicate in a simple, direct manner.
- Provide cues for reality orientation.
- Maintain social interaction and self-esteem.

Nutritional Interventions. It is important to support the ongoing nutrition of individuals with dementia, since they may experience decreased hunger and ability to taste food. Problems that occur during feeding may include clients' refusing to open their mouth, pocketing food in their cheeks, refusing to swallow, and coughing or choking while swallowing.

People who demonstrate symptoms of moderate to severe cognitive impairment may benefit from having meals in the same place at the same time each day. Small, frequent, nutritionally dense meals and snacks should be provided. It is important to assess the condition of the teeth and ensure dentures fit well. During later stages of dementia, individuals may need to be reminded to open the mouth and chew. Food should be soft and cut in small pieces. Thin liquids may become difficult to swallow, so serving gelatins, pudding, or ice cream may decrease problems with liquid intake. Coughing during meals is a sign of swallowing difficulties; referral to a speech therapist is recommended.

Mental Interventions. Reality orientation supports failing memory in early stages of dementia and preserves independent functioning for a longer duration. Although written messages and signs may become meaningless to individuals with advancing dementia, pictures often evoke a response. Persons in all stages of dementia benefit from the use of clocks, calendars, and mementos placed in their environment. As the disease progresses, daily orientation to caregivers and daily tasks improves the productivity and responses of older adults with altered thought processes.

Behavioral Interventions. Behaviors are a form of communication and may be the cognitively impaired client's primary method of communicating needs; therefore recognizing behaviors may be the first step in ensuring that appropriate care is provided. Disruptive behaviors are a result of the disease, not a deliberate action on the part of the older person. The caregiver must realize that the patient cannot control the behaviors and cannot be taught to change. The person demonstrating the symptoms may be unaware of their effect on others, while the family or other people involved may be more sensitive to the behaviors. It is important for care providers to learn what to expect as the older person's disease progresses. The effective management of problem behaviors should focus not on trying to change the older person, but on modifying factors that may contribute to these behaviors. Careful and creative observation may identify the message in the behavior and provide opportunities for behavioral intervention (Sutor, Rummans, and Smith, 2001). Various behavior problems, possible antecedents, and strategies specific to these antecedents are listed in Table 29-5.

Because of the potential side effects of pharmacologic interventions, behavioral techniques should be the first line of treatment for older adults with altered thought processes. Use of physical or chemical restraints has demonstrated no benefit in controlling disruptive behaviors or managing disease. Unless the behaviors are upsetting or dangerous, learning how to adjust when these occur will probably result in a less stressful environment.

Social Interventions. Maintaining social interaction and human contact in a variety of ways is beneficial for older persons with cognitive decline. It provides the much needed opportunity for participation in activities that prevent boredom and restlessness. The response from an older adult will be positive if he or she is provided the opportunity to experience success and contribute in a positive way.

Family Interventions. In cases of clients with severe dementing disease, caregivers have been described as the hidden victims of illness. It is important to provide social and emotional support to the family members caring for the individual with cognitive disorders. Day-to-day problems such as

TABLE 29-5 Behavioral Management Techniques

BEHAVIOR	POTENTIAL CAUSES OR ANTECEDENTS	MANAGEMENT STRATEGIES
Wandering	Stress—noise, clutter, crowding	Reduce excessive stimulation
	Lost—looking for someone or something familiar	Provide familiar objects, signs, pictures; offer to help find objects or place; reassure
	Restless, bored—no stimuli	Provide meaningful activity
	Medication side effect	Monitor, reduce, or discontinue medication
	Lifelong pattern of being active or usual coping style	Respond to underlying mood or motivation; provide safe area to move about (e.g., secured circular path)
	Needing to use the toilet	Institute toileting schedule (such as every 2 hr); place signs or pictures on bathroom door
	Environmental stimuli—exit signs, people leaving	Remove or camouflage environmental stimuli; provide identification or alarm bracelets
Difficulty with personal care tasks	Task too difficult or overwhelming	Divide task into small, successive steps
	Caregiver impatience, rushing	Be patient, allow ample time, or try again later
	Cannot remember task	Demonstrate action or task; allow patient to perform parts of the task that can still be accomplished
	Pain involved with movement	Treat underlying condition; consider pain medication or physiotherapy; modify or assist the movement needed
	Cannot understand or follow caregiver instructions	Repeat request simply; state instructions 1 step at a time
	Fear of task—cannot understand need for task or instructions	Reassure, comfort, distract from task with music or conversation; ask patient to help perform task
	Inertia, apraxia; difficulty initiating and completing a task	Set up task sequence by arranging materials (such as clothing) in the order to be used; help begin the task
Suspiciousness, paranoia	Forgot where objects were placed	Offer to help find; have more than 1 of same object available; have a list where objects should be placed; learn favorite hiding places
	Misinterpreting actions or words	Do not argue or try to reason; do not take personally; distract
	Misinterpreting who people are; suspicious of their intentions	Introduce self and role routinely; draw on old memory, connections; do not argue
	Change in environment or routine	Reassure, familiarize, set routine
	Misinterpreting environment	Assess vision, hearing; modify environment as needed; explain misinterpretation simply; distract

Continued

TABLE 29-5 Behavioral Management Techniques—cont'd

BEHAVIOR	POTENTIAL CAUSES OR ANTECEDENTS	MANAGEMENT STRATEGIES
Suspiciousness, paranoia (cont'd)	Physical illness	Evaluate medically
	Social isolation	Encourage and provide familiar social opportunities
	Someone actually taking something from the patient	Verify the situation
Agitation (also "sundowning," catastrophic reactions)	Discomfort, pain	Assess and manage sources of pain, constipation, infection, or full bladder; check clothing for comfort
	Physical illness (such as urinary tract infection)	Evaluate medically; eliminate caffeine and alcohol
	Fatigue	Schedule adequate rest; monitor activity
	Overstimulation—noise, overhead paging, people, radio, television, activities	Reduce noise, stress; remove from situation: use television sparingly; limit crowding (e.g., dining hallways just before meals)
	Mirroring of caregiver's affect	Control affect; model calm with low tone and slow rate; use support system and groups for outlet
	Overextending capabilities (resulting in failure); caregiver expectations too high	Do not put in failure-oriented situations or tasks; understand losses and reduce expectations accordingly
	Patient is being "quizzed" (multiple questions that exceed abilities)	Avoid persistent testing of memory; pose 1 question at a time; eliminate questions that require abstract thought, insight, or reasoning
	Medication side effect	Assess, monitor, and reduce medication if possible; monitor health concerns
	Patient is thwarted from desired activity (e.g., attempting to escape)	Redirect energy to similar activity; ask patient to help with meaningful activity; have diversionary tactics for outbursts; choose battles—assess whether behavior is merely irritating, rather than compromising patient safety or obstructing care
	Lowered stress threshold	Simplify tasks, create calm; lower expectations and demands; avoid arguments and reprimands
	Unfamiliar people or environment; change in schedule or routine	Be consistent; avoid changes, surprises; make change gradually
	Restless	Plan calming music, massage, or meaningful activities; assign tasks that provide exercise
Incontinence	Infection, prostate problem, chronic illness, medication side effect, stress or urge incontinence	Evaluate medically
	Difficulty in finding bathroom	Place signs, picture on door; ensure adequate lighting
	Lack of privacy	Provide for privacy
	Difficulty undressing	Simplify clothing, use elastic waistbands
	Difficulty in seeing toilet	Use contrasting colors on toilet and floor
	Impaired mobility	Evaluate medically, treat associated pain (include physiotherapy); provide a commode; reduce diuretics when possible
	Dependence created by socialized reinforcement	Provide increased attention for continence rather than incontinence; allow independence when possible, even if time-consuming
	Cannot express need	Schedule toileting (such as every 2 hr while awake); reduce diuretics and bedtime liquids when possible
	Task overwhelming	Simplify; establish step-by-step routine

Continued

TABLE 29-5 Behavioral Management Techniques—cont'd

BEHAVIOR	POTENTIAL CAUSES OR ANTECEDENTS	MANAGEMENT STRATEGIES
Sleep disturbance	Illness, pain, medication effect (e.g., causing daytime sleepiness or nocturnal awakening)	Evaluate medically
	Depression	Prescribe antidepressant (consider bedtime sedative such as trazodone)
	Less need for sleep	Schedule later bedtime; allow activities or tasks safely done at night; plan more daytime exercise
	Too hot, too cold	Adjust temperature
	Disorientation from darkness	Use night-lights
	Caffeine or alcohol effect	Reduce or eliminate alcohol; limit caffeine after noon
	Hunger	Provide nighttime snack
	Urge to void	Ensure clear, well-lit pathway to bathroom
	Normal age- and disease-related fragmentation of sleep (like that of an infant or toddler)	Accept; plan for safety
	Daytime sleeping	Eliminate or limit naps, provide activity and exercise instead; for naps, use recliner rather than bed
	Fear of darkness; restless	Provide soft music, massage, night-light
Inappropriate or impulsive sexual behavior	Dementia-related decreased judgment and social awareness	Do not overreact or confront; respond calmly and firmly; distract and redirect
	Misinterpreting caregivers interaction	Do not give mixed sexual message (double entendres and innuendos—even in jest); avoid nonverbal messages; distract while performing personal care, bathing
	Uncomfortable—too warm, clothing too tight; need to void; genital irritation	Check room temperature; assist with comfortable weather-appropriate clothing; ensure that elimination needs are met; examine for groin rash, perineal skin problems, stool impaction
	Need for attention, affection, intimacy	Increase or meet basic need for touch and warmth; model appropriate touch; offer soothing objects (such as stuffed animals); provide hand or back massage
	Self-stimulating, reacting to what feels good	Offer privacy; remove from inappropriate place

From Carlson DL et al: Management of dementia-related behavioral disturbances: a nonpharmacologic approach, *Mayo Clin Proc* 70:1108, 1995.

finances, legal obligations, household chores, self-care needs, troublesome behaviors, and interpersonal conflicts are just a sampling of the difficulties that must be managed. Involving the family in care planning for a family member with dementia assists in family member adjustment and support.

Family members do not always understand role changes and expectations associated with caring for a loved one with a cognitive disorder. One of the most important issues faced is the loss of autonomy, not only for the older person, but also for the caregiver. The encouragement and support of family members are critical to the motivation of a disabled older person. Adjusting to the fact that dementia is irreversible and prolonged places families in situations of dealing with grief over a long period. Nurses need to assist family members in understanding and accepting that each person manages feelings differently. With this understanding, family members can serve as a strong support through the adjustment process.

In addition to client assessment, the nurse must also assess the caregiver's physical health, functional status, medication regimen, nutritional status, and exercise patterns, although these may be assessed informally. The information obtained from this assessment may identify factors contributing to the caregiver's general well-being. Nurses need to encourage caregivers to take time out from their task and participate in self-care and health promotion activities. Referrals to social support groups such as dementia and Alzheimer's support groups may also be beneficial for caregivers and family members.

Environmental Interventions. Individuals with dementia often have difficulty processing information, and the overloading of senses may cause confusion and anxiety. It is essential to consider the visual, auditory, olfactory, and tactile characteristics of the environment to make it more pleasant to the patient (Rasin and Barrick, 2004). Changes in the environment, routines, or setting may exacerbate negative behaviors in individuals with a cognitive disorder. Mealtime, bath time, and activities should be predictable. Consistency is essential when identifying strategies for environmental modification. It is essential to create a feeling of security for the older adult with altered thought processes, but routines should not become so rigid that changes will not be accepted.

Certain routines, such as sitting next to the same person during mealtime or having the same caregiver, are comforting. Changes in the routine should be introduced slowly and a stimulus provided to ensure that feelings of comfort and security are not lost. Environmental modifications may be required to provide security and safety as the disease progresses. Examples of environmental modifications include decreasing stimuli by using soft colors and limiting obstacles. Eliminating access to unsafe locations and unnecessary noises in the environment also may help in managing disruptive behaviors.

Safety and Self-esteem Interventions. The impaired judgment, unpredictable behavior, and decreased cognitive ability in individuals diagnosed with dementia usually lead to job loss if they are working, sometimes even before there is a diagnosis and understanding of what is causing the problem. This will have a negative effect on their financial status and self-esteem, and may psychologically inhibit the person from using preserved abilities. Self-esteem, independence, and autonomy are also affected when the individual with dementia must give up driving for reasons of safety. Wandering can sometimes be managed through environmental changes such as fences or alarm systems and close supervision (Yeaworth, 2002).

Evaluation

Evaluation is a continual process when caring for individuals with altered thought process related to cognitive decline. Behaviors and activities require ongoing assessment to determine variances from the baseline. Careful observation and recording of moods, behaviors, and memory provide clues to minor changes in the individual's condition. Interventions should be evaluated on an ongoing basis for efficacy. Successful and unsuccessful interventions should be communicated to other caregivers and family members to aid in continuity of care.

CHALLENGES IN THE CARE OF OLDER ADULTS WITH COGNITIVE DISORDERS

Individuals with cognitive disorders react differently to those disorders. Because it is difficult to predict these reactions, nurses must be aware of the possible emotional, behavioral, and physical challenges they may face when caring for older persons with cognitive disorders. As a case manager and educator, the nurse also must teach family members and caregivers about potential challenges and introduce a variety of methods for facing these challenges.

Sundown Syndrome

Sundown syndrome is a commonly observed tendency for people with dementia to become more confused and agitated around late afternoon to nightfall. Sundown syndrome may resemble delirium. Along with depleted cognition, other symptoms such as reduced attention, altered sleeping and waking patterns, and disturbed psychomotor behavior are present, and these symptoms tend to be more evident in the evening. There is no specific cause for the occurrence of sundown syndrome; however, some have hypothesized that sundowning may be the result of neurologic damage making it impossible for the demented individual to clearly interpret environmental stimuli. Specific pathophysiologic findings that relate to sundown syndrome behaviors include disturbance in REM sleep, episodes of sleep apnea, and deterioration of the suprachiasmatic nucleus of the hypothalamus.

Sundown syndrome may also be modified through behavioral interventions, including redirection, the provision of companionship and empathy, environmental modifications in lighting, and noise reduction. Because the cause of sundowning may be different for each client, individualized care is essential. The first step in the management of sundowning behavior includes the identification and treatment of any physiologic factors that may be contributing to those behaviors. These may include hunger, thirst, pain, and elimination needs. Nonpharmacologic management strategies for sundown syndrome include:

- Scheduling appointments and activities earlier in the day when the individual is rested
- Reducing environmental stimulation as the day progresses
- Providing activities that are calming in the evening, such as playing soft music
- Increasing lighting levels: turning on room lights before dusk and providing a nightlight at bedtime
- Offering companionship and reassurance during the evening hours
- Providing 1-hour rest periods in either the late morning or the early afternoon

Medication management of these behaviors should be avoided unless the older person is a danger to self or others. If nonpharmacologic interventions are unsuccessful, low doses of specific neuroleptic agents may be indicated.

Wandering

Wandering behaviors have been described as one of the most challenging behaviors to manage in older persons with cognitive impairments. A review of the literature by Lai and Arthur (2003) found the typical wanderer to be a relatively young member of the older population, more cognitively impaired, and more likely to be male. Wanderers might have experienced sleep problems, had a more active lifestyle in their younger years, and used more psychotropic medications within their lifetime. They may wander in response to a need to use the bathroom or to combat boredom.

Some nonpharmacologic interventions for wandering behaviors include:

- Ensuring an environment safe for wandering
- Informing neighbors and police of this potential problem
- Having the person wear a medical alert bracelet
- Observing potential wandering trigger behaviors
- Maintaining a regular activity and exercise program for individuals prone to wandering behavior

Paranoia or Suspiciousness

Paranoid or suspicious behaviors may reflect an individual's basic insecurity about his or her progressive memory and sensory losses. Individuals with dementia may forget where they placed an item and then become suspicious of others and accuse them of stealing that item. Paranoia may occur in response to sensory deficits. As individuals observe others talking but are unable to hear what is being said, they may fear that others are talking about them and cling to or hoard objects, fearing they will be stolen. Nonpharmacologic interventions for suspicious or paranoid behavior include:

- Securing valuables in locked locations
- Avoiding the use of confrontation and the application of logic
- Looking in wastebaskets before emptying
- Not whispering or behaving in a secretive manner
- Marking all personal items with that individual's name

Hallucinations and Delusions

Hallucinations experienced by individuals with dementia are most often visual, but may be auditory. Medical causes of hallucinations should be evaluated, since issues such as overmedication, toxicity, fever, infection, or a combination of causes may trigger this response. If the hallucination is disturbing to the older person, offering protection and security may help calm him or her. Reasoning or logic is ineffective. Delusions occur when an individual believes something to be true when it is illogical or wrong. Depending on the stage of the disease, reality orientation may be appropriate. If the disease has progressed, it may be best to go along with the individual's reality, but attempt to change disturbing behaviors regarding the situation. Behavior modification is the treatment of choice in the management of both hallucinations and delusions; however, if these symptoms place an individual at risk, a short course of an antipsychotic medication may be necessary.

Catastrophic Reactions

Catastrophic reactions are defined as emotional outbursts or overreaction toward minor stresses. These may be precipitated by emotional and sensory overload and aggravated by fatigue, overstimulation, inability to meet expectations, or misinterpretation of actions or words. Signs of impending reaction might include restlessness or refusals to carry out tasks. Nurses and caregivers must assess the environment for potential triggers and remove these triggers. Nonpharmacologic interventions useful in dealing with catastrophic reactions include:

- Removing the individual from the environment where the reaction is occurring
- Providing a calming atmosphere to distract the individual
- Using a calm tone of voice, touch, and reassurance
- Temporarily separating the individual from the causative source

Resources

Physical and mental strain placed on caregivers can be significantly reduced if available resources are identified and used. Community resources become increasingly important as the primary caregiver grows more isolated and overextended. The nurse should identify appropriate community resources available to the client and family and encourage family members to participate as the need becomes critical. These resources may include community mental health centers, adult day care centers, respite services, local Alzheimer's Associations and support groups, medical information and referral programs, and other family support groups specific to the disease type.

Family Support Groups. There has been a significant increase in family support groups providing a network to help families faced with caring for a loved one with dementia. These support groups offer a variety of services ranging from assisting family members in coping with the inevitable losses faced by victims of dementia to emotional support and respite.

Respite Services. Respite is a service provided to family members requiring occasional relief from the pressures of continuous caregiving. Respite services may prevent premature institutionalization of individuals with dementia because of caregiver stress. Respite programs offer relief services ranging from several hours to several weeks. Shared respite care is a form of respite available in some communities where a number of families join together to provide care on a rotating basis. Shared respite family members may watch over a group of clients, which allows free time for other families. Caring for loved ones in the company of others may reduce the social isolation experienced by caregivers.

Adult Day Care. Adult day care centers help keep people with dementia in the community by providing family respite, promoting activity, and encouraging the retention of previously learned skills. Some centers provide specialized social work, nursing, or physical and occupational therapy services. Adult day care centers allow family members to work during the day, do errands, rest, and yet be involved in important areas of their loved ones' lives.

Home Health Care. Home health care can provide nursing, physical and occupational therapies, social workers, and personal care services to clients in their homes in the later stages of dementia. Home health personnel can help with direct care needs, including meals and shopping, medications, cleaning, laundry, transportation, appraisal of a person's condition, and companionship. Unless the individual has skilled nursing or therapy needs, these services are not covered by Medicare.

Legal Services. Legal services are necessary when family members must consider questions related to the person's ability to handle finances and to make decisions. It is important to set up a durable power of attorney for financial matters and a health care proxy for medical matters early in the disease process while the individual can still participate in decision making. Legal guardianship is granted when individuals are no longer capable of making decisions for themselves. This requires that a physician or mental health professional document that the client does not understand the ramifications of decisions or behaviors.

Community Mental Health Centers. Community mental health centers may have specialized geriatric programs, which provide a wide range of services. These services may include comprehensive assessment; psychiatric evaluations; and individual, group, and family counseling. In addition, case management services available in community mental health centers may assist in the identification of other community resources to maintain individuals in the home.

Psychiatric Hospitals. Psychiatric hospitals offer assessment and behavior stabilization. In addition, an increasing number of geriatric psychiatric units can meet the multidimensional physiologic and mental health needs of older adults with cognitive disorders. Psychiatric hospital placement usually occurs when an individual cannot be managed in the community setting and more advanced assessment and behavior management techniques are required. Outcomes of geriatric psychiatric hospital placements may include medication management and behavior modification therapies for the individual's return to the community or may result in long-term care placement.

OTHER COMMON PROBLEMS AND CONDITIONS

Parkinson's Disease

PD is the most common form of parkinsonism (parkinsonian syndrome). PD is a commonly occurring, progressive degenerative disorder of the basal ganglia involving the dopaminergic nigrostriatal pathway (Lewis, Heitkemper, and Dirksen, 2004). PD is characterized by a slowing in the initiation and execution of movement (bradykinesia), increased muscle tone (rigidity), tremor at rest, and impaired postural reflexes (Lewis, Heitkemper, and Dirksen, 2004).

The prevalence of PD is about 160 per 100,000 persons and the incidence is about 20 per 100,000 persons. The risk of PD increases with age, with peak onset in the sixth decade. There is a decline in the incidence of PD after 70 to 75 years of age (Diederich et al, 2003). Onset of PD before the age of 50 is more likely related to a genetic defect. PD is more common in men by a ratio of 3:2 (Lewis, Heitkemper, and Dirksen, 2004), and is second only to stroke as the most common neurologic impairment in older adults.

Motor activity occurs as a result of the integrated actions originating from the cerebral cortex, basal ganglia, and cerebellum. The main area in the brain affected by PD is the basal ganglia. The basal ganglia are a group of neurons located deep within the cerebrum near the lateral ventricles. The basal ganglia control both muscle tone and the process of voluntary movement. This is accomplished through the secretion of the excitatory neurotransmitter acetylcholine (ACh) and the inhibitory neurotransmitter dopamine. Dopamine is a neurotransmitter produced in the substantia nigra and in the adrenal glands. It is then transmitted to the basal ganglia when needed. ACh is produced in the basal ganglia and transmits excitatory messages throughout this area. Dopamine inhibits the function of ACh in the basal ganglia in order to control fine and voluntary movements. Therefore it is the dopaminergic-cholinergic balance that produces normal motor function (Fig. 29-7).

In PD, degeneration of the dopaminergic nigrostriatal pathway causes dopamine depletion in the basal ganglia,

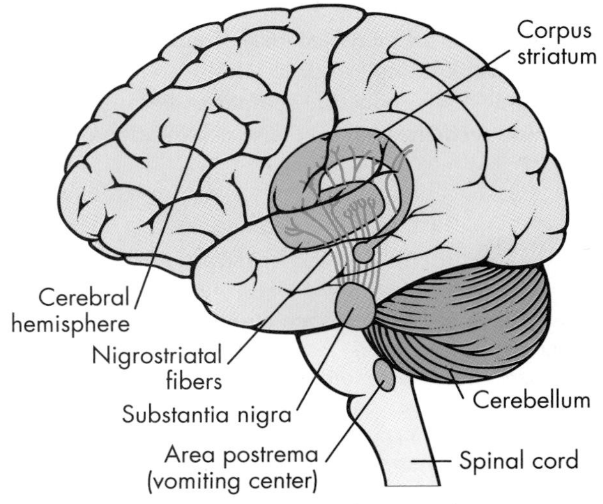

Fig. 29-7 Nigrostriatal disorders producing parkinsonism. (From Lewis SM, Heitkemper MM, Dirksen SR: *Medical surgical nursing: assessment and management of clinical problems*, ed 6, St Louis, 2004, Mosby.)

while the ACh-secreting neurons remain active. This creates an imbalance between excitatory and inhibitory neural activity in neurotransmitters and is the cause of symptoms such as hypertonia (tremor and rigidity) and akinesia in PD.

Risk Factors. PD is an idiopathic syndrome. There is an autosomal-dominant form of parkinsonian syndrome related to a genetic defect of chromosome 4. Environmental factors contributing to PD include postencephalitic parkinsonism, drug-induced weq, toxin-induced parkinsonian syndrome, exposure to agriculture pesticides and herbicides, and trauma to the midbrain. Other related causes include hydrocephalus, hypoxia, infections, stroke, tumor, and traumas (Black, Hawks, and Hogan, 2005).

Clinical Manifestations. Signs and symptoms begin subtly and include manifestations such as fatigue and a slight resting tremor. These may be the only initial symptoms. In a small portion of individuals, dementia may be the presenting symptom. The classic manifestations of PD are tremors at rest, muscle rigidity, bradykinesia, and postural abnormalities.

Balance in PD is affected by postural changes. Individuals with PD may have difficulty getting out of a chair, walking backward, or maneuvering in tight spaces. Fear of falling is a common complaint. Gait changes occur due to the postural changes and a decrease in autonomic balancing reflexes. Common problems with postural and gait changes include festinating gait, freezing, propulsive gait, and retropulsion (Box 29-7).

Muscle rigidity also affects the eyes, mouth, and voice and contributes to the staring gaze. These manifestations may develop alone or in combination. As the disorder progresses, more manifestations become apparent, including uncoordinated movements; short stepped, shuffling, and propulsive gait, which leads to increased risk of falls; postural disturbance; and trunk tilting forward.

Autonomic-neuroendocrine symptoms become noticeable and include seborrhea, an excessive perspiration of face and neck with the absence of perspiration on trunk and extremities. Heat intolerance, constipation, anxiety, depression, sleep disturbances, and dysphagia (difficulty swallowing) are also neuroendocrine manifestations of PD. The course of the disorder is slowly progressive. The person becomes more rigid and more disabled, eventually requiring full assistance with ADLs.

BOX 29-7 Terms for Parkinson's Disease

- **Festinating gait:** occurs when the individual can only take small short steps
- **Freezing:** a phenomenon where the individual appears to be glued to the floor, unable to move
- **Propulsive gait:** occurs when an individual begins walking, then starts running forward, unable to stop until he or she falls or runs into something
- **Retropulsion:** similar to propulsive gait, but the individual is walking and falling backward instead of forward

Diagnostic Studies. No specific studies can be used to diagnose PD. The diagnosis is based primarily on the clinical features of the disorder. Some of the diagnostic and laboratory studies used to assist in the identification of PD include a CBC, which may show anemia. Chemistry profile may show low albumin and protein. Drug screens may be done to rule out toxic causes of the symptoms. An EEG may show a slow pattern and disorganization of electrical activity in the brain. An upper gastrointestinal series may show delayed emptying, distention, and megacolon. A video fluoroscopy may show a slowed response of the cricopharyngeal muscles when swallowing. A diagnosis of PD is confirmed when the individual's symptoms improve with antiparkinsonian drugs (Black, Hawks, and Hogan, 2005; Lewis, Heitkemper, and Dirksen, 2004).

Management. Treatment is aimed at relieving clinical manifestations, increasing the individual's ability to perform ADLs, and decreasing the risk for injury. This is accomplished through the use of medications, surgery, and rehabilitation aimed at optimizing functional level. A team approach is essential to high-quality care of PD clients.

Medication. Medications are used primarily to relieve the symptoms associated with PD. Medications used include monoamine oxidase (MAO) inhibitors, which are used as adjunct therapy; dopaminergics, used to provide dopamine to the basal ganglia; dopamine agonists, used to activate dopamine in the CNS; and anticholinergics, used to block the release of ACh. A new class of drug called catechol *O*-methyltransferase inhibitors can be given with dopaminergics to increase availability of dopamine in the brain (Black, Hawks, and Hogan, 2005). Table 29-6 lists drugs used to treat PD. Unfortunately; these drugs eventually lose their effectiveness. The fluctuating response of individuals to antiparkinsonian drugs is called the on-off response. Antidepressants, especially amitriptyline, are used to treat depression often associated with PD. Propranolol may be used to treat tremors.

Surgical Therapy. Surgical procedures to alleviate symptoms of PD are used in clients who have not responded to medication therapy. The surgical procedures fall into three categories: ablation (destruction), deep brain stimulation (DBS), and transplantation. The ablative and DBS procedures work by reducing the increased neural activity produced by dopamine depletion. Transplantation of fetal neural tissue is designed to provide dopamine-producing cells in the brain of clients with PD. This procedure is still in its experimental phase (Lewis, Heitkemper, and Dirksen, 2004).

TABLE 29-6 Drugs Used to Treat Parkinson's Disease

DRUG CLASSIFICATION AND EXAMPLE	ACTION	INDICATIONS	COMMON SIDE EFFECTS	NURSING IMPLICATIONS
ANTICHOLINERGICS				
Trihexyphenidyl (Artane) Benztropine (Cogentin) Procyclidine (Kemadrin) Ethopropazine (Parsidol)	Inhibit action of endogenous acetylcholine and muscarine agonists to block the excitatory effect of the cholinergic system	Tremor, rigidity, drooling	Dry mouth, constipation, blurred vision, confusion, hallucinations	Usually contraindicated in clients with acute-angle glaucoma and tachycardia; monitor pulse and blood pressure during periods of dosage adjustment; administer with meals; do not withdraw medication suddenly
ANTIHISTAMINES				
Diphenhydramine (Benadryl)	Mild anticholinergic	Tremor, rigidity, insomnia,	Dry mouth, lethargy, confusion	Use with caution in clients with seizures, hypertension, hyperthyroidism, heart and renal disease, and diabetes; administer with meals or antacids
DOPAMINERGICS				
Amantadine (Symmetrel)	Cause release of dopamine in central nervous system	Rigidity, bradykinesia	Dizziness, ataxia, insomnia, leg edema	Monitor client for postural hypotension; do not administer at bedtime
Carbidopa-levodopa		Tremor, rigidity, bradykinesia	Orthostatic hypotension, nausea, hallucinations, dystonia, dyskinesia	Monitor blood pressure; use elastic stockings to increase venous return; monitor client for urinary retention
DOPAMINE AGONISTS				
Bromocriptine (Parlodel)	Activate dopamine receptors in the central nervous system	Fluctuation of manifestations, dyskinesia, dystonia	Hallucinations, mental fogginess, orthostatic hypotension, confusion	Monitor blood pressure and mental status
Pergolide (Permax)			Orthostatic hypotension, nausea, insomnia	Monitor blood pressure; do not administer at bedtime
COMT				
Tolcapone	Enhance effect of dopamine	Adjuvant treatment	Diarrhea, elevated liver enzymes	Monitor liver enzymes
Encapone	Enhance effect of dopamine	Adjuvant treatment	Nausea, headache	Monitor for levodopa side effects
MAO INHIBITORS				
Selegiline (Deprenyl)*	Inhibit monoamine oxidase B, an enzyme that converts chemical by-products in the brain into neurotoxins that prevent substantia nigra cell death	Adjuvant treatment	Nausea, dizziness, confusion, hallucinations, dry mouth	Monitor for levodopa side effects, as selegiline may increase effect of levodopa

From Black JM, Hawks JH, Hogan MA: *Medical-surgical nursing: clinical management for positive outcome,* ed 7, Philadelphia, 2005, Saunders.
COMT, Catechol *O*-methyltransferase; *MAO,* monoamine oxidase.
*One study showed that levodopa in combination with selegiline provided no clinical benefit over levodopa alone in treating early, mild Parkinson's disease. Moreover, mortality was significantly higher when these two drugs were used together.

NURSING MANAGEMENT

Diagnosis

Priority nursing diagnoses for a client with PD include:

- Impaired physical mobility
- Impaired verbal communication
- Altered nutrition: less than body requirements
- High risk for injury

Planning and Expected Outcomes

Expected outcomes for a client with PD include:

1. Client will maintain an effective communication pattern.
2. Client will maintain physical functioning and mobility and will not sustain injury.
3. Client will maintain effective coping by demonstrating use of coping strategies that enhance individual and family functioning.
4. Client will maintain socialization by participation in activities.
5. Client will verbalize satisfactory effects from medications and safely manage the medication schedule.

The care planning and expected outcomes for a client with PD frequently need revision because of changes in the client's status.

Intervention

Nursing care includes teaching clients the importance of performing active range-of-motion exercises twice a day, walking at least 4 times a day, and using assistive device when recommended to prevent injury associated with falls. Because PD leads to rigidity of the facial muscles, mouth, and general function of individuals, assessment of communication skills, speech, and writing is needed.

Consultation with a speech pathologist may be necessary if the client develops dysphagia. Assessment of nutritional status and self-feeding abilities is crucial to prevent aspiration, respiratory complication, and nutritional imbalance. Nurses are also responsible for monitoring the intake of foods high in bulk and fluids.

Client education includes:

- Teaching preventive measures for malnutrition, falls and other environmental hazards, constipation, skin breakdown from incontinence, and joint contractures
- Teaching gait training and exercises for improving ambulation, swallowing, speech, and self-care

Referral to community agencies and resources is also helpful. Some of the resources specifically available to individuals and families affected by PD include the American Parkinson's Disease Association ([800] 223-2732), the National Parkinson Foundation ([800] 327-4545), the Parkinson's Disease Foundation ([800] 457-6676), and the United Parkinson Foundation ([312] 733-1893). Referral to appropriate Internet sites for further information is helpful as well. The nurse should encourage families and clients to communicate with their primary care provider when they have questions about their illness and encourage clients and their families to keep a diary to track symptoms, effects, and side effects of medications.

Evaluation

PD is a progressive terminal disease that has no cure at this time. Therefore the evaluation of nursing interventions should focus on maintenance of function and engagement in activities for as long as possible. Evaluation is based on documentation of achievement of expected outcomes, as evidenced by an older adult client exhibiting intact skin, appropriate body weight, effective communication, effective coping, and knowledge of appropriate self-care practices. Participation of family members in the continued care and rehabilitation is also noted. Specific problems are documented, as is any teaching.

Cerebrovascular Accident or Brain Attack

A CVA (stroke or brain attack) occurs when there is a disruption in the normal blood supply to the brain tissue. CVAs occur suddenly and produce focal neurologic deficits lasting more than 24 hours. They are medical emergencies that should be treated immediately to prevent permanent neurologic deficits and disability. A TIA consists of the same symptoms, but lasts less than 24 hours. Because of the significance of this attack on the brain, the duration of the symptoms are much less important than the cause of the event and actions to be taken to prevent a future attack (Elkin, 2003).

Stroke is the third leading cause of death and the most common cause of disability in the United States. In the past 20 years cases of CVA have decreased by 30%. A CVA may be caused by several pathologic changes. Eighty percent to eight-five percent of brain attacks (stroke) are due to brain ischemia. Of this number, 15% to 20% are divided between subarachnoid hemorrhage and primary intracerebral hemorrhage (Elkin, 2003). Hemorrhagic strokes are the leading risk factor for the development of seizures in older adults. An estimated 730,000 individuals develop stroke every year. In the United States there are an estimated 4.5 million stroke survivors.

Approximately 30% to 50% of those who survive a CVA are left with moderate to severe disability. Sixty percent to seventy-five percent of cases of CVA occur in individuals over the age of 65. Blacks are more likely than whites to have a stroke, perhaps because this population has a higher incidence of hypertension and diabetes. The incidence of stroke is greater in men than women.

In 1996 a national campaign was begun to increase public awareness of CVA (Black, Hawks, and Hogan, 2005; Elkin, 2003; Lewis, Heitkemper, and Dirksen, 2004; Urden, Stacey, and Lough, 2002). The National Institute of Neurologic

Disorders and Stroke (NINDS) conducted a study that was published in 1996 (Barson, 1997), which revolutionized the way we approach and treat acute ischemic stroke (AIS). The major accomplishment is the use of thrombolitic agents (recombinant tissue plasminogen activators [r-TPA]) within a 3-hour window of the onset of signs or symptoms in AIS. Findings from this study demonstrating decreased mortality and morbidity rates have ignited a campaign to make the public aware of the common signs and symptoms associated with "brain attack" and to activate the emergency system for prompt diagnosis and early treatment of stroke.

Cerebral infarctions are ischemic or hemorrhagic in origin. The brain is very sensitive to a decrease in blood supply. As a result, when cerebral blood flow is reduced to a level insufficient to maintain neuronal viability, it causes a state of hypoxia. This hypoxic state leads to tissue ischemia and injury. Short-term ischemias result in TIAs. Long-term ischemia leads to permanent infarction (death of cerebral cells). Cellular events that ensue as a result of the ischemia involve altered cell membrane. As a result, the polarization of the cell membrane changes, allowing an influx of calcium into the cell and altering cellular metabolism. Glutamate is then released, altering the cell's permeability to electrolytes. Electrolytes change the metabolic rate of the cell, leading to cellular acidosis, lactic acid production, vasodilation, and cellular hypoxia. Sustained anoxic events lead to infarct of brain tissue and irreversible neuronal injury. If an infarct occurs, the affected brain softens and liquefies.

The extent of brain infarction depends on factors such as location and size of an occluded vessel and the adequacy of the collateral circulation to the area supplied by the occluded vessel. Cell death and permanent changes can occur within 3 to 10 minutes of anoxia. The most common vessels for ischemic stroke are middle cerebral artery and vertebrobasilar artery (Black, Hawks, and Hogan, 2005). A mean arterial pressure of 50 mm Hg or less can affect brain perfusion.

Symptoms of thrombotic stroke can be sudden but typically progress gradually over minutes to hours. The development of thrombotic strokes causes a syndrome known as stroke-in-evolution. The completed stroke is a CVA that has reached its maximum damage in regards to causing neurologic deficits.

Risk Factors. The risk factors for the development of TIAs include inflammatory arterial disorders, sickle cell anemia, atherosclerotic changes in cerebral vessels, thrombosis, and emboli. An estimated 50,000 Americans a year experience TIAs. Recurrence of symptoms is 30% at 3 months, 60% at 6 months, and 80% at 1 year without definitive treatment. They are frequently precursors to a CVA (McCance and Huether, 2002).

CVAs are caused by two major pathologic events: ischemic and hemorrhagic stroke. Ischemic stroke can be further categorized as thrombotic, cardioembolic, and lacunar. The most common cause for ischemic strokes are atherosclerosis, inflammatory disease process, and a break from a thrombus outside the brain or in the cardiovascular system. Hemorrhagic strokes are divided into subarachnoid and intracerebral hemorrhages, according to site of the hemorrhage. The most common causes for hemorrhagic strokes are hypertension, ruptured aneurysm, vascular malformations, bleeding into a tumor, hemorrhage associated with bleeding disorders or anticoagulation, head trauma, and illicit drug use (McCance and Huether, 2002).

The incidence of deaths from stroke has gradually declined in many industrialized countries over the past 20 years. The aggressive campaign started by NINDS in 1996 to educate the general population regarding the risk factors and forms of prevention has played a pivotal role in decreasing the mortality rate.

Risk factors associated with CVA are nonmodifiable and modifiable. The nonmodifiable risk factors for CVA include gender, age, race, and heredity. Although changes cannot be made in these areas, awareness of the association of stroke could increase clients' involvement in the process of secondary prevention. Advanced age is one of the most significant risk factors for stroke. Modifiable risk factors include hypertension, diabetes mellitus, cardiovascular disease, nonvalvular atrial fibrillation, blood lipid abnormalities, smoking, substance abuse (particularly cocaine), obesity, a sedentary lifestyle, high stress levels, previous CVA or TIA, heavy alcohol use, and sudden discontinuation of antihypertensive medications (causes hemorrhagic stroke). Modifiable risk factors can be reduced or eliminated through lifestyle changes. Hypertension is the most important modifiable risk factor for both ischemic and hemorrhagic stroke. Table 29-7 summarizes the levels of prevention for stroke.

Clinical Manifestations. Specific clinical manifestations of a TIA vary, depending on the vessel involved, the degree of obstruction of the vessel, and collateral blood supply. If the carotid system is involved, the individual may experience blurred vision, gradual visual obstruction, flashes of light, and headaches. If the posterior system is involved, symptoms may include tinnitus, vertigo (dizziness), bilateral sensory and motor symptoms, diplopia, facial weakness, and ataxia.

Early warning signs for thrombotic stroke include transient hemiparesis, loss of speech, and paresthesias (abnormal sensations) involving one side of the body. These findings are referred to as TIAs. Common signs and symptoms that may precede cerebral hemorrhage in hypertensive clients include severe occipital or nuchal (back of neck) headache, vertigo or syncope (fainting), paresthesias, transient paralysis, epistaxis (nose bleed), and retinal hemorrhages.

Common findings that are seen with stroke include headache, vomiting, seizure, mental status changes (including coma), fever, and electrocardiogram (ECG) changes (T-wave changes, shortened P-R interval, prolonged Q-T

TABLE 29-7 Levels of Prevention for Stroke

LEVEL	PREVENTIVE STEPS
Primary prevention	Maintain ideal body weight. Manage of cholesterol levels. Stop smoking. Reduce alcohol consumption. Eliminate illicit drugs.
Secondary prevention	Tightly manage blood pressure. Effectively manage diabetes mellitus. Promptly treat cardiovascular disease, TIA, and atrial fibrillation.
Tertiary prevention	Initiate rehabilitation program early.

interval, premature ventricular contractions, sinus bradycardia, ventricular tachycardia, and supraventricular tachycardia).

Clinical manifestations vary according to cerebral vessel involved:

- Internal carotid: contralateral motor and sensory deficits of the arm, leg, and face. In dominant hemispheric CVA, aphasia. In nondominant hemispheric CVA, apraxia, agnosia, and unilateral neglect and homonymous hemianopia (loss of one half of the visual field in each eye).
- Middle cerebral artery: drowsiness, stupor, coma, contralateral hemiplegia and sensory deficits of arm and face, aphasia, and homonymous hemianopia can be seen.
- Anterior cerebral artery: contralateral weakness or paralysis and sensory loss of the foot and leg, loss of decision making and voluntary action abilities, and urinary incontinence.
- Vertebral artery: pain in face, nose, or eye; numbness or weakness of face on ipsilateral side; problems with gait; dysphagia; and dysarthria (difficulty speaking).

Diagnostic Tests. The characteristic feature of ischemic CVA is persistent clinical manifestations that last longer than 24 hours. Therefore prompt diagnosis and treatment play a pivotal role in decreasing the progression of the injury and complications or disabilities that ensue. With the advent of improved imaging technologies, an individual experiencing any significant manifestation will receive a noncontrast CT scan of the head, a standard MRI or a diffuse-weighted MRI, or diffuse-weighted imaging (DWI). The latter provides signs of the earliest changes associated with ischemia, even before injury or infarction occurs. This makes the DWI a valuable tool in the early detection and treatment of CVAs. DWIs performed with perfusion imaging can also improve precision of diagnosis.

Establishing an accurate diagnosis between hemorrhagic and ischemic stroke is vital. CT scan without contrast is the first step in trying to determine differences in stroke type. Because of the strong correlation between cardiovascular disease and stroke, an ECG is also essential. A chest x-ray study and cardiac monitoring are suggested to rule out cardioembolism or any coexisting conditions such as cardiomegaly associated with valvular disease. Additional studies that may be recommended include a hematologic function laboratory test, electrolytes, glucose levels, and liver and kidney function test. An EEG is done if the client has seizures, and a lumbar puncture is performed if subarachnoid hemorrhage is suspected but not seen in the CT scan.

Management

Medical and Pharmacologic Therapy. As a result of advancements in pharmacologic therapy, clients with ischemic stroke receive thrombolytic agents within 3 hours of the onset of the CVA (Adams et al, 1996; Urden, Stacey, and Lough, 2002). Confirmation of ischemic stroke with CT scan without contrast is essential before r-TPA can be used. NINDS has established exclusion criteria for r-TPA therapy for acute ischemic stroke (Box 29-8). The desired effect of this therapy is to dissolve the clot and reperfuse the compromised brain tissue.

BOX 29-8 Exclusion Criteria for Intravenous r-TPA Therapy for Acute Ischemic Stroke

- Current use of oral anticoagulant or prothrombin time >15 seconds
- Use of heparin in previous 48 hours and a prolonged partial thromboplastin time
- Platelet count < 100,000/mm^3
- Previous stroke or head injury within the past 3 months
- Major surgery within past 14 days
- Pretreatment systolic blood pressure > 185 mm Hg or diastolic blood pressure > 110 mm Hg
- Rapidly improving neurologic signs
- Isolated, mild neurologic deficits such as ataxia alone, sensory loss alone, dysarthria alone, or minimum weakness
- Prior intracranial hemorrhage
- History of urinary bleeding within past 21 days
- Recent myocardial infarction

Clients receiving r-TPA should not receive anticoagulants, antiplatelets, or any type of antithrombotic drug for at least 24 hours after treatment (Adams et al, 1996; Simon et al, 2004). Other drugs used to manage or treat ischemic stroke include anticoagulants (heparin) and antiplatelet therapy (enteric-coated aspirin). The goal of these drugs is to retard the growth of the clot.

Drugs used to treat complications associated primarily with hemorrhagic stroke include anticonvulsants (phenytoin [Dilantin]) and calcium channel blockers (nimodipine). Anticonvulsants help prevent or manage seizures that result from hemorrhagic stroke. Calcium channel blockers help decrease or prevent vasospasm associated with subarachnoid bleeding. Hypertension medications are used cautiously during the early stages of the stroke to prevent interference with compensatory mechanism resulting from the brain insult. If the client did not receive r-TPA, elevated blood pressure is treated to keep it below 180/105 mm Hg. The drug most commonly used in this situation is labetalol. If the blood pressure elevations persist, nitroprusside is used for short-term management. Osmotic diuretics may also be used to help manage increased intracranial cerebral pressure (ICP).

Surgical management includes:

- Endarterectomy
- Extracranial-intracranial bypass
- Management of arteriovenous malformation
- Management of cerebral aneurysms
- Management of intracranial bleeding and evacuation of hematomas

NURSING MANAGEMENT

Diagnosis

Nursing diagnoses for an older adult with a CVA include:

- Altered cerebral tissue perfusion related to hemorrhage and/or increased intracranial pressure
- Ineffective breathing pattern related to changes in mental status
- High risk for aspiration related to loss of muscle tone, airway protection, and dysphagia
- Impaired physical mobility related to arm and/or leg weakness or paralysis (hemiparesis or hemiplegia)
- Impaired verbal communication related to aphasia and dysarthria related to alteration in the speech center
- High risk for injury related to seizures or hemiplegia
- High risk for impaired skin integrity related to prolonged immobility
- Altered patterns of urinary elimination related to immobility
- Tactile and auditory sensory-perceptual alteration related to impaired proprioception and hearing loss
- Eating, bathing, dressing, and toileting self-care deficit related to impairments secondary to CVA
- Knowledge deficit: medication use, rehabilitation, and long-term care for CVA related to lack of exposure

Planning and Expected Outcomes

Outcomes for an older adult with a CVA include:

1. Client will not die.
2. Client will have minimum residual deficits and complications.
3. Client's increased ICP will be reduced.
4. Client will not suffer evolution, extension, or completion of the stroke.

Intervention

Initial nursing interventions include positioning the client at a 30- to 45-degree angle to prevent further elevation of ICP. This position also helps manage or protect the airway of a client with a neurologic deficit. Monitoring of vital signs assists the nurse in detecting signs of increased ICP and in effectively managing the blood pressure. The nurse is responsible for continuous monitoring for signs of complications such as hydrocephalus, vasospasm, and increased neurologic changes.

Additional nursing interventions include:

- Encourage active range of motion on unaffected side and passive range of motion on affected side.
- Turn client every 2 hours.
- Monitor lower extremities for thrombophlebitis resulting from immobilization.
- Encourage use of unaffected arm for ADLs.
- Teach client to put clothing on affected side first.
- Resume oral diet only after client has successfully completing a swallowing evaluation. The client may need thickened liquids or foods the consistency of oatmeal, and may need to chew on the unaffected side of the mouth. This is sometimes referred to as a dysphagia diet.
- Collaborate with occupational and physical therapists for rehabilitation.
- Try alternate methods of communication with clients who have aphasia.
- Teach client with homonymous hemianopia to adapt to the deficit by turning the head side to side to fully scan the visual field.

The nurse also needs to educate the client and family about:

- CVA and CVA prevention
- Community resources
- Physical care and need for psychosocial support
- Medications

Evaluation

Client progress occurs in small increments, and interventions are modified to assist clients in meeting their goals. Evaluation criteria include:

- Maintenance and improvement of cerebral tissue perfusion
- Avoidance of respiratory complications
- Prevention of aspiration from food, fluids, and secretions
- Prevention of contractures
- Prevention of edema in affected extremity
- Maintenance of skin integrity
- Achievement of independence
- Pain management
- Increased ability to communicate, express feelings, and understand others
- Prevention of fecal and urinary incontinence
- Establishment of normal voiding pattern
- Compensation for sensory deficits and physical and intellectual losses
- Participation by family members in rehabilitation process

Hypothermia and Hyperthermia in Older Adults

As aging occurs, thermoregulatory mechanisms undergo physiologic changes, placing the older individual at risk for inability to manage extreme temperatures. The hypothalamus is responsible for regulating the body temperature. Although no significant age-related changes occur in this organ, the hypothalamus depends on the sensorial functions to transmit sensory information. These sensory functions undergo changes with aging, and older persons may be unable to effectively manage changes in temperature.

Hypothermia. Hypothermia is defined as a core body temperature of less than 95° F (35° C). The two categories of hypothermia are primary and secondary. Primary, or exposure, hypothermia follows exposure to low temperature or immersion accidents with intact thermoregulation. Secondary hypothermia is most commonly seen in clients with chronic illnesses, alcohol or substance abuse, and extreme age (Kare and Shneiderman, 2001).

Hypothermia-related deaths in the United States occur in 0.3 out of 100,000 individuals. Approximately half these deaths occur in individuals over 65 years of age. The highest rate of death is in states with cold climate (Kare and Shneiderman, 2001).

At rest, an individual produce 40 to 60 kcal of heat per square meter of body surface area. Heat production increases with movement. Shivering increases the rate of heat production by 2 to 5 times. The body loses heat through a variety of mechanisms. Under dry conditions, heat is loss via radiation (55% to 65%). However, evaporation is the dominant mechanism of heat loss with medical alterations in the body, especially when the person is receiving drugs that hinder perspiration. Conduction and convection account for about 15% of heat loss, and respiration accounts for the remainder (Decker and Li, 2000). Changes in the environment drastically affect the way heat is loss. The hypothalamus controls the mechanism of thermoregulation, and alterations in the CNS may impair this mechanism.

Risk Factors. Primary hypothermia is due to environmental exposure, with no underlying medical conditions contributing to this process. Secondary hypothermia is associated with an underlying medical condition that prevents the body from conducting normal thermoregulation. The causes and risk factors include:

- Accidental immersion in cold water
- Exposure to cold temperature
- Drastic changes in the environmental temperature
- Alcohol and substance abuse
- Excessive heat loss or impaired production
- Burns, psoriasis or other desquamating skin condition that contributes to heat loss
- Surgery and trauma, especially cardiac surgery
- Nutritional deficiency
- Sepsis
- Spinal cord injury with poikilothermy
- Stroke
- Anoxia
- Uremia
- Hypoglycemia
- Adrenal insufficiency and hypothyroidism
- Drugs (benzodiazepines, opiates, alcohol, barbiturates, clonidine, and lithium)

Clinical Manifestations. In its early stages, hypothermia, like other conditions in older adults, presents in a nonspecific manner. Findings include fatigue, apathy, confusion, lethargy, shivering, numbness, slurred speech, impaired coordination, and possible coma. As the core temperature drops below 95° F (35° C), the individual's clinical picture starts to appear more like a disorder. For this reason, nurses need to become familiar with clinical manifestations of hypothermia in the elderly. Early signs of hypothermia include confusion, impaired gait, fatigue, lethargy, and combativeness. As the core temperature drops, the signs and symptoms worsen. When an older adult's temperature drops below 93° F (34° C), cardiac arrhythmias occur, particularly bradyarrhythmias, flattening of the T or P waves, and atrial fibrillation. Death is usually the result of lethal arrhythmias or respiratory arrest (Kare and Shneiderman, 2001). Peripheral vasoconstriction occurring with hypothermia may also lead to increases in kidney perfusion and a subsequent increase in urine output referred to as *cold diuresis*.

Diagnostic Findings. The most objective datum for the diagnosis of hypothermia is a measured core temperature of less than 95° F (35° C). In addition to physical findings, individuals may manifest changes in their acid-base balance. Initially the individual hyperventilates, which leads to respiratory alkalosis. As the hypothermia progresses, metabolic rate drops and metabolic and respiratory acidosis ensues. As a result of these stresses on the body, glucose and white blood cell levels become elevated. Coagulopathy can be seen as a result of prolonged hypothermia. Thyroid-stimulating hormone and corticotropin are also assessed. A toxicology screen is done to rule out the presence of opiates or illicit substances as the causative factor. Chest radiology is necessary to rule out patchy infiltrates or signs of pneumonia. A CT scan of the head is done to rule out concomitant conditions.

Management. The therapeutic management of hypothermia depends on the core temperature. If hypothermia is mild, passive external rewarming with insulated coverings and moving the older adult to a warm environment are indicated. Active external rewarming is useful in mild to moderate hypothermia without cardiac symptoms. This rewarming includes warming blankets, covering of the head, heating lamps, and warm water immersion. Moderate to severe hypothermia requires active core rewarming techniques such as warm intravenous fluids, warm humidified oxygen, and warm gastric and bladder irrigation. Peritoneal dialysis and pleural lavage are reserved for cases with cardiac instability (Kare and Shneiderman, 2001). In older clients with comorbid conditions, the mortality rate after moderate to severe hypothermia may be 50% or greater than in the general population, depending on the severity at presentation and the underlying disease (Kare and Shneiderman, 2001).

Hyperthermia. Hyperthermia is defined as a disorder that affects the thermoregulation mechanism where clients have a core body temperature greater than 105° F (40.6° C). Hyperthermia causes severe CNS dysfunction and hot, dry skin. The most severe and life-threatening heat illness in older persons is heat stroke. This condition is most often seen in debilitated individuals and usually presents differently from the exertional heat stroke seen in the young. The mortality rate in the older population with heat stroke may reach 70% if treatment is delayed more than 2 hours (Kare and Shneiderman, 2001).

To balance core temperature, the body should have the ability to produce and dissipate heat. Core heat develops as a result of cellular metabolism. When environmental temperature exceeds core temperature, the body's thermoregulation mechanism activates heat loss via dissipation. Dissipation occurs via the skin, one of the most important elements in body heat regulation (Simon, 1993).

In response to elevated core temperature, the hypothalamus activates efferent fibers of the autonomic nervous system to stimulate vasodilation of the skin vessels, which leads to perspiration. This form of heat dissipation is achieved via the convection and evaporation mechanisms. Heat in body can only be generated by activity occurring in the muscular system. To increase body temperature, the rate of heat production has to exceed the rate of heat loss. Consequently, hyperthermia occurs when excessive metabolic production of heat, excessive ambient heat, or inability to dissipate heat overwhelms the thermoregulatory mechanism.

Risk Factors. Risk factors leading to hyperthermia are either physiologic or environmental but usually work in combination. Older individuals are unable to increase their cardiac output for heat dissipation. This condition, together with poorly ventilated homes lacking air conditioning during heat waves, increases the probability for heat stroke. Combining environmental conditions with a sedentary lifestyle, disabilities, poor hydration, and prescription medications that impair the ability to tolerate heat (e.g., diuretics, antihypertensives, neuroleptics, and anticholinergics) can also hasten the development of heat stroke (Kare and Shneiderman, 2001). Additional factors that cause or predispose older adults to hyperthermia are:

- Disorders leading to excessive heat production
- Malignant hyperthermia associated with anesthesia
- Thyrotoxicosis (hormonal hyperthermia)
- Salicylic acid intoxication
- Delirium tremens
- Extensive use of occlusive clothing
- Dehydration
- CVA
- Alcohol abuse (ETOH)
- Heat syncope and heat exhaustion

Clinical Manifestations. Anhidrosis (lack of perspiration) is the most common manifestation in hyperthermia other than a core temperature greater than 105° F (40.6° C). Most of the clinical manifestations occur as a result of altered CNS function and range from confusion to coma. Additional neurologic signs of hyperthermia include hallucinations, combativeness, bizarre behaviors, and syncope. Extensive evaluation is required to rule out possible psychiatric alterations contributing to this phenomenon.

Management. It is important to monitor core temperature and perform complete neurologic and physical assessments in older persons with hyperthermia. The main objective is to bring the temperature down immediately. Interventions used to decrease body temperature include:

- Spraying or sponge bathing the individual with cool water (approximately 90° F [32° C])
- Placing a fan near the client to circulate cool air
- Decreasing the room temperature
- Placing ice packs on the groin and axilla together with cooling blankets

It is important for the nurse to use protective cream to prevent skin burn from the cooling blanket and to provide a lightweight gown and bed coverings for client. Bedrest should be maintained to decrease muscle activity and subsequent heat production. Antipyretic medications may be administered as ordered to facilitate client comfort. It is also essential to administer oral and intravenous fluid to maintain adequate hydration.

More invasive medical techniques used in the treatment of hyperthermia include peritoneal and gastric lavage with ice water. Precautions need to be taken before conducting these interventions. The airway needs to be protected and no surgery scheduled. Benzodiazepines may be used to manage shivering (Kare and Shneiderman, 2001). By understanding the risk factors for the development of thermoregulation disorders, the nurse is better equipped to develop strategies to prevent these alterations in older persons.

Home Care

1. Assess sensorimotor function. A decline in this function is the most notable change in older adults and may be the cause of other changes, such as slowed reaction time.
2. Memory impairment may compromise the teaching of homebound clients, requiring the nurse to use alternative approaches and to rely on family and significant others involved in caregiving.
3. Assess for signs of impaired emotional control, diminished initiative, withdrawal, or other changes, which may be initial signs of brain dysfunction.
4. Altered thought processes occur with cognitive decline or disturbances in cognitive function, both of which occur in homebound clients with dementia, depression, delirium, or amnesic disorders.
5. The effects of aging must be considered when interpreting laboratory tests and alerting physicians about abnormal results.
6. Instruct caregivers about dosages and side effects of medications, especially tranquilizers and antidepressants that are used in managing symptoms caused by dementia.
7. Instruct caregivers on methods to manage behavioral problems and caregiver stress.
8. Use social workers to assess community resources for caregivers and clients with dementia.
9. Assess the home environment of the older person with cognitive impairment for safety hazards, and provide caregivers with tips and strategies for reducing and eliminating the identified hazards.

SUMMARY

Many challenges face nurses caring for older adults, especially due to the continuing increase in this population group within the United States and other countries of the Western world. It has been found that a significant percentage of older adults suffer from some form of cognitive impairment, all of whom could benefit from nursing care focusing on the special needs of these people. Without radical changes in the way health care is allocated and delivered in this country, the issues of shrinking health care dollars, accessibility to care, and increasing commercially managed care could threaten the care of older adults. Those with cognitive impairment continue to be at high risk for limited access to appropriate and cost-effective care. This will become especially critical as more state mental health hospitals are closed without adequate community-based treatment facilities to replace them.

Cost-effective models for care should be developed and tested along the continuum of care from prevention of illness to management of acute illness, restoration of function and, finally, to staying in the home environment in the community. Also, most of the time older adults are less active participants in their own care. They trust and accept physician decisions and recommendations without question. This group needs extensive teaching to become informed consumers and partners in health care.

The practice of gerontologic nursing is collaborative and interdisciplinary in scope. This is necessitated by the vast complexity, diversity, an dissimilarity of older adults in terms of their physical and mental conditions, health care needs, past life experiences, current lifestyles, culture, ethnicity, and resources. The family is an extremely important aspect of gerontologic practice, not only because the majority of older adults live within a family setting, but also because the family is becoming a primary provider of care.

The most serious health problems occur in those more than 80 years old, and this group is likely to be cared for by relatives who are more than 65 years of age. The blend of medical-surgical, psychiatric, and community health nursing skills, and expertise required to care for older adults with cognitive impairments provides unique and unlimited opportunities and challenges in practice.

Key Points

- The nervous system is a network of complex structures that change as an individual ages.
- The loss of neurons is not as excessive in the process of aging as previous believed. In actuality, large neurons appear to shrink and few are lost.
- Normal aging is associated with changes in the ability to consciously learn and retain new information *easily*.
- The age-related neurodegenerative and neurochemical changes in the cerebellum are believed to be the underlying cause of decline in motor and cognitive function.
- Sleep disorders are common in aging individuals. Excessive daytime somnolence is not part of normal aging.
- Vision changes that occur with aging are significant. The lens of the eye thickens, becoming yellow, cloudy, and less elastic.
- Presbycusis is the hearing loss associated with the aging process.
- The loss of taste and smell receptors means that food is not appetizing to the older adult.
- It is important to include functional assessment as part of the assessment of older adults.
- Decline in cognitive function is an effect of disease, not an effect of the normal aging process.
- Depression may manifest itself through signs such as fatigue; constipation; psychomotor retardation; depressed mood; loss of interest, energy, libido, or pleasure; changes in appetite, weight, and sleep patterns; and agitation, anxiety, or crying.
- The risk factors for delirium include advanced age, CNS diseases, infection, polypharmacy, hypoalbuminemia, electrolyte imbalances, trauma history, gastrointestinal or

genitourinary disorders, cardiopulmonary disorders, and sensory changes.

- The treatment of delirium is focused on the identification and treatment of the underlying cause.
- Nonpharmacologic approaches for delirium may include removing bladder catheters, improving nutritional intake, using reality orientation, decreasing sensory overstimulation or deprivation, and reassuring the older adult and their family members.
- Dementia is a syndrome of gradual and progressive cognitive decline.
- Although dementia is more common in old age, it is not part of the normal aging process.
- From the time of diagnosis, individuals with AD survive about half as long as those of similar age without dementia.
- Ginkgo biloba, an herbal plant extract, has shown promise in stabilizing and occasionally improving cognitive performance and function in demented older adults for 6 months to a year.
- Management of AD focuses on maintaining cognitive and global function early on in the disease process to postpone the need for institutional care.
- Individuals who have experienced a CVA have an even greater risk of VaD.
- Older adults are at risk for the development of subdural hematomas because of brain atrophy and corresponding vascular changes that occur with normal aging and risk for falls and subsequent head injury.
- The only positive way to diagnose dementia-related disorders is brain tissue biopsy or autopsy of the brain.
- Antipsychotics are useful for the treatment of psychotic symptoms such as a delusions or hallucinations.
- When depression is a concern in a client who is agitated, SSRIs have been helpful in managing agitation.
- Nurses caring for older adults who have symptoms of an acute cognitive disorder need to support existing sensory perception until the cognitive state returns to the previous level of function.
- Public policy has shifted to encourage family members to care for older adults in their homes, thus decreasing health care costs and individualizing care to meet client needs.
- Nursing focus has shifted from the caregiver to care coordinator, teaching and assisting the family members with home care, providing supportive care, and serving as a client advocate.
- The purpose of a comprehensive assessment is to determine problem areas, as well as areas of strength, on which to base a care plan, including education of families and caregivers.
- Persons with cognitive disorders commonly demonstrate problematic behaviors.
- People who demonstrate symptoms of moderate to severe cognitive impairment may benefit from having meals in the same place at the same time each day.
- Persons in all stages of dementia benefit from the use of clocks, calendars, and mementos within the environment.
- The effective management of problem behaviors should focus not on trying to change the older person, but on modifying factors that may be contributing to these behaviors.
- Use of physical or chemical restraints has demonstrated no benefit in controlling disruptive behaviors or managing disease.
- Maintaining social interaction and human contact in a variety of ways is beneficial for older persons with cognitive decline.
- Changes in the routine should be introduced slowly and a stimulus provided to ensure that feelings of comfort and security are not lost.
- Wandering can sometimes be managed through environmental changes such as fences or alarm systems and close supervision.
- Sundown syndrome may also be modified through behavioral interventions, including redirection, the provision of companionship and empathy, and environmental modifications in lighting and noise reduction.
- PD, the most common form of parkinsonism, is a common progressive degenerative disorder of the basal ganglia involving the dopaminergic nigrostriatal pathway.
- A CVA occurs when there is a disruption in the normal blood supply to the brain tissue.
- Stroke is the third leading cause of death and the most common cause of disability in the United States.
- The major accomplishment is the use of thrombolytic agents (r-TPA) within a 3-hour window of the onset of the sign or symptom in AIS.
- Advanced age is one of the most significant risk factors for stroke.
- Modifiable risk factors include hypertension, diabetes mellitus, cardiovascular disease, nonvalvular atrial fibrillation, blood lipid abnormalities, smoking, substance abuse (particularly cocaine), obesity, a sedentary lifestyle, high stress levels, previous CVA or TIA, heavy alcohol use, and sudden discontinuation of antihypertensive medications.
- Hypertension is the most important modifiable risk factor for both ischemic and hemorrhagic stroke.
- As aging occurs, thermoregulatory mechanisms undergo physiologic changes, placing the older individual at risk for inability to manage extreme temperatures.
- Hypothermia is defined as a core body temperature of less than 95° F (35° C).
- Primary hypothermia is due to environmental exposure, with no underlying medical conditions contributing to this process.
- Secondary hypothermia is associated with an underlying medical condition that prevents the body from conducting normal thermoregulation.

- Hyperthermia is defined as a disorder that affects the thermoregulation mechanism and presents with a core body temperature greater than 105° F (40.6° C).
- Anhidrosis (lack of perspiration) is the most common manifestation in hyperthermia other than a core temperature greater than 105° F (40.6° C).

Case Study

Mr. J is 78-year-old black man who arrived in the emergency department lethargic, vomiting, unable to speak clearly, and with weakness on the right side of his body. Mr. J has a medical history of hypertension and diabetes mellitus type 2. His family (wife and daughter) reported that for the past 3 months he has been having right-sided weakness and slurred speech that resolved within an hour of onset. Mr. J also has glaucoma, gout, and a history of atrial fibrillation (managed with medications). Mr. J's family reported that he was taking the following medication at home: digoxin, allopurinol, furosemide (Lasix), NPH insulin twice a day, lisinopril, baby acetylsalicylic acid, potassium chloride, and eyedrops.

Mr. J's wife, a 77-year-old woman, reported that approximately 3 days ago Mr. J stopped taking his blood pressure medications (lisinopril and furosemide) because he had spent the money on a horse race. Two nights ago he started to experience more frequent numbness of the right arm and slurred speech, but she didn't think it was important because it disappeared after several hours. Today she had difficulty waking him up, and her daughter told her to call the ambulance.

Mr. J's blood pressure on admission was 220/120 mm Hg; his heart rate was 126 beats/min; respiratory rate was 28 breath/min; and temperature was 98.9° F (37° C). He had right-sided hemiparesis and hemiplegia. His speech was slurred and at times incomprehensible. Mr. J was able to maintain airway at this time.

Oxygen via nasal cannula is started at 2 L/min, and a peripheral intravenous line is started with intravenous fluid therapy of normal saline at 80 ml/hour. A 12-lead ECG is performed, and Mr. J was sent for a CT scan of the head.

Critical Thinking Questions

1. Which one of Mr. J symptoms supports a diagnosis of stroke?
2. What are the risk factors that Mr. J presents for the development of stroke?
3. Indicate the type of stroke Mr. J most likely had, and support your answer.
4. What evidence is presented to support that Mr. J had experienced previous TIAs?
5. Why is atrial fibrillation a risk factor for embolic stroke?
6. Explain the rationale for each of the interventions conducted for Mr. J.
7. Explain why Mr. J was taking each of the medications prescribed at home.
8. Identify three high-priority nursing diagnoses based on Mr. J's assessment, and develop an appropriate nursing care plan.

REFERENCES

Aarsland D et al: Risk of dementia in Parkinson's disease: a community based, prospective study, *Neurology* 56:730, 2001.

Adams HP et al: Guidelines for thrombolytic therapy for acute stroke: a supplement to the guidelines for the management of patients with acute ischemic stroke, *Circulation* 94(5):1167, 1996.

Administration on Aging: *A profile of older Americans: 2003*, Washington, DC, 2003, US Department of Health and Human Services.

Albert MS: Memory decline: the boundary between aging and age-related disease, *Ann Neurol* 51(3):282, 2002.

Alexopoulos G, Mattis S: Diagnosing cognitive dysfunction in the elderly: primary screening tests, *Geriatrics* 46:33, 1991.

American Psychiatric Association: *Diagnostic and Statistical Manual of Mental Disorders*, ed 4, text revision (DSM-IV-TR), Washington, DC, 2000, The Association.

Arias E et al: *Deaths: final data for 2001*, National Vital Statistics Reports 52(3), DHHS Pub No (DHS) 2003–1120, Hyattsville, Md, 2001, National Center for Health Statistics.

Bak O: Some aspects of measurement by Wechsler Intelligence Scale in the context of mental retardation diagnosis in adults, *Psych Poland* 35(4):635-646, 2001.

Balir BD: Presentation and recognition of common psychiatric disorders in the older adult, *Clin Geriatr* 8:26, 2000.

BarsonW: *Emergency department management of stroke.* Proceedings of the National Symposium on Rapid Identification and treatment of Acute Stroke, December 13, 1996, Washington, DC, 1997, National Institute of Neurological Disorders and Stroke (NINDS).

Birks J et al: Ginkgo biloba for cognitive impairment and dementia, *Cochrane Review*, vol 3, Update Software, Oxford, 2003, Cochrane Library.

Black JM, Hawks JH, Hogan MA: *Medical-surgical nursing: clinical management for positive outcome*, ed 7, Philadelphia, 2005, Saunders.

Carr DB et al: Current concepts in the pathogenesis of Alzheimer's disease, *Am J Med* 103(2S):3S, 1997.

Clare L et al: Cognitive rehabilitation and cognitive training for early-stage Alzheimer's disease and vascular dementia, systematic review, *Cochrane Dementia and Cognitive Improvement Group Cochrane Database of Systematic Reviews*, vol 1, 2004.

Clark CM, Ewbank DC: Performance of the dementia severity rating scale: a caregiver questionnaire for rating severity in Alzheimer's disease, *Alzheimer's Dis Assoc Dis* 10:31, 1996.

Cole M, Pimeau F, McCusker J: Effectiveness of interventions to prevent delirium in hospitalized patients: a systematic review, 1996, *Can Med Assn M* 159(9):1263-1268, 1996.

Cotter VT, Clark CM, Karlawish JHT: Cognitive function assessment in individuals at risk for Alzheimer's disease, *J Am Acad Nurse Pract* 15(2):79, 2003.

Decker W, Li J: *Hypothermia*, 2000. Accessed May 3, 2004, from website: http://www.emedicine.com/emerg/topic279.htm.

Depression in old age, *Harvard Mental Health Letter* 20(3):5, 2003.

Diederich NJ et al: Parkinson disease with old-age onset, *Arch Neurol* 60:529, 2003.

Elkin MS: Stroke in the elderly, *Mount Sinai J Med* 70(1):27, 2003.

Esmonde T, Cooke S: Shunting for normal pressure hydrocephalus (NPH), systematic review, *Cochrane Dementia and Cognitive Improvement Group Cochrane Database of Systematic Reviews*, vol 1, 2004.

Federal Interagency Forum on Aging-Related Statistics: *Older Americans 2000: key indicators of well-being*, Hyattsville, Md, 2000, National Center for Health Statistics, website: www.agingstats.gov.

Folstein MF, Folstein SE, McHugh PR: "Mini-Mental State": a practical method for grading the cognitive states of patients for the clinician, *J Psych Res* 12:189, 1975.

Foreman MD et al: Delirium in elderly patients: an overview of the state of the science, *J Gerontol Nurs* 27:4, April 2001.

Geller LN et al: Alzheimer's disease: biological aspects. In Reichel W, editor: *Care of the elderly clinical aspects of aging,* ed 4, Baltimore, 1995, Williams & Wilkins.

Green RC et al: MIRAGE Study Group: risk of dementia among white and African American relatives of patients with Alzheimer's disease, *JAMA* 287:329, 2002.

Grossberg GT: Psychiatric symptoms of Alzheimer's disease: focus on agitation and aggression, *Alzheimer's Dis Manage Today* 1(1):4, 1998.

Grossman M: Frontotemporal dementia: a review, *J Int Neuropsychol Soc* 8:566, 2002.

Hebert LE et al: Alzheimer disease in the U.S. population: prevalence estimates using the 2000 Census, *Arch Neurol* 60(8):1119, 2003.

Inouye SK: Risk factors for delirium and intervention protocols, *N Engl J Med* 340(9):669, 1999.

Inouye SK, Charpentier PA: Predicting factors for delirium in hospitalized elderly persons, *JAMA* 275: 852, 1996.

Inouye SK et al: Clarifying confusion: the confusion assessment method, *Ann Intern Med* 113:941-948, 1990.

Insel KC, Badger TA: Deciphering the 4 D's: cognitive decline, delirium, depression and dementia—a review, *J Adv Nurs* 38(4):360, 2002.

Jorm A, Jacob P: The informant questionnaire on cognitive decline in elderly (IQOCDE): socio-demographic correlates, reliability, validity and norms, *Psychol Med* 19:1015, 1989.

Kalra S, Bergeron C, Lang AE: Lewy body disease and dementia: a review, *Arch Intern Med* 156:487, 1996.

Kare JA, Shneiderman A: Hyperthermia and hypothermia in the older population, *Topics Emerg Med* 23(3):39, 2001.

Knopman DS: The initial recognition and diagnosis of dementia, *Am J Med* 104:2S, 1998.

Knopman DS, Boeve BJ, Petersen RC: Essentials of the proper diagnoses of mild cognitive impairment, dementia, and major subtypes of dementia, *Mayo Clin Proc* 78(10)1290-1308, 2003.

Lai CKY, Arthur DG: Wandering behaviour in people with dementia, *J Adv Nurs* 44(2):173, 2003.

Lantz MS, Buchalter EN: Psychiatry rounds: practical management of Lewy body dementia, *Clin Geriatr* 10(12):18, 2002.

Larson EB et al: Survival after initial diagnosis of Alzheimer disease, *Ann Intern Med* 140(7):501-509, 2004.

Levkoff S, Besdine R, Wetle T: Acute confusional states (delirium) in hospitalized elderly, *Ann Rev Gerontol Geriatr* 6:1-26, 1986.

Lewin Group: *Medicare and Medicaid costs for people with Alzheimer's disease,* Washington, DC, April 2001, Lewin Group.

Lewis SM, Heitkemper MM, Dirksen SR: *Medical surgical nursing: assessment and management of clinical problems,* ed 6, St Louis, 2004, Mosby.

Lonergan E, Luxenberg J, Colford J: Haloperidol for agitation in dementia, *Cochrane Database Syst Rev,* vol 4, CD002852, 2001.

Lopez-Arrieta JM, Birks J: Nimodipine for primary degenerative, mixed and vascular dementia, *Cochrane Dementia and Cognitive Improvement Group Cochrane Database of Systematic Reviews,* vol 1, 2004.

Malouf R, Birks J: Donepezil for vascular cognitive impairment, *Cochrane Database of Systematic Reviews,* vol 1, CD004395, 2004.

Malouf R, Areosa Sastre A: Vitamin B_{12} for cognition, *Cochrane Database of Systematic Reviews,* vol 1, 2004.

Malouf R, Grimley Evans J, Areosa Sastre A: Folic acid with or without vitamin B_{12} for cognition and dementia, *Cochrane Database of Systematic Reviews,* vol 1, 2004.

McCance KL, Huether SE: *Pathophysiology: the biologic basis for disease in adults and children,* ed 4, St Louis, 2002, Mosby.

McKeith I et al: Efficacy of rivastigmine in dementia with Lewy bodies: a randomized double blind, placebo controlled international study, *Lancet* 356:2031, 2000.

McKhann GM et al: Clinical and pathological diagnosis of frontotemporal dementia: report of the work group on frontotemporal dementia and Pick's disease, *Arch Neurol* 58:1803, 2001.

Miller DB, O'Callaghan JP: Effects of aging and stress on hippocampal structures and function, *Metabolism* 52(10):17, 2003.

Nagley SJ: Predicting and preventing confusion in your patients, *J Gerontol Nurs* 12(3):27-31, 1986.

Neelon VJ, Champagne M: Managing cognitive impairment: the current basis for practice. In Funk S et al, editors: *Key aspects of elder care managing falls, incontinence, and cognitive impairment,* New York, 1992, Springer Publishing.

Neelon VJ et al: The NEECHAM confusion scale: construction, validation and clinical testing, *Nurs Res* 45:324, 1996.

Plassman BL et al: Documented head injury in early childhood and risk of Alzheimer's disease and other dementias, *Neurology* 55:1158, 2000.

Preston JE: Ageing choroid plexus–cerebrospinal fluid system, *Microscopy Res Techniques* 52(1):31, 2001.

Rasin J, Barrick AL: Living with illness—bathing patients with dementia: concentrating on the patient's needs rather than merely the task, *Am J Nurs* 104(3):30, 2004.

Roman GC: Vascular dementia: distinguishing characteristics, treatment, and prevention, *J Am Geriatr Soc* 51(5):S296, 2003.

Seshadri S et al: Plasma homocysteine as a risk factor for dementia and Alzheimer's disease, *N Engl J Med* 14(346):476, 2002.

Simon HB: Hyperthermia, *N Engl J Med* 329(7):483, 1993.

Simon JE et al: Is intravenous recombinant tissue plasminogen activator (r-TPA) safe for use in patients over 80 years old with acute ischaemic stroke?—the Calgar experience, *Age Ageing* 33:143, 2004.

Sutor B, Rummans TA, Smith GE: Assessment and management of behavioral disturbances in nursing home patients with dementia, *Mayo Clin Proc* 76(5):540, 2001.

Tabet N, Feldmand H: Ibuprofen for Alzheimer's disease, *Cochrane Dementia and Cognitive Improvement Group Cochrane Database of Systematic Reviews,* vol 1, 2004.

Tabet N et al: Vitamin E for Alzheimer's disease, *Cochrane Dementia and Cognitive Improvement Group Cochrane Database of Systematic Reviews,* vol 1, 2004.

Trzepacz PT, Baker RW, Greenhouse J: A symptom rating scale for delirium, *Psych Res* 23:89-97, 1988.

Urden LD, Stacey KM, Lough ME: *Thelan's critical care nursing: diagnosis and management,* ed 3, St Louis, 2002, Mosby.

Vermeersch P: Development of a scale to measure confusion in hospitalized adults, doctoral dissertation, Case Western Reserve University, *Dissertation Abstr Int* 47(09B):3709, 1986.

Vermeersch P: Clinical assessment of confusion. In Funk S et al, editors: *Key aspects of elder care managing falls, incontinence, and cognitive impairment,* New York, 1992, Springer Publishing.

Vij S, Gentili A: *Sleep disorders, geriatric,* 2002. Accessed May 3, 2004, from website: http://www.emedicine.com/med/topic3179.htm.

Ward NS, Frackowiak SJ: Age related changes in the neural correlates of motor performance, *Brain* 126(4):873, 2003.

Yeaworth RC: Dementia: common types, interventions and advocacy, *Neb Nurse* 35(3):28, 2002.

Yesavage JA et al: Development and validation of a geriatric depression screening scale: a preliminary report, *J Psych Res* 17:37, 1983.

Internet Addresses

DEMENTIA AND ALZHEIMER'S DISEASE

Alzheimer's Association
225 North Michigan Avenue, Floor 17
Chicago, IL 60601-7633
(800) 272-3900 or (312) 335-8700
Fax: (312) 335-1110
www.alz.org

Alzheimer's Disease Education & Referral Center
P.O. Box 8250
Silver Spring, MD 20907-8250
(800) 438-4380
www.alzheimers.org

American Association for Geriatric Psychiatry
7910 Woodmont Avenue, Suite 1050
Bethesda, MD 20814-3004
(301) 654-7850
Fax: (301) 654-4137
www.aagponline.org

National Family Caregivers Association
10400 Connecticut Avenue, Suite 500
Kensington, MD 20895-3944
(800) 896-3650
Fax: (301) 942-2302
www.nfcacares.org

CHRONIC NEUROLOGIC DISORDERS AND PARKINSON'S DISEASE

American Association of Neuroscience Nurses
4700 West Lake Avenue
Glenview, IL 60025-1485
(888) 557-2266 or (847) 375-4733
Fax: (847) 734-8677
www.aann.org

American Parkinson Disease Association
1250 Hylan Boulevard, Suite 4B
Staten Island, NY 10305-1946
(800) 223-2732
Fax: (781) 981-4399
www.apdaparkinson.com

Association of Rehabilitation Nurses (ARN)
4700 West Lake Avenue
Glenview, IL 60025-1485
(800) 229-7530 or (847) 375-4710
Fax: (877) 734-9384
www.rehabnurses.org

STROKE

American Stroke Association
American Heart Association National Center
7272 Greenville Avenue
Dallas, TX 75231
(888) 4-STROKE or (888) 478-7653
www.strokeassociation.org

National Institute of Neurological Disorders and Stroke
P.O. Box 5801
Bethesda, MD 20824
(800) 352-9424 or (301) 496-5751
www.ninds.nih.gov

National Stroke Association
9707 East Easter Lane
Englewood, CO 80112
800-STROKES or 303-649-9299
Fax: 303-649-1328
www.stroke.org

Stroke Clubs International
805 12th Street
Galveston, TX 77550
(409) 762-1022
strokeclubs@earthlink.net

30 Integumentary Function

SABRINA FRIEDMAN, MSN, PhD, FNP

Learning Objectives

On completion of this chapter, the reader will be able to:

1. Discuss the primary functions of the integumentary system.
2. Identify normal age-related skin changes.
3. Discuss four common skin problems and conditions experienced by older adults and their associated nursing implications.
4. Describe three types of skin cancer that affect older adults.
5. Differentiate between the three types of lower leg ulcers.
6. Describe the risk factors for pressure ulcer development.
7. Identify five pressure ulcer preventive strategies endorsed by the Agency for Healthcare Research and Quality clinical guidelines.
8. State three principles necessary for successful wound healing.
9. Conduct an assessment for a client with impaired skin integrity.
10. Determine when to appropriately use antiseptics.
11. Discuss six types of dressings, including indications, contraindications, advantages, and drawbacks.

The skin is an organ that provides the protective outer covering of the body. The skin, hair, nails, and glands make up what is called the integumentary system. The integumentary system is the largest organ of the body. The primary function of the skin is to serve as a barrier against harmful bacteria and other threatening agents, making skin the first line of defense for the immune system. Other major functions of the integumentary system include (1) preventing fluid loss or dehydration, (2) protecting the body from ultraviolet (UV) rays and other external environmental hazards, and (3) protecting underlying organs from injury. In addition, the skin provides thermal regulation of body temperature. Radiation, conduction, convection, and evaporation are facilitated by sensory perceptions that occur in the skin's nerve endings. Blood vessels in the skin assist in regulating blood pressure because of the amount of blood that can be stored within the system. The integumentary system also reveals emotions such as anger, fear, or embarrassment through vasodilation, which reddens the skin tissue. In the presence of the sun's UV rays, the skin synthesizes vitamin D, which is then used by other parts of the body. Subcutaneous fat, the deepest layer of the integumentary system, provides insulation and acts as a caloric reservoir. Hair serves as body insulation and provides unique physical characteristics by virtue of its varying textures, shades, patterns, and colors.

A careful and thorough assessment of the integumentary system is essential when performing a physical assessment on a patient. Skin assessment can help determine hydration status, potential for or actual infection, and other information about the individual (e.g., sun exposure, attention to personal appearance, scars). Palpation of the skin can identify tender areas, nodules, and masses (see Assessments in Chapter 4).

The value of the integumentary system is demonstrated by the high morbidity and mortality rates associated with extensive burns when all functions of the skin are greatly compromised. The overall state of health is affected by physical or emotional insults to this system, such as loss of thermal regulation or fluid, impaired barrier protection, and other catastrophic changes in physical appearance and functioning. The integumentary system provides valuable information for comprehending its complexities.

AGE-RELATED CHANGES IN SKIN STRUCTURE AND FUNCTION

The integumentary system reflects the normal aging process, which includes graying hair, increased number and depth of wrinkles, loss of elasticity, and discoloration and thickening of the nails. Box 30-1 describes basic age-related skin changes.

Epidermis

The epidermis is the outermost layer of the skin. The replacement rate of the stratum corneum, the first layer of epidermis, declines by 50% as a person ages. This decline results in slower healing, reduced barrier protection, and delayed absorption of medications and chemicals placed on the skin. The area of contact between the epidermis and dermis decreases with age, resulting in easy separation of these

BOX 30-1 Age-Related Skin Changes

- Loss of thickness, elasticity, vascularity, and strength that can delay healing process and increase risk of skin tears and bruising
- Increased lentigines (brown-pigmented spots, or age spots)
- Loss of subcutaneous tissue causing wrinkling and sagging of skin, which can affect self-esteem, temperature control, and drug efficacy
- Loss of hair follicles along with thinning and graying
- Increased hair density in nose and ears, particularly in men, which can clog external ear canals and impair hearing
- Thicker nails with longitudinal lines
- Decreased sebaceous and sweat gland activity, which affects thermoregulation and decreases sweating
- Higher incidence of benign and malignant skin growths

layers. Therefore skin tears occur from harmless activities such as removing a bandage or pulling an older client up in the bed. Bruising occurs more easily as a result of these age-related skin changes. A thinner epidermis allows more moisture to escape and may compound previously existing skin problems. The number of melanocytes, which provide pigment and hair color, decreases with age, giving older adults less protection from UV rays, paler skin, and graying hair. Melanocytes also produce uneven pigmentation, causing the development of lentigines, also known as "age spots" or "liver spots."

Dermis

The dermis decreases in thickness by approximately 20% with aging. It consists of strong connective tissue that contains the sweat glands, blood vessels, and nerve endings. With aging the number of sweat glands, blood vessels, and nerve endings also decreases. These changes lead to diminished thermoregulatory function and inflammatory response, decreased tactile sensation, reduced pain perception, and development of wrinkles and sagging skin as a result of loss of underlying tissue. Collagen, a fibrous protein that provides tensile strength within the dermis, stiffens and becomes less soluble.

Subcutaneous Fat

Aging results in a decreased amount of subcutaneous tissue and a redistribution of fat to the abdomen and thighs. Breast tissue also changes and becomes more granular and atrophic. As a result of a loss of padding supplied by subcutaneous tissues, there is a greater risk of hypothermia, skin shearing (see Pressure Ulcers, later in this chapter, for the definition and negative results of shearing), and blunt trauma injury. The loss of this protective padding increases vulnerability of pressure points. Topical medication and dermal medication patch absorption can increase due to the changes in the subcutaneous tissue.

Appendages

As an individual ages, fewer eccrine glands (sweat glands of the palms, feet, and forehead) and apocrine sweat glands (sweat glands of the axilla, scalp, face, and genital areas) exist, resulting in decreased body odor and reduced evaporative heat loss because of decreased sweating. There is less need for antiperspirants and deodorants. However, older adults are at greater risk of heat stroke as a result of a compromised cooling mechanism. Older adults should avoid heat exposure over long periods and in areas of high humidity. Hats with wide brims and cool, light, breezy clothing should be worn when outdoors. It is important that older adults drink extra fluid (minimum of 2000 ml/day, unless contraindicated by a medical condition, such as renal failure or congestive heart failure [CHF]) to maintain adequate hydration, particularly during the summer and in hot climates (Ebersole, Hess, and Luggen, 2004).

Sebum oils the skin and provides an antimicrobial property. The sebaceous glands and pores become larger with aging. Nevertheless, many older adults experience dry skin, which places them at a greater risk of infection as a result of an impaired immune response.

Hair thins, and its growth declines. A progressive loss of melanin occurs, resulting in graying of the hair. Heredity influences when this graying process begins. Older women may have increased lip and chin hair while experiencing a thinning of hair on the head, axilla, and perineal area. Men lose scalp and beard hair, yet experience increased growth over eyebrows and in ears and nostrils. The increased hair in ears predisposes men to cerumen impaction, which leads to impaired hearing (see Chapter 31). Changes in patterns of hair growth and distribution as a person ages are thought to be hormone related. Nails grow more slowly with age and become thicker, more brittle (may split or break easily), and dull; they also develop longitudinal striation with ridges (Ebersole, Hess, and Luggen, 2004). These changes can affect a person's body image and self-concept (see Cultural Awareness box).

COMMON PROBLEMS AND CONDITIONS

Benign Skin Growths

Cherry Angiomas. Cherry angiomas are common, bright red, 1- to 5-mm superficial vascular lesions that begin around age 30 and increase in number with age. The cause of these lesions is unknown. They are red or deep purple dome-shaped papules. Although they are most commonly found on the trunk, they can be located anywhere on the body and vary in number. Because cherry angiomas are new growths,

Cultural Awareness

BIOCULTURAL VARIATIONS IN INTEGUMENTARY SYSTEM DURING HEALTH AND ILLNESS

Normal skin color ranges vary widely, and health care practitioners have attempted to describe the variations seen by labeling observations with some of the following adjectives: copper, olive, tan, and various shades of brown (light, medium, dark). The term *ashen* is sometimes used to describe pallor.

Normal Biocultural Variations

Mongolian spots, irregular areas of deep blue pigmentation, are usually located in the sacral and gluteal areas but sometimes occur on the abdomen, thighs, shoulders, or arms. Mongolian spots are present in 90% of blacks, 80% of Asian-Americans and Native Americans, and 9% of whites.

Vitiligo, a condition in which the melanocytes become nonfunctional in some areas of the skin, is characterized by unpigmented skin patches. Vitiligo affects more than 2 million Americans, primarily dark-skinned individuals. Older adults with vitiligo also have a statistically higher-than-normal chance of developing pernicious anemia, diabetes mellitus, and hyperthyroidism.

Cyanosis

Cyanosis is the most difficult clinical sign to observe in darkly pigmented people. Because peripheral vasoconstriction can prevent cyanosis, environmental conditions such as air conditioning, mist tents, and other factors that may lower the room temperature should be noted. For an older adult to manifest clinical evidence of cyanosis, the blood must contain 5 g of reduced hemoglobin in 1.5 g of methemoglobin per 1 dl of blood.

Given that most conditions causing cyanosis also cause decreased oxygenation of the brain, other clinical symptoms, such as changes in level of consciousness, are evident. Cyanosis usually is accompanied by increased respiratory rate, use of accessory muscles of respiration, nasal flaring, and other manifestations of respiratory distress. When assessing people of Mediterranean descent, the nurse should be aware that the circumoral region is normally dark blue.

Jaundice

In both light- and dark-skinned clients, jaundice is best observed in the sclera. Many darkly pigmented people (e.g., blacks, Filipino Americans) have heavy deposits of subconjunctival fat that contain high levels of carotene in sufficient quantities to mimic jaundice. The fatty deposits become denser as the distance from the cornea increases. The portion of the sclera that is revealed naturally by the palpebral fissure is the best place to assess color accurately. If the palate does not have heavy melanin pigmentation, jaundice can be detected there in the early stages (i.e., when serum bilirubin is 2 to 4 mg/dl). The absence of a yellowish tint of the palate when the sclera are yellow indicates carotene pigmentation of the sclera rather than jaundice. Light or clay-colored stools and dark golden urine often accompany jaundice in both light- and dark-skinned clients.

Pallor

When assessing for pallor in darkly pigmented older adults, the nurse may experience difficulty because the underlying red tones that give brown or black skin its luster are absent. The brown-skinned individual manifests pallor with a more yellowish brown color, and the black-skinned person appears ashen or gray. Generalized pallor can be observed in the mucous membranes, lips, and nail beds. The palpebral conjunctiva and nail beds are preferred sites for assessing the pallor of anemia. When inspecting the conjunctiva, the nurse should lower the lid sufficiently to visualize the conjunctiva near both the outer canthus and the inner canthus. The coloration is often lighter near the inner canthus.

In addition to changes in skin color, the pallor of impending shock is accompanied by other clinical manifestations such as increasing pulse rate, oliguria, apprehension, and restlessness. Anemias, particularly chronic iron deficiency anemia, may be apparent by the characteristic "spoon" nails, which have a concave shape. A lemon-yellow tint of the face and slightly yellow sclera accompany pernicious anemia, which is also manifested by neurologic deficits and a red, painful tongue. The nurse will also note the following symptoms in the presence of most severe anemias: fatigue, exertional dyspnea, rapid pulse, dizziness, and impaired mental function.

Erythema

Erythema (redness) is commonly associated with localized inflammation and is characterized by increased skin temperature. When assessing inflammation in dark-skinned clients, it is often necessary to palpate the skin for increased warmth, tautness or tightly pulled surfaces that may indicate edema, and hardening of deep tissues or blood vessels.

The erythema associated with rashes is not always accompanied by noticeable increases in skin temperature. Macular, papular, and vesicular skin lesions are identified by a combination of palpation and inspection, combined with the client's description of symptoms. For example, people with macular rashes usually complain of itching, and evidence of scratching will be apparent. When the skin is only moderately pigmented, a macular rash may become recognizable if the skin is gently stretched. Stretching the skin decreases the normal red tone, thus providing more contrast and making the macules appear brighter. In some skin disorders with generalized rash, the hard and soft palates are the locations where the rash is most readily visible.

The increased redness that accompanies carbon monoxide poisoning and the blood disorders collectively known as the polycythemias can be observed in the lips of dark-skinned clients. Because lipstick masks the actual color of the lips, older adult women should be asked to remove it with a tissue.

Petechiae

In dark-skinned clients petechiae are best visualized in the areas of lighter melanization such as the abdomen, buttocks, and volar surface of the forearm. When the skin is black or very

Cultural Awareness—cont'd

dark brown, petechiae cannot be seen. Most of the diseases that cause bleeding and microembolus formation, such as thrombocytopenia, subacute bacterial endocarditis, and other septicemias, are characterized by the presence of petechiae in the mucous membranes and skin. Petechiae are most easily visualized in the mouth, particularly the buccal mucosa, and in the conjunctiva of the eye.

Ecchymotic lesions caused by systemic disorders are found in the same locations as petechiae, although their larger size makes them more apparent on dark-skinned individuals. When differentiating petechiae and ecchymosis from erythema in the mucous membrane, the nurse should note that pressure on the tissue momentarily blanches erythema but not petechiae or ecchymosis.

clients are often concerned that they are malignant or indicate a serious health problem. Clients need to be reassured that cherry angiomas are benign growths resulting from increased vascularity in the dermis and occur in most people.

Seborrheic Keratoses. Seborrheic keratoses are benign lesions, sometimes called the "barnacles of old age" (Luggen, 2003). These are scaly growths that have a "stuck-on," crumbly appearance that varies in color from tan to brown to black. The lesions may be elevated and range in diameter from 2 to 3 mm. Characterized by slow growth, these lesions begin to appear later in life. The borders may be round and smooth or irregular and notched. To the untrained eye, these lesions can resemble a malignant melanoma, particularly when dark brown or black. They have a greasy feeling and often occur in sun-exposed areas (face, neck, or trunk) but can appear anywhere on the body. In an Australian study of the relationship between sun exposure and the prevalence of seborrheic keratoses, the median number of lesions in those who had them increased with age from 6 per person among 15- to 25-year-olds to 69 per person in those more than 75 years of age. The growths are usually removed for cosmetic reasons (often related to self-esteem) or if irritated. If the lesion is "picked off," it will recur. Therefore it is best to have a physician remove the growth if it is bothersome to a client. Cryotherapy is effective, and the lesion usually sloughs off in a few weeks. Clients should be reassured that the growths are benign and are a commonly occurring skin manifestation.

Skin Tags (Acrochordons). Skin tags are common stalklike, benign tumors often found on the neck, axilla, eyelids, and groin, although they can be located anywhere on the body. Beginning as early as age 20, these are tiny, flesh-colored or brown excrescences that develop into a long, narrow stalk (up to 1 cm). As they mature, they can be easily removed with scissors, electrocautery, or liquid nitrogen. Skin tags are usually excised only on the request of the client, usually for cosmetic reasons.

Inflammatory Dermatoses

Seborrheic Dermatitis. Seborrheic dermatitis is a common, chronic inflammation of the skin. The scalp, ear canals, eyebrows, eyelashes, nasolabial folds, axilla, breasts, chest, and groin are common sites. The cause is generally unknown, but it is thought to be an inflammatory reaction to the lipid-loving yeast *Pityrosporum ovale* (Helm and Marks, 1998). It is more common in clients who have Parkinson's disease or who have suffered a stroke.

In differentiating between dandruff and seborrheic dermatitis, note that dandruff is scaling without inflammation, and seborrheic dermatitis is an inflammatory response sometimes associated with scaling. With inadequate management, dandruff can evolve into seborrheic dermatitis. Seborrheic dermatitis appears as a white or yellow scale with a plaquelike appearance. An erythematous red base, indicating an inflammatory process, is *always* present. Mild itching is not uncommon. The usual pattern of distribution begins with the scalp and moves down toward the eyebrows, progressing to the chest with a bilateral, symmetric presentation.

Intertrigo. Intertrigo is a form of seborrheic dermatitis. It results from the friction of opposing skin surfaces and the irritation this causes. It is usually found in the armpits, inner aspects of the thighs, skin folds of the breasts, and abdominal folds. The area is erythematous and may itch. Intertrigo occurs more often in aging clients who are obese or diabetic. Medical management usually includes losing weight, applying topical hydrocortisone cream, and keeping the skin clean and dry.

Psoriasis

Psoriasis is a common chronic inflammatory dermatosis affecting approximately 2% of the population in the United States (Helm and Marks, 1998). The condition may affect persons of any age, although it often begins during early adulthood. Psoriasis is sometimes associated with other diseases such as arthritis, myopathy, enteropathy, spondylitic heart disease, and acquired immunodeficiency syndrome (AIDS). Psoriasis has a tendency to be genetically inherited, with approximately one third of clients having a positive family history; it has been classed as an autoimmune disorder (Helm and Marks, 1998). Once psoriasis begins, there are periods of remission and relapse with varying degrees of intensity. There is no known cure.

Clinically, psoriatic lesions are typically seen as well-circumscribed, pink plaques covered with silver-white, loosely adherent scales. These scaly plaques result from the accelerated replication of the dermis and epidermis over certain parts of the body. Psoriasis frequently affects the skin of the elbows, knees, scalp, lumbosacral areas, intergluteal cleft, and glans penis. Changes in the nails occur in approximately 30% of clients and consist of yellow-brown discoloration with pitting, dimpling, separation of the nail plate from the underlying bed (oncolysis), thickening, and crumbling. Psoriasis is a reactive disorder. Triggers such as infection, smoking, climate, and hormonal factors may exacerbate an attack; other factors such as sunlight may decrease the severity of an attack.

Psoriasis can be a cause of a total body erythema and scaling termed *erythroderma*. Another variant of psoriasis is the pustular type, which manifests as multiple small pustules forming the erythematous plaques. Pustular psoriasis may be benign and localized or life-threatening and generalized. In the more generalized form, the client will also have fever, leukocytosis, arthralgias, diffuse cutaneous and mucosal pustules, secondary infection, and electrolyte disturbances.

NURSING MANAGEMENT

Assessment

Nursing assessment consists of recognizing the inflammatory dermatitis and noting its location, degree of erythema, itching, and scaling. The dermatitis should be examined for an erythematous base with yellow, white, or silvery scales or plaques. The nurse should inquire about itching; usual hygienic habits; and steps the client has taken to control the scaly, erythemic dermatitis. Bedbound individuals are more prone to develop seborrheic dermatitis; therefore targeting these clients for assessment, in addition to thorough cleansing of scalp, hair, and skin, is a preventive strategy.

Diagnosis

Nursing diagnoses for a client with inflammatory dermatitis include:

- Impaired skin integrity related to immunologic deficit (psoriasis)
- Impaired skin integrity related to bedbound state (seborrheic dermatitis)
- Impaired skin integrity related to physiologic disease process (intertrigo)
- Body image disturbance related to the psoriatic lesions

Planning and Expected Outcomes

The goal of nursing management is control of the inflammatory process with maintenance therapy using topical agents and shampoo as prescribed. Client comfort is evidenced when medical treatment is done according to advice. Expected outcomes include:

1. Skin lesions will remain free from infection.
2. Client will experience resolution of the inflammatory process.
3. Client will demonstrate increased knowledge of the condition as evidenced by:
   - Verbalizing rationale for regular and consistent skin care
   - Verbalizing knowledge of maintenance therapy
   - Verbalizing triggers to inflammatory dermatitis
   - Correctly demonstrating application of topical medications

Intervention

One crucial aspect of nursing management is to ensure proper use of an antiseborrheic shampoo containing zinc pyrithione, selenium sulfide, or ketoconazole. One successful strategy is to wet hair, chest, axilla, and affected areas; apply selenium shampoo; and then proceed with the rest of the bath or shower. After cleansing the affected areas, the client should apply hydrocortisone 1% cream or another prescribed steroid cream, which decreases the inflammation and irritated red appearance of the skin. Low-dose steroid creams or the newer nonsteroidal cream, such as pimecrolimus cream (Elidel), must be used on the face to prevent scarring, atrophy, or acne. After inflammation and scaling have resolved, the client should continue selenium shampoo on the scalp twice weekly as preventive maintenance therapy.

Nursing interventions for a client with psoriasis consist of reinforcing the directions of the physician or advanced practice nurse (APN) to optimize treatment and identify client-specific triggers that may be avoided to decrease the severity of flare episodes. Since psoriasis varies in type and severity, treatment plans may use both prescription and over-the-counter topical ointments. As with seborrheic dermatitis, a common therapy used to treat psoriasis is a topical steroid. Topical steroids may be over-the-counter or prescription strength and are not recommended for use on the face. Coal tar has been used topically for many years to relieve the itching and scaling in minor cases of psoriasis. These compounds are messy and can make the skin more sensitive to UV and sunlight. A topical vitamin D_3 ointment, calcipotriene skin ointment (Dovonex), is used for moderate cases of psoriasis. It is available by prescription only and has few known side effects. Dovonex should not be used on the face, and photosensitivity is likely. Tazarotene (Tazorac) is a *retinoid*, a group of drugs related to vitamin A. It should be applied only to the affected areas, and contact should be avoided with the eyes, eyelids, and mouth. Because the medication may result in photosensitivity, exposure to sunlight should be avoided.

Light therapy using ultraviolet B (UVB) rays has been shown to be beneficial when used in prescription light boxes. It is currently thought that ultraviolet A (UVA) light therapy used in combination with psoralen (an oral or topical medication) is the preferred method (called PUVA). The UV dosage is carefully monitored for the amount of exposure, since there is a limit on the total exposure time. With UVA light therapy, it is important to be aware of the potential risk of developing skin cancer. There are also a number of reports that foods may trigger psoriasis attacks; therefore approaches to diet modification and other homeopathic remedies abound in client resource literature. Clients should be encouraged to discuss with their health care team any and all remedies used. The nurse should teach the older adult client, family members, and staff the causes of inflammatory dermatitis to alleviate anxiety and misconceptions. Explanation of treatment measures and the importance of follow-through will increase compliance and involvement in care. Symptom management is an area where nurses can have a positive effect on an older adult's quality of life.

Evaluation

Nursing accountability and evaluation are supported through accurate, comprehensive charting that describes physical assessment and maintenance interventions. A weekly assessment of the lesions with a description of response to treatment, including maintenance therapy, is recorded. In addition, the nurse should address the response to teaching (e.g., verbalized understanding) as measured by client, family, or staff compliance with treatment.

Pruritus

Pruritus is another term for itching that is so intense it causes the client to scratch. The most common cause of itching is dry skin, or xerosis. The mechanism of itching is not fully understood, but histamine is a known mediator of pruritus. Itching can be precipitated by heat, sudden temperature changes, sweating, clothing, cleaning products such as soap, fatigue, and emotional stress; it is usually more severe in the winter (Ebersole, Hess, and Luggen, 2004). Pruritus can be related either to a skin disorder or systemic disease; therefore the complaint should not be dismissed and warrants a complete assessment (Box 30-2). Often pruritus is associated with dry skin, but it can be associated with scabies, eczema, drug reaction, liver or renal disease, hyperglycemia, thyroid disease, prodromal symptoms of herpes zoster, venous stasis, or anemia (Golkar and Eichenfield, 1998).

BOX 30-2 Possible Sources of Pruritus

SKIN DISORDERS
- Atopic eczema
- Contact dermatitis
- Urticaria or allergic reactions
- Seborrheic dermatitis
- Exfoliative dermatitis
- Psoriasis
- Bullous pemphigoid

INFESTATIONS
- Scabies
- Pediculosis
- Fleas, bedbugs, or mites

INFECTIONS
- Herpes zoster
- Candidiasis
- Folliculitis
- Impetigo

MISCELLANEOUS
- Liver disease or failure
- Renal disease (uremia)
- Diabetes (hyperglycemia)
- Thyroid disease
- Venous stasis
- Xerosis (dry skin)
- Abdominal cancer (visceral malignancies)
- CNS tumors (visceral malignancies)

DRUGS
- Opiates and derivatives
- Phenothiazines
- Tolbutamide
- Erythromycin
- Estrogen
- Progestins
- Testosterone
- Aspirin
- Quinidine
- Vitamin B complex

Modified from Bernhard JD. In Moschella SL, Hurley HJ, editors: *Dermatology*, ed 3, Philadelphia, 1992, WB Saunders; Ebersole P, Hess P: *Toward healthy aging: human needs and nursing response,* ed 5, St Louis, 1998, Mosby.

NURSING MANAGEMENT

Assessment

A full skin assessment is warranted when a client complains of pruritus. The client is interviewed to determine the location, intensity, and onset of itching. The nurse should inquire about any patterns of behavior that precipitate itching (e.g., anxiety, environmental exposures, friction [rubbing the skin with a towel]) and obtain information about bathing practices and kinds of soaps, detergents, and skin products used. The nurse should also look for rashes, vesicles, scaling, and erythema; any of these suggests a skin disorder.

Diagnosis

Nursing diagnoses for a client with pruritus include:
- High risk for impaired skin integrity related to scratching
- Pain related to persistent burning and itching

Client/Family Teaching

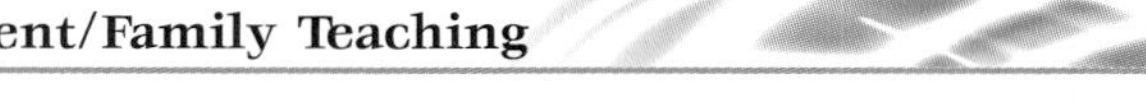

PREVENTION AND TREATMENT OF DRY SKIN (XEROSIS)

Bathing or showering with warm water should not exceed a frequency of every other day. Pat skin dry to avoid irritation. In the winter, when the air is drier, one bath or shower a week is sufficient, with a daily sponge bath to underarms, perineal area, and skinfolds.

Bath oil can be used in a basin when sponge bathing, but not in the tub or shower. To avoid risk of slipping in the tub or shower, apply oil after bathing.

Avoid the use of harsh soaps (e.g., Zest, Ivory, Dial); instead use a superfatted soap (e.g., Dove, Basis, Tone, Cetaphil) in limited quantities with only one lathering.

Use heavy emollient lotions or creams containing urea or lactic acid (e.g., Lubriderm, Nivea, Eucerin, Aveeno) after bathing when skin is moist. Mineral oil, petroleum jelly, and shortening are less expensive alternatives.

Never use alcohol or other drying rubs on skin because these deplete natural skin oils.

Drink at least 1500 to 2500 ml of water a day to ensure adequate hydration, if not contraindicated by other medical conditions (e.g., CHF).

Avoid tight-fitting clothes that rub against the skin.

Modified from Davis C. In Carnevali DL, Patrick M, editors: *Nursing management for the elderly,* ed 3, Philadelphia, 1993, JB Lippincott; Ebersole P, Hess P, Luggen AS: *Toward healthy aging: human needs and nursing response,* ed 6, St Louis, 2004, Mosby; Newman DK, Smith DAJ: *Geriatric care plans,* Springhouse, Pa, 1991, Springhouse.

- Anxiety related to role strain, family crisis, or other sources of client's anxiety
- Risk for infection related to impaired skin integrity

Planning and Expected Outcomes

The goal of nursing management is resolution of pruritus without injury from scratching. Time should be planned to teach the client and family about etiologic factors and the importance of not scratching. Expected outcomes include:

1. Skin will remain intact.
2. Client will experience adequate periods of rest without symptoms of scratching.
3. Client will obtain adequate pain relief as evidenced by verbalization of comfort and pain relief.

Intervention

Nursing interventions are influenced by the cause of the pruritus. If dry, scaly skin (xerosis) is present with no lesions or erythema, the nurse should suggest that the client apply emollients (e.g., Lubriderm, Moisturel, or Eucerin lotion or cream), which have more lanolin or oily substances than many commercial lotions. Emollients should be applied at least twice daily and immediately after bathing to trap moisture. The client should gently pat skin dry and avoid brisk drying with a towel. If the client is unable to apply lotion, the nurse should instruct the caregiver in its use. The client should decrease the frequency of baths to a maximum of every other day (see Client/Family Teaching box). Antihistamines may be needed to relieve itching and to prevent tissue breakdown from scratching. However, cautious use of these agents in older adults is warranted as a result of the anticholinergic side effects of confusion, urinary retention, and constipation (Ebersole, Hess, and Luggen, 2004).

A diagnostic workup may be conducted to identify any systemic cause (e.g., cancer, diabetes) for persistent pruritus. Anxiety or stress may be the source of itching. If so, the nurse should assess the client's self-esteem and coping strategies and identify any family or role strain or other factors that may lead to anxiety. He or she should also discuss stress management strategies and assist the client in determining effective strategies. A referral to a community agency or professional such as an APN, psychologist, or psychiatrist may be needed for continued support and guidance.

The older adult client, family members, and staff need to be taught the management of pruritus and the need to prevent skin trauma from scratching. Treatment measures should also be explained to increase compliance and involvement in care. The causes of pruritus may be difficult to determine, and the expected effects of topical agents may be diminished as a result of the delayed absorption of medications placed on aging skin.

Evaluation

Evaluation of interventions focuses on symptom relief, prevention of secondary complications, and, when possible, identification of the source of the pruritus. Nursing accountability is demonstrated through documentation of physical presentation, such as erythema, intact skin with no lesions, hives, or rash; the response to treatment measures; client comprehension of teaching; and other nursing interventions.

Candidiasis

Candidiasis is an inflammatory process of the epidermis caused by the yeastlike fungus *Candida albicans. C. albicans* is a normally occurring flora in the mouth, vagina, and gut (moist habitats). Pregnancy, oral contraception, antibiotics, diabetes, topical and inhalant steroids, skin maceration, and immunocompromised conditions create an environment that fosters the development of yeast infections such as candidiasis. Candidiasis is most commonly seen in diaper-clad infants, incontinent clients, and bedbound individuals and in moisture-prone areas of the body (e.g., skin folds, axilla).

Candidiasis is characterized by erythematous, denuded, or raw skin usually surrounded by satellite papules or pustules.

Satellite lesions are a helpful diagnostic clue. Red, erythematous areas on the buttocks, perineum, or intertriginous areas of incontinent clients also have diagnostic significance. Scaling may also be present, usually at the borders.

NURSING MANAGEMENT

Assessment

Nursing assessment includes inspection of skin, particularly under any fat folds where moisture will accumulate. A hallmark of candidiasis is a bright-red erythema with satellite papules or pustules. Any breaks in the skin, which place the client at greater risk for infection or further breakdown, should be noted. The client may be the one to alert the nurse to the infection. The nurse should conduct a medication assessment to identify any medications that may precipitate this fungal infection, such as antibiotics or steroids. If the client has diabetes, hyperglycemia may be present; therefore the nurse should conduct a diet assessment to evaluate compliance and should check blood sugar. For some individuals with type 2 diabetes, a candidiasis infection may be the first clinical manifestation of hyperglycemia. Therefore a thorough health history is warranted when a candidiasis infection is present.

Diagnosis

Nursing diagnoses for a client with candidiasis include:

- Impaired skin integrity related to poor control of moisture
- Self-care deficit: toileting
- Total incontinence

Planning and Expected Outcomes

The goal of nursing management is prevention and resolution of candidiasis and, consequently, increased client comfort. Expected outcomes include:

1. Skin lesions will be without evidence of infection and will be healing.
2. Client will perform self-care practices (within limitations) for keeping skin dry and clean.
3. Skin will regain usual appearance without evidence of candidiasis.

Intervention

The main nursing intervention is keeping the skin dry, especially the intertriginous areas. A client's discomfort, costs, and nursing time could be minimized through preventive strategies such as drying the skin well (particularly the skinfolds) after bathing or sweating episodes and changing the sheets as soon as possible after an incontinent episode. After changing linens, the nurse should cleanse and dry skin well and apply a zinc-based cream (such as Desitin) to the buttocks and perineal area. Cornstarch or powder, whether medicated or scented, is not recommended because of clumping and hence limited long-term skin protection. Creams are much more effective and efficient.

The nurse should teach the older adult client, family members, and support staff to pat skin dry and should educate the staff and provide scientific rationale for changing linen, cleansing the affected area, and using a moisture barrier such as zinc oxide or Desitin. The importance of prompt delivery of care following an incontinent event must be stressed. It is important to keep topical antifungal agents on the infected area until healing is complete, which may take 2 to 3 weeks. If the yeast infection does not improve, the physician or APN should be informed so that an alternative agent can be considered.

Management protocols can be developed and approved by the employee's institution and medical and nursing staff with the intent of empowering the professional nurse to act immediately when candidiasis is present. This promotes high-quality care, client comfort, a sense of professional pride, and a team approach. Nursing management is key in resolving a candidiasis infection.

Evaluation

Evaluation of nursing management focuses on treatment efficacy and rate of recurrence. The nurse must document how the infection responds to medical treatment, as well as maintenance therapy of keeping skin dry and applying a moisture barrier. The effectiveness of client care can be supported with positive outcomes, compliance with preventive actions, and verbalized comprehension. If little improvement is seen in 2 weeks, the nurse should ensure that moisture control and application of antifungal cream are being maintained. Consultation with the physician or APN is needed when there is a poor response to therapy; another agent may be ordered.

Herpes Zoster (Shingles)

Herpes zoster, also known as shingles, is caused by the reactivation of latent varicella zoster (chickenpox) virus. The virus remains in the dorsal nerve endings after an episode of chickenpox, which is usually experienced in childhood. The main reason for recurrence is an immune system deficiency. Conditions that may impair the immune system are advanced age, stress or emotional upset, fatigue, or radiotherapy. An immunocompromised state caused by disease (e.g., human immunodeficiency virus, lymphoma, leukemia, other malignancies) or drugs (e.g., chemotherapy, steroids) can also activate the latent virus. Chickenpox is highly contagious because it is an airborne virus. Herpes zoster is not as infectious, since it is related to reactivation of latent varicella zoster. Therefore it is not necessary to isolate a client with herpes zoster. Cases of contracting shingles after personal exposure have been reported, but these have been in individuals who have not had chickenpox. Consequently, clients with herpes zoster should be cared for only by health care personnel who have had chickenpox or have positive serum varicella titers (Habif, 2004). As always, universal precautions should be exercised.

Approximately 50% of herpes zoster cases involve the thoracic region, 15% involve the cranial dermatomes, and 10% affect the cervical and lumbar regions. Ophthalmic herpes zoster is referred to an ophthalmologist for evaluation and treatment, since blindness could result from corneal scarring.

Herpes zoster often has prodromal symptoms of tingling, hyperesthesia, tenderness, and burning or itching pain along the affected dermatome. The prodromal symptoms are followed by vesicles with an erythematous base occurring within 3 to 5 days. A unilateral bandlike erythematous, maculopapular rash first occurs along the involved dermatome and rarely crosses the midline of the body. The rash develops into clustered vesicles (usually on an erythematous base) that become purulent, rupture, and crust. These vesicles are vulnerable to secondary bacterial infections. Some lesions become necrotic or hemorrhagic. This occurs more often in older adults. It may take up to 1 month for the crusting lesions to heal, with mild cases resolving in 7 to 10 days. The average duration for herpes zoster is 3 weeks. Scarring and permanent or temporary pigment discoloration may occur, especially in severe cases. Lymphadenopathy is not uncommon with an occasional temperature elevation. Postinfection paresthesias and meningoencephalitis may occur for 2 to 4 weeks when motor neurons and the central nervous system (CNS) are involved (Habif, 2004).

The incidence of herpes zoster increases with age, most likely as a consequence of diminishing immune function. The older adult is also at a greater risk of developing postherpetic segmental pain. Dissemination is often seen in older adults or immunosuppressed clients. Disseminated herpes zoster, which is rare and occurs in only 2% to 5% of clients, is more serious because of its systemic nature. In disseminated herpes zoster, satellite lesions appear outside the affected dermatome within 4 to 6 days after the initial eruption. Dissemination may be associated with fever, lymphadenopathy, headache, neck rigidity, and an increased risk of serious complications such as encephalitis, hepatitis, and pneumonitis. Disseminated herpes zoster may occur in as many as 15% to 50% of clients with active Hodgkin's disease, and 10% to 25% of these clients die (Habif, 2004).

One of the major complications from this acute viral infection is postherpetic neuralgia, pain that persists along the affected dermatome after resolution of vesicular lesions. Postherpetic neuralgia can last less than 1 year, but it may last a lifetime with little pain relief. It affects approximately 33% of clients age 40, and by age 70 the risk increases to 74%. Postherpetic neuralgia is more common in persons with trigeminal nerve involvement (Habif, 2004).

NURSING MANAGEMENT

Assessment

Nursing assessment begins with interviewing the client to identify prodromal symptoms, such as burning, itching, or tingling along a dermatome before rash development. The nurse should obtain pertinent health history that addresses chickenpox history, medications, diabetes, malignancy with recent chemotherapy or radiotherapy, and AIDS and other immunocompromised states. The nurse should also identify persons with whom the client has had close physical contact who have not had chickenpox or the chickenpox vaccine, since they may be at risk of infection. He or she should inspect the area of discomfort for the characteristic unilateral, bandlike, erythemic, maculopapular rash that may have clustered vesicles. Initially, the area may be a raised, erythemic rash before the vesicles appear. Intense pain is often associated with the rash, particularly in older adults. Based on the lesions and prescribed treatments, the nurse must determine the effect on the client's mobility and capacity for activities of daily living. Recommended treatment measures may require the assistance of another person.

Diagnosis

Nursing diagnoses for a client with herpes zoster include:

- Impaired skin integrity related to immunologic deficit
- Risk for infection related to impaired skin integrity
- Sleep pattern disturbance related to impaired skin integrity or to pain
- Pain related to inadequate pain relief from analgesia
- Knowledge deficit: disease process and treatment related to lack of previous exposure

Planning and Expected Outcomes

The goals of nursing management are prevention of secondary infection and scarring, as well as pain relief. Local skin care treatments may need to be taught to the client or caregiver. The nurse must be alert to the possibility of long-term pain (postherpetic neuralgia) and the resulting depression that can occur. Expected outcomes include:

1. Skin lesions will remain free from necrotic tissue and infection.
2. Client will experience adequate periods of restful sleep, as evidenced by:
   - No requests for pain medication during the night
   - Reports of uninterrupted sleep during the night and feeling well rested on arising
3. Client will obtain adequate pain relief, as evidenced by:
   - Verbalizing comfort and pain relief after taking analgesic
   - Augmenting analgesic pain relief with use of relaxation exercises, music diversion tapes, or guided imagery
4. Client will demonstrate increased knowledge of condition as evidenced by:
   - Verbalizing significant and reportable signs and symptoms of infection
   - Verbalizing rationale for regular, consistent use of analgesics
   - Correctly performing return demonstration of lesion care and dressing change procedure

Intervention

Nursing interventions consist of notifying the physician or APN as soon as the characteristic rash and vesicles are identified, especially if they follow a dermatomal pattern. After a diagnosis is made, follow-through with medical and nursing management is paramount to client comfort. Lesions should be monitored closely for the development of secondary bacterial infections, as evidenced by erythema, tenderness, or purulent discharge. If satellite lesions develop outside the dermatome, especially if the client is also experiencing headache, neck rigidity, or pulmonary congestion, the physician or APN must be notified immediately, since this is indicative of disseminated herpes zoster.

The nurse should teach the older adult client, family members, and staff the cause of shingles so that anxiety and misconceptions can be alleviated, and he or she should explain the treatment measures to increase compliance and involvement in care. Herpes zoster can be very painful, so prompt administration of pain medications is crucial for client comfort. For optimum pain control, clients should be instructed to inform the nurse when they experience the initial onset of pain, before the pain becomes well entrenched. Effective pain management is one area where nurses can have a positive effect on a client's quality of life (see Chapter 15). If postherpetic neuralgia occurs, antidepressants are used as adjuncts to analgesics for control of pain.

Evaluation

Evaluation of interventions focuses on pain control, with documented results of analgesics and adjunct therapies, and on prevention of secondary infection by frequent monitoring of site. Many barriers to effective pain management in older adults exist, leading to frequent underrecognition and undertreatment of pain (see Chapter 15). If pain is not relieved, the physician or APN should be consulted to obtain an alternative analgesic agent or adjunct drug therapy. The inflammatory response in an older adult may be diminished, even in the presence of severe infection, so the nurse should be alert to even slight symptoms of secondary bacterial infection. If evidence of cellulitis is noted, the physician or APN should be informed to implement topical or oral antibiotic therapy. Documentation of assessment, response to treatment measures, client comprehension of teaching, and other nursing interventions demonstrates nursing accountability (see the Nursing Care Plan).

Nursing Care Plan
Herpes Zoster

Clinical Situation: Mrs. R. is a 71-year-old woman who lives in her own home. She has severe rheumatoid arthritis and hypertension. She takes methotrexate, prednisone, lisinopril, and hydrochlorothiazide. She has had both hips replaced in the past 5 years.

Mrs. R. began to experience a burning with pain 2 days ago and this morning awoke with clustered vesicles on the left side of her torso extending from the midback around to the midline of the anterior aspect of her chest. She went in to see her primary care physician. The physician ordered acyclovir, analgesics as needed for pain, and a topical antibiotic to prevent secondary infection.

Nursing Diagnoses

High risk for infection related to herpes zoster and open lesions

Outcomes

Client will experience no secondary infection, as evidenced by no fever and other vital signs within normal limits, and will practice habits that decrease the risk of infection.

Interventions

Instruct client not to scratch or rub affected area in order not to break vesicles, which would increase risk of secondary infection.

Assess vital signs, mental status, and skin lesions every shift to identify signs of infection (fever, tachycardia, erythema, tenderness, purulent discharge, confusion).

If client is febrile, ensure adequate hydration, since fever increases hydration needs.

Tachycardia could precipitate CHF from decreased cardiac output; monitor for shortness of breath, rales, edema, and other signs of cardiovascular compromise.

If vesicle lesions rupture, implement topical treatment, noting response.

Ensure adequate nutrition to foster healing.

Monitor food intake, and ensure food preferences are being met.

Teach client the need to eat at least 2000 calories and drink a minimum of 1500 ml of liquid per day.

Be alert for vesicles outside of involved dermatome, which could indicate disseminated herpes zoster; if vesicles appear, contact physician or nurse practitioner immediately.

Teach client, staff, and visitors the value of hand washing and proper disposal of dressing and treatment material as an infection control standard.

Identify staff and visitors who have no known history of chickenpox or vaccine and inform them that they are not able to provide care for the client because they may not have an immunity to the varicella virus; isolation is not required; the infection control strategy is to take universal precautions.

PREMALIGNANT SKIN GROWTHS: ACTINIC KERATOSIS

Actinic keratosis is a premalignant lesion of the epidermis that is caused by long-term exposure to UV rays. This precancerous lesion is more common in light-complexioned individuals and occurs most commonly on the dorsum of the hands, scalp, outer ears, face, and lower arms. Actinic keratosis may evolve into squamous cell carcinoma (SCC) if not treated, so it should receive prompt attention (Habif, 2004).

Actinic keratosis begins in vascular areas as a reddish macule or papule that has a rough, yellowish brown scale that may itch or cause discomfort. During assessment the nurse should be attuned to the rough surface of the lesion and its location and be particularly alert if a suspicious lesion is on a sun-exposed area. Accumulation of keratin can also lead to the formation of a cutaneous horn that tends to develop on the outer ear. Because of an abundant vascular supply, removal of the crust may cause bleeding. Induration, inflammation, or oozing may be indicative of malignancy and merit prompt referral (Habif, 2004).

NURSING MANAGEMENT

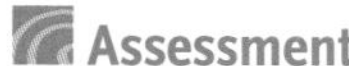

Assessment

Nursing assessment begins with the client interview to determine risk factors, such as frequency of activities with sun exposure and use of preventive practices (e.g., wearing a hat and long sleeves while outside). The skin should be inspected and any rough lesions palpated and noted for location and texture. If hand lotion is used frequently, a roughness will not be present; therefore the nurse should look for an erythemic macule or papule. The nurse should refer clients to their primary care provider whenever a suspicious lesion is found. The nurse should also explain the value of treating skin cancer early, which can minimize scarring and disfigurement.

Diagnosis

Nursing diagnoses for a client with actinic keratosis include:

- Impaired skin integrity related to removal of a lesion
- High risk for infection related to break in skin integrity
- Body image disturbance related to disfigurement and scarring resulting from removal of lesion

Planning and Expected Outcomes

The goal of nursing management after the removal of premalignant lesions is the prevention of secondary infection and assistance in coping with any body image disturbance. Expected outcomes include:

1. Site of lesion removal will heal without evidence of secondary infection.
2. Client will demonstrate no changes in body image perception.
3. Client will demonstrate behavior change through adoption of preventive skin care practices.

Intervention

Nursing intervention consists of reinforcing the treatment regimen with the client and family, monitoring the treated site to prevent secondary infection, providing support, and teaching preventive strategies. To lower a client's anxiety and assist with body image changes, the nurse should explain the treatment, stressing that erythema and crusting are temporary. The resulting body image trauma from treatment of many facial lesions can isolate an individual. The nurse can identify the client's fears and discuss them in an open, reassuring manner.

Wounds should be assessed for development of a bacterial infection, as seen by increased tenderness, increasing erythema around the treated site, purulent discharge, and possibly fever. Topical management with an antibiotic ointment may be implemented prophylactically.

The nurse should teach older adult clients and family members preventive strategies necessary to prevent recurrence and stress the need to wear hats with wide brims and long-sleeved shirts to protect the skin from sun exposure. If an individual is going to be in the sun, a sunscreen with a sun protection factor of at least 15 should be applied (Habif, 2004).

Evaluation

Evaluation of nursing management is supported with documentation addressing treatment progress, which includes physical description, client comprehension of educational information, and identification of and coping with any body image disturbances.

MALIGNANT SKIN GROWTHS

Basal Cell Carcinoma

Basal cell carcinoma (BCC) is the most common skin cancer and is more prevalent in fair-skinned, blond, or red-headed individuals with extensive previous sun exposure. BCC rarely occurs in black persons because the darker skin pigmentation plays a protective role against UVB radiation, the spectrum thought to be causative in the development of skin cancer (Johnson, Moy, and White, 1998). It occurs more often in men than women; however, this gender difference has decreased in recent years. BCC is most commonly found on the face and scalp, less often on the trunk, and rarely on the hands. It may also arise from scars or burns, particularly in older adults who have experienced chronic sun damage. BCC usually does not metastasize, but if left untreated, it may metastasize to the bone, lungs, and brain (Habif, 2004).

Typically, BCC appears as a pearly papule with a depression in the center, giving the lesion a doughnut-like appearance with telangiectasia on or around the lesion. BCC can also appear as a blue-black pearly nodule (pigmented basal cell) or a red, scaly, or eczematous-appearing macule that is usually on the thoracic area (superficial spreading BCC). BCC can grow aggressively but follows the path of least resistance and usually does not infiltrate bone, cartilage, or muscle (Habif, 2004).

NURSING MANAGEMENT

Assessment

Nursing assessment begins with an interview focusing on length of time lesion has been present, presence of risk factors such as chronic sun exposure, and history of previous skin lesions. A skin assessment is conducted, with the nurse being alert for pearly, doughnut-shaped lesions with telangiectasia. A magnifying glass may be useful to closely examine any lesion. The nurse should inspect and palpate the lesion, surrounding tissue, and lymph nodes (to identify possible metastasis). When a suspicious lesion is identified, the client is referred to the primary care provider for prompt treatment. The nurse should explain to the client that early treatment lessens the extent of scarring and lowers the risk of metastasis.

Diagnosis

Nursing diagnoses for a client with BCC include:

- Impaired skin integrity related to removal of a cancerous lesion
- High risk for infection related to break in skin integrity and surgical wound
- Body image disturbance related to disfigurement and scarring resulting from removal of cancerous lesion
- Fear of cancer, pain, or death related to having a cancerous skin lesion

Planning and Expected Outcomes

The goal of nursing management is to facilitate referral and treatment of suspicious lesions for removal without secondary infection. Time should be planned to discuss the client's and family's feelings about having a cancerous lesion to identify any need for a community referral or educational material. In addition, client education regarding preventive strategies should be included in the plan. Expected outcomes include:

1. Site of BCC will heal without evidence of infection.
2. Client will demonstrate no disturbance in body image.
3. Client will verbalize concerns regarding diagnosis and will be able to articulate feelings and concerns related to the diagnosis.
4. Client will adopt preventive strategies into lifestyle.
5. Client will demonstrate increased knowledge of condition.

Intervention

Nursing interventions include reinforcement of the treatment regimen and monitoring the wound for secondary infection (e.g., erythema, tenderness, and purulent discharge). The nurse should explain procedures, emphasizing that a wound or erosion can occur that may require a dressing. He or she should teach the client or family about dressing care and signs of infection. Removal can result in scarring, especially if the lesion is large; consequently, reassurance should be provided and feelings addressed regarding having a cancerous lesion and the associated body image changes. Focus is placed on comfort, education, and emotional support.

The nurse must identify and discuss the client's feelings about having a cancerous lesion, with referral to appropriate community resources if the client is having difficulty coping or has a high anxiety level. The nurse should explain that the risk of metastasis is low and refer the client to the American Cancer Society (ACS), a local library, or the Internet for information. Preventive strategies such as wearing long sleeves and hats with wide brims and using sunscreens should also be taught.

Evaluation

Evaluation of interventions focuses on monitoring for infection, pain control measures, comprehension of client education, and discussions related to body image changes and fear of cancer. If there is poor pain control or development of an infection, the physician or APN is contacted for an alternative strategy. Documentation of assessment, response to treatment measures, client comprehension of teaching, and other nursing interventions demonstrates nursing accountability.

Squamous Cell Carcinoma

SCC is skin cancer arising from the epidermis and is found most often on the scalp, outer ears, lower lip, and dorsum of the hands. SCC can also develop in chronic leg ulcers or open fractures with a 20% incidence of metastasis, generally to regional lymph nodes (Helm and Marks, 1998). SCC accounts for 90% of lip lesions. The etiologic factors of SCC can be UV rays, chemical carcinogens, and x-rays. SCC is more common in men and older adults, with the incidence increasing with geographic proximity to the equator. SCC is the most common skin cancer in blacks, in whom the majority of SCCs are found in areas that have not been exposed to the sun The opposite is true in whites, in whom 65% of SCCs are found on sun-exposed skin (Helm and Marks, 1998; Johnson, Moy, and White, 1998).

Symptoms of SCC usually include a thick, adherent scale with a soft, movable tumor that has well-defined borders. The center is often ulcerated or crusted. At first glance, SCC may even look like a wart. The base may be inflamed and red, and usually bleeds easily. SCC can arise from actinic keratosis, which supports early detection and removal of such lesions. If tumors are ignored or left unattended, they may enlarge, creating significant disfigurement after surgical excision.

NURSING MANAGEMENT

Assessment

Nursing assessment begins with interviewing the client, focusing on length of time lesion has been present, risk factors such as chronic sun exposure, and history of previous skin lesions. The nurse should inspect and palpate the lesion, surrounding tissue, and lymph nodes (to identify possible metastasis). A magnifying glass may be useful to closely examine any lesion. When a suspicious lesion is identified, especially if the lip is involved, the nurse should refer the client to the primary care provider for prompt treatment. He or she should also explain to the client that early treatment lessens the extent of scarring and, in the event of a cancerous lesion, lowers the risk of metastasis.

Diagnosis

Nursing diagnoses for a client with SCC include:

- Impaired skin integrity related to removal of a lesion
- High risk for infection related to break in skin integrity and surgical wound
- Body image disturbance related to disfigurement and scarring resulting from removal of cancerous lesion
- Fear related to cancer, pain, or death

Planning and Expected Outcomes

The goal of nursing management is to facilitate referral and treatment of suspicious lesions for removal without secondary infection. Time should be planned to discuss the client's and family's feelings about having a cancerous lesion to identify the need for a community referral or educational material. In addition, preventive strategies should be included in client education. Expected outcomes include:

1. Skin lesions will remain free from necrotic tissue and infection.
2. Skin lesions will heal with minimum scarring.
3. Client will demonstrate positive adaptation to body image changes, as evidenced by verbalization of feelings of acceptance.
4. Client will verbalize acceptance of the diagnosis and seek appropriate care.

Intervention

Nursing intervention is the same as with BCC; however, more disfigurement may be present after removal. If the lesion is large and extensive, more intense emotional and social support may be needed. The nurse should identify and discuss the client's feelings about having a cancerous lesion, with referral to appropriate community resources (e.g., therapist or support group) if the client is having difficulty coping or is experiencing high levels of anxiety. The nurse should explain that the risk of metastasis is low and refer the client to the ACS, Internet, and local library for additional information and literature. The client may experience greater anxiety about long-term quality-of-life issues if metastasis is present.

The nurse should teach the older adult client and family methods to care for the wound after removal of the lesion, signs of infection, preventive strategies, and the appearance of questionable skin lesions that warrant examination by the primary care provider.

Evaluation

Evaluation, supported by documentation, focuses on the appearance of wound infection, the client's coping response to changes in body image, and comprehension of teaching. If assessment reveals the development of an infection, the physician or APN should be contacted so that therapy can be implemented. Return demonstrations of dressing changes assist in evaluating the client's comprehension and technique. In addition, the nurse should obtain verbal confirmation of teaching by asking the client to repeat or list preventive activities (e.g., ways of protecting skin from UV rays).

Melanoma

Melanoma is a malignant neoplasm of pigment-forming cells that is capable of metastasizing to any organ of the body, even before the lesion is noted; therefore early detection is crucial. Melanoma represents 2% of all cancers and 1% of cancer-related deaths, and it is the second most common cause of death in men ages 30 to 49. After excision, primary, "thin" (less than 76 mm thick) melanoma has a 5-year survival rate of approximately 98%. The survival rate for other stages is 83%.

Melanoma incidence is rising. This is most likely a result of thinning of the ozone layer, combined with increased recreational sun exposure. A genetic predisposition to melanoma also exists, with 10% of clients having a parent or sibling with a history of melanoma. Individuals with a family history of melanoma should perform monthly skin self-examinations and have a professional skin evaluation at regular intervals (Habif, 2004).

Individuals at high risk are fair skinned, have a tendency to sunburn rather than tan, have red or blond hair, have multiple nevi, and have a tendency to freckle. Blacks, Asians, and dark-skinned whites are at less risk of developing melanoma; however, the majority of melanomas found in these populations were in skin not exposed to the sun, especially the periungual, palmar, and plantar surfaces (Johnson, Moy, and White, 1998). An individual with one melanoma is at risk for having another (Habif, 2004).

Melanoma's clinical hallmark is an irregularly shaped nevus (mole), papule, or plaque that has undergone a change, particularly in color. The characteristic signs of a majority of malignant melanomas are referred to as the *ABCDs*: **a**symmetry, **b**order irregularity, **c**olor variation (red, white, blue), and **d**iameter greater than 6 mm (Helm and Marks, 1998). The lesion may itch or bleed; however, this is usually a later sign. Any mole or lesion that has irregularly shaped borders and has had a color change, usually to a darker color, should be examined by a dermatologist or family physician.

All melanomas grow both vertically and radially. During the radial (lateral) growth phase, metastasis occurs infrequently, which reinforces the need for early detection and professional examination (Habif, 2004).

There are four types of melanoma, the most common of which is the *superficial spreading melanoma*, which is slower growing. Superficial spreading melanoma accounts for 70% of all melanomas, occurring most commonly on the back in males and the extremities in females. The mean age of diagnosis is the mid-40s. Superficial melanoma is a flat, slightly elevated, pigmented papule or patch that has irregular borders and varied colors within the lesion. Fortunately, superficial spreading melanoma usually enlarges slowly in a radial (lateral) fashion (Habif, 2004).

Nodular melanoma occurs in 15% to 30% of the clients with melanoma and has the worst prognosis because it grows vertically at an early stage. Nodular melanoma is not often found on the head, neck, and trunk, and it is more common in black and dark-skinned individuals. The mean age at diagnosis is the fifth or sixth decade of life. Nodular melanoma is a hard, usually dark nodule arising from a preexisting mole (Habif, 2004).

Lentigo melanoma occurs in 5% to 10% of all melanoma clients and is more prevalent in women. Of these lesions, 30% to 50% arise in individuals with lentigo maligna. Therefore thorough skin assessment and instruction in self-examination is important in people with lentigo maligna. The mean age of occurrence is 70. Lentigo maligna melanoma is a brown-tannish macular lesion with varied pigmentation and highly irregular borders (Habif, 2004).

Acral-lentiginous melanoma (10% of all melanomas) usually occurs on the palms, soles, fingers, and toes. It is more common in older adults, with a mean age of 60 at the time of diagnosis. It is the most common melanoma found in blacks and Asians; therefore inspection of the foot soles, palms, and hands is warranted when caring for black and Asian-American clients. Acral-lentiginous melanoma resembles lentigo melanoma with its flat, irregular, discolored borders (Habif, 2004; Johnson, Moy, and White, 1998).

NURSING MANAGEMENT

Assessment

Nursing assessment begins with interviewing the client to determine how long the lesion has been present and to identify risk factors such as chronic sun exposure and family history. The nurse should inspect and palpate the suspicious lesion, surrounding tissue, and lymph nodes (to identify possible metastasis). A magnifying glass may be useful to closely examine any lesion. When a suspicious lesion is identified, the nurse should promptly refer the client to the primary care provider. He or she should also explain that early treatment lessens the extent of scarring and possibly intervenes before metastasis. Because this is an aggressive cancerous lesion, the nurse should discuss the client's feelings and fears about cancer.

Diagnosis

Nursing diagnoses for a client with melanoma include:

- Impaired skin integrity related to removal of a cancerous lesion
- Fear of cancer, pain, or death related to having a cancerous skin lesion
- High risk for infection related to break in skin integrity and surgical wound
- Body image disturbance related to disfigurement and scarring resulting from removal of cancerous lesion

Planning and Expected Outcomes

The goals of nursing management are to facilitate referral and treatment of suspicious lesions for removal without secondary infection and metastasis and to address fears and feelings related to cancer, with referral to community resources as indicated. The nurse must discuss the client's and family's feelings about having a cancerous lesion to identify the need for a community referral or educational material. Expected outcomes include:

1. Site of excision will heal without evidence of infection.
2. Client will verbalize fears related to the diagnosis and actively seek information and clarification.
3. Client will identify community resources for support and additional information.
4. Client will verbalize understanding of the treatment plan.
5. Client will demonstrate increased knowledge of condition, as evidenced by adoption of preventive strategies.

Intervention

Nursing management includes reinforcement of the treatment regimen by monitoring the wound for secondary infection (e.g., erythema, tenderness, purulent discharge) and reinforcement of the caring component of nursing by discussing the client's and family's feelings related to cancer. The nurse should identify and discuss the client's and family's feelings about having a cancerous lesion, with referral to appropriate community resources if the client is having difficulty coping or has a high level of anxiety. He or she should also explain that there is a risk of metastasis and refer the client to the ACS, Internet, or local library for additional information.

The nurse should teach the client or family dressing care and signs of infection. Removal can result in scarring, especially if the lesion was large; consequently, reassurance must be provided and feelings related to body image changes addressed; the focus is on comfort, education, and emotional support. Preventive strategies such as wearing hats with wide brims, wearing long sleeves, and using sunscreen should also be taught to both client and family. In addition, the client and family members should have annual skin assessments, since a hereditary tendency for occurrence exists.

Evaluation

Evaluation of nursing interventions focuses on monitoring for infection, the effectiveness of pain control measures, comprehension of client education, and discussions related to body image changes and fears about cancer. If there is poor pain control or development of an infection, the physician or APN should be contacted for an alternative strategy. Documentation of assessment, response to treatment measures, client comprehension of teaching, and other nursing interventions demonstrates nursing accountability.

LOWER EXTREMITY ULCERS

Chronic leg ulcers are a common problem in older adults, occurring primarily from three causes: arterial insufficiency, diabetic neuropathy, and venous hypertension (Table 30-1). A brief overview of each etiologic factor and treatment follows. Greater emphasis is placed on venous ulcers because these are more prevalent in older adults and more challenging as a result of their chronicity.

Arterial Ulcers

Arterial or ischemic ulcers result from arterial insufficiency and are not as prevalent as venous ulcers. Clients with arterial insufficiency, also referred to as peripheral vascular disease (PVD), have 9 times the risk of amputation compared with those who only have venous disease (Arnold et al, 1994). Arteriosclerosis—thickening and hardening of the arterial wall—is the primary cause for the decreased blood flow that results in ischemia and eventually tissue death. The term *arteriosclerosis obliterans* is used when atheromatous lesions develop in the lower extremities below the abdominal aorta. Several risk factors, including smoking, diabetes, hyperlipoproteinemia, and hypertension, can lead to arteriosclerosis obliterans.

Pain with exercise, at night, or while resting is the most common sign of arterial insufficiency. Pain at rest indicates severely restricted arterial blood flow. The area proximal to (above) the painful area is usually the site of restricted blood flow. Pulses distal to the restriction may be present as a result of collateral circulation. The client may also complain of cramping, burning, or aching. As the disease advances, the extremity develops a cyanotic hue and becomes cool. The skin becomes thin, shiny, and dry, with an associated loss of hair and thickened toenails, all resulting from the diminished blood supply. Tissue anoxia leads to necrosis and poor healing. Arterial ulcers are usually located on the feet and toes. The causes must be corrected so that oxygen and other nutrients are available to promote healing of necrotic wounds. Treatment is usually surgical intervention with revascularization; if the disease is too advanced, amputation may be necessary.

TABLE 30-1 Leg Ulcer Differentiation

TYPE	PRIMARY CAUSE	CHARACTERISTICS
Arterial	Arterial insufficiency; PVD	Located on toes, feet, or lower third of leg; irregularly shaped wound; thin, shiny, cool skin with cyanotic hue, loss of hair, thickened toenails; pain with activity, rest, or at night
Diabetic neuropathy	Neuropathy	Located on plantar surface of foot; circular, often deep wounds; decreased or absent vibratory sensation; painful; paresthesia
Venous	Venous hypertension	Located on medial aspect of lower third of leg; irregularly shaped wound; either flat or shallow crater; discoloration, varicosities, edema, and exudate; pain relieved with activity

Diabetic Neuropathic Ulcers

Risk factors for developing a diabetic foot ulcer are smoking, hypertension, lipoprotein abnormalities (particularly elevated low-density lipoprotein), chronic hyperglycemia, absent vibratory sensation in the lower extremities, PVD, and poor outpatient diabetes education (Levin, 1997). Older adults who live alone or have mental confusion are at an increased risk for foot ulcer because they may not have the means to recognize an ulcer or to follow up with appropriate treatment. A risk factor for lower extremity amputation is neuropathy, which is implicated in approximately 90% of diabetic foot ulcers. This sensory loss is associated with a 15.5% relative risk of amputation. Therefore individuals with diabetes and neuropathy are at risk of developing lower leg ulcers, which may lead to an amputation.

Pain and temperature are usually the first sensations affected by neuropathy. The loss of the peripheral sensory feedback system impairs the client's ability to feel tissue damage, inflammation, or injury. Ulcers resulting from diabetic peripheral neuropathy tend to be bilateral, symmetric, and located on the plantar surface of the foot. Clients usually complain of pain and paresthesias; however, they also have diminished or absent vibratory and temperature sensation of the affected extremities. Pain relieved by walking is one diagnostic sign of neuropathy. Neuropathic ulcers are usually well perfused, yet a client with diabetes may have arterial insufficiency, which compromises healing abilities.

Treatment can vary, depending on the etiologic factors and wound condition. Client education regarding how to minimize the risk of chemical, thermal, and mechanical trauma is the first-line defense for diabetic foot ulcers. Physical examination of the foot should include testing for neuropathy and the identification of high foot pressures. An easy and inexpensive device for establishing neuropathy is the Semmes-Weinstein monofilament. Inability to feel the 5.07 monofilament indicates the client is at risk for ulceration and needs orthotics (specially fitted shoes designed to prevent ulcers and to decrease callous formation by redistributing weight) to off-load pressure (Birke and Rolfsen, 1998). The nurse should stress to clients with diabetes, particularly if they have PVD, that any trauma to the lower leg, ankles, or feet can lead to an ulcer and possible amputation. They must protect feet and lower legs with proper shoes and foot care. Orthotics may be helpful in preventing mechanical trauma. When an ulcer is present, a total contact cast may be applied to redistribute weight and minimize trauma. Casting is contraindicated when cellulitis, sinus tracts, or excessive exudate is present (Armstrong, Lavery, and Bushman, 1998). Some physicians use hyperbaric oxygenation in hopes of increasing oxygenation to the affected area; however, this treatment is controversial because of its questionable effectiveness in wounds with compromised circulation, such as diabetic ulcers. The success of this strategy depends on the amount of circulation present in the affected area.

Venous Ulcers

Venous ulcer, or venous dermatitis, has been recognized for more than 2000 years. The cause of this chronic, costly condition is not completely known, but it has been attributed to chronic venous insufficiency. Venous ulcers affect 1% to 1.3% of the general population, with a higher incidence (3.5%) in older adults. Chronic venous leg ulcers usually have an onset in early adulthood; however, peak prevalence is seen in people ages 70 and older. Venous ulcers occur more often in women (3:1) than in men. Epidemiologic studies have revealed that 57% to 80% of all lower leg ulcers are related to venous insufficiency, with 10% to 25% having a combination of venous and arterial insufficiency.

Homans stated in 1917 that venous ulcers were related to venous stagnation, which led to anoxia and ulceration. Consequently, the term *venous stasis ulcer* or *dermatitis* was established. The concept of stasis was challenged in 1929 when research revealed higher oxygenation in limbs with venous ulcers. The correct term now is *venous ulcer,* since the cause is not related to stasis. Browse and Burnand (1982) revealed the most current etiologic factor: an enlarged capillary bed from venous hypertension that causes leakage of fibrinogen into interstitial tissue, creating a fibrin cuff (Burton, 1994). Falanga and Eaglstein (1993) are now proposing that the fibrin cuff facilitates the trapping of growth factors, which impedes healing (Vowden, 1998).

Venous hypertension is the primary cause of venous ulcer. Valvular incompetence of the deep or perforating veins of the lower leg is present in the majority of venous ulcer cases. Venous hypertension leads to a tortuous capillary system, which causes an accumulation of fibrinogen, leukocytes, and erythrocytes. The accumulation of erythrocytes in the tissue produces a brownish skin discoloration caused by the release of hemoglobin. Often the discoloration and thickening of the skin (liposclerosis) is the first indication of venous hypertension. Capillary occlusion caused by trapping of white blood cells results in the release of proteolytic enzymes, which foster fibrinogen leakage. This excessive fibrinogen forms a fibrin cuff that impairs diffusion of oxygen, nutrients, and possibly growth factors (Harris, Brown-Etris, and Troyer-Caudle, 1996). The fibrin cuff creates a barrier that prevents or delays exchange of oxygen and other nutrients, resulting in cell death. Anoxia and trapping of growth factors are the primary causes of ulceration and poor healing. The fibrin cuff is irreversible, which sets the stage for frequent recurrence and makes venous ulcer a chronic disorder.

The diagnosis of venous ulcer is commonly based on clinical presentation. Venous ulcers are usually on the medial aspect of the lower leg, with flat or shallow craters and irregular borders, accompanied by varicosities, liposclerosis (brown-ruddy color and thickened skin), and itching. Venous ulcers generate a large amount of exudate and are usually surrounded by erythema and edema. It is difficult at times to differentiate between cellulitis and typical venous ulcer presentation, since both have erythema, tenderness, and induration (Harris, Brown-Etris, and Troyer-Caudle, 1996).

It is well recognized that venous ulcers heal with prolonged elevation of the affected extremity; however, compliance is difficult. Research has demonstrated that compression therapy of at least 20 to 30 mm Hg at the ankle and distal lower leg decreases edema by compressing fluid through the fibrin cuff (Fletcher, Sheldon, and Cullum, 1997). The most common cause of recurrence is noncompliance with compression therapy. It is important to remember that compression therapy is intended for ambulatory clients. The older adult with dependent edema, not primary venous disease, does not tolerate compression well. Compression therapy is not a management option for arterial insufficiency; pain and cyanosis will occur from further impaired circulation.

NURSING MANAGEMENT

Assessment

Nursing assessment begins with determining the location and characteristics of lower leg ulcers. The nurse should determine ulcer dimensions, depth, and amount of exudate; palpate popliteal pulses at least every day if the client is in acute care and at every visit if he or she is in an ambulatory or home setting; and note any discoloration and edema. The nurse should also ascertain if the client experiences any pain or itching and how it has been managed. A nutritional assessment should be conducted, which includes the client's weight, 24-hour diet recall, chewing abilities, and food preparation abilities. The nurse should determine if shopping assistance is needed.

Diagnosis

Nursing diagnoses for a client with lower extremity ulcers include:

- Impaired skin integrity related to altered circulation
- High risk for infection related to open, chronic wounds

Planning and Expected Outcomes

The goal of nursing management is to facilitate healing without infection by promoting treatment compliance and by providing client education regarding the disease process and treatment, stressing that venous ulcers are a chronic process. Time for client education will be needed. Expected outcomes include:

1. Skin lesions will remain free from necrotic tissue and infection.
2. Edema in lower extremities will be controlled.
3. Skin lesions will heal with minimum scarring.
4. Client will be able to maintain a healed state for at least 6 months.

Intervention

Nursing interventions consist of keeping legs elevated above the heart; implementing compression therapy; administering wound care; and educating the client regarding venous ulcer cause and its chronic nature, the strategy of compression therapy, and specific wound care. The nurse must stress the need to maintain compression therapy to facilitate healing of ulcers and avoid further breakdown. Infection is difficult to determine, since venous ulcers often have erythemic bases with induration; however, if the client develops a fever and tenderness surrounding the ulcer, the physician or APN should be contacted. The nurse should determine if any community services such as Meals on Wheels, grocery shopping assistance, and other support services are needed. He or she should also identify and discuss the client's feelings regarding chronicity and body image changes; teach the client that venous ulcers generate a large amount of exudate; and instruct on dressing changes and how to place 15 to 20 cm blocks at the foot of the bed at home for long-term edema management.

Evaluation

Evaluation of nursing interventions focuses on prevention of further ulcer deterioration and infection, as well as the effectiveness of client education. Return demonstration of compression therapy application and wound care is a concrete evaluation and ensures client comprehension. Nursing accountability is demonstrated by documentation of assessment, response to treatment measures, client comprehension of teaching, and other nursing interventions.

PRESSURE ULCERS

Pressure ulcers (also known as bedsores, decubitus, or pressure sores) have plagued humans for centuries. Hippocrates devised a débridement treatment with healing by secondary closure. Ambroise Paré, a sixteenth-century surgeon, published strategies for healing skin ulcers that challenged the existing practice of pouring hot oil on the wound. These included increased nutrition and mobility, débridement, and application of dressings (Levine, 1992).

It was not until the twentieth century that scientific research began to determine the cause and appropriate management of pressure ulcers. In 1930 Landis determined that the average capillary pressure before which ischemia occurs is below 32 mm Hg. In the 1950s Kosiak (1958) found that pressure applied to rabbits' ears over 2 hours would result in ulceration. Thus the universal recommendation of turning every 2 hours was established. The first pressure ulcer risk assessment tool was designed and tested by Doreen Norton (1989) in the late 1950s, but not disseminated until 1962 when she presented study findings at a conference.

In 1962 researchers first demonstrated that moisture, applied with occlusive dressings, increases epithelialization (healing process) (Krasner, 1991). In 1972 a plastic occlusive dressing was shown to cut epithelialization time in half, which led to film dressings, followed by hydrocolloidal dressings.

This information explosion has resulted in varied terminology and beliefs. As a result, leading experts in pressure ulcer management and research formed the National Pressure Ulcer Advisory Panel (NPUAP) in 1987, with the intent of improving prevention and management through education, legislation, standardization of staging criteria, and identification of research needs. The NPUAP held consensus conferences beginning in May 1988, the outcome of which included standardized staging criteria that are endorsed by the International Association for Enterostomal Therapists and the Agency for Healthcare Research and Quality (AHRQ) (formerly the Agency for Health Care Policy and Research [AHCPR]). Also, to standardize terms and to more accurately reflect the cause of pressure damage, NPUAP decreed that *pressure ulcer* is a more appropriate term than *pressure sore* or *decubitus*. Therefore the term *pressure ulcer* is used throughout this discussion.

In December 1989 the Omnibus Budget Reconciliation Act (OBRA) established the AHCPR. Based on reviews of current research and practice, this agency was charged with developing clinical practice guidelines that appropriately and effectively prevent, diagnose, treat, and manage clinically relevant disorders and diseases (AHCPR, 1992). Pressure ulcer prevention and management was one of the first three areas reviewed by the AHCPR. As a result, *Pressure Ulcers in Adults: Prediction and Prevention* was published in May 1992, and *Treatment of Pressure Ulcers* was published in February 1994. These comprehensive references are guides for the following discussion.

Epidemiology of Pressure Ulcers

The epidemiology of pressure ulcers has been difficult to quantify and varies based on sample size, definition of terms, and type of facility. Despite methodologic limitations, incidence (new cases) and prevalence (over a specific period) rates of pressure ulcers are sufficiently high to generate concern.

The incidence of pressure ulcers in hospitals ranges from 2.7% to as high as 60%. The prevalence rate in hospitals ranges from 3.5% to 29.5%. Several studies have identified high-risk groups of hospitalized clients: quadriplegic clients, older clients with hip fractures, orthopedic clients who are immobile, and critical care clients (AHCPR, 1992).

The prevalence rate of pressure ulcers in long-term care facilities ranges from 2.4% to 23%. Incidence rates vary among nursing care facilities because of the heterogeneous case-mix and staffing patterns. Better data are needed to determine the degree of the problem in long-term care (AHCPR, 1992). It is believed that OBRA regulations have been instrumental in decreasing the incidence of pressure ulcers in nursing facilities.

Etiology of Pressure Ulcers

Pressure on soft tissue over bony prominences or other hard surfaces is the primary causative factor in pressure ulcer formation. However, other contributing factors exist and explain why some individuals break down within 30 minutes of lying in the same position, whereas others do not break down for hours.

Pressure ulcers begin at the point of contact between soft tissue and a hard surface (e.g., bone). Consequently, an upside-down cone-shaped wound develops with the largest area of breakdown being near the bone. Common bony prominences susceptible to pressure ulcer development are the sacrum, ischial tuberosity (especially in an upright sitting position in a chair or bed), lateral malleolus, trochanter, and heels. However, any pressure point is vulnerable when pressure is intense and prolonged (Allman, 1997) (Fig. 30-1).

The intensity of pressure that leads to capillary closure, compounded by the duration of pressure and tissue tolerance, results in tissue anoxia, ischemia, edema, and eventually tissue necrosis. Immobility, decreased activity, and decreased sensory perception place individuals at risk for unrelieved pressure that generates tissue ischemia and death. Tissue tolerance is influenced by extrinsic factors—moisture, friction, and shearing—and intrinsic factors—poor nutrition, advanced age, hypotension, emotional stress, smoking, and skin temperature (Cox, Laird, and Brown, 1998). The development of pressure ulcers is a complex, synergistic phenomenon that makes prevention a challenge (Fig. 30-2).

Capillary pressure ensures the movement of blood through the capillary membrane, maintaining oxygenation and tissue nutrition. Exact capillary pressure is not known. Various studies have identified ranges from 10 to 14 mm Hg in the venous limb system to 32 to 40 mm Hg in the arteriolar limb system (Landis, 1930). Capillary collapse can result from intense and prolonged pressure, which leads to tissue anoxia, ischemia, reactive hyperemia (erythema), leakage of plasma into interstitial tissue, and microvascular hemorrhage observable by nonblanchable erythema. If pressure persists, tissue death results. It is assumed that capillary pressure, which varies depending on location and individual, ranging from 10 to 40 mm Hg, must be exceeded to impair circulation.

Individuals with normal sensation regularly shift their weight, voluntarily and involuntarily, in response to the discomfort from capillary closure and resulting tissue anoxia (Allman, 1997). People with sensory impairment (paralysis or sedation), however, do not have this normal protective reflex, which can explain the higher incidence of pressure ulcers among paralyzed individuals or those undergoing long surgical procedures. Clients with altered mental status as a consequence of disease (e.g., dementia) or medication may have decreased pain or tissue anoxia perception. These individuals are at risk for pressure ulcer development.

Tissue tolerance, another major contributing factor in the development of a pressure ulcer, is defined as the ability of

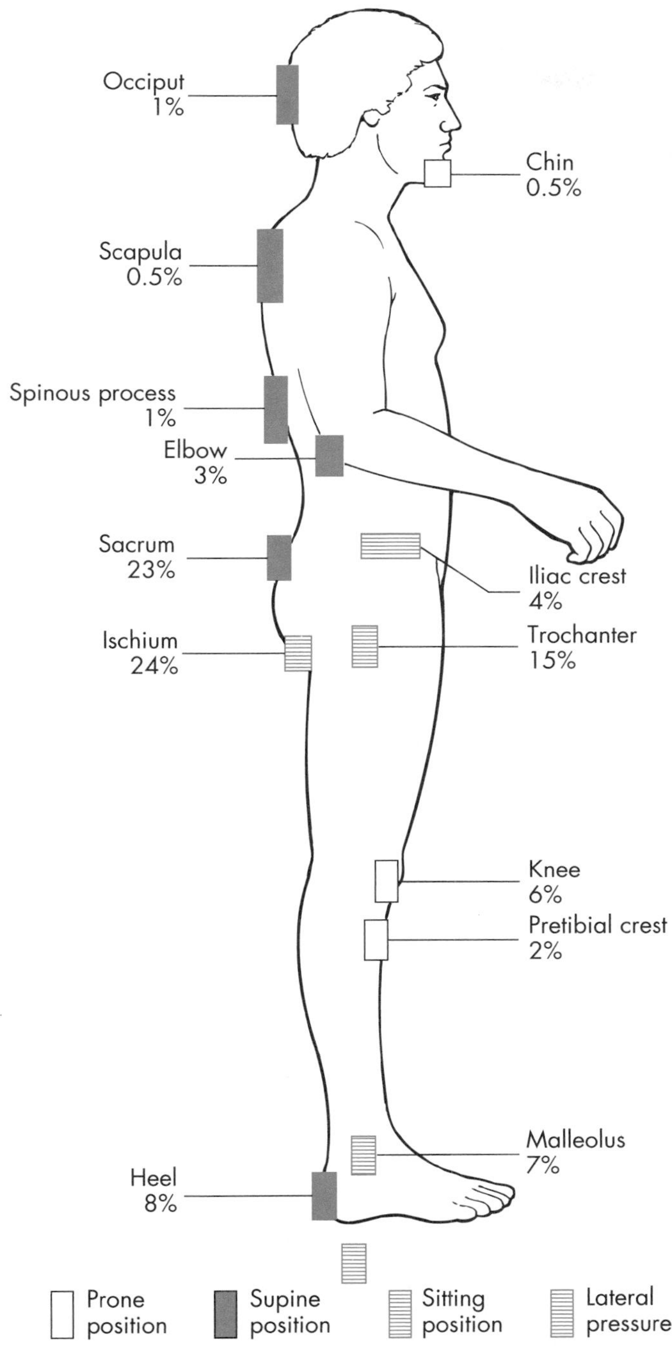

Fig. 30-1 Common sites for pressure ulcers and frequency of ulceration per site. (Artwork by John A. Craig, MD, from Clinical Symposia, vol 31, No 5. Used as a reference with permission from Icon Learning Systems, a division of MediMedia USA, Inc. All rights reserved.)

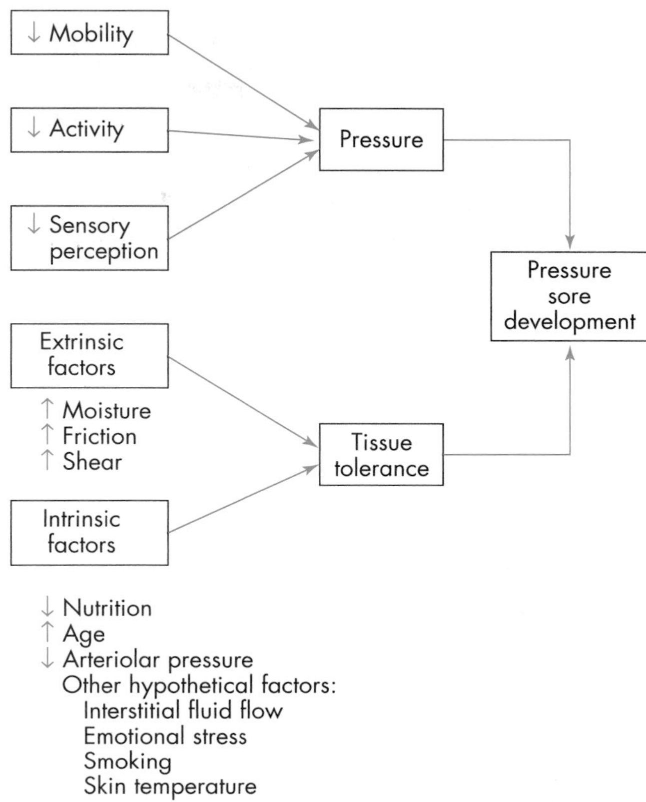

Fig. 30-2 Factors contributing to the development of pressure ulcers. (Reprinted with permission from Braden B, Bergstrom N: A conceptual schema for the study of the etiology of pressure sores, *Rehabil Nurs* 12[1]:8, 1987. Copyright 1987 by the Association of Rehabilitation Nurses.)

the skin and supporting structures to endure the effects of pressure. The integumentary structures, blood vessels, interstitial fluid, and collagen function as "springs" that transmit pressure load from the skin's surface to skeletal structures (Maklebust, 1997). It is apparent, then, that poor tissue tolerance makes one more vulnerable to pressure intensity and duration, thus increasing the response to pressure. Shearing, friction, age-related changes in the integumentary system, low blood pressure, and nutritional status all influence the integrity of tissue tolerance.

Shearing, the sliding of parallel surfaces, causes stretching and occlusion of arterial supply, which is usually of the fascia and muscle. Shearing forces can decrease blood supply, leading to tissue ischemia and necrosis. The most common position for shearing is when the head of the bed is elevated, causing the body to slide downward (Fig. 30-3). Resistance keeps the skin in place while gravity pulls the body toward the foot of the bed. It is believed that shearing forces cause more damage than is recognized, with as many as 40% of pressure ulcers resulting from shearing rather than pressure (Bryant et al, 1992).

Friction, the rubbing of skin against another surface, primarily affects the epidermal and dermal layers, causing a superficial abrasion (e.g., sheet burn) (Maklebust, 1997). Restless clients or those with persistent movements are at risk for friction injuries. However, when friction occurs concurrently with gravitational forces, shearing is the outcome.

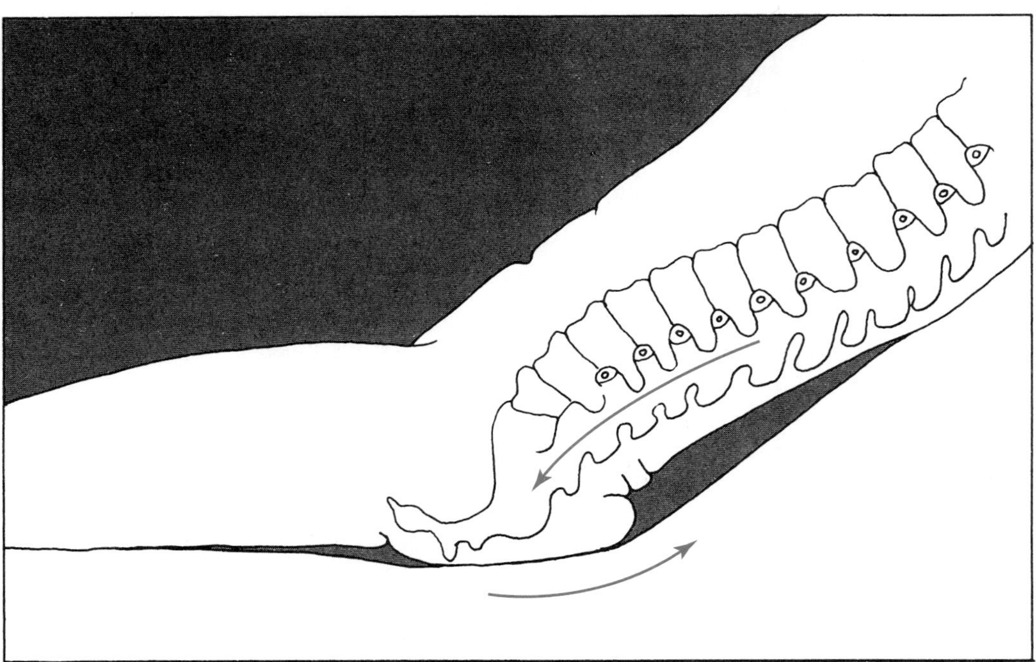

Fig. 30-3 Shearing force. (From Loeper JM et al: *Therapeutic positioning and skin care*, Minneapolis, 1986, Sister Kenny Institute.)

Moisture from incontinence or profuse sweating can decrease tensile strength, alter skin resiliency to external forces, and exacerbate friction and shearing forces (Cox, Laird, and Brown, 1998). Some experts believe that friction and shearing forces are increased in the presence of mild to moderate moisture and decreased in the presence of profuse moisture (Bryant et al, 1992). Therefore urinary incontinence may not be as significant in pressure ulcer development as was once thought. Regardless, efforts should be made to keep skin dry.

As many studies have revealed, nutritional status greatly influences the development of pressure ulcers. Protein deficiency weakens tissue tolerance (i.e., the spring between the skin surface and bony prominences), making soft tissue more susceptible to breakdown when pressure intensity is prolonged. Hypoproteinemia changes osmotic equilibrium, which leads to edema. Consequently, sluggish oxygenation and transportation create an environment for tissue breakdown and poor healing. Serum albumin levels below 3.5 g/dl have a correlation with pressure ulcer development and poor wound healing (Thomas, 1997). Proteins are also needed for collagen formation, granulation tissue formation, and immunologic response.

The incidence of pressure ulcers is increased in older adults, particularly in those over age 70. With aging, the epidermis thins, elasticity decreases, and vessels degenerate, resulting in reduced blood flow. Collagen fibers stiffen and the immune response becomes sluggish (Habif, 2004). These age-related changes impair the early warning sign of erythema, delay crucial early immunologic responses, and impede the healing process, thereby making older adults at risk for pressure ulcer development.

Low blood pressure and dehydration can reduce circulation, especially in the microvasculature, which eventually leads to tissue ischemia. Diastolic blood pressure below 60 mm Hg has been found to be a risk factor for pressure ulcer formation, presumably because of decreased peripheral circulation and subsequent ischemia (Braden and Bryant, 1990).

Other intrinsic factors are stress, smoking, and elevated body temperature. Emotional stress with reduction in effective coping mechanisms leads to release of cortisol from the adrenal glands. The effects of cortisol are not completely understood but are believed to alter the skin's ability to absorb mechanical loads, such as pressure. In addition, cortisone may affect cellular metabolism between capillary beds and cells, making the skin vulnerable to breakdown and poor healing. A relationship between cigarette smoking and pressure ulcer development is becoming evident, especially in spinal cord–injured clients. The reason is not clear but is thought to be related to vasoconstriction. Elevated temperature, especially in older adults, is associated with pressure ulcer formation, possibly caused by increased oxygen demands in anoxic tissue (Bryant et al, 1992).

The formation of a pressure ulcer is a complex process involving many variables within the nurse's control (e.g., pressure, shearing, moisture), as well as variables out of the nurse's control (e.g., smoking, malnutrition, low blood pressure, paralysis). The principal mechanisms of injury are loss of microcirculation through pressure compressing the microvessels, or intrinsic factors causing soft tissue to become more vulnerable to lost blood supply.

Risk Assessment Tools

The success of pressure ulcer prevention depends on early identification of at-risk clients. As recommended by the AHCPR clinical guidelines, a valid, research-based assessment tool should be used. To establish consistency and accuracy, there should be written protocols specifying how to use the risk assessment tool, when to use it, and which health care team members should use it. A risk assessment should be conducted on all individuals who are bedbound, chairbound, incontinent, frail, disabled, or nutritionally compromised or who have demonstrated altered mental status (AHCPR, 1992). An assessment should be conducted on clients admitted to an acute care facility, rehabilitation hospital, nursing facility, home care agency, or other health care facility. Identified high-risk individuals should be reassessed at regular intervals if mobility or activity is impaired. Whenever a client's condition changes (e.g., decreased mobility, eating less, change in serum albumin), the risk assessment should be repeated and the care plan modified accordingly.

Numerous instruments have been designed to identify clients at risk for pressure ulcer formation. However, many tools have not been subjected to vigorous evaluation of reliability and validity testing. The Braden and Norton risk assessment tools, according to AHCPR clinical guidelines, have undergone the most extensive evaluations.

The Norton Risk Assessment Scale was the first such tool designed for use in a study investigating geriatric nursing problems in hospitals. Consequently, it has set the stage for more comprehensive assessment tools. The study began in the late 1950s, but results were not disseminated until a conference in 1962. At that time it was believed that pressure ulcers were the result of poor nursing care; however, additional research has revealed the problem to be much more complex. The Norton scale is simple to use and has only five assessment categories. Although the original research assessed nutritional status, it was not included in the scale because it was believed that the client's general health was a reflection of nutritional status. Norton (1989) indicates that nutritional status, including eating behaviors, would have been an important parameter to include. Clients with a score of 16 or lower on the Norton scale are considered to be at risk for pressure ulcer development (Table 30-2).

The Braden Scale for Predicting Pressure Sore Risk has been shown to be highly reliable when used by registered nurses and is the most rigorously tested risk assessment tool (AHCPR, 1992; Bergstrom et al, 1987). The Braden scale assesses sensory perception rather than mental status. Assessing sensory perception is thought to be a more precise risk indicator, since impaired sensation prevents an individual from sensing the need to change positions, which in turn decreases pressure intensity (Braden and Bergstrom, 1987). As a rule, a client scoring below 18 on the Braden scale is considered to be at high risk for skin breakdown (Table 30-3) (see Research box).

Another tool discussed in the literature is Gosnell's scale, designed in the mid-1980s. Gosnell's scale paralleled Norton's; however, it added nutritional and other medical variables such as medications, vital signs, and hydration status. Risk scoring has been revised from the original work, with higher scores reflecting greater risk (Gosnell, 1989). The tool requires more data collection but includes more in-depth assessment of intrinsic factors such as blood pressure and hydration. Although this tool has undergone some reliability and validity testing, AHCPR still endorsed the Braden and Norton scales because these tools have been more extensively tested.

Preventive Strategies

Prevention is the first line of defense for pressure ulcers, which are costly health care problems that adversely affect

TABLE 30-2 Norton Risk Assessment Scale

		PHYSICAL CONDITION	MENTAL CONDITION	ACTIVITY	MOBILITY	INCONTINENT	TOTAL SCORE
		Good 4 Fair 3 Poor 2 Very bad 1	Alert 4 Apathetic 3 Confused 2 Stupor 1	Ambulant 4 Walk/help 3 Chairbound 2 Bed 1	Full 4 Sl. Limited 3 V. limited 2 Immobile 1	Not 4 Occasionally 3 Usually/urine 2 Doubly 1	
Name	Date						

Reprinted with permission from Norton D, McLaren R, Exton-Smith AN: *An investigation of geriatric nursing problems in hospital,* Edinburgh, 1975, Churchill Livingstone.

TABLE 30-3 Braden Scale for Predicting Pressure Sore Risk

Patient's Name________________ Evaluator's Name__________________ Date of Assessment

SENSORY PERCEPTION Ability to respond meaningfully to pressure-related discomfort	**1. Completely Limited:** Unresponsive (does not moan, flinch, or gasp) to painful stimuli, due to diminished level of consciousness or sedation. OR limited ability to feel pain over most of body surface.	**2. Very Limited:** Responds only to painful stimuli. Cannot communicate discomfort except by moaning or restlessness, OR has a sensory impairment which limits the ability to feel pain or discomfort over 1/2 of body.	**3. Slightly Limited:** Responds to verbal commands but cannot always communicate discomfort or need to be turned, OR has some sensory impairment which limits ability to feel pain or discomfort in 1 or 2 extremities.	**4. No Impairment:** Responds to verbal commands. no sensory deficit which would limit ability to feel or voice pain or discomfort.				
MOISTURE Degree to which skin is exposed to moisture	**1. Constantly Moist:** Skin is kept moist almost constantly by perspiration, urine, etc. Dampness is detected every time patient is moved or turned.	**2. Moist:** Skin is often but not always moist. Linen must be changed at least once a shift.	**3. Occasionally Moist:** Skin is occasionally moist, requiring an extra linen change approximately once a day.	**4. Rarely Moist:** Skin is usually dry; linen requires changing only at routine intervals.				
ACTIVITY Degree of physical activity	**1. Bedfast:** Confined to bed.	**2. Chairfast:** Ability to walk severely limited or nonexistent. Cannot bear own weight and/or must be assisted into chair or wheelchair.	**3. Walks Occasionally:** Walks occasionally during day but for very short distances, with or without assistance. Spends majority of each shift in bed or chair.	**4. Walks Frequently:** Walks outside the room at least twice a day and inside room at least once every 2 hours during waking hours.				
MOBILITY Ability to change and control body position	**1. Completely Immobile:** Does not make even slight changes in body or extremity position without assistance.	**2. Very Limited:** Makes occasional slight changes in body or extremity position but unable to make frequent or significant changes independently.	**3. Slightly Limited:** Makes frequent though slight changes in body or extremity position independently.	**4. No Limitations:** Makes major and frequent changes in position without assistance.				
NUTRITION Usual food intake pattern	**1. Very Poor:** Never eats a complete meal. Rarely eats more than 1/3 of any food offered. Eats 2 servings or less of protein (meat or dairy products) per day. Takes fluids	**2. Probably Inadequate:** Rarely eats a complete meal and generally eats only about 1/2 of any food offered. Protein intake includes only 3 servings of meat	**3. Adequate:** Eats over half of most meals. Eats a total of 4 servings of protein (meat, dairy products) each day. Occasionally will refuse a meal, but will usually take a	**4. Excellent:** Eats most of every meal. Never refuses a meal. Usually eats a total of 4 or more servings of meat and dairy products. Occasionally				
				Total score				

Continued

TABLE 30-3 Braden Scale for Predicting Pressure Sore Risk—cont'd

Patient's Name________________ Evaluator's Name________________ Date of Assessment

NUTRITION—*Cont'd*	poorly. Does not take a liquid dietary supplement. OR is NPO and/or maintained on clear liquids or IVs for more than 5 days.	or dairy products per day. Occasionally will take a dietary supplement, OR receives less than optimum amount of liquid diet or tube feeding.	supplement if offered, OR is on a tube feeding or TPN regimen, which probably meets most of nutritional needs.	eats between meals. Does not require supplementation.				
FRICTION AND SHEAR	1. Problem: Requires moderate to maximum assistance in moving. Complete lifting without sliding against sheets is impossible. Frequently slides down in bed or chair, requiring frequent repositioning maximum assistance. Spasticity, contractures, or agitation leads to almost constant friction.	2. Potential Problem: Moves feebly or requires minimum assistance. During a move skin probably slides to some extent against sheets, chair, restraints, or other devices. Maintains relatively good position in chair or bed most of the time but occasionally slides down.	3. No Apparent Problem: Moves in bed and in chair independently and has sufficient muscle strength to lift up completely during move. Maintains good position in bed or chair at all times.					
				Total score				

NPO, Nothing by mouth; *IVs,* intravenous feedings; TPN, total parenteral nutrition.

a client's quality of life. The professional nurse has a responsibility to identify clients at risk for pressure ulcers and to implement research-based preventive strategies. Nurses as front-line providers and managers of care are key health care team members who can influence the prevalence of pressure ulcers and enhance the client's quality of life. Nurses can mobilize the health care team when needs are identified by seeking a dietary consultation and alerting the physician or APN when a client is not eating sufficiently or when a client develops nonblanchable erythema. Written preventive protocols, endorsed (and embraced) by the health care team and institution, can empower the professional nurse to act independently and immediately when vulnerable clients are identified.

All at-risk individuals identified through use of a risk assessment tool should have a daily skin inspection with close attention to bony prominences as recommended by AHCPR clinical guidelines. This routine assessment should be documented to demonstrate professional accountability and evaluate preventive strategy outcomes. Another skin-related activity recommended by AHCPR clinical guidelines is to cleanse the skin of an incontinent client with a mild, nonirritating cleanser using warm, not hot, water at the time of soiling to minimize skin irritation and dryness. Moisturizers, such as emollient lotions, should be used to keep the skin from drying and cracking. It is best to apply the lotion immediately after bathing to increase moisture absorbed by the skin. Skin should not be rubbed or massaged over bony prominences because it may cause further deep tissue damage, especially if erythema is present (which already indicates injury) (AHCPR, 1992).

Proper turning and placement reduce the effects of pressure but not the intensity. It has been standard practice to turn clients a minimum of every 2 hours, which was endorsed in the AHCPR clinical guidelines. However, capillary closing pressure varies with each individual; therefore the ideal strategy is to determine the turning schedule based on development of erythema, which may precede ischemia (Bergstrom, 1987). For many reasons this ideal strategy may not be possible, but it should be done when staffing and

Research

SAMPLE AND SETTING

Three different reliability studies were conducted on a rehabilitation unit, on a cardiovascular and neurologic unit, and in a skilled nursing facility. A total of 124 subjects, ranging in age from 37 to 100, were involved. Two different prospective validity studies were conducted on two 28-bed medical-surgical units in a large hospital. A total of 99 clients, ranging in age from 14 to 102, were involved.

METHODS

To determine interrater reliability when registered nurses (RNs), licensed practical nurses (LPNs), and nursing assistants (NAs) used the tool, a graduate research nursing student directly observed the staff and conducted chart reviews over a period of weeks. Validity was tested by defining the sensitivity and specificity of the scale. All clients who were free from skin breakdown when admitted to participating medical-surgical units were included in the prospective validity study. Staff members were educated on use of the risk assessment tool, and they then used the tool to rate the client weekly and at time of discharge, death, or transfer.

FINDINGS

The Braden scale was found to be highly reliable when used by RNs, primary nurses, and graduate students. There was nearly perfect agreement between raters and RNs. The interrater reliability between LPNs and NAs was satisfactory but not as good as for the more educated health care team members.

IMPLICATIONS

RNs would be the best professionals to use the assessment tool. Institutional protocols establishing a procedure for tool use will improve the reliability of the tool.

Bergstrom N et al: The Braden scale for predicting pressure sore risk, *Nurs Res* 36(4):205, 1987.

client condition allow a turning schedule based on the clinical presentation of erythema, particularly in frail, vulnerable clients.

Clients should be turned only at a 30-degree oblique angle, rather than a lateral, side-lying 90-degree angle, to decrease pressure intensity over the trochanter and lateral malleolus prominences. It is also easier to turn a person at a 30-degree angle (Colin et al, 1996) (Fig. 30-4). To decrease pressure intensity on the heels, a client should have a pillow or pillows under the calves to lift the feet and heels off the bed. Commercial devices also exist to suspend the heel, maintain or correct foot-ankle position, and protect the client from neurosensory damage.

At-risk individuals should be placed on a pressure-reducing device in hopes of preventing development of a pressure ulcer by decreasing pressure intensity. Pressure-reducing support surfaces, such as mattress overlays, chair cushions or overlays, and specialized beds, redistribute weight over a larger area and reduce tissue-interface pressure. Tissue-interface pressure is the amount of pressure between the skin and resting surface (e.g., mattress). It has been thought that if the tissue-interface pressure is 32 mm Hg or lower, capillary closure will not occur. However, this logic may be questioned because capillary closing pressures vary from one individual to another.

Mattress overlays reduce pressure, are usually economical with only a one-time charge, and are accessible in most environments. Overlays can be static (e.g., foam, gel, water, air, and low air loss) or dynamic (e.g., alternating air). Because the overlays are placed on top of a mattress, the height of the bed is increased, making it more difficult for clients to get in and out of the bed, which is a common client and nurse complaint. The overlay may also decrease the protective height of bed side rails because the effective mattress height has increased. Some mattress overlays trap moisture and heat, which can be uncomfortable. Foam overlays should have a base height of at least 4 inches from the bottom to the

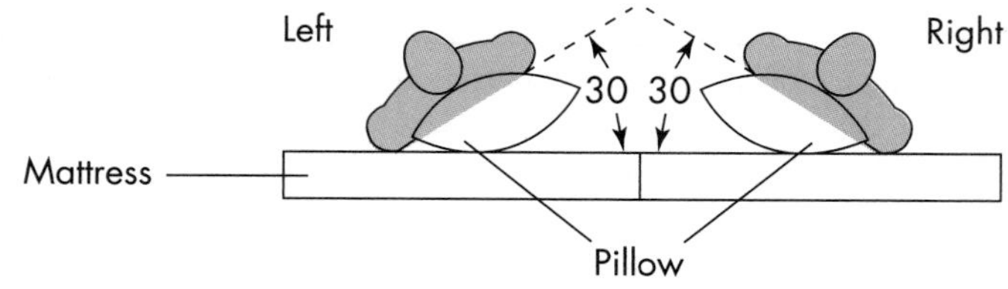

Right: _____ AM/PM _____ AM/PM _____ AM/PM _____ AM/PM _____ AM/PM _____ AM/PM

Left: _____ AM/PM _____ AM/PM _____ AM/PM _____ AM/PM _____ AM/PM _____ AM/PM

Flat: _____ AM/PM _____ AM/PM _____ AM/PM _____ AM/PM _____ AM/PM _____ AM/PM

Fig. 30-4 Repositioning schedule. Begin with the person on his or her back. Reposition by placing pillows underneath the person's shoulder blades, buttocks, and thighs. Adjust the pillows so that the person is at a 30-degree angle to the mattress. Alternate the position from right to left. Elevating the head of the bed increases the risk for ulcer development and should be avoided. Avoid placing persons at high risk for ulcer development flat on their backs. (Modified from Seiler WO and Stahelin HB: *Geriatrics* 40:30, 1985. Reprinted with permission from *Fam Pract Recertifica* 12:104, 1990.)

beginning of the convolutions, not to the peak, and a stiffness of 25% of indentation load deflection (AHCPR, 1992). Foam overlays must also be examined regularly to assess for continued effectiveness (i.e., no obvious sagging) because their use is limited. Static air and water overlays must be checked regularly for proper inflation and cleaned periodically.

Specialty beds such as air-fluidized beds (Clinitron) or low–air loss beds (KinAir or Flexicair) are generally used for individuals who have multiple stage III and IV pressure ulcers or who are at high risk, that is, after posterior grafts or flap procedures. These beds can actually overheat a client and can elevate the body temperature if not adequately controlled. Multiple hybrids of the air-fluidized and low–air loss beds exist, enabling the nurse to better match a bed with client needs. Specialty beds do not eliminate the need for meticulous nursing care. Clients must still be repositioned, assessed, and kept clean and dry.

Skin moisture, whether the result of incontinence of urine or feces, perspiration, or wound exudate, should be minimized. If necessary, absorbent underpads or diapers can be used to maintain a dryer skin surface. Topical barriers, such as zinc oxide, can be applied after cleansing and gently drying the skin (AHCPR, 1992). Indwelling Foley catheters should be used only on a short-term basis and avoided if at all possible because of the risk of urinary tract infection. Thought must be given as to the reason for a catheter and whether the benefit of placement outweighs the risk of infection. Although most orders are for turning and repositioning every 2 hours, the primary care provider may need to be contacted to implement consistent scheduled checks before the 2-hour intervals. With implementation of regular checks to keep skin clean and dry and the use of absorbent pads and topical barriers, catheter placement can be avoided, thus reducing client risk.

Skin injury from friction or shearing forces can be avoided by using proper turning techniques and proper placement. Friction injuries can be prevented by using proper transfer techniques and a draw sheet. Lubricants, topical barrier creams, film or hydrocolloid dressings, or protective padding can be used to reduce damage when skin moves across a coarse or hard surface. Shearing occurs when the body shifts and slides downward; therefore most shearing injuries can be eliminated with proper placement. For example, not elevating the head of the bed greater than 30 degrees and elevating the knees slightly when the head is elevated prevent slipping down in bed. When the client is sitting in a chair, placing the feet on a stool prevents sliding downward (AHCPR, 1992).

Nutritional status must be closely monitored by assessing caloric intake, weight, serum albumin, cholesterol, and total lymphocyte count (TLC). Accurate food intake should be monitored routinely to identify both the need for changes before a compromised state develops and nutritionally at-risk clients. Hydration status is another important nutritional component, since dehydration can contribute to development of a pressure ulcer. An older adult requires a minimum of 2000 to 2500 ml of water a day unless contraindicated, such as in CHF or renal failure. The use of an air-fluidized or low–air loss bed increases daily fluid needs because insensible loss is increased. When the professional nurse recognizes a pattern of decreased food or water intake, a full assessment addressing food preferences, dentition, and swallowing difficulties is warranted. The client should also be evaluated for constipation or fecal impaction, which decreases appetite. A dietary consultation and nutritional supplements may be needed. Weight changes slowly; therefore weighing the client monthly is sufficient and is needed more frequently only when assessing cardiovascular status. A weight loss of 5% to 10% is significant, and a weight loss of one third of the ideal body weight is an ominous sign (Stotts and Wipke-Tevis, 1996).

A serum albumin of 3 g/dl or lower is associated with protein malnutrition and increased morbidity and mortality (Stotts and Wipke-Tevis, 1996). Malnutrition is also correlated with a low TLC. A TLC of 800 to 1200/mm^3 is indicative of moderate malnutrition, and a count below 800/mm^3 is classified as severely malnourished (Pinchcofsky-Devin and Kaminski, 1986). Pinchcofsky-Devin and Kaminski (1986) demonstrated a relationship between pressure ulcers and a TLC below 1200/mm^3. Serum protein and TLC are valid nutritional indicators for pressure ulcer development. Serum cholesterol is another nutritional parameter to monitor. Several studies have demonstrated a positive correlation between nursing facility residents' and hospitalized clients' mortality rates and serum cholesterol below 120 to 150 mg/dl (Strauss and Margolis, 1996). Therefore a serum cholesterol below 150 mg/dl warrants aggressive nutritional support.

Because of multiple risk factors and their synergistic effect on pressure ulcer development, prevention is a nursing challenge, offering an opportunity to demonstrate the impact of nursing by recognizing at-risk clients, immediately implementing preventive strategies, and preventing a costly health care problem. Most of all, preventive measures promote high-quality client care, which is the primary goal of nursing (Box 30-3).

Pressure Ulcer Management

Nurses play a key role in pressure ulcer management because they are the professionals responsible for wound care and often the first team members to identify wound changes. In addition, the professional nurse, especially in long-term care, is perceived by physicians as an expert in pressure ulcer management. It is not uncommon for physicians to say, "Do whatever treatment you think is best." Often the physician or APN, when assessing medical management, asks the nurse to describe and evaluate the treatment. Therefore it is important for the professional nurse to comprehend the healing process, to understand treatment strategies, and to maintain

BOX 30-3 Pressure Ulcer Prevention Points

RISK ASSESSMENT

1. Consider all bedbound or chairbound persons, or those whose ability to reposition is impaired, to be at risk for pressure ulcers.
2. Select and use a method of risk assessment (e.g., Norton scale, Braden scale) that ensures systematic evaluation of individual risk factors.
3. Assess all at-risk clients at the time of admission to health care facilities and at regular intervals thereafter.
4. Identify all individual risk factors (e.g., decreased mental status, moisture, incontinence, nutritional deficits) to direct specific preventive treatments. Modify care according to the individual factors.

SKIN CARE AND EARLY TREATMENT

1. Inspect the skin at least daily, and document assessment results.
2. Individualize bathing frequency. Use a mild cleansing agent. Avoid hot water and excessive friction.
3. Assess and treat incontinence. When incontinence cannot be controlled, cleanse skin at time of soiling, use a topical moisture barrier, and select underpads or briefs that are absorbent and provide a quick-drying surface to the skin.
4. Use moisturizers for dry skin. Minimize environmental factors leading to dry skin such as low humidity and cold air.
5. Avoid massage over bony prominences.
6. Use proper positioning, transferring, and turning techniques to minimize skin injury from friction and shear forces.
7. Use dry lubricants (cornstarch) or protective coverings to reduce friction injury.
8. Identify and correct factors compromising protein and calorie intake and consider nutritional supplementation or support for nutritionally compromised persons.
9. Institute a rehabilitation program to maintain or improve mobility and activity status.
10. Monitor and document interventions and outcomes.

MECHANICAL LOADING AND SUPPORT SURFACES

1. Reposition bedbound persons at least every 2 hours and chairbound persons every hour.
2. Use a written repositioning schedule.
3. Place at-risk persons on a pressure-reducing mattress or chair cushion. Do not use doughnut-type devices.
4. Consider postural alignment, distribution of weight, balance and stability, and pressure relief when positioning persons in chairs or wheelchairs.
5. Teach chairbound persons who are able to shift their weight every 15 minutes.
6. Use lifting devices (e.g., trapeze, bed linen) to move rather than drag persons during transfers and position changes.
7. Use pillows or foam wedges to keep bony prominences such as knees and ankles from making direct contact with each other.
8. Use devices that totally relieve pressure on the heels (e.g., place pillows under the calf to raise the heels off the bed).
9. Avoid positioning directly on the trochanter when using the side-lying position (use the 30-degree lateral inclined position).
10. Elevate the head of the bed as little (maximum 30-degree angle) and for as short a time as possible.

EDUCATION

1. Implement educational programs for the prevention of pressure ulcers that are structured; organized; comprehensive; and directed at all levels of health care providers, clients, family, and caregivers.
2. Include information on the following:
   - Etiology of and risk factors for pressure ulcers
   - Risk assessment tools and their application
   - Skin assessment
   - Selection and use of support surfaces
   - Development and implementation of individualized programs of skin care
   - Demonstration of positioning to decrease risk of tissue breakdown
   - Accurate documentation of pertinent data
3. Include built-in mechanisms to evaluate program effectiveness in preventing pressure ulcers.

From National Pressure Ulcer Advisory Panel's Summary of the AHCPR Clinical Practice Guideline: *Pressure ulcers in adults: prediction and prevention,* AHCPR Pub No 92-0047, Rockville, Md, May 1992.

a current knowledge base. The following discussion reviews the healing trajectory and treatment options, which include nutritional management. It is hoped that the professional nurse will become empowered, promote a positive image for nursing, and, most important, be able to deliver more successful client care by comprehending the healing process physiology and the logic for treatment strategies.

Physiology of Wound Healing. An understanding of the healing process is necessary to critically analyze pressure ulcer care and determine the best management strategy. Pressure ulcer research has expanded our understanding of the etiology of pressure ulcers and the healing process. There are three major stages of wound healing: the inflammatory stage; the proliferative, or granulation, stage; and the maturation, or matrix formation, stage.

The *inflammatory stage,* characterized by redness, heat, pain, and swelling, lasts approximately 4 to 5 days. The inflammatory stage initiates the healing process by stabilizing the wound through platelet activity that stops bleeding and triggers the immune system. Neutrophils, monocytes, and macrophages arrive within 24 hours of the insult to control bacteria, remove dead tissue, and secrete angiogenesis factor (AGF) and other growth factors, which stimulate the development of granulation tissue. Bradykinin and histamine, released from injured cells, cause vasodilation, which leads to swelling. This creates the red, swollen, tender, clinical presentation often seen in wounds (Schaffer and Barbul, 1998). The inflammatory stage is crucial for successful healing, with a delayed or altered response possibly contributing to the development of chronic, stagnant wounds if appropriate growth factors and responses were not mobilized when the client was first injured. Medications (e.g., steroids), decreased tissue oxygenation, poor nutritional status, and age-related changes (e.g., decreased response of the immune system) can impair this stage.

The *proliferative,* or *granulation, stage* begins 24 hours after injury and continues for up to 22 days. Three significant events occur: epithelialization, granulation, and collagen synthesis. Epithelialization, via a microscopic epithelial layer, seals and protects the wound from bacteria and fluid loss. This microscopic layer, which is fostered by a moist environment, is extremely fragile and can easily be washed away with aggressive wound irrigation or harsh wiping of the involved area. Granulation, also known as neovascularization, is the formation of new capillaries that generate and feed new tissue, creating a beefy-red tissue bed that bleeds easily. Collagen synthesis creates a support matrix that provides strength to the new tissue. Oxygen, iron, vitamin C, zinc, magnesium, and amino acids are necessary for collagen synthesis. Fibroblasts, stimulated in the first phase by AGF, are necessary for collagen production (Calvin, 1998). This phase rebuilds the injured area and can easily be influenced by the effectiveness of the inflammation stage and wound environment.

The *maturation stage,* also known as the *differentiation* or *remodeling phase,* is the final stage. It does not begin until 21 days after injury and can take years to complete. During this stage maximum tensile strength is generated through collagen deposits that make the wound thicker and more compact. These collagen deposits contract until closure is attained. Initially, the scarred area is a dark, scarlet red that fades over time to a silvery white. Tensile strength reaches only 80% of preinjury capacity; therefore the "scarred" area is more vulnerable to breakdown or injury (Hunt, 1988).

Definition of Terms and Staging Criteria. A *pressure ulcer* is "any lesion caused by unrelieved pressure resulting in damage of underlying tissue" and is usually over bony prominences (AHCPR, 1992).

The recommended staging criteria established by the NPUAP in 1989 were adopted by AHCPR clinical practice guidelines (Box 30-4). If an ulcer is covered with eschar, a stage cannot be determined until the eschar is removed. Box 30-5 provides definitions of relevant terms.

Basic Principles of Pressure Ulcer Management. Three basic principles guide successful pressure ulcer management:

1. Eliminate or minimize precipitating factors such as pressure, friction, shearing, and poor nutrition.
2. Provide nutritional support and monitor nutritional status.
3. Create and maintain a clean, moist wound environment with adequate circulation and oxygenation.

Pressure ulcer preventive strategies must be implemented, or wound care efforts are futile (see Box 30-3). Through institutional policy and protocol, the professional nurse applies an appropriate mattress overlay without waiting for a physician's order. The professional nurse ensures that proper technique is used by all staff members when repositioning a client to minimize shearing and friction forces. As leader of the nursing team, the professional nurse is responsible for observing nursing aides or other support team members who deliver hands-on care to identify specific learning needs so that pressure, shearing, and friction are minimized. Teaching the logic for such techniques can motivate staff members to exercise more diligence in performing proper preventive actions. The nurse must rely on teaching principles such as repetition of key information in a nonthreatening manner. He or she should reinforce appropriate activity with positive feedback. Preventive strategies then become a routine, which demonstrates and enhances the power of nursing (Xakellis and Frantz, 1998).

Nutritional status should be monitored with the physician or APN monitoring serum albumin levels, prealbumin levels, weight, and food consumption so that needs can be identified immediately. This also promotes a collaborative effort among health care providers. When food intake is first noted to decrease, the professional nurse should identify reasons, such as not meeting food preferences, sore mouth, the client's being rushed to eat, conflict with staff, depression, or pain.

For closure of the wound or ulcer, a clean, moist environment must be created and maintained. This principle, which has been scientifically established, is the key to successful healing and should guide the professional nurse and practitioner. Consequently, necrotic tissue must be removed and any infectious process (as seen by erythema, induration, and tenderness in the periwound skin; pus; or a pale wound bed) resolved to implement a dressing strategy that fosters rapid epithelialization and granulation.

It is important to know when to culture a wound because of the expense to the client and the health care system. Also, inappropriate antibiotic use is decreased when wounds are cultured appropriately. All wounds are contaminated; therefore all cultures grow surface bacteria, and the true pathogen may not be identified. A culture is warranted only when cellulitis (e.g., erythema, induration, tenderness) or wound infection (evident by pale wound bed, pus, increased tenderness, persistent exudate, or no new growth) exists. To obtain an accurate culture, the nurse should obtain both anaerobic and aerobic cultures. The most accurate method, consid-

BOX 30-4 Staging Criteria

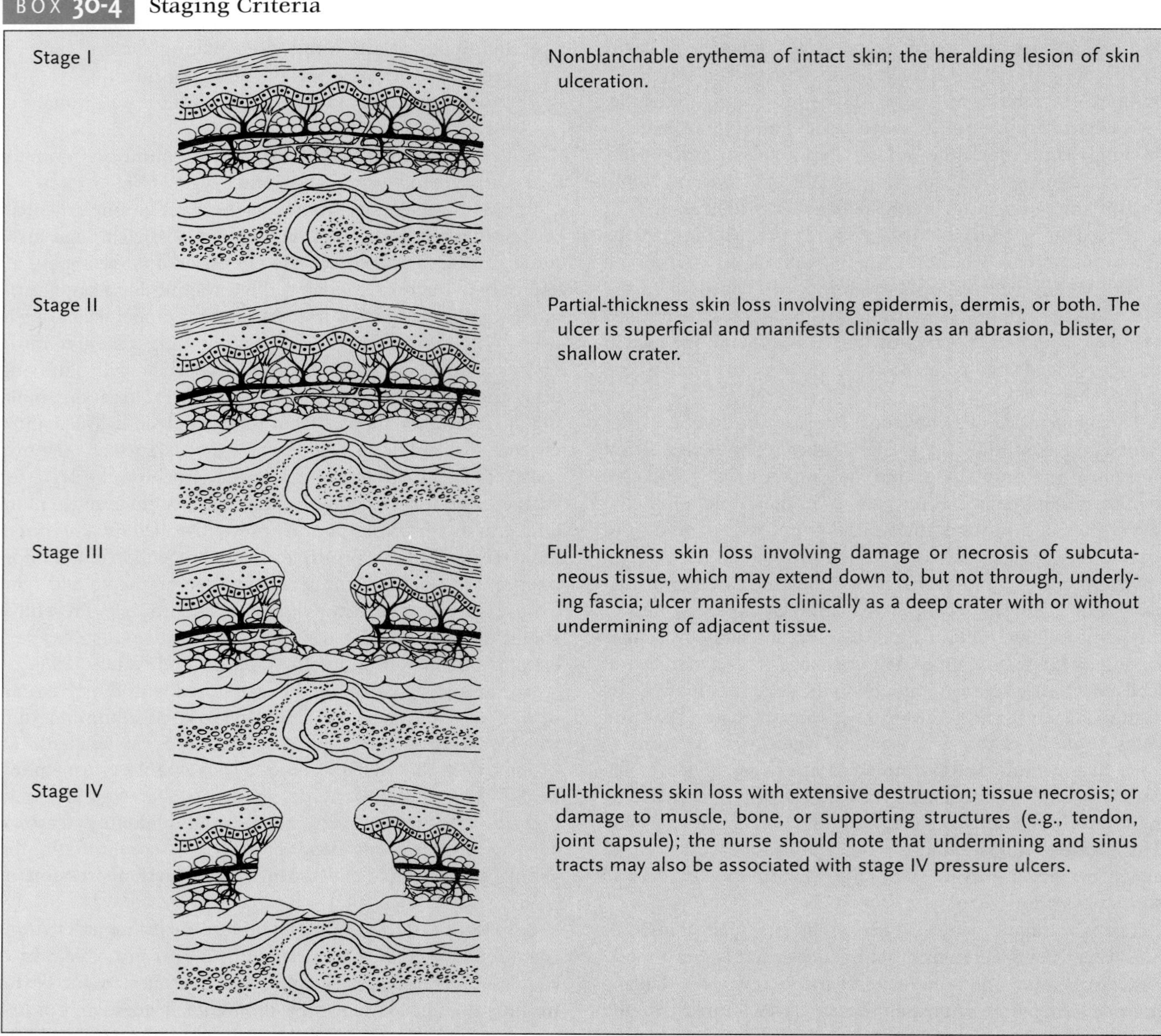

From Agency for Health Care Policy and Research: *Pressure ulcers in adults: prediction and prevention,* Clinical Practice Guideline No 3, Rockville, Md, 1992, US Department of Health and Human Services.

ered the gold standard for pressure ulcer cultures, is to obtain a tissue or needle aspiration biopsy (Robson, 1997). According to the AHCPR treatment guidelines, an ulcer is *not* to be cultured using a culturette, since colonized bacteria may be obtained instead of the offending pathogen. An infected wound is managed either topically, with antiseptics, or systemically, depending on the severity and risk of osteomyelitis.

Great controversy exists regarding the use of antiseptic solutions such as povidone-iodine (Betadine) or acetic acid because of their cytotoxic effects. Antiseptic solutions should be used only when the wound is obviously infected, never on a healthy, granulating ulcer. Infection and associated stress on the wound are as destructive—maybe more so—as any antiseptic. The management goal must be kept in mind: to obtain a clean wound bed. If an antiseptic can facilitate the achievement of this wound environment, it should be tried, especially if it means a client does not have to be admitted to a hospital or receive intravenous antibiotic therapy. The key to successful use of any antiseptic agent is discontinuing it when purulent discharge or signs of infection have resolved so that tissue destruction is minimal.

BOX 30-5 Definitions of Terms

Autolysis: Self-débridement of necrotic tissue by white blood cells, which is fostered by a dressing that retains moisture (e.g., transparent film); a yellowish brown fluid is generated from the white blood cells and breakdown of tissue
Débridement: Removal of dead, damaged tissue
Epithelialization: Growth of a microscopic layer that covers an open wound, which creates a barrier that protects from fluid loss and bacterial assault and that is highly fragile and easily destroyed
Eschar: Thick, necrotic, devitalized tissue; often black, but can be yellowish
Exudate: Wound discharge that can be serosanguineous, serous, or purulent
Friction: Rubbing of skin against another surface (e.g., sheets, bed, chair)
Granulation tissue: New capillary growth that creates a beefy-red color and tissue that bleeds easily (friable)
Interface pressure: Force exerted between body and support surface (e.g., mattress)
Pressure ulcer: Lesion caused by unrelieved pressure that causes tissue damage and death; usually occurs over bony prominences or other pressure points (e.g., tubing, foreign material in bed)
Reactive hyperemia: Transient, blanching erythema from tissue anoxia, which generates a compensatory mechanism resulting in dilated vessels
Shearing force: Sliding of parallel surfaces when skeletal frame and deep fascia slide downward; the superficial fascia remains attached to the dermis, thus stretching or occluding the arterial supply to fascia and muscle, which can lead to tissue anoxia and damage; most common position for this occurrence is when the head of the bed is elevated and the body slides downward
Sinus tract: Vertical tunnel connecting one anatomic compartment with another
Tissue tolerance: The skin's (i.e., blood vessels, interstitial fluid, collagen, other structures) ability to endure the effects of pressure without adverse consequences
Undermining: Separation of tissue under the dermis creating a horizontal tunnel; length can be measured by inserting a cotton-tipped applicator into the tunnel, marking length on applicator, and then placing next to a tape measure

Modified from Bryant RA et al: Pressure ulcers. In Bryant RA, editor: *Acute and chronic wounds: nursing management,* St Louis, 1992, Mosby; Agency for Health Care Policy and Research: *Pressure ulcers in adults: prediction and prevention,* Clinical Practice Guideline No 3, Rockville, Md, 1992, US Department of Health and Human Services; Sanders SL: Pressure ulcers, part II, Management strategies, *J Am Acad Nurse Pract* 4(3):101, 1992.

Antiseptic solutions are used with wet-to-dry dressings, which also provide some mechanical débridement. At times, a wound may be irrigated with the antiseptic; however, a rinse with normal saline should follow. The most common antiseptics are povidone-iodine, acetic acid, hydrogen peroxide, and sodium hypochlorite (also known as Dakin's solution or Clorpactin). All four solutions are cytotoxic and destroy fragile epithelial tissue and fibroblasts. Povidone-iodine, when used *long term* or *undiluted,* can cause systemic iodine toxicity, which is evidenced by an unpleasant brassy taste, burning in the mouth or throat, sore gums and teeth, increased salivation, head and cold symptoms (rhinitis), gastric irritation, diarrhea, and occasional fever; it has been known to lead to death (Goodman, Thomas, and Rappaport, 1990). The keys to successful use of povidone-iodine are dilution; short-term use (3 to 5 days); and never using it on a healthy, granulating wound bed. Acetic acid is recommended for wounds infected with *Pseudomonas* organisms, evidenced by a malodorous, green discharge or positive culture. Hydrogen peroxide provides some débridement by effervescent action. It would be prudent to not use hydrogen peroxide in a sinus tract or deep, cavernous wound. Sodium hypochlorite, which is essentially diluted bleach, can affect clotting abilities and also burn intact healthy tissue not protected by zinc oxide. Second-degree burns have been witnessed from Dakin's solution that was inadvertently splashed on the skin surrounding a wound. Regardless of the solution, it should be used only during time of infection and wound stress. If the professional nurse notices that antiseptic use has continued for longer than 1 week, a reminder or question should be posed to the physician or APN.

The first step in pressure ulcer wound care is to thoroughly assess the wound to determine the most effective strategy and dressing. The professional nurse is usually the first person to identify a need for change; therefore this assessment should be an ongoing process. The nurse should examine the wound, noting its color; any discharge, bleeding, or odor; degree of undermining or presence of a sinus tract (can be measured using a cotton-tipped applicator); any necrotic tissue; pain or tenderness; and amount of erythema surrounding wound edges. Limited erythema around the wound is a normal phenomenon that signifies increased circulation to provide nutrients; however, if the erythema extends, infection or candidiasis should be suspected and the wound closely monitored. Ideally, the wound base should be a beefy-red color, which is indicative of granulation. However, some hydrogel and hydrocolloid dressings generate a pale pink wound bed, which ordinarily would mean an "ill" wound bed. If the bed is pale pink and not associated with a purulent discharge or cellulitis, the wound environment is most likely clean and should just be observed. Note that granulation tissue has a rich capillary supply and bleeds easily and profusely when disturbed (e.g., when it is irrigated or a dressing changed). Thus, if a tunneling wound bleeds, it can be deduced that granulation tissue exists, although it is not visible as a result of the tunneling.

The wound assessment should be ongoing and supported with documentation. All new wounds should be described, including location, color, discharge, tenderness, amount of necrotic tissue or undermining, dimensions, and stage. The wound measurements should include length, width, and depth. When measuring undermining, the nurse should use a cotton-tipped applicator, marking depth on the applicator and placing it next to a tape measure to obtain dimension and to note position (e.g., 4 cm at 2 o'clock). It is not imperative that all dimensions or locations of undermining be documented. The nurse should record only the greatest length because the wound cannot be deemed healed until closed. It is recommended that facilities develop a written procedure stating how dimensions should be obtained and documented (e.g., length by width by depth, undermining) to establish continuity and minimize confusion regarding the procedure.

Débridement. Moist, necrotic tissue provides a perfect medium for bacteria and delays the inflammatory response and the accompanying arrival of tissue reparative factors, negatively affecting the healing trajectory (Steed et al, 1996). Therefore necrotic tissue must be débrided as soon as possible, and measures (such as wet-to-dry dressings or topical antimicrobials) taken to resolve bacterial insults, until purulent discharge has dissipated. If necrotic tissue is not débrided, the nurse's efforts are futile and the client's comfort and quality of life are affected.

The removal of dry, hard eschar should be considered, since its presence slows the migration of epithelial cells and delays healing, except for stable heel ulcers, in which case dry eschar should be left intact (AHCPR, 1994). At times this dry eschar can serve as an efficient and comfortable dressing, but the area must be watched for development of infection. If the client has diabetes or has an ischemic wound with a dry, hard, intact eschar, it may be more prudent to leave the eschar in place. It serves as a barrier and does not place the client at risk for any possible problems from frequent dressing changes (e.g., infection, skin tears, and candidiasis). However, the eschar and periwound skin must be monitored. If the eschar becomes soft and mushy, tissue liquefaction is most likely accumulating and must be removed. This is especially true if the wound is tender or has periwound erythema indicating infection.

Four methods of débridement are mechanical, autolytic, chemical, and surgical. Mechanical débridement (wet-to-dry dressings or whirlpool) is effective for removing slimy or stringy exudate that cannot be removed surgically or chemically (because of damage to viable tissue). If mechanical débridement using wet-to-dry dressings is employed, the nurse should protect wound borders from maceration with zinc oxide or stoma adhesive. Using a whirlpool or a handheld pulsed irrigation system once or twice daily can mechanically débride and should be reserved for large, exuding wounds; this should be discontinued after the wound is clean or demonstrates stability. Mechanical débridement requires more nursing time, is more uncomfortable for the client, and may destroy fragile epithelial cells. For these reasons, a more efficient method should be sought first.

Autolytic débridement is effective for removing stringy slough when less than 50% of the wound bed is involved and there is no evidence of infection in the periwound skin. Autolytic débridement involves using the body's own enzymes to provide additional débriding and cleansing. Hydrocolloid or hydrogel dressings can soften and facilitate removal of eschar if the wound is not infected. It should be noted that autolysis creates a larger-appearing wound because debris is being removed. Autolysis generates a brownish yellow fluid that may have some pus in it as a result of dead cells and neutrophils. The nurse should not become alarmed unless there is clinical evidence of infection (e.g., erythema, tenderness, heat, and swelling). Autolytic débridement may be used in conjunction with mechanical methods to further shorten the time to wound cleansing.

Chemical débridement is costly ($20 to over $60 per tube) and time consuming; however, it can be effective on small, necrotic areas or for removing yellow, tender eschar that is difficult to remove surgically. Chemical débridement is primarily used in the home setting or nursing facility where appropriately educated or certified professionals are not readily accessible to surgically débride at the bedside. Chemical débridement may save the client from hospital admission. If used, the chemical enzyme must *not* be applied on healthy, viable tissue because the enzyme will destroy granulation tissue and epithelial cells. Clients should be certain to read storage instructions for débriding enzymatics; some have to be refrigerated.

If the wound has a dry, rubbery eschar, surgical débridement is recommended over chemical débridement because chemical débridement takes much longer. The main principle that guides surgical débridement is to stop when bleeding occurs, indicating that viable, healthy tissue has been reached. Because the wound is dirty, aseptic technique is appropriate. To prevent "showering" of bacteria from surgical débridement and to assist in cleaning up the wound, wet-to-dry dressings moistened with an antiseptic such as povidone-iodine can be applied every shift for 1 to 3 days, depending on the wound condition.

Wound Care Principles and Dressing Types. The wound care market is a multibillion-dollar business and has created many dressing options. Therefore the professional nurse must understand the healing trajectory to select the best treatment option. The major goal is to create an environment that supports healing—a clean, moist (hydrated, not wet) ulcer bed. If no growth is evident in weekly measurements after 2 to 4 weeks, consideration should be given to changing the dressing strategy. Table 30-4 provides a brief

TABLE 30-4 Type of Dressings

ADVANTAGES	DRAWBACKS	CONTRAINDICATIONS
GAUZE		
Allows for mechanical débridement via wet-to-dry dressing method Protects dry, healing wounds Serves as filler dressing for dead space Absorbs exudate Assists with cleaning up wound; manages exudates	Requires more frequent dressing changes Requires securing with tape or film Requires loose packing or it may create pressure and possibly enlarge the wound Destroys fragile epithelial cells and slows down healing, especially when gauze dries out	Use on healthy, granulating wound unless moistened with saline or other noncytotoxic solution; even then fragile epithelial cells may be destroyed. Use on dry, necrotic tissue, unless keeping eschar in place for protection (appropriate only when no signs of infection exist).
NONADHERENT DRESSING OR SEMIPERMEABLE POLYURETHANE FOAM		
Decreases trauma to wound base and fragile epithelial cells because does not adhere to tissue or wound base Protects dry, healing wound Has minimum to moderate absorption ability, particularly the foam type, which can prevent or decrease maceration Insulates wound (particularly the foam type [provides comfort])	Requires securing with tape or film Usually requires daily to every-shift dressing changes	Not appropriate for mechanical débridement because it does not adhere. Use on a healthy, granulating wound unless a topical agent (e.g., bacitracin) is used. Use on dry, necrotic tissue, unless keeping eschar in place for protection (appropriate only when no signs of infection exist).
TRANSPARENT FILM DRESSING		
Retains moisture and is semipermeable and comfortable Is water resistant; thus can seal and secure other dressings Allows easy inspection to monitor for complications Fosters autolysis as a result of moisture retention Minimizes friction injury when applied to vulnerable areas (e.g., elbows, coccyx, heels)	Can be difficult to apply Can leak	Use on infected or cellulitic wounds. Use on thin, friable skin surrounding wound edges that cannot be protected with stoma adhesive (risk of creating other open wounds or skin tear). Use on exuding wounds.
HYDROCOLLOIDAL DRESSING		
Retains moisture, which facilitates granulation and is comfortable Provides a water and bacteria barrier, which protects wound Requires less frequent dressing changes, which promotes efficient use of nursing time and comfort to client Promotes removal of dry necrotic eschar when left in place for several days	Melt-out occurs, creating foul odor and possible leakage Unable to visibly monitor wound Can cause hypergranulation tissue (leafy, friable, beefy-red granulation tissue), which impedes healing and usually requires débridement or removal with sharp instrument or silver nitrate Is expensive but requires fewer dressing changes	Use on infected or cellulitic wounds. Use on thin, friable skin surrounding wound edges (more damage may be created when wafer removed). Use on heavy, exuding wounds.

TABLE 30-4 Type of Dressings—cont'd

ADVANTAGES	DRAWBACKS	CONTRAINDICATIONS
HYDROGEL		
Provides moisture, which facilitates granulation Facilitates some débridement for wounds with thin, stringy yellow eschar Promotes removal of dry necrotic eschar when dressing left in place for several days Nonadherent surface, which provides comfort to client Requires less frequent dressing changes, which promotes efficient use of nursing time and comfort to client	Must use another product to keep in place and secure with tape or film Can cause hypergranulation tissue (leafy, friable, beefy-red granulation tissue), which impedes healing and usually requires débridement or removal with sharp instrument or silver nitrate Is expensive but requires fewer dressing changes	Use on heavy, exuding wounds. Use on cellulitic wounds. Use on wounds with purulent discharge.

overview of the various dressing categories and general treatment principles.

With each dressing change, all open wounds should be *gently* irrigated with approximately 20 to 50 ml of normal saline using either a catheter-tip syringe, butterfly tubing with the needle cut off and connected to a Luer-Lok syringe, or a syringe with a 19-gauge needle. After irrigation, the wound can be assessed.

It is prudent to always write the date and time of the dressing change on the outside of the dressing itself. This practice reflects professional accountability and assists in problem solving. For example, a wound may have more discharge or a significant change because the dressing was not changed soon enough or, inadvertently, not changed at all.

If the wound border has candidiasis, evidenced by a fire-red erythema usually with satellite lesions and denuded skin, a zinc oxide/nystatin (50/50) mixture can be applied on affected areas, and then the dressing applied. Because candidiasis flourishes in a moist environment, a thoughtful assessment should be done to identify the reason for excess moisture. Is a moist dressing, such as gauze, overlapping the wound edges? Is the film dressing generating so much fluid retention and maceration that candidiasis is occurring? If so, the zinc oxide/nystatin cream could be applied and the wound monitored. It may be that the dressing type must be changed. After the candidiasis has resolved, a stoma adhesive wafer can be placed around the wound to protect the skin from future problems. Stoma adhesive is recommended over a hydrocolloid dressing because tape and film dressings do not stick to the stoma adhesive barrier as they do to a hydrocolloid wafer. If no infection exists, another alternative that decreases maceration is to apply petroleum jelly (Vaseline) or zinc oxide around the wound borders and then to apply the dressing.

Gauze dressings have been used for many years with success; however, there has been an explosion of scientific information regarding pressure ulcers and wound care since 1962, when moisture was first identified as a facilitator of healing. This discovery has generated many other effective, efficient, and comfortable options. Thus gauze is primarily used for débriding and cleaning up a wound bed, except when used for protecting closed surgical wounds. However, when a wound has tunneling or undermining, saline-moistened gauze, *loosely* packed into the wound, can maintain a moist environment. Caution should be exercised not to pack tightly or have the moistened gauze touching the healing surface surrounding the ulcer to avoid additional damage and maceration. If gauze is being used on a clean wound, the strategy should be wet-to-moist dressing to prevent drying of epithelial cells. The nurse should slightly moisten the gauze touching the wound bed with normal saline and place dry gauze or an abdominal pad over the moist gauze and secure with tape; this should keep the wound moist at all times.

Some gauze is impregnated with material such as saline, povidone-iodine, or Vaseline. The hypertonic saline gauze (Mesalt) is an exudate absorber and assists in cleaning wounds. After the exudate has diminished, a less harsh wound care product should be employed (e.g., a hydrogel). Gauze ribbons impregnated with povidone-iodine (iodoform gauze) are effective for cleaning up a tunneling wound that has purulent or foul exudate. However, the povidone-iodine gauze should be stopped when the purulent foul exudate has resolved so that healthy tissue is not destroyed. Vaseline gauze is a good, inexpensive method for keeping a wound from drying out and protecting the wound and surrounding tissue. Vaseline gauze secured with Kerlix wrapped around the extremity, changed every 2 to 4 days and as needed, is an effective strategy for healing skin tears. The Vaseline keeps the wound moist and protects from further insults.

Nonadherent dressings such as Telfa are used when the wound bed must be protected and epithelial cells left undisturbed. Nonadherent dressings are suitable for skin tears, skin grafts, or other wounds that require minimum insult. Often, an antibiotic ointment is applied to the wound bed (which keeps it moist), and then the bed is covered with a nonadherent dressing, which is changed once or twice a day.

Foam dressings, which are nonadherent, absorbent dressings, protect an ulcer and assist in minimizing maceration of ulcer edges. Foam dressings have also been used around tracheal tubes; they are beneficial when candidiasis exists around tracheal stomas, acting to absorb moisture. Foam dressings are secured with tape or film and may be used in combination with other topical agents or primary dressings.

Transparent films are used for stage I or II pressure ulcers (superficial wounds) to secure dressings, to protect vulnerable areas (e.g., elbows) from friction, and to facilitate autolysis. Transparent films, such as Opsite or Tegaderm, are semipermeable, thus allowing exchange of air. Film dressings can be left on for 3 to 7 days but should be checked a minimum of once a day. Film dressings facilitate autolysis, which causes fluid buildup and can consequently lead to maceration of good tissue and dressing leakage. Vaseline or zinc oxide applied around the ulcer edges before placement of the film may prevent maceration. A nonadherent dressing or alginate may also be used under the film to assist with exudate management.

Hydrocolloids such as DuoDERM are sticky, nonpermeable wafers containing a hydrocolloid material that eventually melts, combines with natural body fluids, and keeps the wound bed moist. The nonpermeable wafer also serves as a barrier and creates a hypoxic wound environment that stimulates granulation, as long as peripheral circulation provides enough oxygen. Hydrocolloid dressings should not be used if candidiasis exists. Hydrocolloid wafers are usually changed every 3 to 7 days. It should be noted that a foul, sour odor is generated by hydrocolloid dressings, which is considered normal. Infection is present when erythema, warmth, tenderness, or purulent discharge exists. Hydrocolloid dressings should *never* be applied to ulcers that are infected, have purulent discharge, or have a suspected infection. The occlusive, moist environment provides a perfect medium for bacterial growth and may worsen the infection.

Hydrogels consist primarily of water and are effective in maintaining a moist ulcer bed, which fosters healing. Hydrogel dressings can be obtained in a sheet form suitable for superficial wounds or as an amorphous gel that can be applied and spread into deep, cavity wounds. Hydrogel dressings should not be used on infected wounds because they retain humidity, thus facilitating autolytic débridement. The cover dressing should be chosen based on the health of the surrounding skin and the degree of wound exudate. Examples of cover dressings include gauze, foam, and transparent films. Dressings using a hydrogel can be left in place for 1 day or up to 5 to 7 days, depending on the setting, product, and ulcer state (Table 30-5; see Nursing Care Plan).

Alginates are a category of exudate management dressings. The alginate dressings are manufactured from seaweed and are applied to wounds that are moderately to heavily exudative. In most cases the alginates are safe to use on infected wounds. These dressings have excellent exudate handling properties and are useful in wounds and around drainage tubes when the wound fluid is causing periwound skin maceration.

TABLE 30-5 General Pressure Ulcer Care Guidelines

STAGE	ACTIONS	DRESSING OPTIONS
I	Implement preventive strategies (e.g., mattress overlay; nutritional assessment; reinforcement of value of turning, keeping dry, and minimizing friction)	Can protect with film or hydrocolloid
II and III	Implement preventive strategies, assess for infection, débride necrotic tissue, conduct nutritional assessment, and provide appropriate nutritional support	Can use film, if clean, depending on depth; hydrocolloid; hydrogel, wet-to-moist dressing; if infected, manage topically with antiseptic and wet-to-dry dressing until infection is resolved
IV	Same as above; specialized bed may be considered	If clean, hydrogel, hydrocolloid paste and wafer, or wet-to-moist dressing; if infected, manage topically with antiseptic and wet-to-dry dressing until infection is resolved (but no longer than 5 days)

Nursing Care Plan
Pressure Ulcer

Clinical Situation: Mr. F. is an 78-year-old man who developed stage IV pressure ulcers on his sacral area and left ischium while recently hospitalized for acute renal failure. His decreased appetite and poor food intake, a 10-pound weight gain, and his not being initially placed on an eggcrate mattress led to the development of the pressure ulcers. Mr. F. was discharged home with home health care.

The sacral and ischial pressure ulcers are clean, beginning to granulate, managed with a hydrogel, covered with a foam dressing to lessen maceration, and sealed with a transparent dressing that is changed every other day. It is estimated that complete healing will take 6 to 8 months as long as nutritional status and other preventive strategies are maintained.

Nursing Diagnosis

Impaired skin integrity related to alteration in nutritional state, altered circulation, and immobilization

Outcome

Client will have intact skin, as evidenced by clean, healing wounds; maintenance of circulation to skin; and laboratory values within normal limits.

Interventions

Implement pressure ulcer preventive strategies to create an environment that will foster healing and prevent further development of ulcers:
- Place mattress overlay on bed and obtain appropriate pressure-relieving chair cushion to decrease ischial pressure.
- Teach client and family to lay client at 30-degree angle and support extremities with pillows when lying in bed to lessen trochanter pressure.
- Teach client, family, and nurse's aide to avoid hot baths and harsh soaps, to use moisturizers for dry skin, and not to massage over bony prominences.
- Teach client not to sit at 45- to 90-degree angle when in bed or on couch to minimize shearing forces.
- Assess and treat incontinence by cleansing skin at the time of soiling; use a topical moisture barrier and (if necessary) absorbent undergarments or briefs to maintain a dry surface and decrease risk of additional skin breakdown.

Inspect skin during home visits, observing for any pressure points, as seen by erythema or skin breakdown. If stage I or II ulcer is present but site is not infected, apply film or hydrocolloidal dressing to protect from further breakdown.

Assess pressure ulcer when changing dressing, noting wound bed and border color, discharge, and general condition.

Document each assessment and measure weekly. If wound bed is infected or cellulitic, as seen by erythema, tenderness, pale granulation tissue, or purulent discharge, change dressing to wet-to-dry with an antiseptic, but only until wound is improved and no longer than 5 to 7 days to minimize damage to viable tissue.

If wound is stagnant, as documented by serial dimensions over 3 to 6 weeks, consider changing to another dressing strategy.

Monitor nutritional status, since it can influence skin integrity and healing process:
- Monitor weight gains or losses monthly.
- Take 24-hour diet recall with each visit to assess eating habits and nutritional intake.
- Teach client and family the role nutrition plays in healing and general health status.
- If weight loss is experienced, interview client to determine reason (e.g., food preferences not met, food cold or aesthetically unappealing).
- Examine oral cavity and, if appropriate, denture fit.

Maintain a clean, moist wound environment to foster healing.
- If necrotic tissue is present, facilitate débridement by arranging for physician, nurse practitioner, or certified enterostomal therapist to perform bedside débridement.
- If there is only a small amount of necrotic tissue, attempt chemical or mechanical débridement.

Select most comfortable and efficient dressing, such as a hydrogel or hydrocolloidal dressing, with the intent of maintaining a moist wound environment, which fosters granulation and thus healing.

Use clean technique for dressing care; sterile technique is not necessary because the wound is dirty.

Gently irrigate wound with normal saline to clean wound, make appropriate assessment, and measure wound dimensions weekly.

Teach client and family dressing care and changing technique to involve them in the care and to promote self-care.

SUMMARY

Pressure ulcers are a costly health care problem, not only in terms of dollars, but also in nursing time and human lives. Prevention is the first line of defense for pressure ulcer development. Nurses have an opportunity to demonstrate the profession's power and accountability by implementing preventive strategies, thereby having a positive effect on a client's quality of life while preventing a costly health care problem. It is imperative that the nurse conduct pressure ulcer risk assessments, use mattress overlays, teach support staff prevention and management techniques, monitor the client's nutritional status, and serve as a role model by focusing on prevention. With expanded pressure ulcer knowledge and the publication of the AHCPR clinical guidelines, preventive measures are a nurse's responsibility.

Home Care

1. Regularly assess for signs and symptoms of skin breakdown in homebound older adults who are at high risk for the development of a pressure ulcer.
2. Assess for and instruct caregivers and homebound older adults on factors that predispose clients to the development of a pressure ulcer.
3. Use the services of a wound care clinical nurse specialist in assessing, planning, and recommending appropriate wound care management techniques.
4. Prevention is the first-line strategy for pressure ulcer care. Teach caregivers of at-risk homebound older adults the techniques for preventing a pressure ulcer—focusing on preventing moisture, avoiding friction and shearing, changing position frequently, and ensuring excellent nutritional intake.

Vital to successful healing is for the nurse to establish a collaborative relationship with the physician and APN so that the most efficient and effective strategies can be used. Collaboration develops trust and professional maturity and is necessary for growth in our strained health care system.

Successful pressure ulcer management requires the application of the principles of healing, which should guide selection of treatment strategies. Frequent review of the healing trajectory, when reinforced with clinical examples, facilitates comprehension of this complex process. Pressure ulcer management is a science and an art that requires experience.

Key Points

- As a result of normal, age-related changes in the skin, older adults are more susceptible to skin tears and bruising caused by thinning of skin.
- Older adults are at greater risk for hypothermia, shearing, pressure damage, and blunt trauma as a result of decreased subcutaneous tissue.
- Older adults can experience altered medication absorption as a result of an age-related decrease in fatty tissue and dermis blood supply.
- Older adults are at increased risk of heatstroke as a result of the compromised cooling mechanism from decreased sweating.
- Typical locations for seborrheic dermatitis are the scalp margins, progressing downward to eyebrows, base of eyelashes, around nose in a butterfly pattern, ears, and sternum.
- Psoriasis is a common disorder affecting the epidermis and the dermis. It can be recognized by erythematous, scaly, and itchy patches on various parts of the body. A number of triggers exacerbate the condition.
- Pruritus warrants a full skin assessment because it can be indicative of many diseases, drug reactions, and possibly cancer. The nurse should determine location, intensity, alleviating and aggravating events, onset, and what the client is doing to control it.
- Candidiasis, recognized by fire-red, denuded skin with satellite macules or pustules, develops in moist intertriginous areas.
- Herpes zoster is characterized by prodromal symptoms of itching or burning along a dermatome, followed by a unilateral, bandlike maculopapular rash and vesicles, which rarely cross the midline.
- The nurse should notify the physician or APN if the following suspected lesions are found on assessment of actinic keratosis: BCC, SCC, or melanoma.
- Venous hypertension leads to the formation of a capillary fibrin cuff, which causes chronic edema, decreased circulation, and recurring medial lower leg ulcers.
- Arterial ulcers are usually located on toes or feet and are associated with pain during activity, nighttime, and rest. The cause of decreased arterial blood flow must be corrected for ulcers to heal.
- Diabetic neuropathic ulcers are usually located on the plantar foot and result from loss of protective sensation in the foot, which leads to abnormal gait and increased pressure on the foot. Bony deformities may develop and further change foot pressures, increasing the likelihood of trauma and subsequent ulceration.
- Pressure ulcers are a costly health care problem, not only in terms of dollars, but also in nursing time and human lives. Prevention is the first-line strategy for pressure ulcer care.
- The nurse should assess the nutritional status of clients with pressure ulcers with monthly weight and laboratory parameters.
- To minimize friction, the nurse should use sheets to lift and pull the client up in bed and apply a film dressing or dimethicone-containing lotion to vulnerable areas such as elbows, coccyx, and heels.
- To minimize shearing forces, the nurse should not elevate the head of the bed greater than 30 to 45 degrees.
- Antiseptic solutions should be used only when the wound is infected; they should never be used on a clean, healthy wound because they are cytotoxic and destructive to tissue.
- Surface cultures have been shown to grow different organisms than what is in underlying tissues and blood cultures; thus routine wound cultures are not appropriate.

Critical Thinking Exercises

1. Outline major teaching points that would be beneficial to maintaining the integumentary health of older individuals.
2. A 72-year-old black man has a history of SCC. After having a lesion removed from his upper back 3 years ago, he has been extremely anxious about other skin lesions and skin changes. What approach would you take to help your

client reduce his anxiety and yet remain active in the prevention and early recognition of skin cancer?

3. Your 84-year-old client suffered a stroke 1 year ago and is cared for at home. The client is dependent for position changes, is unable to communicate the need to be turned, must be fed, and has a stage II pressure ulcer on his sacral area. Develop a teaching plan for the family to ensure that the client's needs will be met.

References

Agency for Health Care Policy and Research: *Treatment of pressure ulcers,* Clinical Practice Guideline No 15, Rockville, Md, 1994, US Department of Health and Human Services.

Agency for Health Care Policy and Research: *Pressure ulcers in adults: prediction and prevention,* Clinical Practice Guideline No 3, Rockville, Md, 1992, US Department of Health and Human Services.

Allman RM: Pressure ulcer prevalence, incidence, risk factors, and impact, *Clin Geriatr Med* 31:421, 1997.

Armstrong DG, Lavery LA, Bushman TR: Peak foot pressures influence the healing time of diabetic foot ulcers treated with total contact casts, *J Rehabil Res Dev* 35:1, 1998.

Arnold TE et al: Prospective multicenter study of managing lower extremity venous ulcers, *Ann Vasc Surg* 8:356, 1994.

Bergstrom N et al: The Braden Scale for predicting pressure sore risk, *Nurs Res* 36(4):205-210, 1987.

Birke JA, Rolfsen RJ: Evaluation of self-administered sensory testing tool to identify patients at risk of diabetes-related foot problems, *Diabetes Care* 21:23, 1998.

Braden BJ, Bergstrom N: Clinical utility of the Braden scale for predicting pressure sore risk, *Decubitus* 2(3):44, 1987.

Braden BJ, Bryant R: Innovation to prevent and treat pressure ulcers, *Gerontol Nurs* 182-186, 1990.

Browse RA, Burnand KG: The cause of venous ulceration, *Lancet* 2(8292):243-245, 1982.

Bryant RA et al: Pressure ulcers. In Bryant RA, editor: *Acute and chronic wounds nursing management,* St Louis, 1992, Mosby.

Burton CS: Venous ulcers, *Am J Surg* 167(1A):375-405, 1994.

Calvin M: Cutaneous wound repair, *Wounds* 10:12, 1998.

Colin D et al: Comparison of 90 degrees and 30 degrees laterally inclined positions in the prevention of pressure ulcers using transcutaneous oxygen and carbon dioxide pressures, *Adv Wound Care* 9:35, 1996.

Cox KR, Laird M, Brown JM: Predicting and preventing pressure ulcers in adults, *Nurs Manage* 29(7):41, 1998.

Ebersole P, Hess P, Luggen, AS: *Toward healthy aging: human needs and nursing response,* ed 6, St Louis, 2004, Mosby.

Falanga V, Eaglstein WH: The "trap" hypothesis of venous ulceration, *Lancet* 34(8851):1006-1007, 1993.

Fletcher A, Sheldon TA, Cullum N: A systematic review of compression treatment for venous leg ulcers, *Br Med J* 6315:576, 1997.

Golkar L, Eichenfield LF: Are you undertreating your dry skin patients? *Skin Aging* 6(2):35, 1998.

Goodman T, Thomas C, Rappaport N: Skin ulcers: overview of nursing implications, *AORN J* 52(1):24-28, 30-31, 33-37, 1990.

Gosnell DJ: Pressure sore risk assessment: a critic, part I, The Gosnell scale, *Decubitus* 2(3):32, 1989.

Habif TP: *Clinical dermatology,* ed 4, St Louis, 2004, Mosby.

Harris AH, Brown-Etris M, Troyer-Caudle J: Managing vascular leg ulcers. Part 1: Assessment, *Am J Nurs* 96:38-43, 1996.

Helm KF, Marks JG: *Atlas of differential diagnosis in dermatology,* New York, 1998, Churchill Livingstone.

Hunt TK: The physiology of wound healing, *Ann Emerg Med* 17:1265-1273, 1988.

Johnson BL, Moy RL, White GM: *Ethnic skin,* St Louis, 1998, Mosby.

Kosiak M: Etiology and pathology of ischemic ulcers, *Arch Phys Med Rehabil* 40(2):62, 1958.

Krasner D: Resolving the dressing dilemma: selecting wound dressings by category, *Ostomy Wound Manage* 35(4):62, 1991.

Landis EM: Micro-injection studies of capillary blood pressure in human skin, *Heart* 15(209), 1930.

Levine JM: Historical notes on pressure ulcers: the cure of Ambrose Pare, *Decubitus* 5(2):23-26, 1992.

Levin M: Diabetic foot wounds: pathogenesis and management, *Adv Wound Care* 10(2):24, 1997.

Luggen AS: Wrinkles and beyond: skin problems in older adults, *Adv Nurse Pract* 9:55, 2003.

Maklebust J: Pressure ulcers: decreasing the risk for older adults, *Geriatr Nurs* 18:250, 1997.

Norton D: Calculation of the risk: reflections on the Norton scale, *Decubitus* 2(3):24, 1989.

Pinchcofsky-Devin G, Kaminski M: Correlation of pressure sores and nutritional status, *J Am Geriatr Soc* 34:435, 1986.

Robson MC: Wound infection: A failure of would healing caused by an imbalance of bacteria, *Surg Clin North Am* 77:637-650, 1997.

Schaffer M, Barbul A: Lymphocyte function in wound healing and following injury, *Br J Surg* 85:444, 1998.

Steed DL et al: Effect of extensive debridement and treatment on the healing of diabetic foot ulcers, *J Am Coll Surg* 183:61-64, 1996.

Stotts NA, Wipke-Tevis D: Nutrition, perfusion, and wound healing: an inseparable triad, *Nutrition* 12:733-734, 1996.

Strauss EA, Margolis DJ: Malnutrition in patients with pressure ulcers: morbidity, mortality, and clinically practical assessments, *Adv Wound Care* 9(5):37-40, 1996.

Thomas DR: Specific nutritional factors in wound healing, *Adv Wound Care* 10:40-43, 1997.

Vowden P: The investigation and assessment of venous disease, *J Wound Care* 7:143, 1998.

Xakellis G, Frantz RA: Cost-effectiveness of an intensive pressure ulcer prevention protocol in long-term care, *Adv Wound Care* 11:22, 1998.

31 Sensory Function

SABRINA FRIEDMAN, MSN, PhD, EdD, FNP

Learning Objectives

On completion of this chapter, the reader will be able to:

1. Describe age-related changes in the senses.
2. Compare and contrast cataracts and glaucoma and the associated nursing interventions.
3. Compare and contrast retinal disorders and the medical and nursing management of each disorder.
4. Identify nursing interventions for older persons with low vision.
5. Describe the proper method for instilling eye medications.
6. Describe the proper method for removing impacted cerumen.
7. Identify safety measures for clients with vertigo.
8. Identify nursing interventions for clients with xerostomia.
9. Describe potential hazards for older persons with diminished senses of vision, hearing, and touch.
10. Conduct sensory system assessment and describe the normal findings.
11. Describe aural rehabilitation methods to use with persons who are hearing impaired.
12. Identify how activities of daily living are affected by sensory changes.

The senses connect the human body to the environment. They allow individuals to be aware of and interpret various stimuli, thus enabling interaction with the environment. Sensory changes can have a dramatic effect on the quality of life for older adults. Visual and hearing impairments may interfere with communication, social interactions, and mobility, leading to social isolation. Olfactory, gustatory, and tactile deprivations can lead to nutritional problems and safety hazards. It is important to understand the sensory changes associated with aging to help older adults adapt and function as independently as possible.

In the past, five senses were recognized: sight, hearing, taste, smell, and touch. Today, additional senses are recognized and categorized into two major groups: general and special. General senses include the senses of touch, pressure, pain, temperature, vibration, and proprioception (position sense). These have relatively simple receptors, which are located all over the body. Theses senses are further classified as somatic (those providing sensory information about the body and the environment) or visceral (those supplying information about the internal organs). Special senses are produced by highly localized organs and specialized sensory cells. These include the senses of sight, hearing, taste, smell, and balance.

Sensation is a conscious or unconscious awareness of external and internal stimuli. Perception is the interpretation of conscious sensations. The brain receives stimuli from both inside and outside the body. Conscious sensation occurs via action potentials generated by receptors that reach the cerebral cortex.

VISION

Vision plays an integral part in a person's ability to function in the environment. Visual acuity (ability to see clearly) is an important part of performing activities of daily living (ADLs); dressing, grooming, cooking, sewing, driving, and reading are all tasks that involve the use of eyesight.

Age-Related Changes in Structure and Function

Normal age-related changes in the external and internal eye have been well documented. The eyelids lose tone and become lax, which may result in ptosis of the eyelids, redundancy of the skin of the eyelids, and malposition of the eyelids. Eyebrows may turn gray and become coarser in men, with outer thinning in both men and women. The conjunctiva thins and yellows in appearance. In addition, this membrane may become dry because of diminished quantity and quality of tear production. The sclera may develop brown spots. The cornea yellows and develops a noticeable surrounding ring, made up of fat deposits, called the arcus senilis. The pupil decreases in size and loses some of its ability to constrict. Aging changes that decrease the size of the pupil and limit the amount of light entering the eye also occur in the iris. The lens increases in density and rigidity, affecting the eye's ability to transmit and focus light. Peripheral vision decreases, night vision diminishes, and sensitivity to glare increases (Roach, 2001). The yellowing of the lens results in difficulty identifying certain colors, especially cool colors such as blue, green, and violet (Lueckenotte, 1998).

Ophthalmoscopic examination of the retina may reveal the following changes: blood vessels narrow and straighten; arteries seem opaque and gray; and drusen, localized areas of hyaline degeneration, may be noted as gray or yellow spots near the macula (Lueckenotte, 1998). Two common complaints of older adults, floaters and dry eyes, are discussed in the following section.

Common Complaints

Floaters and Flashers. Floaters appear as dots, wiggly lines, or clouds that a person may see moving in the field of vision. They become more pronounced when a person is looking at a plain background. Floaters occur more often after the age of 50 as tiny clumps of gel or cellular debris float in the vitreous humor in front of the retina. They are caused by degeneration of the vitreous gel and are more common in older adults who have undergone cataract operations or yttrium-aluminum-garnet (YAG) laser surgery.

In general, floaters are normal and harmless, but they may be a warning sign of a more serious condition, especially if they increase in number and if changes in the type of floater, light flashes, or visual hallucinations are noted. These symptoms may indicate a vitreous or retinal tear, which could lead to detachment. In addition, visual hallucinations have been associated with a brain tumor or cortical ischemia. Therefore any of these symptoms warrants a complete eye examination by an ophthalmologist.

Flashers occur when the vitreous fluid inside the eye rubs or pulls on the retina and produces the illusion of flashing lights or lightning streaks. Flashers that appear as jagged lines, last 10 to 20 minutes, and are present in both eyes are likely to be caused by a spasm of blood vessels in the brain called a migraine. These flashers commonly occur with advancing age, but they warrant prompt medical attention if they increase in number, if a large number of new floaters appears, or if partial loss of side vision is noted (Kollarits, 1998).

The nurse should refer a client who experiences any of the above symptoms to an ophthalmologist for a comprehensive eye examination. If no cause is found for the floaters and flashers, the nurse should teach the client about the condition and how to live with it. Clients should be taught to look up and down to get the floaters out of the field of vision. In addition, the nurse should provide the client with the printed information instruction sheet titled "Aging and Your Eyes" so he or she may learn more about floaters and flashers (Kollarits, 1998) (Box 31-1).

Dry Eyes. Dry eyes result as the quantity and quality of tear production diminish with aging. Stinging, burning, scratchiness, and stringy mucus are some of the symptoms. Although this may seem surprising, increased tearing may be a symptom of dry eyes. If tear secretion is below normal, excess tears are produced by the lacrimal gland in response to irritation. If no foreign body is found, the condition is called dry eye syndrome. Tear production decreases with age, and menopausal women are most often afflicted. Also, dry eyes may be associated with arthritis and the use of certain medications.

Treatment consists of tear replacement or conservation. Tears can be replaced by instilling an over-the-counter artificial tear preparation to lubricate the eye and replace missing moisture. This type of preparation may be used as often as necessary, especially before activities that require significant eye movement. Solid inserts that gradually release lubricants throughout the day are also available. An ophthalmologist can conserve the naturally produced tears by temporarily or permanently closing the lacrimal drainage system. Other methods of conservation include use of a humidifier when

BOX 31-1 Aging and Your Eyes

1. Use bright light when performing tasks such as sewing, reading, and cooking; avoid fluorescent light.
2. Use a magnifying glass, if necessary, for close work.
3. See your health care provider regularly to detect health problems (e.g., diabetes, hypertension) that might affect your eyes.
4. Have your eyes examined and a glaucoma test performed by a qualified specialist every 1 to 2 years. Have your eyes examined more frequently if you have a disease or condition that is known to affect your vision.
5. Symptoms that require an immediate call to your health care provider or eye care specialist include pain, discharge, redness or swelling, and loss of vision (no matter how slight).
6. The use of a humidifier in the home or artificial tears may relieve dry eyes, which is a common condition. Check with your health care provider or eye care specialist before using any such over-the-counter preparations.
7. Excessive tearing can be a benign condition, or it may reflect a more serious problem. See your health care provider or eye care specialist if you are troubled by this problem.
8. Floaters, a common occurrence in older persons, are just spots or flecks that literally "float" across your field of vision. They usually occur gradually and are most noticeable in a brightly lit environment. If they occur in association with light flashes in your visual field, call your health care provider or eye care specialist.
9. Cataracts are a normal part of the aging process. They develop gradually and without pain. However, when tasks become increasingly difficult and fatiguing because of the vision changes that cataracts produce, see your health care provider or eye care specialist to discuss treatment options.

Data from US Department of Health and Human Services: *Aging and your eyes,* Bethesda, Md, 2002, National Institute on Aging.

the heat is on, wraparound glasses to reduce evaporation of eye moisture caused by wind, and avoidance of smoke (Kollarits, 1998).

Common Problems and Conditions

Common problems related to the aging eye include presbyopia, ectropion and entropion, blepharitis, glaucoma, cataracts, retinal disorders, eye injuries, and visual impairment. Presbyopia is a normal change that occurs with aging. The other problems are eye diseases that are more prominent in older adults.

Presbyopia. The most common complaint of adults older than 40 is a diminished ability to focus clearly on close objects (arm's length), such as a newspaper. In presbyopia the lens loses its ability to focus on close objects. Accommodation is impaired as the lens thickens and loses its elasticity. The ciliary muscles weaken the lens's ability to contract. Treatment involves wearing reading glasses or bifocals (two-part lenses that correct near and distant vision); there is an excellent prognosis for corrected vision.

Nursing care is aimed at encouraging the client to adjust to the glasses by wearing them and following up with a visit to the ophthalmologist every 2 years. Clients can be provided with an "Aging and Your Eyes" pamphlet (see Box 31-1) for information about presbyopia. Also, clients and their families can be taught eye health promotion and prevention techniques (see Health Promotion/Illness Prevention box).

Ectropion and Entropion. Ectropion and entropion are external eye conditions, specifically malpositions of the lower lid, which irritate the eye. Both conditions are due to tissue laxity and scarring of the eyelids from infection. Ectropion (turning outward) prevents normal closure and causes redness and tearing of the eyeball. Ectropion interferes with draining of the tears, and increased tearing may occur (Roach, 2001). Entropion (turning inward) results in the eyelashes rubbing against the eye, causing corneal abrasion. The lower lashes may not be visible and can cause watering and redness of the eye. Both can be treated by minor same-day outpatient surgery performed by an ophthalmologist. The prognosis for complete recovery and cessation of symptoms is excellent.

Blepharitis. Blepharitis is a chronic inflammation of the eyelid margins that is commonly found in older adults. It can be caused by seborrheic dermatitis or infection. The use of antihistamines, anticholinergics, antidepressants, and diuretics can exacerbate this condition because of the drying effects of the medications. In addition, the deficiency in tear production with aging can lead to infection. The symptoms include red, swollen eyelids; matting and crusting along the base of the eyelash at the margins; small ulcerations along the lid margins; and complaints of irritation, itching, burning, tearing, and photophobia. Treatment is aimed at removing the bacteria and healing the affected areas. Physicians may prescribe topical antibiotics or steroids. However, the nurse can play a large role in the treatment of this condition by teaching a client the following interventions.

The client must be taught scrupulous eye hygiene, including good hand-washing habits. Mild soap (e.g., Ivory, Neutrogena) should be used. Contact lens wearers must be taught proper cleaning and storage techniques to prevent contamination of the eye, lens, lens solution, and lens case. Since cosmetics are a common source of bacterial contamination, eye makeup products should be replaced every 3 to 6 months to avoid bacterial growth. It is also important that clients know how to apply makeup with cotton balls and cotton-tipped applicators and understand the importance of discarding the applicators after each use. Mascara should be water resistant, free of lash-extending fibers, and not applied to the base of the lashes. Eyeliner should be a medium-hard pencil and not be applied to the inner margin of the eyelid. Clients should avoid the use of aerosol hairsprays because these can irritate the eyes. The inflammation caused by blepharitis and the client's comfort level will improve after a week of these hygienic practices.

Glaucoma. Glaucoma is the second leading cause of blindness in the United States and the first cause of blindness among blacks. Although glaucoma can occur at any age, those most at risk are adults older than age 60 (Roach, 2001). The most common form has few, if any, symptoms and may cause partial vision loss before it is detected.

Glaucoma results from a blockage in the drainage of the fluid (the aqueous humor) in the anterior chamber of the eye.

Health Promotion/Illness Prevention

The Eye

HEALTH PROMOTION

- Notify health care provider of any pain, discharge, redness, swelling, or loss of vision.
- Take measures for detection and appropriate treatment of vision difficulties and eye disease (e.g., cataracts, glaucoma, diabetic retinopathy, macular degeneration).
- Maintain prescribed corrective lenses, low-vision aids, and medications.

PREVENTION OF DISEASE

- Have a yearly eye examination and screening (including a glaucoma test) for eye disease and vision problems.
- Use a bright light when sewing, reading, and cooking; avoid fluorescent light.
- Have an ultraviolet filter coating on spectacle lenses and sunglasses for outdoor activities.

Normally this fluid drains through Schlemm's canal and is transported to the venous circulation system. If the fluid is formed faster than it can be eliminated, eye pressure increases. Pressure is then transferred to the optic nerve, where irreparable damage, possibly even total blindness, can result. Three types of glaucoma are found in older adults: chronic open-angle glaucoma, closed-angle glaucoma, and secondary glaucoma.

Chronic Open-Angle Glaucoma. Chronic open-angle glaucoma, the most common type (making up 90% of all primary glaucoma), develops slowly. Degenerative changes in Schlemm's canal obstruct the escape of aqueous humor, resulting in increased intraocular pressure. This type of glaucoma can damage vision so gradually and painlessly that a person is unaware of a problem until the optic nerve is badly damaged. Visual loss begins with deteriorating peripheral vision.

Closed-Angle Glaucoma. This is acute glaucoma that occurs suddenly as a result of complete blockage. It requires prompt medical attention to avoid severe vision loss or blindness. The following symptoms of closed-angle glaucoma occur rapidly (Kollarits, 1998):

- Severe eye pain
- Redness in the eye
- Clouded or blurred vision
- Nausea and vomiting
- Bradycardia
- Rainbow halos surrounding lights
- Pupil dilation
- Steamy appearance of cornea

Secondary Glaucoma. Secondary glaucoma occurs when the drainage angle is damaged by eye injury or other specific conditions, such as medication use (e.g., use of steroids), tumors, inflammation, or abnormal blood vessels.

NURSING MANAGEMENT

Assessment

Clients with glaucoma may complain of dull eye pain, or they may experience no early symptoms. Visual field testing reveals a loss of peripheral vision (tunnel vision), and increased intraocular pressure is seen on ophthalmologic examination.

Diagnosis

Potential nursing diagnoses for the client with glaucoma include:

- Sensory/perceptual alterations (visual) related to decreased peripheral vision
- Knowledge deficit: glaucoma causes and treatments related to lack of exposure and inexperience
- Pain related to increased intraocular pressure
- Potential for infection related to eyedrop instillation
- Dressing and grooming self-care deficit related to visual impairment

Planning and Expected Outcomes

Expected outcomes for the client with glaucoma include:

1. Client will have no further loss of vision.
2. Client will follow prescribed glaucoma care guidelines daily.
3. Client will state that eye pain is decreased.
4. Client will be free from eye infection.
5. Client will be able to perform ADLs safely and independently.

Intervention

Nursing management is aimed at teaching the client that glaucoma is a chronic condition requiring lifelong medical treatment. Any current visual loss is permanent, but further loss can be prevented by following the care guidelines outlined in Box 31-2. If medication is unable to control rising intraocular pressure, surgical intervention may be necessary.

Trabeculoplasty is usually performed on an outpatient basis. It requires an intraocular pressure check 3 to 4 hours after surgery. A sudden rise in intraocular pressure can occur

BOX 31-2 The Client With Glaucoma

1. Medical follow-up and eye medication will be required for the rest of your life.
2. Eyedrops *must* be continued as long as prescribed, even in the absence of symptoms.
   a. Blurred vision decreases with prolonged use.
   b. Avoid driving for 1 to 2 hours after administration of miotics.
3. To prevent complications:
   a. Press lacrimal duct for 1 minute after eyedrop insertion to prevent rapid systemic absorption.
   b. Have a reserve bottle of eyedrops at home.
   c. Carry eyedrops on person (not in luggage) when traveling.
   d. Carry card or wear Medic-Alert bracelet identifying glaucoma and the eyedrops solution prescribed.
4. Bright lights and darkness are not harmful.
5. There is no apparent relationship between vascular hypertension and ocular hypertension.
6. Report any reappearance of symptoms immediately to the ophthalmologist.
7. If admitted to the hospital for a different medical condition, alert staff of continued need to use prescribed eyedrops.
8. Avoid the use of mydriatic or cycloplegic drugs (e.g., atropine) that dilate the pupils.

From Phipps WJ: The patient with eye problems. In Long BC, Phipps WJ, Cassmeyer VS, editors: *Medical-surgical nursing: a nursing process approach,* ed 3, St Louis, 1993, Mosby.

immediately after surgery. A 4- to 8-week wait is necessary to determine if the procedure was effective. However, continual use of glaucoma medications is necessary.

Trabeculectomy requires overnight hospitalization. Postoperative nursing care for the client who has had a trabeculectomy includes (1) routine postanesthesia care; (2) protection of the operative eye with an eye patch or a shield, proper positioning of the client on the back or on the side of the inoperative eye, and the use of a call light and side rails; (3) administration of pain medications and cold eye compresses to maintain comfort; (4) monitoring of the eye for increased intraocular pressure, bleeding, or infection; and (5) assistance and teaching of safe, independent performance of ADLs (Phipps, 1993).

Evaluation

Evaluation includes documentation of the achievement of the expected outcomes, no further vision loss, and the independent performance of ADLs. It is imperative that the client and family understand the chronic nature of this disease and its treatment. The client must be able to state the name and dosage of the prescribed eye medications and describe their daily use, even during periods of travel or hospitalization. The client must also be able to identify the significant signs and symptoms in order to report correct information to the ophthalmologist.

Cataracts. Cataracts are the most common disorder found in the aging adult. The highest incidence is found in adults over the age of 55; cataracts are found in virtually all adults over the age of 80.

A cataract is a clouding of the normally clear and transparent lens of the eye. The lens focuses light on the retina to produce a sharp image. When a cataract forms, the lens can become so opaque that light cannot be transmitted to the retina. Cataracts result from changes in the chemical composition of the lens; these changes can be caused by aging, eye injuries, certain diseases, and heredity. In addition, there are different types of cataracts. The normal aging process may cause the lens to harden and turn cloudy. These cataracts are called senile cataracts and can occur as early as age 40. Eye injuries, such as a hard blow, puncture, cut, or burn, can damage the lens and result in a traumatic cataract. Secondary cataracts can be caused by certain infections, drugs, or diseases (e.g., diabetes).

The size and location of a cataract determine the amount of interference with clear sight. A cataract located near the center of the lens produces more noticeable symptoms, such as:

- Dimmed, blurred, or misty vision
- The need for brighter light to read
- Glare and light sensitivity
- Loss of color perception
- Recurrent eyeglass prescription changes

These symptoms develop slowly and at different rates in each eye.

NURSING MANAGEMENT

Assessment

Subjective complaints include having trouble reading and the necessity of cleaning glasses (the vision difficulties are thought to be caused by dirty glasses). Lens opacity may be visible on external or internal eye examination.

Diagnosis

Nursing diagnoses for the client with cataracts include:

- Sensory/perceptual alterations (visual) related to a hard and cloudy lens
- Anxiety related to uncertain surgical outcome
- Knowledge deficit: cataracts related to lack of exposure
- Potential for injury related to changes in visual acuity
- Dressing/grooming self-care deficit related to inability to see body and face clearly enough to maintain appearance of clothes and cosmetics

Planning and Expected Outcomes

Expected outcomes for a client with cataracts include:

1. Client will have cataract surgery when it is recommended by an ophthalmologist.
2. Client will ask questions about preoperative and postoperative care and report satisfaction with information.
3. Client's affected eye will be free from increased intraocular pressure, stress on the suture line, hemorrhage, and infection.
4. Client will verbalize appropriate home care activities to avoid and activities to do after cataract surgery.
5. Client will demonstrate correct administration of eyedrops.
6. Client will avoid falling, bumping into objects, and having automobile accidents before and after surgery.
7. Client will dress and groom self when vision returns.

Intervention

Nursing management for a client with cataracts focuses mainly on preoperative and postoperative surgical care, since surgery is the only method for treating cataracts. However, asymptomatic clients do not require referral. Most cataract surgery is performed as outpatient surgery with the administration of a local anesthetic; this makes preoperative teaching difficult because clients arrive just hours before surgery. Many ambulatory centers conduct preoperative assessment and teaching by phone a week before surgery. Preoperative care involves administering eyedrops and a sedative as ordered. Postoperative care requires teaching the client and family home care procedures for the period after cataract surgery (see Client/Family Teaching box), including the method for instilling eyedrops. The home care instructions need to include special precautions recommended by the

Client/Family Teaching 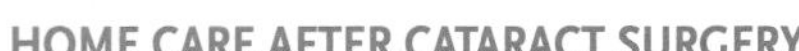

HOME CARE AFTER CATARACT SURGERY

Activities Not to Do

Avoid rubbing or pressing on the eye.

Avoid bending at the waist or lifting heavy objects for at least 1 month:

- To pick objects up from the floor, kneel while keeping head erect.
- To put on stockings or tie shoes, sit and raise foot to reach hand while keeping head erect.
- Use long pick-up "reachers" to pick up small objects from the floor.

Avoid straining with bowel movements (stool softener may be necessary).

Avoid taking showers and shampooing hair (soap may irritate eye) for specified time as instructed.

Limit reading (back and forth movement may loosen stitches).

Activities to Do

Sleep on back or unaffected side for prescribed time frame (3 to 4 weeks).

Apply metal eye shield at night or when napping to protect eye.

Wear glasses indoors (all day) and sunglasses with side shields outdoors.

Wash hands before instilling eyedrops, and follow the correct procedure for eyedrop instillation.

Follow steps for eye pad:

- Wash hands before changing eye pad.
- Use two oval eye pads.
- Tape pad snugly and diagonally from above nose to lower cheek.

Modified from Phipps WJ: The patient with eye problems. In Long BC, Phipps WJ, Cassmeyer VS, editors: *Medical-surgical nursing: a nursing process* approach, ed 3, St Louis, 1993, Mosby.

ophthalmologist based on the type of surgery performed. If a lens implant has not been inserted, clients need to wear contact lenses or cataract glasses. Clients wearing cataract glasses experience loss of depth perception and distorted peripheral and color vision. They need to be taught that objects are magnified by 25% and appear larger and closer than they really are; this requires home safety measures and the modification of dressing and cosmetic application after surgery (see Nursing Care Plan).

Evaluation

Evaluation includes documentation of the achievement of the expected outcomes. Clients who have had successful cataract surgery will be free from complications and have improved vision. Additionally, they will report performance of their usual daily activities with the use of lens implants, contact lenses, or corrective glasses. The client and family will arrange assistance with ADLs for the first 24 to 48 hours after surgery, or they will notify the home health agency.

Retinal Disorders. Three common disorders that affect the retina of an older adult are macular degeneration, diabetic retinopathy, and retinal detachment.

Age-Related Macular Degeneration. Age-related macular degeneration (AMD) is the leading cause of blindness among older adults in the United States. It does not cause total blindness but results in loss of close vision. AMD is a poorly understood disease that causes damage to the macula, the key focusing area of the retina. The cells within the macula diminish in functional ability with age, and replacement of the damaged cells is decreased, causing irreversible damage to the macula (Roach, 2001). As a result, there is a decline in central visual acuity that makes daily tasks requiring close vision nearly impossible. Peripheral vision is retained.

Types of AMD include:

- **Dry macular degeneration.** Also known as involutional macular degeneration, this condition is caused by breakdown or thinning of macular tissue related to the aging process. Vision loss is gradual.
- **Wet macular degeneration.** Also known as exudative macular degeneration, this type of AMD results when abnormal blood vessels form and hemorrhage on the retina. Vision loss may be rapid and severe.

AMD is almost exclusively a disorder of whites and is more common in women than in men. Cases tend to cluster in families. Smoking, low dietary intake of antioxidant vitamins and zinc, and sun exposure are some modifiable risk factors (Taylor, 2002).

Symptoms of macular degeneration include:

- Difficulty performing tasks that require close central vision, such as reading and sewing
- Decreased color vision (i.e., colors look dim)
- Dark or empty area in the center of vision
- Straight lines appearing wavy or crooked
- Words on a page looking blurred

Diabetic Retinopathy. Loss of visual function is one of the most common complications of diabetes. Altered circulation to the eye may result in retinal edema, degeneration, or detachment. This condition is a complication of diabetes that affects the retinal capillary circulation. Ballooning of these tiny vessels leads to hemorrhaging, scarring, and blindness. These vascular changes in and around the retina lead to macular edema, which causes the retina to swell. There are no symptoms of early retinal changes, and no symptoms may be apparent even when the retinopathy is advanced. Early detection requires a complete ophthalmoscopic examination; therefore clients with diabetes should have a yearly examination by an ophthalmologist.

Retinal Detachment. Studies have shown that 6% of the population has small holes or tears in the retina. Aging tends

Nursing Care Plan
Cataracts

Clinical Situation: Mrs. S is a 75-year-old retired nurse who has been admitted to the skilled nursing unit of a local hospital for rehabilitation therapy following repair of a right hip fracture. She is accompanied by her daughter. Mrs. S has no significant medical history, but a fall in her home resulted in the break in her hip. She states that she has been having trouble with her eyes and she tripped on the stairs. Since her admission to the hospital, a vision screening detected cataracts in both eyes and surgery was recommended once she recovers. Mrs. S requires assistance with all ADLs except eating. She is unable to bear weight on her right leg, so assistance is needed to transfer to the toilet, chair, or bed. She also needs help bathing and dressing the lower half of her body because she cannot reach her legs or feet. Mrs. S states that her biggest concern is fear of falling again.

Nursing Diagnosis

Sensory/perceptual alteration (visual) related to hard and cloudy lens
Potential for injury related to altered visual acuity
Partial self-care deficit: bathing and hygiene, dressing and grooming, and toileting related to immobility
Anxiety related to fear of falling

Outcomes

Client will verbalize questions and concerns regarding cataracts and recommended surgical treatment.
Client will have cataract surgery when appropriate.
Client will not fall.
Client will assist with self-care to the fullest extent possible as evidenced by fulfilling needs for cleanliness, grooming, and toileting.
Client will report reduced anxiety, as evidenced by relaxed state and learning about cataract surgery.

Interventions

Provide client with printed information sheet, "Aging and Your Eyes" (see Box 31-1) and the client education sheet "Home Care After Cataract Surgery" (see Client/Family Teaching box, p. 734).
Encourage client and family member to speak with an ophthalmologist about recommended surgery.
Explain preoperative and postoperative procedures related to recommended surgery.
Provide a safe environment (e.g., bed in low position, side rails as needed, call light and personal items in reach).
Assist with transfers until client demonstrates safe transfer while unassisted.
Assess client's home for factors that hinder or support vision changes.
Administer pain medication as needed before performing self-care.
Encourage client to perform as much of own care as possible to help restore independence.
Provide assistance, supervision, and teaching with the use of assistive devices as needed to perform self-care. Assess factors in the client's home that support or hinder self-care.
Encourage expression of fears of falling.
Use therapeutic communication to gain insight into client's fears and give realistic feedback.
Increase attention to client when he or she is feeling anxious.

From McFarland GK, McFarlane EA: *Nursing diagnosis and intervention: planning for patient care*, ed 3, St Louis, 1997, Mosby.

to weaken these spots (Kollarits, 1998). Retinal detachment occurs when the sensory layer of the retina separates from the pigmented layer. Tears or holes occur in the retina as a result of trauma, aging (degeneration), hemorrhage, or tumor. When a tear occurs, fluid seeps between the layers, causing detachment. The usual symptoms include:

- Light flashes
- Shower of floaters that resemble spots, bugs, or spider webs
- Loss of vision
- Veil or curtain obstructing vision

NURSING MANAGEMENT

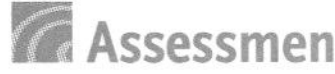

Assessment

There are no early symptoms of diabetic retinopathy and sometimes no symptoms with advanced retinopathy. Clients with macular degeneration may complain that they are unable to thread a needle or that the words on a page look blurred, making it difficult to read. Clients with retinal detachment notice flashes of light followed by floating spots before the eye and progressive loss of vision. The specific area of vision loss depends on where the detachment is located. When detachment occurs quickly and is extensive, the client may feel that a curtain has been drawn before the eyes.

Ongoing nursing assessment involves monitoring the client's subjective statements about changes in vision and observing for signs of anxiety. All three retinal disorders are diagnosed by ophthalmoscopic examination.

Diagnosis

Nursing diagnoses are determined by analysis of the client assessment. Possible nursing diagnoses for a client with a retinal disorder include:

- Sensory/perceptual alterations (visual) related to damaged macula or retina
- Knowledge deficit: effect of diabetes on eyes caused by lack of exposure to accurate information
- Knowledge deficit: retinal detachment condition, surgery, preoperative and postoperative care, and home care after surgery
- Anxiety related to fear of blindness

Planning and Expected Outcomes

Expected outcomes for an older person with a retinal disorder include:

1. Client will adjust successfully to vision loss by using low-vision aids.
2. Client will state in own words the effect of diabetes on eyes.
3. Client will see an ophthalmologist yearly.
4. Client will ask questions about preoperative and postoperative retinal surgery care and report satisfaction with information.
5. Client's affected eye will be free from further retinal detachment, infection, or hemorrhaging.
6. Client will verbalize appropriate home care activities to participate in after retinal surgery.
7. Client will demonstrate correct administration of eyedrops.
8. Client will report reduced anxiety.

Intervention

Clients with macular degeneration and diabetic retinopathy must learn to cope with chronic, gradual vision loss. Clients with macular degeneration are often taught to self-monitor their central vision using an Amsler chart, a small printed grid. The appearance of an increase in waves or curves on the grid may indicate worsening disease. Clients must be taught how to obtain and use low-vision aids (Box 31-3). Teaching about the condition and encouraging yearly follow-up visits with an ophthalmologist help clients understand the disease and how it affects their eyes (see Box 31-1).

Clients with retinal detachment require the immediate care of bedrest in a proper position (i.e., retinal hole in most dependent position) and eye patches (may be prescribed for one or both eyes) until surgery is performed. Safety precautions and means of communicating are essential for the client at this point. Postoperative care includes administration of eye medication, pain medication, antiemetics as needed, and cough medication as needed. Cold compresses are applied to reduce swelling and promote comfort. Clients must be instructed to avoid jerking movements of the head, such as coughing, sneezing, and vomiting. If the eyes are patched, safety precautions, such as keeping call lights, side rails, and necessary items within reach, must be instituted. Finally, assistance must be provided with ADLs and walking as needed to promote comfort and safety. Home care instructions to teach the client and family include (1) report increases in floaters, flashes of light, decreased vision, drainage, or increased pain to an ophthalmologist; (2) administer eyedrops; (3) limit physical activity for 1 to 2 weeks, and resume active sports and heavy lifting as indicated by a physician; and (4) make follow-up appointments with the ophthalmologist.

Clients with any retinal disorder may experience anxiety about the loss of vision and possible blindness. The opportunity for clients to discuss their concerns needs to be provided. Nurses must also be knowledgeable of available resources.

BOX 31-3 Low-Vision Aids

- Prisms, mirrors
- Magnifying devices
- Glasses
- Magnifying television screen
- Large-print books, magazines, telephone pads, clocks, watches, and playing cards
- Computers
- Reading machines
- Talking books, clocks, and wristwatches
- Closed-circuit television, video units, and computers
- Special lighting, including high-intensity reading lamps
- Special lenses
  —Telescopic for distance vision
  —Microscopic for close vision
- Reading aids
  —Angled book stands and book racks
  —Prismatic glasses

Modified from Redford JB: Assistive devices. In Duthie EH, Katz PR, editors: *Practice of geriatrics*, ed 3, Philadelphia, 1998, WB Saunders.

Evaluation

Evaluation includes documentation of the achievement of the expected outcomes. Clients with macular degeneration and diabetic retinopathy will describe the condition and report use of low-vision aids. These clients will also follow up with annual visits to the ophthalmologist. Clients who have had detachment surgery will experience no complications and gradual improvement in vision. Clients will limit their physical activity for 1 to 2 weeks with the help of significant others or home health care. Clients with macular degeneration will monitor their central vision with an Amsler chart and report changes to the ophthalmologist. Clients with any retinal disorder will report reduced anxiety as evidenced by their ability to learn about and cope with their disease.

Visual Impairment. Visual impairment is the most common sensory problem faced by older adults. The visually impaired population includes those with low vision (20/50 to 20/200) and those who are legally blind (visual acuity of

20/200 or worse in the better eye with the aid of the best possible spectacle or contact lens correction) (Kollarits, 1998). Blindness in older persons results from diabetic retinopathy, glaucoma, cataracts, and macular degeneration, and its incidence has increased as the number of persons ages 65 and older grows.

Sudden vision loss is considered a medical emergency and should be evaluated immediately. It may be caused by retinal detachment or an eye injury (see Emergency Treatment box). The medical management of vision loss depends on the type, cause, and amount experienced. Any client with a visual disability that cannot be improved by corrective lenses or surgery should be referred to a low-vision specialist or center.

NURSING MANAGEMENT

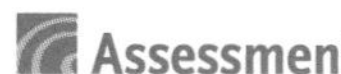

Assessment

It is important to assess nursing home residents and those living alone, since the impact of visual acuity is far reaching (Roach, 2001). Nursing assessment of the client with impaired vision requires an understanding of the client's response to the vision loss. The older adult who becomes blind suddenly usually has a harder time adjusting to the disability than a person who was born blind. Loss of vision may result in a self-esteem disturbance, leading to social isolation.

> **EMERGENCY TREATMENT**
>
> **EYE INJURIES**
>
> Burns (chemical or flame)
> - Flush eye immediately with cool water or any available nontoxic liquid.
> - Seek medical assistance.
>
> Foreign body (loose substance on conjunctiva such as dirt or an insect)
> - Pull upper lid down over lower lid to produce tearing and dislodge substance.
> - Irrigate eye with water if needed.
> - Do *not* rub eye.
> - Seek medical assistance if above interventions are unsuccessful.
>
> Contact injury (e.g., hematoma, ecchymosis, laceration)
> - If no laceration is present, apply cold compresses.
> - If laceration is present, cover eye and seek medical assistance.
>
> Penetrating objects
> - Do not remove object.
> - Place protective shield (e.g., paper cup) over eye and cover.
> - Seek medical assistance.
>
> Modified from Phipps WJ: The patient with eye problems. In Phipps WJ, Sands J, Marek J: *Medical-surgical nursing: concepts and clinical practice,* ed 6, St Louis, 1999, Mosby.

A self-esteem disturbance leads to decreased self-confidence, which can affect interactions with others, the ability to carry out normal daily activities, job performance, and the desire to engage in familiar hobbies. Grief and mourning occur over the loss of vision and result in reactions similar to those experienced with death, such as denial, anger, guilt, hopelessness, and depression. The client's ability to cope with the loss depends on the type, amount, and duration of the vision loss as well as the client's support system and coping style. Over time, persons with vision loss are able to compensate by increasing sensitivity in other senses, such as hearing, taste, touch, and balance.

Diagnosis

Potential nursing diagnoses for the client with visual impairment include:

- Self-esteem disturbance related to sudden loss of vision
- Social isolation related to impaired communication
- Ineffective individual coping related to sudden loss of vision
- Feeding, bathing and hygiene, dressing and grooming, and toileting self-care deficits related to visual impairment
- Impaired physical mobility related to visual impairment
- Risk for injury related to impaired vision

Planning and Expected Outcomes

Expected outcomes for a client with visual impairment include:

1. Client will perceive himself or herself positively by making positive statements about self.
2. Client will participate successfully in activities with others.
3. Client will demonstrate increased objectivity and ability to solve problems, make decisions, and communicate needs.
4. Client will safely provide self-care by using low-vision aids and environmental strategies.
5. Client will demonstrate the safe and correct use of adaptive devices.

Intervention

Counseling provides an opportunity for persons who have become visually impaired to talk about their feelings, concerns, and anxieties. Once these emotions have been identified, clients can be given assistance in identifying their strengths and resources. Problem solving can lead to alternative ways to complete the tasks of everyday living and participate in recreational activities.

The nurse who is interacting with a visually impaired client must rely heavily on various techniques and methods when communicating with that person. See Boxes 31-4 and 31-5 for tips and aids that facilitate communicating and

BOX 31-4 Signs and Behaviors That May Indicate Vision Problems

CLIENT MAY REPORT:
- Pain in eyes
- Difficulty seeing in darkened area
- Double or distorted vision
- Migraine headaches coupled with blurred vision
- Flashes of light
- Halos surrounding lights

STAFF MAY NOTICE THE CLIENT:
- Getting lost
- Bumping into objects
- Straining to read or not reading
- Spilling food on clothing
- Withdrawing socially
- Making less eye contact
- Displaying placid facial expressions
- Viewing the television at close range
- Suffering from a decreased sense of balance
- Mismatching clothes

From McNeely E, Griffin-Shirley M, Hubbard A: Teaching caregivers to recognize diminished vision among nursing home residents, *Geriatr Nurs* 13(6):332, 1992.

BOX 31-5 Communicating with and Caring for Visually Impaired Nursing Facility Residents

- Always identify yourself clearly.
- Always make it clear when you are leaving the room.
- Make sure you have the resident's attention before you start to talk.
- Try to minimize the number of distractions.
- Whenever possible, choose bright clothes with bold contrasts.
- Check to see that the best possible lighting is available.
- Assess your position in relation to the resident. One eye or ear of resident may be better than the other.
- Try not to move items in the resident's room. Narrate your actions.
- Try to keep the resident between you and the window or you will appear as a dark shadow.
- Use some means to identify residents who are known to be visually impaired.
- Use the analogy of clock hands to help the resident locate objects.
- Keep color and texture in mind when buying clothes.
- *Be careful about labeling residents as confused! They may be making mistakes because of poor vision.*
- Obtain and encourage the use of low-vision aids.

Modified from McNeely E, Griffin-Shirley M, Hubbard A: Teaching caregivers to recognize diminished vision among nursing home residents, *Geriatr Nurs* 13(6):332, 1992.

caring for the visually impaired. Keep in mind that these tips can be used in any setting—home care, acute care, or long-term care.

Strategies to increase adaptation to daily living include (1) organizing the environment, (2) encouraging the use of the clock method of eating, and (3) using a sighted guide to assist in ambulation (Box 31-6). Organizing the environment means placing items of clothing in specific drawers or closets to facilitate selection and placing furniture in specific locations to facilitate mobility. Additionally, the use of color-contrast and color-coding schemes helps the client locate items; bright, sharply contrasting colors make furniture and personal items visually distinct. For example, a bright red toothbrush shows up well against a white sink. Coding schemes that facilitate independent living include applying fluorescent tape around light switches, thermostats, and keyholes. Coding with colored paper, textured paper such as sandpaper, or rubber bands can help the client differentiate among medications. The clock method assists the client at meals because the location of food on the plate is described in terms of a clock face (e.g., beans at the top of the plate are at the 12 o'clock position; potatoes at the bottom of the plate are at the 6 o'clock position). In addition, the client can use a piece of bread or roll to push food onto the fork. Sighted guides, who lead persons with visual impairments from place to place, can help a client walk confidently (see Box 31-6). The use of a cane or a seeing-eye dog can also promote independence in mobility, especially when the client is in an unfamiliar environment.

BOX 31-6 The Sighted Guide

1. Ask the older adult if he or she would like to walk with a sighted guide.
2. If assistance is accepted, offer your elbow or arm. The older adult should grasp your arm just above the elbow. If necessary, physically assist the older adult by guiding his or her hand to your arm or elbow.
3. You will then go a half-step ahead and slightly to the side of the older adult. The older adult's shoulder should be directly behind your shoulder. (Note: If the older adult is frail, locate the hand on your forearm. When this modified grasp is used, the older adult will be positioned laterally to your body.)
4. You and the older adult should be relaxed and walk at a comfortable pace. When approaching doorways or a narrow space, tell the older adult. The older adult should then go directly behind you. Some modifications may be needed for frail older adults; be sure the modifications are safe and comfortable.
5. Describe the surroundings to the older adult as you walk to augment mobility and enrich experience.

Modified from McNeely E, Griffin-Shirley M, Hubbard A: Teaching caregivers to recognize diminished vision among nursing home residents, *Geriatr Nurs* 13(6):332, 1992.

The home health or community health nurse can assist with referral to a social worker who has information on local, state, and federal services available. Services for persons with visual impairments include counseling, mobility training, vocational rehabilitation, self-care skills training, special education, and financial assistance. Low-vision aids such as "talking books," tapes, and tape players are available from public libraries, the National Federation of the Blind, the American Foundation for the Blind, the National Association for Visually Handicapped, the National Braille Association, and the U.S. Library of Congress. Legal blindness entitles a person to some federal assistance, based on need. Blind persons can also claim an additional tax deduction on their federal income tax returns.

Evaluation

Evaluation includes documentation of the achievement of the expected outcomes, demonstrated by the client actively participating in self-care and social activities. Clients who display signs and symptoms of depression or social isolation require further counseling to talk about their feelings, strengths, and resources. In addition, alternative visual aids and strategies will need to be identified to increase communication and promote self-care.

HEARING AND BALANCE

The organs of hearing and balance can be divided into three parts: the external ear, the middle ear, and the inner ear. The external ear and middle ear are involved only in hearing; the inner ear is involved in both hearing and balance. The external ear consists of the auricle and the external auditory canal, a passageway from the outside to the eardrum. The middle ear is an air-filled space that contains the tympanic membrane, the eardrum, and the auditory ossicles. The inner ear contains the sensory organs for hearing and balance. It is made up of interconnecting, fluid-filled tunnels and chambers in the petrous portion of the temporal bone.

The organs of balance are located within the inner ear and can be divided into two parts. The vestibule contains the membranous labyrinth, which consists of the utricle and saccule. This portion evaluates the position of the head relative to gravity or linear acceleration and deceleration. The second part is located in the semicircular canals and is called the kinetic labyrinth. This labyrinth evaluates movements of the head.

Age-Related Changes in Structure and Function

Age-related changes in the external ear can be seen in the auricle, which appears larger because of continued cartilage formation and loss of skin elasticity. The lobule of the auricle becomes elongated, with a wrinkled appearance. The periphery of the auricle becomes covered with coarse, wirelike hairs. Compared with women, men have larger tragi, which are laterally situated in the external canal. These tragi become larger and coarser with age. The auditory canal narrows as a result of inward collapsing. The hairs lining the canal become coarser and stiffer. In addition, cerumen glands atrophy, causing the cerumen to be much drier. In the middle ear, age-related changes to the tympanic membrane result in a dull, retracted, and gray appearance. Degeneration of ossicular joints in the middle ear has also been noted. Finally, changes within the inner ear result in decreased vestibular sensitivity.

Age-related balance decline is caused by a combination of decreased sensory input, slowing of motor responses, and musculoskeletal limitations. Numerous studies comparing healthy younger and older adults have reported an increase in postural sway in older adults. Despite this increase, most healthy older adults have enough sensory function reserve to maintain postural control. However, deprivation in more than one system is likely to lower the balance threshold. In addition, under conditions in which balance is maximally stressed, such as climbing up or down steps or curbs and getting in and out of a bathtub, maintaining balance becomes more difficult.

Common Problems and Conditions

Pruritus. Pruritus, itching within the external auditory canal, is related to age-related atrophic changes in the skin. Atrophy of the epithelium and epidermal sebaceous glands results in dryness. Often, chronic pruritus of the ear canal results from an itch-scratch-itch cycle initiated by the dry skin. The problem may be exacerbated by efforts to retard and remove dry earwax buildup. Several drops of glycerine or mineral oil instilled in the ear canal daily will add moisture to the external ear. More resistant conditions can be treated by instilling steroid-containing medications in the external canal.

Cerumen Impaction. Cerumen impaction is a reversible, often overlooked cause of conductive hearing loss. With increasing age, atrophic changes in the sebaceous and apocrine glands lead to drier cerumen. These changes in the cerumen coupled with a narrowed auditory canal and stiffer, coarser hairs lining the canal lead to cerumen impaction. The cerumen blockage may interfere with the passage of sound vibrations through the external auditory canal to the middle and inner ear, affecting a person's ability to hear and communicate. This impaired communication may then lead to social isolation and depression.

Common symptoms of cerumen impaction include hearing loss, feeling of fullness in the ear, itching, and tinnitus (ringing in the ears). Identification and removal of the impaction can restore hearing acuity and relieve symptoms associated with impaction.

NURSING MANAGEMENT

Assessment

Clients with cerumen buildup may complain of ear fullness, itching, and difficulty hearing. An otoscopic examination shows that the external ear canal is obstructed by cerumen and that the tympanic membrane is not visible.

Diagnosis

Potential nursing diagnoses for a client with the aforementioned assessment findings include:

- Sensory/perceptual alterations (auditory) related to cerumen impaction
- Social isolation related to difficulty communicating with family and friends

Planning and Expected Outcomes

Expected outcomes for a client with cerumen impaction include:

1. Client will be free from cerumen impaction.
2. Client will follow proper instillation of softening agents.
3. Client will report satisfactory level of involvement with family and friends.

Intervention

The nurse must assess clients for signs of hearing impairment that may indicate cerumen impaction, including (1) difficulty understanding the spoken word (clients may ask why others are mumbling or deliberately excluding them from conversation), (2) loud radio and television volume, (3) withdrawal from social activities and accompanying depression, and (4) possible confusion and paranoia. Once an otoscopic examination reveals an impaction, the nurse should follow the protocol for cerumen removal. For clients living in the community, both clients and their families should be taught how to instill the softening agent. In addition, clients should be instructed to notify their health care provider if they experience a decrease in hearing, pain, or a ringing or a crackling in their ear.

The protocol for cerumen removal includes the following steps (Meador, 1995):

1. Clip and remove hairs in the ear canal.
2. Instill a softening agent, mineral oil, or a carbamide peroxide and glycerin solution (Debrox, a nonprescription otic solution) twice daily for several days until wax softens.
3. Irrigate the ear by using a bulb syringe, a plastic syringe (2 to 4 oz), or a WaterPik device (on its low setting).
4. Use a solution of 3 oz of 3% hydrogen peroxide in 1 qt of water warmed to 98° to 100° F. If the client is sensitive to hydrogen peroxide, use sterile, normal saline solution.
5. Place a towel around the client's neck and tip his or her head to the side being drained, with the emesis basin kept under the ear to catch drainage.
6. Tip the client's head to side that is being irrigated.
7. Place the tip of the irrigating device just inside the external meatus with the tip visible.
8. Straighten the auditory meatus by gently drawing the pinna up and back.
9. The flow of irrigating fluid should be steady; as fluid passes the plug, small to large pieces of cerumen will be forced out of the canal. Lavage continues until the cerumen is removed.
10. Drain excessive fluid from the ear by tilting the head toward the affected side. Wipe with a cotton-tipped applicator and alcohol (70% isopropyl).
11. Firmly impacted cerumen must be manually extracted by a physician or advanced practice nurse with an otoscope and a curette.

Evaluation

The client will be free from cerumen impaction and verbalize a decrease in ear fullness and an increase in the ability to hear. The cerumen removal should be documented, noting the method of irrigation, the amount and type of debris removed, and the client's response. The client will demonstrate the proper method to instill the softening agent. The client will also state ear symptoms to report to his or her health care provider.

Tinnitus. Tinnitus is an annoying combination of both conductive and sensorineural hearing loss. It is a subjective sensation of noise in the ear, defined as a ringing, buzzing, or hissing. Individuals at any age may experience tinnitus, but its prevalence increases with advancing age. For many older adults it is a chronic condition with which they must cope. For others it is an indication of permanent hearing loss or a tumor.

The most common causes of tinnitus are noise or toxin damage to the hair receptors of the cochlear nerve and age-related changes in the organs of hearing and balance. Tinnitus is not a disease but a symptom associated with many diseases, conditions, and medical treatments. Tinnitus can be classified as subjective or objective. Subjective tinnitus is audible only to the client. It is characterized as ringing, buzzing, or humming. Objective tinnitus, although rare, is audible to both the client and the examiner. It is more likely to be low pitched and is often associated with an identifiable cause, such as muscle spasms or vascular and musculoskeletal cranial disorders. An additional important classification of tinnitus is whether it is bilateral or unilateral. Unilateral tinnitus is associated with more serious diseases, such as Meniere's disease, tumors, or vascular problems, and requires an extensive workup.

NURSING MANAGEMENT

Assessment

The Tinnitus Questionnaire and Tinnitus Handicap Inventory should be used to gather necessary subjective data (Boxes 31-7 and 31-8). Objectively, the client will have signs of subjective or objective unilateral or bilateral ringing in the ear.

Diagnosis

Potential nursing diagnoses for the client with tinnitus include:

- Altered health maintenance related to lack of knowledge about tinnitus prevention practices
- Sensory/perceptual alterations (auditory) related to ringing in the ears
- Anxiety related to coping with chronic condition of ringing in the ears

BOX 31-7 Tinnitus Questionnaire

1. How long have you had ringing (or other sounds) in your ears?
2. Describe as nearly as possible the sound you hear.
3. Is the sound in the left, right, or both ears? Is it constant or occasional?
4. Does the sound change with exercise, climbing stairs, or fast walking?
5. Do you have a hearing problem?
6. Do you have ear pain, discharge, or an infection?
7. When is the sound in your ears worse: daytime, evening, or night?
8. Does this sound interfere with sleep, television, radio, crowds, or conversation?
9. Do you grind your teeth or clench your jaws at times?
10. Have you recently had: dental problems or treatments? Ear pain? Excessive ear wax? Ear discharge or infection? Cold or flu? Recent head or neck injury? Headaches? Dizziness? Balance difficulty? Visual problems? Swallowing problems? Speaking problems? Numbness or weakness anywhere?
11. Do you: smoke? Drink coffee, tea, chocolate, cola or other carbonated drinks with caffeine, or alcoholic or quinine water drinks?
12. What prescription medications do you take? What other medications do you take: aspirin, aspirin-containing medications, or ibuprofen (Advil) for headaches, joint pain or congestion; sleeping aids; or diet pills?
13. Do you experience considerable sudden or intense noise at work, home, or recreation that involves the use of motors or firearms?
14. Have you or any family member had allergies? Arthritis? Anemia? Diabetes? High blood pressure? Thyroid problems?

From Ross V, Echevarria KH, Robinson B: Geriatric tinnitus: causes, clinical treatment and prevention, *Gerontol Nurs* 17(10):6, 1991.

Planning and Expected Outcomes

Expected outcomes for the client with tinnitus include:

1. Client will follow tinnitus prevention practices.
2. Client will use home masking measures and a hearing aid or tinnitus masker to relieve tinnitus.
3. Client will cope with anxiety independently by using relaxation techniques.

Intervention

Nursing interventions are outlined in Box 31-9. Clients should be taught prevention practices, including (1) treating correctable problems (e.g., cerumen impaction, ear infection) that cause tinnitus; (2) softening loud sounds through improved acoustics; (3) using protective ear plugs; and (4) avoiding ototoxic substances in foods, drinks, and drugs. Teach clients about the following home masking measures that produce a variety of distracting sounds:

- Portable radio tuned between stations
- Loud ticking clock
- Soft, pleasant music
- Electric fan
- Sleeping with head elevated on two pillows

Recommend that clients be evaluated for aids or a specially designed masker to lessen tinnitus. Coping strategies to relieve anxiety and stress, such as relaxation training, biofeedback, and counseling, should also be taught.

Evaluation

Achievement of the expected outcomes is evidenced by clients following recommended tinnitus interventions and strategies to cope with the chronic ringing in their ears. The Tinnitus Handicap Inventory (see Box 31-8) should be administered to determine the client's improvement in symptoms. Clients noting no improvement or an increase in symptoms should be referred to a multidisciplinary team (specializing in tinnitus) composed of an otolaryngologist, audiologist, and psychiatrist for evaluation and counseling. Clients taking medications will be free from side effects. Those displaying adverse side effects should report to their health care provider for dosage modification, alternative drug therapy, or discontinuation of medication.

Hearing Loss

It is estimated that 7 million to 10 million adults ages 65 and older in the United States have some type of hearing impairment. Hearing loss is not a normal part of the aging process and should be further evaluated for proper treatment.

Hearing impairment is classified as conductive, sensorineural, or mixed. Conductive hearing loss results from interruption of the transmission of sound through

BOX 31-8 **Tinnitus Handicap Inventory**

The purpose of the scale is to identify the problems your tinnitus may be causing you. Check "Yes," "Sometimes," or "No" for each question. Do not skip a question.

	Yes	Sometimes	No
1. Because of your tinnitus is it difficult for you to concentrate?			
2. Does the loudness of your tinnitus make it difficult for you to hear people?			
3. Does your tinnitus make you angry?			
4. Does your tinnitus make you feel confused?			
5. Because of your tinnitus do you feel desperate?			
6. Do you complain a great deal about your tinnitus?			
7. Because of your tinnitus do you have trouble falling asleep at night?			
8. Do you feel as though you cannot escape your tinnitus?			
9. Does your tinnitus interfere with your ability to enjoy social activities (e.g., going out to dinner or to the movies)?			
10. Because of your tinnitus do you feel frustrated?			
11. Because of your tinnitus do you feel that you have a terrible disease?			
12. Does your tinnitus make it difficult for you to enjoy life?			
13. Does your tinnitus interfere with your job or household responsibilities?			
14. Because of your tinnitus do you find that you are often irritable?			
15. Because of your tinnitus is it difficult for you to read?			
16. Does your tinnitus make you upset?			
17. Do you feel that your tinnitus problem has placed stress on your relationship with members of your family and friends?			
18. Do you find it difficult to focus your attention away from your tinnitus and on other things?			
19. Do you feel that you have no control over your tinnitus?			
20. Because of your tinnitus do you often feel tired?			
21. Because of your tinnitus do you feel depressed?			
22. Does your tinnitus make you feel anxious?			
23. Do you feel that you can no longer cope with your tinnitus?			
24. Does your tinnitus get worse when you are under stress?			
25. Does your tinnitus make you feel insecure?			

From Newman CW, Jacobson GP, Spitzer JB: Development of the tinnitus handicap inventory, *Arch Otolaryngol Head Neck Surg* 122:142, Feb 1996.

the external auditory canal and middle ear. Conditions that may result in conductive hearing loss are cerumen impaction, otitis media, and otosclerosis (fixation of auditory ossicles).

Sensorineural hearing loss results when the inner ear, auditory nerve, brainstem, or cortical auditory pathways do not function properly so that sound waves are not interpreted correctly. Mixed hearing loss is a conductive hearing loss superimposed on a sensorineural hearing loss.

Presbycusis. Presbycusis, a sensorineural hearing loss, is the most common form of hearing loss in older adults. Typically, the loss is bilateral, resulting in difficulty hearing high-pitched tones and conversational speech. It affects men more than women. The cause of presbycusis remains unclear. Studies designed to identify a direct cause have proven no clear correlation. Therefore the diagnosis is one of exclusion by ruling out other causes of hearing loss:

- Noise-induced hearing loss (i.e., prolonged exposure to loud noise)
- Infection
- Head injury
- Metabolic disease (of the pancreas or kidneys)
- Vascular disease
- Heart disease
- Genetic factors

Signs and symptoms displayed by the client include:

- Increasing volume on television or radio
- Tilting head toward person speaking
- Cupping hand around one ear
- Watching speaker's lips
- Speaking loudly
- Not responding when spoken to

NURSING MANAGEMENT

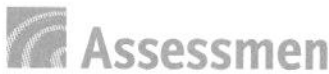

Assessment

Subjective data that should be obtained from a client suffering from hearing loss include onset, type, and progression of hearing loss, including differences in either ear; family history of hearing loss; presence of other symptoms,

BOX 31-9 Chronic Tinnitus Interventions

MILD TINNITUS (DOES NOT AFFECT ADLs)

- Reassure older adult that tinnitus is not life threatening.
- Instruct client to avoid ototoxic substances in foods, drinks, and drugs.
  —Avoid quinine, aspirin, and antiinflammatory drug compounds.
  —Avoid caffeine, sodium, chocolate, tea, and alcohol.

MODERATE TINNITUS (INTERFERES WITH SLEEP AND ADLs)

- Teach simple home masking measures to relieve tinnitus:
  —Radio tuned between stations
  —Clocks that tick
  —Soft, pleasant, distracting music
  —Semielevated head position to sleep
- Recommend evaluation for properly fitted hearing aid; may relieve tinnitus even if hearing loss is mild.
- More sophisticated, commercial tinnitus maskers and instruments may be matched to the individualized pitch of one's tinnitus.
- Use habituation therapy (exposing clients to low-level broad-band noise produced by wearable noise generators).
- Medication (e.g., amitriptyline [Elavil], alprazolam [Xanax], diazepam [Valium], and histamines) may be used, but with caution, since they may cause drowsiness and mental confusion.

SEVERE TINNITUS

- Refer client for extensive counseling and education.
- Apply all moderate tinnitus interventions.
- Teach relaxation methods to cope with stress and promote sleep; combined with biofeedback, this has proved to be beneficial for long-term sufferers of tinnitus.
- Perform electrical stimulation.
- Perform acupuncture.
- Perform surgery (rare for those clients with objective tinnitus or those who have no auditory function and perceive tinnitus as originating from nonfunctioning ear).
- Contact local self-help tinnitus support groups (for information, contact the American Tinnitus Association, PO Box 5, Portland, OR 97207).

Compiled from Ross V, Schevarria K, Robinson B: Geriatric tinnitus: causes, clinical treatment, and prevention, *J Gerontol Nurs* 17(10):6, 1991; Seidman MD, Jacobson GP: Update on tinnitus, *Otolaryngol Clin North Am* 29(3):455, 1996.

such as pressure or pain in ears, ringing in ear, or dizziness; history of head injury or noise exposure; and current medications with known ototoxic effects. Objectively, the client may display some behavioral symptoms of hearing loss (Box 31-10). A complete hearing evaluation should be conducted.

Diagnosis

Nursing diagnoses based on analysis of the client's hearing loss include:

- Sensory/perceptual alterations (auditory) related to sensorineural hearing loss
- Social isolation related to hearing loss
- Self-esteem disturbance related to hearing loss

Planning and Expected Outcomes

Expected outcomes for a client with a hearing loss include:

1. Client will effectively use aural rehabilitative techniques.
2. Client will maintain satisfactory social contacts and activities with others.
3. Client will perceive himself or herself positively as evidenced by positive self-talk and behaviors.

Intervention

Interventions for the client with a hearing impairment focus on aural rehabilitation and facilitation of communication. Clients often deny their hearing loss and need much encouragement and support to explore the various methods to improve hearing. The nurse should provide clients with a printed information sheet on hearing loss (Box 31-11).

Aural rehabilitation includes auditory training, speech and reading training, and hearing aids. Auditory training helps the person with a hearing impairment listen to a speaker by differentiating among gross sounds. Speech and reading training includes lip reading and speech skills. Lip reading requires understanding of verbal communication by integrating lip movements, facial expressions, gestures, and environmental

BOX 31-10 Behavioral Clues Indicating Difficulty Hearing

- Difficulty hearing over the telephone
- Trouble following conversation when two or more persons are talking at the same time
- Turning up the volume on the television
- Leaning forward to hear better or straining to understand conversations
- Shunning large-group and small-group audience situations
- Complaining about people mumbling
- Difficulty understanding women and children talking
- Asking for frequent repetition and answering questions inappropriately
- Losing sense of humor or becoming grim

Data from US Department of Health and Human Services: *Age page: hearing and older people*, Bethesda, Md, 1995, National Institute on Aging.

BOX 31-11 Hearing and Older Adults

1. Presbycusis is the normal hearing loss associated with aging. Changes in the structure and function of the inner ear make it difficult to understand certain types of speech sounds and produce an intolerance for loud noise. The sounds that are usually lost first are f, s, th, ch, and sh. As hearing loss progresses, the ability to hear the sounds of b, t, p, k, and s is also impaired.
2. Some of the most common signs and symptoms of hearing loss include:
   a. Difficulty understanding speech
   b. Certain sounds being overly annoying or loud
   c. Difficulty discriminating speech; another person's speech sounding slurred or mumbled
   d. Trouble hearing at large gatherings, especially where there is background noise
   e. Constant ringing or hissing background noise
3. Do not be afraid to tell your family and friends to face you and to speak at a normal rate, in lower tones (not necessarily louder), and with greater clarity. If you do not understand, ask the person to repeat. Listen carefully while watching the person's face and lips.
4. If you are having a hearing problem, see your health care provider. A hearing problem may be caused by a serious medical condition that your health care provider may be able to diagnose and treat, or your health care provider may wish to refer you to a specialist (otolaryngologist or audiologist) for further evaluation.
5. A hearing aid may be recommended. Seek professional guidance in obtaining the best aid suited to your needs. Find a reputable dealer by checking with the Better Business Bureau. Because of the high cost of hearing aids and their upkeep, it is wise to choose carefully.

Data from US Department of Health and Human Services: *Age page: hearing and older people,* Bethesda, Md, 1995, National Institute on Aging.

Client/Family Teaching

STRATEGIES TO IMPROVE COMMUNICATION WHEN THERE IS HEARING LOSS

Provide good visual contact with clients. Hearing-impaired individuals need to supplement hearing with lip reading. They need to be able to see the speaker's face and lips. Avoid situations where there is glare or shadows on the client's field of vision.

Reduce or eliminate background noise.

Speak at a normal rate and volume. Do not overarticulate or shout.

Use short sentences, and pause at the end of each sentence.

Use facial expressions or gestures to give useful clues.

Ask how you can help the listener.

Be patient, and stay positive and relaxed.

Data from US Department of Health and Human Services: *Age page: hearing and older people,* Bethesda, Md, 1995, National Institute on Aging.

Client/Family Teaching

ASSISTED-LISTENING DEVICES

These devices are designed to amplify sound or transform sound into tactile or visual signals. These systems allow a hearing impaired person to communicate more effectively and function more independently.

- Microphones placed close to sound source
- Amplifiers for the telephone, television, or radio
- Closed-captioned television
- Teletypewriters
- Doorbell and telephone that light as well as ring
- Flashing smoke detectors and alarm clocks
- Burglar alarms that both light up and sound (Patt, 1998)

clues. This process is extremely difficult without auditory clues. Speech skills must be conserved with the reduced auditory feedback experienced by the client with impaired hearing. Persons who have hearing impairments must learn to work intelligently with inefficient communication and decreased speech (see Client/Family Teaching box). Hearing aids amplify sound but do not improve the ability to hear. Technologic advances currently offer clients a wide variety of amplification options to suit their changing environmental needs (i.e., quiet to noisy). Clients and their families should be instructed on the basics of hearing aid use and care (see Client/Family Teaching box). All nurses and nursing assistants should have a basic understanding of how to work with a hearing aid to assist the client who is unable to care for the aid. Clients and their families should be taught where to obtain and how to use assisted-listening devices (see Client/Family Teaching box and Health Promotion/Illness Prevention box).

Evaluation

Evaluation is based on documentation of the achievement of expected client outcomes as evidenced by the client using aural rehabilitation techniques and devices to enhance communication. The client and family will demonstrate the proper use, cleaning, and troubleshooting of the hearing aid. The client will remain actively involved with others and the environment. Those clients displaying signs and symptoms of depression and social isolation will require further encouragement and support to explore other methods to improve hearing.

Client/Family Teaching

HEARING AID ASSESSMENT TOOL FOR CLEANING, INSERTING, AND TROUBLESHOOTING

COMPONENT	LOOK	LISTEN
Earmold or in-the-ear aid	Opening clear? Cracks or rough areas? Check fit.	Use sounds *(a/u/c/s)*.
Battery	Using battery tester, check voltage (replace at 1.1 or below). Compartment clean? Battery contacts clean? Battery inserted properly (match + on battery to + on battery compartment)? Is battery compartment shut all the way?	
Case	Cracks? Separating?	Press case gently.
Microphone	Clean? Visible damage?	Interruption in amplification?
Dials	Clean? Easily rotated?	Rotate. Reasonable gain variation? Static?
Switches	Clean? Easy to move?	Turn on and off. Static?
Cord (body aid)	Cracked? Frayed? Connection plugs clean?	Run fingers down cord. Clean? Interruption in amplification? Connections tight?
Tubing (behind-ear aid)	Cracks? Good connection to earmold and aid? Moisture? Debris?	Cover opening of earmold and turn to maximum gain. Feedback? Distortion? Static?
Receiver (body aid)	Cracks? Firmly attached to earmold snap?	Reduced gain? Substitute spare receiver and recheck. Five speech sounds clearly amplified?
Volume control	Smooth, gradual increase	Clear quality?
Distortion		Turn to maximum gain to check.
Feedback	Recheck receiver snap, tubing, and earmold.	External feedback? Internal?

Health Promotion/Illness Prevention

The Ear

HEALTH PROMOTION

- Notify physician of any pain, discharge, redness, swelling, dizziness, ringing in ears, or loss of hearing.
- See physician for early detection and appropriate treatment for hearing difficulties and ear disease (e.g., cerumen impaction, tinnitus, presbycusis, vertigo).
- Maintain prescribed hearing aids, assistive listening devices, and medications.

PREVENTION OF DISEASE

- Have periodic ear examination and screening for ear disease and hearing problems.
- Avoid exposure to hazardous noise.
- Use protective earplugs in high-risk occupations and activities.

Common Problems and Conditions of Balance

Dizziness and Dysequilibrium. Dizziness and dysequilibrium are common complaints of older adults. Although there is a general decrease in vestibular sensitivity with aging, the symptoms of dizziness or imbalance should not be considered a normal part of aging. Balance disorders contribute to deficits in ambulation that may interfere with an older person's ability to carry out normal ADLs. The five age-related conditions of dysequilibrium that have been documented in older adults are:

1. **Benign paroxysmal positional vertigo:** severe episodes of vertigo precipitated by a particular change in head position
2. **Ampullary dysequilibrium:** vertigo or dysequilibrium associated with rotational head movements
3. **Macular dysequilibrium:** vertigo precipitated by a change of head position in relation to the direction of gravitational force (e.g., severe dizziness when rising from bed)
4. **Vestibular ataxia of aging:** constant feeling of imbalance with ambulation (Tideiksaar, 1998)
5. **Meniere's disease:** an uncommon disease seen most often in older women, characterized by severe vertigo

accompanied and usually preceded by tinnitus and progressive low-frequency sensorineural hearing loss

Although the vestibular system of the inner ear is the most common source of dizziness and balance disorders, the following causes must also be considered:

- Visual disturbances
- Musculoskeletal disorders
- Neurologic dysfunctions
- Metabolic abnormalities
- Cardiovascular disease
- Medications

Signs and symptoms vary for each disorder but may include any of the following:

- Whirling dizziness when the head is moved in a certain position
- Dizziness or imbalance when the head is moved quickly to the right, left, up, or down
- Constant feeling of imbalance when walking

Meniere's Disease. Meniere's disease is caused by pressure within the labyrinth of the inner ear, which is a result of excess endolympha that causes swelling in the cochlea. What causes the excess fluid is unclear. The three major characteristics are vertigo, tinnitus, and hearing loss. Other associated symptoms include loss of balance, nausea and vomiting, and spasmodic eye movement.

NURSING MANAGEMENT

Assessment

Subjective data include a description of vertigo episodes (including frequency and duration); a list of accompanying symptoms, such as nausea and vomiting, hearing loss, or tinnitus; a history of balance problems; and a drug history. Objective data include a complete assessment of hearing and balance.

Diagnosis

Potential nursing diagnoses for the client with vertigo and Meniere's disease include:

- Sensory/perceptual alterations (kinesthetic) related to vertigo and imbalance
- Potential for injury related to acute onset of vertigo
- Knowledge deficit: cause of vertigo and its treatment related to lack of exposure and inexperience
- Knowledge deficit: preoperative and postoperative surgical care for Meniere's disease related to lack of exposure
- Anxiety related to uncertainty of future vertigo attacks

Planning and Expected Outcomes

Expected outcomes for the client include:

1. Client will accurately follow prescribed medication regimen and exercise protocol.
2. Client will safely follow measures to reduce dizziness and prevent falls.
3. Client will state the causes and treatment of vertigo.
4. Client will ask questions about surgical care for Meniere's disease.
5. Client will meet own self-care needs as evidenced by reports of normal appetite, sleep, and activity.

Intervention

Pharmacologic treatment includes antivertiginous drugs such as meclizine (Antivert) or diphenhydramine (Benadryl). Meclizine may cause drowsiness; clients should be instructed to avoid alcoholic beverages while taking this drug. Clients with a history of asthma, glaucoma, or enlargement of the prostate gland must be monitored carefully while taking meclizine because of its anticholinergic action. Diphenhydramine, an antihistamine, is likely to cause dizziness, sedation, and hypotension in older clients. A diuretic such as hydrochlorothiazide (HydroDIURIL) and a low-sodium diet help remove excess endolympha fluid. Clients undergoing diuretic therapy need to be monitored for evidence of fluid or electrolyte imbalance.

Vestibular rehabilitation therapy is conducted by a physical therapist, who designs an exercise program consisting of oculomotor and postural tasks that are taught to the client and incorporated into daily living (Patt, 1998).

Surgery may be performed for Meniere's disease to prevent further damage and sensorineural hearing loss. A client undergoing ear surgery is given a local anesthetic. Preoperative care includes giving instructions for postoperative care and sedating the client. Postoperative care includes (1) positioning the operative ear up for 4 hours after surgery; (2) medicating for pain and vertigo; (3) following safety precautions (e.g., side rails up, call light in reach, assistance with ambulation); (4) monitoring the client for changes in hearing, vertigo, neurologic symptoms (e.g., headache), or facial paralysis; and (5) instructing the client to keep his or her mouth open when sneezing or coughing.

There is no complete cure for vertigo. Therefore clients must be taught the following measures to reduce dizziness: (1) move slowly; (2) avoid bright, glaring lights (a quiet, darkened room is best); and (3) if vertigo occurs during ambulation, lie down immediately and hold the head still. The client with vertigo must be taught the causes of vertigo and the pharmacologic treatment, vestibular exercises, and measures to reduce vertigo and promote safety during an acute attack.

Evaluation

Evaluation includes achievement of the expected outcomes as evidenced by clients accurately following the prescribed medication regimen and exercise protocol. Clients displaying adverse side effects will report these to their health care provider for a modification in their medication regimen.

Clients will be free from falls by following measures to reduce dizziness. Those with reported falls will be evaluated with a fall assessment tool and taught alternative safety measures.

TASTE AND SMELL

The senses of taste and smell detect the aesthetics and safety of the environment. There is some evidence that the senses of smell and taste diminish with aging. Loss of smell and taste can affect an older person's food choices and intake and subsequently impair nutritional and immune status, which can exacerbate disease states. A decreased sensitivity to odors puts the older person at risk for noxious chemicals and poisonings (e.g., a person may fail to detect the odor of smoke or leaking gas).

Age-Related Changes in Structure and Function

Age-related changes in the senses of smell and taste are related to alterations in the oral mucosa and tongue and the pathologic state of the nasal cavity. During aging, anatomic and physiologic changes occur (e.g., reductions in cell number, damage to cells, diminished levels of neurotransmitters). In healthy older adults, olfactory losses result from normal aging, medications, viral infections, long-term exposure to toxic fumes, and head trauma. The majority of studies indicate a dramatic decline in sensitivity to airborne chemical stimuli with aging. Additionally, recognition of odors declines dramatically with age.

The cause of taste changes in normal aging is not fully understood. Studies of anatomic losses in the structures of the taste system in older adults report conflicting findings. Taste losses result from disease states of the nervous and endocrine systems, nutritional and upper respiratory conditions, viral infections, and medications.

Common Problems and Conditions

Xerostomia. Xerostomia, commonly referred to as dry mouth, is a subjective sensation of abnormal oral dryness. Reduced salivary flow is a common complaint of older adults. Longitudinal studies have established that salivary flow from the parotid gland is unchanged with advancing age. Factors leading to a dry mouth include disease states (e.g., Alzheimer's disease, depression, Sjögren's syndrome), conditions (e.g., radiotherapy of the head and neck, mouth breathing), and medications (e.g., sedatives, antihistamines, antidepressants, diuretics, chemotherapy, anticholinergics).

Dry mouth in the elderly can lead to an increased risk of serious respiratory infection, impaired nutritional status, and reduced ability to communicate. Complaints of abnormal taste sensations, burning of the oral tissues and tongue, and cracking of the lips are common. The oral mucosa is dry, thin, and smooth, and the tongue may have a thick, white, foul-smelling coating. The decrease in salivary flow interferes with chewing and swallowing. Clients with dentures may complain of sore gums and tissues and denture slippage from the loss of saliva flow, which forms a mechanical barrier.

NURSING MANAGEMENT

Assessment

Subjective assessment should include a health history of factors leading to a decrease in salivary flow and the client's oral complaints. Objectively, the lips of a client with xerostomia appear red, inflamed, cracked, and dry, and they may bleed. The tongue has red areas and a coated base; it appears thicker, with prominent lingual groove and papillae. The mucous membranes of the palate and the lining of the mouth and gums appear dry, red, and edematous. The saliva is scant, ropy, and viscid. The amount of moisture in the oral cavity can be assessed by running a gloved finger over the oral mucosa to evaluate stickiness, which indicates dry mucous membranes. The client's voice may be dry and raspy, and he or she may complain of difficulty articulating words. Taste testing is performed to evaluate taste sensation, which may be diminished.

Diagnosis

Potential nursing diagnoses for the client with xerostomia include:

- Sensory/perceptual alterations (gustatory) related to decrease in salivary flow
- Altered oral mucous membrane related to changes induced by xerostomia
- Altered nutritional status related to changes induced by xerostomia

Planning and Expected Outcomes

Expected outcomes for the client with xerostomia include:

1. Client will verbalize an increase in taste sensation.
2. Client will exhibit unimpaired oral mucosa tissue integrity as evidenced by moist, pink, smooth mucosal surfaces.
3. Client will verbalize no oral discomfort.
4. Client will state contributing factors, symptoms, and treatment of xerostomia.
5. Client will demonstrate correct oral hygiene regimen.

Intervention

Nursing interventions for the client with xerostomia focus on attaining an intact oral mucosa tissue integrity. Teaching clients about the factors leading to a decrease in salivary flow, as well as the associated symptoms, is key to the prevention and treatment of xerostomia. The treatment regimen focuses on increasing salivary flow. Clients need to be taught the basic oral hygiene of brushing teeth twice daily with a soft toothbrush and a nonabrasive fluoride toothpaste, as well as daily flossing. Fluid balance is vital to maintain moisture in the oral cavity. Clients need to take in 2 to 3 L of fluid per day, if not contraindicated. Also, foods prepared with gravy or sauces contain moisture and should be included in the diet, if not contraindicated. Additional methods to teach clients for increasing salivary flow include the use of artificial saliva, sugar-free hard candy, and gum.

Evaluation

Evaluation of the interventions is based on the appearance of the oral mucous membranes, the client's relief of symptoms, and an increased level of comfort through effective daily treatment practices.

TOUCH

At birth, touch is the most developed sense. Touch involves tactile information on pressure, vibration, and temperature. Although touch, pressure, and vibration are commonly classified as separate sensations, they are detected by the same types of receptors. The only differences among these three are (1) touch sensation usually results from stimulation of receptors in the skin or in tissues immediately beneath the skin, (2) pressure sensation generally results from deformation of deeper tissues, and (3) vibration sensation results from rapidly repetitive sensory signals.

Sensitivity to light touch diminishes in older adults and may be related to a decreased density of cutaneous receptors for touch sensation. Tactile vibratory thresholds progressively increase with age, most likely because of changes in pacinian corpuscle receptor sensitivity. Studies to evaluate the influence of age on thermal perception report conflicting findings. The warm-cold difference threshold increases with age.

The most common disorders affecting tactile information include cerebrovascular accident (CVA), peripheral vascular disease (PVD), and diabetic neuropathy. All three conditions involve changes in the vascular system that result in decreased blood flow to various parts of the body. Signs and symptoms of a CVA depend on the cerebral artery affected and the portion of the brain supplied by that artery. In PVD and diabetic neuropathy the impaired blood flow manifests as a loss of sensation most commonly noted in the lower extremities.

The common thread among these disorders is the alteration of peripheral tissue perfusion. Nursing interventions are directed toward preventing accidental trauma and injury in the affected limbs. Client education focuses on skin, leg, and foot care. The effectiveness of nursing interventions is determined by the absence of trauma, especially in the lower extremities.

Home Care

1. Sensory changes can lead to social isolation in homebound older adults (e.g., not being able to interact effectively with family members as a result of visual or hearing deficits).
2. Sensory changes increase safety hazards (e.g., burning or falling) for homebound older adults.
3. Instruct caregivers and homebound older adults about signs and symptoms of age-related sensory changes. Instruct them to report to their physician or home care nurse any signs and symptoms that interfere with independent function or present safety hazards.
4. Instruct caregivers and homebound older adults about prescribed treatments or surgical procedures (e.g., preoperative and postoperative care of cataract surgery, eyedrops, eardrops, antibiotics).
5. Assist caregivers and homebound older adults in organizing the environment to accommodate any decreased sensory function (e.g., use of color contrast, bold print books, hearing aid on the telephone).

SUMMARY

The senses of older adults are the key to their interaction with the environment. As these senses decline because of normal age-related changes or pathologic conditions, nurses in every setting must adapt interventions to promote the highest level of independent functioning.

The focus of gerontologic nursing care is illustrated in the following poem by Lillian Morrison (1987):

Body

I have lived with it for years,
this big cat, developed an
affection for it. Though it is
aging now, I cannot abandon it
nor do I want to. I would love
to throw it about in play but
must be careful. It cannot summon
that agile grace of old. Yet
it's really pleasant to be with,
familiar, faithful, complaining
a little, continually going
about its business, loving to lie down.

Lillian Morrison

Key Points

- Studies have documented age-related changes in the senses of vision and hearing.
- Age-related changes remain questionable in the senses of taste and smell.
- A cataract is opacity of the lens and requires surgery for successful treatment.
- Glaucoma is increased intraocular pressure and requires lifelong treatment with medications to lower the pressure.

- Retinal detachment requires immediate medical attention and can be repaired only by surgical intervention.
- Wet macular degeneration and diabetic retinopathy can be treated successfully with laser surgery.
- Organizing the environment, using the clock method of eating, and assisting ambulation with a sighted guide help a person who is visually impaired maintain independence.
- Hearing loss affects an older person's ability to communicate and can lead to depression, social isolation, and loss of self-esteem.
- Prevention and treatment of cerumen impaction is an important nursing function in the care of older adults, especially in the long-term care setting.
- Vertigo can be a chronic and annoying condition, but the use of proper safety measures and methods of reducing dizziness can facilitate daily functioning.
- Xerostomia can cause pain in the oral mucosa, gums, and tongue, leading to alterations in taste. Treatment includes a daily oral care regimen and methods to increase salivary production.
- Older persons with a diminished sense of touch are at risk for injury, especially in the affected limbs.

Critical Thinking Exercises

1. A 65-year-old woman has tinnitus and episodes of imbalance. Her son and daughter-in-law are concerned about having to leave her alone during the day while they are at work. What strategies could you suggest to the family regarding safety measures in the home?
2. Discuss how loss of sensory function in the elderly affects their self-esteem, performance of ADLs, safety, independence, and interactions with others.

References

Kollarits CR: The aging eye. In Duthie EH, Katz PR, editors: *Practice of geriatrics,* ed 3, Philadelphia, 1998, Saunders.

Lueckenotte AG: *Pocket guide to gerontologic assessment,* ed 3, St Louis, 1998, Mosby.

McFarland GK, McFarlane EA: *Nursing diagnosis and intervention: planning for patient care,* ed 3, St Louis, 1997, Mosby.

Meador JA: Cerumen impaction in the elderly, *J Gerontol Nurs* 21(12):43, 1995.

Morrison L: Body. In Martz S, editor: *When I am an old woman I shall wear purple,* ed 2, Watsonville, Calif, 1987, Papier-Mache Press.

Patt BS: Otologic disorders. In Duthie EH, Katz PR, editors: *Practice of geriatrics,* ed 3, Philadelphia, 1998, Saunders.

PhippsWJ: The patient with eye problems. In Long BC, Phipps WJ, Cassmeyer VS, editors: *Medical-surgical nursing: a nursing process approach,* St Louis, 1993, Mosby.

Roach S: *Introductory gerontological nursing,* Philadelphia, 2001, Lippincott Williams & Wilkins.

Taylor, RA: *Manual of family practice,* ed 2, Philadelphia, 2002, Lippincott Williams & Wilkins.

Tideiksaar R: Disturbances of gait, balance, and the vestibular system. In Tallis RC, Fillit HM, Brocklehurst JC, editors: *Brocklehurst's textbook of geriatric medicine and gerontology,* ed 5, London, 1998, Churchill Livingstone.

Index

Page numbers followed by f indicate figures; t, tables; b, boxes.

D

E

F

O